COMPLETE GUIDE TO
SYMPTOMS, ILLNESS & SURGERY
FOR PEOPLE OVER 50

COMPLETE GUIDE TO
SYMPTOMS, ILLNESS & SURGERY FOR PEOPLE OVER 50

H. Winter Griffith, M.D.

**Surgical Illustrations
by Mark Pederson**

THE
BODY PRESS
PERIGEE

The Body Press/Perigee Books
are published by
The Berkley Publishing Group
200 Madison Avenue
New York, NY 10016

Book produced by
Summerlin Publishing Group
P.O. Box 32012, Tucson, AZ 85751-2012

Library of Congress Cataloging-in-Publication Data

Griffith, H. Winter (Henry Winter).
    Complete guide to symptoms, illness & surgery for people over 50 /
H. Winter Griffith.
        p. cm.
    Includes index.
    ISBN 0-399-51749-9

    1. Aged—Diseases—Handbooks, manuals, etc. 2. Aged— Health and
hygiene—Handbooks, manuals, etc. I. Title.
    [DNLM: 1. Diagnosis—in middle age—handbooks. 2.—Diagnosis—in
old age—handbooks. 3. Medicine—handbooks. 4. Surgery, Operative—
in middle age. 5. Surgery, Operative—in old age—handbooks. WB
39 G853ca]
RA777.6.G75 1992   91-44129 CIP
618.97—dc20
DNLM/DLC
for Library of Congress

Printed in the United States of America

8   9   10   11   12   13   14   15

Contents

About the Author

H. Winter Griffith, M.D., is a prolific author of many medical books, including the best-selling *Complete Guide to Prescription & Non-Prescription Drugs, Complete Guide to Sports Injuries, Complete Guide to Symptoms, Illness & Surgery,* and *Complete Guide to Pediatric Symptoms, Illness & Medications,* all from The Body Press/Perigee Books. Other books include *Vitamins, Minerals and Supplements* and *Medical Tests—Doctor-Ordered and Do-It-Yourself.*

Dr. Griffith received his medical degree from Emory University in 1953 and spent 20 years in private practice in Florida, where he first recognized the need for better communication between physicians and patients. He joined the faculty at Florida State University and subsequently became an Associate Professor of Family and Community Medicine at the University of Arizona College of Medicine, where he pursued his goals for patient education. Dr. Griffith now devotes all of his time to writing, continuing his commitment to the concept of physician-patient education and communication.

Technical Consultants

Ruth M. Schaller, R.N., Nurse Family Practitioner

Faculty, University of Arizona College of Medicine
Faculty, University of Arizona College of Nursing
Faculty, University of Phoenix
Nurse Practitioner, Tucson Unified School District

Constance W. Clark, M.A. (GER)

Graduate degree in gerontology from Tulane University
Director, Division of Elderly Services, Our Lady of the Lake Regional Medical Center,
    Baton Rouge, Louisiana

William C. Farr, M.D., Ph.D.

Private medical practice confined to geriatrics, Tucson, Arizona

Dear Readers:

As we get older, most of us have fears about our health, especially when sickness occurs. This book can help you overcome some of those fears and let you know that in most cases your health can improve. You want to know if and when you should see a doctor, what the long-term health effects of an illness will be and whether you can care for yourself instead of depending on others.

You must know if your lifestyle needs to be changed and how the medicines being prescribed will work. Your doctor or nurse can answer many of your questions, but so often, you think of questions after you leave your doctor's office or the hospital. The information in this book is always available to answer many of your medical questions.

Educating yourself about your health and your body is a lifetime project. As you age, physical and emotional changes take place that you need to understand so you can optimize your health.

Older adults respond to an illness or a surgical procedure in different ways than a younger person. It's important for both patients and health care providers to recognize the differences and work together to achieve the best results possible.

Maintaining your health and making sure you have the best treatment when you are sick is a combined team effort by you, your family and medical professionals. By educating yourself about an illness or surgical procedure, you can be an active, knowledgeable and involved team member in making the best decisions about your health care.

Knowing what your symptoms mean, how serious an illness is and why medical treatment or surgery is needed are all important questions that need to be addressed. This book will help you find usable answers.

Sincerely,

H. Winter Griffith, M.D.

H. Winter Griffith, M.D.

Health Care for the Aging Patient

A tragic mistake in caring for older people is for the patient, the care-giver or the doctor to assume that any illness that comes along in an aging patient is there only because someone is "aging." So when an older patient shows signs of departure from a usual state of health, the first assumption that should be made is that this departure represents an illness or injury and that it is not the result of aging alone.

The pursuit of a specific diagnosis and competent treatment is exactly as important in older people as it is in any other age group. Many of the same illnesses, common in younger years, also affect aging patients. The causes may be the same, but the signs and symptoms and treatment may vary because of some changes that take place with aging that we cannot control.

In many individuals some physiological processes decline with age—for example, the flow of blood through the kidneys may be slower and maximal heart rate with exercise will be slower. On the other hand, liver function, total lung capacity and many other functions may remain the same.

As a patient or as a care-giver to an aging patient, you can and should share responsibility with your doctor for medical treatment and care. Just knowing some of the basic information about an illness may enable you to get maximum benefit from your medical treatment and prevent or recognize recurrence early.

FIVE MAJOR INFORMATION SECTIONS

There are five major information sections in this book: Symptoms, Illnesses & Disorders, Surgeries, Medications and Appendices. The information for each section is organized in chart or list form and has been tailored where possible to specific needs of the older patient. This information provides introductory knowledge about these topics. It will not always provide you with a precise diagnosis, but it will provide important information for you to remember during treatment after you and your doctor have arrived at a working diagnosis. The chart formats vary. The section beginning on page x explains how to read and use the information charts and lists in the book.

The Appendices provide information that does not fit the chart or list format. This section includes special diets, forms of physical therapy and short essays on important topics relating to health care of older people.

DOCTOR-PATIENT COMMUNICATION

It is extremely important that a patient and doctor have sufficient and clear communication about the patient's symptoms, illness and possible treatments. This book cannot be a substitute for that communication, although it can help prepare patients and care-givers to better understand all aspects of health care.

Only the patient can know what his or her signs and symptoms feel like, and only through discussion with the doctor can a complete diagnosis and approach to treatment be attained. This book is intended as an *introduction* and a *supplement* to what the patient's doctor may discover.

GETTING OLDER—AND STAYING HEALTHY

If we acknowledge that "older" doesn't necessarily mean "sicker," we must also recognize that the aging patient usually does have an intense interest in understanding his or her ailments and what can be done about them to make the quality of life better. This book, first of all, will help you *understand* the nature of your illness.

It will also help you determine when you should consult your doctor, and it will supply you with *preventative* measures to combat disease before it happens or recurs.

This book attempts to provide the accepted general consensus among a majority of experts. Doctors do not always agree on the best course of treatment for a particular illness in a particular patient. If your doctor's recommendations differ from those presented here, you should assume that your doctor's opinions are valid. Nevertheless, you should feel free to discuss all options and ask questions. Your doctor should welcome and answer your questions. If not, consider consulting another doctor.

Your best chance to age in good health is greatly enhanced if you participate fully in taking care of yourself. This book has been written to help you reach that goal.

Using the Symptoms Section

Each of the symptom lists is designed to suggest one or more illnesses and disorders that a specific symptom or a group of symptoms might indicate. Each list focuses on one prominent, common symptom. As an example, review the symptom list for **ABDOMINAL PAIN, RECURRENT ATTACKS** on the facing page.

These lists do not include every possible sign or symptom the human body can experience, but they represent the most familiar and easily recognizable ones.

The lists provide a guide for how serious symptoms are. They give you clues as to what symptoms can mean. They refer you to the Illnesses & Disorders section of the book for further information. *However, they are not intended as self-diagnosis guides.* No book should replace a competent doctor's diagnosis! The lists are only to help you decide how to proceed when you or someone else develops symptoms.

Refer to the numbers on the sample symptom list for an explanation of each heading described below.

1—NAME OF SYMPTOM

The lists are titled and arranged alphabetically by the name that is most common or that best describes the symptom (**ABDOMINAL PAIN, RECURRENT ATTACKS**).

In cases in which the symptom name is ambiguous or the symptom can apply to several parts of the body, the body part is part of the title. For example, the symptom **SWELLING** appears as separate lists titled **ABDOMINAL SWELLING; ANKLES, SWOLLEN; SWELLING OR LUMP;** and **TESTICLES OR PENIS, PAINFUL OR SWOLLEN.** One list, **SWELLING OR LUMP**, is alphabetized by the symptom name, **SWELLING.** The rest are alphabetized by the body part the swelling affects.

If you can't find your symptom under its own name, refer to the Index or check alphabetically for the main part of the body it affects.

2—SYMPTOMS & FACTORS

The main symptom is grouped in the first column with other symptoms or factors that frequently accompany it. Each group may indicate a separate illness or disorder. Recurrent abdominal pain can mean many things, depending on what other symptoms appear with it.

Read through the groups of symptoms and find the group that most closely matches your particular symptoms. Then refer to the second column for the name of a possible illness or problem.

Sometimes none of the symptom groups will perfectly match the symptoms of your present problem. Your doctor can ask about your medical history, perform a physical examination and order laboratory tests. Any or all of these may be necessary to establish a precise diagnosis.

3—POSSIBLE PROBLEM

The second column provides a list of illnesses, disorders or other medical problems that a symptom group can indicate. If the possible problem is listed as the name of the illness or disorder, you can find additional information in the Illnesses & Disorders section of the book under that name. If the possible problem is something other than an illness or disorder, a recommendation is listed under the name of the problem.

No attempt has been made to include every possible illness or disorder signaled by a symptom group. The identifications are based on illnesses that are *most obvious, most common or most serious.* For similar reasons, some rare

ABDOMINAL PAIN, RECURRENT ATTACKS

(Find your closest combination of symptoms in left-hand column; see possible problem in right-hand column. You may not experience all symptoms listed.)

SYMPTOMS & FACTORS	POSSIBLE PROBLEM
• Flushed skin on the head and neck. • Watery eyes. • Diarrhea with abdominal cramps. • Respiratory symptoms similar to those of asthma. • Irregular heartbeat. • Nausea and vomiting. • Unexplained weight loss.	**CARCINOID SYNDROME** (Refer to Illnesses section)
Early symptoms include: • Pain in the left side of the abdomen that improves after bowel movements. • Episodes of bloody diarrhea with mucus, alternating with symptom-free intervals. **During an acute attack:** (THIS IS AN EMERGENCY; SEEK MEDICAL CARE IMMEDIATELY!) • Increased bloody diarrhea (up to 10 to 20 bowel movements a day). • Severe cramps and pain around the rectum. • Appetite and weight loss. • Bloated abdomen. • Fever as high as 104F (40C). • Rapid heartbeat.	**COLITIS, ULCERATIVE** (Refer to Illnesses section)
• Cramping abdominal pain—especially after eating. The pain is sometimes in the right lower abdomen, mimicking appendicitis. • Nausea and diarrhea; general ill feeling; fever. • Appetite and weight loss. • Abdominal tenderness; abdominal mass that can be felt. • Bloody stools (sometimes).	**CROHN'S DISEASE** (Refer to Illnesses section)
Diverticulosis symptoms: • Mild cramping, bloated feeling or tenderness in the left side of the abdomen that is relieved by passing gas or moving bowels. • Occasional bright red blood in the stool. Non-infected diverticulae sometimes bleed. • Constipation or diarrhea (sometimes). **Diverticulitis symptoms:** • Intermittent cramping; abdominal pain that becomes constant. • Fever. • Nausea. • Tenderness over the affected area of the colon.	**DIVERTICULAR DISEASE** (Refer to Illnesses section)
• Cramping pain in the upper right of the abdomen. Pain may also occur in the chest (imitating a heart attack), in the upper back or the right shoulder. These symptoms frequently follow a meal rich in fats. • Tenderness in the upper abdomen. • Nausea and vomiting. • Belching. • Slight fever. If high fever and chills occur, a bacterial infection is present. • Jaundice (yellow skin and eyes) sometimes. • Pale stools (sometimes). • Itching skin (sometimes).	**GALLBLADDER, INFECTION OF** (Refer to Illnesses section)

(ABDOMINAL PAIN, RECURRENT ATTACKS, continued on next page)

illnesses described on the illness charts in this book have not been referred to on symptom lists.

If anyone develops dramatic symptoms that you think represent life-threatening danger, *call for emergency help*. Dial 0 or 911 and report your address or location, along with directions.

In extreme situations, render what first aid you can, such as giving cardiopulmonary resuscitation (CPR). Yell for help from anyone within range.

Using the Illnesses & Disorders Section

The information about illnesses and disorders is organized in condensed, easy-to-read charts. Each illness or disorder is described in a one-page format shown in the sample chart **THYROID, OVERACTIVE** on page xv. Major sections of the chart format are numbered and explained in the next few pages.

Most of the charts in this section refer to illnesses. In some cases, however, charts refer to disorders or problems that are not really illnesses. An example would be **EARWAX BLOCKAGE**.

1—NAME OF ILLNESS OR DISORDER

The charts are arranged alphabetically by the most common name for the illness, disorder or medical problem. Other names for these appear in parentheses following the main heading. **THYROID, OVERACTIVE** is also known as **Hyperthyroidism, Thyrotoxicosis and Toxic Goiter**, and its chart lists both.

Sometimes the names for medical problems vary in different geographic regions. All names in this book, including alternate names, are cross-referenced in the Index.

To find information about a medical problem, check the Index under the name by which you know the problem. You may also look up its major symptom in the symptom lists. If you can't find the illness chart you want, ask your doctor or nurse for alternate names by which the disorder is known.

2—BASIC INFORMATION FOR OLDER ADULTS

This section includes *Description, Special Considerations for Aging, Signs & Symptoms, Causes & Risk Factors* and *Doctor's Treatment & Diagnostic Tests.* Each is discussed separately below.

3—DESCRIPTION

A short description of the illness or disorder is provided. This description may also include information of general interest, such as how common an illness or disorder is or whether it is contagious, cancerous or inherited.

4—SPECIAL CONSIDERATIONS FOR AGING

Here will be a listing of factors that come into play in aging patients that is keyed to the particular illness or disorder on the chart.

5—SIGNS AND SYMPTOMS

Signs are observed. *Symptoms* are felt or experienced. A sign may be observed by the patient or by someone else, or it may represent physical findings determined by laboratory tests, x-rays and other diagnostic measures. Symptoms are feelings only the patient can describe.

Refer to the chart. The first item under this heading—hyperactivity—is a sign. It can be observed by the patient and others around him or her. The next three items—feeling warm or hot all the time, tremors, and sweating—are signs *and* symptoms. They can be observed by others *and* they can be felt by the patient. The fifth—itching skin—is a symptom that only the patient can feel and describe.

Signs and symptoms are listed together in this book; no attempt is made to separate the two. On most charts, a wide range of possible signs and symptoms is listed. *It is unlikely that any patient will have all, or even most, of the possible signs and symptoms.* The presence or absence of signs and symptoms may vary according to:
- The age and sex of the patient.
- The extent of the illness.
- The stage of the illness.

- The patient's medical and family history.
- The patient's current state of health.

6—CAUSES & RISK FACTORS

Many times the cause of an illness or disorder is unknown. The causes for most medical problems include the following:
- Inherited (congenital) defects.
- Infections from bacteria, viruses, parasites, yeasts or fungi. All of these are sometimes referred to as "germs," but most people associate "germs" with bacteria only.
- Physical injury.
- Toxins (poisons) from a wide range of sources, such as contaminated food, environmental pollution and bites from poisonous snakes or insects.
- Allergies.
- Tumors. These may be benign or malignant. Benign tumors do not spread to adjacent or distant organs and threaten life. Malignant (cancerous) tumors can.
- Endocrine disorders. These occur when too many or too few hormones are produced by the pituitary gland, thyroid gland, parathyroid gland, pancreas, adrenal glands, ovaries, testicles or thymus gland.
- Mental or emotional disorders, such as anxiety, depression or schizophrenia.
- Defects in the body's immune system. These include hypersensitivity, which can cause such illnesses and disorders as rheumatoid arthritis, systemic lupus erythematosus, hives and many others.

Many illnesses and disorders have known risk factors that can trigger the problem, make it more likely to occur or increase its duration and intensity. The most common risk factors include:
- Stress—either physical or emotional.
- Anxiety, depression and other mental or emotional problems.
- Fatigue or overwork.
- Poor nutrition due to improper diet or disease.
- Obesity.

- Recent or chronic illness that can lower resistance to other illnesses.
- Recent surgery or injury.
- Genetic factors, such as a family or ethnic tendency toward a particular illness or disorder.
- The use of drugs of abuse, such as alcohol, tobacco, caffeine, narcotics, psychedelics, hallucinogens, marijuana, sedatives, hypnotics or cocaine.
- Advanced aging.
- The use of medications, whether prescription or non-prescription. Even necessary medications cause adverse reactions and side effects that can complicate the treatment and affect the outcome of a medical problem.
- Exposure to allergens, environmental pollutants or poisons.
- Geographic area.
- Crowded or unsanitary living conditions.
- Socioeconomic factors.

7—DOCTOR'S TREATMENT & DIAGNOSTIC TESTS

A doctor's care is often necessary, not only to diagnose and prescribe treatment for a medical problem, but to supervise self-care (or hospitalization, when necessary) and to provide additional medical treatment such as surgery or special diagnostic procedures.

In addition, even the simplest medical problems sometimes develop complications that require a doctor's care. In those cases, a doctor's treatment can be appropriate even though it applies to a small fraction of cases.

Find a competent personal doctor who communicates well with you and with whom you can establish mutual respect.

Psychotherapy, counseling or biofeedback training may be the only useful type of health care for a medical problem caused mainly by stress or emotional problems. Counseling and therapy are also helpful in providing personal and family support, especially for illnesses that are terminal or

THYROID, OVERACTIVE
(Hyperthyroidism; Thyrotoxicosis; Toxic Goiter)

BASIC INFORMATION FOR OLDER ADULTS

DESCRIPTION—Hyperthyroidism is the overactivity of the thyroid, an endocrine gland that regulates all body functions. Body parts involved: The thyroid gland, a hormone-producing organ at the base of the neck next to the trachea (windpipe), and most other body organs, especially the endocrine system, which includes the pituitary gland, parathyroid glands, pancreas, adrenal glands and ovaries or testicles.

SPECIAL CONSIDERATIONS FOR AGING—Usual signs and symptoms may be absent and be replaced by symptoms of confusion, dizziness, failure to thrive, falling, incontinence, increasing dementia, refusal to eat or drink, weight loss, depression, paranoia, hypochondriasis, psychosis or threats of suicide.

SIGNS & SYMPTOMS
- Hyperactivity.
- Feeling warm or hot all the time.
- Tremors.
- Sweating.
- Itching skin.
- Pounding, rapid, irregular heartbeat.
- Weight loss despite overeating.
- Marked anxiety and restlessness.
- Sleeplessness.
- Fatigue and weakness.
- Protruding eyes (exophthalmos) and double vision (sometimes).
- Diarrhea (sometimes).
- Hair loss (sometimes).
- Goiter (sometimes).

CAUSES & RISK FACTORS
Causes include:
- Grave's disease.
- Thyroid nodules or tumors.
- Thyroid infection or inflammation (goiter).
- Pituitary disorders.
- Ovarian disorders.
Risk factors include:
- A family history of hyperthyroidism.
- Stress.

DOCTOR'S TREATMENT & DIAGNOSTIC TESTS
- Medical history and physical exam.
- Laboratory blood studies, including radioimmunoassays (see Glossary).
- ECG (see Glossary).
- Self-care instructions focused on the older patient.
- Surgery to remove part of the thyroid if medication does not control the disorder. Advancing age alone is not a deterrent.

HOME TREATMENT BY SELF OR CARE-GIVER

GENERAL INSTRUCTIONS—Since this condition develops gradually, the symptoms may be difficult to recognize. If your family members and friends mention changes in your behavior or appearance, consult your doctor.

MEDICATION (ADJUSTED FOR AGING)
- Your doctor may prescribe:
  Antithyroid drugs to depress thyroid activity.
  Beta-adrenergic blockers to decrease a rapid heartbeat.
  Radioactive iodine, which selectively destroys thyroid cells.
- *Note:* Adverse reactions and side effects may be more frequent and severe in older persons. Remind your doctor of any medicines you already take.

ACTIVITY FOR OLDER PATIENTS
- Rest in bed as much as possible until the disorder is cured.
- Ask your doctor to recommend activity levels as you adjust to the medication and improve.

FOOD & BEVERAGE
- Eat a diet that is high in protein to replace tissue lost from thyroid overactivity.
- See Appendix 1 regarding good nutrition for people over 50.

FUTURE CONSIDERATIONS FOR THE AGING ADULT

POSSIBLE COMPLICATIONS
- Congestive heart failure.
- "Thyroid storm," a sudden worsening of all symptoms. *This is a life-threatening emergency!*
- Misdiagnosis as a psychiatric anxiety reaction.

PROBABLE OUTCOME—Usually curable with medication or surgery. Allow 6 months of treatment for the condition to stabilize. Some forms may return to normal without treatment.

PREVENTING RECURRENCE—There are no specific preventive measures.

CALL YOUR DOCTOR IF

- You have symptoms of overactive thyroid.
- The symptoms worsen suddenly, especially after surgery.
- New, unexplained symptoms develop. The drugs used in treatment may produce side effects.

8

9

10

11

12

13

14

15

16

17

represent major lifestyle adjustments.

Rehabilitation is often helpful for illnesses or injuries that cause temporary or permanent disability. Rehabilitation may be provided by trained physical therapists or physiatrists (medical doctors who specialize in physical therapy). If rehabilitation is mentioned as appropriate health care, ask your doctor for information specific to your disability.

Your own observation of symptoms is usually the first—and often the most important—diagnostic measure. It is the first step toward medical treatment. For that reason, it is listed under this heading on many of the illness charts. Exceptions are made for a few medical problems, such as those that are signaled by unconsciousness, in which self-observation is impossible.

A medical history and physical exam by a doctor are almost universal requirements before treatment for any illness or disorder can begin. Even if a medical problem is usually treated at home, a history and exam will be necessary if complications develop that require medical treatment.

Additional diagnostic measures include laboratory studies and other medical tests. The most common include:

- X-ray examination.
- Studies of body fluids, such as blood, serum, plasma or spinal fluid.
- Microscopic and chemical examination of excreted material, such as urine or stools.
- CAT (computerized axial tomography) scans of the affected body part.
- MRI (magnetic resonance imaging).
- ECG (electrocardiogram), EEG (electroencephalogram) and EMG (electromyogram).
- Therapeutic trial of medication. This is used sometimes for a critically ill patient without a specific diagnosis while the doctor is awaiting laboratory results.

You may not undergo every diagnostic test listed on the chart; conversely, you may undergo tests that are *not* listed on the chart. Some tests are performed only if previous tests have not provided enough information. Others are performed only when complications develop. All medical diagnostic tests mentioned in this book are defined in the Glossary.

8—HOME TREATMENT BY SELF OR CARE-GIVER

This section includes *General Instructions, Medication (Adjusted for Aging), Activity for Older Patients* and *Food & Beverage.*

9—GENERAL INSTRUCTIONS

The instructions under this heading apply to home treatment. They cover common matters, such as the application of prescribed drops or ointments, the use of soaks for skin problems, how to bathe an affected part of the body, etc. In some cases they include instructions for emergency treatment by care-givers.

These instructions are not complete and may not apply to everybody, but they provide a good review of general measures that are helpful for most patients.

Self-care or home care is an important part of care for almost all disorders. Sometimes total self-care suffices if you have had previous experience with a medical problem and have a source to use to review important points in treatment.

Usually, however, a medical problem should be diagnosed by a doctor before you attempt self-care. Once your doctor diagnoses an illness or disorder and outlines a treatment program, self-care or home care is often important.

The treatment measures outlined in this book are designed to guide you whether you are caring for yourself or are taking care of someone else.

Effective self-care includes maintaining a positive attitude about yourself and being determined to improve or heal. During illness, a sense of humor and a positive outlook are just as helpful as medication or other treatment measures.

The information given here should not replace your doctor's instructions, because treatments vary a great deal between individuals.

If the instructions don't seem to fit your problem, ask your doctor or nurse for answers that apply uniquely to you.

10—MEDICATION (ADJUSTED FOR AGING)

The information under this heading generally describes medications of two types—those your doctor may prescribe and non-prescription medications you can take safely.

Prescription medications are named by generic name or family name. A brief description of a medication's purpose and effect is given. For more information about a specific medication, see the Index. It contains entries for brand names and generic names for the families of medications contained in the Medications section of this book.

For additional information, you may refer to my book *Complete Guide to Prescription and Non-Prescription Drugs*, which is published by The Body Press/Perigee Books.

For general instructions about the safe use of medications, see Appendix 21.

11—ACTIVITY FOR OLDER PATIENTS

Patients are often confused about whether they must stay in bed during an illness. They are often concerned about returning to regular activities and wonder whether their activity will be restricted after recovery. These questions are answered under this heading.

Additionally, guidelines are given for resuming sexual relations—an important subject that patients are sometimes reluctant to mention. If the illness has been life-threatening, as with a heart attack, or if it involves abdominal or genital organs, this is particularly pertinent information.

Exercise references are often included. When not otherwise specified, references to regular physical exercise mean *aerobic* exercise (see Appendix 20).

12—FOOD & BEVERAGE

Information on diet can vary from "no special diet is required" to references to special diets included in the Appendix, such as the following:
- A regular, well-balanced diet that is high in fiber.
- A milk-restricted diet.
- A gluten-restricted diet.
- An allergy diet.
- A liquid diet.
- A low-fat diet.
- A low-salt diet.
- A weight-loss diet.
- A soft diet.
- Others.

For additional specialized diets, consult your doctor or a dietitian.

13—FUTURE CONSIDERATIONS FOR THE AGING ADULT

This section includes *Possible Complications, Probable Outcome* and *Preventing Recurrence*.

14—POSSIBLE COMPLICATIONS

Complications are additional medical problems triggered by or resulting from the original illness. Complications sometimes occur, despite accurate diagnosis and competent treatment. Some are preventable, a few are inevitable— but most are rare.

15—PROBABLE OUTCOME

A very important concern in any illness is the patient's question, "What is going to happen to me? How will this illness or disorder affect my life?" No one can completely predict the outcome of an accident or illness. The predictions in this section are guesses based on averages.

Patients and doctors work toward optimal results, but medicine is an inexact science. Response to treatment depends on many variables, and there are many unanswered questions about health and illness. This is particularly true with older patients.

Some illnesses are considered incurable at present. The term "incurable" is a general one that can be applied to everything from insignificant conditions that are mere annoyances to fatal illnesses that bring certain death in a short time. For that reason, additional information about life expectancy is usually included for incurable illnesses. Again, individual variations are common, but the predictions are an attempt to answer a patient's most important questions. They help you adopt optimistic but realistic expectations.

In almost all cases—no matter how serious the illness—the symptoms can be relieved or controlled to minimize pain and discomfort.

16—PREVENTING RECURRENCE

Prevention can be of two types— prevention of the initial illness or prevention of a relapse or recurrence after recovery.

Prevention of any medical problem is the *best treatment*. Researchers continue to discover ways to prevent, delay or diminish some types of illness, pain and disability as well as untimely deaths. These are included whenever available.

The causes and risk factors for an illness often provide the best clues for prevention. Many illnesses, however, cannot be prevented at present.

17—CALL YOUR DOCTOR IF

For most medical problems, a phone call or visit to your doctor is recommended to establish a diagnosis.

After diagnosis, when the course of an illness departs from what is expected, your doctor wants to know. Many developing complications can be averted with prompt medical treatment. Specific symptoms are listed that indicate complications.

Of course, if any other symptoms begin that you believe are related to your illness or the medications you take, you should call your doctor about them, too.

Using the Surgeries Section

The information about common surgeries is organized in charts with a format similar to that used for the charts in the Illnesses & Disorders section (see the sample chart on page xv). In addition, an illustration is included for each surgical procedure.

Generally, the surgeries discussed in this section are those commonly performed to treat an illness or disorder, such as thyroid gland removal, or to make a diagnosis, such as dilatation and curettage.

Sometimes a surgery is mentioned on an illness chart as part of treatment. For instance, thyroid gland removal is mentioned on the chart for **THYROID, OVERACTIVE** (the previous sample chart) as a treatment for patients whose disorder does not respond to other treatment.

Each major heading on the surgery charts is numbered in the sample chart on page xxi, and the numbered sections are explained in the next few pages.

1—NAME OF SURGERY

The charts are arranged alphabetically by the name that most simply describes the surgical procedure. In some cases, medical professionals refer to the surgery by a more technical name. The technical name appears in parentheses below the main title.

Thyroid gland removal is clearly understood by everyone, but your surgeon may refer to it as *thyroidectomy*. Both names are included on the chart, and the surgery appears in the Index under both names.

2—BASIC INFORMATION

This section includes *Description, Body Parts Involved, Reasons for Surgery, Special Considerations for Older Patients* and *Surgical Risk Increases With*. Each topic is discussed separately.

3—DESCRIPTION

A short description of the surgery may include information about how common the procedure is and whether or not the medical problem requiring surgery is caused by illness or injury. The illustration also explains the procedure.

4—BODY PARTS INVOLVED

Body parts can refer to specific organs, such as the brain, or to body systems, such as the central nervous system. The body parts are often defined in the text and shown in the illustration depicting the surgery. Further information is available in the Glossary.

5—REASONS FOR SURGERY

This section lists the most common reasons for a surgical procedure. (Of course, it cannot include *all* possible reasons).

If the medical problems listed are unfamiliar to you, refer to the Index. Some have separate charts in the Illnesses and Disorders section, and the rest are explained in the Glossary.

6—SPECIAL CONSIDERATIONS FOR OLDER PATIENTS

Listed here will be some of the factors related to surgical diagnoses or procedures that aging can affect.

7—SURGICAL RISK INCREASES WITH

Risk factors make a surgery more complicated or delay healing. The following are common risk factors for most surgeries:
- Stress, anxiety, depression or other emotional problems.
- Poor nutrition from any cause.
- Chronic illness.
- Recent illness, surgery or injury.
- Genetic factors.

- Obesity.
- Smoking.
- Alcoholism.
- Advanced aging (usually because other medical problems are present).
- The use of drugs of abuse, such as narcotics, psychedelics, hallucinogens, marijuana, sedatives, hypnotics or cocaine.
- The use of some medications, whether prescription or non-prescription. The medicines most likely to increase surgical risk include antihypertensives, muscle relaxants, tranquilizers, sleep inducers, insulin, sedatives, cortisone, beta-adrenergic blockers, calcium channel blockers and antibiotics. These same medications, of course, are lifesaving for some serious illnesses, but they can complicate treatment and outcome of other medical or surgical problems.

8—BEFORE SURGERY

This section includes *Who Operates, Diagnostic Tests, Anesthesia* and *Description of Operation*. Each topic is discussed separately below.

9—WHO OPERATES

A routine surgery is often performed by a general surgeon or by a doctor who specializes in the body system involved. For instance, either a general surgeon or an obstetrician-gynecologist might remove an ovarian cyst. Highly complicated surgeries, such as a heart transplant, are usually done by surgeons with much additional specialized training.

We have included the type of surgeon most likely to perform the procedure, but variations can occur. In many communities general surgeons perform operations that are customarily performed elsewhere by a surgical subspecialist.

Your surgeon should not be uneasy about discussing his or her previous experience and education with you before surgery. Most competent surgeons welcome and sometimes recommend a second opinion when the surgery to be performed is elective rather than an emergency.

This section also includes information on where the surgery is performed. A surgical procedure may be performed in any of the following places:
- A doctor's office.
- An independent outpatient surgical facility.
- A hospital outpatient surgical facility.
- The operating room of a hospital.
- An emergency room.

10—DIAGNOSTIC TESTS

Laboratory studies are helpful in diagnosis and in providing necessary anatomical information prior to surgery. Many tests are the same as those discussed earlier in the description of the Illnesses and Disorders section.

Some tests are especially useful in surgery. Examples include:
- Special x-ray studies of the brain, skeletal system and gastrointestinal tract (upper GI series or lower GI series).
- Intravenous studies of the kidneys and the urinary tract (intravenous pyelogram and retrograde pyelogram).
- Coronary angiographies (x-ray studies of the coronary arteries performed during a cardiac catheterization procedure).
- Biopsy (a microscopic study of tissue) before surgery to establish a diagnosis prior to extensive surgery (usually for cancer) and biopsy afterward of tissue removed during the surgical procedure.

11—ANESTHESIA

Anesthesia makes surgery possible without pain. Recent great advances in anesthesia knowledge and techniques have made many more surgical procedures possible and safe for older patients.

Prior to giving anesthesia, most surgeons prescribe preoperative medications. These generally consist of:

THYROID GLAND REMOVAL
(Thyroidectomy)

 BASIC INFORMATION

DESCRIPTION—Removal of part or all of the thyroid gland.

BODY PARTS INVOLVED—Thyroid gland, the organ in the neck below the Adam's apple that controls the body's metabolism.

REASONS FOR SURGERY
- Benign or cancerous tumors of the thyroid.
- Thyroglossal cysts (see Glossary).
- To treat thyrotoxicosis (excess thyroid hormone).
- Goiter that causes swallowing difficulties.

SPECIAL CONSIDERATIONS FOR OLDER PATIENTS
- Advancing age alone does not preclude surgery.
- More likely to experience respiratory and kidney problems, confusion and blood clots after surgery.
- Characteristic signs and symptoms of many surgical disorders and complications are frequently atypical, changed or absent.
- Surgical repair is complete and effective, but healing takes longer.

SURGICAL RISK INCREASES WITH
- Obesity.
- Smoking.
- Poor nutrition.
- Untreated hyperthyroidism.

Use of antithyroid medication and iodides before surgery decreases risk. Ask your doctor.

 BEFORE SURGERY

WHO OPERATES—General surgeon, usually in hospital.

DIAGNOSTIC TESTS—Blood studies; sonograms; CT scan; needle biopsy; radioactive-iodine uptake and scan (see Glossary).

ANESTHESIA—General anesthesia by inhalation and injection, with an airway tube placed in the windpipe.

DESCRIPTION OF OPERATION
- An incision is made in the neck following natural skin lines.
- Blood supply to the thyroid gland is clamped.
- All or part of the thyroid gland is cut free and removed, and a drain is left in place. In certain cases, some normal thyroid gland tissue is left intact.

- The skin is closed with sutures or clips, which can usually be removed in 2 to 10 days after surgery.

 AFTER SURGERY

POSSIBLE COMPLICATIONS
- Hoarseness if vocal cord nerves are damaged during surgery.
- Hypothyroidism.
- Hypoparathyroidism.
- Excessive bleeding.
- Surgical wound infection.

AVERAGE HOSPITAL STAY—6 to 8 days.

PROBABLE OUTCOME FOR OLDER PATIENTS—Underlying problem cured in most patients. Cancer that is present but has not spread may require radiation treatment. Allow about 6 weeks for recovery from surgery.

GUIDE TO RECUPERATION FOR PEOPLE OVER 50
- Use warm heat packs and massage to relieve pain and discomfort.
- Bathe as usual. Wash incision gently.
- See Appendix 9.

MEDICATIONS & TESTS—Your doctor may prescribe:
- Pain relievers. Follow dosage schedule.
- Thyroid hormones.

ACTIVITY FOR OLDER PATIENTS—Ask your doctor for personalized instructions.

Typical times for resuming:
Bathing . . . . Immediately.
Exercise . . . . 4 weeks.
Driving . . . . 4 weeks.
Sexual activity . . . . When able.
Work . . . . Variable.

FOOD & BEVERAGES—No special diet.

 CALL YOUR DOCTOR IF

- Pain, swelling, redness, drainage or bleeding increases in the surgical area.
- You develop signs of infection: headache, muscle aches, dizziness or a general ill feeling and fever.
- You develop symptoms of hypothyroidism: excessive weakness, fatigue, intolerance of cold, menstrual irregularities, constipation, or dry and coarse skin and hair.

- Tranquilizers or sedatives to help reduce apprehension.
- Pain relievers (frequently narcotic drugs such as morphine) to reduce apprehension and decrease the amount of anesthesia needed.
- An anticholinergic medication, such as scopolamine or atropine, to decrease the secretions of the nose, throat and lungs during the operation.

The type of anesthesia used depends on the surgical problem, the age and general condition of the patient, and sometimes the availability of personnel to administer the anesthesia.

If an operation can be performed with any of several types of anesthesia, you have a right to know the advantages and disadvantages of each. If you wish, you have the right to participate in the selection. Don't hesitate to ask questions.

If a chart lists several anesthesia options for a surgery, you will have one of them, but not all.

The various types of anesthesia include:

Local Anesthesia—This is usually an injectable form of a drug ending in "caine," such as novocaine or xylocaine. Local anesthesia is frequently injected into an injury site, such as a fracture, and bleeding from the injury disperses the anesthetic to all pain-sensitive parts of the injury. Local anesthesia may also be used to block a specific nerve bundle, allowing a pain-free procedure such as a tooth extraction. Local anesthetics are sometimes combined with epinephrine to reduce the bleeding in certain procedures, such as dental surgery or the removal of superficial skin lesions.

Before you have an injection of local anesthesia, tell your doctor or dentist about any allergic responses you have had to local anesthesia in the past. Also inform him or her about any prescription or non-prescription medications you take and about any cardiovascular disease, heartbeat irregularities or peripheral vascular disease you have. The use of local anesthetics with epinephrine under these circumstances can sometimes complicate the disorder.

Spinal Anesthesia—An injection of local anesthetic into the spinal canal above the level of the surgery site is known as spinal anesthesia. It relieves pain satisfactorily for many procedures below the waist, such as surgery of the rectum, genitourinary tract or lower extremities.

A special type of low spinal anesthesia is called caudal or "saddle block" anesthesia as it affects the body area that comes into contact with a horse's saddle.

General Anesthesia—This form of anesthesia involves the injection of a short-acting hypnotic or sedative into a vein. It quickly produces light sleep and allows the placement of an airway tube (endotracheal tube) without discomfort. The tube is connected to hoses that lead to gas machines.

The anesthesiologist controls the flow of anesthesia gases and monitors many body functions, such as blood pressure, breathing rate, pulse and ECG, while you sleep.

When you awaken, the endotracheal tube may still be in place—or it may have been removed. Unless respiration needs continued machine support, the endotracheal tube is usually removed in the recovery room.

The tube will make your throat sore for about 24 hours. This is normal and requires no treatment.

12—DESCRIPTION OF OPERATION

The surgical procedure is described in brief, non-technical terms, and the illustration for each procedure shows what occurs during surgery. Individual surgeons may use slightly varying techniques, but the basic steps are included and only details vary. New surgical methods are constantly being developed that may not be explained here.

If you want additional information, your surgeon can give more details or a librarian can suggest resource materials with fuller descriptions and explanations.

During some surgeries of the gastrointestinal tract, a hollow tube (Levin tube) is passed through your nose into your stomach after you are asleep. The tube will probably be in place when you awaken in the recovery room. The purpose of the tube is to keep the stomach empty to prevent the vomiting or aspiration of material while you are asleep. It also keeps the stomach decompressed until normal muscular movement of the gastrointestinal tract can resume after surgery. An empty stomach is more comfortable and helps prevent complications that may arise if the stomach becomes distended with air or gas.

The average time in surgery and in the recovery room are not listed because variations are too great. Factors that affect the time in surgery include:

- The exact techniques chosen.
- The experience and preference of the surgeon.
- The availability and experience of assistants and operating room personnel.
- The presence or absence of complications during surgery.
- The age and condition of the patient prior to surgery.

Don't hesitate to ask your surgeon to estimate the time your operation will require. This is particularly important for family members who may be waiting for the outcome.

13—AFTER SURGERY

This section includes *Possible Complications, Average Hospital Stay, Probable Outcome for Older Patients, Guide to Recuperation for People Over 50, Medications & Tests, Activity for Older Patients, Food & Beverage* and *Call Your Doctor If.*

14—POSSIBLE COMPLICATIONS

Complications are additional medical problems related to the surgery that occur during or after the procedure.

They sometimes happen despite accurate diagnosis, skillful surgery, competent assistance and well-equipped operating rooms. Some complications are preventable, and some occur frequently—but most are rare.

15—AVERAGE HOSPITAL STAY

This estimate is based on an average for people over 50. It varies according to how healing and recuperation progress and whether complications develop before, during or after surgery. It is also influenced by the amount Medicare and private insurance companies will allow as reimbursement for specific procedures.

16—PROBABLE OUTCOME FOR OLDER PATIENTS

This heading relates to the surgery's effect on the underlying disorder and the average length of time required to recover from surgery. Estimates are based on the assumption that complications do not occur and healing proceeds normally. Complications can alter the course of healing dramatically. A positive outlook following surgery is an important factor that facilitates a good outcome and rapid healing.

17—GUIDE TO RECUPERATION FOR PEOPLE OVER 50

This section generally provides instructions for self-care during recuperation after hospitalization. It should serve as a reminder of instructions given you by your surgeon. It should not replace your doctor's instructions.

Some questions are almost universal following surgery. Most patients are unsure how to care for a surgical wound. They have questions about pain, bathing, stitches, clothing and other matters. These questions are answered in this section.

18—MEDICATIONS & TESTS

The medications usually prescribed or suggested after surgery are described, along with brief instructions for their use. Important post-operative tests are also listed.

19—ACTIVITY FOR OLDER PATIENTS

Resumption of activity is a strong area of concern for post-surgical patients. In this section is information on what types of exercise are appropriate, and average times are provided for when to resume sexual relations, when to resume driving, when to resume bathing and when to return to work. These will differ greatly depending on each individual's health condition.

20—FOOD & BEVERAGE

During surgery with general anesthesia, the gastrointestinal tract is kept empty. After the patient awakens, the gastrointestinal tract may be temporarily quiet or inactive. Clear liquids are usually provided until the gastrointestinal tract begins to function again. When appropriate, this information is included in the surgery charts. Additional diet instructions usually refer to special diets in the Appendix section.

21—CALL YOUR DOCTOR IF

You should call your doctor if healing and recuperation after surgery don't follow the usual course of events. Excessive bleeding and general or surgical wound infection are common dangers after most surgical procedures, and these are always mentioned on surgery charts when appropriate.

Other reasons listed for which you should call your doctor can serve as reminders of possible complications. If you develop symptoms you believe are related to your surgery—even if they don't appear on the chart—call your doctor about them.

Using the Medications Section

The information about medications in this book is organized in condensed, easy-to-read charts. Every medication is known by a brand name (e.g., Actidil), a generic name (e.g., TRIPROLIDINE) or a family name (e.g., antihistamine). The medication charts in this book are arranged alphabetically by the family name of the medication in most cases. Both prescription and non-prescription medications are included. Each major heading on the charts is numbered on the sample chart on page xxvii, and these numbered sections are explained below.

1—FAMILY NAME OF MEDICATION

This is the family name for a group of medications that are generally used for the same purpose. The sample chart is for antihistamines. If you are not sure what the family name is for a medication you want to read about, look in the index for either the brand name or the generic name.

2—BRAND & GENERIC NAMES

Brand names are those given to a particular medication by the manufacturer. In this list, they begin with a capital letter followed by lower-case letters. Generic names are the official chemical names for the medication. In this list, the generic names are written with all capital letters. All listings are in alphabetical order. In some instances brand names are so numerous that there is not sufficient space in this book to list them all, so only the most common are listed.

3—USES

This section lists the illness or disorder for which the medication is prescribed.

Most uses listed are approved by the U.S. Food and Drug Administration.

Some uses may be listed if ongoing experiments and clinical trials indicate that the medication may be used with effectiveness and safety. Still other uses are included for which the medication may not be officially sanctioned, but for which doctors may prescribe the medication anyway.

The use for which your doctor prescribes the medication may not be listed. You and your doctor should discuss the reason for any prescription medication you take. You alone will probably decide whether to take a non-prescription medication. The information on these charts may help you make a decision.

4—POSSIBLE ADVERSE REACTIONS OR SIDE EFFECTS

Adverse reactions or side effects are symptoms that may occur when you take a medication. They are the effects on the body other than the desired therapeutic effect. Some are important, and some are insignificant.

Some adverse reactions and side effects can be prevented, which is one reason the information is included in the book. Most adverse reactions and side effects are minor and last only a short time. With many medications, the reactions that occur will frequently diminish in intensity as time passes.

As recommended in the charts, you should consult a doctor if any of the listed side effects or adverse reactions occurs (or if you experience any new symptoms that are not listed).

The majority of medications, when they are used properly for valid reasons, offer benefits that outweigh the potential hazards of some of the adverse reactions and side effects.

5—WARNINGS & PRECAUTIONS

Read these entries for special information that may apply to you.

6—AGE-RELATED FACTORS

These are special considerations that apply to older adults. Changes associated with age may have a bearing on the way a medication reacts in the body. Doctors should always consider the age of a patient in determining the proper dosage level of any medication being prescribed.

7—POSSIBLE INTERACTIONS WITH OTHER DRUGS

This section does not list all the possible interactions, but serves as a reminder that there are often interactions between two or more medications that you take. This includes non-prescription as well as prescription medications. Some interactions can be dangerous. If you take two or more medications, remind your doctor or pharmacist of this before you take them.

8—OVERDOSE

This section lists symptoms of an overdose and what emergency action to take.

9—SYMPTOMS

The symptoms listed here are most likely to develop with accidental or purposeful overdose. An overdose patient may not show all the symptoms listed. Sometimes the symptoms are identical to ones listed as side effects or adverse reactions. The difference is their intensity and severity. You will have to judge. Consult a doctor or poison control center if you have any doubt.

10—WHAT TO DO

If you suspect an overdose (even if there are no symptoms), follow the instructions in this section. Expanded instructions for emergency procedures are at the end of this book.

ANGIOTENSIN-CONVERTING ENZYME (ACE) INHIBITORS

BRAND & GENERIC NAMES

Commonly prescribed brand names (start with a Capital) and generic names (all CAPITALS) include CAPTOPRIL, Capoten, ENALAPRIL, LISINOPRIL, Prinivil, Vasotec and Zestril.

USES

- Treats high blood pressure.
- Treats congestive heart failure.

POSSIBLE ADVERSE REACTIONS OR SIDE EFFECTS

If any of the following occurs, consult a doctor:
- Hives.
- Rash.
- Intense itching.
- Faintness soon after a dose.
- Difficulty breathing.
- Loss of taste.
- Swelling of mouth, face, hands or feet.
- Dizziness.
- Chest pain.
- Fast or irregular heartbeat.
- Coughing.
- Sore throat.
- Cloudy urine.
- Fever.
- Chills.
- Nausea.
- Vomiting.
- Indigestion.
- Abdominal pain.

WARNINGS & PRECAUTIONS

- Avoid heavy exercise in hot weather.
- Before taking this medicine, consult your doctor if you have diabetes mellitus (sugar diabetes), heart disease, blood vessel disease, kidney disease, liver disease, systemic lupus erythematosus or have recently had a heart attack, stroke or kidney transplant.
- Don't drive or try risky physical activity until you know how drug affects you.
- See Appendix 21.

AGE-RELATED FACTORS

- Older patients are more likely to have age-related kidney or liver function impairment. This may lead to the need for reduction of the usual dosage.
- Aging does not affect expected results.
- Your doctor or care-giver should carefully monitor your response to this drug.

POSSIBLE INTERACTION WITH OTHER DRUGS

- If you are using or taking any other drug (prescription or non-prescription), ask your doctor or pharmacist if there are possible interactions.
- Angiotensin-converting enzyme inhibitors cannot safely be taken with some drugs.
- Angiotensin-converting enzyme inhibitors taken with some drugs may require dosage adjustment.

Do not drink alcoholic beverages or use cocaine, marijuana or tobacco while taking this medicine. These may decrease the effectiveness of the medicine or cause uncomfortable or dangerous adverse reactions.

OVERDOSE

SYMPTOMS
Fever; chills; sore throat; fainting; convulsions; coma.

WHAT TO DO
- Dial 911 (emergency) or 0 (operator) for an ambulance or medical help. Then give first aid immediately.
- If patient is unconscious and not breathing, give mouth-to-mouth breathing. If there is no heartbeat, use cardiac massage and mouth-to-mouth breathing (CPR). Don't try to make patient vomit. If you can't get help quickly, take patient to nearest emergency facility.

Symptoms

ABDOMINAL PAIN, RECURRENT ATTACKS

(Find your closest combination of symptoms in left-hand column; see possible problem in right-hand column. You may not experience all symptoms listed.)

SYMPTOMS & FACTORS	POSSIBLE PROBLEM
• Flushed skin on the head and neck. • Watery eyes. • Diarrhea with abdominal cramps. • Respiratory symptoms similar to those of asthma. • Irregular heartbeat. • Nausea and vomiting. • Unexplained weight loss.	**CARCINOID SYNDROME** (Refer to Illnesses section)

Early symptoms include:
- Pain in the left side of the abdomen that improves after bowel movements.
- Episodes of bloody diarrhea with mucus, alternating with symptom-free intervals.

During an acute attack:
(THIS IS AN EMERGENCY; SEEK MEDICAL CARE IMMEDIATELY!)
- Increased bloody diarrhea (up to 10 to 20 bowel movements a day).
- Severe cramps and pain around the rectum.
- Appetite and weight loss.
- Bloated abdomen.
- Fever as high as 104F (40C).
- Rapid heartbeat.

COLITIS, ULCERATIVE
(Refer to Illnesses section)

- Cramping abdominal pain—especially after eating. The pain is sometimes in the right lower abdomen, mimicking appendicitis.
- Nausea and diarrhea; general ill feeling; fever.
- Appetite and weight loss.
- Abdominal tenderness; abdominal mass that can be felt.
- Bloody stools (sometimes).

CROHN'S DISEASE
(Refer to Illnesses section)

Diverticulosis symptoms:
- Mild cramping, bloated feeling or tenderness in the left side of the abdomen that is relieved by passing gas or moving bowels.
- Occasional bright red blood in the stool. Non-infected diverticulae sometimes bleed.
- Constipation or diarrhea (sometimes).

Diverticulitis symptoms:
- Intermittent cramping; abdominal pain that becomes constant.
- Fever.
- Nausea.
- Tenderness over the affected area of the colon.

DIVERTICULAR DISEASE
(Refer to Illnesses section)

- Cramping pain in the upper right of the abdomen. Pain may also occur in the chest (imitating a heart attack), in the upper back or the right shoulder. These symptoms frequently follow a meal rich in fats.
- Tenderness in the upper abdomen.
- Nausea and vomiting.
- Belching.
- Slight fever. If high fever and chills occur, a bacterial infection is present.
- Jaundice (yellow skin and eyes) sometimes.
- Pale stools (sometimes).
- Itching skin (sometimes).

GALLBLADDER, INFECTION OF
(Refer to Illnesses section)

(ABDOMINAL PAIN, RECURRENT ATTACKS, continued on next page)

SYMPTOMS & FACTORS	POSSIBLE PROBLEM
• Colicky (intermittent) pain in the upper right abdomen or between the shoulder blades. • Nausea and vomiting. • Bloating or belching. • Intolerance of fatty foods (indigestion, bloating and belching). • Jaundice (yellow skin and eyes). • No symptoms in about 40% of cases.	**GALLSTONES** (Refer to Illnesses section)
The following signs are worse at night: • Belching or slight regurgitation of stomach contents into the mouth, producing an acid taste. • Heavy, burning or uncomfortable sensation in the chest. • Difficulty swallowing. • Mild abdominal pain.	**HEARTBURN** (Refer to Illnesses section)
• No symptoms in the early stages (frequently). • Bloody or black, tarry stools. • Cramping abdominal pain. • Feeling of fullness. • Change in bowel habits, such as diarrhea, constipation or narrow-caliber stools. • Unexplained weight loss. • Pain in the rectum. • Anemia. • Loss of bowel control (sometimes).	**LARGE INTESTINE, CANCER OF** (Refer to Illnesses section)
• Rapid, unexplained weight loss. • Pain in the back or upper abdomen that is often relieved by bending forward. • Blood clots in veins anywhere, especially the arms and legs. This is often an early sign. • Jaundice (yellow skin and eyes) from blockage of the nearby bile duct. Jaundice is usually accompanied by intense itching.	**PANCREAS, CANCER OF** (Refer to Illnesses section)
Severe acute pancreatitis: **(THIS IS AN EMERGENCY; SEEK MEDICAL CARE IMMEDIATELY!)** • Extreme abdominal pain. • Vomiting. • Abdominal swelling and gas. • Fever. • Muscle aches. **Chronic pancreatitis:** • Persistent, mild or severe pain, often after meals, in the upper abdomen, sometimes radiating to the back or generalized. Pain is aching, burning, gnawing or stabbing. Pain episodes may last days or weeks, but rarely less than 1 day. • Mild jaundice (yellow skin and eyes) sometimes. • Rapid weight loss.	**PANCREATITIS** (Refer to Illnesses section)
Symptoms vary, depending on which organ is affected by the decreased blood supply. The most common include: • Chest pain (heart involvement). • Shortness of breath (lung involvement). • Abdominal pain (intestinal and liver involvement). • Blood in the urine (kidney involvement). • Numbness and tingling of the hands and feet (nerve involvement).	**POLYARTERITIS** (Refer to Illnesses section)

(ABDOMINAL PAIN, RECURRENT ATTACKS, continued on next page)

SYMPTOMS & FACTORS	POSSIBLE PROBLEM
• Cramp-like pain in the middle or to one side of the lower abdomen. Pain is usually relieved with bowel movements. • Nausea. • Bloating and gas. • Headache. • Rectal pain. • Backache. • Occasional appetite loss that may lead to weight loss. • Diarrhea or constipation, usually alternating. • Fatigue. • Depression. • Anxiety.	**SPASTIC COLON** (Refer to Illnesses section)
Early stages: • Vague symptoms of indigestion, such as fullness, burping, nausea and poor appetite. **Later stages:** • Unexplained weight loss. • Vomiting blood. • Black stools. • Fullness after eating small amounts. • Pain in the upper abdomen. • Mass in the upper abdomen that can be felt (sometimes).	**STOMACH CANCER** (Refer to Illnesses section)
• Abdominal pain and cramps. • Vomiting (occasionally). • Appetite loss. • Fever. • Weakness. • Swollen abdomen. • Sharp, dull or annoying pain in the chest. • Acid taste in the mouth. • Mild nausea and diarrhea (rare). • Belching or gaseousness.	**STOMACH INFLAMMATION** (Refer to Illnesses section)
• Nausea that sometimes causes vomiting. • Diarrhea that ranges from 2 or 3 loose stools to many watery stools. • Abdominal cramps, pain or tenderness. • Appetite loss. • Fever. • Weakness.	**STOMACH & INTESTINAL INFLAMMATION** (Refer to Illnesses section)
Early stages (usually begin in 7 to 10 days): • Appetite loss, nausea, vomiting, diarrhea and abdominal cramps. **Later stages:** • Puffy eyelids and face. • Muscle pain. • Itching, burning skin. • Sweating. • High fever (102F to 104F or 38.9C to 40C).	**TRICHINOSIS** (Refer to Illnesses section)

(ABDOMINAL PAIN, RECURRENT ATTACKS, continued on next page)

SYMPTOMS & FACTORS	POSSIBLE PROBLEM
• Burning, boring or gnawing pain, usually in the upper abdomen, but occasionally below the breastbone. The pain is often interpreted as heartburn, indigestion or hunger and may be relieved by drinking milk, eating, resting or taking antacids. • Pain lasts 30 minutes to 3 hours. It may occur immediately after eating or hours later. It frequently awakens one at night. • Pain comes and goes. Weeks of intermittent pain may alternate with short pain-free periods. • Appetite and weight loss. • Recurrent vomiting. • Blood in the stool. • Anemia. • Belching and bloating.	**ULCER, DUODENAL** (Refer to Illnesses section)
• Burning, gnawing pain in the upper abdomen or the lower chest below the breastbone. The pain is often interpreted as indigestion, heartburn or hunger and may be relieved temporarily with milk, antacids or bland food. • Pain lasts 30 minutes to 3 hours. It may occur immediately after eating or hours later. • Pain comes and goes. Weeks of intermittent pain may alternate with short pain-free periods. • Loss of appetite. • Weight loss. • Anemia. • Occasional vomiting.	**ULCER, STOMACH** (Refer to Illnesses section)

ABDOMINAL PAIN, SUDDEN ATTACK

(Find your closest combination of symptoms in left-hand column; see possible problem in right-hand column. You may not experience all symptoms listed.)

SYMPTOMS & FACTORS	POSSIBLE PROBLEM
Symptoms vary according to which artery is affected: • Thoracic (chest) aneurysm produces pain in the chest, neck, back and abdomen. The pain may be sudden and sharp. It also causes hoarseness and swallowing difficulty. • Abdominal aneurysm produces back pain (sometimes severe), appetite and weight loss and a pulsating mass in the abdomen.	**ANEURYSM** (Refer to Illnesses section) (THIS IS AN EMERGENCY; SEEK MEDICAL CARE IMMEDIATELY!)
• Pain that begins close to the navel and migrates toward the right lower abdomen. Pain becomes persistent and well localized. It worsens with moving, breathing deeply, coughing, sneezing, walking or being touched. • Nausea and sometimes vomiting. • Constipation and inability to pass gas. • Diarrhea (occasionally). • Low fever (under 102F or 38.9C), beginning after other symptoms. • Tenderness in the right lower abdomen, usually about a third of the distance from the navel to the top of the hip bone. (This description applies only if the appendix is in its normal position. In some cases, the tip of the appendix is located elsewhere, making diagnosis difficult.) • Abdominal swelling (late stages).	**APPENDICITIS** (Refer to Illnesses section) (THIS IS AN EMERGENCY; SEEK MEDICAL CARE IMMEDIATELY!)

(ABDOMINAL PAIN, SUDDEN ATTACK, continued on next page)

SYMPTOMS & FACTORS	POSSIBLE PROBLEM
• Burning and stinging on urination. • Frequent urination, especially at night, although the urine amount may be small. • Increased urge to urinate. • Pain in the lower part of abdomen over the bladder. • Low back pain. • Low-grade fever (under 101F or 38.3C). • Bad-smelling urine. • Painful sexual intercourse. • Lack of urinary control (sometimes).	**BLADDER INFECTION** (Refer to Illnesses section)
• Colicky (intermittent) pain in the upper right abdomen or between the shoulder blades. • Nausea and vomiting. • Bloating or belching. • Intolerance of fatty foods (indigestion, bloating and belching). • Jaundice (yellow skin and eyes). • No symptoms in about 40% of cases.	**GALLSTONES** (Refer to Illnesses section)
• Mild nausea. • Heartburn. • Upper abdominal pain. • Gas or belching. • Bloated or full feeling. • Acid taste.	**INDIGESTION** (Refer to Illnesses section)
• Abdominal pain and cramps. • Nausea and vomiting. In the advanced stage, vomit resembles feces. • Weakness, dizziness or fainting. • Little or no urine due to fluid loss. • Audible noises from the abdomen in early stages. • Abdominal bloating, swelling and gas. • Fever (sometimes). • Diarrhea (partial obstruction only). • Rectal bleeding (sometimes). • Inability to pass gas or stool.	**INTESTINAL OBSTRUCTION** (Refer to Illnesses section) (THIS IS AN EMERGENCY; SEEK MEDICAL CARE IMMEDIATELY!)
Sudden onset of: • Fever and shaking chills. • Burning, frequent urination. • Cloudy urine or blood in the urine. • Aching (sometimes severe) in one or both sides of the lower back. • Abdominal pain.	**KIDNEY INFECTION, ACUTE** (Refer to Illnesses section)
• Episodes of severe, colicky (intermittent) pain every few minutes. The pain usually appears first in the back, just below the ribs. Over several hours or days, the pain follows the stone's course through the ureter toward the groin. Pain stops when the stone passes. • Frequent nausea.	**KIDNEY STONES** (Refer to Illnesses section) (THIS IS AN EMERGENCY; SEEK MEDICAL CARE IMMEDIATELY!)
Some produce no symptoms. Others produce any of the following: • Swelling without pain in the lower abdomen. • Painful sexual intercourse. • Stinging or burning on urination (if the cyst presses on the bladder). • Difficulty emptying the bladder completely. • Brownish vaginal discharge. • Increased hairiness (if the cyst produces excess hormones).	**OVARIAN CYSTS** (Refer to Illnesses section)

(ABDOMINAL PAIN, SUDDEN ATTACK, continued on next page)

SYMPTOMS & FACTORS	POSSIBLE PROBLEM
Severe acute pancreatitis: (THIS IS AN EMERGENCY; SEEK MEDICAL CARE IMMEDIATELY!) • Extreme abdominal pain. • Vomiting. • Abdominal swelling and gas. • Fever. • Muscle aches. **Chronic pancreatitis:** • Persistent mild or severe pain, often after meals, in the upper abdomen, sometimes radiating to the back or generalized. Pain is aching, burning, gnawing or stabbing. Pain episodes may last days or weeks, but rarely less than 1 day. • Mild jaundice (yellow skin and eyes) sometimes. • Rapid weight loss.	**PANCREATITIS** (Refer to Illnesses section)
Early symptoms (up to 1 week): • Painful sexual intercourse. • Bad-smelling vaginal discharge. • Low fever. • Frequent, painful urination. **Later symptoms (1 to 3 weeks):** • Severe pain and tenderness in the lower abdomen on one or both sides. • High fever. • Increased bad-smelling vaginal discharge.	**PELVIC INFLAMMATORY DISEASE** (Refer to Illnesses section)
• Pain in one area or throughout the abdomen. Pain usually starts suddenly and becomes increasingly severe. Pain may be cramping at first, and then steady. The patient often prefers to lie quietly on the back because movement or pressure on the abdomen increases pain. • Shoulder pain (sometimes). • Chills and fever (often high). • Dizziness and weakness. • Rapid heartbeat. • Low blood pressure.	**PERITONITIS** (Refer to Illnesses section) (THIS IS AN EMERGENCY; SEEK MEDICAL CARE IMMEDIATELY!)
• Diarrhea, often accompanied by abdominal cramps. In mild cases, diarrhea may be only 2 or 3 loose bowel movements a day. In severe cases, it may be watery diarrhea as often as every 10 or 15 minutes. • Vomiting (occasionally); fever. • Blood in the stool (sometimes). A relatively mild salmonella infection may be mistaken for simple gastroenteritis.	**SALMONELLA INFECTION** (Refer to Illnesses section)
• Painful red blisters anywhere on the body. Blisters appear 4 to 5 days after early symptoms begin. The blisters appear on a broad streak of reddened skin along sensory nerve routes to a particular area of skin. They occur most often on the chest and spread only on one side of the body. • Mild chills and fever. • General ill feeling. • Mild nausea, abdominal cramps or diarrhea. • Chest pain, face pain or burning pain in the skin of the abdomen, depending on the affected area.	**SHINGLES** (Refer to Illnesses section)

(ABDOMINAL PAIN, SUDDEN ATTACK, continued on next page)

SYMPTOMS & FACTORS	POSSIBLE PROBLEM
• Abdominal pain and cramps. • Vomiting (occasionally). • Appetite loss. • Fever. • Weakness. • Swollen abdomen. • Sharp, dull or annoying pain in the chest. • Acid taste in the mouth. • Mild nausea and diarrhea (rare). • Belching or gas.	**STOMACH INFLAMMATION** (Refer to Illnesses section)
• Nausea that sometimes causes vomiting. • Diarrhea that ranges from 2 or 3 loose stools to many watery stools. • Abdominal cramps, pain or tenderness. • Appetite loss. • Fever. • Weakness.	**STOMACH & INTESTINAL INFLAMMATION** (Refer to Illnesses section)

If you experience SUDDEN ATTACK OF ABDOMINAL PAIN plus the following:

• Mild pain in lower abdomen. • Constipation or gas. • Recent diet change such as adding more fiber.	**WHAT TO DO:** Call doctor if discomfort persists longer than 3 hours. Symptoms together probably do not represent any disorder.
• Pain in lower abdomen in females with unexplained vaginal bleeding.	**WHAT TO DO:** See Unexpected Vaginal Bleeding (in Symptoms section).

ABDOMINAL SWELLING

(Find your closest combination of symptoms in left-hand column; see possible problem in right-hand column. You may not experience all symptoms listed.)

SYMPTOMS & FACTORS	POSSIBLE PROBLEM
• Flushed skin on the head and neck. • Watery eyes. • Diarrhea with abdominal cramps. • Respiratory symptoms similar to those of asthma. • Irregular heartbeat. • Nausea and vomiting. • Unexplained weight loss.	**CARCINOID SYNDROME** (Refer to Illnesses section)
Early stages: • Fatigue; weakness. • Poor appetite; nausea; weight loss. • Enlarged liver. • Red palms. **Late stages:** • Jaundice (yellow skin and eyes). • Dark yellow or brown urine. • Spider blood vessels of the skin (fine vessels which spread out from a central point). • Hair loss. • Breast enlargement in men. • Fluid accumulation in the abdomen and legs. • Enlarged spleen. • Diarrhea; stool may be black or bloody. • Bleeding and bruising. • Mental confusion; coma.	**CIRRHOSIS OF THE LIVER** (Refer to Illnesses section)

(ABDOMINAL SWELLING, continued on next page)

SYMPTOMS & FACTORS	POSSIBLE PROBLEM
• Shortness of breath, especially with exertion or when lying flat in bed. • Fatigue, weakness or faintness. • Cough (usually with sputum). • Wheezing (sometimes). • Swelling of the abdomen, legs and ankles. • Rapid or irregular heartbeat.	**CONGESTIVE HEART FAILURE** (Refer to Illnesses section)
• Hard mass in the right upper abdomen. • Unexplained weight loss and appetite loss. • Jaundice (yellow skin and eyes) rarely. • Abdominal discomfort that resembles a pulled muscle. • Low blood sugar (weakness, sweating, hunger, tremor and headache). • Fever. • Fluid in the abdomen; enlarged spleen. • Bleeding tendency in the gastrointestinal tract and other sites.	**HEPATOMA** (Refer to Illnesses section)
• Abdominal pain and cramps. • Nausea and vomiting. In the advanced stage, vomit resembles feces. • Weakness, dizziness or fainting. • Little or no urine due to fluid loss. • Audible noises from the abdomen in early stages. • Abdominal bloating, swelling and gas. • Fever (sometimes). • Diarrhea (partial obstruction only). • Rectal bleeding (sometimes). • Inability to pass gas or stool.	**INTESTINAL OBSTRUCTION** (Refer to Illnesses section) **(THIS IS AN EMERGENCY; SEEK MEDICAL CARE IMMEDIATELY!)**
Early stages: • Repeated kidney infections. • A mass in the abdomen. • Hypertension. • No symptoms (frequently) until the cysts replace so much normal kidney structure that kidney failure occurs. **Symptoms of kidney failure:** • Pain in the lower back. • Frequent urination. • Increasing fatigue and weakness. • Headache • Bad breath. • Nausea, vomiting or diarrhea. • Fluid retention, especially swelling around the ankles or eyes. • Shortness of breath. • Chest pain. • Itching skin.	**KIDNEY, POLYCYSTIC** (Refer to Illnesses section)
• Loss of appetite and weight loss. • Tender mass in the right upper abdomen. • Pain in the upper abdomen. • Low-grade fever, usually less than 101F (38.3C). • Jaundice (yellow eyes and skin) sometimes. • Swollen abdomen from fluid retention (sometimes). • Mental status changes, such as confusion or forgetfulness.	**LIVER CANCER** (Refer to Illnesses section)

(ABDOMINAL SWELLING, continued on next page)

SYMPTOMS & FACTORS	POSSIBLE PROBLEM
Frequently no symptoms occur until the tumor becomes large. **Early symptoms:** • Vague discomfort in the lower abdomen. • Gastrointestinal upsets. • Irregular menstrual periods. **Later symptoms:** • Deep voice. • Excessive hair growth. • Unexplained weight loss. • An enlarged, hard and sometimes tender mass in the lower abdomen. • Painful sexual intercourse. • Anemia.	**OVARIAN CANCER** (Refer to Illnesses section)
Some produce no symptoms. Others produce any of the following: • Swelling without pain in the lower abdomen. • Painful sexual intercourse. • Stinging or burning on urination (if the cyst presses on the bladder). • Difficulty emptying the bladder completely. • Brownish vaginal discharge. • Increased hairiness (if the cyst produces excess hormones).	**OVARIAN CYSTS** (Refer to Illnesses section)

ANKLE PAIN

(Find your closest combination of symptoms in left-hand column; see possible problem in right-hand column. You may not experience all symptoms listed.)

SYMPTOMS & FACTORS	POSSIBLE PROBLEM
Slow or sudden onset of: • Redness, aching, pain, warmth and tenderness in any or all active joints in the hands, wrists, elbows, shoulders, knees, feet, ankles, jaw or spine. • Morning stiffness; muscular atrophy. • Low-grade fever. • Nodules under the skin (sometimes). • Pale skin. • Appetite loss.	**ARTHRITIS, RHEUMATOID** (Refer to Illnesses section)
• Pain and swelling at the fracture site. • Tenderness close to the fracture. • Paleness and deformity (sometimes). • Loss of pulse below the fracture, usually in an extremity. **(THIS IS AN EMERGENCY; SEEK MEDICAL CARE IMMEDIATELY!)** • Numbness, tingling or paralysis below the fracture (rare). **(THIS IS AN EMERGENCY; SEEK MEDICAL CARE IMMEDIATELY!)** • Bleeding or bruising at the site. • Weakness and inability to bear weight.	**FRACTURES, BONE** (Refer to Illnesses section)
• Sudden onset of severe pain in the inflamed joint, usually at the base of the big toe or larger joints. • Involved joints are red, hot, swollen and very tender. Skin over the joint is red and shiny. • Fever (sometimes).	**GOUT** (Refer to Illnesses section)

(ANKLE PAIN, continued on next page)

(ANKLE PAIN, continued from previous page)

SYMPTOMS & FACTORS	POSSIBLE PROBLEM
• Joint stiffness and pain, including backache. Weather changes, especially cold, damp weather, may increase aching. • Limited movement and loss of dexterity in affected joints. • Redness, heat or fever in affected joints (sometimes). • Swelling of affected joints (sometimes), especially finger joints. • Cracking or grating sounds with joint movement (sometimes).	**OSTEOARTHRITIS** (Refer to Illnesses section)
• Pain or tenderness in the area of injury; severity varies with the extent of injury. • Swelling of the affected joint. • Redness or bruising in the area of injury, either immediately or several hours after injury. • Loss of normal mobility in the injured joint.	**SPRAINS & STRAINS** (Refer to Illnesses section)

If you experience ANKLE PAIN plus the following:

• Affected joints red, warm or swollen.	**WHAT TO DO:** Call doctor now.
• Fever; general ill feeling.	**WHAT TO DO:** Call doctor now.
• Recent illness, such as sore throat or skin infection.	**WHAT TO DO:** Call doctor now.

ANKLES, SWOLLEN

(Find your closest combination of symptoms in left-hand column; see possible problem in right-hand column. You may not experience all symptoms listed.)

SYMPTOMS & FACTORS	POSSIBLE PROBLEM
If cardiomyopathy is extensive enough to cause congestive heart failure, the following symptoms may occur: • Irregular or rapid heartbeat. • Shortness of breath with activity. • Swelling of the feet and ankles. • Fatigue. • Cough with frothy, bloody sputum. **(THIS IS AN EMERGENCY; SEEK MEDICAL CARE IMMEDIATELY!)** • Appetite loss. • Loss of sex drive. • Chest pain.	**CARDIOMYOPATHY** (Refer to Illnesses section)
• Shortness of breath, especially with exertion or when lying flat in bed. • Fatigue, weakness or faintness. • Cough (usually with sputum). • Wheezing. • Swelling of the abdomen, legs and ankles. • Rapid or irregular heartbeat. • Low blood pressure. • Distended neck veins. • Enlarged liver.	**CONGESTIVE HEART FAILURE** (Refer to Illnesses section)

(ANKLES, SWOLLEN, continued on next page)

SYMPTOMS & FACTORS	POSSIBLE PROBLEM

Mild glomerulonephritis produces no symptoms. Diagnosis is possible only with urine studies. Severe glomerulonephritis produces the following:

- Smoky or slightly red urine.
- General ill feeling.
- Drowsiness.
- Nausea or vomiting.
- Headaches.
- Fever (sometimes).
- Appetite loss.
- Decreased urination.
- Fluid accumulation in the body, especially puffy eyes and ankles.
- Shortness of breath.
- High blood pressure.
- Protein in the urine.
- Disturbed vision.

GLOMERULONEPHRITIS
(Refer to Illnesses section)

- Chest pain (angina pectoris).
- Heart rhythm irregularity.
- Fainting.
- Shortness of breath.
- Swollen feet and ankles.
- Distended neck veins.
- Heart failure.
- Heart murmur (see Glossary).

IDIOPATHIC HYPERTROPHIC SUBAORTIC STENOSIS
(Refer to Illnesses section)

- Fatigue.
- Shortness of breath.
- Irregular heartbeat.
- Fever.
- Other symptoms caused by the underlying disorder.

If myocarditis causes congestive heart failure, the following symptoms may also occur:

- Swollen feet and ankles.
- Distended neck veins.
- Rapid heartbeat, even when at rest.
- Difficulty breathing while resting or lying down.

MYOCARDITIS
(Refer to Illnesses section)

Early stages:
- No symptoms (usually).

Later stages:
- Weakness and fatigue.
- Shortness of breath with exertion.
- Frequent fainting.
- Swelling of the ankles and feet caused by fluid retention.
- Distended neck veins.
- Bluish skin.
- Chest pain.
- Enlarged liver and swollen abdomen.

OBTRUCTIVE PULMONARY DISEASE, CHRONIC
(Refer to Illnesses section)

- Confusion.
- Restlessness and anxiety.
- Weakness.
- Muscle cramps (usually in the legs).
- Changes in pulse rate and blood pressure.
- Tissue swelling (edema).
- Stupor or coma (if severe imbalance). **(THIS IS AN EMERGENCY; SEEK MEDICAL CARE IMMEDIATELY!)**

Sodium imbalance may be part of a disease with other symptoms that predominate, such as fever, vomiting, diarrhea or excessive sweating.

SODIUM, TOO MUCH OR TOO LITTLE IN BLOOD
(Refer to Illnesses section)

(ANKLES, SWOLLEN, continued on next page)

(ANKLES, SWOLLEN, continued from previous page)

SYMPTOMS & FACTORS	POSSIBLE PROBLEM
• Pain or tenderness in the area of injury; severity varies with the extent of injury. • Swelling of the affected joint. • Redness or bruising in the area of injury, either immediately or several hours after injury. • Loss of normal mobility in the injured joint.	**SPRAINS & STRAINS** (Refer to Illnesses section)
• Swelling and pain in the area drained by the vein, usually the ankle, calf or thigh. Swelling in the leg includes everything below the clot, extending to the toes. • Tenderness and redness of the affected parts. • Soreness or pain when walking. The soreness does not disappear with rest. • Pain when raising the leg and flexing the foot (sometimes). • Fever (sometimes). • Increased heartbeat (sometimes).	**THROMBOSIS, DEEP-VEIN** (Refer to Illnesses section)

If you experience SWOLLEN ANKLES plus the following:

• Injury to ankle in last 4 months and pain recurs.	**WHAT TO DO:** Call doctor soon.
• Recent confinement for several hours, such as in a car, bus, train or airplane.	**WHAT TO DO:** Elevate legs. When possible, avoid prolonged sitting or standing. Move around frequently.
• Swelling persists more than 48 hours.	**WHAT TO DO:** Call doctor soon.

ANXIETY & NERVOUSNESS

(Find your closest combination of symptoms in left-hand column; see possible problem in right-hand column. You may not experience all symptoms listed.)

SYMPTOMS & FACTORS	POSSIBLE PROBLEM
Early stages: • Low tolerance for anxiety. • Need for alcohol at the beginning of the day or at times of stress. • Insomnia; nightmares. • Habitual Monday-morning hangovers and frequent absences from work. • Preoccupation with obtaining alcohol and hiding drinking from family and friends. • Guilt or irritability when others suggest drinking is excessive. **Late stages:** • Frequent blackouts; memory loss. • Delirium tremens (tremors; hallucinations; confusion; sweating; rapid heartbeat). These occur most often with alcohol withdrawal. • Liver disease (jaundice; internal bleeding; bloating). • Neurological impairment (numbness and tingling in hands and feet; declining sexual interest and potency; confusion; coma). • Congestive heart failure (shortness of breath; swelling of feet).	**ALCOHOLISM** (Refer to Illnesses section)

(ANXIETY & NERVOUSNESS, continued on next page)

SYMPTOMS & FACTORS	POSSIBLE PROBLEM
• Feeling that something undesirable or harmful is about to happen. • Dry mouth; swallowing difficulty or hoarseness. • Rapid breathing and heartbeat. • Twitching or trembling. • Muscle tension; headaches. • Sweating. • Cold, clammy hands. • Nausea; diarrhea; weight loss. • Sleeplessness; nightmares. • Irritability. • Fatigue. • Memory problems. • Sexual impotence.	**ANXIETY** (Refer to Illnesses section)
• Rash, itching or hives. • Jaundice (yellow skin and eyes). • Flushed skin. • Facial swelling. • Anxiety. • Many other possible symptoms.	**DRUG HYPERSENSITIVITY** (Refer to Illnesses section)
• Rapid breathing. • Numbness and tingling around the mouth, hands and feet. • Weakness or faintness. • Muscle spasm or contractions in the hands and feet. • Fainting (occasionally). • Marked anxiety.	**HYPERVENTILATION SYNDROME** (Refer to Illnesses section)
Anxiety and persistent reports of symptoms involving any body part. Concern about heart disease or cancer is common. Symptoms may change, but the person's belief that a serious condition exists does not. Frequently reported symptoms include insomnia, sexual dysfunction and gastrointestinal discomfort, such as bloating, belching and cramps.	**HYPOCHONDRIASIS** (Refer to Illnesses section)
• Confusion. • Restlessness and anxiety. • Weakness. • Muscle cramps (usually in the legs). • Changes in pulse rate and blood pressure. • Tissue swelling (edema). • Stupor or coma (if severe imbalance). **(THIS IS AN EMERGENCY; SEEK MEDICAL CARE IMMEDIATELY!)** Sodium imbalance may be part of a disease with other symptoms that predominate, such as fever, vomiting, diarrhea or excessive sweating.	**SODIUM, TOO MUCH OR TOO LITTLE IN BLOOD** (Refer to Illnesses section)
• Hyperactivity. • Feeling warm or hot all the time. • Tremors. • Sweating. • Itching skin. • Pounding, rapid, irregular heartbeat. • Weight loss, despite overeating. • Marked anxiety and restlessness. • Sleeplessness. • Fatigue and weakness. • Protruding eyes (exophthalmos) and double vision (sometimes). • Diarrhea (sometimes). • Hair loss (sometimes). • Goiter (sometimes).	**THYROID, OVERACTIVE** (Refer to Illnesses section)

(ANXIETY & NERVOUSNESS, continued on next page)

(ANXIETY & NERVOUSNESS, continued from previous page)

SYMPTOMS & FACTORS	POSSIBLE PROBLEM
If you experience ANXIETY & NERVOUSNESS plus the following:	
• Use of prescription or non-prescription drugs.	**WHAT TO DO:** Discontinue non-prescription drugs and call doctor now regarding prescription drugs.
• Recent withdrawal from tobacco, alcohol or drugs, such as sleeping pills.	**WHAT TO DO:** Call doctor about drug withdrawal.
• Anxiety about any of following: enclosed spaces; airplanes; crowds; heights; "going crazy"; infection; death.	**WHAT TO DO:** Call doctor when convenient.

APPETITE LOSS

(Find your closest combination of symptoms in left-hand column; see possible problem in right-hand column. You may not experience all symptoms listed.)

SYMPTOMS & FACTORS	POSSIBLE PROBLEM
• Weakness and fatigue. • Gastrointestinal disturbances (nausea, vomiting, abdominal pain, diarrhea, appetite and weight loss). • Low blood pressure causing faintness and dizziness. • Brownish skin (looks suntanned) with white patches. • Darkening of freckles, scars and breast nipples. • Hair loss. • Feeling cold all the time. • Dramatic behavior or mood changes, including aggression or depression. • Confusion. • Coma.	**ADDISON'S DISEASE** (Refer to Illnesses section)
• Lethargy. • Appetite loss. • Vomiting and diarrhea. • Dehydration and thirst. • Irregular heartbeat. • Depression, delirium, confusion. • Seizures or coma (worst cases only). (THIS IS AN EMERGENCY; SEEK MEDICAL CARE IMMEDIATELY!)	**CALCIUM, TOO MUCH** (Refer to Illnesses section)
Early stages: • Poor appetite; nausea; weight loss. • Fatigue; weakness. • Enlarged liver. • Red palms. **Late stages:** • Jaundice (yellow skin and eyes). • Dark yellow or brown urine. • Spider blood vessels of the skin (fine vessels which spread out from a central point). • Hair loss. • Breast enlargement in men. • Fluid accumulation in the abdomen and legs. • Enlarged spleen. • Diarrhea; stool may be black or bloody. • Bleeding and bruising. • Mental confusion; coma.	**CIRRHOSIS OF THE LIVER** (Refer to Illnesses section)

(APPETITE LOSS, continued on next page)

SYMPTOMS & FACTORS	POSSIBLE PROBLEM
Mild glomerulonephritis produces no symptoms. Diagnosis is possible only with urine studies. Severe glomerulonephritis produces the following: • Appetite loss. • Smoky or slightly red urine. • General ill feeling. • Drowsiness. • Nausea or vomiting. • Headaches. • Fever (sometimes). • Decreased urination. • Fluid accumulation in the body, especially puffy eyes and ankles. • Shortness of breath. • High blood pressure. • Protein in the urine. • Disturbed vision.	**GLOMERULONEPHRITIS** (Refer to Illnesses section)
Early stages: • Flu-like symptoms, such as fever, fatigue, nausea, vomiting, diarrhea and loss of appetite. **Several days later:** • Jaundice (yellow eyes and skin) caused by a buildup of bile in the blood. • Dark urine from bile spilling over into the urine. • Light, "clay-colored" or whitish stools.	**HEPATITIS, ACUTE VIRAL** (Refer to Illnesses section)
• Loss of appetite and weight loss. • Tender mass in the right upper abdomen. • Pain in the upper abdomen. • Low-grade fever, usually less than 101F or 38.3C. • Yellow eyes and skin (sometimes). • Swollen abdomen from fluid retention (sometimes). • Mental status changes, such as confusion or forgetfulness.	**LIVER CANCER** (Refer to Illnesses section)
• Loss of appetite. • Nausea and vomiting. • Spinning sensation. • Weakness and unsteadiness.	**MOTION SICKNESS** (Refer to Illnesses section)
• Abdominal pain and cramps. • Vomiting (occasionally). • Appetite loss. • Fever. • Weakness. • Swollen abdomen. • Sharp, dull or annoying pain in the chest. • Acid taste in the mouth. • Mild nausea and diarrhea (rare). • Belching or gas.	**STOMACH INFLAMMATION** (Refer to Illnesses section)
• Nausea that sometimes causes vomiting. • Diarrhea that ranges from 2 or 3 loose stools to many watery stools. • Abdominal cramps, pain or tenderness. • Appetite loss. • Fever. • Weakness.	**STOMACH & INTESTINAL INFLAMMATION** (Refer to Illnesses section)

(APPETITE LOSS, continued on next page)

(APPETITE LOSS, continued from previous page)

SYMPTOMS & FACTORS	POSSIBLE PROBLEM
Two or more of the following: • Poor appetite. • Poor growth. • Sensations of unpleasant tastes and odors and decreased senses of taste and smell. • Decreased sex drive. • Darkening of skin all over the body. • Sparse hair growth. • Deformed nails.	**ZINC DEFICIENCY** (Refer to Illnesses section)

If you experience APPETITE LOSS plus the following:

• Use of vitamins or prescription or non-prescription drugs, especially anticancer drugs; digitalis; aminophylline; narcotics; antihistamines; ephedrine; methylphenidate; diphenylhydantoin; amphetamines.	**WHAT TO DO:** Call doctor now about prescription drugs and discontinue use of non-prescription drugs.
• Weight loss. • Vague feeling of illness and fatigue.	**WHAT TO DO:** Call doctor now. These may be symptoms of several disorders.

ARM OR HAND PAIN

(Find your closest combination of symptoms in left-hand column; see possible problem in right-hand column. You may not experience all symptoms listed.)

SYMPTOMS & FACTORS	POSSIBLE PROBLEM
Any of the following: • Tightness, squeezing, pressure or mild ache in the chest (more during exercise). • Sudden difficulty breathing (sometimes). • Frequent chest pain similar to that of indigestion. • A choking feeling in the throat. • Chest pain that radiates to the jaw, teeth or earlobes. • Heaviness, numbness, tingling or ache in the arm, shoulder, elbow or hand—usually on the left side. • Pain between the shoulder blades. • Paleness and sweating.	**ANGINA PECTORIS** (Refer to Illnesses section)
Slow or sudden onset of: • Redness, aching, pain, warmth and tenderness in any or all active joints in the hands, wrists, elbows, shoulders, knees, feet, ankles, jaw or spine. • Morning stiffness; muscular atrophy. • Low-grade fever. • Nodules under the skin (sometimes). • Pale skin. • Appetite loss.	**ARTHRITIS, RHEUMATOID** (Refer to Illnesses section)
• Pain, tenderness and limited movement in the affected area. • When shoulder involved, radiation of pain into the neck, arm or fingertips. • Severe pain with movement of the arm. • Fever (sometimes).	**BURSITIS** (Refer to Illnesses section)

(ARM OR HAND PAIN, continued on next page)

17

SYMPTOMS & FACTORS	POSSIBLE PROBLEM
• Tingling or numbness in part of the hand. • Sharp pains that shoot from the wrist up the arm, especially at night. • Burning sensations in the fingers. • Morning stiffness or cramping of hands. • Thumb weakness. • Frequent dropping of objects. • Inability to make a fist. • Shiny, dry skin on the hand.	**CARPAL TUNNEL SYNDROME** (Refer to Illnesses section)
Early stages: • No symptoms (often). **Later stages:** • Angina pectoris (discomfort or pain in the chest coming on with exercise and disappearing with rest). • Heart attack.	**CORONARY ARTERY DISEASE** (Refer to Illnesses section)
• Sudden onset of severe pain in the inflamed joint, usually at the base of the big toe or larger joints. • Involved joints are red, hot, swollen and very tender. Skin over the joint is red and shiny. • Fever (sometimes).	**GOUT** (Refer to Illnesses section)
• Pain or tenderness in the injury area. • Gradual stiffening or contraction of the injured muscle. • Swelling, redness or bruising at the injury site.	**MUSCLE, PULLED OR TORN** (Refer to Illnesses section)
• Joint stiffness and pain, including backache. Weather changes, especially cold, damp weather, may increase aching. • Limited movement and loss of dexterity in affected joints. • No redness, heat or fever in affected joints (usually). • Swelling of affected joints (sometimes), especially finger joints. • Cracking or grating sounds with joint movement (sometimes).	**OSTEOARTHRITIS** (Refer to Illnesses section)
• Fever. Sometimes this is the only symptom. • Pain, swelling, redness, warmth and tenderness in the area over the infected bone, especially when moving a nearby joint. Nearby joints—especially the knee—may also be red, warm and swollen. • Pus drainage through a skin abscess, without fever or severe pain (chronic osteomyelitis only).	**OSTEOMYELITIS** (Refer to Illnesses section)
• Fingers—Hardening and thickening of the skin, stiffness, poor circulation, numbness and fingertip ulceration. • Digestive system—Swallowing difficulty, poor food absorption, bloating after eating, weight loss, heartburn and a feeling that food sticks in the chest. • Skin—Hardening and thickening, especially in the face, which becomes tight and loses its elasticity. • Muscle aches. • Weakness and fatigue. • Joint pain, stiffness and swelling.	**SCLERODERMA** (Refer to Illnesses section)
• Pain or tenderness in the area of injury; severity varies with the extent of injury. • Swelling of the affected joint. • Redness or bruising in the area of injury, either immediately or several hours after injury. • Loss of normal mobility in the injured joint.	**SPRAINS & STRAINS** (Refer to Illnesses section)

(ARM OR HAND PAIN, continued on next page)

SYMPTOMS & FACTORS	POSSIBLE PROBLEM
• Restricted movement, tenderness and swelling around the inflamed tendon. Common sites are the shoulder, elbow, Achilles' tendon or hamstring. • Weakness in the tendon caused by calcium deposits that often accompany tendinitis.	**TENDINITIS** (Refer to Illnesses section)
• Pain and tenderness over the elbow. • Weak grip. • Pain when twisting the hand and arm, as in using a screwdriver, lifting a heavy object or playing tennis.	**TENNIS ELBOW** (Refer to Illnesses section)

If you experience ARM OR HAND PAIN plus the following:

• Severe pain in arm following injury or obvious fracture with misshapen arm.	**WHAT TO DO:** Call doctor now.

BACKACHE

(Find your closest combination of symptoms in left-hand column; see possible problem in right-hand column. You may not experience all symptoms listed.)

SYMPTOMS & FACTORS	POSSIBLE PROBLEM
Lower back: • Severe pain in the low back or back of one leg, buttock or foot (sciatica). Pain usually affects one side and worsens with movement, coughing, sneezing, lifting or straining. • Weakness, numbness or muscular wasting of the affected leg. **Neck:** • Pain in the neck or shoulder or down one arm. Pain worsens with movement. • Weakness, numbness or muscular wasting of the affected arm.	**DISK, RUPTURED** (Refer to Illnesses section)
Sudden onset of: • Fever and shaking chills. • Burning, frequent urination. • Cloudy urine or blood in the urine. • Aching (sometimes severe) in one or both sides of the lower back. • Abdominal pain.	**KIDNEY INFECTION, ACUTE** (Refer to Illnesses section)
• Pain or tenderness in the injury area. • Gradual stiffening or contraction of the injured muscle. • Swelling, redness or bruising at the injury site.	**MUSCLE, PULLED OR TORN** (Refer to Illnesses section)
• Joint stiffness and pain, including backache. Weather changes, especially cold, damp weather, may increase aching. • Limited movement and loss of dexterity in affected joints. • Redness, heat or fever in affected joints (sometimes). • Swelling of affected joints (sometimes), especially finger joints. • Cracking or grating sounds with joint movement (sometimes).	**OSTEOARTHRITIS** (Refer to Illnesses section)
Early symptoms: • Backache. • No symptoms (often). **Late symptoms:** • Sudden back pain with a cracking sound indicating fracture. • Deformed spinal column with humps. • Loss of height. • Fractures occurring with minor injury, especially of the hip or arm.	**OSTEOPOROSIS** (Refer to Illnesses section)

(BACKACHE, continued on next page)

SYMPTOMS & FACTORS	POSSIBLE PROBLEM
• Depression. • Rapid, unexplained weight loss. • Pain in the back or upper abdomen that is often relieved by bending forward. • Blood clots in veins anywhere, especially the arms and legs. This is often an early sign. • Jaundice (yellow skin and eyes) from blockage of the nearby bile duct. Jaundice is usually accompanied by intense itching.	**PANCREAS, CANCER OF** (Refer to Illnesses section)
• Progressive weakness, numbness and wasting of muscles whose nerve supply comes from the affected area of the spinal cord. • Difficult urination or bowel movements; incontinence. • Chronic back pain.	**SPINAL CORD TUMOR** (Refer to Illnesses section)
• Lump in front or back of the vagina or projecting outside it. • Vague discomfort in the pelvic region. • Backache that worsens with lifting. • Discomfort with urinating. • Occasional stress incontinence (urine leakage when laughing, sneezing or coughing).	**UTERINE PROLAPSE** (Refer to Illnesses section)

If you experience BACKACHE plus the following:

• Sudden backache.	**WHAT TO DO:** Call doctor now.
• Recent fall or injury to back with any of the following: difficulty moving arm or leg; loss of bladder or bowel control; numbness or tingling in extremities.	**WHAT TO DO:** Call doctor now. Don't move injured person until help arrives because there may be spinal cord damage.
• Any of the following: overweight; use of chair too high or too low for desk; recent heavy lifting or strenuous exercise; recent use of jackhammer or other heavy equipment.	**WHAT TO DO:** See Appendix 15 for suggestions for back care.

BOWEL, LACK OF CONTROL

(Find your closest combination of symptoms in left-hand column; see possible problem in right-hand column. You may not experience all symptoms listed.)

SYMPTOMS & FACTORS	POSSIBLE PROBLEM
• Cramping abdominal pain. • Loose, watery or unformed bowel movements. • Lack of bowel control (sometimes). • Fever (sometimes).	**DIARRHEA, ACUTE** (Refer to Illnesses section)
• Absence of normal bowel movements. • Sense of fullness in the rectum, but inability to pass stool. • Lack of urinary control. • A firm mass in the lower left abdomen (sometimes). • Pain or cramps (sometimes). Impaction often develops slowly without discomfort. • Thin, watery discharge from the rectum.	**FECAL IMPACTION** (Refer to Illnesses section)

(BOWEL, LACK OF CONTROL, continued on next page)

(BOWEL, LACK OF CONTROL, continued from previous page)

SYMPTOMS & FACTORS	POSSIBLE PROBLEM
Mild hypoglycemic reaction: • Excessive hunger. • Weakness. • Nervousness. • Emotional instability. • Difficulty concentrating. • Sweating. • Headache. **Moderate hypoglycemic reaction:** • Increased weakness. • Excessive sweating. • Cold, clammy skin. • Numbness around the mouth or fingers. • Pounding heartbeat. • Memory loss. • Double vision. • Staring expression. • Difficulty walking. • Increasing confusion. **Severe hypoglycemic reaction:** • Lack of urinary and bowel control. • Muscle twitching. • Unconsciousness. • Convulsions.	**HYPOGLYCEMIA OF DIABETES** (Refer to Illnesses section) (THIS IS AN EMERGENCY; SEEK MEDICAL CARE IMMEDIATELY!)
• No symptoms in the early stages (frequently). • Bloody or black, tarry stools. • Cramping abdominal pain. • Feeling of fullness. • Change in bowel habits, such as diarrhea, constipation or narrow-caliber stools. • Unexplained weight loss. • Pain in the rectum. • Anemia. • Loss of bowel control (sometimes).	**LARGE INTESTINE, CANCER OF** (Refer to Illnesses section)
The following symptoms may vary according to the site of brain damage: • Loss of bowel and bladder control. • Inability to speak. • Inability to move part of the body. • Loss of consciousness.	**STROKE** (Refer to Illnesses section) (THIS IS AN EMERGENCY; SEEK MEDICAL CARE IMMEDIATELY!)

If you experience LACK OF BOWEL CONTROL plus the following:

• Convulsions or unconsciousness.	**WHAT TO DO:** Call doctor now. These may be symptoms of stroke, epilepsy or brain tumor.
• Any of the following: recent vaginal surgery; history of rectal surgery; anal fissure or fistula; hemorrhoids.	**WHAT TO DO:** Call doctor now.

BREAST PAIN OR LUMPS

(Find your closest combination of symptoms in left-hand column; see possible problem in right-hand column. You may not experience all symptoms listed.)

SYMPTOMS & FACTORS	POSSIBLE PROBLEM
No symptoms in early stages, but may be detected even then by mammogram. Later symptoms include: • Swelling or lump in the breast. • Vague discomfort in the breast without true pain. • Retraction of the nipple. • Distorted breast contour. • Dimpled or pitted skin in the breast. • Enlarged nodes under the arm (late). • Bloody discharge from the nipple (rare).	**BREAST CANCER** (Refer to Illnesses section)
• Lumps in the breasts, usually on both sides. Solitary lumps may occur, but multiple lumps are common. • Lumps offer resistance when pressed with fingertips; they may be tender. • Lumps may be accompanied by generalized breast pain. • Lumps come in different sizes; when relatively large and near the surface, they can be moved freely within the breast. • Lumps deep within the breast may be indistinguishable from breast cancer.	**FIBROCYSTIC BREAST DISEASE** (Refer to Illnesses section)

BREATH, BAD

(Find your closest combination of symptoms in left-hand column; see possible problem in right-hand column. You may not experience all symptoms listed.)

SYMPTOMS & FACTORS	POSSIBLE PROBLEM
• Excessive thirst that is difficult to satisfy. • Passage of large amounts (up to 15 quarts a day) of dilute, colorless urine. • Dry hands. • Constipation. • Unusual breath odor—sometimes described as "orangy."	**DIABETES MELLITUS, INSULIN-DEPENDENT OR NON-INSULIN-DEPENDENT** (Refer to Illnesses section)
• No symptoms in the early stages (often). • Shortness of breath that increases in severity over several years. • Wheezing and coughing that produces scant sputum. • Occasional recurrent infections of the lungs or bronchial tubes. • Barrel-shaped chest. • Swelling in legs and feet (edema). • Bad breath	**EMPHYSEMA** (Refer to Illnesses section)
• Chest pain. Pain varies from vague discomfort to stabbing pain. It is often worse with coughing or breathing. Pain may extend to the lower chest wall or abdomen. • Rapid, shallow breathing. • Chills. • Fever. • Extreme fatigue. • Bad breath. • Weight loss.	**EMPYEMA** (Refer to Illnesses section)

(BREATH, BAD, continued on next page)

SYMPTOMS & FACTORS	POSSIBLE PROBLEM
No symptoms or few until 60% to 75% of kidney filtration fails. Then, 1 or more of the following: • Listlessness, mental confusion and drowsiness. • High blood pressure. • Shortness of breath. • Bad breath. • Inflamed, bleeding gums and mouth ulcers. • Abdominal pain. • Itching skin. • Numbness, tingling and burning in the legs and feet. • Muscle cramps. • Decreased sex drive. • Anemia with paleness and fatigue. • Unusual bleeding. • Muscle and bone pain. Bones break easily.	**KIDNEY FAILURE, CHRONIC** (Refer to Illnesses section)
• Cough with sputum. The sputum is pus-like, often blood-streaked and sometimes smells bad. • Bad breath. • Sweating. • Fever to 101F (38.3C) or higher. • Chills. • Weight loss. • Chest pain (sometimes).	**LUNG ABSCESS** (Refer to Illnesses section)
• Unpleasant taste in the mouth. • Bad breath. • Loosening of teeth in the sockets. • Aching teeth and gums when eating hot, cold or sweet food. • If an abscess develops, tenderness, swelling, pain and fever will also occur.	**PERIODONTITIS** (Refer to Illnesses section)
• Persistent toothache or throbbing, extreme pain upon biting or chewing. • Swelling and tenderness in the neck glands and on the side of the face. • Earache. • Fever. • General ill feeling. • Foul taste and bad breath (if the abscess opens spontaneously).	**TOOTH ABSCESS** (Refer to Illnesses section)
• Tooth sensitivity to heat and cold. • Tooth discomfort after eating sugar. • Darkening on or between the teeth (cavity) when the decay has progressed enough to be seen. The most common tooth cavity sites are the gum line, biting surfaces and surfaces between adjacent teeth. • Unpleasant taste in the mouth and bad breath because of stagnant food and bacteria trapped in the cavity. • Persistent tooth pain (in the final stages of decay when the pulp becomes inflamed).	**TOOTH DECAY** (Refer to Illnesses section)

If you experience BAD BREATH plus the following:

• Fever.	**WHAT TO DO:** See Fever (in Symptoms section).
• Sore mouth or tongue.	**WHAT TO DO:** See Sore Mouth (in Symptoms section).
• Recent consumption of garlic, onions or alcohol.	**WHAT TO DO:** Nothing. Breath will return to normal.

BREATHING DIFFICULTY

(Find your closest combination of symptoms in left-hand column; see possible problem in right-hand column. You may not experience all symptoms listed.)

SYMPTOMS & FACTORS	POSSIBLE PROBLEM
Any of the following may occur within seconds or a few minutes after exposure to a substance to which you are very allergic: • Tingling or numbness around the mouth. • Sneezing. • Itching all over, particularly soles and palms and often accompanied by hives. • Redness around ears, resembling recent sunburn. • Watery eyes. • Tightness in the chest; difficulty breathing; coughing. • Swelling or itching in the mouth or throat. • Pounding heart. • Faintness. • Shivering. • Dilated pupils. • Loss of consciousness. Not all symptoms occur in every case. Seek immediate help for any.	**ANAPHYLAXIS** (Refer to Illnesses section) **(THIS IS AN EMERGENCY; SEEK MEDICAL CARE IMMEDIATELY!)**
Any of the following: • Tightness, squeezing, pressure or mild ache in the chest (more during exercise). • Sudden breathing difficulty (sometimes). • Frequent chest pain similar to that from indigestion. • A choking feeling in the throat. • Chest pain that radiates to the jaw, teeth or earlobes. • Heaviness, numbness, tingling or ache in the arm, shoulder, elbow or hand—usually on the left side. • Pain between the shoulder blades. • Paleness and sweating.	**ANGINA PECTORIS** (Refer to Illnesses section)
• Feeling that something undesirable or harmful is about to happen. • Dry mouth; swallowing difficulty or hoarseness. • Rapid breathing and heartbeat. • Twitching or trembling. • Muscle tension; headaches. • Sweating. • Cold, clammy hands. • Nausea; diarrhea; weight loss. • Sleeplessness; nightmares. • Irritability. • Fatigue. • Memory problems. • Sexual impotence.	**ANXIETY** (Refer to Illnesses section)
• Cough that produces little or no sputum initially, but does later on. • Low fever (usually less than 101F or 38.3C). • Burning chest discomfort or feeling of pressure behind the breastbone. • Wheezing or uncomfortable breathing (sometimes).	**BRONCHITIS, ACUTE** (Refer to Illnesses section)
• Frequent cough or coughing spasms. • Shortness of breath. • Sputum that is thick and difficult to cough up. Sputum production varies according to whether infection is present. • Barrel chest (in the late.stages). • Chest pain (rare).	**BRONCHITIS, CHRONIC** (Refer to Illnesses section)

(BREATHING DIFFICULTY, continued on next page)

24

SYMPTOMS & FACTORS	POSSIBLE PROBLEM
If cardiomyopathy is extensive enough to cause congestive heart failure, the following symptoms may occur: • Irregular or rapid heartbeat. • Shortness of breath with activity. • Swelling of the feet and ankles. • Fatigue. • Cough with frothy, bloody sputum. • Chest pain.	**CARDIOMYOPATHY** (Refer to Illnesses section)
Early stages: • No symptoms (often). **Later stages:** • Angina pectoris (discomfort or pain in the chest coming on with exercise and disappearing with rest). • Heart attack. (THIS IS AN EMERGENCY; SEEK MEDICAL CARE IMMEDIATELY!)	**CORONARY ARTERY DISEASE** (Refer to Illnesses section)
Early dumping syndrome: • Weakness and fainting. • Sweating. • Irregular or rapid heartbeat. • Decreased blood pressure. • Flushing of skin. • Dizziness. • Shortness of breath. • Vomiting. • Explosive diarrhea and abdominal cramps. **Late dumping syndrome:** • Sweating, anxiety and tremors. • Exhaustion and faintness. • Decreased blood pressure. • Headache.	**DUMPING SYNDROME** (Refer to Illnesses section)
• No symptoms in the early stages (often). • Shortness of breath that increases in severity over several years. • Wheezing and coughing that produces scant sputum. • Occasional recurrent infections of the lungs or bronchial tubes. • Barrel-shaped chest. • Swelling in legs and feet (edema).	**EMPHYSEMA** (Refer to Illnesses section)
• Chest pain. Pain varies from vague discomfort to stabbing pain. It is often worse with coughing or breathing. Pain may extend to the lower chest wall or abdomen. • Rapid, shallow breathing. • Chills. • Fever. • Extreme fatigue. • Bad breath. • Weight loss.	**EMPYEMA** (Refer to Illnesses section)
• Chest pain or ''heavy, squeezing or crushing'' feeling in the chest. • Sweating. • Cold, clammy, wet skin. • Pain that radiates from the mid-chest over the breastbone to the jaw, neck, either arm, the area between the shoulder blades or the upper abdomen (sometimes). • Feeling of impending doom. • Shortness of breath. • Nausea and vomiting.	**HEART ATTACK** (Refer to Illnesses section) (THIS IS AN EMERGENCY; SEEK MEDICAL CARE IMMEDIATELY!)

(BREATHING DIFFICULTY, continued on next page)

SYMPTOMS & FACTORS	POSSIBLE PROBLEM
• Rapid breathing. • Numbness and tingling around the mouth, hands and feet. • Weakness or faintness. • Muscle spasm or contractions in the hands and feet. • Fainting (occasionally). • Marked anxiety.	**HYPERVENTILATION SYNDROME** (Refer to Illnesses section)
• Chest pain (angina pectoris). • Heart rhythm irregularity. • Fainting. • Shortness of breath.	**IDIOPATHIC HYPERTROPHIC SUBAORTIC STENOSIS (IHSS)** (Refer to Illnesses section)
• General ill feeling. • Headache. • Chills and fever up to 105F (40.6C). • Muscle aches. • Cough without sputum that progresses to one with gray or blood-streaked sputum. • Nausea, vomiting, diarrhea. • Disorientation. • Shortness of breath.	**LEGIONNAIRE'S DISEASE** (Refer to Illnesses section)
• Frequent coughing with bad-smelling green or yellow sputum (sometimes flecked with blood). • Repeated lung infections. • Shortness of breath. • General ill feeling. • Frequent fatigue. • Anemia (frequently).	**LUNG DISEASE, CHRONIC** (Refer to Illnesses section)
Lupus symptoms frequently flare up and then subside. Episodes generally include fever and fatigue, plus any 4 of the following: • Rash, usually on the cheeks. • Ulcers in the mouth. • Red palms and hands. • Joint pain with redness, swelling and tenderness—but no deformity. • Swelling of the face and legs. • Shortness of breath. • Rapid or irregular heartbeat. • Chest pain. • Hair loss. • Swelling of the lymph glands. • Protein in the urine. • Increased sensitivity to the sun. • Mental changes, including psychosis.	**LUPUS ERYTHEMATOSUS, SYSTEMIC** (Refer to Illnesses section)
• Fatigue. • Shortness of breath. • Irregular heartbeat. • Fever. • Other symptoms caused by the underlying disorder. If myocarditis causes congestive heart failure, the following symptoms may also occur: • Swollen feet and ankles. • Distended neck veins. • Rapid heartbeat, even when at rest. • Difficulty breathing while resting or lying down.	**MYOCARDITIS** (Refer to Illnesses section)

(BREATHING DIFFICULTY, continued on next page)

SYMPTOMS & FACTORS	POSSIBLE PROBLEM
• Obstruction of air through the nose (chronic "stuffy nose" feeling). • Impaired sense of smell. • Feelings of fullness in the face. • Nasal discharge (sometimes). • Facial pain (sometimes). • Headaches (sometimes).	**NASAL POLYPS** (Refer to Illnesses section)
Early stages: • No symptoms (usually). **Later stages:** • Weakness and fatigue. • Shortness of breath with exertion. • Frequent fainting. • Swelling of feet and ankles. • Distended neck veins. • Chest pain. • Enlarged liver and swollen abdomen.	**OBSTRUCTIVE PULMONARY DISEASE, CHRONIC** (Refer to Illnesses section)
• High fever (over 102F or 38.9C) and chills. • Shortness of breath. • Cough with sputum that may contain blood or blood streaks. • Rapid breathing. • Chest pain that worsens with inhalation. • Abdominal pain. • Fatigue. • Bluish lips and nails (rare).	**PNEUMONIA, BACTERIAL** (Refer to Illnesses section) (THIS IS AN EMERGENCY; SEEK MEDICAL CARE IMMEDIATELY!)
• Cough (with or without sputum). • Fever. • Labored breathing. • Chest pain. • Abdominal pain. • Bluish skin (severe cases).	**PNEUMONIA, MYCOPLASMA** (Refer to Illnesses section)
• Fever and chills. • Muscle aches and fatigue. • Cough or "croup," with or without sputum. • Rapid, labored breathing (sometimes). • Chest pain. • Sore throat. • Loss of appetite. • Enlarged lymph glands in the neck.	**PNEUMONIA, VIRAL** (Refer to Illnesses section)
The following symptoms vary according to the degree of lung collapse and extent of underlying lung disease. Symptoms may be less acute if the pneumothorax develops slowly: • Sharp chest pain. Pain may extend to a shoulder or across the chest or abdomen. • Shortness of breath. • Dry, hacking cough with or without bloody sputum (occasionally).	**PNEUMOTHORAX** (Refer to Illnesses section) (THIS IS AN EMERGENCY; SEEK MEDICAL CARE IMMEDIATELY!)
Symptoms vary depending on which organ is affected by the decreased blood supply. The most common include: • Chest pain (heart involvement). • Shortness of breath (lung involvement). • Abdominal pain (intestinal and liver involvement). • Blood in the urine (kidney involvement). • Numbness and tingling of the hands and feet (nerve involvement).	**POLYARTERITIS** (Refer to Illnesses section)

(BREATHING DIFFICULTY, continued on next page)

SYMPTOMS & FACTORS	POSSIBLE PROBLEM
• Sudden shortness of breath. • Faintness or fainting. • Pain in the chest. • Cough (sometimes with bloody sputum). • Rapid heartbeat. • Low fever. These symptoms are often preceded by swelling and pain in the leg.	**PULMONARY EMBOLISM** (Refer to Illnesses section) (THIS IS AN EMERGENCY; SEEK MEDICAL CARE IMMEDIATELY!)

If you experience BREATHING DIFFICULTY plus the following:

• Noisy breathing.	**WHAT TO DO:** See Wheezing (in Symptoms section).
• Breathing difficulty soon after taking any medicine.	**WHAT TO DO:** Discontinue non-prescription drugs and notify doctor now regarding prescription drugs.
• Breathing difficulty soon after eating shellfish or other food likely to cause food allergy.	**WHAT TO DO:** Call doctor now.
• Possible aspiration of food or other foreign body.	**WHAT TO DO:** Call doctor now.

BRUISING OR BLOOD SPOTS UNDER THE SKIN, UNEXPLAINED

(Find your closest combination of symptoms in left-hand column; see possible problem in right-hand column. You may not experience all symptoms listed.)

SYMPTOMS & FACTORS	POSSIBLE PROBLEM
• Paleness. • Weakness, tiredness, faintness and breathlessness. • Frequent infections. • Spontaneous bleeding from the nose, mouth, rectum, vagina, gums and other sites. • Red dots of bleeding under the skin. • Unexplained bruising. • Ulcers in the mouth, throat and rectum.	**ANEMIA, APLASTIC** (Refer to Illnesses section)
Few or no symptoms until 60% to 75% of kidney filtration fails. Then 1 or more of the following: • Listlessness, mental confusion and drowsiness. • High blood pressure. • Shortness of breath. • Bad breath. • Inflamed, bleeding gums and mouth ulcers. • Abdominal pain. • Itching skin. • Numbness, tingling and burning in the legs and feet. • Muscle cramps. • Decreased sex drive. • Anemia with paleness and fatigue. • Unusual bleeding. • Muscle and bone pain. Bones break easily.	**KIDNEY FAILURE, CHRONIC** (Refer to Illnesses section)

(BRUISING OR BLOOD SPOTS UNDER THE SKIN, UNEXPLAINED, continued on next page)

(BRUISING OR BLOOD SPOTS UNDER THE SKIN, UNEXPLAINED, continued from previous page)

SYMPTOMS & FACTORS	POSSIBLE PROBLEM
• Fever. • Tiredness. • Anemia. • Increasing paleness. • General ill feeling. • Easy bruising and spontaneous bleeding (nosebleeds, bleeding from the gums or gastrointestinal tract). • Enlarged spleen and abdominal pain. • Susceptibility to infection, especially pneumonia. • Mouth infections with ulcers and sores. • Headache and lethargy if meninges (brain membranes) are affected.	**LEUKEMIA, ACUTE** (Refer to Illnesses section)
• Abnormal bleeding in the mouth. • A rash of pinpoint-size dots that doesn't fade when the skin is pressed. • Unexplained bruising. • Spontaneous nosebleeds. • Blood in the urine. • Unexplained vaginal bleeding. • Black, tarry stools. • Signs of anemia: weakness, fatigue, paleness (if bleeding is prolonged).	**THROMBOCYTOPENIA** (Refer to Illnesses section) **(THIS IS AN EMERGENCY; SEEK MEDICAL CARE IMMEDIATELY!)**
• Swollen, bleeding gums. • Nosebleeds. • Loss of teeth. • Rough skin. • Bleeding or bruising under the skin or into joints. • Weakness and fatigue. • Mental changes, including hallucinations and bizarre behavior. • Increased susceptibility to infection.	**VITAMIN C DEFICIENCY** (Refer to Illnesses section)
• Unusual bleeding, such as from the gums, nose or gastrointestinal tract. • Unexplained bruising.	**VITAMIN K DEFICIENCY** (Refer to Illnesses section)

If you experience UNEXPLAINED BRUISING OR BLOOD SPOTS UNDER THE SKIN plus the following:

• Fever. • Pain in affected area. • Headache. • Weakness. • General ill feeling.	**WHAT TO DO:** Call doctor now. These symptoms may represent a serious contagious illness.
• Use of prescription or non-prescription drugs, such as anticoagulants; aspirin; sulfa drugs; digitoxin; quinine; quinidine; antihistamines; phenothiazines; antidepressants; local anesthetics; penicillin; mercury; bismuth; cortisone drugs; anticonvulsants.	**WHAT TO DO:** Discontinue non-prescription drugs and notify doctor now regarding prescription drugs.
• Violent coughing, vomiting or choking.	**WHAT TO DO:** Call doctor now.

BUMPS ON SKIN

(Find your closest combination of symptoms in left-hand column; see possible problem in right-hand column. You may not experience all symptoms listed.)

SYMPTOMS & FACTORS	POSSIBLE PROBLEM
• Unsightly red, thickened skin on the nose and cheeks. Small blood vessels are visible on the skin surface. • Papules (small raised bumps) and pustules (small, white blisters with pus) on the affected skin (sometimes).	**ACNE ROSACEA** (Refer to Illnesses section)
• A domed nodule that is painful, tender and red and has pus on the surface. Boils can appear suddenly and ripen in 24 hours. They are usually 1-1/2cm to 3cm in diameter; some are larger. • Fever (rare). • Swelling of the closest lymph glands.	**BOILS** (Refer to Illnesses section)
• Corn—A small, tender and painful raised bump on the side or over the joint of a toe. Corns are usually 3mm to 10mm in diameter and have hard centers. • Callus—A rough, thickened area of skin that appears after repeated pressure or irritation.	**CORN OR CALLUS** (Refer to Illnesses section)
Itchy papules (small, raised bumps) on skin with the following characteristics: • Papules swell and produce pink or red lesions called wheals. Wheals have clearly defined edges and flat tops. They measure 1cm to 5cm in diameter. • Wheals join together quickly and form larger raised, flat, skin-colored lesions called plaques. • Wheals and plaques change shape, resolve and reappear in minutes or hours. This rapid change is unique to hives.	**HIVES** (Refer to Illnesses section)
Papules (small, raised bumps) on skin with the following characteristics: • Papules are flat-topped with well-defined borders. • Young papules are relatively flat and light brown. More advanced papules are dark brown or black. • Papules are wider than tall, and they appear "stuck on." • Papules measure 5mm to 20mm in diameter. They are distributed on the chest, back, face and arms. • Papules don't itch or hurt. • Papules vary in number, from only I or 2 papules up to 100.	**KERATOSIS, SEBORRHEIC** (Refer to Illnesses section)
Plaques (red, raised skin lesions) with the following characteristics: • Plaques are 1cm to 4cm in diameter and have clearly defined borders. • Plaques may appear anywhere on the face, but the cheeks and jawline are the most common sites. Some people describe them as "butterfly" lesions when two lesions of unequal size appear on both sides of the nose. • Plaques sometimes appear on the scalp with localized patches of hair loss. • Plaques scar as they heal.	**LUPUS ERYTHEMATOSUS, DISCOID** (Refer to Illnesses section)

(BUMPS ON SKIN, continued on next page)

SYMPTOMS & FACTORS	POSSIBLE PROBLEM
First stage: • A red papule (small, raised bump) on the skin of the thighs, buttocks or armpits that grows as large as 5cm. **Later stages:** Any or some of the following: • Muscle aches and pains. • Fatigue and lethargy. • Chills and fever. • Stiff neck with headache. • Backache. • Nausea and vomiting. • Sore throat. • Enlargement of the spleen and lymph glands. • Migrating joint pain, eventually accompanied by redness and warmth. • Enlarged heart and heart rhythm disturbances.	**LYME DISEASE** (Refer to Illnesses section)
A flat or slightly raised skin lesion that can be black, brown, blue, red, white or a mixture of all colors. Its borders are often irregular and may bleed.	**MELANOMA, MALIGNANT** (Refer to Illnesses section)
A small skin lesion that does not heal in 3 weeks with the following characteristics: • The lesion appears flat and "pearly." Its edges are translucent and rounded or rolled. The edges may have small, curvy, new blood vessels. The ulcer in the center is dimpled. Lesion size varies from 4mm to 6mm, but it may grow larger if untreated. • The lesion occurs on skin that is exposed to the sun and shows evidence of sun damage. • The lesion grows slowly. It does not hurt or itch.	**SKIN CANCER, BASAL-CELL** (Refer to Illnesses section)
A small, disfiguring, scaling, raised bump on the skin with a crusting ulcer in the center. The bump doesn't hurt or itch.	**SKIN CANCER, SQUAMOUS-CELL** (Refer to Illnesses section)
Benign skin lesions fall into the following categories: • Tags—Soft, flesh-colored buds, often on stalks, found on the neck, armpits or groin. • Moles—Flat or raised lesions with clearly defined borders. Moles may be black, blue, red, yellow or brown. • Cherry spots—Pinhead-sized, bright-red lesions on the chest or back. • Strawberry marks—Bright red raised areas in infants that grow until they are removed. • Keloids—Thick, pale, irregular growths that begin at the site of a scar and gradually increase in size. • Dermatofibromas—Rounded nodules, usually brownish and usually on the legs. • Freckles—Flat, brownish spots of pinhead size or larger.	**SKIN LESIONS, BENIGN** (Refer to Illnesses section)
A small, raised bump on the skin with the following characteristics: • Warts begin very small (1mm to 3mm) and grow larger. • Warts have a rough surface and clearly defined borders. • They are usually the same color as the skin, but sometimes darker. • Warts often appear in clusters around a "mother wart." • If you cut into the wart surface, it contains small black dots or bleeding points. • Warts are painless and don't itch.	**WARTS** (Refer to Illnesses section)

(BUMPS ON SKIN, continued on next page)

SYMPTOMS & FACTORS	POSSIBLE PROBLEM
• Pinhead-sized bump that grows to 2mm or 3mm. Shaving off the top reveals small black dots, pinpoint bleeding and an underlying translucent core. • Pain on walking. The wart compresses underlying tender tissue.	**WARTS, PLANTAR** (Refer to Illnesses section)
Venereal warts have the following characteristics: • They appear on moist surfaces, especially the penis, entrance to the vagina and entrance to the rectum. • They are thin, flexible, solid elevations of the skin, growing in stalks or clusters. They are taller than they are wide. • Each wart measures 1mm to 2mm in diameter, but clusters may be quite large. • They don't hurt or itch.	**WARTS, VENEREAL** (Refer to Illnesses section)

If you experience BUMPS ON SKIN plus the following:

• Rash or fever.	**WHAT TO DO:** See Rash with Fever (in Symptoms section).

BURPING OR GAS

(Find your closest combination of symptoms in left-hand column; see possible problem in right-hand column. You may not experience all symptoms listed.)

SYMPTOMS & FACTORS	POSSIBLE PROBLEM
• Colicky (intermittent) pain in the upper right abdomen or between the shoulder blades. • Nausea and vomiting. • Bloating or belching. • Intolerance of fatty foods (indigestion, bloating and belching). • Jaundice (yellow skin and eyes). • No symptoms in about 40% of cases.	**GALLSTONES** (Refer to Illnesses section)
The following signs are worse at night: • Belching or slight regurgitation of stomach contents into the mouth, producing an acid taste. • Heavy, burning or uncomfortable sensation in the chest. • Swallowing difficulty. • Mild abdominal pain.	**HEARTBURN** (Refer to Illnesses section)
• Mild nausea. • Heartburn. • Upper abdominal pain. • Gas or belching. • Bloated or full feeling. • Acid taste.	**INDIGESTION** (Refer to Illnesses section)
• Rumbling abdominal sounds, abdominal cramps and diarrhea. • Gas and bloating. • Nausea. • Headaches. • Diarrhea.	**LACTOSE INTOLERANCE** (Refer to Illnesses section)
• Diarrhea. • Weakness. • Weight loss. • Gas and vague abdominal discomfort. • Bad-smelling, copious stools.	**MALABSORPTION** (Refer to Illnesses section)

(BURPING OR GAS, continued on next page)

SYMPTOMS & FACTORS	POSSIBLE PROBLEM
• Cramp-like pain in the middle or to one side of the lower abdomen. Pain is usually relieved with bowel movements. • Nausea. • Bloating and gas. • Headache. • Rectal pain. • Backache. • Occasional appetite loss that may lead to weight loss. • Diarrhea or constipation, usually alternating. • Fatigue. • Depression. • Anxiety.	**SPASTIC COLON** (Refer to Illnesses section)

If you experience BURPING OR GAS plus the following:
• High-fiber diet.

WHAT TO DO:
Nothing. Improves eventually without diet change.

CHEST PAIN

(Find your closest combination of symptoms in left-hand column; see possible problem in right-hand column. You may not experience all symptoms listed.)

SYMPTOMS & FACTORS	POSSIBLE PROBLEM
Any of the following: • Tightness, squeezing, pressure or mild ache in the chest (more during exercise). • Sudden breathing difficulty (sometimes). • Frequent chest pain similar to that from indigestion. • A choking feeling in the throat. • Chest pain that radiates to the jaw, teeth or earlobes. • Heaviness, numbness, tingling or ache in the arm, shoulder, elbow or hand—usually on the left side. • Pain between the shoulder blades. • Paleness and sweating.	**ANGINA PECTORIS** (Refer to Illnesses section)
Sudden, major collapse of lung: • Chest pain. • Shortness of breath; rapid breathing. • Shock (severe weakness, paleness of skin, rapid heartbeat). • Dizziness.	**ATELECTASIS** (Refer to Illnesses section)
• Cough that produces little or no sputum initially, but does later on. • Low fever (usually less than 101F or 38.3C). • Burning chest discomfort or feeling of pressure behind the breastbone. • Wheezing or uncomfortable breathing (sometimes).	**BRONCHITIS, ACUTE** (Refer to Illnesses section)
If cardiomyopathy is extensive enough to cause congestive heart failure, the following symptoms may occur: • Irregular or rapid heartbeat. • Shortness of breath with activity. • Swelling of the feet and ankles. • Fatigue. • Cough with frothy, bloody sputum. (THIS IS AN EMERGENCY; SEEK MEDICAL CARE IMMEDIATELY!) • Chest pain.	**CARDIOMYOPATHY** (Refer to Illnesses section)

(CHEST PAIN, continued on next page)

SYMPTOMS

SYMPTOMS & FACTORS	POSSIBLE PROBLEM
Early stages: • No symptoms (often). **Later stages:** • Angina pectoris (discomfort or pain in the chest coming on with exercise and disappearing with rest). • Heart attack. **(THIS IS AN EMERGENCY; SEEK MEDICAL CARE IMMEDIATELY!)**	**CORONARY ARTERY DISEASE** (Refer to Illnesses section)
• Chest pain. Pain varies from vague discomfort to stabbing pain. It is often worse with coughing or breathing. Pain may extend to the lower chest wall or abdomen. • Rapid, shallow breathing. • Chills. • Fever. • Extreme fatigue. • Bad breath. • Weight loss.	**EMPYEMA** (Refer to Illnesses section)
• Pain and swelling at the fracture site. • Tenderness close to the fracture. • Paleness and deformity (sometimes). • Loss of pulse below the fracture, usually in an extremity. **(THIS IS AN EMERGENCY; SEEK MEDICAL CARE IMMEDIATELY!)** • Numbness, tingling or paralysis below the fracture (rare). **(THIS IS AN EMERGENCY; SEEK MEDICAL CARE IMMEDIATELY!)** • Bleeding or bruising at the site. • Weakness and inability to bear weight.	**FRACTURES, BONE** (Refer to Illnesses section)
• Chest pain or "heavy, squeezing or crushing" feeling in the chest. • Sweating. • Cold, clammy, wet skin. • Pain that radiates from the mid-chest over the breastbone to the jaw, neck, either arm, the area between the shoulder blades or upper abdomen (sometimes). • Feeling of impending doom. • Shortness of breath. • Nausea and vomiting.	**HEART ATTACK** (Refer to Illnesses section) **(THIS IS AN EMERGENCY; SEEK MEDICAL CARE IMMEDIATELY!)**
The following signs are worse at night: • Belching or slight regurgitation of stomach contents into the mouth, producing an acid taste. • Heavy, burning or uncomfortable sensation in the chest. • Swallowing difficulty. • Mild abdominal pain.	**HEARTBURN** (Refer to Illnesses section)
• Chest pain (angina pectoris). • Heart rhythm irregularity. • Fainting. • Shortness of breath.	**IDIOPATHIC HYPERTROPHIC SUBAORTIC STENOSIS (IHSS)** (Refer to Illnesses section)
• Pain or tenderness in the injury area. • Gradual stiffening or contraction of the injured muscle. • Swelling, redness or bruising at the injury site.	**MUSCLE, PULLED OR TORN** (Refer to Illnesses section)

(CHEST PAIN, continued on next page)

SYMPTOMS & FACTORS	POSSIBLE PROBLEM
• Dull or sharp pain in the front of the chest, radiating to the neck and shoulder. The pain worsens with movement and eases when sitting up or leaning forward. • Rapid breathing. • Cough. • Fever and chills. • Weakness. • Anxiety. • The most important signs are apparent only with medical examination: friction rub heard through a stethoscope; elevated white blood cell count; rapid sedimentation rate (see Glossary); abnormal ECG (see Glossary).	**PERICARDITIS, ACUTE** (Refer to Illnesses section)
• Sudden chest pain that worsens with breathing and coughing. The pain varies from vague discomfort that occurs only with deep breathing or coughing to intense, stabbing pain. Pain is usually over the area of pleura inflammation, but it may also occur in the lower chest or abdomen. • Fever (sometimes). • Discomfort on moving the affected side. • Rapid, shallow breathing. If fluid develops at the site of inflammation between the two membrane layers, the liquid is called pleural effusion. When this happens, the pleurisy pain usually subsides, but breathlessness worsens.	**PLEURISY** (Refer to Illnesses section)
Early symptoms: • Shortness of breath. • Cough that produces flecks of blood, but little or no sputum. • General ill feeling. **Late symptoms:** • Fitful sleep. • Appetite and weight loss. • Chest pain. • Hoarseness; coughing blood. • Symptoms of congestive heart failure. • Bluish nails. • Shadows on the lungs (visible with chest x-rays).	**PNEUMOCONIOSIS** (Refer to Illnesses section)
• High fever (over 102F or 38.9C) and chills. • Shortness of breath. • Cough with sputum that may contain blood or bloody streaks. • Rapid breathing. • Chest pain that worsens with inhalations. • Abdominal pain. • Fatigue. • Bluish lips and nails (rare).	**PNEUMONIA, BACTERIAL** (Refer to Illnesses section) **(THIS IS AN EMERGENCY; SEEK MEDICAL CARE IMMEDIATELY!)**
• Cough (with or without sputum). • Fever. • Labored breathing. • Chest pain. • Abdominal pain. • Bluish skin (severe cases).	**PNEUMONIA, MYCOPLASMA** (Refer to Illnesses section)
• Fever and chills. • Muscle aches and fatigue. • Cough or "croup," with or without sputum. • Rapid, labored breathing (sometimes). • Chest pain. • Sore throat. • Loss of appetite. • Enlarged lymph glands in the neck.	**PNEUMONIA, VIRAL** (Refer to Illnesses section)

(CHEST PAIN, continued on next page)

SYMPTOMS & FACTORS	POSSIBLE PROBLEM
The following symptoms vary according to the degree of lung collapse and extent of underlying lung disease. Symptoms may be less acute if the pneumothorax develops slowly: • Sharp chest pain. Pain may extend to a shoulder or across the chest or abdomen. • Shortness of breath. • Dry, hacking cough with or without bloody sputum (sometimes).	**PNEUMOTHORAX** (Refer to Illnesses section) (THIS IS AN EMERGENCY; SEEK MEDICAL CARE IMMEDIATELY!)
Symptoms vary depending on which organ is affected by the decreased blood supply. The most common include: • Chest pain (heart involvement). • Shortness of breath (lung involvement). • Abdominal pain (intestinal and liver involvement). • Blood in the urine (kidney involvement). • Numbness and tingling of the hands and feet (nerve involvement).	**POLYARTERITIS** (Refer to Illnesses section)
• Sudden shortness of breath. • Faintness or fainting. • Pain in the chest. • Cough (sometimes with bloody sputum). • Rapid heartbeat. • Low fever. These symptoms are often preceded by swelling and pain in the leg.	**PULMONARY EMBOLISM** (Refer to Illnesses section) (THIS IS AN EMERGENCY; SEEK MEDICAL CARE IMMEDIATELY!)
• Painful red blisters anywhere on the body. Blisters appear 4 to 5 days after early symptoms begin. The blisters appear on a broad streak of reddened skin along sensory nerve routes to a particular area of skin. They occur most often on the chest, and spread only on one side of the body. • Mild chills and fever. • General ill feeling. • Mild nausea, abdominal cramps or diarrhea. • Chest pain, face pain, or burning pain in the skin of the abdomen, depending on the affected area.	**SHINGLES** (Refer to Illnesses section)

CONFUSION

(Find your closest combination of symptoms in left-hand column; see possible problem in right-hand column. You may not experience all symptoms listed.)

SYMPTOMS & FACTORS	POSSIBLE PROBLEM
• Headaches that worsen when lying down. • Vomiting with nausea or sudden vomiting without nausea. • Vision disturbances, including double vision. • Weakness on one side of the body. • Lack of balance; dizziness. • Loss of sense of smell. • Memory loss. • Personality changes. • Seizures. (THIS IS AN EMERGENCY; SEEK MEDICAL CARE IMMEDIATELY!)	**BRAIN TUMOR** (Refer to Illnesses section)

(CONFUSION, continued on next page)

SYMPTOMS & FACTORS	POSSIBLE PROBLEM
• Lethargy. • Appetite loss. • Vomiting and diarrhea. • Dehydration and thirst. • Irregular heartbeat. • Depression; delirium; confusion. • Seizures or coma (worst cases only). **(THIS IS AN EMERGENCY; SEEK MEDICAL CARE IMMEDIATELY!)**	**CALCIUM, TOO MUCH** (Refer to Illnesses section)
• Dry mouth and lips. • Decreased or absent urination. • Sunken eyes. • Dry, wrinkled skin with poor resilience. • Confusion; coma. • Low blood pressure. • Severe thirst. • Increase in heart rate and breathing. • Light-headedness.	**DEHYDRATION** (Refer to Illnesses section)
• Forgetfulness, especially of recent events. • Unpredictable, sometimes violent, behavior. • Confusion. • Loss of interest in normal activities. • Disorientation, especially at night. • Poor personal hygiene and appearance. • Depression. • Poor judgment. • Staggering gait. • Incoherent speech.	**DEMENTIA** (Refer to Illnesses section)
The following may indicate either: • Dry mouth. • Wrinkled skin. • Increased, decreased or absent urination. • Fatigue. • Puffy legs, hands, face or abdomen. • Lung congestion. • Weakness and confusion. • Heartbeat irregularities. • Light-headedness.	**FLUID & ELECTROLYTE DISORDERS** (Refer to Illnesses section)
The following vary greatly in frequency and severity: • Weakness or faintness. • Sweating. • Excessive hunger. • Nervousness and trembling hands. • Heartbeat irregularities. • Headache. • Confusion. • Personality changes. • Loss of consciousness. • Seizures (sometimes).	**HYPOGLYCEMIA, FUNCTIONAL** (Refer to Illnesses section)
Mild hypoglycemic reaction: • Excessive hunger. • Weakness. • Nervousness. • Emotional instability. • Difficulty concentrating. • Sweating. • Headache.	**HYPOGLYCEMIA OF DIABETES** (Refer to Illnesses section) **(THIS IS AN EMERGENCY; SEEK MEDICAL CARE IMMEDIATELY!)**

(CONFUSION, continued on next page)

SYMPTOMS & FACTORS	POSSIBLE PROBLEM

Moderate hypoglycemic reaction:
- Increased weakness.
- Excessive sweating.
- Cold, clammy skin.
- Numbness around the mouth or fingers.
- Pounding heartbeat.
- Memory loss.
- Double vision.
- Staring expression.
- Difficulty walking.
- Increasing confusion.

Severe hypoglycemic reaction:
- Muscle twitching.
- Unconsciousness.
- Convulsions.
- Lack of urinary control.

HYPOGLYCEMIA OF DIABETES (continued)
(Refer to Illnesses section)
(THIS IS AN EMERGENCY; SEEK MEDICAL CARE IMMEDIATELY!)

- Confusion.
- Restlessness and anxiety.
- Weakness.
- Muscle cramps (usually in the legs).
- Changes in pulse rate and blood pressure.
- Tissue swelling (edema).
- Stupor or coma (if severe imbalance).

Sodium imbalance may be part of a disease with other symptoms that predominate, such as fever, vomiting, diarrhea or excessive sweating.

SODIUM, TOO MUCH OR TOO LITTLE IN BLOOD
(Refer to Illnesses section)

The following symptoms may vary according to the site of brain damage:
- Inability to speak.
- Inability to move part of the body.
- Loss of consciousness.

STROKE
(Refer to Illnesses section)
(THIS IS AN EMERGENCY; SEEK MEDICAL CARE IMMEDIATELY!)

- Recurrent headaches that worsen each day.
- Fluctuating drowsiness, dizziness, mental changes or confusion.
- Weakness or numbness on one side of the body.
- Vision disturbances.
- Vomiting without nausea.
- Pupils of different sizes (sometimes).

SUBDURAL HEMORRHAGE & HEMATOMA
(Refer to Illnesses section)
(THIS IS AN EMERGENCY; SEEK MEDICAL CARE IMMEDIATELY!)

Early symptoms:
- Poor muscle coordination.
- Confusion.
- Shivering and low body temperature (95F to 98F or 35C to 36.7C) rectally.
- Slow pulse.
- Sleepiness.

Late symptoms:
- Rigid muscles.
- Temperature drop to 77F to 84F (25C to 28.9C).
- Purple fingers, toes and nail beds.
- Loss of consciousness.

TEMPERATURE, TOO LOW
(Refer to Illnesses section)
(THIS IS AN EMERGENCY; SEEK MEDICAL CARE IMMEDIATELY!)

The following symptoms are brief, lasting from several minutes to a few hours.
- Loss of muscle function on one side of the body.
- Headache.
- Dizziness.
- Tingling in the arms and legs.
- Numbness.
- Vision disturbance or temporary blindness in one eye.
- Confusion.
- Faintness without loss of consciousness.
- Slurred speech or inability to speak.

TRANSIENT ISCHEMIC ATTACK (TIA)
(Refer to Illnesses section)

(CONFUSION, continued on next page)

(CONFUSION, continued from previous page)

SYMPTOMS & FACTORS	POSSIBLE PROBLEM
If you experience CONFUSION plus the following:	
• Unusually long time since eating or use of insulin or oral hypoglycemic drug.	**WHAT TO DO:** Drink sweet drink or eat sweet snack. If confusion lasts longer than 10 minutes, call doctor.
• Signs of physical illness, such as fever, cough or loss of bladder control.	**WHAT TO DO:** Call doctor now.
• Recent head injury.	**WHAT TO DO:** Call doctor now.
• Fever of 103F (39.4C) or higher.	**WHAT TO DO:** Call doctor now.
• Heart disease, lung disease or diabetes.	**WHAT TO DO:** Call doctor now. These symptoms may represent a complication of an underlying disorder.
• Agitation, delirium, disorientation, hallucinations or inability to recognize others.	**WHAT TO DO:** Call doctor now.
• Use of prescription or non-prescription drugs, such as antihistamines; appetite suppressants; muscle relaxants; pain killers; sedatives; tranquilizers; mind-altering drugs (marijuana; cocaine; LSD; heroin).	**WHAT TO DO:** Discontinue non-prescription drugs and call doctor now regarding prescription drugs.
• Alcohol consumption, either alone or with drug.	**WHAT TO DO:** Call doctor and stop drinking alcohol.

CONSTIPATION, CHRONIC

(Find your closest combination of symptoms in left-hand column; see possible problem in right-hand column. You may not experience all symptoms listed.)

SYMPTOMS & FACTORS	POSSIBLE PROBLEM
• Cramp-like pain in the middle or to one side of the lower abdomen. Pain is usually relieved with bowel movements. • Nausea. • Bloating and gas. • Headache. • Rectal pain. • Backache. • Occasional appetite loss that may lead to weight loss. • Diarrhea or constipation, usually alternating. • Fatigue. • Depression. • Anxiety.	**COLITIS, ULCERATIVE** (Refer to Illnesses section)
People vary widely in bowel activity. Any of the following may be a sign of constipation: • Infrequent bowel movements, sometimes accompanied by abdominal swelling. • Hard feces. • Straining during bowel movements. • Pain or bleeding with bowel movements. • Sensation of continuing fullness after a bowel movement.	**CONSTIPATION** (Refer to Illnesses section)

(CONSTIPATION, CHRONIC, continued on next page)

SYMPTOMS & FACTORS	POSSIBLE PROBLEM

Diverticulosis symptoms:
- Mild cramping, bloated feeling or tenderness in the left side of the abdomen that is relieved by passing gas or moving bowels.
- Occasional bright red blood in the stool. Non-infected diverticulae sometimes bleed.
- Constipation or diarrhea (sometimes).

Diverticulitis symptoms:
- Intermittent cramping, abdominal pain that becomes constant.
- Fever.
- Nausea.
- Tenderness over the affected area of the colon.

DIVERTICULAR DISEASE
(Refer to Illnesses section)

- Rectal bleeding. Bright red blood may appear as streaks on toilet paper adhering to fecal residue, or it may be a slow trickle for a short while following bowel movements.
- Pain, itching or mucus discharge after bowel movements.
- A lump that can be felt in the anus.
- A sensation that the rectum has not emptied completely after a bowel movement (large hemorrhoids only).

HEMORRHOIDS
(Refer to Illnesses section)

- No symptoms in the early stages (frequently).
- Bloody or black, tarry stools.
- Cramping abdominal pain.
- Feeling of fullness.
- Change in bowel habits, such as diarrhea, constipation or narrow-caliber stools.
- Unexplained weight loss.
- Pain in the rectum.
- Anemia.
- Loss of bowel control (sometimes).

LARGE INTESTINE, CANCER OF
(Refer to Illnesses section)

It is unlikely one person will have all the following symptoms, but most will have several:
- Decreased tolerance of cold.
- Decreased sweating.
- Decreased appetite.
- Constipation.
- Chest pain.
- Coarse or slow-growing hair.
- Slow, rapid or irregular heartbeat.
- Weight gain or extreme thinness.
- Placidity or nervousness.
- Sleepiness or insomnia.
- Mental impairment, including depression, psychosis or poor memory.
- Fluid retention, especially around the eyes.
- Dull facial expression and droopy eyelids.
- Coarse skin.
- Decreased tolerance of medication.
- Decreased sex drive and infertility.
- Anemia.
- Numbness and tingling of the hands and feet.
- Deepened or hoarse voice.

THYROID, UNDERACTIVE
(Refer to Illnesses section)

(CONSTIPATION, CHRONIC, continued on next page)

SYMPTOMS & FACTORS	POSSIBLE PROBLEM
If you experience CONSTIPATION plus the following:	
• Use of prescription or non-prescription drugs.	**WHAT TO DO:** Discontinue non-prescription drugs and call doctor now regarding prescription drugs.
• Dieting.	**WHAT TO DO:** Include more fiber in your diet. For a balanced diet, see Appendix 1.

COUGH

(Find your closest combination of symptoms in left-hand column; see possible problem in right-hand column. You may not experience all symptoms listed.)

SYMPTOMS & FACTORS	POSSIBLE PROBLEM
• Chest tightness and shortness of breath. Sense of suffocation. • Wheezing upon breathing out. • Coughing, especially at night, with little or no sputum. • Rapid, shallow breathing that is easier with sitting up. • Breathing difficulty—neck muscles tighten. **Severe symptoms of acute attack:** (THIS IS AN EMERGENCY; SEEK MEDICAL CARE IMMEDIATELY!) • Bluish skin. • Exhaustion. • Grunting respiration. • Inability to speak. • Mental changes, including restlessness or confusion.	**ASTHMA** (Refer to Illnesses section)
• Cough that produces little or no sputum initially, but more later on. • Low fever (usually less than 101F or 38.3C). • Burning chest discomfort or feeling of pressure behind the breastbone. • Wheezing or uncomfortable breathing (sometimes).	**BRONCHITIS, ACUTE** (Refer to Illnesses section)
• Frequent cough or coughing spasms. • Shortness of breath. • Sputum that is thick and difficult to cough up. Sputum production varies according to whether infection is present. • Barrel chest (in the late stages). • Chest pain (rare).	**BRONCHITIS, CHRONIC** (Refer to Illnesses section)
• Runny or stuffy nose. Nasal discharge is watery at first, then becomes thick and greenish yellow. • Sore throat. • Hoarseness. • Cough that produces little or no sputum. • Low-grade fever. • Fatigue. • Watering eyes. • Appetite loss. • Aching muscles and bones. • Headache. • Chills.	**COLD, COMMON** (Refer to Illnesses section)

(COUGH, continued on next page)

SYMPTOMS & FACTORS	POSSIBLE PROBLEM
• Shortness of breath, especially with exertion or when lying flat in bed. • Fatigue, weakness or faintness. • Cough (usually with sputum). • Wheezing (sometimes). • Swelling of the abdomen, legs and ankles. • Rapid or irregular heartbeat.	**CONGESTIVE HEART FAILURE** (Refer to Illnesses section)
• No symptoms in the early stages (often). • Shortness of breath that increases in severity over several years. • Wheezing and coughing that produces scant sputum. • Occasional recurrent infections of the lungs or bronchial tubes. • Barrel-shaped chest. • Swelling in legs and feet (edema).	**EMPHYSEMA** (Refer to Illnesses section)
In persons sensitive to the fungus, the following appear 4 to 8 hours after exposure to hay. Symptoms usually diminish in a few hours, but may last up to 2 weeks: • Breathlessness (sometimes with wheezing). • Dry cough. • Chest pain. • Chills and fever. • Headache and muscle aches. The following occur with repeated episodes over many years. All these are similar to emphysema and chronic obstructive pulmonary disease (COPD) from any cause: • Increasing shortness of breath with wheezing on exertion. • Cough with sputum. • Fatigue. • Weight loss.	**FARMER'S LUNG** (Refer to Illnesses section)
• Chills and moderate to high fever. • Muscle aches, including backache. • Cough, usually with little or no sputum. • Sore throat. • Hoarseness. • Runny nose. • Headache. • Fatigue. • Loss of appetite. • Chest pain.	**INFLUENZA** (Refer to Illnesses section)
• Cough with sputum. The sputum is pus-like, often blood-streaked and sometimes smells bad. • Bad breath. • Sweating. • Fever to 101F (38.3C) or higher. • Chills. • Weight loss. • Chest pain (sometimes).	**LUNG ABSCESS** (Refer to Illnesses section)
• Persistent cough. • Sputum that may contain blood. • Wheezing. • Chest pain. • Fatigue and weakness. • Weight loss.	**LUNG CANCER** (Refer to Illnesses section)

(COUGH, continued on next page)

SYMPTOMS & FACTORS	POSSIBLE PROBLEM

- Frequent coughing with bad-smelling, green or yellow sputum (sometimes flecked with blood).
- Repeated lung infections.
- Shortness of breath.
- General ill feeling.
- Frequent fatigue.
- Anemia (frequently).

LUNG DISEASE, CHRONIC
(Refer to Illnesses section)

- Dull or sharp pain in the front of the chest, radiating to the neck and shoulder. The pain worsens with movement and eases when sitting up or leaning forward.
- Rapid breathing.
- Cough.
- Fever and chills.
- Weakness.
- Anxiety.
- The most important signs are apparent only with medical examination: friction rub heard through a stethoscope; elevated white blood cell count; rapid sedimentation rate (see Glossary); abnormal ECG (see Glossary).

PERICARDITIS, ACUTE
(Refer to Illnesses section)

Early stages:
- No symptoms (often).
- Symptoms that resemble those of influenza.

Second stages:
- Low fever.
- Weight loss.
- Chronic fatigue.
- Heavy sweating, especially at night.

Later stages:
(THIS IS AN EMERGENCY; SEEK
MEDICAL CARE IMMEDIATELY!)
- Cough with sputum that becomes progressively bloody, yellow, thick or gray.
- Chest pain.
- Shortness of breath.
- Reddish or cloudy urine (sometimes).

TUBERCULOSIS (TB)
(Refer to Illnesses section)

The infection is usually so mild that it produces no symptoms. In a few cases the symptoms may be quite severe. They include:
- Cough.
- Sore throat.
- Chills and fever.
- Chest pain.
- Headache.
- Muscle and joint aches.
- Shortness of breath.
- Skin rash.
- General ill feeling.
- Depression.
- Sweating at night.
- Weight loss.
- Stiff neck (sometimes).

VALLEY FEVER
(Refer to Illnesses section)

(COUGH, continued on next page)

SYMPTOMS & FACTORS	POSSIBLE PROBLEM
If you experience COUGH plus the following:	
• Shortness of breath.	**WHAT TO DO:** See Breathing Difficulty (in Symptoms section).
• Lack of sputum, hoarseness or voice loss.	**WHAT TO DO:** See Voice Loss or Hoarseness (in Symptoms section).

COUGH WITH BLOOD

(Find your closest combination of symptoms in left-hand column; see possible problem in right-hand column. You may not experience all symptoms listed.)

SYMPTOMS & FACTORS	POSSIBLE PROBLEM
If cardiomyopathy is extensive enough to cause congestive heart failure, the following symptoms may occur: • Irregular or rapid heartbeat. • Shortness of breath with activity. • Swelling of the feet and ankles. • Fatigue. • Cough with frothy, bloody sputum. (THIS IS AN EMERGENCY; SEEK MEDICAL CARE IMMEDIATELY!) • Chest pain.	**CARDIOMYOPATHY** (Refer to Illnesses section)
• Cough with sputum. The sputum is pus-like, often blood-streaked and sometimes smells bad. • Bad breath. • Sweating. • Fever to 101F (38.3C) or higher. • Chills. • Weight loss. • Chest pain (sometimes).	**LUNG ABSCESS** (Refer to Illnesses section)
• Persistent cough. • Sputum that may contain blood. • Wheezing. • Chest pain. • Fatigue and weakness. • Weight loss.	**LUNG CANCER** (Refer to Illnesses section)
Early symptoms: • Shortness of breath. • Cough that produces flecks of blood, but little or no sputum. • General ill feeling. **Late symptoms:** (THIS IS AN EMERGENCY; SEEK MEDICAL CARE IMMEDIATELY!) • Fitful sleep. • Appetite and weight loss. • Chest pain. • Hoarseness; coughing blood. • Symptoms of congestive heart failure. • Bluish nails. • Shadows on the lungs (visible with chest x-rays).	**PNEUMOCONIOSIS** (Refer to Illnesses section)

(COUGH WITH BLOOD, continued on next page)

SYMPTOMS & FACTORS	POSSIBLE PROBLEM
• High fever (over 102F or 38.9C) and chills. • Shortness of breath. • Cough with sputum that may contain blood or blood streaks. • Rapid breathing. • Chest pain that worsens with inhalation. • Abdominal pain. • Fatigue. • Bluish lips and nails (rare).	**PNEUMONIA, BACTERIAL** (Refer to Illnesses section) **(THIS IS AN EMERGENCY; SEEK MEDICAL CARE IMMEDIATELY!)**
The following symptoms vary according to the degree of lung collapse and extent of underlying lung disease. Symptoms may be less acute if the pneumothorax develops slowly: • Sharp chest pain. Pain may extend to a shoulder or across the chest or abdomen. • Shortness of breath. • Dry, hacking cough with or without bloody sputum (occasionally).	**PNEUMOTHORAX** (Refer to Illnesses section) **(THIS IS AN EMERGENCY; SEEK MEDICAL CARE IMMEDIATELY!)**
The following symptoms often begin suddenly in the middle of the night and worsen rapidly: • Extreme shortness of breath, sometimes with wheezing. • Rapid breathing. • Restlessness and anxiety. • Paleness. • Sweating. • Bluish nails and lips. • Low blood pressure. • Cough. This may be unproductive at first, but later it can produce a frothy, blood-stained sputum.	**PULMONARY EDEMA** (Refer to Illnesses section) **(THIS IS AN EMERGENCY; SEEK MEDICAL CARE IMMEDIATELY!)**
• Sudden shortness of breath. • Faintness or fainting. • Pain in the chest. • Cough (sometimes with bloody sputum). • Rapid heartbeat. • Low fever. These symptoms are often preceded by swelling and pain in the leg.	**PULMONARY EMBOLISM** (Refer to Illnesses section) **(THIS IS AN EMERGENCY; SEEK MEDICAL CARE IMMEDIATELY!)**
Early stages: • No symptoms (often). • Symptoms that resemble those of influenza. **Second stages:** • Low fever. • Weight loss. • Chronic fatigue. • Heavy sweating, especially at night. **Later stages:** **(THIS IS AN EMERGENCY; SEEK MEDICAL CARE IMMEDIATELY!)** • Cough with sputum that becomes progressively bloody, yellow, thick or gray. • Chest pain. • Shortness of breath. • Reddish or cloudy urine (sometimes).	**TUBERCULOSIS (TB)** (Refer to Illnesses section)

(COUGH WITH BLOOD, continued on next page)

SYMPTOMS & FACTORS	POSSIBLE PROBLEM
If you experience COUGH WITH BLOOD plus the following:	
• Persisting cough with blood following recent cold or flu.	**WHAT TO DO:** Call doctor now. May be symptom of active bleeding in breathing passages which may become difficult to control.

DEPRESSION

(Find your closest combination of symptoms in left-hand column; see possible problem in right-hand column. You may not experience all symptoms listed.)

SYMPTOMS & FACTORS	POSSIBLE PROBLEM
Early stages: • Low tolerance of anxiety. • Need for alcohol at the beginning of the day or at times of stress. • Insomnia; nightmares. • Habitual Monday-morning hangovers and frequent absences from work. • Preoccupation with obtaining alcohol and hiding drinking from family and friends. • Guilt or irritability when others suggest drinking is excessive. **Late stages:** • Frequent blackouts; memory loss. • Delirium tremens (tremors; hallucinations; confusion; sweating; rapid heartbeat). These occur most often with alcohol withdrawal. • Liver disease (jaundice; internal bleeding; bloating). • Neurological impairment (numbness and tingling in hands and feet; declining sexual interest and potency; confusion; coma). • Congestive heart failure (shortness of breath; swelling of feet).	**ALCOHOLISM** (Refer to Illnesses section)
• Rapid, unexplained weight loss. • Pain in the back or upper abdomen that is often relieved by bending forward. • Blood clots in veins anywhere, especially the arms and legs. This is often an early sign. • Jaundice (yellow skin and eyes) from blockage of the nearby bile duct. Jaundice is usually accompanied by intense itching. **(THIS IS AN EMERGENCY; SEEK MEDICAL CARE IMMEDIATELY!)**	**PANCREAS, CANCER OF** (Refer to Illnesses section)
It is unlikely one person will have all the following symptoms, but most will have several: • Decreased tolerance of cold. • Decreased sweating. • Decreased appetite. • Constipation. • Chest pain. • Coarse or slow-growing hair. • Slow, rapid or irregular heartbeat. • Weight gain or extreme thinness. • Placidity or nervousness. • Sleepiness or insomnia. • Mental impairment, including depression, psychosis or poor memory. • Fluid retention, especially around the eyes.	**THYROID, UNDERACTIVE** (Refer to Illnesses section)

(DEPRESSION, continued on next page)

(DEPRESSION, continued from previous page)

SYMPTOMS & FACTORS	POSSIBLE PROBLEM
• Dull facial expression and droopy eyelids. • Coarse skin. • Decreased tolerance of medication. • Decreased sex drive and infertility. • Anemia. • Numbness and tingling of the hands and feet. • Deepened or hoarse voice.	**THYROID, UNDERACTIVE (continued)** (Refer to Illnesses section)

If you experience DEPRESSION plus the following:

• Three or more of the following: loss of energy or fatigue; difficulty sleeping, waking up or daytime sleepiness; reduced sex drive; loss of pleasure in usual activities; poor appetite or unexplained weight loss; overeating and weight gain; feelings of excessive guilt, worthlessness or self-reproach; decreased ability to think, concentrate or make decisions; recurrent thoughts of death, suicide or suicide attempt; crying or tearfulness; decline in social activity or talkativeness; hallucinations.	**WHAT TO DO:** See Depression in Illnesses section.
• Recent virus infection with fever such as flu, Epstein-Barr or hepatitis.	**WHAT TO DO:** Call doctor if depression worsens or lasts longer than 2 weeks. These symptoms commonly occur for 3 to 6 months following serious infection.
• Traumatic or sad event such as death in family.	**WHAT TO DO:** See Depression in Illnesses section.

DIARRHEA

(Find your closest combination of symptoms in left-hand column; see possible problem in right-hand column. You may not experience all symptoms listed.)

SYMPTOMS & FACTORS	POSSIBLE PROBLEM
• Fatigue. • Unexplained weight loss. • Recurrent respiratory and skin infections. • Fever. • Swollen lymph glands throughout the body. • Genital changes. • Enlarged spleen. • Diarrhea. • Night sweats. • Positive laboratory tests.	**AIDS (Acquired Immune Deficiency Syndrome)** (Refer to Illnesses section)
• Intermittent diarrhea with bad-smelling and sometimes bloody stools. • Diarrhea is often preceded by constipation in early stages. • Gas and abdominal bloating. • Severe abdominal cramps and tenderness. • Fever over 101F or 38.3C. • Mucus and blood in the stool (sometimes). • Fatigue. • Muscle and joint aches. **If the liver is involved:** • Tenderness over the liver and right side of the abdomen. • Jaundice (yellow skin and eyes) sometimes.	**AMOEBA INFECTIONS** (Refer to Illnesses section)

(DIARRHEA, continued on next page)

SYMPTOMS & FACTORS	POSSIBLE PROBLEM
Early symptoms include: • Pain in the left side of the abdomen that improves after bowel movements. • Episodes of bloody diarrhea with mucus, alternating with symptom-free intervals. **During an acute attack:** (THIS IS AN EMERGENCY; SEEK MEDICAL CARE IMMEDIATELY!) • Increased bloody diarrhea (up to 10 to 20 bowel movements a day). • Severe cramps and pain around the rectum. • Appetite and weight loss. • Bloated abdomen. • Fever as high as 104F or 40C. • Rapid heartbeat.	**COLITIS, ULCERATIVE** (Refer to Illnesses section)
• Cramping abdominal pain. • Loose, watery or unformed bowel movements. • Lack of bowel control (sometimes). • Fever (sometimes).	**DIARRHEA, ACUTE** (Refer to Illnesses section)
Early dumping syndrome: • Weakness and fainting. • Sweating. • Irregular or rapid heartbeat. • Decreased blood pressure. • Flushing of skin. • Dizziness. • Shortness of breath. • Vomiting. • Explosive diarrhea and abdominal cramps. **Late dumping syndrome:** • Sweating, anxiety and tremors. • Exhaustion and faintness. • Decreased blood pressure. • Headache.	**DUMPING SYNDROME** (Refer to Illnesses section)
• Abdominal cramps. • Fever. • Diarrhea (up to 20 or 30 watery bowel movements in 1 day). • Blood, mucus or pus in the stool. • Nausea or vomiting. • Muscle aches or pain. • White blood cell count lower than normal at the onset (sometimes).	**DYSENTERY, BACILLARY** (Refer to Illnesses section) (THIS IS AN EMERGENCY; SEEK MEDICAL CARE IMMEDIATELY!)
• Sudden diarrhea and abdominal cramping. Some persons have only mild diarrhea and indigestion. • Loose, bulky, bad-smelling stools. • Slight fever (uncommon).	**GIARDIASIS** (Refer to Illnesses section)
• Watery diarrhea (sometimes bloody) with abdominal cramps. • Fever. • High white blood cell count. • Drop in blood pressure, sometimes to shock levels, with weak pulse and rapid heartbeat. (THIS IS AN EMERGENCY; SEEK MEDICAL CARE IMMEDIATELY!) • Nausea and vomiting. • Disorientation.	**PSEUDOMEMBRANOUS ENTEROCOLITIS** (Refer to Illnesses section)

(DIARRHEA, continued on next page)

(DIARRHEA, continued from previous page)

SYMPTOMS & FACTORS	POSSIBLE PROBLEM
• Diarrhea, often accompanied by abdominal cramps. In mild cases, diarrhea may be only 2 or 3 loose bowel movements a day. In severe cases, it may be watery diarrhea as often as every 10 or 15 minutes. • Vomiting (occasionally); fever. • Blood in the stool (sometimes). A relatively mild salmonella infection may be mistaken for simple gastroenteritis.	**SALMONELLA INFECTIONS** (Refer to Illnesses section)
• Cramp-like pain in the middle or to one side of the lower abdomen. Pain is usually relieved with bowel movements. • Nausea. • Bloating and gas. • Headache. • Rectal pain. • Backache. • Occasional appetite loss that may lead to weight loss. • Diarrhea or constipation, usually alternating. • Fatigue. • Depression. • Anxiety.	**SPASTIC COLON** (Refer to Illnesses section)
• Abdominal pain and cramps. • Vomiting (occasionally). • Appetite loss. • Fever. • Weakness. • Swollen abdomen. • Sharp, dull or annoying pain in the chest. • Acid taste in the mouth. • Mild nausea and diarrhea (rare). • Belching or gas.	**STOMACH INFLAMMATION** (Refer to Illnesses section)
• Nausea that sometimes causes vomiting. • Diarrhea that ranges from 2 or 3 loose stools to many watery stools. • Abdominal cramps, pain or tenderness. • Appetite loss. • Fever. • Weakness.	**STOMACH & INTESTINAL INFLAMMATION** (Refer to Illnesses section)
• Diarrhea. In mild cases, this may be only 2 or 3 loose bowel movements a day. In severe cases, it may be watery diarrhea as often as every 10 or 15 minutes. • Vomiting. • Fever. • Headache. • Muscle aches. • Rose-colored skin rash on the abdomen. • Abdominal cramps (sometimes). • Blood in the stool (sometimes). A relatively mild attack may be mistaken for simple gastroenteritis.	**TYPHOID FEVER** (Refer to Illnesses section)

If you experience DIARRHEA plus the following:

• Use of prescription or non-prescription drugs.	**WHAT TO DO:** Discontinue non-prescription drugs and call doctor now regarding prescription drugs.
• Recurrent attacks or pain in lower abdomen.	**WHAT TO DO:** See Recurrent Abdominal Pain (in Symptoms section).

DIZZINESS

(Find your closest combination of symptoms in left-hand column; see possible problem in right-hand column. You may not experience all symptoms listed.)

SYMPTOMS & FACTORS	POSSIBLE PROBLEM
• No symptoms (sometimes). • Continuously irregular heartbeat in which no two beats are of equal strength or duration. You may perceive them as ''flip- flops.'' • Weakness, dizziness or faintness (sometimes). • Chest pain (sometimes).	**ATRIAL FIBRILLATION** (Refer to Illnesses section)
• Hearing loss (to varying degrees). • A plugged feeling in the ear. • Severe pain in ears, over cheekbones or forehead. • Dizziness. • Ringing noises in the ear.	**BAROTITIS MEDIA** (Refer to Illnesses section)
• Sudden pain in the ear. • Partial hearing loss. • Bleeding or discharge from the ear. The discharge may resemble pus within 24 to 48 hours after rupture. • Ringing in the ear. • Dizziness.	**EARDRUM, RUPTURED** (Refer to Illnesses section)
• No symptoms (sometimes) for less severe forms. • Slow, irregular heartbeat. • Dizziness. • Sudden loss of consciousness. **(THIS IS AN EMERGENCY; SEEK MEDICAL CARE IMMEDIATELY!)** • Convulsions (sometimes).	**HEART BLOCK** (Refer to Illnesses section)
• Awareness of one's own heartbeat, including whether it skips; is always fast, slow or irregular; or suddenly changes rhythm. • Shortness of breath. • Sudden faintness or weakness. • No symptoms (frequently).	**HEART RHYTHM IRREGULARITY** (Refer to Illnesses section)
• No symptoms (sometimes). • Fatigue and weakness. • Dizziness or fainting. • Chest pain. • Shortness of breath. • Lung congestion. • Heart rhythm irregularities. • Heart murmurs (abnormal heart sounds heard by the doctor through a stethoscope). • Abnormal blood pressure (high or low).	**HEART VALVE DISEASE** (Refer to Illnesses section)
Heat stroke: • Sudden dizziness, weakness, faintness and headache. • Skin that is hot and dry without sweating. • High body temperature. • Rapid heartbeat. • Muscle cramps. **Heat exhaustion:** • Skin that is cool and moist. • Pale or gray skin color. • Slow pulse. • Confusion. • Muscle cramps. • Low or normal body temperature. • Dark yellow or orange urine.	**HEAT STROKE OR HEAT EXHAUSTION** (Refer to Illnesses section) **(THIS IS AN EMERGENCY; SEEK MEDICAL CARE IMMEDIATELY!)**

(DIZZINESS, continued on next page)

50

SYMPTOMS & FACTORS	POSSIBLE PROBLEM
• Extreme dizziness—especially with head movement—that begins gradually and peaks in 48 hours. • Involuntary eye movement. • Nausea and vomiting (sometimes). • Loss of balance, especially falling toward the affected side. • Temporary hearing loss (sometimes).	**LABYRINTHITIS** (Refer to Illnesses section)
The following occur with every acute attack: • Severe dizziness. • Noises in the affected ear, such as ringing or buzzing. • Hearing loss that increases with each attack. **Possible accompanying symptoms:** • Vomiting. • Sweating. • Jerky eye movements. • Loss of balance.	**MENIERE'S DISEASE** (Refer to Illnesses section)
• Pain in one area or throughout the abdomen. Pain usually starts suddenly and becomes increasingly severe. Pain may be crampy at first, and then steady. The patient often prefers to lie quietly on the back because movement or pressure on the abdomen increases pain. • Shoulder pain (sometimes). • Chills and fever (often high). • Dizziness and weakness. • Rapid heartbeat. • Low blood pressure.	**PERITONITIS** (Refer to Illnesses section) (THIS IS AN EMERGENCY; SEEK MEDICAL CARE IMMEDIATELY!)
Some patients have no symptoms. Others have any of the following: • Fatigue; headache; drowsiness; dizziness. • Itching or flushed skin. • Enlarged spleen. • Unexplained bleeding.	**POLYCYTHEMIA** (Refer to Illnesses section)
• Recurrent headaches that worsen each day. • Fluctuating drowsiness, dizziness, mental changes or confusion. • Weakness or numbness on one side of the body. • Vision disturbances. • Vomiting without nausea. • Pupils of different sizes (sometimes).	**SUBDURAL HEMORRHAGE & HEMATOMA** (Refer to Illnesses section) (THIS IS AN EMERGENCY; SEEK MEDICAL CARE IMMEDIATELY!)
• Red skin rash, sometimes with small blisters, in areas exposed to sunlight. • Fever. • Fatigue or dizziness.	**SUN POISONING** (Refer to Illnesses section)
The following symptoms are brief, lasting from several minutes to a few hours. • Loss of muscle function on one side of the body. • Headache. • Dizziness. • Tingling in the arms and legs. • Numbness. • Vision disturbance or temporary blindness in one eye. • Confusion. • Faintness without loss of consciousness. • Slurred speech or inability to speak.	**TRANSIENT ISCHEMIC ATTACK (TIA)** (Refer to Illnesses section)

(DIZZINESS, continued on next page)

SYMPTOMS & FACTORS	POSSIBLE PROBLEM
If you experience DIZZINESS plus the following:	
• Use of prescription or non-prescription drugs.	**WHAT TO DO:** Discontinue non-prescription drugs and call doctor now regarding prescription drugs.
• Dizziness happens when standing up suddenly.	**WHAT TO DO:** Avoid rising suddenly. Dizziness may be caused by a temporary drop in blood pressure.

EAR, RINGING OR BUZZING SOUNDS IN

(Find your closest combination of symptoms in left-hand column; see possible problem in right-hand column. You may not experience all symptoms listed.)

SYMPTOMS & FACTORS	POSSIBLE PROBLEM
• Hearing loss (to varying degrees). • A plugged feeling in the ear. • Severe pain in ears, over cheekbones or in forehead. • Dizziness. • Ringing noises in the ear.	**BAROTITIS MEDIA** (Refer to Illnesses section)
• Difficulty discriminating (listening selectively) to environmental sounds. • Ringing in the ears. • Dizziness. • Difficulty understanding speech of others, especially with distracting background noise.	**HEARING IMPAIRMENT OR LOSS** (Refer to Illnesses section)
The following occur with every acute attack: • Severe dizziness. • Noises in the affected ear, such as ringing or buzzing. • Hearing loss that increases with each attack. **Possible accompanying symptoms:** • Vomiting. • Sweating. • Jerky eye movements. • Loss of balance.	**MENIERE'S DISEASE** (Refer to Illnesses section)
If you experience RINGING OR BUZZING SOUNDS IN THE EAR plus the following:	
• Strange, loud ear noises or severe, uncomfortable tickling.	**WHAT TO DO:** Call doctor now. Symptoms suggest an insect in the outer ear canal.

EARACHE

(Find your closest combination of symptoms in left-hand column; see possible problem in right-hand column. You may not experience all symptoms listed.)

SYMPTOMS & FACTORS	POSSIBLE PROBLEM
• Hearing loss (to varying degrees). • A plugged feeling in the ear. • Severe pain in ears, over cheekbones or in forehead. • Dizziness. • Ringing noises in the ear.	**BAROTITIS MEDIA** (Refer to Illnesses section)

(EARACHE, continued on next page)

SYMPTOMS & FACTORS	POSSIBLE PROBLEM
• Irritability. • Pain in ear, either sharp or aching. • Feeling of fullness in the ear. • Hearing loss. • Fever. • Discharge or leakage from the ear. • Diarrhea; vomiting (sometimes).	**EAR INFECTION, MIDDLE** (Refer to Illnesses section)
• Ear pain that worsens when the earlobe is pulled. • Slight fever (sometimes). • Discharge of pus from the ear. • Temporary loss of hearing on the affected side.	**EAR INFECTION, OUTER** (Refer to Illnesses section)
• Sudden pain in the ear. • Partial hearing loss. • Bleeding or discharge from the ear. The discharge may resemble pus within 24 to 48 hours after rupture. • Ringing in the ear. • Dizziness.	**EARDRUM, RUPTURED** (Refer to Illnesses section)
• Decreased hearing. • Ear pain. • Plugged feeling in the ear. • Ringing in the ear.	**EARWAX BLOCKAGE** (Refer to Illnesses section)
• Dull, aching pain on one side of the jaw (below the ear) that radiates to the temples, the back of the head and along the jawline. • Tenderness of the muscles used to chew. • "Clicking" or "popping" sounds when opening the mouth. • Inability to open the jaw completely. • Headache.	**TEMPOROMANDIBULAR JOINT SYNDROME (TMJ)** (Refer to Illnesses section)
• Persistent toothache or throbbing, extreme pain upon biting or chewing. • Swelling and tenderness in the neck glands and on the side of the face. • Earache. • Fever. • General ill feeling. • Foul taste and bad breath (if the abscess opens spontaneously).	**TOOTH ABSCESS** (Refer to Illnesses section)

EYE DISCOMFORT

(Find your closest combination of symptoms in left-hand column; see possible problem in right-hand column. You may not experience all symptoms listed.)

SYMPTOMS & FACTORS	POSSIBLE PROBLEM
• Eye pain, usually severe. • Sensitivity to bright light. • Eyelid spasm. • Tearing. • Blurred vision. • Redness in the white of the eye.	**CORNEAL ABRASION OR ULCER** (Refer to Illnesses section) (THIS IS AN EMERGENCY; SEEK MEDICAL CARE IMMEDIATELY!)

(EYE DISCOMFORT, continued on next page)

SYMPTOMS & FACTORS	POSSIBLE PROBLEM
• Severe pain, irritation and redness in the eye. • Foreign body visible with the naked eye (usually). Sometimes the foreign body is very small, trapped under the eyelid and invisible except with medical examination. • Scratchy feeling with blinking. • Symptoms may improve with foreign body still present.	**EYE, FOREIGN BODY IN** (Refer to Illnesses section) **(THIS IS AN EMERGENCY; SEEK MEDICAL CARE IMMEDIATELY!)**
• Swelling, redness, tenderness, pain, bleeding or bruising ("black eye") in or around the eye. • Change in ability to see clearly.	**EYE INJURIES** (Refer to Illnesses section) **(THIS IS AN EMERGENCY; SEEK MEDICAL CARE IMMEDIATELY!)**
Inflammation of the eye (swelling, redness, pain and excessive tears) caused when the inward-turning eyelid and lashes rub against the cornea.	**EYELID, INWARD-TURNING** (Refer to Illnesses section)
• Outward turning of the lower eyelid, causing an unattractive facial appearance. • Inflammation (pain, redness and swelling) in the affected eyelid. • Inadequate eye lubrication, caused when lubricating tears run down the cheek instead of into the eye.	**EYELID, OUTWARD-TURNING** (Refer to Illnesses section)
• A painless swelling on the eyelid, which at first may resemble a sty. The eyelid may swell, and the eye may feel irritated. • After a few days, these early symptoms disappear, leaving a painless, slow-growing, firm lump in the eyelid. Skin over the lump can be moved loosely.	**EYELID EDGE, INFECTION OF** (Refer to Illnesses section)
• Bulging eyes, which creates a staring or frightened look. • Double vision. • Blurred vision. • Pain (sometimes). • Infrequent blinking (sometimes).	**EYES, BULGING** (Refer to Illnesses section)
• Severe, throbbing eye pain and headache. • Redness in the eye. • Blurred vision or halos around lights. • Tender, firm eyeball. • Dilated, fixed pupil. • Swollen upper eyelid. • Vomiting and weakness (due to severe eye pain).	**GLAUCOMA, ACUTE** (Refer to Illnesses section) **(THIS IS AN EMERGENCY; SEEK MEDICAL CARE IMMEDIATELY!)**
Sudden onset: • Severe eye pain. • Photophobia (sensitivity to light). • Eye redness. • Smaller pupil in the affected eye (sometimes). • Tears. • Blurred vision. **Gradual onset:** • Eye pain. • Photophobia (sensitivity to light). • Floating spots in the field of vision. • Blurred vision.	**IRIS, INFLAMMATION & INFECTION OF** (Refer to Illnesses section)

(EYE DISCOMFORT, continued on next page)

SYMPTOMS (side tab, vertical)

SYMPTOMS & FACTORS	POSSIBLE PROBLEM
• Fever. • Headache. • Irritability. • Eyes that are sensitive to light. • Stiff neck. • Vomiting. • Confusion, lethargy and drowsiness.	**MENINGITIS, ASEPTIC** (Refer to Illnesses section)
• Fever, chills and sweating (may be absent in critically ill persons). • Headache. • Irritability. • Eyes sensitive to light; pupils may be of different sizes. • Stiff neck. • Vomiting. • Red or purple skin rash. • Confusion, lethargy, drowsiness or unconsciousness. • Sore throat or other signs of respiratory illness may precede other symptoms.	**MENINGITIS, BACTERIAL** (Refer to Illnesses section) **(THIS IS AN EMERGENCY; SEEK MEDICAL CARE IMMEDIATELY!)**
The following symptoms may affect one or both eyes: • Clear, green or yellow discharge from the eye. • After sleeping, crusts on lashes that cause eyelids to stick together. • Eye pain. • Swollen eyelids. • Sensitivity to bright light. • Redness and gritty feeling in the eye. • Intense itching (allergic conjunctivitis only).	**PINKEYE** (Refer to Illnesses section)
Early stages: • Nasal congestion with green-yellow (sometimes blood-tinged) discharge. • Feeling of pressure inside the head. • Eye pain. • Headache that is worse in the morning or when bending forward. • Cheek pain that may resemble a toothache. • Post-nasal drip. • Cough (sometimes) that is usually non-productive. • Disturbed sleep (sometimes). • Fever (sometimes). **Late stages:** • Complete blockage of the sinus openings, blocking the discharge and increasing pain.	**SINUS INFECTION** (Refer to Illnesses section)
• Redness, swelling, warmth, tenderness or pain on the edge of the top or bottom eyelid. The head of the sty is usually on the outside, but it may be on the underside of the lid. • Increased tear production. • Sensitivity to bright light. • A gritty feeling in the eye.	**STY** (Refer to Illnesses section)

If you experience EYE DISCOMFORT plus the following:

• Recent eye injury with visible damage, or loss of vision.	**WHAT TO DO:** THIS IS AN EMERGENCY; SEEK MEDICAL CARE IMMEDIATELY!
• Redness or gritty feeling in the eye.	**WHAT TO DO:** Use non-prescription artificial tears. Call doctor if discomfort lasts longer than 2 days.

FACE PAIN

(Find your closest combination of symptoms in left-hand column; see possible problem in right-hand column. You may not experience all symptoms listed.)

SYMPTOMS & FACTORS	POSSIBLE PROBLEM
Early stages: • No symptoms (often). **Later stages:** • Angina pectoris (discomfort or pain in the chest with radiating pain to jaw and lower face that comes on with exercise and disappears with rest). • Heart attack.	**CORONARY ARTERY DISEASE** (Refer to Illnesses section)
• Chest pain or "heavy, squeezing or crushing" feeling in the chest. • Sweating. • Cold, clammy, wet skin. • Pain that radiates from the midchest over the breastbone to the jaw, neck, either arm, the area between the shoulder blades or upper abdomen (sometimes). • Feeling of impending doom. • Shortness of breath. • Nausea and vomiting.	**HEART ATTACK** (Refer to Illnesses section) (THIS IS AN EMERGENCY; SEEK MEDICAL CARE IMMEDIATELY!)
The following symptoms may resemble those of an infection such as influenza. • Low fever. • Muscle stiffness, aches and pains—especially in the morning. The muscles involved are usually those of the trunk, upper arms and legs. • Severe, throbbing headache (usually in one temple). • Redness, swelling, tenderness and pulsating nodules along the temporal artery on one side of the head. • Appetite loss.	**POLYMYALGIA RHEUMATICA OR TEMPORAL ARTERITIS** (Refer to Illnesses section) (THIS IS AN EMERGENCY; SEEK MEDICAL CARE IMMEDIATELY!)
• Painful red blisters anywhere on the body. Blisters appear 4 to 5 days after early symptoms begin. The blisters appear on a broad streak of reddened skin along sensory nerve routes to a particular area of skin. They occur most often on the chest and spread only on one side of the body. • Mild chills and fever. • General ill feeling. • Mild nausea, abdominal cramps or diarrhea. • Chest pain, face pain, or burning pain in the skin of the abdomen, depending on the affected area.	**SHINGLES** (Refer to Illnesses section)
Early stages: • Nasal congestion with green-yellow (sometimes blood-tinged) discharge. • Feeling of pressure inside the head. • Eye pain. • Headache that is worse in the morning or when bending forward. • Cheek pain that may resemble a toothache. • Post-nasal drip. • Cough that is usually nonproductive (sometimes). • Disturbed sleep (sometimes). • Fever (sometimes). **Late stages:** • Complete blockage of the sinus openings, blocking the discharge and increasing pain.	**SINUS INFECTION** (Refer to Illnesses section)

(FACE PAIN, continued on next page)

SYMPTOMS & FACTORS	POSSIBLE PROBLEM
Severe face pain, described as "jabbing" or "searing." Pain is often triggered by touching or stroking the face, brushing teeth, shaving, exposure to wind or chewing. Bouts of pain usually last 1 to 15 minutes. Attacks may occur several times a day or may disappear for weeks or months. Between bouts, there is little or no discomfort.	**TIC DOULOUREUX** (Refer to Illnesses section)
• Dull, aching pain on one side of the jaw (below the ear) that radiates to the temples, the back of the head and along the jawline. • Tenderness of the muscles used to chew. • "Clicking" or "popping" sounds when opening the mouth. • Inability to open the jaw completely. • Headache.	**TEMPOROMANDIBULAR JOINT SYNDROME (TMJ)** (Refer to Illnesses section)
• Persistent toothache or throbbing, extreme pain upon biting or chewing. • Swelling or tenderness in the neck glands and on the side of the face. • Earache. • Fever. • General ill feeling.	**TOOTH ABSCESS** (Refer to Illnesses section)
• Frequent contraction of muscles on the side of the face. • Annoying, tooth-grinding noises at night. These may be loud enough to awaken others. • Damaged teeth, supporting gums and bone (apparent in a dental exam). • Headaches.	**TOOTH GRINDING** (Refer to Illnesses section)

FACIAL SKIN PROBLEMS

(Find your closest combination of symptoms in left-hand column; see possible problem in right-hand column. You may not experience all symptoms listed.)

SYMPTOMS & FACTORS	POSSIBLE PROBLEM
• Unsightly red, thickened skin on the nose and cheeks. Small blood vessels are visible on the skin surface. • Papules (small raised bumps) and pustules (small, white blisters with pus) on the affected skin (sometimes).	**ACNE ROSACEA** (Refer to Illnesses section)
• Breakout may be preceded by tingling in the lips. • Eruptions of very small, painful blisters—usually around the mouth, but sometimes on the genitals. The blisters are grouped together, and each is surrounded by a red ring. They fill with fluid, then dry up and disappear within a week. • If the eye is infected, eye pain and redness; feeling that something is in the eye; sensitivity to light; tearing.	**COLD SORES** (Refer to Illnesses section)
• Itching rash in areas where heat and moisture are retained, such as skin creases of elbows, knees, neck, face, hands, feet, groin, genitals and around the anus. • Uncontrolled scratching (frequently unconscious).	**DERMATITIS, ALLERGIC** (Refer to Illnesses section)
Brownish or reddish scaly patches on exposed areas of skin. The patches are painless.	**KERATOSIS, ACTINIC** (Refer to Illnesses section)
A flat or slightly raised skin lesion that can be black, brown, blue, red, white or a mixture of all colors. Its borders are often irregular and may bleed.	**MELANOMA, MALIGNANT** (Refer to Illnesses section)

(FACIAL SKIN PROBLEMS, continued on next page)

SYMPTOMS & FACTORS	POSSIBLE PROBLEM
• Painful red blisters anywhere on the body. Blisters appear 4 to 5 days after early symptoms begin. The blisters appear on a broad streak of reddened skin along sensory nerve routes to a particular area of skin. They occur most often on the chest and spread only on one side of the body. • Mild chills and fever. • General ill feeling. • Mild nausea, abdominal cramps or diarrhea. • Chest pain, face pain, or burning pain in the skin of the abdomen, depending on the affected area.	**SHINGLES** (Refer to Illnesses section)
• A red rash with many small blisters. Some blisters contain pus, and yellow-brown crusts form when they break. The blisters don't hurt but may itch. • Enlarged, hard lymph glands (sometimes).	**SKIN, BACTERIAL INFECTIONS OF** (Refer to Illnesses section)
A small skin lesion that does not heal in 3 weeks with the following characteristics: • The lesion appears flat and ''pearly.'' Its edges are translucent and rounded or rolled. The edges may have small, curvy, new blood vessels. The ulcer in the center is dimpled. Lesion size varies from 4mm to 6mm, but it may grow larger if untreated. • The lesion occurs on skin that is exposed to the sun and shows evidence of sun damage. • The lesion grows slowly. It does not hurt or itch.	**SKIN CANCER, BASAL-CELL** (Refer to Illnesses section)
A small, disfiguring, scaling, raised bump on the skin with a crusting ulcer in the center. The bump doesn't hurt or itch.	**SKIN CANCER, SQUAMOUS-CELL** (Refer to Illnesses section)
Benign skin lesions fall into the following categories: • Tags—Soft, flesh-colored buds, often on stalks, found on the neck, armpits or groin. • Moles—Flat or raised lesions with clearly defined borders. Moles may be black, blue, red, yellow or brown. • Cherry spots—Pinhead-sized, bright red lesions on the chest or back. • Strawberry marks—Bright red raised areas in infants that grow until they are removed. • Keloids—Thick, pale, irregular growths that begin at the site of a scar and gradually increase in size. • Dermatofibromas—Rounded nodules, usually brownish and usually on the legs. • Freckles—Flat, brownish spots of pinhead size or larger.	**SKIN LESIONS, BENIGN** (Refer to Illnesses section)
Macules (small areas of different skin color) or patches with the following characteristics: • They are flat, white and can't be felt with fingers. • They spread to form very large, irregularly shaped areas without pigmentation. • They are usually on both sides of the body in approximately the same place. • Their size varies from 2mm or 3mm to several centimeters in diameter. • They don't hurt or itch.	**VITILIGO** (Refer to Illnesses section)

FAINTING OR FAINTNESS

(Find your closest combination of symptoms in left-hand column; see possible problem in right-hand column. You may not experience all symptoms listed.)

SYMPTOMS & FACTORS	POSSIBLE PROBLEM
Any of the following may occur within seconds or a few minutes after exposure to a substance to which you are very allergic: • Tingling or numbness around the mouth. • Sneezing. • Itching all over, particularly soles and palms and often accompanied by hives. • Redness around ears, resembling recent sunburn. • Watery eyes. • Tightness in the chest; difficult breathing; coughing. • Swelling or itching in the mouth or throat. • Pounding heart. • Faintness. • Shivering. • Dilated pupils. • Loss of consciousness. Not all symptoms occur in every case. Seek immediate help for any.	**ANAPHYLAXIS** (Refer to Illnesses section) (THIS IS AN EMERGENCY; SEEK MEDICAL CARE IMMEDIATELY!)
• Weakness, especially in the arms and legs. • Sore tongue. • Nausea, appetite loss and weight loss. • Bleeding gums. • Numbness and tingling in the hands and feet. • Difficulty maintaining proper balance. • Pale lips, tongue and gums. • Yellow eyes and skin. • Shortness of breath. • Depression. • Confusion and dementia. • Headache. • Poor memory.	**ANEMIA, PERNICIOUS** (Refer to Illnesses section)
• Feeling that something undesirable or harmful is about to happen. • Dry mouth; difficulty swallowing or hoarseness. • Rapid breathing and heartbeat. • Twitching or trembling. • Muscle tension; headaches. • Sweating. • Cold, clammy hands. • Nausea; diarrhea; weight loss. • Sleeplessness; nightmares. • Irritability. • Fatigue. • Memory problems. • Sexual impotence.	**ANXIETY** (Refer to Illnesses section)
• No symptoms (sometimes). • Continuously irregular heartbeat in which no two beats are of equal strength or duration. You may perceive them as "flip-flops." • Weakness, dizziness or faintness (sometimes). • Chest pain (sometimes).	**ATRIAL FIBRILLATION** (Refer to Illnesses section)
• Brief dizziness, followed by fainting and unconsciousness. • No pulse. No breathing. • Bluish-white skin. Dilated pupils. • Seizures. • Loss of bowel and bladder control (sometimes). Simple fainting may resemble cardiac arrest, but pulse and breathing continue.	**CARDIAC ARREST** (Refer to Illnesses section) (THIS IS AN EMERGENCY; SEEK MEDICAL CARE IMMEDIATELY!)

(FAINTING OR FAINTNESS, continued on next page)

SYMPTOMS & FACTORS	POSSIBLE PROBLEM
• Shortness of breath, especially with exertion or when lying flat in bed. • Fatigue, weakness or faintness. • Cough (usually with sputum). • Wheezing (sometimes). • Swelling of the abdomen, legs and ankles. • Rapid or irregular heartbeat.	**CONGESTIVE HEART FAILURE** (Refer to Illnesses section)
Early dumping syndrome: • Weakness and fainting. • Sweating. • Irregular or rapid heartbeat. • Decreased blood pressure. • Flushing of skin. • Dizziness. • Shortness of breath. • Vomiting. • Explosive diarrhea and abdominal cramps. **Late dumping syndrome:** • Sweating, anxiety and tremors. • Exhaustion and faintness. • Decreased blood pressure. • Headache.	**DUMPING SYNDROME** (Refer to Illnesses section)
• No symptoms (sometimes) for less severe forms. • Slow, irregular heartbeat. • Dizziness. • Sudden loss of consciousness. • Convulsions (sometimes). **(THIS IS AN EMERGENCY; SEEK MEDICAL CARE IMMEDIATELY!)**	**HEART BLOCK** (Refer to Illnesses section)
• Heart pounding or palpitations. The pulse at the wrist or neck will be 100 to 180 beats per minute, which is much faster than normal. • Faintness or feeling of impending death. • Chest pain. • Involuntary cough. • Breathlessness.	**HEARTBEAT, RAPID** (Refer to Illnesses section)
• Awareness of one's own heartbeat, including whether it skips; is always fast, slow or irregular; or suddenly changes rhythm. • Shortness of breath. • Sudden faintness or weakness. • No symptoms (frequently).	**HEART RHYTHM IRREGULARITY** (Refer to Illnesses section)
Heat stroke: • Sudden dizziness, weakness, faintness and headache. • Skin that is hot and dry without sweating. • High body temperature. • Rapid heartbeat. • Muscle cramps. **Heat exhaustion:** • Skin that is cool and moist. • Pale or gray skin color. • Slow pulse. • Confusion. • Muscle cramps. • Low or normal body temperature. • Dark yellow or orange urine.	**HEAT STROKE OR HEAT EXHAUSTION** (Refer to Illnesses section) **(THIS IS AN EMERGENCY; SEEK MEDICAL CARE IMMEDIATELY!)**

(FAINTING OR FAINTNESS, continued on next page)

SYMPTOMS & FACTORS	POSSIBLE PROBLEM
• Rapid breathing. • Numbness and tingling around the mouth, hands and feet. • Weakness or faintness. • Muscle spasm or contractions in the hands and feet. • Fainting (sometimes). • Marked anxiety.	**HYPERVENTILATION SYNDROME** (Refer to Illnesses section)
The following vary greatly in frequency and severity: • Weakness or faintness. • Sweating. • Excessive hunger. • Nervousness and trembling hands. • Heartbeat irregularities. • Headache. • Confusion. • Personality changes. • Loss of consciousness. • Seizures (sometimes).	**HYPOGLYCEMIA, FUNCTIONAL** (Refer to Illnesses section)
Mild hypoglycemic reaction: • Excessive hunger. • Weakness. • Nervousness. • Emotional instability. • Difficulty concentrating. • Sweating. • Headache. **Moderate hypoglycemic reaction:** • Increased weakness. • Excessive sweating. • Cold, clammy skin. • Numbness around the mouth or fingers. • Pounding heartbeat. • Memory loss. • Double vision. • Staring expression. • Difficulty walking. • Increasing confusion. **Severe hypoglycemic reaction:** • Muscle twitching. • Unconsciousness. • Convulsions. • Lack of urinary control.	**HYPOGLYCEMIA OF DIABETES** (Refer to Illnesses section) (THIS IS AN EMERGENCY; SEEK MEDICAL CARE IMMEDIATELY!)
• Chest pain (angina pectoris). • Heart rhythm irregularity. • Fainting. (THIS IS AN EMERGENCY; SEEK MEDICAL CARE IMMEDIATELY!) • Shortness of breath.	**IDIOPATHIC HYPERTROPHIC SUBAORTIC STENOSIS (IHSS)** (Refer to Illnesses section)
The following symptoms may vary according to the site of brain damage: • Inability to speak. • Inability to move part of the body. • Loss of consciousness.	**STROKE** (Refer to Illnesses section) (THIS IS AN EMERGENCY; SEEK MEDICAL CARE IMMEDIATELY!)

(FAINTING OR FAINTNESS, continued on next page)

SYMPTOMS & FACTORS	POSSIBLE PROBLEM
The following symptoms are brief, lasting from several minutes to a few hours. • Loss of muscle function on one side of the body. • Headache. • Dizziness. • Tingling in the arms and legs. • Numbness. • Vision disturbance or temporary blindness in one eye. • Confusion. • Faintness without loss of consciousness. • Slurred speech or inability to speak.	**TRANSIENT ISCHEMIC ATTACK (TIA)** (Refer to Illnesses section)

If you experience FAINTING OR FAINTNESS plus the following:

• An unusually long time since eating.	**WHAT TO DO:** Drink sweetened juice or beverage or eat something sugary or starchy. Symptoms suggest low blood sugar.
• Use of prescription or non-prescription drugs.	**WHAT TO DO:** Discontinue non-prescription drug and call doctor now regarding prescription drugs.
• Dizziness.	**WHAT TO DO:** See Dizziness in Symptoms section.
• Faintness occurs when standing up suddenly or following bed confinement.	**WHAT TO DO:** Avoid rising suddenly. Symptoms suggest a temporary drop in blood pressure.
• Shortness of breath prior to faintness.	**WHAT TO DO:** Call doctor if it happens repeatedly. Symptoms suggest a temporary change in blood chemistry.
• Recent strenuous exercise.	**WHAT TO DO:** Call doctor if it happens repeatedly. Symptoms suggest a temporary change in blood chemistry.

FATIGUE

(Find your closest combination of symptoms in left-hand column; see possible problem in right-hand column. You may not experience all symptoms listed.)

SYMPTOMS & FACTORS	POSSIBLE PROBLEM
• Weakness and fatigue. • Gastrointestinal disturbances (nausea, vomiting, abdominal pain, diarrhea and appetite and weight loss). • Low blood pressure causing faintness and dizziness. • Brownish skin (looks suntanned) with white patches. • Darkening of freckles, scars and breast nipples. • Hair loss. • Feeling cold all the time. • Dramatic behavior or mood changes, including aggression or depression. • Confusion. • Coma. (THIS IS AN EMERGENCY; SEEK MEDICAL CARE IMMEDIATELY!)	**ADDISON'S DISEASE** (Refer to Illnesses section)

(FATIGUE, continued on next page)

(FATIGUE, continued from previous page)

SYMPTOMS & FACTORS	POSSIBLE PROBLEM
• Fatigue. • Unexplained weight loss. • Recurrent respiratory and skin infections. • Fever. • Swollen lymph glands throughout the body. • Genital changes. • Enlarged spleen. • Diarrhea. • Night sweats. • Positive laboratory tests.	**AIDS (Acquired Immune Deficiency Syndrome)** (Refer to Illnesses section)
• Paleness. • Weakness, tiredness, faintness and breathlessness. • Frequent infections. • Spontaneous bleeding from the nose, mouth, rectum, vagina, gums and other sites. • Red dots of bleeding under the skin. • Unexplained bruising. • Ulcers in the mouth, throat and rectum.	**ANEMIA, APLASTIC** (Refer to Illnesses section)
• Fatigue and weakness. • Red, sore, glazed tongue. • Paleness. • Shortness of breath. • Nausea, vomiting and diarrhea (rare). • Abdominal distention.	**ANEMIA, FOLIC ACID-DEFICIENCY** (Refer to Illnesses section)
• Fatigue. • Shortness of breath. • Irregular heartbeat. • Jaundice (yellow skin and eyes; dark urine). • Enlarged spleen.	**ANEMIA, HEMOLYTIC** (Refer to Illnesses section)
Signs of pronounced anemia include: • Tiredness, weakness and headache. • Paleness, especially in the hands and lining of the lower eyelids. **Less common signs include:** • Tongue inflammation. • Sore mouth or tongue. • Fainting. • Breathlessness. • Rapid heartbeat. • Appetite loss. • Abdominal discomfort. • Cravings for ice, paint or dirt. • Susceptibility to infection.	**ANEMIA, IRON-DEFICIENCY** (Refer to Illnesses section)
• Weakness, especially in the arms and legs. • Sore tongue. • Nausea, appetite loss and weight loss. • Bleeding gums. • Numbness and tingling in the hands and feet. • Difficulty maintaining proper balance. • Pale lips, tongue and gums. • Jaundice (yellow eyes and skin). • Shortness of breath. • Depression. • Confusion and dementia. • Headache. • Poor memory.	**ANEMIA, PERNICIOUS** (Refer to Illnesses section)

(FATIGUE, continued on next page)

SYMPTOMS & FACTORS	POSSIBLE PROBLEM
• Feeling that something undesirable or harmful is about to happen. • Dry mouth; difficulty swallowing or hoarseness. • Rapid breathing and heartbeat. • Twitching or trembling. • Muscle tension; headaches. • Sweating. • Cold, clammy hands. • Nausea; diarrhea; weight loss. • Sleeplessness; nightmares. • Irritability. • Fatigue. • Memory problems. • Sexual impotence.	**ANXIETY** (Refer to Illnesses section)
Symptoms are often absent until atherosclerosis reaches advanced stages. Symptoms depend on what part of the body has a decreased blood flow and the extent of disease. Common symptoms include: • Muscle cramps if atherosclerosis involves vessels in the legs. • Angina pectoris or heart attack if it involves blood vessels to the heart. • Stroke or transient ischemic attack if it involves vessels to the neck and brain. • Headache.	**ATHEROSCLEROSIS** (Refer to Illnesses section)
• Headaches that worsen when lying down. • Vomiting with nausea or sudden vomiting without nausea. • Vision disturbances, including double vision. • Weakness on one side of the body. • Lack of balance; dizziness. • Loss of sense of smell. • Memory loss. • Personality changes. • Seizures. (THIS IS AN EMERGENCY; SEEK MEDICAL CARE IMMEDIATELY!)	**BRAIN TUMOR** (Refer to Illnesses section)
If cardiomyopathy is extensive enough to cause congestive heart failure, the following symptoms may occur: • Irregular or rapid heartbeat. • Shortness of breath with activity. • Swelling of the feet and ankles. • Fatigue. • Cough with frothy, bloody sputum. (THIS IS AN EMERGENCY; SEEK MEDICAL CARE IMMEDIATELY!) • Chest pain.	**CARDIOMYOPATHY** (Refer to Illnesses section)
Early stages: • Fatigue; weakness. • Poor appetite; nausea; weight loss. • Enlarged liver. • Red palms. **Late stages:** • Jaundice (yellow skin and eyes). • Dark yellow or brown urine. • Spider blood vessels of the skin (fine vessels which spread out from a central point). • Hair loss. • Breast enlargement in men. • Fluid accumulation in the abdomen and legs. • Enlarged spleen.	**CIRRHOSIS OF THE LIVER** (Refer to Illnesses section)

(FATIGUE, continued on next page)

SYMPTOMS & FACTORS	POSSIBLE PROBLEM
• Diarrhea; stool may be black or bloody. • Bleeding and bruising. • Mental confusion; coma. (THIS IS AN EMERGENCY; SEEK MEDICAL CARE IMMEDIATELY!)	**CIRRHOSIS OF THE LIVER (continued)** (Refer to Illnesses section)
Early stages: • No symptoms (often). **Later stages:** • Angina pectoris (discomfort or pain in the chest coming on with exercise and disappearing with rest). • Heart attack.	**CORONARY ARTERY DISEASE** (Refer to Illnesses section)
• Loss of interest in life; boredom. • Listlessness and fatigue. • Insomnia; excessive or disturbed sleeping. • Social isolation. • Appetite loss or overeating. • Loss of sex drive. • Constipation. • Difficulty making decisions or concentrating. • Unexplained crying bouts. • Intense guilt feelings over minor or imaginary misdeeds. • Irritability. • Various pains, such as headache or chest pain, without evidence of disease. • Anxiety or agitation. • Thoughts of death or suicide.	**DEPRESSION** (Refer to Illnesses section)
• No symptoms (sometimes). • Fatigue and weakness. • Dizziness or fainting. • Chest pain. • Shortness of breath. • Lung congestion. • Heart rhythm irregularities. • Heart murmurs (abnormal heart sounds heard by the doctor through a stethoscope). • Abnormal blood pressure (high or low).	**HEART VALVE DISEASE** (Refer to Illnesses section)
• Persistent cough. • Sputum that may contain blood. • Wheezing. • Chest pain. • Fatigue and weakness. • Weight loss.	**LUNG CANCER** (Refer to Illnesses section)
• Frequent coughing with bad-smelling green or yellow sputum (sometimes flecked with blood). • Repeated lung infections. • Shortness of breath. • General ill feeling. • Frequent fatigue. • Anemia (frequently).	**LUNG DISEASE, CHRONIC** (Refer to Illnesses section)
First stage: • A red papule (small, raised bump) on the skin of the thighs, buttocks or armpits that grows as large as 5cm.	**LYME DISEASE** (Refer to Illnesses section)

(FATIGUE, continued on next page)

SYMPTOMS & FACTORS	POSSIBLE PROBLEM

Later stages:
Any or some of the following:
- Muscle aches and pains.
- Fatigue and lethargy.
- Chills and fever.
- Stiff neck with headache.
- Backache.
- Nausea and vomiting.
- Sore throat.
- Enlargement of the spleen and lymph glands.
- Migrating joint pain, eventually accompanied by redness and warmth.
- Enlarged heart and heart rhythm disturbances.

LYME DISEASE (continued)
(Refer to Illnesses section)

The first episode of the following symptoms usually occurs about 8 to 30 days after the mosquito bite:
- Headache.
- Fatigue.
- Nausea.
- Hard, shaking chills with fever for 12 to 24 hours.
- Rapid breathing.
- Heavy sweating, accompanied by a drop in temperature.

Episodes may recur every 2 or 3 days until the disease is treated. Without treatment, the disease can continue for years.

MALARIA
(Refer to Illnesses section)

- Fatigue.
- Shortness of breath.
- Irregular heartbeat.
- Fever.
- Other symptoms caused by the underlying disorder.

If myocarditis causes congestive heart failure, the following symptoms may also occur:

- Swollen feet and ankles.
- Distended neck veins.
- Rapid heartbeat, even when at rest.
- Breathing difficulty while resting or lying down.

MYOCARDITIS
(Refer to Illnesses section)

It is unlikely one person will have all the following symptoms, but most will have several:
- Decreased tolerance of cold.
- Decreased sweating.
- Decreased appetite.
- Constipation.
- Chest pain.
- Coarse or slow-growing hair.
- Slow, rapid or irregular heartbeat.
- Weight gain or extreme thinness.
- Placidity or nervousness.
- Sleepiness or insomnia.
- Mental impairment, including depression, psychosis or poor memory.
- Fluid retention, especially around the eyes.
- Dull facial expression and droopy eyelids.
- Coarse skin.
- Decreased tolerance of medication.
- Decreased sex drive and infertility.
- Anemia.
- Numbness and tingling of the hands and feet.
- Deepened or hoarse voice.

THYROID, UNDERACTIVE
(Refer to Illnesses section)

(FATIGUE, continued on next page)

SYMPTOMS & FACTORS	POSSIBLE PROBLEM
If you experience FATIGUE plus the following:	
• Use of prescription or non-prescription drugs.	**WHAT TO DO:** Discontinue non-prescription drugs and call doctor now regarding prescription drugs.
• You are a woman at menopause or post-menopause.	**WHAT TO DO:** Call doctor. Fatigue is a normal occurrence for many women due to decreasing hormone levels. Your doctor may recommend ERT (estrogen replacement therapy).

FEVER

(Find your closest combination of symptoms in left-hand column; see possible problem in right-hand column. You may not experience all symptoms listed.)

SYMPTOMS & FACTORS	POSSIBLE PROBLEM
• Fatigue. • Unexplained weight loss. • Recurrent respiratory and skin infections. • Fever. • Swollen lymph glands throughout the body. • Genital changes. • Enlarged spleen. • Diarrhea. • Night sweats. • Positive laboratory tests.	**AIDS (Acquired Immune Deficiency Syndrome)** (Refer to Illnesses section)
• Burning and stinging on urination. • Frequent urination, especially at night, although the urine amount may be small. • Increased urge to urinate. • Pain in the lower part of abdomen over the bladder. • Low back pain. • Low-grade fever (under 101F or 38.3C). • Bad-smelling urine. • Painful sexual intercourse. • Lack of urinary control (sometimes).	**BLADDER INFECTION** (Refer to Illnesses section)
• Cough that produces little or no sputum initially, but does later on. • Low fever (usually less than 101F or 38.3C). • Burning chest discomfort or feeling of pressure behind the breastbone. • Wheezing or uncomfortable breathing (sometimes).	**BRONCHITIS, ACUTE** (Refer to Illnesses section)
• Sudden tenderness, swelling and redness in an area of the skin. The area of cellulitis is initially 5cm to 20cm in diameter and grows rapidly in the first 24 hours. A thin, red line often extends from the middle of the cellulitis toward the heart. Cellulitis does not develop into a boil. • Fever, sometimes accompanied by chills and sweats. • General ill feeling. • Swollen lymph glands nearest the cellulitis (sometimes).	**CELLULITIS** (Refer to Illnesses section)

(FEVER, continued on next page)

SYMPTOMS & FACTORS	POSSIBLE PROBLEM
• Runny or stuffy nose. Nasal discharge is watery at first, then becomes thick and greenish yellow. • Sore throat. • Hoarseness. • Cough that produces little or no sputum. • Low-grade fever. • Fatigue. • Watering eyes. • Appetite loss. • Aching muscles and bones. • Headache. • Chills.	**COLD, COMMON** (Refer to Illnesses section)
Fever (measured rectally) for at least 2 weeks. Fever may be intermittent.	**FEVER OF UNDETERMINED ORIGIN (FUO)** (Refer to Illnesses section)
Heat stroke: • Sudden dizziness, weakness, faintness and headache. • Skin that is hot and dry without sweating. • High body temperature. • Rapid heartbeat. • Muscle cramps. **Heat exhaustion:** • Skin that is cool and moist. • Pale or gray skin color. • Slow pulse. • Confusion. • Muscle cramps. • Low or normal body temperature. • Dark yellow or orange urine.	**HEAT STROKE OR HEAT EXHAUSTION** (Refer to Illnesses section)
Early stages: • Flu-like symptoms, such as fever, fatigue, nausea, vomiting, diarrhea and loss of appetite. **Several days later:** • Jaundice (yellow eyes and skin) caused by a buildup of bile in the blood. • Dark urine from bile spilling over into the urine. • Light, "clay-colored" or whitish stools.	**HEPATITIS, ACUTE VIRAL** (Refer to Illnesses section)
• Chills and moderate to high fever. • Muscle aches, including backache. • Cough, usually with little or no sputum. • Sore throat. • Hoarseness. • Runny nose. • Headache. • Fatigue. • Loss of appetite. • Chest pain.	**INFLUENZA** (Refer to Illnesses section)
Sudden onset of: • Fever and shaking chills. • Burning, frequent urination. • Cloudy urine or blood in the urine. • Aching in one or both sides of the lower back (sometimes severe). • Abdominal pain.	**KIDNEY INFECTION, ACUTE** (Refer to Illnesses section)

(FEVER, continued on next page)

(FEVER, continued from previous page)

SYMPTOMS & FACTORS	POSSIBLE PROBLEM
• Fever. • Headache. • Irritability. • Eyes that are sensitive to light. • Stiff neck. • Vomiting. • Confusion, lethargy and drowsiness.	**MENINGITIS, ASEPTIC** (Refer to Illnesses section)
• Fever, chills and sweating (may be absent in critically ill persons). • Headache. • Irritability. • Eyes sensitive to light; pupils may be of different sizes. • Stiff neck. • Vomiting. • Red or purple skin rash. • Confusion, lethargy, drowsiness or unconsciousness. • Sore throat or other signs of respiratory illness may precede other symptoms.	**MENINGITIS, BACTERIAL** (Refer to Illnesses section) (THIS IS AN EMERGENCY; SEEK MEDICAL CARE IMMEDIATELY!)
• Fatigue. • Shortness of breath. • Irregular heartbeat. • Fever. • Other symptoms caused by the underlying disorder. If myocarditis causes congestive heart failure, the following symptoms may also occur: • Swollen feet and ankles. • Distended neck veins. • Rapid heartbeat, even when at rest. • Difficulty breathing while resting or lying down.	**MYOCARDITIS** (Refer to Illnesses section)
• High fever (over 102F or 38.9C) and chills. • Shortness of breath. • Cough with sputum that may contain blood or blood streaks. • Rapid breathing. • Chest pain that worsens with inhalation. • Abdominal pain. • Fatigue. • Bluish lips and nails (rare).	**PNEUMONIA, BACTERIAL** (Refer to Illnesses section) (THIS IS AN EMERGENCY; SEEK MEDICAL CARE IMMEDIATELY!)
• Cough (with or without sputum). • Fever. • Labored breathing. • Chest pain. • Abdominal pain. • Bluish skin (severe cases). (THIS IS AN EMERGENCY; SEEK MEDICAL CARE IMMEDIATELY!)	**PNEUMONIA, MYCOPLASMA** (Refer to Illnesses section)
• Fever and chills. • Muscle aches and fatigue. • Cough or "croup," with or without sputum. • Rapid, labored breathing (sometimes). • Chest pain. • Sore throat. • Loss of appetite. • Enlarged lymph glands in the neck.	**PNEUMONIA, VIRAL** (Refer to Illnesses section)

(FEVER, continued on next page)

SYMPTOMS & FACTORS	POSSIBLE PROBLEM
If you experience FEVER plus the following:	
• Cough. • Shortness of breath, even when resting.	**WHAT TO DO:** See Pneumonia (in Illnesses section).
• Use of prescription or non-prescription drugs.	**WHAT TO DO:** Discontinue non-prescription drugs and call doctor now regarding prescription drugs.
• Rash.	**WHAT TO DO:** See Rash with Fever (in Symptoms section).

FOOT PROBLEMS

(Find your closest combination of symptoms in left-hand column; see possible problem in right-hand column. You may not experience all symptoms listed.)

SYMPTOMS & FACTORS	POSSIBLE PROBLEM
Slow or sudden onset of: • Redness, aching, pain, warmth and tenderness in any or all active joints in the hands, wrists, elbows, shoulders, knees, feet, ankles, jaw or spine. • Morning stiffness; muscular atrophy. • Low-grade fever. • Nodules under the skin (sometimes). • Pale skin. • Appetite loss.	**ARTHRITIS, RHEUMATOID** (Refer to Illnesses section)
• Moist, soft, gray-white or red scales on feet, especially between toes. • Dead skin between toes. • Itching in inflamed areas. • Damp, musty foot odor. • Small blisters on the feet (sometimes).	**ATHLETE'S FOOT** (Refer to Illnesses section)
• Intermittent pain in the instep or the leg when exercising. The pain improves with rest. • Pain, blueness, heat and tingling in the legs when exposed to cold. • Painful ulcers on the toes and fingertips (sometimes).	**BUERGER'S DISEASE** (Refer to Illnesses section)
• An inward-turned great toe that may overlap the second—and sometimes the third—toe. • Thickened skin over the bony protrusion at the base of the great toe. • Fluid accumulation under the thickened skin (sometimes). • Foot pain and stiffness.	**BUNION** (Refer to Illnesses section)
• Pain, tenderness and limited movement in the affected area. • When shoulder involved, radiation of pain into the neck, arm, fingertips. • Severe pain with movement of the arm. • Fever (sometimes).	**BURSITIS** (Refer to Illnesses section)

(FOOT PROBLEMS, continued on next page)

SYMPTOMS & FACTORS	POSSIBLE PROBLEM
• Pain and swelling at the fracture site. • Tenderness close to the fracture. • Paleness and deformity (sometimes). • Loss of pulse below the fracture, usually in an extremity. **(THIS IS AN EMERGENCY; SEEK MEDICAL CARE IMMEDIATELY!)** • Numbness, tingling or paralysis below the fracture (rare). **(THIS IS AN EMERGENCY; SEEK MEDICAL CARE IMMEDIATELY!)** • Bleeding or bruising at the site. • Weakness and inability to bear weight.	**FRACTURES, BONE** (Refer to Illnesses section)
• Sudden onset of severe pain in the inflamed joint, usually at the base of the big toe or larger joints. • Involved joints are red, hot, swollen and very tender. Skin over the joint is red and shiny. • Fever (sometimes).	**GOUT** (Refer to Illnesses section)
Pain and tenderness in the sole of the foot under the heel bone.	**HEEL SPUR** (Refer to Illnesses section)
• Severe, unexplained foot pain when standing or walking. Pain disappears when the load is taken off the feet. • Swelling and increased warmth and tenderness over the painful area.	**MARCH FRACTURE** (Refer to Illnesses section)
• Joint stiffness and pain, including backache. Weather changes, especially cold, damp weather, may increase aching. • Limited movement and loss of dexterity in affected joints. • Redness, heat or fever in affected joints (sometimes). • Swelling of affected joints, especially finger joints (sometimes). • Cracking or grating sounds with joint movement (sometimes).	**OSTEOARTHRITIS** (Refer to Illnesses section)
• Pinhead-sized bump that grows to 2mm or 3mm. Shaving off the top reveals small black dots, pinpoint bleeding and an underlying translucent core. • Pain on walking. The wart compresses underlying tender tissue.	**WARTS, PLANTAR** (Refer to Illnesses section)

If you experience FOOT PROBLEMS plus the following:

• Bottom of foot has painful, red, swollen area on sole.	**WHAT TO DO:** Call doctor. You may need tetanus protection if these symptoms represent a penetrating wound or splinter.
• Excessively dry, thick skin on bottom of feet.	**WHAT TO DO:** Apply lubricating ointment.
• Excessively sweaty feet.	**WHAT TO DO:** Wash and dry feet twice a day and apply talcum powder. Wear cotton socks.

HAIR GROWTH IN WOMEN, EXCESSIVE

(Find your closest combination of symptoms in left-hand column; see possible problem in right-hand column. You may not experience all symptoms listed.)

SYMPTOMS & FACTORS	POSSIBLE PROBLEM
• Round face and puffy eyes. • Ruddy complexion. • Growth of facial hair in women. • Fat accumulation over the upper back and trunk, accompanied by purple "stretch marks." • High blood pressure. • Mental and emotional changes, including psychosis. • Enlarged clitoris. • Diabetes mellitus. • Peptic ulcers. • Osteoporosis. • Low resistance to infection. • Insomnia. • Thin, easily bruised skin.	**CUSHING'S SYNDROME** (Refer to Illnesses section)
Frequently no symptoms occur until the tumor becomes large. **Earliest symptoms include:** • Vague discomfort in the lower abdomen. • Gastrointestinal upsets. • Irregular menstrual periods. **Later symptoms:** • Deep voice. • Excessive hair growth. • Unexplained weight loss. • An enlarged, hard and sometimes tender mass in the lower abdomen. • Painful sexual intercourse. • Anemia.	**OVARIAN CANCER** (Refer to Illnesses section)
Some produce no symptoms. Others produce any of the following: • Swelling without pain in the lower abdomen. • Painful sexual intercourse. • Stinging or burning on urination (if the cyst presses on the bladder). • Difficulty emptying the bladder completely. • Brownish vaginal discharge. • Increased hairiness (if the cyst produces excess hormones).	**OVARIAN CYSTS** (Refer to Illnesses section)
May not cause symptoms. If symptoms occur, they may include: • Mild pelvic pain. • Pain in the lower back. • Discomfort with sexual intercourse. • Abnormal menstruation, including changes in menstrual flow, length of periods and intervals between periods. • Excessive hair growth, deep voice and weight gain (sometimes). If a large ovarian tumor twists or ruptures, the following will occur in the lower abdomen: • Severe pain. • Rigid muscles. • Swelling.	**OVARIAN TUMOR, BENIGN** (Refer to Illnesses section)

(HAIR GROWTH IN WOMEN, EXCESSIVE, continued on next page)

SYMPTOMS & FACTORS	POSSIBLE PROBLEM

If you experience EXCESSIVE HAIR GROWTH (IN WOMEN) plus the following:

- Use of prescription or non-prescription drugs.

WHAT TO DO:
Discontinue non-prescription drugs and call doctor now regarding prescription drugs.

- Growth occurs on face and ovaries were recently removed.

WHAT TO DO:
Call doctor soon. Also consult cosmetologist for removal of unwanted hair.

HAIR LOSS

(Find your closest combination of symptoms in left-hand column; see possible problem in right-hand column. You may not experience all symptoms listed.)

SYMPTOMS & FACTORS	POSSIBLE PROBLEM

- Feeling that something undesirable or harmful is about to happen.
- Dry mouth; difficulty swallowing or hoarseness.
- Rapid breathing and heartbeat.
- Twitching or trembling.
- Muscle tension; headaches.
- Sweating.
- Cold, clammy hands.
- Nausea; diarrhea; weight loss.
- Sleeplessness; nightmares.
- Irritability.
- Fatigue.
- Memory problems.
- Sexual impotence.

ANXIETY
(Refer to Illnesses section)

- Sudden hair loss in sharply defined oval or circular patches.
- No itching or pain.
- Denuded site becomes white.
- In rare cases loss of body hair may be total.

BALDNESS
(Refer to Illnesses section)

- In men, hair loss occurs on top of the head and in the temple areas of the scalp.
- In women, hair loss usually occurs only on top of the head.
- In both sexes, some scattered loss may also occur.

BALDNESS, PATTERN
(Refer to Illnesses section)

Plaques (red, raised skin lesions) with the following characteristics:
- Plaques are 1cm to 4cm in diameter and have clearly defined borders.
- Plaques may appear anywhere on the face, but the cheeks and jawline are the most common sites. Some people describe them as "butterfly" lesions when two lesions of unequal size appear on both sides of the nose.
- Plaques sometimes appear on the scalp with localized patches of hair loss.
- Plaques scar as they heal.

LUPUS ERYTHEMATOSUS, DISCOID
(Refer to Illnesses section)

Lesions that itch (sometimes) and have the following characteristics:
- On the scalp, lesions cause patchy hair loss and scaling scalp.
- On body skin, lesions are red, circular, flat, scaling and have well-defined borders.
- On the bearded area of the face, lesions cause an itchy, scaling rash under the beard.
- On the feet—See Athlete's Foot in the Illnesses section.
- Of the nails—See Paronychia in the Illnesses section.

RINGWORM
(Refer to Illnesses section)

(HAIR LOSS, continued on next page)

SYMPTOMS & FACTORS	POSSIBLE PROBLEM
• Hair loss at 4 to 5 times the normal rate. Normal hair loss is approximately 400 hairs a day, mostly during washing or brushing. • No itching or pain.	**TELOGEN EFFLUVIUM** (Refer to Illnesses section)

If you experience HAIR LOSS plus the following:

• Use of prescription or non-prescription drugs, especially for cancer or circulatory disorders.	**WHAT TO DO:** Discontinue non-prescription drugs and call doctor now regarding prescription drugs.
• Frequent use of any of following hair-care products or hairstyles: dyes; bleaches; straighteners; permanent waves; curling irons or hot rollers; tight braids; ponytails; cornrows.	**WHAT TO DO:** Change hairstyle and avoid damaging products or styles. Call doctor if hair loss persists.
• It has been 2 to 3 months following serious illness and high fever.	**WHAT TO DO:** Nothing need be done since this is a temporary effect of illness. Hair should return to normal within a few months.

HALLUCINATIONS

(Find your closest combination of symptoms in left-hand column; see possible problem in right-hand column. You may not experience all symptoms listed.)

SYMPTOMS & FACTORS	POSSIBLE PROBLEM
Early stages: • Low tolerance of anxiety. • Need for alcohol at the beginning of the day, or at times of stress. • Insomnia; nightmares. • Habitual Monday-morning hangovers and frequent absences from work. • Preoccupation with obtaining alcohol and hiding drinking from family and friends. • Guilt or irritability when others suggest drinking is excessive. **Late stages:** • Frequent blackouts; memory loss. • Delirium tremens (tremors; hallucinations; confusion; sweating; rapid heartbeat). These occur most often with alcohol withdrawal. • Liver disease (jaundice; internal bleeding; bloating). • Neurological impairment (numbness and tingling in hands and feet; declining sexual interest and potency; confusion; coma). • Congestive heart failure (shortness of breath; swelling of feet).	**ALCOHOLISM** (Refer to Illnesses section)
• Forgetfulness, especially of recent events. • Unpredictable, sometimes violent, behavior. • Confusion. • Loss of interest in normal activities. • Disorientation, especially at night. • Poor personal hygiene and appearance. • Depression. • Poor judgment. • Staggering gait. • Incoherent speech.	**DEMENTIA** (Refer to Illnesses section)

(HALLUCINATIONS, continued on next page)

(HALLUCINATIONS, continued from previous page)

SYMPTOMS & FACTORS	POSSIBLE PROBLEM
Depends on the substance of abuse. Most produce: • A temporary pleasant mood. • Relief from anxiety. • False feelings of self-confidence. • Increased sensitivity to sights and sounds (including hallucinations). • Altered activity levels—either stupor and sleep-like states or frenzies. **(THIS IS AN EMERGENCY; SEEK MEDICAL CARE IMMEDIATELY!)** • Unpleasant or painful symptoms when the abused substance is withdrawn. **(THIS IS AN EMERGENCY; SEEK MEDICAL CARE IMMEDIATELY!)**	**DRUG ABUSE & ADDICTION** (Refer to Illnesses section)

If you experience HALLUCINATIONS plus the following:

• Use of prescription or non-prescription drugs.	**WHAT TO DO:** Discontinue non-prescription drugs and call doctor now regarding prescription drugs.
• Excessive alcohol consumption or use of mind-altering drugs.	**WHAT TO DO:** Discontinue use of alcohol or drug. Call doctor if hallucinations last longer than 4 hours.
• Hearing voices that accuse you of real or imagined misdeeds; feelings of guilt.	**WHAT TO DO:** Call doctor. These symptoms suggest severe neurosis, psychosis or brain damage.
• Seeing or hearing close relative or friend who has recently died.	**WHAT TO DO:** Call doctor if hallucinations last longer than 6 weeks. They should cease eventually.
• Hallucinations occur when falling asleep or just before waking.	**WHAT TO DO:** Nothing need be done. This is a common occurrence at these times.

HEADACHE

(Find your closest combination of symptoms in left-hand column; see possible problem in right-hand column. You may not experience all symptoms listed.)

SYMPTOMS & FACTORS	POSSIBLE PROBLEM
• Feeling that something undesirable or harmful is about to happen. • Dry mouth; difficulty swallowing or hoarseness. • Rapid breathing and heartbeat. • Twitching or trembling. • Muscle tension; headaches. • Sweating. • Cold, clammy hands. • Nausea; diarrhea; weight loss. • Sleeplessness; nightmares. • Irritability. • Fatigue. • Memory problems. • Sexual impotence.	**ANXIETY** (Refer to Illnesses section)

(HEADACHE, continued on next page)

SYMPTOMS & FACTORS	POSSIBLE PROBLEM
Usually no symptoms unless disease is severe. Following are symptoms of a hypertensive crisis: • Headache; drowsiness; confusion. • Numbness and tingling in the hands and feet. • Coughing blood; nosebleeds. • Severe shortness of breath. • Seizures. (THIS IS AN EMERGENCY; SEEK MEDICAL CARE IMMEDIATELY!)	**BLOOD PRESSURE, TOO HIGH** (Refer to Illnesses section)
The following symptoms usually appear gradually over several hours. They resemble symptoms of a brain tumor or stroke: • Pain in the back if the infection is in the covering of the spinal cord. • Headache and drowsiness. • Nausea and vomiting. • Weakness, numbness, or paralysis of one side of the body. • Irregular gait. • Convulsions. • Fever. • Confusion or delirium. • Speaking difficulty.	**BRAIN OR EPIDURAL ABSCESS** (Refer to Illnesses section) (THIS IS AN EMERGENCY; SEEK MEDICAL CARE IMMEDIATELY!)
• Headaches that worsen when lying down. • Vomiting with nausea or sudden vomiting without nausea. • Vision disturbances, including double vision. • Weakness on one side of the body. • Lack of balance; dizziness. • Loss of sense of smell. • Memory loss. • Personality changes. • Seizures. (THIS IS AN EMERGENCY; SEEK MEDICAL CARE IMMEDIATELY!)	**BRAIN TUMOR** (Refer to Illnesses section)
• Severe headache. • Stiff neck. • Fever. • Blurred vision. • Protein in the urine. • Mental disturbances, such as confusion, depression, agitation or inappropriate speech or dress. • Cough. • Drowsiness.	**CRYPTOCOCCOSIS** (Refer to Illnesses section)
• Loss of interest in life; boredom. • Listlessness and fatigue. • Insomnia; excessive or disturbed sleeping. • Social isolation. • Appetite loss or overeating. • Loss of sex drive. • Constipation. • Difficulty making decisions or concentrating. • Unexplained crying bouts. • Intense guilt feelings over minor or imaginary misdeeds. • Irritability. • Various pains, such as headache or chest pain, without evidence of disease. • Anxiety or agitation. • Thoughts of death or suicide.	**DEPRESSION** (Refer to Illnesses section)

(HEADACHE, continued on next page)

SYMPTOMS & FACTORS	POSSIBLE PROBLEM
These symptoms develop within 24 to 96 hours after a head injury: • Headache that steadily worsens. • Drowsiness or unconsciousness. • Nausea or vomiting. • Inability to move arms and legs. • Change in the size of eye pupils. • Seizures.	**EXTRADURAL HEMORRHAGE** (Refer to Illnesses section) (THIS IS AN EMERGENCY; SEEK MEDICAL CARE IMMEDIATELY!)
• Severe, throbbing eye pain and headache. • Redness in the eye. • Blurred vision or halos around lights. • Tender, firm eyeball. • Dilated, fixed pupil. • Swollen upper eyelid. • Vomiting and weakness (due to severe eye pain).	**GLAUCOMA, ACUTE** (Refer to Illnesses section) (THIS IS AN EMERGENCY; SEEK MEDICAL CARE IMMEDIATELY!)
Symptoms depend on the extent of injury. The presence or absence of swelling at the injury site is not related to the seriousness of injury. Signs and symptoms include any or all of the following: • Drowsiness or confusion. • Vomiting and nausea. • Blurred vision. • Pupils of different sizes. • Loss of consciousness—either temporarily or for long periods. **(THIS IS AN EMERGENCY; SEEK MEDICAL CARE IMMEDIATELY!)** • Amnesia or memory lapses. • Irritability. • Headache. • Bleeding of the scalp if the skin is broken.	**HEAD INJURY** (Refer to Illnesses section)
The nature of attacks varies between persons and from time to time in the same person. Symptoms of a classic migraine attack appear in the following sequence: • Inability to see clearly, followed by seeing bright spots and zigzag patterns. Visual disturbances may last several minutes or several hours, but they disappear once the headache begins. • Dull, boring pain in the temple that spreads to the entire side of the head. Pain becomes intense and throbbing. • Nausea and vomiting. In other types of migraine attacks, the above symptoms (vision disturbances, headache or vomiting) may be absent, or other symptoms may be present. Some persons become pale, with bloodshot eyes and a runny nose or eyes.	**MIGRAINE HEADACHE** (Refer to Illnesses section)
Any of the following: • Moderate pain in the front or back of the head accompanied by tight muscles in the neck or scalp. • Constant pain over the temples accompanied by the feeling that a vise is over the back of the head. • Throbbing pain all over the head. • Nausea and vomiting (sometimes).	**HEADACHE, TENSION OR VASCULAR** (Refer to Illnesses section)
• Rumbling abdominal sounds, abdominal cramps and diarrhea. • Gas and bloating. • Nausea. • Headaches. • Diarrhea.	**LACTOSE INTOLERANCE** (Refer to Illnesses section)

(HEADACHE, continued on next page)

SYMPTOMS & FACTORS	POSSIBLE PROBLEM
The first episode of the following symptoms usually occurs about 8 to 30 days after the mosquito bite:	**MALARIA** (Refer to Illnesses section)

The first episode of the following symptoms usually occurs about 8 to 30 days after the mosquito bite:
- Headache.
- Fatigue.
- Nausea.
- Hard, shaking chills with fever for 12 to 24 hours.
- Rapid breathing.
- Heavy sweating accompanied by a drop in temperature.

Episodes may recur every 2 or 3 days until the disease is treated. Without treatment, the disease can continue for years.

MALARIA
(Refer to Illnesses section)

- Fever.
- Headache.
- Irritability.
- Eyes that are sensitive to light.
- Stiff neck.
- Vomiting.
- Confusion, lethargy and drowsiness.

MENINGITIS, ASEPTIC
(Refer to Illnesses section)

- Fever, chills and sweating (may be absent in critically ill persons).
- Headache.
- Irritability.
- Eyes sensitive to light; pupils may be of different sizes.
- Stiff neck.
- Vomiting.
- Red or purple skin rash.
- Confusion, lethargy, drowsiness or unconsciousness.
- Sore throat or other signs of respiratory illness may precede other symptoms.

MENINGITIS, BACTERIAL
(Refer to Illnesses section)
(THIS IS AN EMERGENCY; SEEK MEDICAL CARE IMMEDIATELY!)

- Blurred vision, double vision, dizziness or a drooping eyelid caused by tumor pressure on nerves to the eye.
- Headache in the forehead.
- Nausea and vomiting.
- Seizures.
- Runny nose.
- Excessive thirst.
- Menstrual changes.
- Unexplained weight gain.
- Retarded or excessive growth in children.
- Low blood sugar.
- Low blood pressure.
- Loss of peripheral vision.
- Symptoms of abnormalities in other endocrine glands. See Thyroid, Overactive; Parathyroid, Overactive; Cushing's Disease; and Ovarian Tumor (all in Illnesses section).

PITUITARY TUMOR
(Refer to Illnesses section)

Early stages:
- Nasal congestion with green-yellow (sometimes blood-tinged) discharge.
- Feeling of pressure inside the head.
- Eye pain.
- Headache that is worse in the morning or when bending forward.
- Cheek pain that may resemble a toothache.
- Post-nasal drip.
- Cough that is usually nonproductive (sometimes).
- Disturbed sleep (sometimes).
- Fever (sometimes).

Late stages:
- Complete blockage of the sinus openings, blocking the discharge and increasing pain.

SINUS INFECTION
(Refer to Illnesses section)

(HEADACHE, continued on next page)

(HEADACHE, continued from previous page)

SYMPTOMS & FACTORS	POSSIBLE PROBLEM
If you experience HEADACHE plus the following: • Recently taken prescription or non-prescription drugs.	**WHAT TO DO:** Discontinue non-prescription drugs and call doctor now regarding prescription drugs.
• Unusually long time since eating. • Excessive alcohol consumption. • Stuffy, smoky or noisy room. • Exposure to strong sunlight.	**WHAT TO DO:** Use a non-prescription pain reliever, such as acetaminophen. There is probably no underlying disorder.
• It is after excessive alcohol consumption and there is nausea or vomiting.	**WHAT TO DO:** Use a non-prescription pain reliever, such as acetaminophen, and try taking a tablespoon of honey. These are probably effects of a hangover.

HEARING LOSS

(Find your closest combination of symptoms in left-hand column; see possible problem in right-hand column. You may not experience all symptoms listed.)

SYMPTOMS & FACTORS	POSSIBLE PROBLEM
• Ear pain that worsens when the earlobe is pulled. • Slight fever (sometimes). • Discharge of pus from the ear. • Temporary loss of hearing on the affected side.	**EAR INFECTION, OUTER** (Refer to Illnesses section)
• Decreased hearing. • Ear pain. • Plugged feeling in the ear. • Ringing in the ear.	**EARWAX BLOCKAGE** (Refer to Illnesses section)
• Extreme dizziness—especially with head movement—that begins gradually and peaks in 48 hours. • Involuntary eye movement. • Nausea and vomiting (sometimes). • Loss of balance, especially falling toward the affected side. • Temporary hearing loss (sometimes).	**LABYRINTHITIS** (Refer to Illnesses section)
The following occur with every acute attack: • Severe dizziness. • Noises in the affected ear, such as ringing or buzzing. • Hearing loss that increases with each attack. **Possible accompanying symptoms:** • Vomiting. • Sweating. • Jerky eye movements. • Loss of balance.	**MENIERE'S DISEASE** (Refer to Illnesses section)
• Slow, progressive hearing loss. • Ringing in the ears. • Hearing that is better in noisy environments than quiet ones.	**OTOSCLEROSIS** (Refer to Illnesses section)
If you experience HEARING LOSS plus the following: • Earache.	**WHAT TO DO:** See Earache (in Symptoms section).

HEARTBEAT IRREGULARITY

(Find your closest combination of symptoms in left-hand column; see possible problem in right-hand column. You may not experience all symptoms listed.)

SYMPTOMS & FACTORS	POSSIBLE PROBLEM
• Feeling that something undesirable or harmful is about to happen. • Dry mouth; difficulty swallowing or hoarseness. • Rapid breathing and heartbeat. • Twitching or trembling. • Muscle tension; headaches. • Sweating. • Cold, clammy hands. • Nausea; diarrhea; weight loss. • Sleeplessness; nightmares. • Irritability. • Fatigue. • Memory problems. • Sexual impotence.	**ANXIETY** (Refer to Illnesses section)
• No symptoms (sometimes). • Continuously irregular heartbeat in which no two beats are of equal strength or duration. You may perceive them as "flip-flops." • Weakness, dizziness or faintness (sometimes). • Chest pain (sometimes).	**ATRIAL FIBRILLATION** (Refer to Illnesses section)
Usually no symptoms unless disease is severe. Following are symptoms of a hypertensive crisis: • Headache; drowsiness; confusion. • Numbness and tingling in the hands and feet. • Coughing blood; nosebleeds. • Severe shortness of breath. • Seizures. **(THIS IS AN EMERGENCY; SEEK MEDICAL CARE IMMEDIATELY!)**	**BLOOD PRESSURE, TOO HIGH** (Refer to Illnesses section)
• Muscle spasms, twitching or cramps. • Numbness and tingling in the arms, legs, hands and feet. • Seizures. **(THIS IS AN EMERGENCY; SEEK MEDICAL CARE IMMEDIATELY!)** • Irregular heartbeat. • High blood pressure. • Lack of adequate sunshine.	**CALCIUM, TOO LITTLE** (Refer to Illnesses section)
• Lethargy. • Appetite loss. • Vomiting and diarrhea. • Dehydration and thirst. • Irregular heartbeat. • Depression; delirium; confusion. • Seizures or coma (worst cases only). **(THIS IS AN EMERGENCY; SEEK MEDICAL CARE IMMEDIATELY!)**	**CALCIUM, TOO MUCH** (Refer to Illnesses section)
If cardiomyopathy is extensive enough to cause congestive heart failure, the following symptoms may occur: • Irregular or rapid heartbeat. • Shortness of breath with activity. • Swelling of the feet and ankles. • Fatigue. • Cough with frothy, bloody sputum. **(THIS IS AN EMERGENCY; SEEK MEDICAL CARE IMMEDIATELY!)** • Chest pain.	**CARDIOMYOPATHY** (Refer to Illnesses section)

(HEARTBEAT IRREGULARITY, continued on next page)

SYMPTOMS & FACTORS	POSSIBLE PROBLEM
• Shortness of breath, especially with exertion or when lying flat in bed. • Fatigue, weakness or faintness. • Cough (usually with sputum). • Wheezing (sometimes). • Swelling of the abdomen, legs and ankles. • Rapid or irregular heartbeat.	**CONGESTIVE HEART FAILURE** (Refer to Illnesses section)
• Sudden lightheadedness. • General weakness, then falling. • Blurred vision (sometimes). • Nausea (sometimes). • Paleness and sweating. • Rapid heartbeat and rapid breathing. If heartbeat or breathing is not present, this may be cardiac arrest rather than fainting. **(THIS IS AN EMERGENCY; SEEK MEDICAL CARE IMMEDIATELY!)**	**FAINTING** (Refer to Illnesses section)
The following may indicate either: • Dry mouth. • Wrinkled skin. • Increased, decreased or absent urination. • Fatigue. • Puffy legs, hands, face or abdomen. • Lung congestion. • Weakness and confusion. • Heartbeat irregularities. • Lightheadedness.	**FLUID & ELECTROLYTE DISORDERS** (Refer to Illnesses section)
• No symptoms for less severe forms (sometimes). • Slow, irregular heartbeat. • Dizziness. • Sudden loss of consciousness. • Convulsions (sometimes).	**HEART BLOCK** (Refer to Illnesses section)
• Heart pounding or palpitations. The pulse at the wrist or neck will be 100 to 180 beats per minute, which is much faster than normal. • Faintness or feeling of impending death. • Chest pain. • Involuntary cough. • Breathlessness.	**HEARTBEAT, RAPID** (Refer to Illnesses section)
• Awareness of one's own heartbeat, including whether it skips; is always fast, slow or irregular; or suddenly changes rhythm. • Shortness of breath. • Sudden faintness or weakness. • No symptoms (frequently).	**HEART RHYTHM IRREGULARITY** (Refer to Illnesses section)
• No symptoms (sometimes). • Fatigue and weakness. • Dizziness or fainting. • Chest pain. • Shortness of breath. • Lung congestion. • Heart rhythm irregularities. • Heart murmurs (abnormal heart sounds heard by the doctor through a stethoscope). • Abnormal blood pressure (high or low).	**HEART VALVE DISEASE** (Refer to Illnesses section)
• Chest pain (angina pectoris). • Heart rhythm irregularity. • Fainting. • Shortness of breath.	**IDIOPATHIC HYPERTROPHIC SUBAORTIC STENOSIS (IHSS)** (Refer to Illnesses section)

(HEARTBEAT IRREGULARITY, continued on next page)

SYMPTOMS & FACTORS	POSSIBLE PROBLEM
Lupus symptoms frequently flare up and then subside. Episodes generally include fever and fatigue, plus any 4 of the following: • Rash, usually on the cheeks. • Ulcers in the mouth. • Red palms and hands. • Joint pain with redness, swelling and tenderness—but no deformity. • Swelling of the face and legs. • Shortness of breath. • Rapid or irregular heartbeat. • Chest pain. • Hair loss. • Swelling of the lymph glands. • Protein in the urine. • Increased sensitivity to the sun. • Mental changes, including psychosis.	**LUPUS ERYTHEMATOSUS, SYSTEMIC** (Refer to Illnesses section)
• Fatigue. • Shortness of breath. • Irregular heartbeat. • Fever. • Other symptoms caused by the underlying disorder. If myocarditis causes congestive heart failure, the following symptoms may also occur: • Swollen feet and ankles. • Distended neck veins. • Rapid heartbeat, even when at rest. • Breathing difficulty while resting or lying down.	**MYOCARDITIS** (Refer to Illnesses section)
• Pain in one area or throughout the abdomen. Pain usually starts suddenly and becomes increasingly severe. Pain may be crampy at first, and then steady. The patient often prefers to lie quietly on the back because movement or pressure on the abdomen increases pain. • Shoulder pain (sometimes). • Chills and fever (often high). • Dizziness and weakness. • Rapid heartbeat. • Low blood pressure.	**PERITONITIS** (Refer to Illnesses section) **(THIS IS AN EMERGENCY; SEEK MEDICAL CARE IMMEDIATELY!)**
For above-normal levels (hyperkalemia): • Weakness and paralysis. • Dangerously rapid, irregular heartbeat or slow heartbeat (sometimes). • Nausea and diarrhea. **For below-normal levels (hypokalemia):** • Weakness and paralysis. • Low blood pressure. • Life-threatening rapid, irregular heartbeat. This is more severe than with hyperkalemia. **(THIS IS AN EMERGENCY; SEEK MEDICAL CARE IMMEDIATELY!)**	**POTASSIUM IMBALANCE** (Refer to Illnesses section)
• Hyperactivity. • Feeling warm or hot all the time. • Tremors. • Sweating. • Itching skin. • Pounding, rapid, irregular heartbeat. • Weight loss, despite overeating. • Marked anxiety and restlessness. • Sleeplessness.	**THYROID, OVERACTIVE** (Refer to Illnesses section)

(HEARTBEAT IRREGULARITY, continued on next page)

SYMPTOMS & FACTORS	POSSIBLE PROBLEM
• Fatigue and weakness. • Protruding eyes (exophthalmos) and double vision (sometimes). • Diarrhea (sometimes). • Hair loss (sometimes). • Goiter (sometimes).	**THYROID, OVERACTIVE (continued)** (Refer to Illnesses section)

If you experience HEARTBEAT IRREGULARITY plus the following:

• Use of prescription or non-prescription drugs, such as thyroid medication; digitalis preparations; diuretics; diet pills; stimulants; caffeine; decongestants; cold remedies, including nasal sprays; illegal drugs, including marijuana, cocaine, psychedelics or amphetamines.	**WHAT TO DO:** Discontinue non-prescription drugs and notify doctor now regarding prescription drugs.
• Excessive smoking or consumption of caffeine-containing beverages such as coffee, cola, tea or cocoa.	**WHAT TO DO:** Decrease nicotine or caffeine use.
• Fever.	**WHAT TO DO:** See Fever (in Symptoms section).

IMPOTENCE, MALE SEXUAL

(Find your closest combination of symptoms in left-hand column; see possible problem in right-hand column. You may not experience all symptoms listed.)

SYMPTOMS & FACTORS	POSSIBLE PROBLEM
Early stages: • Low tolerance of anxiety. • Need for alcohol at the beginning of the day or at times of stress. • Insomnia; nightmares. • Habitual Monday-morning hangovers and frequent absences from work. • Preoccupation with obtaining alcohol and hiding drinking from family and friends. • Guilt or irritability when others suggest drinking is excessive. **Late stages:** • Frequent blackouts; memory loss. • Delirium tremens (tremors; hallucinations; confusion; sweating; rapid heartbeat). These occur most often with alcohol withdrawal. • Liver disease (jaundice; internal bleeding; bloating). • Neurological impairment (numbness and tingling in hands and feet; declining sexual interest and potency; confusion; coma). • Congestive heart failure (shortness of breath; swelling of feet).	**ALCOHOLISM** (Refer to Illnesses section)
• Feeling that something undesirable or harmful is about to happen. • Dry mouth; swallowing difficulty or hoarseness. • Rapid breathing and heartbeat. • Twitching or trembling. • Muscle tension; headaches. • Sweating. • Cold, clammy hands. • Nausea; diarrhea; weight loss. • Sleeplessness; nightmares. • Irritability. • Fatigue. • Memory problems. • Sexual impotence.	**ANXIETY** (Refer to Illnesses section)

(IMPOTENCE, MALE SEXUAL, continued on next page)

SYMPTOMS & FACTORS	POSSIBLE PROBLEM
Symptoms are often absent until atherosclerosis reaches advanced stages. Symptoms depend on what part of the body has a decreased blood flow and the extent of disease. Common symptoms include: • Muscle cramps if atherosclerosis involves vessels in the legs. • Angina pectoris or heart attack if it involves blood vessels to the heart. • Stroke or transient ischemic attack if it involves vessels to the neck and brain. • Headache.	**ATHEROSCLEROSIS** (Refer to Illnesses section)
Early stages: • Fatigue; weakness. • Poor appetite; nausea; weight loss. • Enlarged liver. • Red palms. **Late stages:** • Jaundice (yellow skin and eyes). • Dark yellow or brown urine. • Spider blood vessels of the skin (fine vessels which spread out from a central point). • Hair loss. • Breast enlargement in men. • Fluid accumulation in the abdomen and legs. • Enlarged spleen. • Diarrhea; stool may be black or bloody. • Bleeding and bruising. • Mental confusion; coma.	**CIRRHOSIS OF THE LIVER** (Refer to Illnesses section)
• Loss of interest in life; boredom. • Listlessness and fatigue. • Insomnia; excessive or disturbed sleeping. • Social isolation. • Appetite loss or overeating. • Loss of sex drive. • Constipation. • Difficulty making decisions; concentration difficulty. • Unexplained crying bouts. • Intense guilt feelings over minor or imaginary misdeeds. • Irritability. • Various pains, such as headache or chest pain, without evidence of disease. • Anxiety or agitation. • Thoughts of death or suicide.	**DEPRESSION** (Refer to Illnesses section)
• Fatigue; excess thirst. • Increased appetite *and* weight loss. • Frequent urination. • Itching around the genitals. • Increased susceptibility to infections, especially urinary tract infections and yeast infections of the skin, mouth or vagina. • Deterioration of vision (advanced stages). • Loss of energy and easy fatiguability.	**DIABETES MELLITUS, INSULIN-DEPENDENT** (Refer to Illnesses section)
• Overweight. • Fatigue and loss of energy. • Excess thirst. • Increased appetite. • Frequent urination. • Decreased resistance to infection, especially urinary tract infections and yeast infections of the skin, mouth or vagina.	**DIABETES MELLITUS, NON-INSULIN-DEPENDENT** (Refer to Illnesses section)

(IMPOTENCE, MALE SEXUAL, continued on next page)

SYMPTOMS & FACTORS	POSSIBLE PROBLEM
• Increased urinary urgency and frequency, especially at night. • Weak urinary stream. • Straining and dribbling on urination. • Feeling that the bladder cannot be emptied completely. • Urine of abnormal color. • Impotence (sometimes). • Burning on urination.	**PROSTATE, ENLARGED** (Refer to Illnesses section)
• Impotence; infertility. • Low blood sugar and weakness; low blood pressure. • Cold intolerance. • Mental changes, including psychosis. • Extreme lethargy. • Persistent headaches.	**PITUITARY GLAND, UNDERACTIVE** (Refer to Illnesses section)
It is unlikely one person will have all the following symptoms, but most will have several: • Decreased tolerance of cold. • Decreased sweating. • Decreased appetite. • Constipation. • Chest pain. • Coarse or slow-growing hair. • Slow, rapid or irregular heartbeat. • Weight gain or extreme thinness. • Placidity or nervousness. • Sleepiness or insomnia. • Mental impairment, including depression, psychosis or poor memory. • Fluid retention, especially around the eyes. • Dull facial expression and droopy eyelids. • Coarse skin. • Decreased tolerance of medication. • Decreased sex drive and infertility. • Anemia. • Numbness and tingling of the hands and feet. • Deepened or hoarse voice.	**THYROID, UNDERACTIVE** (Refer to Illnesses section)
Two or more of the following: • Poor appetite. • Poor growth. • Sensations of unpleasant tastes and odors and decreased senses of taste and smell. • Decreased sex drive. • Darkening of skin all over the body. • Sparse hair growth. • Deformed nails.	**ZINC DEFICIENCY** (Refer to Illnesses section)

If you experience MALE SEXUAL IMPOTENCE plus the following:

• Use of prescription or non-prescription drugs, such as antihypertensives; amphetamines; narcotics; cocaine; antidepressants; antihistamines; antiulcer medicines; diuretics; hormones; beta-adrenergic blockers; tranquilizers; reserpine; marijuana; digitalis; skeletal muscle relaxants; sedatives; hypnotics; phenothiazines.	**WHAT TO DO:** Discontinue non-prescription drugs and call doctor now regarding prescription drugs.
• Acute illness with fever.	**WHAT TO DO:** Nothing usually need be done. Sexual function should return when illness subsides.

ITCHING

(Find your closest combination of symptoms in left-hand column; see possible problem in right-hand column. You may not experience all symptoms listed.)

SYMPTOMS & FACTORS	POSSIBLE PROBLEM
• Sharp pain with passage of a hard or bulky stool. • Streaks of blood on the toilet paper or underwear. • Itching around the rectum.	**ANAL FISSURE** (Refer to Illnesses section)
• Itching rash in areas where heat and moisture are retained, such as skin creases of elbows, knees, neck, face, hands, feet, groin, genitals and around the anus. • Dry, thickened skin in affected areas. • Uncontrolled scratching (frequently unconscious). • Chronic fatigue from loss of sleep due to severe itching.	**DERMATITIS, ALLERGIC** (Refer to Illnesses section)
• Itching (sometimes). • Slight redness. • Cracks and fissures in the skin. • Bright red, weeping areas (severe cases).	**DERMATITIS, CONTACT** (Refer to Illnesses section)
• Rash, itching or hives. • Jaundice (yellow skin and eyes). • Flushed skin. • Facial swelling. • Many other possible symptoms.	**DRUG HYPERSENSITIVITY** (Refer to Illnesses section)
• Rectal bleeding. Bright red blood may appear as streaks on toilet paper adhering to fecal residue, or it may be a slow trickle for a short while following bowel movements. • Pain, itching or mucus discharge after bowel movements. • A lump that can be felt in the anus. • A sensation that the rectum has not emptied completely after a bowel movement (large hemorrhoids only).	**HEMORRHOIDS** (Refer to Illnesses section)
Few or no symptoms until 60% to 75% of kidney filtration fails. Then, 1 or more of the following: • Listlessness, confusion and drowsiness. • High blood pressure. • Shortness of breath. • Bad breath. • Inflamed, bleeding gums and mouth ulcers. • Abdominal pain. • Itching skin. • Numbness, tingling and burning in the legs and feet. • Muscle cramps. • Decreased sex drive. • Anemia, with paleness and fatigue. • Unusual bleeding. • Muscle and bone pain. Bones break easily.	**KIDNEY FAILURE, CHRONIC** (Refer to Illnesses section)
Early stages: • Little or no urine output. **Later stages:** • Nausea, vomiting, diarrhea and appetite loss. • Mental changes, including irritability, drowsiness, stupor or coma. • Convulsions. • Severe itching. • High or low blood pressure. • Unexplained bruising, bleeding spots under the skin or spontaneous bleeding. • Pale skin and weak pulse.	**KIDNEY FAILURE, ACUTE** (Refer to Illnesses section) (THIS IS AN EMERGENCY; SEEK MEDICAL CARE IMMEDIATELY!)

(ITCHING, continued on next page)

SYMPTOMS & FACTORS	POSSIBLE PROBLEM
• Itching and scratching, sometimes intense and usually in hair-covered areas. • Eggs ("nits") on hair shafts. • Scalp inflammation and matted hair. • Enlarged lymph glands at the back of the scalp or in the groin (sometimes). • Red bite marks and hives.	**LICE** (Refer to Illnesses section)
• Skin irritation and painful itching around the anus, especially during sleep. • Restless sleep. • Vaginal discharge, itching and discomfort if pinworms migrate into the vaginal opening. • Poor appetite and stomach pain (rare). • Paleness (sometimes).	**PINWORMS** (Refer to Illnesses section)
Some patients have no symptoms. Others have any of the following: • Fatigue; headache; drowsiness; dizziness. • Itching or flushed skin. • Enlarged spleen. • Unexplained bleeding.	**POLYCYTHEMIA** (Refer to Illnesses section)
Lesions that itch (sometimes) and have the following characteristics: • Lesions on the scalp cause patchy hair loss and scaling scalp. • Lesions on body skin are red, circular, flat, scaling and have well-defined borders. • Lesions on the bearded area of the face cause an itchy, scaling rash under the beard. • Lesions on the feet—See Athlete's Foot in the Illnesses section. • Lesions of the nails—See Paronychia in the Illnesses section.	**RINGWORM** (Refer to Illnesses section)
• Hyperactivity. • Feeling warm or hot all the time. • Tremors. • Sweating. • Itching skin. • Pounding, rapid, irregular heartbeat. • Weight loss, despite overeating. • Marked anxiety and restlessness. • Sleeplessness. • Fatigue and weakness. • Protruding eyes (exophthalmos) and double vision (sometimes). • Diarrhea (sometimes). • Hair loss (sometimes). • Goiter (sometimes).	**THYROID, OVERACTIVE** (Refer to Illnesses section)
Severity of the following symptoms varies between women and from time to time in the same woman: • Vaginal discharge that has an unpleasant odor. • Genital itching. • Vaginal discomfort. • Change in vaginal color from pale pink to red. • Discomfort during sexual intercourse.	**VAGINITIS, BACTERIAL OR NON-SPECIFIC** (Refer to Illnesses section)
Severity of the following symptoms varies greatly between women and from time to time in the same woman. • Bad-smelling vaginal discharge. The discharge is usually thin, whitish and sometimes tinged with blood. • Genital pain and itching. • Discomfort during sexual intercourse. • Change in vaginal color from pale pink to red.	**VAGINITIS, POST-MENOPAUSAL** (Refer to Illnesses section)

(ITCHING, continued on next page)

SYMPTOMS & FACTORS	POSSIBLE PROBLEM
• Foul-smelling, frothy vaginal discharge. • Vaginal itching and pain. • Redness of the vaginal lips (labia) and vagina. • Painful urination if urine touches inflamed tissue. The severity of discomfort varies greatly from woman to woman and from time to time in the same woman. Infected men may have no symptoms.	**VAGINITIS, TRICHOMONAL** (Refer to Illnesses section)

If you experience ITCHING plus the following:

• Use of prescription or non-prescription drugs.	**WHAT TO DO:** Discontinue non-prescription drugs and call doctor now regarding prescription drugs.
• New clothing or new soap product used.	**WHAT TO DO:** Wash new clothing prior to wearing and discontinue use of soap product.

KNEE PAIN

(Find your closest combination of symptoms in left-hand column; see possible problem in right-hand column. You may not experience all symptoms listed.)

SYMPTOMS & FACTORS	POSSIBLE PROBLEM
• Chills and fever (sometimes high). • Redness, swelling, tenderness, heat and pain (often throbbing) in the affected joint. Pain sometimes spreads to other joints. It worsens with movement. • Pain in the buttocks, thighs, groin or end of bone near a joint (sometimes).	**ARTHRITIS, INFECTIOUS** (Refer to Illnesses section)
Slow or sudden onset of: • Redness, aching, pain, warmth and tenderness in any or all active joints in the hands, wrists, elbows, shoulders, knees, feet, ankles, jaw and spine. • Morning stiffness; muscular atrophy. • Low-grade fever. • Nodules under the skin (sometimes). • Pale skin. • Appetite loss.	**ARTHRITIS, RHEUMATOID** (Refer to Illnesses section)
• Pain, tenderness and limited movement in the affected area. • When shoulder involved, radiation of pain into the neck; arm; fingertips. • Severe pain with movement of the arm. • Fever (sometimes).	**BURSITIS** (Refer to Illnesses section)
• Sudden onset of severe pain in the inflamed joint, usually at the base of the big toe or larger joints. • Involved joints are red, hot, swollen and very tender. Skin over the joint is red and shiny. • Fever (sometimes).	**GOUT** (Refer to Illnesses section)
• Sudden joint pain, swelling or deformity after an injury. • Limited or absent movement around a joint.	**JOINT DISLOCATION OR SUBLUXATION** (Refer to Illnesses section)

(KNEE PAIN, continued on next page)

(KNEE PAIN, continued from previous page)

SYMPTOMS & FACTORS	POSSIBLE PROBLEM
• Joint stiffness and pain, including backache. Weather changes, especially cold, damp weather, may increase aching. • Limited movement and loss of dexterity in affected joints. • No redness, heat or fever in affected joints (usually). • Swelling of affected joints, especially finger joints (sometimes). • Cracking or grating sounds with joint movement (sometimes).	**OSTEOARTHRITIS** (Refer to Illnesses section)
• Fever. Sometimes this is the only symptom. • Pain, swelling, redness, warmth and tenderness in the area over the infected bone, especially when moving a nearby joint. Nearby joints—especially the knee—may also be red, warm and swollen. • Pus drainage through a skin abscess, without fever or severe pain (chronic osteomyelitis only).	**OSTEOMYELITIS** (Refer to Illnesses section)
• Pain or tenderness in the area of injury (severity varies with the extent of injury). • Swelling of the affected joint. • Redness or bruising in the area of injury, either immediately or several hours after injury. • Loss of normal mobility in the injured joint.	**SPRAINS & STRAINS** (Refer to Illnesses section)

If you experience KNEE PAIN plus the following:

• Recent injury to leg.	**WHAT TO DO:** Call doctor now.
• Increased physical activity, such as exercise, biking or walking.	**WHAT TO DO:** Use massage on knee, and rest with the leg elevated.

LEG PAIN

(Find your closest combination of symptoms in left-hand column; see possible problem in right-hand column. You may not experience all symptoms listed.)

SYMPTOMS & FACTORS	POSSIBLE PROBLEM
Symptoms are often absent until atherosclerosis reaches advanced stages. Symptoms depend on what part of the body has a decreased blood flow and the extent of disease. Common symptoms include: • Muscle cramps if atherosclerosis involves vessels in the legs. • Angina pectoris or heart attack if it involves blood vessels to the heart. • Stroke or transient ischemic attack if it involves vessels to the neck and brain. • Headache.	**ATHEROSCLEROSIS** (Refer to Illnesses section)
• Intermittent pain in the instep or the leg when exercising. The pain improves with rest. • Pain, blueness, heat and tingling in the legs when exposed to cold. • Painful ulcers on the toes and fingertips (sometimes).	**BUERGER'S DISEASE** (Refer to Illnesses section)
Lower back: • Severe pain in the low back or back of one leg, buttock or foot (sciatica). Pain usually affects one side and worsens with movement, coughing, sneezing, lifting or straining. • Weakness, numbness or muscular wasting of the affected leg. **Neck:** • Pain in the neck or shoulder or down one arm. Pain worsens with movement. • Weakness, numbness or muscular wasting of the affected arm.	**DISK, RUPTURED** (Refer to Illnesses section)

(LEG PAIN, continued on next page)

SYMPTOMS & FACTORS	POSSIBLE PROBLEM
• Pain in the affected bone. The pain is severe, boring and deep. If the bone collapses, pain spreads to other parts of the body. • Weight loss. • Symptoms of anemia, such as weakness, paleness, tiredness and breathlessness.	**MULTIPLE MYELOMA** (Refer to Illnesses section)
• Pain or tenderness in the injury area. • Gradual stiffening or contraction of the injured muscle. • Swelling, redness or bruising at the injury site.	**MUSCLE, PULLED OR TORN** (Refer to Illnesses section)
• Fever. Sometimes this is the only symptom. • Pain, swelling, redness, warmth and tenderness in the area over the infected bone, especially when moving a nearby joint. Nearby joints—especially the knee—may also be red, warm and swollen. • Pus drainage through a skin abscess, without fever or severe pain (chronic osteomyelitis only).	**OSTEOMYELITIS** (Refer to Illnesses section)
• Hardness of a superficial vein (feels like a cord). • Redness, tenderness, swelling and pain in the affected area. • Fever (sometimes).	**THROMBOPHLEBITIS, SUPERFICIAL** (Refer to Illnesses section)
• Swelling and pain in the area drained by the vein, usually the ankle, calf or thigh. Swelling in the leg includes everything below the clot, extending to the toes. • Tenderness and redness of the affected parts. • Soreness or pain when walking. The soreness does not disappear with rest. • Pain when raising the leg and flexing the foot (sometimes). • Fever (sometimes). • Increased heartbeat (sometimes).	**THROMBOSIS, DEEP-VEIN** (Refer to Illnesses section)
The following depend on where the embolus lodges: • Brain—Temporary blindness, difficulty speaking, partial paralysis, hearing loss, headache and dizziness. • Extremities—Pain in the arm or calf after exercise (subsides with rest); weakness, numbness, burning and tingling sensations; weak or absent pulse beyond the blocked blood flow. These symptoms subside with rest. • Intestine—Abdominal pain; nausea; vomiting; shock.	**THROMBOSIS & EMBOLUS, ARTERIAL** (Refer to Illnesses section) **(THIS IS AN EMERGENCY; SEEK MEDICAL CARE IMMEDIATELY!)**
• Enlarged, disfiguring, snakelike, bluish veins that are visible under the skin upon standing. They appear most often in the back of the calf or on the inside of the leg from ankle to groin. • Vague discomfort and aching in the legs, especially after standing. • Fatigue. • Swelling of feet and legs. • Persistent itching of skin.	**VARICOSE VEINS** (Refer to Illnesses section)

If you experience LEG PAIN plus the following:

• Recent injury to leg.	**WHAT TO DO:** Call doctor now.
• Increased physical activity, such as exercise, biking or walking.	**WHAT TO DO:** Use massage on painful area, and rest with the leg elevated.

MEMORY PROBLEMS

(Find your closest combination of symptoms in left-hand column; see possible problem in right-hand column. You may not experience all symptoms listed.)

SYMPTOMS & FACTORS | **POSSIBLE PROBLEM**

Early stages:
- Low tolerance of anxiety.
- Need for alcohol at the beginning of the day or at times of stress.
- Insomnia; nightmares.
- Habitual Monday-morning hangovers and frequent absences from work.
- Preoccupation with obtaining alcohol and hiding drinking from family and friends.
- Guilt or irritability when others suggest drinking is excessive.

Later stages:
- Frequent blackouts; memory loss.
- Delirium tremens (tremors; hallucinations; confusion; sweating; rapid heartbeat). These occur most often with alcohol withdrawal.
- Liver disease (jaundice; internal bleeding; bloating).
- Neurological impairment (numbness and tingling in hands and feet; declining sexual interest and potency; confusion; coma).
- Congestive heart failure (shortness of breath; swelling of feet).

ALCOHOLISM
(Refer to Illnesses section)

Early stages:
- Forgetfulness of recent events.
- Increasing difficulty performing intellectual tasks, such as accustomed work, balancing a checkbook or maintaining a household.
- Personality changes, including narrow range of interest, rigidity in views or beliefs, distrust, restlessness, poor impulse control and poor judgment.

Later stages:
- Difficulty doing simple tasks, such as choosing clothing and problem solving.
- Failure to recognize familiar persons.
- Disinterest in personal hygiene or appearance.
- Difficulty feeding self.
- Belligerence and denial that anything is wrong.
- Loss of usual sexual inhibitions.

Advanced stages:
- Complete loss of memory, speech and muscle function (including bladder and bowel control) necessitating total care and supervision.
- Extreme belligerence and hostility.
- Sleeplessness.

ALZHEIMER'S DISEASE
(Refer to Illnesses section)

- Feeling that something undesirable or harmful is about to happen.
- Dry mouth; difficulty swallowing or hoarseness.
- Rapid breathing and heartbeat.
- Twitching or trembling.
- Muscle tension; headaches.
- Sweating.
- Cold, clammy hands.
- Nausea; diarrhea; weight loss.
- Sleeplessness; nightmares.
- Irritability.
- Fatigue.
- Memory problems.
- Sexual impotence.

ANXIETY
(Refer to Illnesses section)

(MEMORY PROBLEMS, continued on next page)

91

SYMPTOMS & FACTORS	POSSIBLE PROBLEM
• Forgetfulness, especially of recent events. • Unpredictable, sometimes violent, behavior. • Confusion. • Loss of interest in normal activities. • Disorientation, especially at night. • Poor personal hygiene and appearance. • Depression. • Poor judgment. • Staggering gait. • Incoherent speech.	**DEMENTIA** (Refer to Illnesses section)
• Loss of interest in life; boredom. • Listlessness and fatigue. • Insomnia; excessive or disturbed sleeping. • Social isolation. • Appetite loss or overeating. • Loss of sex drive. • Constipation. • Difficulty making decisions and concentrating. • Unexplained crying bouts. • Intense guilt feelings over minor or imaginary misdeeds. • Irritability. • Various pains, such as headache or chest pain, without evidence of disease. • Anxiety or agitation. • Thoughts of death or suicide.	**DEPRESSION** (Refer to Illnesses section)
Symptoms depend on the extent of injury. The presence or absence of swelling at the injury site is not related to the seriousness of injury. Signs and symptoms include any or all of the following: • Drowsiness or confusion. • Vomiting and nausea. • Blurred vision. • Pupils of different sizes. • Loss of consciousness—either temporarily or for long periods. **(THIS IS AN EMERGENCY; SEEK MEDICAL CARE IMMEDIATELY!)** • Amnesia or memory lapses. • Irritability. • Headache. • Bleeding of the scalp if the skin is broken.	**HEAD INJURY** (Refer to Illnesses section)
One or several of the following deficiencies may exist at the same time: **B-1 deficiency (beriberi)** • Tingling or loss of sensation in the legs. • Weakness. • Congestive heart failure. • Mental changes, including poor memory or psychosis. • Lack of urinary control. • Abdominal pain. **B-2 deficiency** • Cracked lips. • Pallor. • Sore tongue. **Niacin deficiency (pellagra)** • Fatigue and weakness. • Poor appetite. • Inflamed skin that may blister, weep and split. • Sore, burning mouth and tongue. • Indigestion.	**VITAMIN B DEFICIENCY** (Refer to Illnesses section)

(MEMORY PROBLEMS, continued on next page)

(MEMORY PROBLEMS, continued from previous page)

SYMPTOMS & FACTORS	POSSIBLE PROBLEM
• Nausea. • Vomiting and diarrhea. • Mental changes, including confusion and psychosis.	**VITAMIN B DEFICIENCY (continued)** (Refer to Illnesses section)

B-6 deficiency
- Dermatitis.
- Sore mouth and tongue.
- Abdominal pain, vomiting and diarrhea.
- Convulsions.

B-12 deficiency
- See Pernicious Anemia in Illnesses section.

If you experience MEMORY PROBLEMS plus the following:

• Inability to remember a period of time.	**WHAT TO DO:** Call doctor soon.
• Use of prescription or non-prescription drugs.	**WHAT TO DO:** Discontinue non-prescription drugs and call doctor now regarding prescription drugs.
• Gradual decline over past 10 years in ability to remember everyday things.	**WHAT TO DO:** Call doctor soon. Also write lists to help your memory. This is not necessarily the beginning of serious mental decline.
• Inability to remember a period of time and you have had any of the following: epileptic seizure; diabetic coma; surgery; serious, feverish illness such as meningitis or pneumonia.	**WHAT TO DO:** Nothing. This may be a common occurrence following these situations.

MOUTH, SORE

(Find your closest combination of symptoms in left-hand column; see possible problem in right-hand column. You may not experience all symptoms listed.)

SYMPTOMS & FACTORS	POSSIBLE PROBLEM
• Paleness. • Weakness, tiredness, faintness and breathlessness. • Frequent infections. • Spontaneous bleeding from the nose, mouth, rectum, vagina, gums and other sites. • Red dots of bleeding under the skin. • Unexplained bruising. • Ulcers in the mouth, throat and rectum.	**ANEMIA, APLASTIC** (Refer to Illnesses section)
• Fatigue and weakness. • Red, sore, glazed tongue. • Paleness. • Shortness of breath. • Nausea, vomiting and diarrhea (rare). • Abdominal distention.	**ANEMIA, FOLIC ACID-DEFICIENCY** (Refer to Illnesses section)

(MOUTH, SORE, continued on next page)

SYMPTOMS & FACTORS	POSSIBLE PROBLEM
Mouth ulcers with the following characteristics: • Ulcers are small, very painful, shallow, covered by a gray membrane, and surrounded by an intense red halo. • Ulcers appear on lips, gums, inner cheeks, tongue, palate and throat; 2 or 3 ulcers usually appear during an attack, but 10 to 15 ulcers are not uncommon. • Ulcers may be so painful during first 2 or 3 days that they interfere with eating or speaking. • Ulcers are preceded by tingling or burning for 24 hours (sometimes).	**CANKER SORES** (Refer to Illnesses section)
• Breakout may be preceded by tingling in the lips. • Eruptions of very small, painful blisters—usually around the mouth, but sometimes on the genitals. The blisters are grouped together, and each is surrounded by a red ring. They fill with fluid, then dry up and disappear within a week. • If the eye is infected, eye pain and redness; feeling that something is in the eye; sensitivity to light; tearing.	**COLD SORES** (Refer to Illnesses section)
• Dry mouth and lips. • Decreased or absent urination. • Sunken eyes. • Dry, wrinkled skin with poor resilience. • Confusion; coma. (THIS IS AN EMERGENCY; SEEK MEDICAL CARE IMMEDIATELY!) • Low blood pressure. • Severe thirst. • Increase in heart rate and breathing. • Lightheadedness.	**DEHYDRATION** (Refer to Illnesses section)
• Fever. • Tiredness. • Anemia. • Increasing paleness. • General ill feeling. • Easy bruising and spontaneous bleeding (nosebleeds, bleeding from the gums or gastrointestinal tract). • Enlarged spleen and abdominal pain. • Susceptibility to infection, especially pneumonia. • Mouth infections with ulcers and sores. • Headache and lethargy if meninges (brain membranes) are affected. (THIS IS AN EMERGENCY; SEEK MEDICAL CARE IMMEDIATELY!)	**LEUKEMIA, ACUTE** (Refer to Illnesses section)
In early stages, the following appear gradually: • Fatigue and general weakness. • Mild to moderate anemia. • Firm, enlarged lymph nodes. • Unexplained weight loss. • Enlarged liver and spleen. • Susceptibility to infection. • Skin nodules (sometimes). • Low-grade fever and sweating at night. **In late stages:** • Inability to resist bacterial, viral or fungal infections. • Incapacitating weakness.	**LEUKEMIA, CHRONIC LYMPHOCYTIC** (Refer to Illnesses section)
• Sensitivity to hot and spicy food. • A small white patch in the mouth. The patch feels firm, rough and stiff. • No symptoms in the early stages.	**LEUKOPLAKIA** (Refer to Illnesses section)

(MOUTH, SORE, continued on next page)

SYMPTOMS & FACTORS	POSSIBLE PROBLEM
Lupus symptoms frequently flare up and then subside. Episodes generally include fever and fatigue, plus any 4 of the following: • Rash, usually on the cheeks. • Ulcers in the mouth. • Red palms and hands. • Joint pain with redness, swelling and tenderness—but no deformity. • Swelling of the face and legs. • Shortness of breath. • Rapid or irregular heartbeat. • Chest pain. • Hair loss. • Swelling of the lymph glands. • Protein in the urine. • Increased sensitivity to the sun. • Mental changes, including psychosis.	**LUPUS ERYTHEMATOSUS, SYSTEMIC** (Refer to Illnesses section)
Patches appear in the mouth with the following characteristics: • Patches are white to creamy yellow and slightly raised. They are similar to milk curds, but they don't wipe off. • Patches are not painful unless they are rubbed off. Then they leave small, painful ulcers. • The mouth is dry.	**THRUSH** (Refer to Illnesses section)
• Painful gums. • Gums that bleed when pressed. • Excess salivation. • Bad breath. • Ulcers covered with gray membrane on the gums. • Difficulty swallowing and speaking.	**TRENCH MOUTH** (Refer to Illnesses section)
One or several of the following deficiencies may exist at the same time: **B-1 deficiency (beriberi)** • Tingling or loss of sensation in the legs. • Weakness. • Congestive heart failure. • Mental changes, including poor memory or psychosis. • Lack of urinary control. • Abdominal pain. **B-2 deficiency** • Cracked lips. • Pallor. • Sore tongue. **Niacin deficiency (pellagra)** • Fatigue and weakness. • Poor appetite. • Inflamed skin that may blister, weep and split. • Sore, burning mouth and tongue. • Indigestion. • Nausea. • Vomiting and diarrhea. • Mental changes, including confusion and psychosis. **B-6 deficiency** • Dermatitis. • Sore mouth and tongue. • Abdominal pain, vomiting and diarrhea. • Convulsions. **B-12 deficiency** • See Pernicious Anemia in Illnesses section.	**VITAMIN B DEFICIENCY** (Refer to Illnesses section)

(MOUTH, SORE, continued on next page)

SYMPTOMS & FACTORS	POSSIBLE PROBLEM

If you experience SORE MOUTH plus the following:

- Use of prescription or non-prescription drugs.

WHAT TO DO:
Discontinue non-prescription drugs and call doctor now regarding prescription drugs.

MUSCLE ACHE OR CRAMP

(Find your closest combination of symptoms in left-hand column; see possible problem in right-hand column. You may not experience all symptoms listed.)

SYMPTOMS & FACTORS	POSSIBLE PROBLEM

Symptoms are often absent until atherosclerosis reaches advanced stages. Symptoms depend on what part of the body has a decreased blood flow and the extent of disease. Common symptoms include:
- Muscle cramps if atherosclerosis involves vessels in the legs.
- Angina pectoris or heart attack if it involves blood vessels to the heart.
- Stroke or transient ischemic attack if it involves vessels to the neck and brain.
- Headache.

ATHEROSCLEROSIS
(Refer to Illnesses section)

- Intermittent pain in the instep or the leg when exercising. The pain improves with rest.
- Pain, blueness, heat and tingling in the legs when exposed to cold.
- Painful ulcers on the toes and fingertips (sometimes).

BUERGER'S DISEASE
(Refer to Illnesses section)

- Muscle spasms, twitching or cramps.
- Numbness and tingling in the arms, legs, hands and feet.
- Seizures. (THIS IS AN EMERGENCY; SEEK MEDICAL CARE IMMEDIATELY!)
- Irregular heartbeat.
- High blood pressure.
- Lack of adequate sunshine.

CALCIUM, TOO LITTLE
(Refer to Illnesses section)

- Stiffness and weakness.
- Sudden, painful muscle spasms ("charley horse") that worsen with activity.
- Nodules or localized areas that are tender to the touch (trigger points).
- Painful muscle areas.
- Fatigue.
- Difficulty remaining asleep.

FIBROSITIS
(Refer to Illnesses section)

Heat stroke:
- Sudden dizziness, weakness, faintness and headache.
- Skin that is hot and dry without sweating.
- High body temperature.
- Rapid heartbeat.
- Muscle cramps.

Heat exhaustion:
- Skin that is cool and moist.
- Pale or gray skin color.
- Slow pulse.
- Confusion.
- Muscle cramps.
- Low or normal body temperature.
- Dark yellow or orange urine.

HEAT STROKE OR HEAT EXHAUSTION
(Refer to Illnesses section)
(THIS IS AN EMERGENCY; SEEK MEDICAL CARE IMMEDIATELY!)

(MUSCLE ACHE OR CRAMP, continued on next page)

SYMPTOMS & FACTORS	POSSIBLE PROBLEM
First stage: • A red papule (small, raised bump) on the skin of the thighs, buttocks or armpits that grows as large as 5cm. **Later stages:** Any or some of the following: • Muscle aches and pains. • Fatigue and lethargy. • Chills and fever. • Stiff neck with headache. • Backache. • Nausea and vomiting. • Sore throat. • Enlargement of the spleen and lymph glands. • Migrating joint pain, eventually accompanied by redness and warmth. • Enlarged heart and heart rhythm disturbances.	**LYME DISEASE** (Refer to Illnesses section)
• Confusion. • Restlessness and anxiety. • Weakness. • Muscle cramps (usually in the legs). • Changes in pulse rate and blood pressure. • Tissue swelling (edema). • Stupor or coma (if severe imbalance). **(THIS IS AN EMERGENCY; SEEK MEDICAL CARE IMMEDIATELY!)** Sodium imbalance may be part of a disease with other symptoms that predominate, such as fever, vomiting, diarrhea or excessive sweating.	**SODIUM, TOO MUCH OR TOO LITTLE IN BLOOD** (Refer to Illnesses section)
• Muscle pain, irritability and frequent, severe spasms. • Severe difficulty swallowing. • Fever. • Difficulty using chest muscles to breathe. • Stiffness in abdominal and back muscles.	**TETANUS** (Refer to Illnesses section) **(THIS IS AN EMERGENCY; SEEK MEDICAL CARE IMMEDIATELY!)**
The following depend on where the embolus lodges: • Brain—Temporary blindness; difficulty speaking; partial paralysis; hearing loss; headache; dizziness. • Extremities—Pain in the arm or calf after exercise (subsides with rest); weakness, numbness, burning and tingling sensations; weak or absent pulse beyond the blocked blood flow. These symptoms subside with rest. • Intestine—Abdominal pain; nausea; vomiting; and shock.	**THROMBOSIS & EMBOLUS, ARTERIAL** (Refer to Illnesses section) **(THIS IS AN EMERGENCY; SEEK MEDICAL CARE IMMEDIATELY!)**

If you experience MUSCLE ACHE OR CRAMP plus the following:

• Use of prescription or non-prescription drugs.	**WHAT TO DO:** Discontinue non-prescription drug and call doctor now regarding prescription drugs.
• Sitting in awkward position; exercising; relaxed or resting in bed.	**WHAT TO DO:** Massage muscle and use heat to relieve pain. These symptoms usually do not indicate an underlying disorder.

NECK PAIN

(Find your closest combination of symptoms in left-hand column; see possible problem in right-hand column. You may not experience all symptoms listed.)

SYMPTOMS & FACTORS	POSSIBLE PROBLEM
Any of the following: • Pain in the neck radiating to the shoulder blades, top of the shoulders, upper arms, hands or back of the head. • Crunching sounds with movement of the neck or shoulder muscles. • Numbness and tingling in the arms, hands and fingers; some loss of feeling in the hands; and impairment of reflexes. • Muscle weakness and deterioration; diminished reflexes. • Neck stiffness. • Headache. • Dizziness; unsteady gait. • Double vision. • With advanced disease, loss of bladder control and leg weakness.	**ARTHRITIS, NECK** (Refer to Illnesses section)
Mild cases: • No symptoms (sometimes). • Fever. • General ill feeling. **Severe cases:** • Vomiting. • Headache. • Stiff neck. • Pupils of different sizes. • Unconsciousness. • Personality changes. • Seizures. • Occasional weakness or paralysis of an arm or leg. • Double vision. • Speech impairment. • Hearing loss. • Drowsiness that progresses to coma. • Sensitivity to light.	**BRAIN INFECTION, VIRAL** (Refer to Illnesses section)
Lower back: • Severe pain in the low back or back of one leg, buttock or foot (sciatica). Pain usually affects one side and worsens with movement, coughing, sneezing, lifting or straining. • Weakness, numbness or muscular wasting of the affected leg. **Neck:** • Pain in the neck or shoulder or down one arm. Pain worsens with movement. • Weakness, numbness or muscular wasting of the affected arm.	**DISK, RUPTURED** (Refer to Illnesses section)
• Dull or sharp pain in the front of the chest radiating to the neck and shoulder. The pain worsens with movement and eases when sitting up or leaning forward. • Rapid breathing. • Cough. • Fever and chills. • Weakness. • Anxiety. • The most important signs are apparent only with medical examination: friction rub heard through a stethoscope; elevated white blood cell count; rapid sedimentation rate (see Glossary); abnormal ECG (see Glossary).	**PERICARDITIS, ACUTE** (Refer to Illnesses section)

(NECK PAIN, continued on next page)

98

(NECK PAIN, continued from previous page)

SYMPTOMS & FACTORS	POSSIBLE PROBLEM
• Acute, severe headache, often followed by unconsciousness. • Drowsiness, dizziness, convulsions or coma. • Eye pain with extreme sensitivity to light. • Vomiting. • Rapid heartbeat and breathing. • Stiff neck with pain on movement. • Fever. • Numbness, weakness or inability to move an arm or leg.	**SUBARACHNOID HEMORRHAGE** (Refer to Illnesses section) **(THIS IS AN EMERGENCY; SEEK MEDICAL CARE IMMEDIATELY!)**
• Pain, numbness and tingling in the neck, shoulders, arms and hands. • Weakness in the arms and hands. • Poor blood circulation characterized by coldness, swelling and blueness in the hands and fingers (rare). • No pulse in the wrist when raising the arm and turning the head toward the opposite shoulder.	**THORACIC OUTLET OBSTRUCTION SYNDROME** (Refer to Illnesses section)
The following may be permanent or intermittent: • Head that turns sideways and bends down. • Neck muscle spasm that is sometimes painful.	**TORTICOLLIS** (Refer to Illnesses section)
• Pain or stiffness in the front and back of the neck—either immediately following or up to 24 hours after injury. • Dizziness. • Headache. • Nausea and vomiting (sometimes).	**WHIPLASH** (Refer to Illnesses section)

If you experience NECK PAIN plus the following:

• Recent strong jolt. • Difficulty controlling arms or legs. • Loss of bowel or bladder control.	**WHAT TO DO:** These symptoms may indicate a damaged spinal cord. **THIS IS AN EMERGENCY; SEEK MEDICAL CARE IMMEDIATELY!**

NIGHTMARES

(Find your closest combination of symptoms in left-hand column; see possible problem in right-hand column. You may not experience all symptoms listed.)

SYMPTOMS & FACTORS	POSSIBLE PROBLEM
Early stages: • Low tolerance of anxiety. • Need for alcohol at the beginning of the day or at times of stress. • Insomnia; nightmares. • Habitual Monday-morning hangovers and frequent absences from work. • Preoccupation with obtaining alcohol and hiding drinking from family and friends. • Guilt or irritability when others suggest drinking is excessive. **Late stages:** • Frequent blackouts; memory loss. • Delirium tremens (tremors; hallucinations; confusion; sweating; rapid heartbeat). These occur most often with alcohol withdrawal. • Liver disease (jaundice; internal bleeding; bloating). • Neurological impairment (numbness and tingling in hands and feet; declining sexual interest and potency; confusion; coma). • Congestive heart failure (shortness of breath; swelling of feet).	**ALCOHOLISM** (Refer to Illnesses section)

(NIGHTMARES, continued on next page)

SYMPTOMS & FACTORS	POSSIBLE PROBLEM
• Feeling that something undesirable or harmful is about to happen. • Dry mouth; difficulty swallowing or hoarseness. • Rapid breathing and heartbeat. • Twitching or trembling. • Muscle tension; headaches. • Sweating. • Cold, clammy hands. • Nausea; diarrhea; weight loss. • Sleeplessness; nightmares. • Irritability. • Fatigue. • Memory problems. • Sexual impotence.	**ANXIETY** (Refer to Illnesses section)

If you experience NIGHTMARES plus the following:

• Use of prescription or non-prescription drugs.	**WHAT TO DO:** Discontinue non-prescription drugs and call doctor now regarding prescription drugs.
• Physical illness with fever.	**WHAT TO DO:** Treatment for the underlying illness will help the nightmares.
• Recent withdrawal of drug, such as sleeping pills.	**WHAT TO DO:** Nothing. Dreams should return to normal in several days.
• No other symptoms.	**WHAT TO DO:** Nothing. Usually of no significance.

NOSE, STUFFY OR RUNNY

(Find your closest combination of symptoms in left-hand column; see possible problem in right-hand column. You may not experience all symptoms listed.)

SYMPTOMS & FACTORS	POSSIBLE PROBLEM
• Runny or stuffy nose. Nasal discharge is watery at first, then becomes thick and greenish yellow. • Sore throat. • Hoarseness. • Cough that produces little or no sputum. • Low-grade fever. • Fatigue. • Watering eyes. • Appetite loss. • Aching muscles and bones. • Headache. • Chills.	**COLD, COMMON** (Refer to Illnesses section)
• Chills and moderate to high fever. • Muscle aches, including backache. • Cough, usually with little or no sputum. • Sore throat. • Hoarseness. • Runny nose. • Headache. • Fatigue. • Loss of appetite. • Chest pain.	**INFLUENZA** (Refer to Illnesses section)

(NOSE, STUFFY OR RUNNY, continued on next page)

SYMPTOMS & FACTORS	POSSIBLE PROBLEM
• An apparently crooked nose. • Obstruction of air through the nostrils. • Nasal discharge.	**HYDROCEPHALUS, NORMAL-PRESSURE** (Refer to Illnesses section)
• Itching, watery eyes. • Frequent sneezing in sudden attacks; stuffy nose with a clear, watery discharge. • Itching in the roof of the mouth. • Wheezing (sometimes). • Sore throat (sometimes). • Headaches (worse at night).	**NASAL ALLERGY** (Refer to Illnesses section)
Early stages: • Nasal congestion with green-yellow (sometimes blood-tinged) discharge. • Feeling of pressure inside the head. • Eye pain. • Headache that is worse in the morning or when bending forward. • Cheek pain that may resemble a toothache. • Post-nasal drip. • Cough that is usually nonproductive (sometimes). • Disturbed sleep (sometimes). • Fever (sometimes). **Late stages:** • Complete blockage of the sinus openings, blocking the discharge and increasing pain.	**SINUS INFECTION** (Refer to Illnesses section)

NUMBNESS, TINGLING OR PRICKLING

(Find your closest combination of symptoms in left-hand column; see possible problem in right-hand column. You may not experience all symptoms listed.)

SYMPTOMS & FACTORS	POSSIBLE PROBLEM
Any of the following may occur within seconds or a few minutes after exposure to a substance to which you are very allergic: • Tingling or numbness around the mouth. • Sneezing. • Itching all over, particularly on soles and palms and often accompanied by hives. • Redness around ears resembling recent sunburn. • Watery eyes. • Tightness in the chest; difficult breathing; coughing. • Swelling or itching in the mouth or throat. • Pounding heart. • Faintness. • Shivering. • Dilated pupils. • Loss of consciousness. Not all symptoms occur in every case. Seek immediate help for any.	**ANAPHYLAXIS** (Refer to Illnesses section) **(THIS IS AN EMERGENCY; SEEK MEDICAL CARE IMMEDIATELY!)**

(NUMBNESS, TINGLING OR PRICKLING, continued on next page)

SYMPTOMS & FACTORS	POSSIBLE PROBLEM
Any of the following: • Pain in the neck radiating to the shoulder blades, top of the shoulders, upper arms, hands or back of the head. • Crunching sounds with movement of the neck or shoulder muscles. • Numbness and tingling in the arms, hands and fingers; some loss of feeling in the hands; and impairment of reflexes. • Muscle weakness and deterioration; diminished reflexes. • Neck stiffness. • Headache. • Dizziness; unsteady gait. • Double vision. • With advanced disease, loss of bladder control and leg weakness.	**ARTHRITIS, NECK** (Refer to Illnesses section)
• Muscle spasms, twitching or cramps. • Numbness and tingling in the arms, legs, hands and feet. • Seizures. • Irregular heartbeat. • High blood pressure. • Lack of adequate sunshine.	**CALCIUM, TOO LITTLE** (Refer to Illnesses section)
• Tingling or numbness in part of the hand. • Sharp pains that shoot from the wrist up the arm, especially at night. • Burning sensations in the fingers. • Morning stiffness or cramping of hands. • Thumb weakness. • Frequent dropping of objects. • Inability to make a fist. • Shiny, dry skin on the hand.	**CARPAL TUNNEL SYNDROME** (Refer to Illnesses section)
Lower back: • Severe pain in the low back or back of one leg, buttock or foot (sciatica). Pain usually affects one side and worsens with movement, coughing, sneezing, lifting or straining. • Weakness, numbness or muscular wasting of the affected leg. **Neck:** • Pain in the neck or shoulder or down one arm. Pain worsens with movement. • Weakness, numbness or muscular wasting of the affected arm.	**DISK, RUPTURED** (Refer to Illnesses section)
• Rapid breathing. • Numbness and tingling around the mouth, hands and feet. • Weakness or faintness. • Muscle spasm or contractions in the hands and feet. • Fainting (occasionally). • Marked anxiety.	**HYPERVENTILATION SYNDROME** (Refer to Illnesses section)
Symptoms usually appear gradually over many months: • Tingling and numbness that begins in the hands and feet and spreads gradually. • Gradual muscle weakness throughout the body—often in same place on both sides. • Shooting pains that are often worse at night. Pains are aggravated by touch or temperature changes. • Painless ulcers on the toes or fingers. • Pale, dry skin that becomes sensitive to touch. • Weight loss. • Severe back pain or loss of bladder or bowel control if caused by intervertebral disk disease.	**PERIPHERAL NEUROPATHY** (Refer to Illnesses section)

(NUMBNESS, TINGLING OR PRICKLING, continued on next page)

SYMPTOMS & FACTORS	POSSIBLE PROBLEM
Symptoms vary depending on which organ is affected by the decreased blood supply. The most common include: • Chest pain (heart involvement). • Shortness of breath (lung involvement). • Abdominal pain (intestinal and liver involvement). • Blood in the urine (kidney involvement). • Numbness and tingling of the hands and feet (nerve involvement).	**POLYARTERITIS** (Refer to Illnesses section)
Early symptoms: • Fingers that turn pale when exposed to cold or stress. Paleness is followed by a bluish tinge and then redness. Numbness and tingling accompany the color changes, and symptoms are relieved by warmth. **Late symptoms:** • Ulcers on the fingertips caused by lack of normal blood flow to the fingers. • Chronic infections under and around fingernails and toenails.	**RAYNAUD'S PHENOMENON** (Refer to Illnesses section)
• Pain, numbness and tingling in the neck, shoulders, arms and hands. • Weakness in the arms and hands. • Poor blood circulation characterized by coldness, swelling and blueness in the hands and fingers (rare). • No pulse in the wrist when raising the arm and turning the head toward the opposite shoulder.	**THORACIC OUTLET OBSTRUCTION SYNDROME** (Refer to Illnesses section)
The following symptoms are brief, lasting from several minutes to a few hours. • Loss of muscle function on one side of the body. • Headache. • Dizziness. • Tingling in the arms and legs. • Numbness. • Vision disturbance or temporary blindness in one eye. • Confusion. • Faintness without loss of consciousness. • Slurred speech or inability to speak.	**TRANSIENT ISCHEMIC ATTACK (TIA)** (Refer to Illnesses section)

If you experience TINGLING OR PRICKLING NUMBNESS plus the following:

• Use of prescription or non-prescription drugs.	**WHAT TO DO:** Discontinue non-prescription drugs and call doctor now regarding prescription drugs.
• Sitting or resting in awkward position causing blocked blood vessels or nerves to arms or legs.	**WHAT TO DO:** Nothing. Symptoms should stop when position is changed.

PUPILS OF DIFFERENT SIZES

(Find your closest combination of symptoms in left-hand column; see possible problem in right-hand column. You may not experience all symptoms listed.)

SYMPTOMS & FACTORS	POSSIBLE PROBLEM
Symptoms vary according to which artery is affected: • Thoracic (chest) aneurysm produces pain in the chest, neck, back and abdomen. The pain may be sudden and sharp. It also causes hoarseness and swallowing difficulty. • Abdominal aneurysm produces back pain (sometimes severe), appetite and weight loss and a pulsating mass in the abdomen.	**ANEURYSM** (Refer to Illnesses section)

(PUPILS OF DIFFERENT SIZES, continued on next page)

SYMPTOMS & FACTORS	POSSIBLE PROBLEM

- Aneurysm in a leg artery causes poor circulation in the leg, with weakness and pallor or swelling and bluish color. A pulsating mass may appear in the groin or behind the knee.
- Aneurysm in a brain artery produces headaches (often throbbing), weakness, paralysis or numbness, pain behind the eye, vision change or partial blindness and unequal pupils. A brain aneurysm may be present for many years without producing symptoms.
- Aneurysm in a heart muscle causes heartbeat irregularities and symptoms of congestive heart failure.

ANEURYSM (continued)
(Refer to Illnesses section)

Mild cases:
- No symptoms (sometimes).
- Fever.
- General ill feeling.

Severe cases:
- Vomiting.
- Headache.
- Stiff neck.
- Pupils of different sizes.
- Unconsciousness.
- Personality changes.
- Seizures.
- Occasional weakness or paralysis of an arm or leg.
- Double vision.
- Speech impairment.
- Hearing loss.
- Drowsiness that progresses to coma.
- Sensitivity to light.

BRAIN INFECTION, VIRAL
(Refer to Illnesses section)

- Headache that worsens when lying down.
- Vomiting, with or without nausea.
- Vision disturbances, including double vision.
- Weakness on one side of the body.
- Lack of balance; dizziness.
- Loss of sense of smell.
- Memory loss.
- Personality change.
- Seizures.

BRAIN TUMOR
(Refer to Illnesses section)

The following symptoms usually appear gradually over several hours. They resemble symptoms of a brain tumor or stroke:
- Pain in the back if the infection is in the covering of the spinal cord.
- Headache and drowsiness.
- Nausea and vomiting.
- Weakness, numbness or paralysis of one side of the body.
- Irregular gait.
- Convulsions.
- Fever.
- Confusion or delirium.
- Difficulty speaking.

BRAIN OR EPIDURAL ABSCESS
(Refer to Illnesses section)
(THIS IS AN EMERGENCY; SEEK MEDICAL CARE IMMEDIATELY!)

Symptoms depend on the extent of injury. The presence or absence of swelling at the injury site is not related to the seriousness of injury. Signs and symptoms include any or all of the following:
- Drowsiness or confusion.
- Vomiting and nausea.
- Blurred vision.
- Pupils of different sizes.

HEAD INJURY
(Refer to Illnesses section)

(PUPILS OF DIFFERENT SIZES, continued on next page)

(PUPILS OF DIFFERENT SIZES, continued from previous page)

SYMPTOMS & FACTORS	POSSIBLE PROBLEM
• Loss of consciousness—either temporarily or for long periods. (THIS IS AN EMERGENCY; SEEK MEDICAL CARE IMMEDIATELY!) • Amnesia or memory lapses. • Irritability. • Headache. • Bleeding of the scalp if the skin is broken.	**HEAD INJURY** (Refer to Illnesses section)
• Recurrent headaches that worsen each day. • Fluctuating drowsiness, dizziness, mental changes or confusion. • Weakness or numbness on one side of the body. • Vision disturbances. • Vomiting without nausea. • Pupils of different sizes (sometimes).	**SUBDURAL HEMORRHAGE & HEMATOMA** (Refer to Illnesses section) (THIS IS AN EMERGENCY; SEEK MEDICAL CARE IMMEDIATELY!)

If you experience PUPILS OF DIFFERENT SIZES plus the following:

• Decreased sweating on side with dilated pupil and drooping eyelid.	**WHAT TO DO:** Call doctor now. These symptoms may indicate a chest tumor.
• No other symptoms.	**WHAT TO DO:** Nothing as long as pupils return to normal.

RASH WITH FEVER

(Find your closest combination of symptoms in left-hand column; see possible problem in right-hand column. You may not experience all symptoms listed.)

SYMPTOMS & FACTORS	POSSIBLE PROBLEM
• Fever, chills and sweating (may be absent in critically ill persons). • Headache. • Irritability. • Eyes sensitive to light; pupils may be of different sizes. • Stiff neck. • Vomiting. • Red or purple skin rash. • Confusion, lethargy, drowsiness or unconsciousness. • Sore throat or other signs of respiratory illness may precede other symptoms.	**MENINGITIS, BACTERIAL** (Refer to Illnesses section) (THIS IS AN EMERGENCY; SEEK MEDICAL CARE IMMEDIATELY!)
The following occur 2 to 5 days after a tick bite: • Fever, often high, with chills. • Red skin rash that begins on hands and feet and spreads to ankles, wrists, legs, trunk and abdomen. • Headache. • Muscle aches and weakness; stiff back. • Nausea and vomiting. • Confusion; coma. (THIS IS AN EMERGENCY; SEEK MEDICAL CARE IMMEDIATELY!)	**ROCKY MOUNTAIN SPOTTED FEVER** (Refer to Illnesses section)

(RASH WITH FEVER, continued on next page)

SYMPTOMS & FACTORS	POSSIBLE PROBLEM

- Diarrhea. In mild cases, this may be only 2 or 3 loose bowel movements a day. In severe cases, it may be watery diarrhea as often as every 10 or 15 minutes.
- Vomiting.
- Fever.
- Headache.
- Muscle aches.
- Rose-colored skin rash on the abdomen.
- Abdominal cramps (sometimes).
- Blood in the stool (sometimes).

A relatively mild attack may be mistaken for simple gastroenteritis.

TYPHOID FEVER
(Refer to Illnesses section)

If you experience RASH WITH FEVER plus the following:

- Use of prescription or non-prescription drugs.

WHAT TO DO:
Discontinue non-prescription drugs and call doctor now regarding prescription drugs.

- Possible exposure to childhood disease such as measles or chickenpox.

WHAT TO DO:
Call doctor now.

RASH WITHOUT FEVER

(Find your closest combination of symptoms in left-hand column; see possible problem in right-hand column. You may not experience all symptoms listed.)

SYMPTOMS & FACTORS	POSSIBLE PROBLEM

- Itching rash in areas where heat and moisture are retained, such as skin creases of elbows, knees, neck, face, hands, feet, groin, genitals and around the anus.
- Dry, thickened skin in affected areas.
- Uncontrolled scratching (frequently unconscious).
- Chronic fatigue from loss of sleep due to severe itching.

DERMATITIS, ALLERGIC
(Refer to Illnesses section)

- Itching (sometimes).
- Slight redness.
- Cracks and fissures in the skin.
- Bright red, weeping areas (severe cases).

DERMATITIS, CONTACT
(Refer to Illnesses section)

- Rash, itching or hives.
- Jaundice (yellow skin and eyes).
- Flushed skin.
- Facial swelling.
- Many other possible symptoms.

DRUG HYPERSENSITIVITY
(Refer to Illnesses section)

- Fatigue; excess thirst.
- Increased appetite *and* weight loss.
- Frequent urination.
- Itching around the genitals.
- Increased susceptibility to infections, especially urinary tract infections and yeast infections of the skin, mouth or vagina.
- Deterioration of vision (advanced stages).
- Loss of energy and easy fatiguability.

DIABETES MELLITUS, INSULIN-DEPENDENT
(Refer to Illnesses section)

(RASH WITHOUT FEVER, continued on next page)

SYMPTOMS & FACTORS	POSSIBLE PROBLEM
• Overweight. • Fatigue and loss of energy. • Excess thirst. • Increased appetite. • Frequent urination. • Decreased resistance to infection, especially urinary tract infections and yeast infections of the skin, mouth or vagina.	**DIABETES MELLITUS, NON-INSULIN-DEPENDENT** (Refer to Illnesses section)
Pustules (small, white blisters with pus inside) with the following characteristics: • Pustules are yellow-white and surrounded by narrow red rings. • Pustules are 1mm to 2mm in size; there may be few or many. • Pustules discharge a blood-stained pus made from dead cells. • Some pustules are pierced by hair; others may be adjacent to hair follicles.	**FOLLICULITIS, BACTERIAL** (Refer to Illnesses section)
Plaques (patches or flat areas) with clearly defined borders and pustules (small, white blisters with pus inside) on top. Pustules are 1mm to 2mm in diameter and frequently appear in clusters.	**FOLLICULITIS, FUNGAL** (Refer to Illnesses section)
Itchy papules (small, raised bumps) on skin with the following characteristics: • Papules swell and produce pink or red lesions called wheals. Wheals have clearly defined edges and flat tops. They measure 1cm to 5cm in diameter. • Wheals join together quickly and form larger raised, flat, skin-colored lesions called plaques. • Wheals and plaques change shape, resolve and reappear in minutes or hours. This rapid change is unique to hives.	**HIVES** (Refer to Illnesses section)
• Itching (often severe). • Vesicles (small, fluid-filled blisters) of varying size on the skin.	**ID REACTION** (Refer to Illnesses section)
Red lumps in the skin. The lumps usually appear within minutes after the bite or sting, but some don't appear for 6 to 12 hours. Skin reactions fall into 2 categories: • A toxic reaction with pain, such as from bee stings. • A toxic reaction with itching due to the body's release of histamine at the bite site, such as from mosquitoes.	**INSECT BITES & STINGS** (Refer to Illnesses section)
Papules (small, raised bumps) with the following characteristics: • Papules are flat-topped with well-defined borders. • Young papules are relatively flat and light brown. More advanced papules are dark brown or black. • Papules are wider than tall, and they appear "stuck on." • Papules measure 5mm to 20mm in diameter. They are distributed on the chest, back, face and arms. • Papules don't itch or hurt. • Papules vary in number from only I or 2 papules up to 100.	**KERATOSIS, SEBORRHEIC** (Refer to Illnesses section)
Plaques (red, raised skin lesions) with the following characteristics: • Plaques are 1cm to 4cm in diameter and have clearly defined borders. • Plaques may appear anywhere on the face, but the cheeks and jawline are the most common sites. Some people describe them as "butterfly" lesions when two lesions of unequal size appear on both sides of the nose. • Plaques sometimes appear on the scalp with localized patches of hair loss. • Plaques scar as they heal.	**LUPUS ERYTHEMATOSUS, DISCOID** (Refer to Illnesses section)

(RASH WITHOUT FEVER, continued on next page)

SYMPTOMS & FACTORS	POSSIBLE PROBLEM
Lesions that itch (sometimes) and have the following characteristics: • Lesions on the scalp cause patchy hair loss and scaling scalp. • Lesions on body skin are red, circular, flat, scaling and have well-defined borders. • Lesions on the bearded area of the face cause an itchy, scaling rash under the beard. • Lesions on the feet—See Athlete's Foot in the Illnesses section. • Lesions of the nails—See Paronychia in the Illnesses section.	**RINGWORM** (Refer to Illnesses section)
• Small, itchy blisters (usually in a thin line) in several parts of the body. The blisters break easily when scratched. • Broken blisters leave scratch marks and thickened skin crisscrossed by grooves and scaling.	**SCABIES** (Refer to Illnesses section)
• A red rash with many small blisters. Some blisters contain pus, and yellow-brown crusts form when they break. The blisters don't hurt but may itch. • Slight fever (sometimes). • Tiredness. • Enlarged, hard lymph glands (sometimes).	**SKIN, BACTERIAL INFECTION OF** (Refer to Illnesses section)
• Red skin rash, sometimes with small blisters, in areas exposed to sunlight. • Fever. • Fatigue or dizziness.	**SUN POISONING** (Refer to Illnesses section)
Severity of the following symptoms varies between women and from time to time in the same woman: • White, "curdy" vaginal discharge (resembles lumps of cottage cheese). The odor may be unpleasant, but not foul. • Swollen, red, tender, itching vaginal lips (labia) and surrounding skin. • Burning on urination. • Change in vaginal color from pale pink to red.	**VAGINITIS, MONILIAL** (Refer to Illnesses section)

If you experience RASH WITHOUT FEVER plus the following:

• Use of prescription or non-prescription drugs.	**WHAT TO DO:** Discontinue non-prescription drugs and call doctor now regarding prescription drugs.

SEIZURES OR CONVULSIONS

(Find your closest combination of symptoms in left-hand column; see possible problem in right-hand column. You may not experience all symptoms listed.)

SYMPTOMS & FACTORS	POSSIBLE PROBLEM
Usually no symptoms unless disease is severe. Following are symptoms of a hypertensive crisis: • Headache; drowsiness; confusion. • Numbness and tingling in the hands and feet. • Coughing blood; nosebleeds. • Severe shortness of breath. • Seizures. (THIS IS AN EMERGENCY; SEEK MEDICAL CARE IMMEDIATELY!)	**BLOOD PRESSURE, TOO HIGH** (Refer to Illnesses section)

(SEIZURES OR CONVULSIONS, continued on next page)

(SEIZURES OR CONVULSIONS, continued from previous page)

SYMPTOMS & FACTORS	POSSIBLE PROBLEM

Mild cases:
- No symptoms (sometimes).
- Fever.
- General ill feeling.

BRAIN INFECTION, VIRAL
(Refer to Illnesses section)

Severe cases:
- Vomiting.
- Headache.
- Stiff neck.
- Pupils of different sizes.
- Unconsciousness.
- Personality changes.
- Seizures.
- Occasional weakness or paralysis of an arm or leg.
- Double vision.
- Speech impairment.
- Hearing loss.
- Drowsiness that progresses to coma.
- Sensitivity to light.

The following symptoms usually appear gradually over several hours. They resemble symptoms of a brain tumor or stroke:
- Pain in the back if the infection is in the covering of the spinal cord.
- Headache and drowsiness.
- Nausea and vomiting.
- Weakness, numbness, or paralysis of one side of the body.
- Irregular gait.
- Convulsions.
- Fever.
- Confusion or delirium.
- Speaking difficulty.

BRAIN OR EPIDURAL ABSCESS
(Refer to Illnesses section)
(THIS IS AN EMERGENCY; SEEK MEDICAL CARE IMMEDIATELY!)

- Headaches that worsen when lying down.
- Vomiting, with or without nausea.
- Vision disturbances, including double vision.
- Weakness on one side of the body.
- Lack of balance; dizziness.
- Loss of sense of smell.
- Memory loss.
- Personality changes.
- Seizures.

BRAIN TUMOR
(Refer to Illnesses section)

- Muscle spasms, twitching or cramps.
- Numbness and tingling in the arms, legs, hands and feet.
- Seizures. **(THIS IS AN EMERGENCY; SEEK MEDICAL CARE IMMEDIATELY!)**
- Irregular heartbeat.
- High blood pressure.
- Lack of adequate sunshine.

CALCIUM, TOO LITTLE
(Refer to Illnesses section)

- Lethargy.
- Appetite loss.
- Vomiting and diarrhea.
- Dehydration and thirst.
- Irregular heartbeat.
- Depression; delirium; confusion.
- Seizures or coma (worst cases only). **(THIS IS AN EMERGENCY; SEEK MEDICAL CARE IMMEDIATELY!)**

CALCIUM, TOO MUCH
(Refer to Illnesses section)

(SEIZURES OR CONVULSIONS, continued on next page)

SYMPTOMS & FACTORS	POSSIBLE PROBLEM
• Brief dizziness, followed by fainting and unconsciousness. • No pulse. No breathing. • Bluish-white skin. Dilated pupils. • Seizures. • Loss of bowel and bladder control (sometimes). Simple fainting may resemble cardiac arrest, but pulse and breathing continue.	**CARDIAC ARREST** (Refer to Illnesses section) (THIS IS AN EMERGENCY; SEEK MEDICAL CARE IMMEDIATELY!)
These symptoms develop within 24 to 96 hours after a head injury: • Headache that steadily worsens. • Drowsiness or unconsciousness. • Nausea or vomiting. • Inability to move arms and legs. • Change in the size of eye pupils. • Seizures.	**EXTRADURAL HEMORRHAGE** (Refer to Illnesses section) (THIS IS AN EMERGENCY; SEEK MEDICAL CARE IMMEDIATELY!)
• No symptoms (sometimes) for less-severe forms. • Slow, irregular heartbeat. • Dizziness. • Sudden loss of consciousness. • Convulsions (sometimes). **(THIS IS AN EMERGENCY; SEEK MEDICAL CARE IMMEDIATELY!)**	**HEART BLOCK** (Refer to Illnesses section)
Mild hypoglycemic reaction: • Excessive hunger. • Weakness. • Nervousness. • Emotional instability. • Difficulty concentrating. • Sweating. • Headache. **Moderate hypoglycemic reaction:** • Increased weakness. • Excessive sweating. • Cold, clammy skin. • Numbness around the mouth or fingers. • Pounding heartbeat. • Memory loss. • Double vision. • Staring expression. • Difficulty walking. • Increasing confusion. **Severe hypoglycemic reaction:** • Muscle twitching. • Unconsciousness. • Convulsions. • Lack of urinary control.	**HYPOGLYCEMIA OF DIABETES** (Refer to Illnesses section) (THIS IS AN EMERGENCY; SEEK MEDICAL CARE IMMEDIATELY!)
The following vary greatly among people in frequency and severity: • Weakness or faintness. • Sweating. • Excessive hunger. • Nervousness and trembling hands. • Heartbeat irregularities. • Headache. • Confusion. • Personality changes. • Loss of consciousness. • Seizures (sometimes).	**HYPOGLYCEMIA, FUNCTIONAL** (Refer to Illnesses section)

(SEIZURES OR CONVULSIONS, continued on next page)

SYMPTOMS & FACTORS	POSSIBLE PROBLEM
Early stages: • Little or no urine output. **Later stages:** • Nausea, vomiting, diarrhea and appetite loss. • Mental changes, including irritability, drowsiness, stupor or coma. • Convulsions. • Severe itching. • High or low blood pressure. • Unexplained bruising, bleeding spots under the skin or spontaneous bleeding. • Pale skin and weak pulse.	**KIDNEY FAILURE, ACUTE** (Refer to Illnesses section) (THIS IS AN EMERGENCY; SEEK MEDICAL CARE IMMEDIATELY!)
Acute phase: • Tingling fingertips. • Muscle tension and spasms in the hands and feet. • Spasms of the larynx and throat muscles, causing difficulty breathing. **Chronic phase:** • Scaling skin. • Splitting nails. • Seizures. • Psychosis.	**PARATHYROID, UNDERACTIVE** (Refer to Illnesses section)
• Blurred vision, double vision, dizziness or a drooping eyelid caused by tumor pressure on nerves to the eye. • Headache in the forehead. • Nausea and vomiting. • Seizures. • Runny nose. • Excessive thirst. • Menstrual changes. • Unexplained weight gain. • Retarded or excessive growth in children. • Low blood sugar. • Low blood pressure. • Loss of peripheral vision. • Symptoms of abnormalities in other endocrine glands. See Thyroid, Overactive; Parathyroid, Overactive; Cushing's Disease; and Ovarian Tumor (all in Illnesses section).	**PITUITARY TUMOR** (Refer to Illnesses section)

If you experience SEIZURES OR CONVULSIONS plus the following:

• Use of prescription or non-prescription drugs.	**WHAT TO DO:** Discontinue non-prescription drugs and call doctor now regarding prescription drugs.
• Recent withdrawal from alcohol or other drugs, such as barbiturates.	**WHAT TO DO:** Call doctor now.

SEXUAL INTERCOURSE, PAINFUL FOR MAN

(Find your closest combination of symptoms in left-hand column; see possible problem in right-hand column. You may not experience all symptoms listed.)

SYMPTOMS & FACTORS	POSSIBLE PROBLEM
• Burning urination. • Thick green-yellow discharge from the penis. • Little or no fever. • Pain or tenderness with sexual intercourse (sometimes). • Rectal discomfort and discharge (sometimes). • Joint pain. • Rash, especially on palms. • Mild sore throat (sometimes). Males usually have more pronounced symptoms than females.	**GONORRHEA** (Refer to Illnesses section)
• Painful blisters, preceded by itching and irritation, on the penis. After a few days, the blisters rupture and leave painful, shallow ulcers which last 1 to 3 weeks. • Difficult, painful urination. • Enlarged lymph glands. • Fever and a general ill feeling.	**HERPES, GENITAL** (Refer to Illnesses section)
Absent penile erection, or erections that are too weak, brief or painful for sexual intercourse.	**IMPOTENCE, MALE SEXUAL** (Refer to Illnesses section)
• Pain, redness, moistness and swelling of the head of the penis. • Inflammation of the foreskin. • Ulceration of the penis. • Enlarged lymph glands in the groin. • Chills and fever (rare). • Discharge from the penis (rare). • Burning on urination (rare).	**PENIS INFECTION** (Refer to Illnesses section)
• Urgency to urinate. • Burning with urination. • Frequent urination; waking to urinate at night. • Difficulty starting urination and emptying the bladder completely. • Fever; chills. • Pain between the scrotum and anus. • Joint and muscle aches. • Blood in the urine or semen (sometimes). • Low back pain. • Pain with a doctor's rectal examination.	**PROSTATITIS** (Refer to Illnesses section)
• Painful or burning urination with cloudy, yellow-green mucus discharge from the urethra. • Frequent urge to urinate, even when there is not much urine in the bladder. • Painful sexual intercourse or temporary impotence. • Dribbling of urine.	**URETHRITIS** (Refer to Illnesses section)

If you experience PAINFUL SEXUAL INTERCOURSE (FOR MAN) plus the following:

• No other symptoms.	**WHAT TO DO:** See Impotence, Sexual (in Symptoms section).

SEXUAL INTERCOURSE, PAINFUL FOR WOMAN

(Find your closest combination of symptoms in left-hand column; see possible problem in right-hand column. You may not experience all symptoms listed.)

SYMPTOMS & FACTORS	POSSIBLE PROBLEM
• Burning and stinging on urination. • Frequent urination, especially at night, although the urine amount may be small. • Increased urge to urinate. • Pain in the lower part of abdomen over the bladder. • Low back pain. • Low-grade fever (under 101F or 38.3C). • Bad-smelling urine. • Painful sexual intercourse. • Lack of urinary control (sometimes).	**BLADDER INFECTION** (Refer to Illnesses section)
Physical changes (directly associated with decreased blood levels of female hormones): • Menstrual irregularity. • Hot flashes or flushes—sensations of heat spreading from the waist or chest toward the neck, face and upper arms. • Headaches. • Dizziness. • Rapid or irregular heartbeat. • Vaginal itching, burning or discomfort during intercourse, beginning a few years after menopause. • Bloating in the upper abdomen. • Bladder irritability. • Breast tenderness. **Emotional changes** (associated with lower hormone levels *and* conflicting feelings about aging and loss of fertility): • Mood changes. • Pronounced tension and anxiety. • Difficulty sleeping. • Depression or melancholy and fatigue.	**MENOPAUSE & POST-MENOPAUSE** (Refer to Illnesses section)
• Lump in front or back of the vagina or projecting outside it. • Vague discomfort in the pelvic region. • Backache that worsens with lifting. • Discomfort with urinating. • Occasional stress incontinence (urine leakage when laughing, sneezing or coughing).	**UTERINE PROLAPSE** (Refer to Illnesses section)
• Itching. • Abnormal vaginal bleeding. • Discomfort or bleeding with intercourse. • Small or large, firm, ulcerated, painless lesion of the vulva. Cancers on the vulva have thick, raised edges and bleed easily. • Uncomfortable urination if cancer spreads to the bladder. • Rectal bleeding if it spreads to the rectum.	**VAGINA OR VULVA, CANCER OF** (Refer to Illnesses section)
Involuntary contraction of the muscles around the vagina and rectum. The vagina closes so tightly that the penis cannot penetrate for sexual intercourse.	**VAGINISMUS** (Refer to Illnesses section)
Severity of the following symptoms varies greatly between women and from time to time in the same woman: • Bad-smelling vaginal discharge. The discharge is usually thin, whitish and sometimes tinged with blood. • Genital pain and itching. • Discomfort during sexual intercourse. • Change in vaginal color from pale pink to red.	**VAGINITIS, POST-MENOPAUSAL** (Refer to Illnesses section)

(SEXUAL INTERCOURSE, PAINFUL FOR WOMAN, continued on next page)

SYMPTOMS & FACTORS	POSSIBLE PROBLEM

If you experience PAINFUL SEXUAL INTERCOURSE (FOR WOMAN) plus the following:

- Vaginal itching.

WHAT TO DO:
See Vaginal Itching (in Symptoms section).

- Vaginal discharge.

WHAT TO DO:
See Vaginal Discharge (in Symptoms section).

SHOULDER PAIN

(Find your closest combination of symptoms in left-hand column; see possible problem in right-hand column. You may not experience all symptoms listed.)

SYMPTOMS & FACTORS	POSSIBLE PROBLEM

Slow or sudden onset of:
- Redness, aching, pain, warmth and tenderness in any or all active joints in the hands, wrists, elbows, shoulders, knees, feet, ankles, jaw and spine.
- Morning stiffness; muscular atrophy.
- Low-grade fever.
- Nodules under the skin (sometimes).
- Pale skin.
- Appetite loss.

ARTHRITIS, RHEUMATOID
(Refer to Illnesses section)

- Pain, tenderness and limited movement in the affected area.
- When shoulder involved, radiation of pain into the neck; arm; fingertips.
- Severe pain with movement of the arm.
- Fever (sometimes).

BURSITIS
(Refer to Illnesses section)

- Pain and swelling at the fracture site.
- Tenderness close to the fracture.
- Paleness and deformity (sometimes).
- Loss of pulse below the fracture, usually in an extremity. **(THIS IS AN EMERGENCY; SEEK MEDICAL CARE IMMEDIATELY!)**
- Numbness, tingling or paralysis below the fracture (rare). **(THIS IS AN EMERGENCY; SEEK MEDICAL CARE IMMEDIATELY!)**.
- Bleeding or bruising at the site.
- Weakness and inability to bear weight.

FRACTURES, BONE
(Refer to Illnesses section)

- Sudden onset of severe pain in the inflamed joint, usually at the base of the big toe or larger joints.
- Involved joints are red, hot, swollen and very tender. Skin over the joint is red and shiny.
- Fever (sometimes).

GOUT
(Refer to Illnesses section)

- Sudden joint pain, swelling or deformity after an injury.
- Limited or no movement around a joint.

JOINT DISLOCATION OR SUBLUXATION
(Refer to Illnesses section)

- Pain or tenderness in the injury area.
- Gradual stiffening or contraction of the injured muscle.
- Swelling, redness or bruising at the injury site.

MUSCLE, PULLED OR TORN
(Refer to Illnesses section)

(SHOULDER PAIN, continued on next page)

SYMPTOMS & FACTORS	POSSIBLE PROBLEM
• Dull or sharp pain in the front of the chest, radiating to the neck and shoulder. The pain worsens with movement and eases when sitting up or leaning forward. • Rapid breathing. • Cough. • Fever and chills. • Weakness. • Anxiety. • The most important signs are apparent only with medical examination: friction rub heard through a stethoscope; elevated white blood cell count; rapid sedimentation rate (see Glossary); abnormal ECG (see Glossary).	**PERICARDITIS, ACUTE** (Refer to Illnesses section)
Early stages: • Pain in the shoulder, often slight, that progresses to severe pain that interferes with sleep and normal activities. Pain worsens with shoulder movement. • Stiffness in the shoulder that prevents normal movement. Reduced movement increases stiffness. **Later stages:** • Pain in the arm or neck. • Inability to move the shoulder. • Intolerable shoulder pain.	**SHOULDER, FROZEN** (Refer to Illnesses section)
• Pain or tenderness in the area of injury; severity varies with the extent of injury. • Swelling of the affected joint. • Redness or bruising in the area of injury, either immediately or several hours after injury. • Loss of normal mobility in the injured joint.	**SPRAINS & STRAINS** (Refer to Illnesses section)
• Restricted movement, tenderness and swelling around the inflamed tendon. Common sites are the shoulder, elbow, Achilles' tendon or hamstring. • Weakness in the tendon caused by calcium deposits that often accompany tendinitis.	**TENDINITIS** (Refer to Illnesses section)
If you experience SHOULDER PAIN plus the following: • Recent increased physical activity, such as golf.	**WHAT TO DO:** Use massage and ice or heat to relieve discomfort.
• Injury or jolt to the area.	**WHAT TO DO:** Call doctor soon.

SKIN PROBLEMS

(Find your closest combination of symptoms in left-hand column; see possible problem in right-hand column. You may not experience all symptoms listed.)

SYMPTOMS & FACTORS	POSSIBLE PROBLEM
• Sudden tenderness, swelling and redness in an area of the skin. The area of cellulitis is initially 5cm to 20cm in diameter and grows rapidly in the first 24 hours. A thin, red line often extends from the middle of the cellulitis toward the heart. Cellulitis does not develop into a boil. • Fever, sometimes accompanied by chills and sweats. • General ill feeling. • Swollen lymph glands nearest the cellulitis (sometimes).	**CELLULITIS** (Refer to Illnesses section)

(SKIN PROBLEMS, continued on next page)

SYMPTOMS & FACTORS	POSSIBLE PROBLEM

Nodules under the skin with the following characteristics:
- Nodules are dome-shaped and about 2cm to 10cm in diameter. Some grow larger.
- Nodules feel "doughy," smooth and easily movable.
- Only one—or many—lipomas may occur at one time.
- Nodules cause no pain.

LIPOMAS
(Refer to Illnesses section)

First stage:
- A red papule (small, raised bump) on the skin of the thighs, buttocks or armpits that grows as large as 5cm.

Later stages—any or some of the following:
- Muscle aches and pains.
- Fatigue and lethargy.
- Chills and fever.
- Stiff neck with headache.
- Backache.
- Nausea and vomiting.
- Sore throat.
- Enlargement of the spleen and lymph glands.
- Migrating joint pain, eventually accompanied by redness and warmth.
- Enlarged heart and heart rhythm disturbances.

LYME DISEASE
(Refer to Illnesses section)

The following begin 1 to 4 weeks after exposure and progress in order:
- A painless blister on the genitals which ulcerates and heals quickly.
- Enlarged lymph glands in the groin that form large, red, tender masses.
- Multiple areas of deep infection that discharge thick pus and blood-stained material.

Other symptoms include:
- Fever.
- Muscle aches and pain, including backache.
- Headaches.
- Joint pain.
- Appetite loss.
- Vomiting.

LYMPHOGRANULOMA VENEREUM
(Refer to Illnesses section)

A flat or slightly raised skin lesion that can be black, brown, blue, red, white or a mixture of all colors. Its borders are often irregular and may bleed.

MELANOMA, MALIGNANT
(Refer to Illnesses section)

Bacterial infection:
- Pain or tenderness, redness, warmth and swelling of tissue adjacent to the fingernail.
- Central whitish area produced by pus.

Fungal infection:
- Redness and swelling around the fingernail.
- No pain, warmth, itching or pus.

NAIL-BED INFECTION
(Refer to Illnesses section)

- A faint rash—often found in skin creases—of oval or round, pale pink or brown areas. One larger patch (the "herald patch") may appear first.
- Mild fatigue.
- Itching, usually mild.
- Occasional slight fever and headache.

PITYRIASIS ROSEA
(Refer to Illnesses section)

- Skin areas that are slightly raised, have red borders and are covered with large white or silver-white scales. The areas crack and become painful.
- Itching (sometimes).
- Joint pain.

PSORIASIS
(Refer to Illnesses section)

(SKIN PROBLEMS, continued on next page)

SYMPTOMS & FACTORS	POSSIBLE PROBLEM
A cyst with the following characteristics: • The cyst has sloped shoulders or a dome-shaped, nodular appearance and a smooth surface. • The cyst is whitish or skin-colored. • Cysts range from 1cm to 4cm in diameter. • If the cyst becomes injured or infected, it may become bright red and painful.	**SEBACEOUS CYST** (Refer to Illnesses section)
• Painful red blisters anywhere on the body. Blisters appear 4 to 5 days after early symptoms begin. The blisters appear on a broad streak of reddened skin along sensory nerve routes to a particular area of skin. They occur most often on the chest and spread only on one side of the body. • Mild chills and fever. • General ill feeling. • Mild nausea, abdominal cramps or diarrhea. • Chest pain, face pain, or burning pain in the skin of the abdomen, depending on the affected area.	**SHINGLES** (Refer to Illnesses section)
• A red rash with many small blisters. Some blisters contain pus, and yellow-brown crusts form when they break. The blisters don't hurt, but they may itch. • Slight fever (sometimes). • Tiredness. • Enlarged, hard lymph glands (sometimes).	**SKIN, BACTERIAL INFECTION OF** (Refer to Illnesses section)
A small skin lesion that does not heal in 3 weeks with the following characteristics: • The lesion appears flat and "pearly." Its edges are translucent and rounded or rolled. The edges may have small, curvy, new blood vessels. The ulcer in the center is dimpled. Lesion size varies from 4mm to 6mm, but it may grow larger if untreated. • The lesion occurs on skin that is exposed to the sun and shows evidence of sun damage. • The lesion grows slowly. It does not hurt or itch.	**SKIN CANCER, BASAL-CELL** (Refer to Illnesses section)
A small, disfiguring, scaling, raised bump on the skin with a crusting ulcer in the center. The bump doesn't hurt or itch.	**SKIN CANCER, SQUAMOUS-CELL** (Refer to Illnesses section)
Benign skin lesions fall into the following categories: • Tags—Soft, flesh-colored buds, often on stalks, found on the neck, armpits or groin. • Moles—Flat or raised lesions with clearly defined borders. Moles may be black, blue, red, yellow or brown. • Cherry spots—Pinhead-sized, bright-red lesions on the chest or back. • Strawberry marks—Bright-red raised areas in infants that grow until they are removed. • Keloids—Thick, pale, irregular growths that begin at the site of a scar and gradually increase in size. • Dermatofibromas—Rounded nodules, usually brownish and usually on the legs. • Freckles—Flat, brownish spots of pinhead size or larger.	**SKIN LESIONS, BENIGN** (Refer to Illnesses section)

(SKIN PROBLEMS, continued on next page)

SYMPTOMS & FACTORS	POSSIBLE PROBLEM

Early stages:
- A small, movable, non-tender nodule appears under the skin of the fingers. The nodule enlarges slowly, becomes pink and ulcerates.

In a few days or weeks:
- Dark nodules appear along the lymphatic channel that drains the area.
- Cough with sputum begins if the organism reaches the lungs (rare).
- Usually no other symptoms—unlike other fungal diseases, which cause fever, chills, a general ill feeling and appetite loss.

SPOROTRICHOSIS
(Refer to Illnesses section)

Macules (small areas of different skin color) or patches with the following characteristics:
- Macules are flat, white and can't be felt with fingers.
- Macules spread to form very large, irregularly shaped areas without pigmentation.
- Macules are usually on both sides of the body in approximately the same place.
- Macules vary from 2mm or 3mm to several centimeters in diameter.
- They don't hurt or itch.

VITILIGO
(Refer to Illnesses section)

Plaques (patches or flat areas) with the following characteristics:
- Bright red patches with poorly defined borders. They are often 6cm to 12cm in diameter or larger.
- Some plaques are weeping or oozing.
- Skin appears moist and crusted.
- Itching is usually severe.
- Smaller plaques (less than 1mm in size) sometimes surround larger plaques. They rarely form small pustules (small, white blisters with pus inside).

YEAST INFECTION, SKIN
(Refer to Illnesses section)

Two or more of the following:
- Poor appetite.
- Poor growth.
- Sensations of unpleasant tastes and odors and decreased senses of taste and smell.
- Decreased sex drive.
- Darkening of skin all over the body.
- Sparse hair growth.
- Deformed nails.

ZINC DEFICIENCY
(Refer to Illnesses section)

If you experience SKIN PROBLEMS plus the following:
- Use of prescription or non-prescription drugs.

WHAT TO DO:
Discontinue non-prescription drugs and call doctor now regarding prescription drugs.

- Itching rash without fever.

WHAT TO DO:
See Rash Without Fever (in Symptoms section).

- Itching without change in skin appearance.

WHAT TO DO:
See Itching (in Symptoms section).

SLEEPING PROBLEMS

(Find your closest combination of symptoms in left-hand column; see possible problem in right-hand column. You may not experience all symptoms listed.)

SYMPTOMS & FACTORS	POSSIBLE PROBLEM
• Feeling that something undesirable or harmful is about to happen. • Dry mouth; difficulty swallowing or hoarseness. • Rapid breathing and heartbeat. • Twitching or trembling. • Muscle tension; headaches. • Sweating. • Cold, clammy hands. • Nausea; diarrhea; weight loss. • Sleeplessness; nightmares. • Irritability. • Fatigue. • Memory problems. • Sexual impotence.	**ANXIETY** (Refer to Illnesses section)
• Loss of interest in life; boredom. • Listlessness and fatigue. • Insomnia; excessive or disturbed sleeping. • Social isolation. • Appetite loss or overeating. • Loss of sex drive. • Constipation. • Difficulty making decisions or concentrating. • Unexplained crying bouts. • Intense guilt feelings over minor or imaginary misdeeds. • Irritability. • Various pains, such as headache or chest pain, without evidence of disease. • Anxiety or agitation. • Thoughts of death or suicide.	**DEPRESSION** (Refer to Illnesses section)
Symptoms depend on the substance of abuse. Most produce: • A temporary pleasant mood. • Relief from anxiety. • False feelings of self-confidence. • Increased sensitivity to sights and sounds (including hallucinations). • Altered activity levels—either stupor and sleeplike states *or* frenzies. **(THIS IS AN EMERGENCY; SEEK MEDICAL CARE IMMEDIATELY!)** • Unpleasant or painful symptoms when the abused substance is withdrawn. **(THIS IS AN EMERGENCY; SEEK MEDICAL CARE IMMEDIATELY!)**	**DRUG ABUSE & ADDICTION** (Refer to Illnesses section)
• Restlessness when trying to fall asleep. • Brief sleep followed by wakefulness. • Normal sleep until very early in the morning (3 a.m. or 4 a.m.), then wakefulness (often with frightening thoughts). • Periods of sleeplessness alternating with periods of excessive sleep or sleepiness at inconvenient times. • Daytime fatigue. • Irritability.	**INSOMNIA** (Refer to Illnesses section)

(SLEEPING PROBLEMS, continued on next page)

SYMPTOMS & FACTORS	POSSIBLE PROBLEM
Any of the following (10% of people with narcolepsy have all signs): • Sleep attacks that may occur up to 10 times a day. These can occur during conversations or other activities. An attack leaves the person feeling refreshed, but another may occur again quickly. • Vivid dreams, sounds or hallucinations at the beginning of a sleep attack or upon awakening. • Temporary paralysis (sudden loss of muscle strength) when falling asleep or just before complete awakening. • Momentary paralysis not related to sleep when feeling sudden emotion, such as anger, fear or joy. • Irresistible drowsiness during the day.	**NARCOLEPSY** (Refer to Illnesses section)
• Long periods (up to 1 or 2 minutes) of not breathing while asleep. • Choking while asleep caused by obstruction in the back of the throat from the uvula and other loose tissue.	**SLEEP APNEA IN ADULTS** (Refer to Illnesses section)
• Hyperactivity. • Feeling warm or hot all the time. • Tremors. • Sweating. • Itching skin. • Pounding, rapid, irregular heartbeat. • Weight loss, despite overeating. • Marked anxiety and restlessness. • Sleeplessness. • Fatigue and weakness. • Protruding eyes (exophthalmos) and double vision (sometimes). • Diarrhea (sometimes). • Hair loss (sometimes). • Goiter (sometimes).	**THYROID, OVERACTIVE** (Refer to Illnesses section)

If you experience SLEEPING PROBLEMS plus the following:

• Use of prescription or non-prescription drugs.	**WHAT TO DO:** Discontinue non-prescription drugs and call doctor now regarding prescription drugs.
• Recent withdrawal from narcotics, tranquilizers, sleeping pills or alcohol.	**WHAT TO DO:** Nothing. Normal sleep should return within several weeks.
• Eating a late, heavy dinner or consumption of 3 or more alcoholic beverages at night.	**WHAT TO DO:** Eat earlier; consume smaller meals; decrease alcohol consumption.
• Drinking caffeine-containing beverage.	**WHAT TO DO:** Decrease use of caffeine, especially during late afternoon or evening.
• Sedentary lifestyle.	**WHAT TO DO:** See Appendix 20 for exercise recommendations.

STOOL, ABNORMAL APPEARANCE

(Find your closest combination of symptoms in left-hand column; see possible problem in right-hand column. You may not experience all symptoms listed.)

SYMPTOMS & FACTORS	POSSIBLE PROBLEM
• Sharp pain with passage of a hard or bulky stool. • Streaks of blood on the toilet paper or underwear. • Itching around the rectum.	**ANAL FISSURE** (Refer to Illnesses section)
Early symptoms include: • Pain in the left side of the abdomen that improves after bowel movements. • Episodes of bloody diarrhea with mucus, alternating with symptom-free intervals. **During an acute attack:** • Increased bloody diarrhea (up to 10 to 20 bowel movements a day). (THIS IS AN EMERGENCY; SEEK MEDICAL CARE IMMEDIATELY!) • Severe cramps and pain around the rectum. • Appetite and weight loss. • Bloated abdomen. • Fever as high as 104F or 40C. • Rapid heartbeat.	**COLITIS, ULCERATIVE** (Refer to Illnesses section)
Bleeding and hemorrhage from any or several body parts. Bleeding may be heavy. (THIS IS AN EMERGENCY; SEEK MEDICAL CARE IMMEDIATELY!) **Common signs of bleeding:** • Bloody vomit or red or black stools. • Vaginal bleeding. • Red or cloudy urine. • Unexplained bruising. • Severe abdominal or back pain caused by bleeding into body organs. • Convulsions (rare). (THIS IS AN EMERGENCY; SEEK MEDICAL CARE IMMEDIATELY!) • Coma (rare). (THIS IS AN EMERGENCY; SEEK MEDICAL CARE IMMEDIATELY!)	**DIC** (Refer to Illnesses section)
Diverticulosis symptoms: • Mild cramping, bloated feeling or tenderness in the left side of the abdomen that is relieved by passing gas or moving bowels. • Occasional bright red blood in the stool. Non-infected diverticulae sometimes bleed. • Constipation or diarrhea (sometimes). **Diverticulitis symptoms:** • Intermittent cramping abdominal pain that becomes constant. • Fever. • Nausea. • Tenderness over the affected area of the colon.	**DIVERTICULAR DISEASE** (Refer to Illnesses section)
• Cramping pain in the upper right of the abdomen. Pain may also occur in the chest (imitating a heart attack), in the upper back or in the right shoulder. These symptoms frequently follow a meal rich in fats. • Tenderness in the upper abdomen. • Nausea and vomiting. • Belching. • Slight fever. If high fever and chills occur, a bacterial infection is present. • Jaundice (yellow eyes and skin) sometimes. • Pale stools (sometimes). • Itching skin (sometimes).	**GALLBLADDER, INFECTION OF** (Refer to Illnesses section)

(STOOL, ABNORMAL APPEARANCE, continued on next page)

SYMPTOMS & FACTORS	POSSIBLE PROBLEM
• Rectal bleeding. Bright red blood may appear as streaks on toilet paper adhering to fecal residue, or it may be a slow trickle for a short while following bowel movements. • Pain, itching or mucus discharge after bowel movements. • A lump that can be felt in the anus. • A sensation that the rectum has not emptied completely after a bowel movement (large hemorrhoids only).	**HEMORRHOIDS** (Refer to Illnesses section)
• No symptoms in the early stages (frequently). • Bloody or black, tarry stools. • Cramping abdominal pain. • Feeling of fullness. • Change in bowel habits, such as diarrhea, constipation or narrow-caliber stools. • Unexplained weight loss. • Pain in the rectum. • Anemia. • Loss of bowel control (sometimes).	**LARGE INTESTINE, CANCER OF** (Refer to Illnesses section)
• No symptoms (usually). • Rectal bleeding (sometimes). • Mucus discharge from the rectum (sometimes).	**LARGE INTESTINE, POLYP OF** (Refer to Illnesses section)
• Diarrhea. • Weakness. • Weight loss. • Gas and vague abdominal discomfort. • Bad-smelling, copious stools.	**MALABSORPTION** (Refer to Illnesses section)
Early stages: • Vague symptoms of indigestion, such as fullness, burping, nausea and poor appetite. **Later stages:** • Unexplained weight loss. • Vomiting blood. • Black stools. • Fullness after eating small amounts. • Pain in the upper abdomen. • Mass in the upper abdomen that can be felt (sometimes).	**STOMACH CANCER** (Refer to Illnesses section)
• Burning, boring or gnawing pain, usually in the upper abdomen, but occasionally below the breastbone. The pain is often interpreted as heartburn, indigestion or hunger and may be relieved by drinking milk, eating, resting or taking antacids. • Pain lasts 30 minutes to 3 hours. It may occur immediately after eating or hours later. It frequently awakens one at night. • Pain comes and goes. Weeks of intermittent pain may alternate with short pain-free periods. • Appetite and weight loss. • Recurrent vomiting. • Blood in the stool. • Anemia. • Belching and bloating.	**ULCER, DUODENAL** (Refer to Illnesses section)

(STOOL, ABNORMAL APPEARANCE, continued on next page)

(STOOL, ABNORMAL APPEARANCE, continued from previous page)

SYMPTOMS & FACTORS	POSSIBLE PROBLEM
• Burning, gnawing pain in the upper abdomen or the lower chest below the breastbone. The pain is often interpreted as indigestion, heartburn or hunger and may be relieved temporarily with milk, antacids or bland food. • Pain lasts 30 minutes to 3 hours. It may occur immediately after eating or hours later. • Pain comes and goes. Weeks of intermittent pain may alternate with short pain-free periods. • Loss of appetite. • Weight loss. • Anemia. • Occasional vomiting.	**ULCER, STOMACH** (Refer to Illnesses section)

If you experience ABNORMAL APPEARANCE OF STOOLS plus the following:

• Recent consumption of green, leafy vegetables; use of iron supplements; use of Pepto-Bismol.	**WHAT TO DO:** Nothing. These normally turn the stool very dark or black.

SWALLOWING DIFFICULTY

(Find your closest combination of symptoms in left-hand column; see possible problem in right-hand column. You may not experience all symptoms listed.)

SYMPTOMS & FACTORS	POSSIBLE PROBLEM
• Feeling that something undesirable or harmful is about to happen. • Dry mouth; difficulty swallowing or hoarseness. • Rapid breathing and heartbeat. • Twitching or trembling. • Muscle tension; headaches. • Sweating. • Cold, clammy hands. • Nausea; diarrhea; weight loss. • Sleeplessness; nightmares. • Irritability. • Fatigue. • Memory problems. • Sexual impotence.	**ANXIETY** (Refer to Illnesses section)
• Difficulty or pain when swallowing. • Rapid weight loss. • Regurgitation of bloody mucus. • Respiratory infections	**ESOPHAGUS CANCER** (Refer to Illnesses section)
Often no symptoms are felt. When there are symptoms, they usually develop within 1 hour or more after eating and include: • "Heartburn" (a burning sensation in the area of the heart and behind the breastbone). May be confused with heart attack symptoms. • Belching. • Difficulty swallowing (rare). • Gastric reflux.	**ESOPHAGEAL REFLUX** (Refer to Illnesses section)
• Sudden or gradual decrease in the ability to swallow. Gradual difficulty swallowing affects solid foods first, then liquids. • Pain in the mouth and chest after eating. • Increased salivation. • Rapid breathing. • Vomiting, sometimes with mucus or blood. Cancer of the esophagus often causes similar symptoms. • Gastric reflux during sleep.	**ESOPHAGEAL STRICTURE OR CORROSIVE ESOPHAGITIS** (Refer to Illnesses section)

(SWALLOWING DIFFICULTY, continued on next page)

SYMPTOMS & FACTORS	POSSIBLE PROBLEM
• Drooping eyelids. • Double vision. • Loss of normal facial expression. • Difficulty swallowing. • Weakness of the arms and legs. • Difficulty speaking clearly. • Difficulty breathing.	**MYASTHENIA GRAVIS** (Refer to Illnesses section)
• Sore throat. • Difficulty swallowing. • Tickle or ''lump'' in the throat. • Fever. • Swollen glands in the neck (sometimes). • Throat may be red or covered with a grayish membrane (sometimes). • Generalized aching.	**PHARYNGITIS** (Refer to Illnesses section)
A pale lump—usually painless—with a hard rim that appears in any part of the mouth or tongue. Lump has the following characteristics: • Lump enlarges, ulcerates and bleeds easily. • Lump may prevent dentures from fitting properly. • Lump may make the tongue stiff and difficult to control, causing speaking and swallowing difficulty.	**ORAL CANCER** (Refer to Illnesses section)
• Fingers—Hardening and thickening of the skin, stiffness, poor circulation, numbness and fingertip ulceration. • Digestive system—Difficulty swallowing, poor food absorption, bloating after eating, weight loss, heartburn and a feeling that food sticks in the chest. • Skin—Hardening and thickening, especially in the face, which becomes tight and loses its elasticity. • Muscle aches. • Weakness and fatigue. • Joint pain, stiffness and swelling.	**SCLERODERMA** (Refer to Illnesses section)
• Fever. • Rapid onset of throat pain. • Throat pain that is worse when swallowing. • Appetite loss. • Headache. • General ill feeling. • Ear pain when swallowing (sometimes). • Swollen glands in the neck. • Bright red tonsils that may have specks of pus.	**STREP THROAT** (Refer to Illnesses section)

If you experience SWALLOWING DIFFICULTY plus the following:

• Recent swallowing of foreign object, such as fish bone.	**WHAT TO DO:** THIS IS AN EMERGENCY; SEEK MEDICAL CARE IMMEDIATELY!
• Sensation that food gets stuck in throat.	**WHAT TO DO:** Increase fluid intake when eating.

SWEATING, EXCESSIVE

(Find your closest combination of symptoms in left-hand column; see possible problem in right-hand column. You may not experience all symptoms listed.)

SYMPTOMS & FACTORS	POSSIBLE PROBLEM
• Feeling that something undesirable or harmful is about to happen. • Dry mouth; difficulty swallowing or hoarseness. • Rapid breathing and heartbeat. • Twitching or trembling. • Muscle tension; headaches. • Sweating. • Cold, clammy hands. • Nausea; diarrhea; weight loss. • Sleeplessness; nightmares. • Irritability. • Fatigue. • Memory problems. • Sexual impotence.	**ANXIETY** (Refer to Illnesses section)
Early stages: • No symptoms (often). **Later stages:** • Angina pectoris (discomfort or pain in the chest coming on with exercise and disappearing with rest). • Heart attack.	**CORONARY ARTERY DISEASE** (Refer to Illnesses section)
• Chest pain or "heavy, squeezing or crushing" feeling in the chest. • Sweating. • Cold, clammy, wet skin. • Pain that radiates from the midchest over the breastbone to the jaw, neck, either arm, the area between the shoulder blades or the upper abdomen (sometimes). • Feeling of impending doom. • Shortness of breath. • Nausea and vomiting.	**HEART ATTACK** (Refer to Illnesses section) **(THIS IS AN EMERGENCY; SEEK MEDICAL CARE IMMEDIATELY!)**
• Itching all over the body. • Swollen, non-tender, rubbery, distinct lymph glands anywhere in the body—but most commonly in the armpit or groin. • Intermittent fever and night sweats. • Pain in the diseased area after drinking alcohol. • Weight loss. • Jaundice (yellow skin and eyes). • General ill feeling. • Anemia. • Bleeding.	**HODGKIN'S DISEASE** (Refer to Illnesses section)
• Heavy perspiration from underarm area, soles and palms—and to a lesser degree, from other body parts. • Unpleasant odor, which is caused by bacteria in sweat.	**SWEATING, EXCESSIVE** (Refer to Illnesses section)
• Hyperactivity. • Feeling warm or hot all the time. • Tremors. • Sweating. • Itching skin. • Pounding, rapid, irregular heartbeat. • Weight loss, despite overeating. • Marked anxiety and restlessness. • Sleeplessness.	**THYROID, OVERACTIVE** (Refer to Illnesses section)

(SWEATING, EXCESSIVE, continued on next page)

SYMPTOMS & FACTORS	POSSIBLE PROBLEM
• Fatigue and weakness. • Protruding eyes (exophthalmos) and double vision (sometimes). • Diarrhea (sometimes). • Hair loss (sometimes). • Goiter (sometimes).	**THYROID, OVERACTIVE (continued)** (Refer to Illnesses section)

If you experience EXCESSIVE SWEATING plus the following:

• Use of prescription or non-prescription drugs.	**WHAT TO DO:** Discontinue non-prescription drugs and call doctor now regarding prescription drugs.
• Use of synthetic material, such as nylon, for clothing or blankets.	**WHAT TO DO:** Wear natural fibers, such as cotton.

SWELLING OR LUMP

(Find your closest combination of symptoms in left-hand column; see possible problem in right-hand column. You may not experience all symptoms listed.)

SYMPTOMS & FACTORS	POSSIBLE PROBLEM
• Fatigue. • Unexplained weight loss. • Recurrent respiratory and skin infections. • Fever. • Swollen lymph glands throughout the body. • Genital changes. • Enlarged spleen. • Diarrhea. • Night sweats. • Positive laboratory tests.	**AIDS (Acquired Immune Deficiency Syndrome)** (Refer to Illnesses section)
• A domed nodule that is painful, tender and red and has pus on the surface. Boils can appear suddenly and ripen in 24 hours. They are usually 1-1/2cm to 3cm in diameter; some are larger. • Fever (rare). • Swelling of the closest lymph glands.	**BOILS** (Refer to Illnesses section)
No symptoms in early stages, but may be detected even then by mammogram. • Swelling or lump in the breast. • Vague discomfort in the breast without true pain. • Retraction of the nipple. • Distorted breast contour. • Dimpled or pitted skin in the breast. • Enlarged nodes under the arm (late). • Bloody discharge from the nipple (rare).	**BREAST CANCER** (Refer to Illnesses section)
• Lumps are usually in both breasts. Solitary lumps may occur, but multiple lumps are common. • Lumps offer resistance when pressed with fingertips and may be tender. • Lumps may be accompanied by generalized breast pain. • Lumps come in different sizes. When the lumps are relatively large and near the surface, they can be moved freely within the breast. • Lumps deep within the breast may be indistinguishable from breast cancer.	**FIBROCYSTIC BREAST DISEASE** (Refer to Illnesses section)

(SWELLING OR LUMP, continued on next page)

SYMPTOMS

SYMPTOMS & FACTORS	POSSIBLE PROBLEM
• A swelling that usually returns to normal position with gentle pressure or by lying down. • Mild discomfort or pain at the site of the lump (sometimes). • Scrotal swelling, with or without pain.	**HERNIA** (Refer to Illnesses section)
• Sudden pain around the nail. • Redness, swelling and warmth around the nail. • Swelling of the lymph glands nearby, such as in the elbow or armpit. • Groupings of tiny blisters that are barely visible around the nail.	**HERPETIC WHITLOW** (Refer to Illnesses section)
• Itching all over the body. • Swollen, non-tender, rubbery, distinct lymph glands anywhere in the body—but most commonly in the armpit or groin. • Intermittent fever and night sweats. • Pain in the diseased area after drinking alcohol. • Weight loss. • Jaundice (yellow skin and eyes). • General ill feeling. • Anemia. • Bleeding.	**HODGKIN'S DISEASE** (Refer to Illnesses section)
Nodules under the skin with the following characteristics: • Nodules are dome-shaped and about 2cm to 10cm in diameter. Some grow larger. • Nodules feel "doughy," smooth and easily movable. • Only one—or many—lipomas may occur at one time. • Nodules cause no pain.	**LIPOMAS** (Refer to Illnesses section)
First stage: • A red papule (small, raised bump) on the skin of the thighs, buttocks or armpits that grows as large as 5cm. **Later stages—any or some of the following:** • Muscle aches and pains. • Fatigue and lethargy. • Chills and fever. • Stiff neck with headache. • Backache. • Nausea and vomiting. • Sore throat. • Enlargement of the spleen and lymph glands. • Migrating joint pain, eventually accompanied by redness and warmth. • Enlarged heart and heart rhythm disturbances.	**LYME DISEASE** (Refer to Illnesses section)
The following begin 1 to 4 weeks after exposure and progress in order: • A painless blister on the genitals which ulcerates and heals quickly. • Enlarged lymph glands in the groin that form large, red, tender masses. • Multiple areas of deep infection that discharge thick pus and blood-stained material. Other symptoms include: • Fever. • Muscle aches and pain, including backache. • Headaches. • Joint pain. • Appetite loss. • Vomiting.	**LYMPHOGRANULOMA VENEREUM** (Refer to Illnesses section)

(SWELLING OR LUMP, continued on next page)

SYMPTOMS & FACTORS	POSSIBLE PROBLEM
• Swollen, non-tender, rubbery, distinct lymph glands anywhere in the body—but most commonly in the armpit, neck or groin. • Weight loss. • General ill feeling. • Anemia. • Bleeding from the gastrointestinal tract. • Jaundice (yellow skin and eyes).	**LYMPHOMA, NON-HODGKIN'S** (Refer to Illnesses section)
A pale lump—usually painless—with a hard rim that appears in any part of the mouth or tongue. Lump has the following characteristics: • Lump enlarges, ulcerates and bleeds easily. • Lump may prevent dentures from fitting properly. • Lump may make the tongue stiff and difficult to control, causing speaking and swallowing difficulty.	**ORAL CANCER** (Refer to Illnesses section)
• Pain and swelling in the salivary gland (between ear and jaw), especially during meals. • Redness and tenderness in the floor of the mouth and under the jaw. • Swollen, tender lymph glands in the neck or under the jaw. • Fever (if infection is present).	**SALIVARY DUCT STONES** (Refer to Illnesses section)
• Pain and swelling of parotid (behind ear) or sublingual (under tongue) salivary glands. • Pain and swelling of lymph glands in the neck (below jaw). • Bitter pus in the mouth from the infected gland. • Fever.	**SALIVARY GLAND INFECTION** (Refer to Illnesses section)
A soft, painful swelling or firm mass above the angle of either jaw or in the floor of the mouth.	**SALIVARY GLAND TUMOR** (Refer to Illnesses section)

If you experience SWELLING OR LUMP plus the following:

• Recent vaccination, such as tetanus or typhoid.	**WHAT TO DO:** Call doctor now.
• Overuse of a joint.	**WHAT TO DO:** Call doctor now. This may be a ganglion cyst.
• Location in throat that causes swallowing difficulty.	**WHAT TO DO:** Call doctor soon. This may be thyroid goiter.

TESTICLES OR PENIS, PAINFUL OR SWOLLEN

(Find your closest combination of symptoms in left-hand column; see possible problem in right-hand column. You may not experience all symptoms listed.)

SYMPTOMS & FACTORS	POSSIBLE PROBLEM
• Pain, redness, moistness and swelling of the head of the penis. • Inflammation of the foreskin. • Ulceration of the penis. • Enlarged lymph glands in the groin. • Chills and fever (rare). • Discharge from the penis (rare). • Burning on urination (rare).	**BALANITIS** (Refer to Illnesses section)

(TESTICLES OR PENIS, PAINFUL OR SWOLLEN, continued on next page)

(TESTICLES OR PENIS, PAINFUL OR SWOLLEN, continued from previous page)

SYMPTOMS & FACTORS	POSSIBLE PROBLEM
• Enlarged, hardened, painful testicle. • Fever. • Tender scrotal contents. • Tenderness of the second testicle (sometimes). • Acute urethritis (often).	**EPIDIDYMITIS** (Refer to Illnesses section)
• A swelling that usually returns to normal position with gentle pressure or by lying down. • Mild discomfort or pain at the site of the lump (sometimes). • Scrotal swelling, with or without pain.	**HERNIA** (Refer to Illnesses section)
• Painful blisters, preceded by itching and irritation, on the penis. After a few days, the blisters rupture and leave painful, shallow ulcers which last 1 to 3 weeks. • Difficult, painful urination. • Enlarged lymph glands. • Fever and a general ill feeling.	**HERPES, GENITAL** (Refer to Illnesses section)
• Abnormally painful penile erection. • Persistent penile erection.	**PRIAPISM** (Refer to Illnesses section)

If you experience PAINFUL OR SWOLLEN TESTICLES OR PENIS plus the following:

• Painless, rubbery strands on skin that extend up scrotum.	**WHAT TO DO:** Call doctor soon. These probably represent enlarged blood vessels in the scrotum.

THIRST, EXCESSIVE

(Find your closest combination of symptoms in left-hand column; see possible problem in right-hand column. You may not experience all symptoms listed.)

SYMPTOMS & FACTORS	POSSIBLE PROBLEM
• Fatigue and weakness. • Temporary paralysis (sometimes). • Tingling sensations in the arms, legs, hands and feet. • Frequent urination, especially at night. • Thirst. • Severe muscle spasms. • Vision disturbances.	**ALDOSTERONE, EXCESSIVE** (Refer to Illnesses section)
• Lethargy. • Appetite loss. • Vomiting and diarrhea. • Dehydration and thirst. • Irregular heartbeat. • Depression; delirium; confusion. • Seizures or coma (worst cases only). (THIS IS AN EMERGENCY; SEEK MEDICAL CARE IMMEDIATELY!)	**CALCIUM, TOO MUCH** (Refer to Illnesses section)

(THIRST, EXCESSIVE, continued on next page)

SYMPTOMS & FACTORS	POSSIBLE PROBLEM
• Dry mouth and lips. • Decreased or absent urination. • Sunken eyes. • Dry, wrinkled skin with poor resilience. • Confusion; coma. (THIS IS AN EMERGENCY; SEEK MEDICAL CARE IMMEDIATELY!) • Low blood pressure. • Severe thirst. • Increase in heart rate and breathing. • Lightheadedness.	**DEHYDRATION** (Refer to Illnesses section)
• Fatigue; excess thirst. • Increased appetite *and* weight loss. • Frequent urination. • Itching around the genitals. • Increased susceptibility to infections, especially urinary tract infections and yeast infections of the skin, mouth or vagina. • Deterioration of vision (advanced stages). • Loss of energy and easy fatiguability.	**DIABETES MELLITUS, INSULIN-DEPENDENT** (Refer to Illnesses section)
• Overweight. • Fatigue and loss of energy. • Excess thirst. • Increased appetite. • Frequent urination. • Decreased resistance to infection, especially urinary tract infections and yeast infections of the skin, mouth or vagina.	**DIABETES MELLITUS, NON-INSULIN-DEPENDENT** (refer to Illnesses section)
• Blurred vision, double vision, dizziness or a drooping eyelid caused by tumor pressure on nerves to the eye. • Headache in the forehead. • Nausea and vomiting. • Seizures. • Runny nose. • Excessive thirst. • Menstrual changes. • Unexplained weight gain. • Retarded or excessive growth in children. • Low blood sugar. • Low blood pressure. • Loss of peripheral vision. • Symptoms of abnormalities in other endocrine glands. See Thyroid, Overactive; Parathyroid, Overactive; Cushing's Disease; and Ovarian Tumor (all in Illnesses section).	**PITUITARY TUMOR** (Refer to Illnesses section)

If you experience EXCESSIVE THIRST plus the following:

• Use of prescription or non-prescription drugs.	**WHAT TO DO:** Discontinue non-prescription drugs and call doctor now regarding prescription drugs.
• Weather is very hot.	**WHAT TO DO:** Increase amount of fluids, particularly water.

THROAT, SORE

(Find your closest combination of symptoms in left-hand column; see possible problem in right-hand column. You may not experience all symptoms listed.)

SYMPTOMS & FACTORS	POSSIBLE PROBLEM
• Runny or stuffy nose. Nasal discharge is watery at first, then becomes thick and greenish yellow. • Sore throat. • Hoarseness. • Cough that produces little or no sputum. • Low-grade fever. • Fatigue. • Watering eyes. • Appetite loss. • Aching muscles and bones. • Headache. • Chills.	**COLD, COMMON** (Refer to Illnesses section)
Early stages: • Sore throat. • Low-grade fever. • Swollen neck glands. • Skin has yellow spots or sores (sometimes). **Late stages:** • Airway obstruction and breathing difficulty. • Shock (low blood pressure; rapid heartbeat; paleness; cold skin; sweating; anxious appearance).	**DIPHTHERIA** (Refer to Illnesses section) **(THIS IS AN EMERGENCY; SEEK MEDICAL CARE IMMEDIATELY!)**
• Chills and moderate to high fever. • Muscle aches, including backache. • Cough, usually with little or no sputum. • Sore throat. • Hoarseness. • Runny nose. • Headache. • Fatigue. • Loss of appetite. • Chest pain.	**INFLUENZA** (Refer to Illnesses section)
• Itching, watery eyes. • Frequent sneezing in sudden attacks; stuffy nose with a clear, watery discharge. • Itching in the roof of the mouth. • Wheezing (sometimes). • Sore throat (sometimes). • Headaches (worse at night).	**NASAL ALLERGY** (Refer to Illnesses section)
• Sore throat. • Difficulty swallowing. • Tickle or "lump" in the throat. • Fever. • Swollen glands in the neck (sometimes). • Throat may be red or covered with a grayish membrane (sometimes). • Generalized aching.	**PHARYNGITIS** (Refer to Illnesses section)
• Fever. • Rapid onset of throat pain. • Throat pain that is worse when swallowing. • Appetite loss. • Headache. • General ill feeling. • Ear pain when swallowing (sometimes). • Swollen glands in the neck. • Bright red tonsils that may have specks of pus.	**STREP THROAT** (Refer to Illnesses section)

TONGUE, SORE

(Find your closest combination of symptoms in left-hand column; see possible problem in right-hand column. You may not experience all symptoms listed.)

SYMPTOMS & FACTORS	POSSIBLE PROBLEM
• Weakness, especially in the arms and legs. • Sore tongue. • Nausea, appetite loss and weight loss. • Bleeding gums. • Numbness and tingling in the hands and feet. • Difficulty maintaining proper balance. • Pale lips, tongue and gums. • Jaundice (yellow eyes and skin). • Shortness of breath. • Depression. • Confusion and dementia. • Headache. • Poor memory.	**ANEMIA, PERNICIOUS** (Refer to Illnesses section)
Signs of pronounced anemia include: • Tiredness, weakness and headache. • Paleness, especially in the hands and lining of the lower eyelids. **Less common signs include:** • Tongue inflammation. • Sore mouth or tongue. • Fainting. • Breathlessness. • Rapid heartbeat. • Appetite loss. • Abdominal discomfort. • Cravings for ice, paint or dirt. • Susceptibility to infection.	**ANEMIA, IRON-DEFICIENCY** (Refer to Illnesses section)
A lump in any part of the mouth or tongue with the following characteristics: • Lump may ulcerate and bleed. • Lump may interfere with the way dentures fit. • Lump may interfere with speech or swallowing.	**MOUTH OR TONGUE TUMOR, BENIGN** (Refer to Illnesses section)
Any of the following: • Bright red, swollen tongue. • Ulcers on the tongue. • Hairy-looking tongue. • Tongue with red tip and edges.	**TONGUE INFLAMMATION** (Refer to Illnesses section)
If you experience SORE TONGUE plus the following: • Use of prescription or non-prescription drugs.	**WHAT TO DO:** Discontinue non-prescription drugs and call doctor now regarding prescription drugs.
• Discomfort confined to one spot.	**WHAT TO DO:** Call dentist. The problem may be caused by abrasion from dentures or irregular teeth.

TREMBLING OR TWITCHING

(Find your closest combination of symptoms in left-hand column; see possible problem in right-hand column. You may not experience all symptoms listed.)

SYMPTOMS & FACTORS	POSSIBLE PROBLEM
Early stages: • Low tolerance of anxiety. • Need for alcohol at the beginning of the day or at times of stress. • Insomnia; nightmares. • Habitual Monday-morning hangovers and frequent absences from work. • Preoccupation with obtaining alcohol and hiding drinking from family and friends. • Guilt or irritability when others suggest drinking is excessive. **Late stages:** • Frequent blackouts; memory loss. • Delirium tremens (tremors; hallucinations; confusion; sweating; rapid heartbeat). These occur most often with alcohol withdrawal. • Liver disease (jaundice; internal bleeding; bloating). • Neurological impairment (numbness and tingling in hands and feet; declining sexual interest and potency; confusion; coma). • Congestive heart failure (shortness of breath; swelling of feet).	**ALCOHOLISM** (Refer to Illnesses section)
Symptoms appear in the following order: • Muscle twitching and weakness, beginning in the hands and spreading to the arms, shoulders and legs. Weakness eventually affects muscles that control breathing and swallowing. • Stiffening, cramps and spasticity of muscle groups. • Altered speech. • Involuntary laughing or crying.	**AMYOTROPHIC LATERAL SCLEROSIS** (Refer to Illnesses section)
• Feeling that something undesirable or harmful is about to happen. • Dry mouth; difficulty swallowing or hoarseness. • Rapid breathing and heartbeat. • Twitching or trembling. • Muscle tension; headaches. • Sweating. • Cold, clammy hands. • Nausea; diarrhea; weight loss. • Sleeplessness; nightmares. • Irritability. • Fatigue. • Memory problems. • Sexual impotence.	**ANXIETY** (Refer to Illnesses section)
• Tremors, especially when not moving. • General muscle stiffness and slowness. • Awkward or shuffling walk. • Stooped posture. • Loss of facial expression. • Voice changes. The voice becomes weak and high-pitched. • Difficulty swallowing. • Intellectual ability is unchanged until advanced stages, when it deteriorates slowly.	**PARKINSON'S DISEASE** (Refer to Illnesses section)

(TREMBLING OR TWITCHING, continued on next page)

SYMPTOMS & FACTORS	POSSIBLE PROBLEM
• Hyperactivity. • Feeling warm or hot all the time. • Tremors. • Sweating. • Itching skin. • Pounding, rapid, irregular heartbeat. • Weight loss, despite overeating. • Marked anxiety and restlessness. • Sleeplessness. • Fatigue and weakness. • Protruding eyes (exophthalmos) and double vision (sometimes). • Diarrhea (sometimes). • Hair loss (sometimes). • Goiter (sometimes).	**THYROID, OVERACTIVE** (Refer to Illnesses section)

If you experience TREMBLING OR TWITCHING plus the following:

• Use of prescription or non-prescription drugs.	**WHAT TO DO:** Discontinue non-prescription drugs and call doctor now regarding prescription drugs.
• Excessive consumption of caffeine-containing beverages.	**WHAT TO DO:** Decrease use of caffeine.
• Unexpected body jerks when falling asleep.	**WHAT TO DO:** Nothing. These usually represent no underlying disorder.
• No other symptoms.	**WHAT TO DO:** Call doctor soon.

URINATION, FREQUENT

(Find your closest combination of symptoms in left-hand column; see possible problem in right-hand column. You may not experience all symptoms listed.)

SYMPTOMS & FACTORS	POSSIBLE PROBLEM
• Blood in the urine. • Burning urination. • Increased frequency of urination, but passage of only small amounts of urine. • Pain in the pelvic area. • Unexplained weight loss.	**BLADDER TUMOR** (Refer to Illnesses section)
• Fatigue; excess thirst. • Increased appetite *and* weight loss. • Frequent urination. • Itching around the genitals. • Increased susceptibility to infections, especially urinary tract infections and yeast infections of the skin, mouth or vagina. • Deterioration of vision (advanced stages). • Loss of energy and easy fatiguability.	**DIABETES MELLITUS, INSULIN-DEPENDENT** (Refer to Illnesses section)
• Overweight. • Fatigue and loss of energy. • Excess thirst. • Increased appetite. • Frequent urination. • Decreased resistance to infection, especially urinary tract infections and yeast infections of the skin, mouth or vagina.	**DIABETES MELLITUS, NON-INSULIN-DEPENDENT** (Refer to Illnesses section)

(URINATION, FREQUENT, continued on next page)

SYMPTOMS & FACTORS	POSSIBLE PROBLEM
Unintentional loss of urine with lifting, sneezing, singing, coughing, laughing, crying or straining to have a bowel movement.	**INCONTINENCE, STRESS** (Refer to Illnesses section)
• Increased urinary urgency and frequency, especially at night. • Weak urinary stream. • Straining and dribbling on urination. • Feeling that the bladder cannot be emptied completely. • Urine of abnormal color. • Impotence (sometimes). • Burning urination.	**PROSTATE, ENLARGED** (Refer to Illnesses section)
• Increased urgency and frequency of urination, especially at night. • Burning. • Difficulty starting urination and emptying the bladder completely. • Fever; chills. • Pain between the scrotum and anus. • Joint and muscle aches. • Blood in the urine or semen (sometimes). • Low back pain. • Pain with a doctor's rectal examination.	**PROSTATITIS** (Refer to Illnesses section)

If you experience FREQUENT URINATION plus the following:

SYMPTOMS & FACTORS	WHAT TO DO
• Painful urination.	**WHAT TO DO:** see Urination, Painful, (in Symptoms section).
• Excessive consumption of caffeine-containing beverages or alcohol.	**WHAT TO DO:** Decrease consumption of caffeine or alcohol.
• Difficulty in controlling bladder.	**WHAT TO DO:** See Urination, Lack of Control, (in Symptoms section).
• Increased urine production and use of diuretic drug.	**WHAT TO DO:** Nothing. These are expected results of the drug.
• Cold weather, excitement or anxiety.	**WHAT TO DO:** Nothing. This is a normal occurrence.

URINATION, LACK OF CONTROL

(Find your closest combination of symptoms in left-hand column; see possible problem in right-hand column. You may not experience all symptoms listed.)

SYMPTOMS & FACTORS	POSSIBLE PROBLEM
Early stages: • Forgetfulness of recent events. • Increasing difficulty performing intellectual tasks, such as accustomed work, balancing a checkbook or maintaining a household. • Personality changes, including narrow range of interest, rigidity in views or beliefs, distrust, restlessness, poor impulse control and poor judgment.	**ALZHEIMER'S DISEASE** (Refer to Illnesses section)

(URINATION, LACK OF CONTROL, continued on next page)

SYMPTOMS & FACTORS	POSSIBLE PROBLEM
Later stages: • Difficulty doing simple tasks, such as choosing clothing and problem solving. • Failure to recognize familiar persons. • Disinterest in personal hygiene or appearance. • Difficulty feeding self. • Belligerence and denial that anything is wrong. • Loss of usual sexual inhibitions. **Advanced stages:** • Complete loss of memory, speech and muscle function (including bladder and bowel control) necessitating total care and supervision. • Extreme belligerence and hostility. • Sleeplessness.	**ALZHEIMER'S DISEASE (continued)** (Refer to Illnesses section)
• Burning, stinging urination. • Increased urgency and frequency of urination, especially at night, although the urine amount may be small. • Pain in the lower part of abdomen over the bladder. • Low back pain. • Low-grade fever (under 101F or 38.3C). • Bad-smelling urine. • Painful sexual intercourse. • Lack of urinary control (sometimes).	**BLADDER INFECTION** (Refer to Illnesses section)
• Forgetfulness, especially of recent events. • Unpredictable, sometimes violent, behavior. • Confusion. • Loss of interest in normal activities. • Disorientation, especially at night. • Poor personal hygiene and appearance. • Depression. • Poor judgment. • Staggering gait. • Incoherent speech.	**DEMENTIA** (Refer to Illnesses section)
Lower back: • Severe pain in the low back or back of one leg, buttock or foot (sciatica). Pain usually affects one side and worsens with movement, coughing, sneezing, lifting or straining. • Weakness, numbness or muscular wasting of the affected leg. **Neck:** • Pain in the neck or shoulder or down one arm. Pain worsens with movement. • Weakness, numbness or muscular wasting of the affected arm.	**DISK, RUPTURED** (Refer to Illnesses section)
• Increased urinary urgency and frequency, especially at night. • Weak urinary stream. • Straining and dribbling on urination. • Feeling that the bladder cannot be emptied completely. • Urine of abnormal color. • Impotence (sometimes). • Burning urination.	**PROSTATE, ENLARGED** (Refer to Illnesses section)
The following symptoms may vary according to the site of brain damage: • Inability to speak. • Inability to move part of the body. • Loss of consciousness.	**STROKE** (Refer to Illnesses section) **(THIS IS AN EMERGENCY; SEEK MEDICAL CARE IMMEDIATELY!)**

(URINATION, LACK OF CONTROL, continued on next page)

SYMPTOMS & FACTORS	POSSIBLE PROBLEM
• Painful or burning urination with cloudy, yellow-green mucus discharge from the urethra. • Frequent urge to urinate, even when there is not much urine in the bladder. • Painful sexual intercourse or temporary impotence in males. • Dribbling of urine in men.	**URETHRITIS** (Refer to Illnesses section)

If you experience LACK OF CONTROL OF URINATION plus the following:

• Use of prescription or non-prescription drugs.	**WHAT TO DO:** Discontinue non-prescription drugs and call doctor now regarding prescription drugs.
• Increased frequency of urination.	**WHAT TO DO:** See Urination, Frequent, (in Symptoms section).

URINATION, PAINFUL

(Find your closest combination of symptoms in left-hand column; see possible problem in right-hand column. You may not experience all symptoms listed.)

SYMPTOMS & FACTORS	POSSIBLE PROBLEM
• Burning, stinging urination. • Increased urgency and frequency of urination, especially at night, although the urine amount may be small. • Pain in the lower part of abdomen over the bladder. • Low back pain. • Low-grade fever (under 101F or 38.3C). • Bad-smelling urine. • Painful sexual intercourse. • Lack of urinary control (sometimes).	**BLADDER INFECTION** (Refer to Illnesses section)
• Severe abdominal pain, boring in nature. • Shock (sweating; faintness; nausea; panting; rapid pulse; pale, cold, moist skin). • Painful urination or inability to urinate. • Bloody discharge from the urethra. • Bloody urine.	**BLADDER OR URETHRA INJURY** (Refer to Illnesses section) **(THIS IS AN EMERGENCY; SEEK MEDICAL CARE IMMEDIATELY!)**
• Blood in the urine. • Painful urination. • Frequent urge to urinate, particularly at night, even though only small amounts of urine pass. • Dull pain in penis, scrotum; labia; back.	**BLADDER STONES, URINARY** (Refer to Illnesses section)
• Blood in the urine. • Burning urination. • Increased frequency of urination, but passage of only small amounts of urine. • Pain in the pelvic area. • Unexplained weight loss.	**BLADDER TUMOR** (Refer to Illnesses section)

(URINATION, PAINFUL, continued on next page)

SYMPTOMS & FACTORS	POSSIBLE PROBLEM
• Burning urination. • Thick green-yellow discharge from the penis or vagina. • Little or no fever. • Pain or tenderness with sexual intercourse (sometimes). • Rectal discomfort and discharge (sometimes). • Joint pain. • Rash, especially on palms. • Mild sore throat (sometimes). Females often have few or no symptoms. Males usually have more pronounced symptoms.	**GONORRHEA** (Refer to Illnesses section)
• Painful blisters, preceded by itching and irritation, on the vaginal lips or penis. In women, the blisters may extend into the vagina to the cervix and urethra. After a few days, the blisters rupture and leave painful, shallow ulcers which last 1 to 3 weeks. • Difficult, painful urination. • Enlarged lymph glands. • Fever and a general ill feeling.	**HERPES, GENITAL** (Refer to Illnesses section)
Sudden onset of: • Fever and shaking chills. • Burning, frequent urination. • Cloudy urine or blood in the urine. • Aching in one or both sides of the lower back (sometimes severe). • Abdominal pain.	**KIDNEY INFECTION, ACUTE** (Refer to Illnesses section) **(THIS IS AN EMERGENCY; SEEK MEDICAL CARE IMMEDIATELY!)**
• Increased urgency and frequency of urination, especially at night. • Burning urination. • Difficulty starting urination and emptying the bladder completely. • Fever; chills. • Pain between the scrotum and anus. • Joint and muscle aches. • Blood in the urine or semen (sometimes). • Low back pain. • Pain with a doctor's rectal examination.	**PROSTATITIS** (Refer to Illnesses section)
• Painful or burning urination with cloudy, yellow-green mucus discharge from the urethra. • Frequent urge to urinate, even when there is not much urine in the bladder. • Painful sexual intercourse or temporary impotence in males. • Dribbling of urine in men.	**URETHRITIS** (Refer to Illnesses section)
• Lump in front or back of the vagina or projecting outside it. • Vague discomfort in the pelvic region. • Backache that worsens with lifting. • Discomfort urinating. • Occasional stress incontinence (urine leakage when laughing, sneezing or coughing).	**UTERINE PROLAPSE** (Refer to Illnesses section)
Severity of the following symptoms varies between women and from time to time in the same woman: • White, "curdy" vaginal discharge (resembles lumps of cottage cheese). The odor may be unpleasant, but not foul. • Swollen, red, tender, itching vaginal lips (labia) and surrounding skin. • Burning urination. • Change in vaginal color from pale pink to red.	**VAGINITIS, MONILIAL** (Refer to Illnesses section)

(URINATION, PAINFUL, continued on next page)

(URINATION, PAINFUL, continued from previous page)

SYMPTOMS & FACTORS	POSSIBLE PROBLEM
• Foul-smelling, frothy vaginal discharge. • Vaginal itching and pain. • Redness of the vaginal lips (labia) and vagina. • Painful urination if urine touches inflamed tissue. The severity of discomfort varies greatly from woman to woman and from time to time in the same woman. Trichomonal parasite also infects men but may cause no symptoms.	**VAGINITIS, TRICHOMONAL** (Refer to Illnesses section)

If you experience PAINFUL URINATION plus the following:

• Excessive consumption of caffeine-containing beverages or alcohol.	**WHAT TO DO:** Decrease consumption of caffeine or alcohol. They tend to irritate the bladder.
• Use of bubble baths or feminine deodorants.	**WHAT TO DO:** Discontinue using those products.
• Very low fluid intake.	**WHAT TO DO:** Increase fluid intake to help dilute urine.
• Frequent urinary tract infections in a woman.	**WHAT TO DO:** Empty bladder immediately before and after sexual intercourse.

VAGINAL BLEEDING, UNEXPECTED

(Find your closest combination of symptoms in left-hand column; see possible problem in right-hand column. You may not experience all symptoms listed.)

SYMPTOMS & FACTORS	POSSIBLE PROBLEM
• No symptoms (usually). • Increased mucus discharge from the vagina (sometimes). • Unexplained vaginal bleeding (sometimes).	**CERVICAL EROSION** (Refer to Illnesses section)
• Unexpected spotting of blood. • Spotting of blood after sexual intercourse or bowel movements. • Vaginal discharge.	**CERVICAL POLYPS** (Refer to Illnesses section)
In the early, easily treatable stages: • No symptoms. **In later stages:** • Unexplained vaginal bleeding. • Persistent vaginal discharge. • Pain and bleeding after intercourse. **In final stages:** • Abdominal pain. • Leaking of feces and urine through the vagina. • Appetite and weight loss. • Anemia.	**CERVIX, CANCER OF** (Refer to Illnesses section)
Bleeding after menopause.	**ENDOMETRIAL HYPERPLASIA** (Refer to Illnesses section)

(VAGINAL BLEEDING, UNEXPECTED, continued on next page)

SYMPTOMS & FACTORS	POSSIBLE PROBLEM
• No symptoms (often). • Bleeding after menopause. • Painful sexual intercourse or bleeding after intercourse. • Anemia (weakness, fatigue and paleness). • Feelings of pressure on the urinary bladder or rectum. • Increased vaginal discharge (rare).	**FIBROID TUMORS OF THE UTERUS** (Refer to Illnesses section)
Early stages: • Bleeding or spotting, especially after sexual intercourse. This often occurs after menstrual activity has ceased for 12 months or more. A watery or blood-streaked vaginal discharge may precede bleeding or spotting. • Enlarged uterus. It is sometimes a large enough mass to be felt externally. **Later stages:** • Spread to other organs, causing abdominal pain, chest pain and weight loss.	**UTERINE CANCER** (Refer to Illnesses section)
• Itching. • Abnormal vaginal bleeding. • Discomfort or bleeding with intercourse. • Small or large, firm, ulcerated, painless lesion of the vulva. Cancers on the vulva have thick, raised edges and bleed easily. • Uncomfortable urination if cancer spreads to the bladder. • Rectal bleeding if it spreads to the rectum.	**VAGINA OR VULVA, CANCER OF** (Refer to Illnesses section)
• Bleeding from the uterus appearing through the vagina, which may be a light-brown discharge or heavy, red bleeding (with or without clots). Mucus may accompany the bleeding. Bleeding episodes vary in length—there is no expected range. • Pelvic pain.	**VAGINAL BLEEDING, POST-MENOPAUSAL** (Refer to Illnesses section)

If you experience UNEXPECTED VAGINAL BLEEDING plus the following:

• Use of prescription drugs containing estrogen.	**WHAT TO DO:** Call doctor now if bleeding severe. If spotting only, call doctor soon.
• Sexual activity.	**WHAT TO DO:** Try using a lubricant prior to sexual intercourse.

VAGINAL DISCHARGE, ABNORMAL

(Find your closest combination of symptoms in left-hand column; see possible problem in right-hand column. You may not experience all symptoms listed.)

SYMPTOMS & FACTORS	POSSIBLE PROBLEM
• Unexpected spotting of blood. • Spotting of blood after sexual intercourse or bowel movements. • Vaginal discharge.	**CERVICAL POLYPS** (Refer to Illnesses section)
Acute cervicitis: • Thick, yellow vaginal discharge. **Chronic cervicitis:** • Slight—sometimes unnoticeable—vaginal discharge. • Backache. • Discomfort with urination. • Discomfort and bleeding with sexual intercourse.	**CERVICITIS** (Refer to Illnesses section)

(VAGINAL DISCHARGE, ABNORMAL, continued on next page)

SYMPTOMS & FACTORS	POSSIBLE PROBLEM
Extensive chronic cervicitis: • Profuse vaginal discharge. • Spotting or bleeding after sexual intercourse.	**CERVICITIS** (Refer to Illnesses section)
• Burning urination. • Thick green-yellow discharge from the vagina. • Little or no fever. • Pain or tenderness with sexual intercourse (sometimes). • Rectal discomfort and discharge (sometimes). • Joint pain. • Rash, especially on palms. • Mild sore throat (sometimes). Females often have few or no symptoms.	**GONORRHEA** (Refer to Illnesses section)
Early symptoms (up to 1 week): • Pain with intercourse. • Bad-smelling vaginal discharge. • Low fever. • Frequent, painful urination. **Later symptoms (1 to 3 weeks later):** • Severe pain and tenderness in the lower abdomen on one or both sides. • High fever. • Increased bad-smelling vaginal discharge.	**PELVIC INFLAMMATORY DISEASE (PID)** (Refer to Illnesses section)
Severity of the following symptoms varies between women and from time to time in the same woman: • White, "curdy" vaginal discharge (resembles lumps of cottage cheese). The odor may be unpleasant, but not foul. • Swollen, red, tender, itching vaginal lips (labia) and surrounding skin. • Burning urination. • Change in vaginal color from pale pink to red.	**VAGINITIS, MONILIAL** (Refer to Illnesses section)
Severity of the following symptoms varies greatly between women and from time to time in the same woman. • Bad-smelling vaginal discharge. The discharge is usually thin, whitish and sometimes tinged with blood. • Genital pain and itching. • Discomfort during sexual intercourse. • Change in vaginal color from pale pink to red.	**VAGINITIS, POST-MENOPAUSAL** (Refer to Illnesses section)
• Foul-smelling, frothy vaginal discharge. • Vaginal itching and pain. • Redness of the vaginal lips (labia) and vagina. • Painful urination if urine touches inflamed tissue. The severity of discomfort varies greatly from woman to woman and from time to time in the same woman.	**VAGINITIS, TRICHOMONAL** (Refer to Illnesses section)

If you experience ABNORMAL VAGINAL DISCHARGE plus the following:

• Vaginal itching.	**WHAT TO DO:** See Vaginal Itching (in Symptoms section).
• Possibility of a tampon left in too long.	**WHAT TO DO:** Remove tampon if possible; if not, call doctor now.

VAGINAL ITCHING

(Find your closest combination of symptoms in left-hand column; see possible problem in right-hand column. You may not experience all symptoms listed.)

SYMPTOMS & FACTORS	POSSIBLE PROBLEM
• Fatigue; excess thirst. • Increased appetite *and* weight loss. • Frequent urination. • Itching around the genitals. • Increased susceptibility to infections, especially urinary tract infections and yeast infections of the skin, mouth or vagina. • Deterioration of vision (advanced stages). • Loss of energy and easy fatiguability.	**DIABETES MELLITUS, INSULIN-DEPENDENT** (Refer to Illnesses section)
• Overweight. • Fatigue and loss of energy. • Excess thirst. • Increased appetite. • Frequent urination. • Decreased resistance to infection, especially urinary tract infections and yeast infections of the skin, mouth or vagina.	**DIABETES MELLITUS, NON-INSULIN-DEPENDENT** (Refer to Illnesses section)
• Intense itching, sensitivity and irritation in the genital area. The skin may be dry. • Thin white vaginal discharge (sometimes). • Discomfort during sexual intercourse.	**GENITAL ITCHING** (Refer to Illnesses section)
• Painful blisters, preceded by itching and irritation, on the vaginal lips. The blisters may extend into the vagina to the cervix and urethra. After a few days, the blisters rupture and leave painful, shallow ulcers which last 1 to 3 weeks. • Difficult, painful urination. • Enlarged lymph glands. • Fever and a general ill feeling.	**HERPES, GENITAL** (Refer to Illnesses section)
Severity of the following symptoms varies between women and from time to time in the same woman: • White, "curdy" vaginal discharge (resembles lumps of cottage cheese). The odor may be unpleasant, but not foul. • Swollen, red, tender, itching vaginal lips (labia) and surrounding skin. • Burning urination. • Change in vaginal color from pale-pink to red.	**VAGINITIS, MONILIAL** (Refer to Illnesses section)
Severity of the following symptoms varies greatly between women and from time to time in the same woman. • Bad-smelling vaginal discharge. The discharge is usually thin, whitish and sometimes tinged with blood. • Genital pain and itching. • Discomfort during sexual intercourse. • Change in vaginal color from pale pink to red.	**VAGINITIS, POST-MENOPAUSAL** (Refer to Illnesses section)
• Foul-smelling, frothy vaginal discharge. • Vaginal itching and pain. • Redness of the vaginal lips (labia) and vagina. • Painful urination if urine touches inflamed tissue. The severity of discomfort varies greatly from woman to woman and from time to time in the same woman.	**VAGINITIS, TRICHOMONAL** (Refer to Illnesses section)

If you experience VAGINAL ITCHING plus the following:

• Use of bubble bath, chemical spray, ointment, cream or douche.	**WHAT TO DO:** Discontinue use of non-prescription products and call doctor now regarding prescription products.

VISION DISTURBANCE OR LOSS

(Find your closest combination of symptoms in left-hand column; see possible problem in right-hand column. You may not experience all symptoms listed.)

SYMPTOMS & FACTORS	POSSIBLE PROBLEM
• Headache that worsens when lying down. • Vomiting, with or without nausea. • Vision disturbances, including double vision. • Weakness on one side of the body. • Lack of balance; dizziness. • Loss of sense of smell. • Memory loss. • Personality change. • Seizures. **(THIS IS AN EMERGENCY; SEEK MEDICAL CARE IMMEDIATELY!)**	**BRAIN TUMOR** (Refer to Illnesses section)
• Blurred vision that may be worse in bright light. The blurring may first become apparent to one while driving at night, when lights seem to scatter or have halos. • Double vision (occasionally). • Opaque, milky white pupil (advanced stages only). • Color perception changes. • Near vision may have improved recently.	**CATARACT** (Refer to Illnesses section)
• Eye pain, usually severe. • Sensitivity to bright light. • Eyelid spasm. • Tearing. • Blurred vision. • Redness in the white of the eye.	**CORNEAL ABRASION OR ULCER** (Refer to Illnesses section)
• Severe headache. • Stiff neck. • Fever. • Blurred vision. • Protein in the urine. • Mental disturbances, such as confusion, depression, agitation or inappropriate speech or dress. • Cough. • Drowsiness.	**CRYPTOCOCCOSIS** (Refer to Illnesses section)
The following are characteristic of all types: • Possibly no signs in the early stages except occasionally a whitish light reflection in pupil. • Gradual loss of vision. • Bulging eyes (sometimes). Retinoblastoma may have the following additional signs: • Crossed eyes. • Tumor that is visible through the pupil.	**EYE TUMOR** (Refer to Illnesses section)
• Bulging eyes, which create a staring or frightened look. • Double vision. • Blurred vision. • Pain (sometimes). • Infrequent blinking (sometimes).	**EYES, BULGING** (Refer to Illnesses section)
The following apply to the site of injury: • Swelling. • Tenderness, crepitation (a crackly feeling upon touching) or pain. • Redness that becomes multicolored soon after injury. • Loss of sensation in the lips and nose from nerve damage. • Double or blurred vision.	**FACIAL BONES, FRACTURE OF** (Refer to Illnesses section) **(THIS IS AN EMERGENCY; SEEK MEDICAL CARE IMMEDIATELY!)**

(VISION DISTURBANCE OR LOSS, continued on next page)

143

SYMPTOMS & FACTORS	POSSIBLE PROBLEM
• Severe, throbbing eye pain and headache. • Redness in the eye. • Blurred vision or halos around lights. • Tender, firm eyeball. • Dilated, fixed pupil. • Swollen upper eyelid. • Vomiting and weakness (due to severe eye pain).	**GLAUCOMA, ACUTE** (Refer to Illnesses section) (THIS IS AN EMERGENCY; SEEK MEDICAL CARE IMMEDIATELY!)
Early stages: • Loss of peripheral vision in small areas. • Blurred vision on one side toward the nose. **Later stages:** • Larger areas of vision loss, usually in both eyes. **Late stages:** • Hard eyeball. • Halos around lights. • Blind spots. • Poor night vision.	**GLAUCOMA, CHRONIC** (Refer to Illnesses section)
Acute uveitis of sudden onset: • Severe eye pain. • Photophobia (sensitivity to light). • Eye redness. • Smaller pupil in the affected eye (sometimes). • Tears. • Blurred vision. **Uveitis of gradual onset:** • Eye pain. • Photophobia. • Floating spots in the field of vision. • Blurred vision.	**IRIS, INFLAMMATION & INFECTION (UVEITIS)** (Refer to Illnesses section)
The nature of attacks varies between persons and from time to time in the same person. Symptoms of a classic migraine attack appear in the following sequence: • Inability to see clearly, followed by seeing bright spots and zigzag patterns. Visual disturbances may last several minutes or several hours, but they disappear once the headache begins. • Dull, boring pain in the temple that spreads to the entire side of the head. Pain becomes intense and throbbing. • Nausea and vomiting. In other types of migraine attack, the above symptoms (vision disturbances, headache or vomiting) may be absent, or other symptoms may be present. Some persons become pale, with bloodshot eyes and a runny nose or eyes.	**MIGRAINE HEADACHE** (Refer to Illnesses section)
• Blurred vision, double vision, dizziness or a drooping eyelid caused by tumor pressure on nerves to the eye. • Headache in the forehead. • Nausea and vomiting. • Seizures. (THIS IS AN EMERGENCY; SEEK MEDICAL CARE IMMEDIATELY!) • Runny nose. • Excessive thirst. • Menstrual changes. • Unexplained weight gain. • Retarded or excessive growth in children. • Low blood sugar. • Low blood pressure. • Loss of peripheral vision. • Symptoms of abnormalities in other endocrine glands. See Thyroid, Overactive; Parathyroid, Overactive; Cushing's Disease; and Ovarian Tumor (all in Illnesses section).	**PITUITARY TUMOR** (Refer to Illnesses section)

(VISION DISTURBANCE OR LOSS, continued on next page)

SYMPTOMS & FACTORS	POSSIBLE PROBLEM
The following usually affect one eye, but sometimes both are affected: • Light flashes in the field of vision. • Floating spots in the field of vision. • Blurred vision. • Wavy visual images (sometimes). • Gradual loss of vision. This may not be noticed because it is so gradual. • No pain.	**RETINAL DETACHMENT** (Refer to Illnesses section) **(THIS IS AN EMERGENCY; SEEK MEDICAL CARE IMMEDIATELY!)**
The following symptoms may vary according to the site of brain damage: • Inability to speak. • Inability to move part of the body. • Loss of consciousness.	**STROKE** (Refer to Illnesses section) **(THIS IS AN EMERGENCY; SEEK MEDICAL CARE IMMEDIATELY!)**
• Recurrent headaches that worsen each day. • Fluctuating drowsiness, dizziness, mental changes or confusion. • Weakness or numbness on one side of the body. • Vision disturbances. • Vomiting without nausea. • Pupils of different sizes (sometimes).	**SUBDURAL HEMORRHAGE & HEMATOMA** (Refer to Illnesses section) **(THIS IS AN EMERGENCY; SEEK MEDICAL CARE IMMEDIATELY!)**
The following symptoms are brief, lasting from several minutes to a few hours. • Loss of muscle function on one side of the body. • Headache. • Dizziness. • Tingling in the arms and legs. • Numbness. • Vision disturbance or temporary blindness in one eye. • Confusion. • Faintness without loss of consciousness. • Slurred speech or inability to speak.	**TRANSIENT ISCHEMIC ATTACK (TIA)** (Refer to Illnesses section)

If you experience VISION DISTURBANCE OR LOSS plus the following:

• Use of prescription or non-prescription drugs.	**WHAT TO DO:** Discontinue non-prescription drugs and call doctor now regarding prescription drugs.
• Excessive fatigue.	**WHAT TO DO:** Get more rest.
• You have diabetes.	**WHAT TO DO:** Call doctor now.
• New contact lenses or glasses.	**WHAT TO DO:** Get eyes checked now. The prescription may be incorrect.
• Recent head or eye injury.	**WHAT TO DO:** Call doctor now.
• Excessive alcohol consumption.	**WHAT TO DO:** Decrease alcohol use.

VOICE LOSS OR HOARSENESS

(Find your closest combination of symptoms in left-hand column; see possible problem in right-hand column. You may not experience all symptoms listed.)

SYMPTOMS & FACTORS	POSSIBLE PROBLEM
• Feeling that something undesirable or harmful is about to happen. • Dry mouth; difficulty swallowing or hoarseness. • Rapid breathing and heartbeat. • Twitching or trembling. • Muscle tension; headaches. • Sweating. • Cold, clammy hands. • Nausea; diarrhea; weight loss. • Sleeplessness; nightmares. • Irritability. • Fatigue. • Memory problems. • Sexual impotence.	**ANXIETY** (Refer to Illnesses section)
• Hoarseness or loss of voice. • High, trembly, weak voice. • Sore throat; tickling in the back of the throat. • Sensation of a lump in the throat. • Slight fever (sometimes). • Difficulty swallowing (rare).	**LARYNGITIS** (Refer to Illnesses section)
• Hoarseness that does not disappear after resting the voice. • "Lump-in-the-throat" feeling. • Painful or difficult swallowing. • Hard, swollen lymph glands in the neck.	**LARYNX CANCER** (Refer to Illnesses section)
• Swelling or lump in the thyroid gland. • Pain and tenderness in the thyroid gland. • Swallowing difficulty. • Hoarseness. • Breathing difficulty (rare). • Symptoms of underactive or overactive thyroid (both in Illnesses section).	**THYROID TUMOR** (Refer to Illnesses section)
It is unlikely one person will have all the following symptoms, but most will have several: • Decreased tolerance of cold. • Decreased sweating. • Decreased appetite. • Constipation. • Chest pain. • Coarse or slow-growing hair. • Slow, rapid or irregular heartbeat. • Weight gain or extreme thinness. • Placidity or nervousness. • Sleepiness or insomnia. • Mental impairment, including depression, psychosis or poor memory. • Fluid retention, especially around the eyes. • Dull facial expression and droopy eyelids. • Coarse skin. • Decreased tolerance of medication. • Decreased sex drive and infertility. • Anemia. • Numbness and tingling of the hands and feet. • Deepened or hoarse voice.	**THYROID, UNDERACTIVE** (Refer to Illnesses section)

(VOICE LOSS OR HOARSENESS, continued on next page)

(VOICE LOSS OR HOARSENESS, continued from previous page)

SYMPTOMS & FACTORS	POSSIBLE PROBLEM
Persistent hoarseness without pain.	**VOCAL CORD NODULES** (Refer to Illnesses section)

If you experience VOICE LOSS OR HOARSENESS plus the following:

• Inhalation of smoke or fumes from a fire.	**WHAT TO DO:** Call doctor if symptoms last over 2 weeks.
• Injury to the throat.	**WHAT TO DO:** Call doctor now.

VOMITING, RECURRENT ATTACKS

(Find your closest combination of symptoms in left-hand column; see possible problem in right-hand column. You may not experience all symptoms listed.)

SYMPTOMS & FACTORS	POSSIBLE PROBLEM
• Headache that worsens when lying down. • Vomiting, with or without nausea. • Vision disturbances, including double vision. • Weakness on one side of the body. • Lack of balance; dizziness. • Loss of sense of smell. • Memory loss. • Personality change. • Seizures. (THIS IS AN EMERGENCY; SEEK MEDICAL CARE IMMEDIATELY!)	**BRAIN TUMOR** (Refer to Illnesses section)
• Lethargy. • Appetite loss. • Vomiting and diarrhea. • Dehydration and thirst. • Irregular heartbeat. • Depression; delirium; confusion. • Seizures or coma (worst cases only). (THIS IS AN EMERGENCY; SEEK MEDICAL CARE IMMEDIATELY!)	**CALCIUM, TOO MUCH** (Refer to Illnesses section)
• Flushed skin on the head and neck. • Watery eyes. • Diarrhea with abdominal cramps. • Respiratory symptoms similar to those of asthma. • Irregular heartbeat. • Nausea and vomiting. • Unexplained weight loss.	**CARCINOID SYNDROME** (Refer to Illnesses section)
Early dumping syndrome: • Weakness and fainting. • Sweating. • Irregular or rapid heartbeat. • Decreased blood pressure. • Flushing of skin. • Dizziness. • Shortness of breath. • Vomiting. • Explosive diarrhea and abdominal cramps. **Late dumping syndrome:** • Sweating, anxiety and tremors. • Exhaustion and faintness. • Decreased blood pressure. • Headache.	**DUMPING SYNDROME** (Refer to Illnesses section)

(VOMITING, RECURRENT ATTACKS, continued on next page)

SYMPTOMS & FACTORS	POSSIBLE PROBLEM
• Cramping pain in the upper right of the abdomen. Pain may also occur in the chest (imitating a heart attack), in the upper back or the right shoulder. These symptoms frequently follow a meal rich in fats. • Tenderness in the upper abdomen. • Nausea and vomiting. • Belching. • Slight fever. If high fever and chills occur, a bacterial infection is present. • Jaundice (yellow skin and eyes), sometimes. • Pale stools (sometimes). • Itching skin (sometimes).	**GALLBLADDER, INFECTION OF** (Refer to Illnesses section)
• Colicky (intermittent) pain in the upper right abdomen or between the shoulder blades. • Nausea and vomiting. • Bloating or belching. • Intolerance of fatty foods (indigestion, bloating and belching). • Jaundice (yellow skin and eyes). • No symptoms in about 40% of cases.	**GALLSTONES** (Refer to Illnesses section)
The following signs are worse at night: • Belching or slight regurgitation of stomach contents into the mouth, producing an acid taste. • Heavy, burning or uncomfortable sensation in the chest. • Swallowing difficulty. • Mild abdominal pain.	**HEARTBURN** (Refer to Illnesses section)
Early stages: • Flu-like symptoms, such as fever, fatigue, nausea, vomiting, diarrhea and loss of appetite. **Several days later:** • Jaundice (yellow eyes and skin) caused by a buildup of bile in the blood. • Dark urine from bile spilling over into the urine. • Light, "clay-colored" or whitish stools.	**HEPATITIS, ACUTE VIRAL** (Refer to Illnesses section)
• Blurred vision, double vision, dizziness or a drooping eyelid caused by tumor pressure on nerves to the eye. • Headache in the forehead. • Nausea and vomiting. • Seizures. (THIS IS AN EMERGENCY; SEEK MEDICAL CARE IMMEDIATELY!) • Runny nose. • Excessive thirst. • Menstrual changes. • Unexplained weight gain. • Retarded or excessive growth in children. • Low blood sugar. • Low blood pressure. • Loss of peripheral vision. • Symptoms of abnormalities in other endocrine glands. See Thyroid, Overactive; Parathyroid, Overactive; Cushing's Disease; and Ovarian Tumor (all in Illnesses section).	**PITUITARY TUMOR** (Refer to Illnesses section)

(VOMITING, RECURRENT ATTACKS, continued on next page)

SYMPTOMS & FACTORS	POSSIBLE PROBLEM
Early stages: • Vague symptoms of indigestion, such as fullness, burping, nausea and poor appetite. **Later stages:** • Unexplained weight loss. • Vomiting blood. • Black stools. • Fullness after eating small amounts. • Pain in the upper abdomen. • Mass in the upper abdomen that can be felt (sometimes).	**STOMACH CANCER** (Refer to Illnesses section)
• Abdominal pain and cramps. • Vomiting (occasionally). • Appetite loss. • Fever. • Weakness. • Swollen abdomen. • Sharp, dull or annoying pain in the chest. • Acid taste in the mouth. • Mild nausea and diarrhea (rare). • Belching or gas.	**STOMACH INFLAMMATION** (Refer to Illnesses section)
• Recurrent headaches that worsen each day. • Fluctuating drowsiness, dizziness, mental changes or confusion. • Weakness or numbness on one side of the body. • Vision disturbances. • Vomiting without nausea. • Pupils of different sizes (sometimes).	**SUBDURAL HEMORRHAGE & HEMATOMA** (Refer to Illnesses section) (THIS IS AN EMERGENCY; SEEK MEDICAL CARE IMMEDIATELY!)
• Burning, boring or gnawing pain, usually in the upper abdomen, but occasionally below the breastbone. The pain is often interpreted as heartburn, indigestion or hunger and may be relieved by drinking milk, eating, resting or taking antacids. • Pain lasts 30 minutes to 3 hours. It may occur immediately after eating or hours later. It frequently awakens one at night. • Pain comes and goes. Weeks of intermittent pain may alternate with short pain-free periods. • Appetite and weight loss. • Recurrent vomiting. • Blood in the stool. • Anemia. • Belching and bloating.	**ULCER, DUODENAL** (Refer to Illnesses section)
• Burning, gnawing pain in the upper abdomen or the lower chest below the breastbone. The pain is often interpreted as indigestion, heartburn or hunger and may be relieved temporarily with milk, antacids or bland food. • Pain lasts 30 minutes to 3 hours. It may occur immediately after eating or hours later. • Pain comes and goes. Weeks of intermittent pain may alternate with short pain-free periods. • Loss of appetite. • Weight loss. • Anemia. • Occasional vomiting.	**ULCER, STOMACH** (Refer to Illnesses section)

149

(Find your closest combination of symptoms in left-hand column; see possible problem in right-hand column. You may not experience all symptoms listed.)

SYMPTOMS & FACTORS	POSSIBLE PROBLEM
• Pain that begins close to the navel and migrates toward the right lower abdomen. Pain becomes persistent and well localized. It worsens with moving, breathing deeply, coughing, sneezing, walking or being touched. • Nausea and sometimes vomiting. • Constipation and inability to pass gas. • Diarrhea (occasionally). • Low fever (under 102F or 38.9C), beginning after other symptoms. • Tenderness in the right lower abdomen, usually about a third of the distance from the navel to the top of the hip bone. (This description applies only if the appendix is in its normal position. In some cases, the tip of the appendix is located elsewhere, making diagnosis difficult.) • Abdominal swelling (late stages).	**APPENDICITIS** (Refer to Illnesses section) **(THIS IS AN EMERGENCY; SEEK MEDICAL CARE IMMEDIATELY!)**
• Colicky (intermittent) pain in the upper right abdomen or between the shoulder blades. • Nausea and vomiting. • Bloating or belching. • Intolerance of fatty foods (indigestion, bloating and belching). • Jaundice (yellow skin and eyes). • No symptoms in about 40% of cases.	**GALLSTONES** (Refer to Illnesses section)
• Severe, throbbing eye pain and headache. • Redness in the eye. • Blurred vision or halos around lights. • Tender, firm eyeball. • Dilated, fixed pupil. • Swollen upper eyelid. • Vomiting and weakness (due to severe eye pain).	**GLAUCOMA, ACUTE** (Refer to Illnesses section) **(THIS IS AN EMERGENCY; SEEK MEDICAL CARE IMMEDIATELY!)**
Depends on the extent of injury. The presence or absence of swelling at the injury site is not related to the seriousness of injury. Signs and symptoms include any or all of the following: • Drowsiness or confusion. • Vomiting and nausea. • Blurred vision. • Pupils of different sizes. • Loss of consciousness—either temporarily or for long periods. **(THIS IS AN EMERGENCY; SEEK MEDICAL CARE IMMEDIATELY!)** • Amnesia or memory lapses. • Irritability. • Headache. • Bleeding of the scalp if the skin is broken.	**HEAD INJURY** (Refer to Illnesses section)
Early stages: • Flu-like symptoms, such as fever, fatigue, nausea, vomiting, diarrhea and loss of appetite. **Several days later:** • Jaundice (yellow eyes and skin) caused by a buildup of bile in the blood. • Dark urine from bile spilling over into the urine. • Light, "clay-colored" or whitish stools.	**HEPATITIS, ACUTE VIRAL** (Refer to Illnesses section)

(VOMITING, SUDDEN ATTACK, continued on next page)

SYMPTOMS & FACTORS	POSSIBLE PROBLEM
• Abdominal pain and cramps. • Nausea and vomiting. In the advanced stage, vomit resembles feces. • Weakness, dizziness or fainting. • Little or no urine due to fluid loss. • Audible noises from the abdomen in early stages. • Abdominal bloating, swelling and gas. • Fever (sometimes). • Diarrhea (partial obstruction only). • Rectal bleeding (sometimes). • Inability to pass gas or stool.	**INTESTINAL OBSTRUCTION** (Refer to Illnesses section) (THIS IS AN EMERGENCY; SEEK MEDICAL CARE IMMEDIATELY!)
• Extreme dizziness—especially with head movement—that begins gradually and peaks in 48 hours. • Involuntary eye movement. • Nausea and vomiting (sometimes). • Loss of balance, especially falling toward the affected side. • Temporary hearing loss (sometimes).	**LABYRINTHITIS** (Refer to Illnesses section)
The following occur with every acute attack: • Severe dizziness. • Noises in the affected ear, such as ringing or buzzing. • Hearing loss that increases with each attack. **Possible accompanying symptoms:** • Vomiting. • Sweating. • Jerky eye movements. • Loss of balance.	**MENIERE'S DISEASE** (Refer to Illnesses section)
• Fever. • Headache. • Irritability. • Eyes that are sensitive to light. • Stiff neck. • Vomiting. • Confusion, lethargy and drowsiness.	**MENINGITIS, ASEPTIC** (Refer to Illnesses section)
• Fever, chills and sweating (may be absent in critically ill persons). • Headache. • Irritability. • Eyes sensitive to light; pupils may be of different sizes. • Stiff neck. • Vomiting. • Red or purple skin rash. • Confusion, lethargy, drowsiness or unconsciousness. • Sore throat or other signs of respiratory illness may precede other symptoms.	**MENINGITIS, BACTERIAL** (Refer to Illnesses section) (THIS IS AN EMERGENCY; SEEK MEDICAL CARE IMMEDIATELY!)
• Loss of appetite. • Nausea and vomiting. • Spinning sensation. • Weakness and unsteadiness.	**MOTION SICKNESS** (Refer to Illnesses section)
• Nausea that sometimes causes vomiting. • Diarrhea that ranges from 2 or 3 loose stools to many watery stools. • Abdominal cramps, pain or tenderness. • Appetite loss. • Fever. • Weakness.	**STOMACH INFLAMMATION** (Refer to Illnesses section)

(VOMITING, SUDDEN ATTACK, continued on next page)

SYMPTOMS & FACTORS	POSSIBLE PROBLEM
• Acute, severe headache, often followed by unconsciousness. • Drowsiness, dizziness, convulsions or coma. • Eye pain with extreme sensitivity to light. • Vomiting. • Rapid heartbeat and breathing. • Stiff neck with pain on movement. • Fever. • Numbness, weakness or inability to move an arm or leg.	**SUBARACHNOID HEMORRHAGE** (Refer to Illnesses section) **(THIS IS AN EMERGENCY; SEEK MEDICAL CARE IMMEDIATELY!)**

If you experience SUDDEN ATTACK OF VOMITING plus the following:

• Use of prescription or non-prescription drugs.	**WHAT TO DO:** Discontinue non-prescription drugs and call doctor now regarding prescription drugs.
• Recent episodes of vomiting.	**WHAT TO DO:** See Vomiting, Recurrent, in Symptoms section.
• Excessive use of alcohol.	**WHAT TO DO:** Decrease alcohol consumption.

WEIGHT GAIN

(Find your closest combination of symptoms in left-hand column; see possible problem in right-hand column. You may not experience all symptoms listed.)

SYMPTOMS & FACTORS	POSSIBLE PROBLEM
Early stages: • Fatigue; weakness. • Poor appetite; nausea; weight loss. • Enlarged liver. • Red palms. **Late stages:** • Jaundice (yellow skin and eyes). • Dark yellow or brown urine. • Spider blood vessels of the skin (fine vessels which spread out from a central point). • Hair loss. • Breast enlargement in men. • Fluid accumulation in the abdomen and legs. • Enlarged spleen. • Diarrhea; stool may be black or bloody. • Bleeding and bruising. • Mental confusion; coma.	**CIRRHOSIS OF THE LIVER** (Refer to Illnesses section)
• Shortness of breath, especially with exertion or when lying flat in bed. • Fatigue, weakness or faintness. • Cough (usually with sputum). • Wheezing (sometimes). • Swelling of the abdomen, legs and ankles. • Rapid or irregular heartbeat.	**CONGESTIVE HEART FAILURE** (Refer to Illnesses section)

(WEIGHT GAIN, continued on next page)

(WEIGHT GAIN, continued from previous page)

SYMPTOMS & FACTORS	POSSIBLE PROBLEM
• Loss of interest in life; boredom. • Listlessness and fatigue. • Insomnia; excessive or disturbed sleeping. • Social isolation. • Appetite loss or overeating. • Loss of sex drive. • Constipation. • Difficulty making decisions and concentrating. • Unexplained crying bouts. • Intense guilt feelings over minor or imaginary misdeeds. • Irritability. • Various pains, such as headache or chest pain, without evidence of disease. • Anxiety or agitation. • Thoughts of death or suicide.	**DEPRESSION** (Refer to Illnesses section)
Over 25% body fat in women, over 20% in men. Most obese persons have no symptoms except associated emotional problems and poor exercise tolerance. Excess weight increases the heart's work.	**OBESITY** (Refer to Illnesses section)
It is unlikely one person will have all the following symptoms, but most will have several: • Decreased tolerance of cold. • Decreased sweating. • Decreased appetite. • Constipation. • Chest pain. • Coarse or slow-growing hair. • Slow, rapid or irregular heartbeat. • Weight gain or extreme thinness. • Placidity or nervousness. • Sleepiness or insomnia. • Mental impairment, including depression, psychosis or poor memory. • Fluid retention, especially around the eyes. • Dull facial expression and droopy eyelids. • Coarse skin. • Decreased tolerance of medication. • Decreased sex drive and infertility. • Anemia. • Numbness and tingling of the hands and feet. • Deepened or hoarse voice.	**THYROID, UNDERACTIVE** (Refer to Illnesses section)

If you experience WEIGHT GAIN plus the following:

• Use of prescription or non-prescription drugs.	**WHAT TO DO:** Discontinue non-prescription drugs and call doctor now regarding prescription drugs.
• Change from active to sedentary lifestyle.	**WHAT TO DO:** Decrease food consumption and increase physical activity.

WEIGHT LOSS

(Find your closest combination of symptoms in left-hand column; see possible problem in right-hand column. You may not experience all symptoms listed.)

SYMPTOMS & FACTORS	POSSIBLE PROBLEM
• Fatigue. • Unexplained weight loss. • Recurrent respiratory and skin infections. • Fever. • Swollen lymph glands throughout the body. • Genital changes. • Enlarged spleen. • Diarrhea. • Night sweats. • Positive laboratory tests.	**AIDS (Acquired Immune Deficiency Syndrome)** (Refer to Illnesses section)
• Enlarged lymph glands. • Weight loss. • Fevers. • Lethargy and achiness. • Diarrhea (chronic). • Rectal growths. • Thrush.	**ARC (Aids-Related Complex)** (Refer to Illnesses section)
• Feeling that something undesirable or harmful is about to happen. • Dry mouth; difficulty swallowing or hoarseness. • Rapid breathing and heartbeat. • Twitching or trembling. • Muscle tension; headaches. • Sweating. • Cold, clammy hands. • Nausea; diarrhea; weight loss. • Sleeplessness; nightmares. • Irritability. • Fatigue. • Memory problems. • Sexual impotence.	**ANXIETY** (Refer to Illnesses section)
• Blood in the urine. • Burning urination. • Increased frequency of urination, but passage of only small amounts of urine. • Pain in the pelvic area. • Unexplained weight loss.	**BLADDER TUMOR** (Refer to Illnesses section)
• Frequent cough or coughing spasms. • Shortness of breath. • Sputum that is thick and difficult to cough up. Sputum production varies according to whether infection is present. • Barrel chest (in the late stages). • Chest pain (rare).	**BRONCHITIS, CHRONIC** (Refer to Illnesses section)
• Flushed skin on the head and neck. • Watery eyes. • Diarrhea with abdominal cramps. • Respiratory symptoms similar to those of asthma. • Irregular heartbeat. • Nausea and vomiting. • Unexplained weight loss.	**CARCINOID SYNDROME** (Refer to Illnesses section)

(WEIGHT LOSS, continued on next page)

SYMPTOMS & FACTORS	POSSIBLE PROBLEM
• Cramping abdominal pain—especially after eating. The pain is sometimes in the right lower abdomen, mimicking appendicitis. • Nausea and diarrhea; general ill feeling; fever. • Appetite and weight loss. • Abdominal tenderness; abdominal mass that can be felt. • Bloody stools (sometimes).	**CROHN'S DISEASE** (Refer to Illnesses section)
• Loss of interest in life; boredom. • Listlessness and fatigue. • Insomnia; excessive or disturbed sleeping. • Social isolation. • Appetite loss or overeating. • Loss of sex drive. • Constipation. • Difficulty making decisions and concentrating. • Unexplained crying bouts. • Intense guilt feelings over minor or imaginary misdeeds. • Irritability. • Various pains, such as headache or chest pain, without evidence of disease. • Anxiety or agitation. • Thoughts of death or suicide.	**DEPRESSION** (Refer to Illnesses section)
• Fatigue; excess thirst. • Increased appetite *and* weight loss. • Frequent urination. • Itching around the genitals. • Increased susceptibility to infections, especially urinary tract infections and yeast infections of the skin, mouth or vagina. • Deterioration of vision (advanced stages). • Loss of energy and easy fatiguability.	**DIABETES MELLITUS, INSULIN-DEPENDENT** (Refer to Illnesses section)
• Overweight. • Fatigue and loss of energy. • Excess thirst. • Increased appetite. • Frequent urination. • Decreased resistance to infection, especially urinary tract infections and yeast infections of the skin, mouth or vagina.	**DIABETES MELLITUS, NON-INSULIN-DEPENDENT** (Refer to Illnesses section)
• Chest pain. Pain varies from vague discomfort to stabbing pain. It is often worse with coughing or breathing. Pain may extend to the lower chest wall or abdomen. • Rapid, shallow breathing. • Chills. • Fever. • Extreme fatigue. • Bad breath. • Weight loss.	**EMPYEMA** (Refer to Illnesses section)
• Hard mass in the right upper abdomen. • Unexplained weight loss and appetite loss. • Jaundice (yellow skin and eyes) rarely. • Abdominal discomfort that resembles a pulled muscle. • Low blood sugar (weakness, sweating, hunger, tremor and headache). • Fever. • Fluid in the abdomen; enlarged spleen. • Bleeding tendency in the gastrointestinal tract and other sites.	**HEPATOMA** (Refer to Illnesses section)

(WEIGHT LOSS, continued on next page)

SYMPTOMS & FACTORS	POSSIBLE PROBLEM
• No symptoms in the early stages (frequently). • Bloody or black, tarry stools. • Cramping abdominal pain. • Feeling of fullness. • Change in bowel habits, such as diarrhea, constipation or narrow-caliber stools. • Unexplained weight loss. • Pain in the rectum. • Anemia. • Loss of bowel control (sometimes).	**LARGE INTESTINE, CANCER OF** (Refer to Illnesses section)
• Loss of appetite and weight loss. • Tender mass in the right upper abdomen. • Pain in the upper abdomen. • Low-grade fever, usually less than 101F or 38.3C. • Jaundice (yellow skin and eyes) sometimes. • Swollen abdomen from fluid retention (sometimes). • Mental status changes, such as confusion or forgetfulness.	**LIVER CANCER** (Refer to Illnesses section)
• Diarrhea. • Weakness. • Weight loss. • Gas and vague abdominal discomfort. • Bad-smelling, copious stools.	**MALABSORPTION** (Refer to Illnesses section)
• Hyperactivity. • Feeling warm or hot all the time. • Tremors. • Sweating. • Itching skin. • Pounding, rapid, irregular heartbeat. • Weight loss, despite overeating. • Marked anxiety and restlessness. • Sleeplessness. • Fatigue and weakness. • Protruding eyes (exophthalmos) and double vision (sometimes). • Diarrhea (sometimes). • Hair loss (sometimes). • Goiter (sometimes).	**THYROID, OVERACTIVE** (Refer to Illnesses section)
Early stages: • No symptoms (often). • Symptoms that resemble those of influenza. **Second stages:** • Low fever. • Weight loss. • Chronic fatigue. • Heavy sweating, especially at night. **Later stages:** • Cough with sputum that becomes progressively bloody, yellow, thick or gray. **(THIS IS AN EMERGENCY; SEEK MEDICAL CARE IMMEDIATELY!)** • Chest pain. • Shortness of breath. • Reddish or cloudy urine (sometimes).	**TUBERCULOSIS (TB)** (Refer to Illnesses section)

(WEIGHT LOSS, continued on next page)

(WEIGHT LOSS, continued from previous page)

SYMPTOMS & FACTORS	POSSIBLE PROBLEM
If you experience WEIGHT LOSS plus the following:	
• Use of prescription or non-prescription drugs.	**WHAT TO DO:** Discontinue non-prescription drugs and call doctor now regarding prescription drugs.
• Increased physical activity.	**WHAT TO DO:** Call doctor if excessive weight loss continues longer than 2 weeks.

WHEEZING

(Find your closest combination of symptoms in left-hand column; see possible problem in right-hand column. You may not experience all symptoms listed.)

SYMPTOMS & FACTORS	POSSIBLE PROBLEM
• Chest tightness and shortness of breath. Sense of suffocation. • Wheezing upon breathing out. • Coughing, especially at night, with little or no sputum. • Rapid, shallow breathing that is easier with sitting up. • Breathing difficulty—neck muscles tighten. **Severe symptoms of acute attack:** **(THIS IS AN EMERGENCY; SEEK EMERGENCY CARE IMMEDIATELY!)** • Bluish skin. • Exhaustion. • Grunting respiration. • Inability to speak. • Mental changes, including restlessness or confusion.	**ASTHMA** (Refer to Illnesses section)
• Cough that produces little or no sputum initially, but does later on. • Low fever (usually less than 101F or 38.3C). • Burning chest discomfort or feeling of pressure behind the breastbone. • Wheezing or uncomfortable breathing (sometimes).	**BRONCHITIS, ACUTE** (Refer to Illnesses section)
• Frequent cough or coughing spasms. • Shortness of breath. • Sputum that is thick and difficult to cough up. Sputum production varies according to whether infection is present. • Barrel chest (in the late stages). • Chest pain (rare).	**BRONCHITIS, CHRONIC** (Refer to Illnesses section)
• No symptoms in the early stages (often). • Shortness of breath that increases in severity over several years. • Wheezing and coughing that produces scant sputum. • Occasional recurrent infections of the lungs or bronchial tubes. • Barrel-shaped chest. • Swelling in legs and feet (edema).	**EMPHYSEMA** (Refer to Illnesses section)

(WHEEZING, continued on next page)

SYMPTOMS & FACTORS	POSSIBLE PROBLEM
The following symptoms often begin suddenly in the middle of the night and worsen rapidly: • Extreme shortness of breath, sometimes with wheezing. • Rapid breathing. • Restlessness and anxiety. • Paleness. • Sweating. • Bluish nails and lips. • Low blood pressure. • Cough. This may be unproductive at first, but later it can produce a frothy, blood-stained sputum.	**PULMONARY EDEMA** (Refer to Illnesses section) (THIS IS AN EMERGENCY; SEEK MEDICAL CARE IMMEDIATELY!)

If you experience WHEEZING plus the following:

• Use of prescription or non-prescription drugs.	**WHAT TO DO:** Discontinue non-prescription drugs and call doctor now regarding prescription drugs.
• Inhalation of chemicals.	**WHAT TO DO:** THIS IS AN EMERGENCY; SEEK MEDICAL CARE IMMEDIATELY!

Illnesses
&
Disorders

ACNE ROSACEA
("Adult Acne")

BASIC INFORMATION FOR OLDER ADULTS

DESCRIPTION—Acne rosacea is a chronic skin inflammation of the face. Severe nose involvement, mostly in older men, is called rhinophyma. Body part involved: The face, especially the nose and surrounding areas.

SPECIAL CONSIDERATIONS FOR AGING
- The skin is thinner and more easily damaged.
- The fatty layer of tissue under the skin becomes thinner.
- The circulation is less efficient.
- The capillaries are more fragile.
- The elasticity of the skin decreases.

SIGNS & SYMPTOMS
- Unsightly red, thickened skin on the nose and cheeks. Small blood vessels are visible on the skin's surface.
- Papules, (small raised bumps) and pustules (small white blisters with pus) on the affected skin (sometimes).

CAUSES & RISK FACTORS—The cause is unknown. The condition is worsened by stress, warm drinks, hot foods and alcohol. Risk factors include:
- Nervousness and stress.
- A fair complexion.
- Excessive alcohol consumption.
- Genetic predisposition.

DOCTOR'S TREATMENT & DIAGNOSTIC TESTS
- Medical history and physical exam.
- Self-care instructions focused on the older patient.
- Psychotherapy or counseling if disfigurement causes distress.
- Surgery to remove excess tissue (sometimes).

HOME TREATMENT BY SELF OR CARE-GIVER

GENERAL INSTRUCTIONS
- Seek care early if you notice evidence of acne rosacea.
- Don't use oil-based makeup.
- See Appendix 13 for suggestions to reduce stress.

MEDICATION (ADJUSTED FOR AGING)
- Your doctor may prescribe antibiotics or topical medications. These are effective for unknown reasons.
- Don't use cortisone preparations, including non-prescription preparations.

- *Note:* Adverse reactions and side effects may be more frequent and severe in older persons. Remind your doctor of any medicines you already take.

ACTIVITY FOR OLDER PATIENTS
- No restrictions are necessary.
- See Appendix 20 regarding physical fitness for the active older adult.

FOOD & BEVERAGE
- No special diet is required. Avoid spicy foods, alcohol or anything that causes the face to flush.
- See Appendix 1 regarding good nutrition for people over 50.

FUTURE CONSIDERATIONS FOR THE AGING ADULT

POSSIBLE COMPLICATIONS—Psychological distress caused by an unsightly appearance; autoimmune eye disorders (rare).

PROBABLE OUTCOME—The symptoms can be controlled with treatment. Acne rosacea is a disease of remissions and frequent flare-ups.

PREVENTING RECURRENCE—There are no specific preventive measures.

CALL YOUR DOCTOR IF

You have symptoms of acne rosacea.

ADDISON'S DISEASE
(Adrenal Insufficiency)

BASIC INFORMATION FOR OLDER ADULTS

DESCRIPTION—Addison's disease is a disease of the endocrine system caused by underactive adrenal glands. Body parts involved: The adrenal glands (located just above the kidneys).

SPECIAL CONSIDERATIONS FOR AGING
- All hormones are produced in reduced quantities.
- There is less efficient response to physical stress (fright and flight) due to the decreased responsiveness of the adrenal glands.

SIGNS & SYMPTOMS
- Weakness and fatigue; low blood pressure causing faintness and dizziness.
- Gastrointestinal disturbances (nausea, vomiting, abdominal pain, diarrhea and appetite and weight loss).
- Brownish skin (looks suntanned) with white patches; darkening of freckles, scars and breast nipples.
- Hair loss; feeling cold all the time.
- Dramatic behavior or mood changes, including aggression or depression.
- Confusion; coma.

CAUSES & RISK FACTORS—The signs and symptoms are caused by low levels of cortisone-like hormones produced by the adrenal glands. The cause of adrenal insufficiency is usually unknown but is sometimes a complication of:
- Tuberculosis; cancer; pituitary disease.
- The use of cortisone drugs for other conditions; when cortisone is withdrawn, normal adrenal function sometimes does not return.

The risk increases with:
- Stress; diabetes mellitus.
- Injury to the abdomen.

DOCTOR'S TREATMENT & DIAGNOSTIC TESTS
- "Before and after" pictures, which may emphasize the gradual skin change.
- Medical history and physical exam.
- Laboratory blood counts, blood and urine measurement of adrenal hormones and tests of adrenal gland function.
- Self-care instructions focused on the older patient.
- Hospitalization for an "adrenal crisis" (see Possible Complications).

HOME TREATMENT BY SELF OR CARE-GIVER

GENERAL INSTRUCTIONS—This is a lifelong condition. Learn how to care for yourself. Strict attention to medication schedules is vital.
- Learn about adrenal crisis and its relationship to body stress (infection, surgery or injury).
- Advise any doctor or dentist who treats you that you have Addison's disease.
- Wear a Medic Alert bracelet or pendant (see Glossary).
- Stay up-to-date on immunizations, including those for influenza and pneumonia.

MEDICATION (ADJUSTED FOR AGING)
- Your doctor will undoubtedly prescribe a cortisone drug. Follow the medication schedule exactly. Never change, omit or discontinue medication without your doctor's advice.
- *Note:* Adverse reactions and side effects may be more frequent and severe in older persons. Remind your doctor of any medicines you already take.

ACTIVITY FOR OLDER PATIENTS—No restrictions are necessary.

FOOD & BEVERAGE
- Consult your doctor about diet.
- See Appendix 1 regarding good nutrition for people over 50.

FUTURE CONSIDERATIONS FOR THE AGING ADULT

POSSIBLE COMPLICATIONS
- "Adrenal crisis" (pain, weakness, low blood pressure, high or low temperature and fainting) caused by any injury or illness.
- Misdiagnosis as a mental condition.

PROBABLE OUTCOME—The symptoms can be controlled with hormone replacement treatment. Addison's disease is fatal without treatment. The drugs used in treatment may produce side effects such as protruding abdomen, thin extremities, puffy face and eyes, acne and growth of facial hair.

PREVENTING RECURRENCE—Don't discontinue the use of cortisone drugs or change the dosage without consulting your doctor.

CALL YOUR DOCTOR IF

- You have symptoms of Addison's disease—especially an adrenal crisis. Call immediately. Adrenal crisis is an *emergency!*
- Any of the following occurs after diagnosis: Any signs of infection, such as fever, chills, muscle aches, headache and dizziness. Serious injury, such as bone fracture, dislocation or internal injuries.
- You are scheduled for elective surgery or require anesthesia for any reason.
- New, unexplained symptoms develop.

AIDS
(Acquired Immune Deficiency Syndrome)

BASIC INFORMATION FOR OLDER ADULTS

DESCRIPTION—AIDS represents a major failure of the body's immune system (immunodeficiency). This decreases the body's ability to fight infection and suppress the multiplication of abnormal cells, such as cancer. Body parts involved: The immune system, including special blood cells (lymphocytes) and the cells of some organs (the bone marrow, spleen, liver and lymph glands). When healthy, these cells manufacture antibodies to protect against disease and cancer.

SPECIAL CONSIDERATIONS FOR AGING
- Characteristic signs and symptoms of many disorders are frequently changed or absent, including those of AIDS.
- The immune system becomes less effective, opening the way for viral, bacterial and other infections; malignancies; immune disorders; and allergies.

SIGNS & SYMPTOMS
- Fatigue; unexplained weight loss.
- Recurrent respiratory and skin infections.
- Fever; swollen lymph glands throughout the body.
- Genital changes; an enlarged spleen.
- Diarrhea; night sweats.
- Positive laboratory tests.
- Progression of the illness to the development of opportunistic infections (pneumocystic pneumonia or cytomegalovirus infections) or secondary cancers, such as Kaposi's sarcoma and non-Hodgkin's lymphoma.

CAUSES & RISK FACTORS—AIDS is caused by the human immunodeficiency virus (HIV), a newly identified virus (retrovirus) that invades and destroys cells of the immune system, resulting in lowered resistance to infections and some types of cancer. The virus is transmitted by:
- Any sexual contact with an affected person; statistically the risk is much higher in homosexual or bisexual men.
- The use of contaminated needles for intravenous drug use.
- Transfusions of blood or blood products from a person with acquired immune deficiency syndrome.
Note: Day-to-day non-sexual contact does *not* transmit the disease, so a person with AIDS is not a danger to the general population.
The risk of contracting AIDS increases with:
- Multiple homosexual or bisexual sexual partners.
- Multiple heterosexual partners (less likely than with homosexual or bisexual partners).
- Sexual activity with IV drug users.
- Exposure of hospital workers and laboratory technicians to the blood, feces and urine of HIV-positive patients.

DOCTOR'S TREATMENT & DIAGNOSTIC TESTS
- Medical history and physical exam.

- Laboratory studies of blood cells, HIV antibodies test (may not become positive for 6 months after contact) and Western blot test.
- Psychotherapy or counseling to help you cope with anxiety and depression about having the disease and the likelihood of death.
- Hospitalization. Medical schools may provide some free care if you are willing to participate in research.

HOME TREATMENT BY SELF OR CARE-GIVER

GENERAL INSTRUCTIONS—Early diagnosis is helpful. If you are at risk, obtain a medical evaluation—even if you feel well. Contact social agencies in your area about AIDS support groups.

MEDICATION (ADJUSTED FOR AGING)
- Drugs are currently not effective in curing AIDS. However, new drug therapies are under development and some have been found to be effective in treating or managing this chronic disease.
- Your doctor may prescribe antibiotics to prevent infections or control them as they develop; antiviral drugs, such as zidovudine (AZT), to slow progression of the disease.

ACTIVITY FOR OLDER PATIENTS—No restrictions are necessary on normal activity, but refrain from unprotected sexual encounters.

FOOD & BEVERAGE—No special diet.

FUTURE CONSIDERATIONS FOR THE AGING ADULT

POSSIBLE COMPLICATIONS—Serious infection in various body systems; cancer.

PROBABLE OUTCOME—This condition is currently considered incurable. However, the symptoms can be relieved or controlled. AIDS may not develop for years following a positive HIV test. Once a person is ill, survival time averages 2-1/2 years, but it may be shorter or longer.

PREVENTING RECURRENCE—Since AIDS is presently incurable, the main concern is to avoid transmitting it to others. Follow these suggestions:
- Use condoms for all sexual activity.
- Avoid intravenous self-administered drugs.
- Don't donate blood to blood banks.

CALL YOUR DOCTOR IF

- You have symptoms of AIDS.
- Infection occurs after diagnosis. The symptoms include fever, cough, diarrhea, skin rash or eruption or a general ill feeling.

ALCOHOLISM

BASIC INFORMATION FOR OLDER ADULTS

DESCRIPTION—Alcoholism is a psychological and physiological dependence on alcohol that results in chronic disease and disruption of inter-personal, family and work relationships. There are more males than females who demonstrate alcoholism. Body parts involved: The brain, central nervous system, liver and heart.

SPECIAL CONSIDERATIONS FOR AGING
- Older adults absorb alcohol more completely.
- Potential for addiction is greater.
- There is more likelihood of denial that there is a problem.

SIGNS & SYMPTOMS
Early stages:
- A low tolerance for anxiety.
- A need for alcohol at the beginning of the day or at times of stress.
- Insomnia; nightmares.
- Habitual Monday-morning hangovers and frequent absences from work.
- Preoccupation with obtaining alcohol and hiding drinking from family and friends.
- Guilt or irritability when others suggest drinking is excessive.

Late stages:
- Frequent blackouts; memory loss.
- Delirium tremens (tremors; hallucinations; confusion; sweating; rapid heartbeat). These occur most often with alcohol withdrawal.
- Liver disease (jaundice; internal bleeding; bloating).
- Neurological impairment (numbness and tingling in hands and feet; declining sexual interest and potency; confusion; coma).
- Congestive heart failure (shortness of breath; swelling of feet).

CAUSES & RISK FACTORS—The causes are not fully understood but include personality factors, especially dependency, anger, mania, depression, introversion or psychiatric disorders; family influences, especially alcoholic parents; social and cultural pressures to drink; the availability and affordability of alcohol; and body chemistry disturbances (hormonal in women). The risk factors increase with genetic factors (some ethnic groups have high alcoholism rates for either social or biological reasons); the use of recreational drugs; and crisis situations, including unemployment, frequent moves or loss of friends or family members.

DOCTOR'S TREATMENT & DIAGNOSTIC TESTS
- Medical history and physical exam.
- Laboratory studies of blood and liver function.
- EEG (see Glossary).
- Self-care instructions focused on the older patient. The first and most difficult step of treatment is admitting that the problem exists.
- Psychotherapy or counseling.

OTHER—Some employers and health insurance companies pay for treatment.

HOME TREATMENT BY SELF OR CARE-GIVER

GENERAL INSTRUCTIONS
- Keep appointments with doctors and counselors.
- Join a local Alcoholics Anonymous group (see Resources section) and attend regularly.
- Reassess your lifestyle—your friends, work and family—to identify and alter factors that encourage drinking.

MEDICATION (ADJUSTED FOR AGING)
- Your doctor may prescribe disulfiram (Antabuse), which causes several extremely unpleasant physical symptoms when alcohol is consumed.
- *Note:* Adverse reactions and side effects may be more frequent and severe in older persons. Remind your doctor of any medicines you already take.

ACTIVITY FOR OLDER PATIENTS—Don't drink and drive.

FOOD & BEVERAGE
- Eat a normal, well-balanced diet. Vitamin supplements, such as thiamine and folic acid, are often necessary.
- See Appendix 1 regarding good nutrition for people over 50.

FUTURE CONSIDERATIONS FOR THE AGING ADULT

POSSIBLE COMPLICATIONS—Chronic liver disease; gastric erosion with bleeding; stomach inflammation; neuritis, tremors, seizures and brain impairment; inflammation of the pancreas; inflammation of the heart; family members of alcoholics may develop psychological symptoms requiring treatment and support from groups such as Al-Anon.

PROBABLE OUTCOME
Without treatment:
- Progressive brain and liver disease.
- Job loss, divorce and criminal behavior.
- Painful, premature death.

With treatment:
- Alcoholism is often controllable.
- Sexual function improves markedly.

PREVENTING RECURRENCE
- Use alcohol in moderation—if at all.
- Encourage a spouse, friend or co-worker to admit when an alcohol problem exists and seek professional care.

CALL YOUR DOCTOR IF

You or a family member has symptoms of alcoholism.

ALDOSTERONE, EXCESSIVE
(Hyperaldosteronism; Conn's Syndrome)

BASIC INFORMATION FOR OLDER ADULTS

DESCRIPTION—Hyperaldosteronism is a disease of the endocrine system caused by the overproduction of aldosterone, a hormone manufactured by the adrenal glands. Excessive aldosterone causes the kidneys to absorb too much sodium and water and eliminate too much potassium. Body parts involved: The adrenal glands (attached to the upper part of the kidneys), the kidneys and the fluids and electrolytes in the bloodstream and body cells.

SPECIAL CONSIDERATIONS FOR AGING
- The immune system becomes less effective, opening the way for viral, bacterial and other infections; malignancies; immune disorders; and allergies.
- Disease in one organ system leads to problems in another system.
- Incidence of illness and disability increases.

SIGNS & SYMPTOMS
- Fatigue and weakness.
- Temporary paralysis (sometimes).
- Tingling sensations in the arms, legs, hands and feet.
- Urinary frequency, especially at night.
- Thirst.
- Severe muscle spasms.
- Vision disturbances.

CAUSES & RISK FACTORS—Caused by the increased adrenal secretion of aldosterone due to:
- A tumor of the adrenal gland (usually benign).
- High blood pressure or kidney disease causing increased production in the kidneys of a hormone (renin) that controls aldosterone levels.
Risk factors include:
- A diet that contains large amounts of licorice.
- Kidney disease.
- Congestive heart failure.
- Cirrhosis of the liver.
- The use of diuretic drugs that cause potassium loss.

DOCTOR'S TREATMENT & DIAGNOSTIC TESTS
- Medical history and physical exam.
- Laboratory blood studies of electrolyte levels.
- ECG (see Glossary).
- Surgical diagnostic procedures, such as laparoscopy (see Glossary).
- X-rays of the kidneys.
- CT scan (see Glossary) of the kidneys.
- Self-care instructions focused on the older patient.
- Hospitalization.
- Surgery to examine the adrenal glands and remove any tumors. Advancing age alone is not a deterrent.

HOME TREATMENT BY SELF OR CARE-GIVER

GENERAL INSTRUCTIONS
- Weigh daily and keep a record. Report a gain of 3 or more pounds in a 24-hour period.
- Wear a Medic Alert bracelet or pendant (see Glossary).

MEDICATION (ADJUSTED FOR AGING)
- Your doctor may prescribe:
Cortisone drugs to replace adrenal hormones if the adrenal gland is removed. This is essential for life. Don't discontinue or change your dose without consulting your doctor. Spironolactone to decrease the aldosterone effect if surgery is not performed. This drug may cause breast enlargement and sexual impotence in men.
- *Note:* Adverse reactions and side effects may be more frequent and severe in older persons. Remind your doctor of any medicines you already take.

ACTIVITY FOR OLDER PATIENTS
- No restrictions are necessary if surgery is not necessary. If it is, resume your normal activities gradually.
- See Appendix 20 regarding physical fitness for the active older adult.

FOOD & BEVERAGE—Eat a diet that is low in sodium (see Appendix 9) and high in potassium. Foods rich in potassium include dried apricots and peaches, raisins, citrus fruits, lentils and whole-grain cereals. Don't eat licorice.

FUTURE CONSIDERATIONS FOR THE AGING ADULT

POSSIBLE COMPLICATIONS—Congestive heart failure; atherosclerosis; kidney failure.

PROBABLE OUTCOME—If the disorder is caused by an adrenal tumor, it is usually curable with surgery. If it is caused by kidney disease or high blood pressure, medical treatment for these disorders will control the symptoms of hyperaldosteronism.

PREVENTING RECURRENCE—If you have kidney disease or high blood pressure, remain under a doctor's care and adhere strictly to your treatment program—even if you have no symptoms.

CALL YOUR DOCTOR IF

- You have symptoms of excessive aldosterone.
- New, unexplained symptoms develop. The drugs used in treatment may produce side effects.

ALTITUDE ILLNESS

BASIC INFORMATION FOR OLDER ADULTS

DESCRIPTION—Altitude illness is any of several illnesses associated with higher-than-usual altitudes. These illnesses are of several types, including:
- Acute mountain sickness (AMS).
- High-altitude pulmonary edema (HAPE).
- High-altitude cerebral edema (HACE).
- High-altitude retinal hemorrhage (HARH).
- Subacute and chronic mountain sickness (CMS), a complication that represents failure to recover from AMS over a long period of time.

Body parts involved: These illnesses affect most body systems, especially the brain, heart, lungs, gastrointestinal tract, circulatory system and electrolytes. Other altitude-related problems include frostbite, blood clots in the legs and lungs, dehydration and swollen feet and ankles. Pre-existing illnesses that are aggravated by high altitude include sickle-cell disease or trait, chronic heart disease and chronic lung disease.

SPECIAL CONSIDERATIONS FOR AGING
- The vital capacity of the lungs decreases and the transfer of carbon dioxide and oxygen to the bloodstream becomes less efficient.
- Obstruction of the airways becomes more common, especially among people who have smoked tobacco for many years.
- The muscles used for breathing weaken.

SIGNS & SYMPTOMS
- AMS—Headache, nausea, vomiting, shortness of breath and sleep disturbances.
- HAPE—Shortness of breath, cough, weakness, headache and coma.
- HACE—Severe headache, staggering gait, hallucinations and stupor. These indicate swelling of the brain. Death will occur without descent.
- HARH—Visual disturbances, including spots before the eyes. Blood clots and bleeding into the retina occur in 50% of those who go above 17,000 feet.
- CMS—Shortness of breath, fatigue, bloated face and body and congestive heart failure after years of living at high altitude (rare).

CAUSES & RISK FACTORS—Insufficient oxygen at high altitudes. Following are the altitudes at which each type of illness can occur:
- AMS—7,000 to 8,000 feet or higher.
- HAPE—9,000 to 10,000 feet.
- HACE—10,000 to 12,000 feet.
- HARH—17,000 feet.

Additional factors that contribute to development of altitude illness include:
- Fatigue or overwork.
- Previous episodes of altitude illness.
- Chronic illness of any sort, particularly cardiovascular and lung diseases.
- Obesity; excessive alcohol consumption.
- The use of mind-altering drugs, including narcotics and tranquilizers.

DOCTOR'S TREATMENT & DIAGNOSTIC TESTS
- Medical history and physical exam.
- Laboratory blood studies and urinalysis.
- ECG (see Glossary); x-rays of the lungs.
- PET scan (see Glossary); radioactive studies with a gamma emissions camera.
- Self-care instructions focused on the older patient.
- Follow-up outpatient visits to monitor progress and adjustment to treatment.
- Hospitalization (in severe cases).

HOME TREATMENT BY SELF OR CARE-GIVER

GENERAL INSTRUCTIONS
- AMS—Descend to lower altitude if illness lasts 2 or more days.
- HAPE—Oxygen, rest and diuretics help, but rapid descent is usually necessary.
- HACE—Oxygen and corticosteroids help, but rapid descent to lower altitudes is the only certain way to recover.
- HARH—There is no treatment except to descend.
- CMS—Return to lower altitudes if the symptoms persist.

MEDICATION (ADJUSTED FOR AGING)—
Your doctor may prescribe:
- For AMS—Diamox (a carbonic anhydrase inhibitor).
- For HAPE—Oxygen; furosemide (a diuretic); morphine (a narcotic pain reliever).
- For HACE—Corticosteroids.

ACTIVITY FOR OLDER PATIENTS—If any altitude illness occurs, decrease activity until the symptoms disappear. Resume your normal activities gradually upon returning to a normal altitude.

FOOD & BEVERAGE—No special diet is required.

FUTURE CONSIDERATIONS FOR THE AGING ADULT

POSSIBLE COMPLICATIONS—Permanent brain, eye, heart and lung damage. Worst cases of HAPE and HACE can lead to death.

PROBABLE OUTCOME—Usually curable without residual impairment after returning to lower altitudes.

PREVENTING RECURRENCE—Don't ascend to heights that cause symptoms. Get complete physical exam and full instructions before planning to be at any elevation you are not accustomed to. Heart, lungs and musculoskeletal systems must be healthy to sustain even minimal activity at high altitude.

CALL YOUR DOCTOR IF

- You have symptoms of any altitude illness.
- New, unexplained symptoms develop. Drugs used in treatment may produce side effects.

ALZHEIMER'S DISEASE
(Alzheimer-Type Dementia; Presenile Dementia)

BASIC INFORMATION FOR OLDER ADULTS

DESCRIPTION—Alzheimer's disease is a brain disorder similar to senile dementia that is characterized by gradual mental deterioration. A rapidly progressive form begins in adults around ages 36 to 45. A more gradual form, with slow development of symptoms, begins around ages 65 to 70. Other disorders with similar signs and symptoms include chronic organic brain syndrome (associated with small clots to the brain or toxic reactions to drugs), advanced syphilis, stroke, brain tumor, or hypothyroidism. These disorders may be treatable. Alzheimer's disease is not. Body part involved: The brain.

SPECIAL CONSIDERATIONS FOR AGING
- Neurological diseases become more likely.
- 60% of patients with Alzheimer's are 55 or older.

SIGNS & SYMPTOMS
Early stages:
- Forgetfulness of recent events.
- Increasing difficulty performing intellectual tasks such as accustomed work, balancing a checkbook or maintaining a household.
- Personality changes, including narrow range of interest, rigidness in views or beliefs, distrust, restlessness, poor impulse control and poor judgment.
Later stages:
- Difficulty doing simple tasks such as choosing clothing and solving problems.
- Failure to recognize familiar persons.
- Disinterest in personal hygiene or appearance.
- Difficulty feeding oneself.
- Belligerence and denial that anything is wrong.
- Loss of usual sexual inhibitions.
Advanced stages:
- Complete loss of memory, speech and muscle function (including bladder and bowel control) necessitating total care and supervision.
- Extreme belligerence and hostility.
- Sleeplessness.

CAUSES & RISK FACTORS—Caused by irreversible damage to or loss of brain cells for unknown reasons. The risk increases with a family history of Alzheimer's disease.

DOCTOR'S TREATMENT & DIAGNOSTIC TESTS
- Medical history and physical exam.
- X-rays of the brain, including a CT scan or MRI (see Glossary for both) to rule out other conditions.
- Psychotherapy or counseling for family members.
- Care-giver instructions.
- Nursing home care when home care becomes impossible.

HOME TREATMENT BY SELF OR CARE-GIVER

GENERAL INSTRUCTIONS
- If a family member has this disease, don't take his or her hostility personally.
- If you care for a family member with this disease, try to obtain help so you can get away often. Don't feel guilty about needing a respite—even if the patient resents it. A day-care center can provide relief.
- Join or start a support group for families of Alzheimer's victims (see Resources section).
- Beware of persons offering treatments for large sums of money. No legitimate treatment currently exists.

MEDICATION (ADJUSTED FOR AGING)—No medication is currently available to treat Alzheimer's disease, but many medications are being studied. Some are useful to control symptoms such as agitation or sleeplessness.

ACTIVITY FOR OLDER PATIENTS
- Stay as active as possible.
- As the condition progresses, all activity will eventually require supervision.

FOOD & BEVERAGE
- Choline and lecithin supplements are under study. Feeding assistance will eventually be necessary.
- See Appendix 1 regarding good nutrition for people over 50.

FUTURE CONSIDERATIONS FOR THE AGING ADULT

POSSIBLE COMPLICATIONS
- Decreased resistance to infections, especially pneumonia and meningitis.
- Seizures and coma (rare).

PROBABLE OUTCOME—This condition is currently considered incurable and untreatable. It is usually fatal within 5 years without skillful care. Scientific research into causes and treatment continues, so there is hope for eventual treatment and cure.

PREVENTING RECURRENCE—There are no specific preventive measures.

CALL YOUR DOCTOR IF

- You or some family member has symptoms of Alzheimer's disease.
- Signs of infection occur, such as fever, chills, muscle aches or headache.
- You care for someone with Alzheimer's disease and you fear you are about to lose emotional control.

AMOEBA INFECTIONS

BASIC INFORMATION FOR OLDER ADULTS

DESCRIPTION—Amoeba infections are parasitic infections of the large intestine. Body parts involved: The intestinal tract (especially the colon) and the liver (sometimes).

SPECIAL CONSIDERATIONS FOR AGING
- The immune system becomes less effective, opening the way for viral, bacterial and other infections; malignancies; immune disorders; and allergies.
- Usual signs and symptoms may be absent and be replaced by symptoms of confusion, dizziness, failure to thrive, falling, incontinence, increasing dementia, refusal to eat or drink, weight loss, depression, paranoia, hypochondriasis, psychosis or threats of suicide.

SIGNS & SYMPTOMS
- Intermittent diarrhea with bad-smelling and sometimes bloody stools. Diarrhea is often preceded by constipation in early stages.
- Gas and abdominal bloating.
- Severe abdominal cramps and tenderness.
- Fever over 101F.
- Mucus and blood in the stool (sometimes).
- Fatigue.
- Muscle and joint aches.

If the liver is involved:
- Tenderness over the liver and right side of the abdomen.
- Jaundice (sometimes).

CAUSES & RISK FACTORS—Amoeba
infections are caused by a microscopic parasite that is spread by flies, cockroaches and direct contact with hands or food contaminated with feces. The most common sources of infection are food handlers, faulty hotel or factory plumbing and raw vegetables or fruit fertilized with human feces or washed in polluted water. The risk increases with crowded or unsanitary living conditions, travel to a foreign country and a combination of anal and oral sex.

DOCTOR'S TREATMENT & DIAGNOSTIC TESTS
- Medical history and physical exam.
- Laboratory studies of stool and blood serum.
- Sigmoidoscopy (see Glossary).
- X-rays of the lower bowel (barium enema).
- Self-care instructions focused on the older patient.
- Hospitalization (in severe cases only).

OTHER—Many people—especially those who live in temperate climates—harbor the amoeba without symptoms. Symptoms occur when the parasite invades tissues of the colon. The symptoms may be very vague.

HOME TREATMENT BY SELF OR CARE-GIVER

GENERAL INSTRUCTIONS—Be extra careful about personal cleanliness. Bathe frequently, and wash your hands with warm water and soap after each bowel movement and before handling food.

MEDICATION (ADJUSTED FOR AGING)—Your doctor may prescribe anti-amoeba medication such as metronidazole.

ACTIVITY FOR OLDER PATIENTS
- Rest in bed during an acute attack. Resume your normal activities when fever disappears and diarrhea improves.
- See Appendix 20 regarding physical fitness for the active older adult.

FOOD & BEVERAGE
- Consume a soft diet progressing to a normal diet.
- See Appendix 1 regarding good nutrition for people over 50.

FUTURE CONSIDERATIONS FOR THE AGING ADULT

POSSIBLE COMPLICATIONS—Peritonitis; hepatitis or liver abscess; lung abscess; infection of the pericardium; brain abscess.

PROBABLE OUTCOME—In most cases without complications, amoeba infections are curable in 3 weeks with treatment. In the carrier state, this disease may not cause any symptoms. In severe cases, it may cause dysentery that requires hospital treatment.

PREVENTING RECURRENCE
- Wash your hands frequently—*always* before eating.
- If you are in an area where food or water may be contaminated, the following measures are necessary:
  Boil drinking water for 10 to 20 minutes.
  Don't use water that may contain raw sewage for any purpose.
  Don't eat unpeeled fruit or vegetables or raw fish or shellfish.

CALL YOUR DOCTOR IF

- You have symptoms of an amoeba infection.
- The following occur during treatment:
  The abdominal cramps continue longer than 24 hours.
  The diarrhea or blood in the stool increases.
  Vomiting begins.
  Pain begins over the liver or jaundice occurs.
  A skin rash appears.
  Irritability or a severe headache develops.

ILLNESSES & DISORDERS

AMYOTROPHIC LATERAL SCLEROSIS
(ALS; Lou Gehrig's Disease)

BASIC INFORMATION FOR OLDER ADULTS

DESCRIPTION—ALS is a progressive breakdown of the cells of the spinal cord resulting in gradual loss of muscle function. This is not contagious or cancerous and is more common in men. The symptoms may be confused with neurologic complications of Lyme disease. Body parts involved: The central nervous system and the muscle system, especially in the hands, forearms, legs, head and neck.

SPECIAL CONSIDERATIONS FOR AGING
- Neurological diseases become more likely.
- Usual signs and symptoms may be absent and be replaced by symptoms of confusion, falling, weakness and weight loss.
- Symptoms usually appear between ages 50 and 70.

SIGNS & SYMPTOMS—Symptoms appear in the following order:
- Muscle twitching and weakness that begin in the hands and spread to the arms, shoulders and legs. The weakness eventually affects the muscles that control breathing and swallowing.
- Stiffening, cramps and spasticity of various muscle groups.
- Altered speech.
- Involuntary laughing or crying.

CAUSES & RISK FACTORS—The cause is unknown. It is sometimes genetically linked (in fewer than 5% of cases).

DOCTOR'S TREATMENT & DIAGNOSTIC TESTS
- Medical history and physical exam.
- Laboratory studies such as electromyography and muscle biopsy (see Glossary for both).
- Self-care instructions focused on the older patient.
- Psychotherapy or counseling to help you learn to cope with disability.
- Eventual hospitalization or nursing home care.

HOME TREATMENT BY SELF OR CARE-GIVER

GENERAL INSTRUCTIONS—Obtain good nursing care to prevent pressure sores.

MEDICATION (ADJUSTED FOR AGING)
- Your doctor may prescribe antibiotics to fight infection if pneumonia develops.
- *Note:* Adverse reactions and side effects may be more frequent and severe in older persons. Remind your doctor of any medicines you already take.

ACTIVITY FOR OLDER PATIENTS
- Stay as active as possible. Weakness will gradually limit your capability.
- See Appendix 20 regarding physical fitness for the active older adult.

FOOD & BEVERAGE
- Eat soft, easy-to-swallow foods. See Appendix 11.
- See Appendix 1 regarding good nutrition for people over 50.

FUTURE CONSIDERATIONS FOR THE AGING ADULT

POSSIBLE COMPLICATIONS
- Pressure sores caused by immobility.
- Pneumonia caused by swallowing difficulty and choking.

PROBABLE OUTCOME—This condition is currently considered incurable. The intelligence and awareness don't become impaired. It is usually fatal within 20 years. However, the pain can be relieved or controlled. Scientific research into causes and treatment continues, so there is hope for increasingly effective treatment and a cure.

PREVENTING RECURRENCE—Cannot be prevented at present.

CALL YOUR DOCTOR IF

- You have symptoms of amyotrophic lateral sclerosis.
- Coughing, choking or fever occurs after diagnosis.

ANAL FISSURE

BASIC INFORMATION FOR OLDER ADULTS

DESCRIPTION—An anal fissure represents a splitting or tearing of sensitive anal tissue. Body part involved: The anus.

SPECIAL CONSIDERATIONS FOR AGING
- Constipation is much more frequent.
- The skin becomes dryer and rougher.
- The fatty layer of tissue under the skin becomes thinner.

SIGNS & SYMPTOMS
- Sharp pain with the passage of a hard or bulky stool.
- Streaks of blood on toilet paper or underwear.
- Itching around the rectum.

CAUSES & RISK FACTORS—Caused by the stretching of the anus by a large, hard stool. The risk increases with:
- Constipation.
- Multiple pregnancies.
- The use of rectal thermometers or enema nozzles.

DOCTOR'S TREATMENT & DIAGNOSTIC TESTS
- Medical history and physical exam.
- Examination of the anus and rectum with an anoscope or sigmoidoscope to rule out other causes of anal or rectal bleeding.
- Self-care instructions focused on the older patient.
- Surgery (sometimes) to remove the fissure or to alter the muscle that contracts and prevents normal healing.

HOME TREATMENT BY SELF OR CARE-GIVER

GENERAL INSTRUCTIONS
- To relieve muscle spasms and pain around the anus, apply a warm towel to the area.
- Sitz baths also relieve pain. Use 8 inches of very warm water 2 or 3 times a day for 10 to 20 minutes.

MEDICATION (ADJUSTED FOR AGING)
- For minor pain, you may use non-prescription drugs such as acetaminophen or topical anesthetics.
- After sitz baths, apply a non-prescription ointment containing zinc oxide to help heal the fissure.
- *Note:* Adverse reactions and side effects may be more frequent and severe in older persons. Remind your doctor of any medicines you already take.

ACTIVITY FOR OLDER PATIENTS
- No restrictions are necessary. Physical activity reduces the likelihood of constipation.
- See Appendix 20 regarding physical fitness for the active older adult.

FOOD & BEVERAGE
- Eat a high-fiber diet and drink extra fluids to prevent constipation.
- See Appendix 1 regarding good nutrition for people over 50.

FUTURE CONSIDERATIONS FOR THE AGING ADULT

POSSIBLE COMPLICATIONS—Permanent scarring that prevents normal bowel movements.

PROBABLE OUTCOME—Most adults recover with treatment, making surgery unnecessary.

PREVENTING RECURRENCE
- Avoid constipation by:
  Drinking at least 8 glasses of water daily.
  Eating a diet high in fiber.
  Using stool softeners or other laxatives if needed.
- Don't strain when having a bowel movement.

CALL YOUR DOCTOR IF

You have symptoms of an anal fissure—especially pain—that persists despite treatment.

ANAL ITCHING
(Pruritus Ani)

BASIC INFORMATION FOR OLDER ADULTS

DESCRIPTION—Anal itching is itching around the anus and genitals. Body parts involved: The anus; the scrotum in men.

SPECIAL CONSIDERATIONS FOR AGING
- The responsiveness of the skin's immune system decreases.
- The skin becomes thinner.
- Stress from any emotional cause—fear, worry, anxiety, sadness, loneliness or anger—affects all aspects of any illness or disorder.

SIGNS & SYMPTOMS—Itching, often intense and worse at night.

CAUSES & RISK FACTORS
Causes include:
- Coffee (sometimes).
- A yeast infection.
- Contact dermatitis caused by soaps, contraceptive foams or jellies, perfumed toilet paper, deodorant sprays, douches or underwear made of synthetic fabric.
- Various skin disorders, including psoriasis or seborrheic dermatitis.
- Chronic diarrhea.
- Excessive wiping with toilet paper.
- Tight, warm clothing.
- Unknown (often).
Risk factors include:
- Stress.
- Diabetes mellitus.
- Excessive sweating.

DOCTOR'S TREATMENT & DIAGNOSTIC TESTS
- Medical history and physical exam.
- Laboratory studies such as cultures for fungi or microscopic examinations for pinworm eggs or scabies in skin burrows.
- Self-care instructions focused on the older patient.
- Doctor's treatment if self-care is not successful within 2 weeks.

HOME TREATMENT BY SELF OR CARE-GIVER

GENERAL INSTRUCTIONS
- Keep showers or baths brief to minimize dryness and soap irritation. Use plain, unscented soap—if any—and warm water instead of hot.
- Keep the rectal area clean, dry and cool. Wear loose clothing and underclothing. Clean carefully after bowel movements, using moist tufts of cotton. For mild cases, use petroleum jelly after wiping.

- Don't use irritants listed as causes.
- Wear underwear with a cotton crotch or underwear made of cotton rather than nylon or other synthetics.
- A woman may pour a glass of warm water over the genitals when urinating to relieve the burning sensation.

MEDICATION (ADJUSTED FOR AGING)
- You may use non-prescription cortisone ointment or cream. Apply it 3 times a day and rub it in gently until it disappears.
- Use a mild laxative for constipation.
- Your doctor may prescribe:
  More potent topical cortisone drugs.
  Zinc oxide.
- *Note:* Adverse reactions and side effects may be more frequent and severe in older persons. Remind your doctor of any medicines you already take.

ACTIVITY FOR OLDER PATIENTS
- Avoid activities that cause excessive perspiration.
- See Appendix 20 regarding physical fitness for the active older adult.

FOOD & BEVERAGE
- Avoid spicy or highly seasoned foods. These irritate the mucous membranes of the anus.
- See Appendix 1 regarding good nutrition for people over 50.

FUTURE CONSIDERATIONS FOR THE AGING ADULT

POSSIBLE COMPLICATIONS
- Skin damage that allows a secondary bacterial infection to develop.
- Skin thickening and chronic inflammation.
- Fatigue from chronic sleep disturbance.
- In women, anal itching may spread to the vulva.

PROBABLE OUTCOME—The symptoms can be controlled with treatment, even if the cause cannot be determined.

PREVENTING RECURRENCE
- Keep the body clean with regular showers or baths.
- Cleanse carefully after bowel movements with moistened cotton or tissue.
- Avoid contact with substances to which you are sensitive (see Causes).

CALL YOUR DOCTOR IF

- You have symptoms of anal itching that persist despite self-care.
- You develop a fever.
- The irritated area seems infected.

ANAPHYLAXIS
(Allergic Shock)

BASIC INFORMATION FOR OLDER ADULTS

DESCRIPTION—Anaphylaxis is a severe allergic response to medications and many other allergy-causing substances. Body parts involved: The blood vessels and the heart, lungs and skin. **(THIS IS AN EMERGENCY; SEEK MEDICAL CARE IMMEDIATELY!)**

SPECIAL CONSIDERATIONS FOR AGING
- Serious allergies are less likely to occur.
- There is less efficient response to physical stress (fright and flight) due to the decreased responsiveness of the adrenal glands.

SIGNS & SYMPTOMS—Any of the following may occur within seconds or a few minutes after exposure to a substance to which you are very allergic:
- Tingling or numbness around the mouth.
- Sneezing; watery eyes.
- Itching all over, particularly on the soles and palms and often accompanied by hives.
- Redness around ears resembling recent sunburn.
- Tightness in the chest; difficult breathing; coughing.
- Swelling or itching in the mouth or throat.
- Pounding heart; faintness; shivering; dilated pupils; loss of consciousness.

Not all symptoms occur in every case. Seek immediate help for any.

CAUSES & RISK FACTORS—Caused by eating or receiving injections of something to which you are sensitive. The allergic response to neutralize or get rid of the material results in a life-threatening overreaction. Things which cause reactions most often include medications of all types, especially penicillin, iron dextran, hormones and antiserum (injections are much riskier than oral medications); stings or bites from insects such as bees, biting ants and some spiders; injected chemicals used in some types of x-ray studies; foods, especially eggs, beans, seafood and fruit. The risk increases with:
- A previous mild allergic response to any of the things listed above.
- A medical history of eczema, hay fever or asthma.

DOCTOR'S TREATMENT & DIAGNOSTIC TESTS
- Medical history and physical exam.
- Laboratory skin tests to determine sensitivities.

HOME TREATMENT BY SELF OR CARE-GIVER

GENERAL INSTRUCTIONS
- If you observe signs of anaphylaxis in someone and he or she stops breathing: Yell for help. Don't leave the victim. Begin mouth-to-mouth breathing immediately.

If there is no heartbeat, give external cardiac massage.
Have someone call 0 (operator) or 911 (emergency) for an ambulance or medical help. Don't stop CPR until help arrives.
- Be alert to the possibility of a reaction when taking any medicine, and be prepared to respond quickly if symptoms occur. If you have had a previous severe allergic reaction, always carry your anaphylaxis kit.

MEDICATION (ADJUSTED FOR AGING)
- Adrenalin by injection is the only pharmacologically effective immediate treatment. Antihistamines help, but less dramatically.
- Aminophylline, cortisone drugs or antihistamines given after the adrenalin help prevent the return of acute symptoms.
- *Note:* Adverse reactions and side effects may be more frequent and severe in older persons. Remind your doctor of any medicines you already take.

ACTIVITY FOR OLDER PATIENTS—Resume your normal activities as soon as your symptoms improve after an attack. Stay under someone's observation for 24 hours in case the symptoms recur.

FOOD & BEVERAGE—Avoid foods to which you are allergic.

FUTURE CONSIDERATIONS FOR THE AGING ADULT

POSSIBLE COMPLICATIONS—Without prompt treatment, anaphylaxis causes shock, cardiac arrest and death.

PROBABLE OUTCOME—Full recovery with prompt treatment.

PREVENTING RECURRENCE
If you have an allergic history:
- Tell your doctor before accepting any medication. Before you are given a shot, ask what it is.
- Keep an anaphylaxis kit with you at all times. Be sure your family knows how to use the kit if you have a reaction.
- Wear a Medic Alert (see Glossary) bracelet or pendant warning that you are allergic.
- Always remain in your doctor's office 15 minutes after receiving any injection. Report any symptoms immediately.

CALL YOUR DOCTOR IF

- You have symptoms of anaphylaxis. *This is an emergency!*
- New, unexplained symptoms develop. The drugs used in treatment may produce side effects.

ANEMIA, APLASTIC

BASIC INFORMATION FOR OLDER ADULTS

DESCRIPTION—Aplastic anemia is a serious disease characterized by decreased bone marrow production of blood cells. It is more common in males. Body parts involved: The bone marrow, the lymphatic system and the blood.

SPECIAL CONSIDERATIONS FOR AGING
- Blood cell production in the bone marrow decreases beginning at about age 70.
- There is less efficient response to physical stress (fright and flight) due to the decreased responsiveness of the adrenal glands.

SIGNS & SYMPTOMS
- Paleness.
- Weakness, tiredness, faintness and breathlessness.
- Frequent infections.
- Spontaneous bleeding from the nose, mouth, rectum, vagina, gums and other sites.
- Red dots of bleeding under the skin.
- Unexplained bruising.
- Ulcers in the mouth, throat and rectum.

CAUSES & RISK FACTORS—Aplastic anemia is caused by poor bone marrow function. Bone marrow is often infiltrated with fat cells, which supplant areas that manufacture blood cells. Infections occur because of reduced white cells, which normally protect against infection. Half of all cases are caused by drugs, especially immunosuppressive drugs, anticancer drugs, chloramphenicol or chemicals such as benzene (found in gasoline). Other cases probably result from immunodeficiency, severe illness or unidentifiable causes. The risk increases with a family history of aplastic anemia; genetic factors such as those associated with congenital hypoplastic anemia (see Glossary); the use of drugs listed as causes; recent severe illness.

DOCTOR'S TREATMENT & DIAGNOSTIC TESTS
- Medical history and physical exam.
- Laboratory studies of blood and bone marrow.
- Surgery (sometimes) to transplant bone marrow. Advancing age alone is not a deterrent.
- Hospitalization for isolation until the body can resist infection.
- Blood transfusions if serious infections occur.
- Self-care instructions focused on the older patient.

HOME TREATMENT BY SELF OR CARE-GIVER

GENERAL INSTRUCTIONS
- A bone marrow transplant requires a donor with compatible antigens. A twin, brother or sister usually makes the best donor. Donated marrow is injected gradually into the patient's veins to try to replace poorly functioning bone marrow with normal cells.

- Hair loss often accompanies treatment, and you may want to wear a wig temporarily.
- Keep your mouth scrupulously clean to decrease the chance of infection. Brush often with a soft toothbrush. Rinse your mouth with a solution of equal parts hydrogen peroxide and water or use a medicated mouthwash if prescribed.

MEDICATION (ADJUSTED FOR AGING)
- Your doctor may prescribe: Immunosuppressive drugs to prevent rejection if a bone marrow transplant is necessary. Antibiotics to prevent or treat infection. Medicated mouthwash to suppress fungus infections.
- *Note:* Adverse reactions and side effects may be more frequent and severe in older persons. Remind your doctor of any medicines you already take.

ACTIVITY FOR OLDER PATIENTS—Resume your normal activities after treatment.

FOOD & BEVERAGE—No special diet is required. You may need iron and vitamin supplements. Ask your doctor.

FUTURE CONSIDERATIONS FOR THE AGING ADULT

POSSIBLE COMPLICATIONS—Poor response to treatment, resulting in uncontrollable infections and bleeding. Complications are fatal in 50% to 70% of those with severe aplastic anemia.

PROBABLE OUTCOME—If the cause can be identified and treated successfully, the disorder is curable. Anemia caused by immunosuppressive drugs usually improves spontaneously when the drugs are withdrawn. Full recovery often requires 6 to 8 months.

PREVENTING RECURRENCE
- Avoid prolonged exposure to toxic compounds such as benzene that are used in many industrial chemicals.
- Don't use drugs that cause aplastic anemia if substitute drugs are available.

CALL YOUR DOCTOR IF

- You have symptoms of aplastic anemia.
- Any of the following occurs after a bone marrow transplant:
  Fever.
  Any sign of infection, such as swelling anywhere in the body. Redness, tenderness or pain may not be present.
  Skin rash.
  Jaundice (yellow skin and eyes).
  Joint pain.
  Puffy feet and ankles.
  Urinary discomfort.
  Decreased daily urine output.

ANEMIA, FOLIC ACID-DEFICIENCY

BASIC INFORMATION FOR OLDER ADULTS

DESCRIPTION—Folic acid-deficiency anemia is a form of anemia caused by a deficiency of folic acid. It is often accompanied by iron-deficiency anemia. Body parts involved: The blood cells, which transport oxygen to all body parts.

SPECIAL CONSIDERATIONS FOR AGING
- Appetite frequently decreases for no apparent reason.
- Disease in one organ system leads to problems in another system.
- The stomach produces less acid.

SIGNS & SYMPTOMS
- Fatigue and weakness.
- Red, sore, glazed tongue.
- Paleness.
- Shortness of breath.
- Nausea, vomiting and diarrhea (rare).
- Abdominal distention.

CAUSES & RISK FACTORS—Causes include inadequate intake or absorption of foods with a high folic acid content, such as meat, poultry, fish, cheese, milk, eggs, green vegetables, yeast and mushrooms; alcoholism; overcooking of foods, which destroys folic acid; a deficiency of vitamin B-12 or vitamin C; and intestinal parasites. The risk increases with illnesses such as tropical sprue, psoriasis, acne rosacea, eczema or dermatitis herpetiformis; fad diets or general poor nutrition, especially vitamin C deficiency; surgical removal of the stomach; smoking, which decreases vitamin C absorption (vitamin C is necessary for folic acid absorption); the use of certain drugs, such as anti-convulsants, methotrexate or triamterene.

DOCTOR'S TREATMENT & DIAGNOSTIC TESTS
- Medical history and physical exam.
- Laboratory blood studies.
- Self-care instructions focused on the older patient.

HOME TREATMENT BY SELF OR CARE-GIVER

GENERAL INSTRUCTIONS—If you smoke, stop smoking.

MEDICATION (ADJUSTED FOR AGING)
- Your doctor may prescribe:
  Folic acid supplements.
  Iron supplements to take orally.
- *Note:* Adverse reactions and side effects may be more frequent and severe in older persons. Remind your doctor of any medicines you already take.

ACTIVITY FOR OLDER PATIENTS
- No restrictions are necessary.
- See Appendix 20 regarding physical fitness for the active older adult.

FOOD & BEVERAGE
- No special diet is required. Eat foods daily that are high in folic acid. The liver can store folic acid for a limited time only.
- See Appendix 1 regarding good nutrition for people over 50.

FUTURE CONSIDERATIONS FOR THE AGING ADULT

POSSIBLE COMPLICATIONS
- Increased susceptibility to infection.
- Congestive heart failure (severe cases only).

PROBABLE OUTCOME—Usually curable in 3 weeks with an adequate folic acid intake.

PREVENTING RECURRENCE
- Don't drink alcohol.
- Eat well. Include fresh vegetables, meat and other animal proteins. Avoid fad diets. Don't overcook food.
- Don't smoke. Smoking increases vitamin requirements.

CALL YOUR DOCTOR IF

- You have symptoms of anemia.
- Your symptoms don't improve in 2 weeks despite treatment.
- Symptoms of infection (fever, chills and muscle aches) occur during treatment.

ANEMIA, HEMOLYTIC

BASIC INFORMATION FOR OLDER ADULTS

DESCRIPTION—Hemolytic anemia involves the premature destruction of mature red blood cells. The bone marrow cannot produce red blood cells fast enough to compensate for those being destroyed. This is not contagious. Body parts involved: The blood, bone marrow and spleen.

SPECIAL CONSIDERATIONS FOR AGING
- Unusual and unexpected reactions to drugs and medications are more likely.
- The bone marrow responds to stress less efficiently.

SIGNS & SYMPTOMS
- Fatigue.
- Shortness of breath.
- Irregular heartbeat.
- Jaundice (yellow skin and eyes, dark urine).
- Enlarged spleen.

CAUSES & RISK FACTORS—Causes include genetic factors such as hereditary spherocytosis, G6PD deficiency, sickle-cell anemia or thalassemia; antibodies produced by the body to fight infections, which for unknown reason attack red blood cells (a response that is sometimes triggered by blood transfusions; malaria; the use of medications, including non-prescription drugs, that damage the red blood cells. Risk factors include a family history of hemolytic anemia and the use of any medication.

DOCTOR'S TREATMENT & DIAGNOSTIC TESTS
- Medical history and physical exam.
- Laboratory blood studies, including a blood count, examination of bone marrow and measurement with radioactive chromium of red blood cell survival.
- Hospitalization for transfusions during a hemolytic crisis.
- Surgery to remove an enlarged spleen (sometimes). Advancing age alone is not a deterrent.
- Self-care instructions focused on the older patient.

HOME TREATMENT BY SELF OR CARE-GIVER

GENERAL INSTRUCTIONS—If removal of the spleen is required, consult your doctor for an explanation of the surgery and postoperative care.

MEDICATION (ADJUSTED FOR AGING)
- Your doctor may prescribe:
  Immunosuppressive drugs to control the antibody response.

Medication to reduce the pain. For minor discomfort, you may use non-prescription drugs such as acetaminophen.
- *Note:* Adverse reactions and side effects may be more frequent and severe in older persons. Remind your doctor of any medicines you already take.

ACTIVITY FOR OLDER PATIENTS
- After treatment, resume normal activities as soon as possible.
- See Appendix 20 regarding physical fitness for the active older adult.

FOOD & BEVERAGE
- No special diet is required.
- See Appendix 1 regarding good nutrition for people over 50.

FUTURE CONSIDERATIONS FOR THE AGING ADULT

POSSIBLE COMPLICATIONS
- Excessive spleen enlargement, which increases destruction of red blood cells.
- Pain, shock and serious illness caused by hemolysis (the destruction of red blood cells).
- Gallstones.

PROBABLE OUTCOME
- If hemolytic anemia is acquired, it can usually be cured when the cause, such as a drug, is removed. Sometimes the spleen is removed surgically.
- If hemolytic anemia is inherited, it is currently considered incurable. However, the symptoms can be relieved or controlled. Scientific research into causes and treatment continues, so there is hope for increasingly effective treatment and a cure.

PREVENTING RECURRENCE—Don't take any medicine that has previously triggered hemolytic anemia.

CALL YOUR DOCTOR IF

- You have symptoms of hemolytic anemia.
- Any of the following occurs during treatment:
  Fever.
  Cough.
  Sore throat.
  Swollen joints.
  Muscle aches.
  Bloody urine.
  Signs of infection in any part of the body (redness, pain, swelling, fever).
- New, unexplained symptoms develop. The drugs used in treatment may produce side effects.

ANEMIA, IRON-DEFICIENCY

BASIC INFORMATION FOR OLDER ADULTS

DESCRIPTION—Iron-deficiency anemia means there is a decreased number of circulating blood cells or insufficient hemoglobin in the cells. Anemia is a symptom (as in fever) of other disorders. For proper treatment, the cause must be found. Body part involved: The blood, which affects all body cells.

SPECIAL CONSIDERATIONS FOR AGING
- The bone marrow responds to stress less efficiently.
- The appetite becomes poorer.

SIGNS & SYMPTOMS
Signs of pronounced anemia include:
- Tiredness, weakness, headache, breathlessness.
- Paleness, especially in the hands and linings of the lower eyelids.

Less common signs include:
- Tongue inflammation, sore mouth or tongue, appetite loss.
- Rapid heartbeat.
- Abdominal discomfort.
- Cravings for ice, paint or dirt.
- Susceptibility to infection.

CAUSES & RISK FACTORS—Causes include decreased absorption of iron or increased need for iron; inadequate intake of food that is high in iron; diseases that result in malabsorption of nutrients; gastrointestinal diseases with bleeding, including cancer. Risk factors include poverty; recent illness, such as an ulcer, diverticulitis, colitis, hemorrhoids or gastrointestinal tumors; postmenopausal vaginal bleeding; bleeding hemorrhoids.

DOCTOR'S TREATMENT & DIAGNOSTIC TESTS
- Medical history and physical exam.
- Laboratory blood studies, especially of hematocrit (see Glossary), hemoglobin and red blood cell counts.
- X-rays of the gastrointestinal tract.
- Self-care instructions focused on the older patient.

HOME TREATMENT BY SELF OR CARE-GIVER

GENERAL INSTRUCTIONS—The most important part of treatment for iron-deficiency anemia is to correct the underlying cause. Iron deficiency can be treated well with iron supplements. Blood transfusions are sometimes prescribed, but they should be unnecessary, except in rare instances.

MEDICATION (ADJUSTED FOR AGING)
- Your doctor may prescribe iron supplements: Take iron on an empty stomach (at least 1/2 hour before meals) for best absorption. If it upsets your stomach, you may take it with a small amount of food (except milk).
  If you take other medications, wait at least 2 hours after taking iron before taking them. Antacids and tetracyclines especially interfere with iron absorption.
  Liquid iron supplements may discolor your teeth. Drink any liquid iron preparation through a straw. Iron supplements may also cause black bowel movements, diarrhea or constipation.
- Continue iron supplements until 2 to 3 months after blood tests return to normal.
- Too much iron is dangerous. Keep iron supplements out of the reach of children.
- *Note:* Adverse reactions and side effects may be more frequent and severe in older persons. Remind your doctor of any medicines you already take.

ACTIVITY FOR OLDER PATIENTS
- No restrictions are necessary.
- See Appendix 20 regarding physical fitness for the active older adult.

FOOD & BEVERAGE
- Limit milk to 1 pint a day. It interferes with iron absorption.
- Eat protein- and iron-containing foods, including meat, beans and leafy green vegetables.
- Increase dietary fiber to prevent constipation.
- See Appendix 1 regarding good nutrition for people over 50.

FUTURE CONSIDERATIONS FOR THE AGING ADULT

POSSIBLE COMPLICATIONS—Failure to diagnose a bleeding malignancy.

PROBABLE OUTCOME—Usually curable with iron supplements if the underlying cause can be identified and cured.

PREVENTING RECURRENCE—Maintain an adequate iron intake through a well-balanced diet or iron supplements.

CALL YOUR DOCTOR IF

- You have symptoms of anemia.
- Nausea, vomiting, severe diarrhea or constipation occur during treatment.

ANEMIA, PERNICIOUS
(B-12 Deficiency Anemia)

BASIC INFORMATION FOR OLDER ADULTS

DESCRIPTION—Pernicious anemia is a form of anemia caused by inadequate absorption of vitamin B-12. Body parts involved: The blood, which affects all body cells, and the stomach.

SPECIAL CONSIDERATIONS FOR AGING
- The appetite decreases.
- The stomach generates less acid.

SIGNS & SYMPTOMS
- Weakness, especially in the arms and legs.
- Sore tongue.
- Nausea, appetite loss and weight loss.
- Bleeding gums.
- Numbness and tingling in the hands and feet.
- Difficulty maintaining proper balance.
- Pale lips, tongue and gums.
- Yellow eyes and skin.
- Shortness of breath.
- Depression.
- Confusion and dementia.
- Headache.
- Poor memory.

CAUSES & RISK FACTORS—Causes include the absence of intrinsic factor, a chemical secreted by the stomach's membrane lining that makes the absorption of vitamin B-12 possible (the reason for the absence of intrinsic factor is unknown, but it may be a genetic deficiency or autoimmune disorder) and the decreased production of hydrochloric acid, especially following stomach surgery or in combination with the absence of intrinsic factor (hydrochloric acid is also necessary for the absorption of vitamin B-12). The risk increases with improper diet, especially a vegetarian diet lacking vitamin B-12 and without supplements; thyroid disease; previous stomach surgery, stomach cancer or gastritis; bulimia or anorexia nervosa; a family history of pernicious anemia; and genetic factors (the disorder is most common in people of northern European ancestry; it is rare in blacks and Asians).

DOCTOR'S TREATMENT & DIAGNOSTIC TESTS
- Medical history and physical exam.
- Laboratory blood studies.
- Radioactive studies such as the Schilling test using radioactive vitamin B-12.
- Bone marrow test.
- Self-care instructions focused on the older patient.

HOME TREATMENT BY SELF OR CARE-GIVER

GENERAL INSTRUCTIONS—Avoid very hot water and heating pads. Your nervous system may not be able to detect dangerously high temperatures.

MEDICATION (ADJUSTED FOR AGING)
- Your doctor will prescribe vitamin B-12 injections. (Oral B-12 is inadequate treatment.) The amount depends on the extent of your illness. The usual dosage is 1 injection a day for 7 days, then 1 injection a week for 1 month, then once a month for the rest of your life.
- Learn to give yourself vitamin B-12 injections, because oral supplements are inadequate. Lifetime treatment is essential. Even with treatment, your ability to absorb vitamin B-12 will not be normal.
- *Note:* Adverse reactions and side effects may be more frequent and severe in older persons. Remind your doctor of any medicines you already take.

ACTIVITY FOR OLDER PATIENTS
- No restrictions are necessary.
- See Appendix 20 regarding physical fitness for the active older adult.

FOOD & BEVERAGE
- No special diet is required. Raw meat and raw liver are no longer prescribed.
- Iron supplements may be helpful adjuncts.
- See Appendix 1 regarding good nutrition for people over 50.

FUTURE CONSIDERATIONS FOR THE AGING ADULT

POSSIBLE COMPLICATIONS—Congestive heart failure; double vision; greater susceptibility to infections; impotence in males.

PROBABLE OUTCOME—This condition is currently considered incurable. However, regular vitamin B-12 injections will control the symptoms indefinitely and reverse complications. The symptoms should disappear within 6 months after treatment begins and stay away so long as adequate treatment continues.

PREVENTING RECURRENCE—If you have had stomach surgery or gastritis, have regular vitamin B-12 injections.

CALL YOUR DOCTOR IF

- You have symptoms of pernicious anemia.
- Your symptoms don't improve in 2 weeks despite treatment.

ANEURYSM
(Aorta and Other Sites)

 BASIC INFORMATION FOR OLDER ADULTS

DESCRIPTION—An aneurysm is an enlargement or bulge in an artery caused by a weak artery wall. Body parts involved: The arteries. Aneurysms occur most often in the aorta (the major artery in the chest and abdomen), the arteries that supply the brain or legs, or the heart wall after a heart attack. (THIS IS AN EMERGENCY; SEEK MEDICAL CARE IMMEDIATELY!)

SPECIAL CONSIDERATIONS FOR AGING—Major blood vessels become thinner and less elastic.

SIGNS & SYMPTOMS—The symptoms vary according to which artery is affected:
- A thoracic (chest) aneurysm produces pain in the chest, neck, back and abdomen. The pain may be sudden and sharp. It also causes hoarseness and swallowing difficulty.
- An abdominal aneurysm produces back pain (sometimes severe), appetite and weight loss and a pulsating mass in the abdomen.
- An aneurysm in a leg artery causes poor circulation in the leg, with weakness and pallor or swelling and bluish color. A pulsating mass may appear in the groin or behind the knee.
- An aneurysm in a brain artery produces headaches (often throbbing), weakness, paralysis or numbness, pain behind the eye, vision change or partial blindness and unequal pupils. A brain aneurysm may be present for many years without producing symptoms.
- An aneurysm in a heart muscle causes heartbeat irregularities and symptoms of congestive heart failure.

CAUSES & RISK FACTORS—Causes include atherosclerosis (hardening of the arteries); congenitally weak arteries (especially with aneurysms in the blood vessels to the brain); syphilis or an infection in the aorta caused by syphilis (rare); injury. The risk increases with a previous heart attack; high blood pressure; smoking; obesity; a family history of atherosclerosis.

DOCTOR'S TREATMENT & DIAGNOSTIC TESTS
- Medical history and physical exam.
- Laboratory blood studies of clotting.
- ECG (see Glossary).
- X-rays of blood vessels (angiography).
- Special radioactive studies of the brain.
- Hospitalization.
- Surgery to replace the diseased vessel or close off the aneurysm. An aneurysm in the brain requires emergency surgery. Surgery for other types of aneurysms may be scheduled at a convenient time. Advancing age alone is not a deterrent.
- Self-care instructions focused on the older patient.

 HOME TREATMENT BY SELF OR CARE-GIVER

GENERAL INSTRUCTIONS—Early detection and treatment before rupture are essential. See your doctor if you have any signs of an aneurysm—especially a pulsating mass in the abdomen or leg—even if it does not cause symptoms.

MEDICATION (ADJUSTED FOR AGING)
- After surgery, your doctor may prescribe: Anticoagulants to prevent blood clot formation in an aneurysm.
  Pain relievers.
- *Note:* Adverse reactions and side effects may be more frequent and severe in older persons. Remind your doctor of any medicines you already take.

ACTIVITY FOR OLDER PATIENTS—Avoid heavy exertion or straining prior to surgery. After surgery, resume normal activities gradually.

FOOD & BEVERAGE—Before surgery, eat a high-fiber diet so you can avoid straining during bowel movements. After surgery, no special diet is necessary.

 FUTURE CONSIDERATIONS FOR THE AGING ADULT

POSSIBLE COMPLICATIONS
- Stroke.
- Rupture of the aneurysm (symptoms include severe headache; severe knifelike pain in the chest, abdomen or leg; and loss of consciousness).

PROBABLE OUTCOME—Often curable with surgery to replace the diseased vessel with grafts (artificial vessels). Surgery on a heart aneurysm can stabilize the heartbeat and prolong life. Aneurysms sometimes recur.

PREVENTING RECURRENCE
- Follow preventive measures for atherosclerosis.
- Follow your treatment program to control high blood pressure.

 CALL YOUR DOCTOR IF

- You have symptoms of an aneurysm, especially a pulsating mass in your abdomen or leg or pain in your chest or abdomen. *This is an emergency!*
- Call for help and rest in bed until help arrives.
- You have had a heart attack and develop heartbeat irregularity or symptoms of congestive heart failure.
- Any symptoms return after surgery.

ANGINA PECTORIS

BASIC INFORMATION FOR OLDER ADULTS

DESCRIPTION—Angina pectoris is chest pain arising from the heart—usually under the sternum (breastbone)—brought on by exercise, emotional upset or heavy meals in a person who has a heart disorder. Body parts involved: The coronary arteries.

SPECIAL CONSIDERATIONS FOR AGING
- Frequency increases with age.
- Stress from any emotional cause—fear, worry, anxiety, sadness, loneliness or anger—affects all aspects of any illness or disorder.

SIGNS & SYMPTOMS
Any of the following:
- Tightness, squeezing, pressure or mild ache in the chest (more during exercise).
- Sudden breathing difficulty (sometimes).
- Frequent chest pain similar to indigestion.
- A choking feeling in the throat.
- Chest pain that radiates to the jaw, teeth or earlobes.
- Heaviness, numbness, tingling or ache in the arm, shoulder, elbow or hand—usually on the left side.
- Pain between the shoulder blades.
- Paleness and sweating.

CAUSES & RISK FACTORS—The reason for angina pectoris is an insufficient supply of blood and oxygen to the heart muscle. Causes include coronary artery disease with partial blockage or spasm of arteries that supply the heart; anemia; an overactive thyroid gland; a heartbeat that is too fast; heart valve disease. The risk increases with sudden overexertion; smoking; obesity; diabetes mellitus; high blood pressure; high blood cholesterol levels; excessive intake of refined carbohydrates (such as sugar), fat or salt; a sedentary lifestyle; fatigue; overwork or stress; a family history of coronary artery disease; exposure to cold and wind.

DOCTOR'S TREATMENT & DIAGNOSTIC TESTS
- Medical history and physical exam.
- Laboratory studies such as blood tests, stress tests and treadmill.
- ECG (see Glossary).
- X-rays of the heart.
- Therapeutic trial of nitroglycerin. Nitroglycerin relieves the symptoms of angina, but it does not affect the symptoms of other disorders.
- Self-care instructions focused on the older patient.
- Surgery to bypass severely blocked coronary arteries (sometimes). Advancing age alone is not a deterrent.
- Balloon angioplasty (see Glossary) to open blocked coronary arteries (sometimes).

HOME TREATMENT BY SELF OR CARE-GIVER

GENERAL INSTRUCTIONS
- Reduce stress to improve overall health. See Appendix 13.
- Follow suggestions under Preventing Recurrence.

MEDICATION (ADJUSTED FOR AGING)—Your doctor may prescribe medication to widen your arteries temporarily so more blood can reach the heart.

ACTIVITY FOR OLDER PATIENTS—If angina attacks begin suddenly or increase in frequency or severity, you should rest at least 2 weeks. Rest in a chair—not in bed—except for 8 to 10 hours of sleep at night. You may read or watch TV. If you must get up, walk slowly. After this period, resume activity slowly to a level just below that which produced pain. Gradually increase exercise time and pace. Warm up slowly before exercise. Avoid situations that increase the heart's workload, such as anger, temperature extremes, high altitude (except on commercial airline flights) or sudden bursts of activity. Consult your doctor about resuming sexual activity.

FOOD & BEVERAGE—See diet suggestions under Preventing Recurrence.

FUTURE CONSIDERATIONS FOR THE AGING ADULT

POSSIBLE COMPLICATIONS—Heart attack.

PROBABLE OUTCOME—Minor angina can be relieved with rest and the use of nitroglycerin and other drugs. Other treatment may be necessary to correct underlying diseases.

PREVENTING RECURRENCE
- Obtain medical treatment for underlying causes or risks.
- Don't smoke.
- Eat a diet that is low in fat and low in salt. Lose weight if you are overweight.
- Avoid activities that trigger angina attacks. Exercise regularly after consulting your doctor.

CALL YOUR DOCTOR IF

- You have symptoms of angina pectoris.
- Any of the following occurs after diagnosis: An attack of chest pain continues longer than 10 to 15 minutes despite rest and treatment with nitroglycerin.
  You wake from sleep with chest pain that does not go away with 1 nitroglycerin tablet. If these attacks continue, report them to your doctor—even if nitroglycerin relieves them.

ANKYLOSING SPONDYLITIS
(Marie-Strumpell Disease)

BASIC INFORMATION FOR OLDER ADULTS

DESCRIPTION—Ankylosing spondylitis is a chronic, progressive joint disease accompanied by inflammation and stiffening that is characterized by a "bent-forward" posture caused by stiffening of the spine and support structures. Manifestations of this disease may be confused with the arthritis of Lyme disease. Body parts involved: The sacroiliac region; the hip joints; and the lumbar, thoracic and cervical areas of the spine.

SPECIAL CONSIDERATIONS FOR AGING
- Years of weight bearing cause wear and tear on bones, joints and ligaments.
- The percentage of muscle tissue decreases, further decreasing ability to walk efficiently.
- Coordination and balance become impaired.

SIGNS & SYMPTOMS
Early stages:
- Recurrent episodes of low backache. Pain can also occur along the sciatic nerve.
- Stiffness that is worse in the morning.

Later stages:
- Progressive worsening of the symptoms. The pain often spreads from the low back to the middle back or higher in the neck. Joints in the arms, legs, feet and hands are sometimes affected.
- Anemia; fatigue.
- Muscle stiffness.
- Weight loss.
- Painful, red eyes.

CAUSES & RISK FACTORS—The cause of ankylosing spondylitis is unknown, but it may be caused by genetic changes or autoimmune disorder. The risk increases with a a family history of ankylosing spondylitis.

DOCTOR'S TREATMENT & DIAGNOSTIC TESTS
- Medical history and physical exam.
- Laboratory blood studies.
- X-rays of the spine (may appear normal early in the disease).
- Self-care instructions focused on the older patient.
- Surgery to replace a damaged hip or to insert bone grafts in the spine (advanced stages only).
- Physical and respiratory therapy.

HOME TREATMENT BY SELF OR CARE-GIVER

GENERAL INSTRUCTIONS
- Sleep face down on a firm mattress. Use a small pillow or none at all.
- Take hot baths or use heat compresses before exercising or to relieve the pain.
- Avoid excessive rest *or* exhaustion.
- Have regular massages if possible.

MEDICATION (ADJUSTED FOR AGING)—Your doctor may prescribe non-steroidal anti-inflammatory drugs. Don't take narcotics for the pain; they are addictive.

ACTIVITY FOR OLDER PATIENTS
- Stay as active as your strength allows: Exercise to maintain good posture and retain as much upright carriage as possible. Back braces don't help.
  Swim regularly if possible. Your buoyancy in water will allow you to move stiff, painful areas more easily.
  Avoid activity that puts stress on the back.
- See Appendix 20 regarding physical fitness for the active older adult.

FOOD & BEVERAGE
- No special diet is required.
- See Appendix 1 regarding good nutrition for people over 50.

FUTURE CONSIDERATIONS FOR THE AGING ADULT

POSSIBLE COMPLICATIONS
- Congestive heart failure.
- Eye inflammation, rarely causing blindness.
- Amyloidosis (a disease that affects many organ systems of the body).
- Heart valve disease.
- Gastrointestinal disease.
- Lung disease.
- Nerve compression causing numbness in the arms or legs.
- Permanent disability and immobilization.

PROBABLE OUTCOME
- This disease is currently considered incurable. The symptoms progress unpredictably and slowly for 10 to 20 years. However, they can be relieved or controlled. Life expectancy is reduced by the likelihood of complications, not by the disease.
- Medical literature cites instances of unexplained recovery. Scientific research into causes and treatment continues, so there is hope for increasingly effective treatment and a cure.

PREVENTING RECURRENCE—There are no specific preventive measures.

CALL YOUR DOCTOR IF

- You have symptoms of ankylosing spondylitis.
- Any of the following occus during treatment:
  Fever. This may indicate the recurrence of an acute phase.
  Increasing pain and disability despite the measures outlined above.

ILLNESSES & DISORDERS

BASIC INFORMATION FOR OLDER ADULTS

DESCRIPTION—Anxiety is a vague, uncomfortable feeling of fear, dread or danger from an unknown source that lasts a month or longer. Some persons become constantly anxious about everything. Body parts involved: The central nervous system and the endocrine system.

SPECIAL CONSIDERATIONS FOR AGING
- Emotional highs and lows are greater.
- Deaths of friends and family members are more likely.

SIGNS & SYMPTOMS
- A feeling that something undesirable or harmful is about to happen.
- A dry mouth, swallowing difficulty or hoarseness.
- Rapid breathing and heartbeat.
- Twitching or trembling.
- Muscle tension or headaches.
- Sweating.
- Cold, clammy hands.
- Nausea, diarrhea or weight loss.
- Sleeplessness or nightmares.
- Irritability.
- Fatigue.
- Memory problems.
- Sexual impotence.

CAUSES & RISK FACTORS
Causes include:
- Activation of the body's defense mechanisms for fight or flight. Excessive adrenalin is discharged from the adrenal glands, and adrenalin breakdown products (catecholamines) eventually affect various parts of the body.
- Fear.

The risk increases with:
- Stress from any source.
- The use of excessive caffeine and some other drugs.
- A family history of neurosis.
- Fatigue or overwork.
- The recurrence of situations that have been previously stressful or harmful.

DOCTOR'S TREATMENT & DIAGNOSTIC TESTS
- Medical history and physical exam.
- Laboratory studies to rule out medical conditions that produce anxiety, such as hyperthyroidism.
- Self-care instructions focused on the older patient.
- Psychotherapy, counseling or a support group.

HOME TREATMENT BY SELF OR CARE-GIVER

GENERAL INSTRUCTIONS
- Obtain therapy to understand the specific but unconscious threat or source of stress.

- Learn techniques, including biofeedback and relaxation therapy, to reduce muscle tension.
- Follow a regular fitness routine using aerobic exercise.

MEDICATION (ADJUSTED FOR AGING)
- Your doctor may prescribe tranquilizers. These are useful for a short time under the following circumstances:
  During periods of unusually intense anxiety.
  Until psychological insights prevent anxiety from developing.
  Until direct action solves the threatening problem.
- Beware of becoming dependent on the medicines. The long-term use of anti-anxiety agents may lead to severe addiction.
- If you take medicine for anxiety, don't discontinue abruptly. Get instructions for slow withdrawal from your doctor.
- *Note:* Adverse reactions and side effects may be more frequent and severe in older persons. Remind your doctor of any medicines you already take.

ACTIVITY FOR OLDER PATIENTS
- Stay active. Physical exertion helps reduce anxiety.
- See Appendix 20 regarding physical fitness for the active older adult.

FOOD & BEVERAGE
- No special diet is required. Avoid caffeine and other stimulants and alcohol.
- See Appendix 1 regarding good nutrition for people over 50.

FUTURE CONSIDERATIONS FOR THE AGING ADULT

POSSIBLE COMPLICATIONS—Untreated anxiety may lead to neuroses, such as phobias, compulsions or hypochondriasis. A sudden increase in anxiety may lead to panic and violent escape behavior.

PROBABLE OUTCOME—Anxiety can be controlled with psychological therapy. Overcoming anxiety often results in a richer, more satisfying life.

PREVENTING RECURRENCE
- Determine what stressful or potentially harmful situation is causing the anxiety. Deal with it directly.
- Consider lifestyle changes to reduce stress.

CALL YOUR DOCTOR IF

- You have symptoms of anxiety and self-treatment has failed.
- You have a sudden feeling of panic.
- New, unexplained symptoms develop. The drugs used in treatment may produce side effects.

APPENDICITIS

BASIC INFORMATION FOR OLDER ADULTS

DESCRIPTION—Appendicitis is an inflammation of the vermiform appendix, a small intestinal pouch that extends from the cecum, the first part of the large intestine. The appendix has no known function, but it can become diseased. Appendicitis affects 1 in 500 people each year. The symptoms vary widely. Appendicitis should be considered in any person with undiagnosed abdominal pain. Body parts involved: The appendix, cecum and peritoneum (membrane covering the intestinal tract).

SPECIAL CONSIDERATIONS FOR AGING
- Appendicitis is frequently more difficult to diagnose since characteristic signs and symptoms may be absent or changed.
- The immune system becomes less effective, opening the way for viral, bacterial and other infections; malignancies; immune disorders; and allergies.

SIGNS & SYMPTOMS
- Pain that begins close to the navel and migrates toward the right lower abdomen. The pain becomes persistent and localized. It worsens with moving, breathing deeply, coughing, sneezing, walking or being touched.
- Nausea and sometimes vomiting.
- Constipation and inability to pass gas.
- Diarrhea (occasionally).
- A low fever (under 102F) that begins after the other symptoms.
- Tenderness in the right lower abdomen, usually about a third of the distance from the navel to the top of the hip bone. (This description applies only if the appendix is in its normal position. In some cases, the tip of the appendix is located elsewhere, making diagnosis difficult).
- Abdominal swelling (late stages).

CAUSES & RISK FACTORS—Caused by an infection, usually with bacteria from the intestinal tract. Why the infection starts is unknown. The appendix may be obstructed by the material moving through the intestinal tract or by a constricting band of tissue. When infected, it becomes swollen, inflamed and filled with pus. The risk increases with recent illness, especially a roundworm infestation or gastrointestinal virus infection.

DOCTOR'S TREATMENT & DIAGNOSTIC TESTS
- Medical history and physical exam (maybe several) by a doctor.
- Laboratory blood studies. Tests usually show higher levels of white blood cells.
- Urinalysis to rule out a urinary tract infection, which can mimic appendicitis.
- Surgery to remove the appendix. Because appendicitis can be hard to diagnose, surgery is often withheld until the signs and symptoms progress enough to confirm the

diagnosis. Advancing age alone is not a deterrent.
- Self-care instructions focused on the older patient.

HOME TREATMENT BY SELF OR CARE-GIVER

GENERAL INSTRUCTIONS
- While diagnosis is uncertain, take a rectal temperature every 2 hours. Keep a record for your doctor.
- For an explanation of surgery and postoperative care, consult your doctor.

MEDICATION (ADJUSTED FOR AGING)
- Don't take any laxatives, enemas or medicines for the pain. Laxatives may cause rupture and pain, and fever reducers make diagnosis more difficult.
- *Note:* Adverse reactions and side effects may be more frequent and severe in older persons. Remind your doctor of any medicines you already take.

ACTIVITY FOR OLDER PATIENTS
- Rest in a bed or chair until surgery.
- See Appendix 20 regarding physical fitness for the active older adult.

FOOD & BEVERAGE
- Don't eat or drink anything if you suspect appendicitis. Anesthesia for surgery is much safer if the stomach is empty. If you are very thirsty, wash your mouth out with water.
- See Appendix 1 regarding good nutrition for people over 50.

FUTURE CONSIDERATIONS FOR THE AGING ADULT

POSSIBLE COMPLICATIONS
- Rupture of the appendix, abscess formation and peritonitis. This is most common in older persons.
- Misdiagnosis because of few or atypical symptoms.

PROBABLE OUTCOME—Usually curable with surgery. If totally untreated, a ruptured appendix is fatal.

PREVENTING RECURRENCE—There are no specific preventive measures.

CALL YOUR DOCTOR IF

- You have symptoms of appendicitis.
- Any of the following occurs while surgery is pending:
  Fever spikes of 102F (38.9C) or higher.
  Continued vomiting.
  Increased pain in the abdomen.
  Fainting.
  Blood in the stool or vomit.

ARC
(Aids-Related Complex)

BASIC INFORMATION FOR OLDER ADULTS

DESCRIPTION—ARC is a group of chronic signs and symptoms that appear in people with an increased likelihood of developing AIDS, but who don't have typical infections of AIDS patients (such as pneumocystic pneumonia) or other characteristic disorders associated with AIDS, such as Kaposi's sarcoma. ARC affects the immune system just as AIDS does, decreasing the body's ability to fight infection and suppressing the multiplication of abnormal cells, such as cancer. Body parts involved: The immune system, including special blood cells (lymphocytes) and the cells of some organs (the bone marrow, spleen, liver and lymph glands). These cells manufacture antibodies to protect against disease and cancer.

SPECIAL CONSIDERATIONS FOR AGING—The immune system becomes less effective, opening the way for infections, malignancies, immune disorders and allergies.

SIGNS & SYMPTOMS
- Enlarged lymph glands; weight loss.
- Fevers; lethargy and achiness; thrush.
- Diarrhea (chronic); rectal growths.
- Blood abnormalities (discovered in blood tests).

CAUSES & RISK FACTORS—Caused by the human immunodeficiency virus (HIV), a newly identified virus (retrovirus) that invades and destroys cells of the immune system, resulting in lowered resistance to infections and some types of cancer. The virus is transmitted by:
- Sexual contact with an affected person (statistically the risk is much higher in homosexual or bisexual men).
- Sharing contaminated needles for intravenous drug use.
- Transfusions of blood or blood products from a person with AIDS.
Note: Day-to-day non-sexual contact does *not* transmit the disease, so a person with AIDS is not a danger to the general population.
The risk increases with:
- Multiple homosexual or bisexual sexual partners.
- Multiple heterosexual partners (less likely).
- Sexual activity with IV drug users.
- Exposure of hospital workers and laboratory technicians to blood, feces and urine of HIV-positive patients.

DOCTOR'S TREATMENT & DIAGNOSTIC TESTS
- Laboratory studies of blood cells, HIV antibodies test (may not become positive for 6 months after contact) and Western blot test.
- Psychotherapy or counseling to help you cope with anxiety and depression about having the disease and the likelihood of death.

- Hospitalization. Medical schools may provide some free care if you are willing to participate in research.

HOME TREATMENT BY SELF OR CARE-GIVER

GENERAL INSTRUCTIONS—Early diagnosis is helpful. If you are at risk, obtain a medical evaluation—even if you feel well. Contact social agencies in your area about ARC support groups.

MEDICATION (ADJUSTED FOR AGING)
- Drugs are currently not effective in curing ARC. However, new drug therapies are under development and some have been found to be effective in treating or managing this chronic disease.
- Your doctor may prescribe:
  Antibiotics to prevent infections or control them as they develop.
  Antiviral drugs, such as zidovudine (AZT), to slow progression of the disease.

ACTIVITY FOR OLDER PATIENTS—No restrictions are necessary on normal activity, but refrain from unprotected sexual encounters.

FOOD & BEVERAGE—No special diet is required.

FUTURE CONSIDERATIONS FOR THE AGING ADULT

POSSIBLE COMPLICATIONS
- Serious infection in various body systems.
- Progression of the disease to full-blown AIDS.
- Cancer.

PROBABLE OUTCOME—This condition is currently considered incurable. However, the symptoms can be relieved or controlled and scientific research into causes and treatment continues. AIDS may not develop for years.

PREVENTING RECURRENCE—Since ARC is presently incurable, the main concern is to avoid transmitting it to others. Follow these suggestions:
- Use condoms for all sexual activity.
- Avoid intravenous self-administered drugs.
- Don't donate blood to blood banks.

CALL YOUR DOCTOR IF

- You have symptoms of ARC.
- Infection occurs after diagnosis. The symptoms include fever, cough, diarrhea, skin rash or eruption or a general ill feeling.

ARTHRITIS, INFECTIOUS
(Septic Arthritis)

BASIC INFORMATION FOR OLDER ADULTS

DESCRIPTION—Infectious arthritis is an inflammation in a joint resulting from infection. Body parts involved: Any joint can be involved, but this type of arthritis is most common in larger joints, such as the hip, or those subject to trauma, such as the knee or the joints in the hands, elbows, shoulders and hips.

SPECIAL CONSIDERATIONS FOR AGING
- Characteristic signs and symptoms of many disorders are frequently changed or absent.
- Signs and symptoms may differ significantly from those listed below.

SIGNS & SYMPTOMS
- Chills and fever (sometimes high).
- Redness, swelling, tenderness, heat and pain (often throbbing) in the affected joint. The pain sometimes spreads to other joints. It worsens with movement.
- Pain in the buttocks, thighs, groin or end of a bone near a joint (sometimes).

CAUSES & RISK FACTORS—Caused by the entry into a joint of germs, usually bacteria (streptococci, staphylococci, gonococci, hemophili or tubercle bacilli) or fungi. The germs gain entry from an infection elsewhere in the body, as with gonorrhea or tuberculosis; an infection next to the joint, as with skin boils, cellulitis or bone infection; or an injury to the joint, including puncture wounds and skin abrasions. The risk increases with illness that has lowered resistance; sexually transmitted infections; diabetes mellitus; rheumatoid arthritis; the use of immunosuppressive drugs; joint surgery; injections into joints; excessive alcohol consumption; many sexual partners; the use of mind-altering drugs, especially those that are injected; poor hygiene; recent injury.

DOCTOR'S TREATMENT & DIAGNOSTIC TESTS
- Medical history and physical exam.
- Laboratory studies such as blood counts, blood culture and culture of fluid from the infected joint.
- X-rays of affected joints.
- Hospitalization (frequently) for complete rest and intravenous antibiotics.
- Surgery to drain fluid from the affected joints or remove foreign material introduced by an injury.
- Physical therapy after recovery to regain the full use of the joint.
- Self-care instructions focused on the older patient.

OTHER—The use of aspirin and other non-steroidal anti-inflammatory drugs for other disorders may suppress signs of joint inflammation, delaying diagnosis.

HOME TREATMENT BY SELF OR CARE-GIVER

GENERAL INSTRUCTIONS—No specific instructions except those under other headings.

MEDICATION (ADJUSTED FOR AGING)
- Your doctor may prescribe: Antibiotics (often intravenous). Don't discontinue antibiotics until your doctor recommends it. Infection may return after the symptoms disappear. Codeine or narcotics for a short time to relieve the pain.
- *Note:* Adverse reactions and side effects may be more frequent and severe in older persons. Remind your doctor of any medicines you already take.

ACTIVITY FOR OLDER PATIENTS—Splints or casts may be necessary to rest the affected joint completely. Movement delays healing. After cure, physical therapy is often necessary to restore joint function. Resume your normal activities gradually as the symptoms improve.

FOOD & BEVERAGE—No special diet is required. See Appendix 1 regarding good nutrition for people over 50.

FUTURE CONSIDERATIONS FOR THE AGING ADULT

POSSIBLE COMPLICATIONS—Misdiagnosis as gout or another non-infectious condition, delaying antibiotic treatment; blood poisoning; permanent joint damage; destruction of bone.

PROBABLE OUTCOME—Usually curable with early diagnosis and treatment. Recovery takes weeks or months. Treatment delay may result in a badly damaged joint and loss of movement, requiring joint replacement.

PREVENTING RECURRENCE
- Protect exposed joints, such as the knee, during activities involving risk of injury.
- Obtain prompt medical treatment for infections elsewhere in the body.

CALL YOUR DOCTOR IF

- You have symptoms of joint infection. Call immediately.
- Any of the following occurs during the illness: Temperature spikes to 103F (39.4C). Fatigue, headache, muscle aches and sweating.
- New, unexplained symptoms develop. The drugs used in treatment may produce side effects.

ILLNESSES & DISORDERS

ARTHRITIS, NECK
(Cervical Spondylosis; Cervical Musculoskeletal Discomfort; Cervical Radiculopathy)

BASIC INFORMATION FOR OLDER ADULTS

DESCRIPTION—Neck arthritis pertains to degenerative changes of the bones in the neck that place pressure on the nerves and muscles to the arms, legs and bladder. Body parts involved: The bones of the neck, the disks between the bones, the blood vessels to the head and the bladder and lower legs (advanced stages).

SPECIAL CONSIDERATIONS FOR AGING
- The bones become thinner.
- Height decreases 0.5 inches each 20 years.
- The percentage of muscle tissue decreases.
- Years of weight bearing cause wear and tear on bones and ligaments.

SIGNS & SYMPTOMS—Any of the following:
- Pain in the neck that radiates to the shoulder blades, tops of the shoulders, upper arms, hands or back of the head.
- Crunching sounds with movement of the neck or shoulder muscles.
- Numbness and tingling in the arms, hands and fingers; some loss of feeling in the hands; the impairment of reflexes.
- Muscle weakness and deterioration; diminished reflexes.
- Neck stiffness; headache.
- Dizziness; unsteady gait; double vision.
- With advanced disease, loss of bladder control and leg weakness.

CAUSES & RISK FACTORS—Causes include arthritis (the inflammation of a joint); injuries such as automobile accidents with "whiplash" injury, athletic injuries, sudden jerks on the arms or falls; osteoarthritis; and outgrowths of bone that sometimes occur with aging. The risk increases with fatigue, overwork or neck injury.

DOCTOR'S TREATMENT & DIAGNOSTIC TESTS
- Medical history and physical exam, including nerve conduction studies and x-rays of the neck.
- Self-care instructions focused on the older patient.
- Treatment for signs of nerve-root pressure (the symptoms in the head, arms or bladder) or pain.
- Surgery (sometimes) to fuse neck bones, remove a damaged disk or enlarge the spinal cord space. Advancing age alone is not a deterrent.

HOME TREATMENT BY SELF OR CARE-GIVER

GENERAL INSTRUCTIONS
- Wear a soft fabric collar (a Thomas collar; see Glossary) to prevent unexpected neck muscle strain.
- Apply moist heat. Take hot showers twice a day and let the water beat on your neck and shoulders for 10 to 20 minutes. Between showers, apply hot soaks to neck. Soak towel or cloth in hot water, wring out and apply.
- Use dry heat. Sit under a heat lamp for 10 to 15 minutes several times a day.
- Improve your posture. Pull in your chin and abdomen when sitting or standing. Use a firm chair and sit with your buttocks against the back.
- Sleep without a pillow. Instead use a cervical pillow, wear a soft fabric collar or put a small rolled towel under your neck.
- If numbness or pain affects the hands or arms, buy or rent a cervical traction apparatus. To set it up, follow the directions that accompany the apparatus.

MEDICATION (ADJUSTED FOR AGING)
- For minor discomfort or disability, you may use aspirin or acetaminophen.
- For serious discomfort, your doctor may prescribe stronger pain medicine, muscle relaxants or tranquilizers.
- *Note:* Adverse reactions and side effects may be more frequent and severe in older persons. Remind your doctor of any medicines you already take.

ACTIVITY FOR OLDER PATIENTS—No restrictions are necessary. See Appendix 20 regarding physical fitness for the active older adult.

FOOD & BEVERAGE—No special diet is required. See Appendix 1 regarding good nutrition for people over 50.

FUTURE CONSIDERATIONS FOR THE AGING ADULT

POSSIBLE COMPLICATIONS—Reduced neck flexibility after surgery or treatment.

PROBABLE OUTCOME—Minor symptoms usually respond well to treatment and subside slowly. Severe symptoms may persist indefinitely.

PREVENTING RECURRENCE
- Avoid sitting in cramped positions.
- Sleep without pillows. Use a soft fabric collar or towel to support the neck.
- Avoid injury. Wear protective headgear for contact sports. Use seat belts in vehicles and keep headrests at proper height.

CALL YOUR DOCTOR IF
- You have symptoms of neck arthritis.
- The symptoms persist or worsen despite treatment.

ARTHRITIS, RHEUMATOID

BASIC INFORMATION FOR OLDER ADULTS

DESCRIPTION—Rheumatoid arthritis is an illness characterized by joint disease that involves muscles, membrane linings of the joints, and cartilage. Two or three times more common in women, it usually begins between the ages of 30 and 40. Body parts involved: The joints, including the cartilage, synovial membranes, muscles and ligaments and blood vessels; the eyes.

SPECIAL CONSIDERATIONS FOR AGING
- Characteristic signs and symptoms of many disorders are frequently changed or absent.
- The immune system becomes less effective, opening the way for viral, bacterial and other infections; malignancies; immune disorders; and allergies.

SIGNS & SYMPTOMS—Slow or sudden onset of:
- Redness, aching, pain, warmth and tenderness in any or all active joints in the hands, wrists, elbows, shoulders, knees, feet, ankles, jaw or spine.
- Morning stiffness; muscular atrophy.
- Low-grade fever; pale skin; appetite loss.
- Nodules under the skin (sometimes).

CAUSES & RISK FACTORS—The cause is unknown, but it is probably caused by an autoimmune disease or infectious agents. The risk increases with emotional or physical stress, as from accidents, menopause or surgery; a family history of rheumatoid arthritis or other autoimmune disorders; and genetic factors, such as defects in the autoimmune system.

DOCTOR'S TREATMENT & DIAGNOSTIC TESTS
- Medical history and physical exam.
- X-rays of the joints; laboratory blood studies to detect a rheumatoid factor.
- Self-care instructions focused on the older patient.
- Time in an extended-care facility (sometimes) for physical therapy.
- Surgery (joint replacement) to correct deformities. Advancing age alone is not a deterrent.

HOME TREATMENT BY SELF OR CARE-GIVER

GENERAL INSTRUCTIONS
- Wearing splints at night may be helpful to support and protect joints with active disease.
- Wearing gloves at night to retain heat.
- Relieve the pain with heat, including hot soaks, heat lamps, heating pads or whirlpool treatments.
- If you don't have a firm mattress, place 3/4-inch plywood between your bedsprings and mattress to support your back.
- Exercise disabled joints passively to help prevent contractures (muscle shortening).
- Consider moving to a dry climate. Damp weather aggravates the symptoms.

MEDICATION (ADJUSTED FOR AGING)
- Your doctor may prescribe non-steroidal anti-inflammatory drugs, including aspirin and other salicylates; gold compounds; immunosuppressive drugs.
- Cortisone drugs usually relieve the pain dramatically for short periods, but they are less effective for long-term use. They don't prevent progressive joint destruction and they sometimes have hazardous side effects.
- Cortisone injections into joints can temporarily relieve the pain.

ACTIVITY FOR OLDER PATIENTS
- Stay in bed, except to use the bathroom, until fever and other signs of flare-ups disappear.
- Between flare-ups, remain active, but include daily rest periods. Sleep for 10 to 12 hours each night. Don't become overtired.
- Stand, walk and sit erectly.
- When able, exercise actively to preserve strength and joint mobility. Build up slowly to the amount suggested by your doctor.
- Exercise in water when possible.

FOOD & BEVERAGE—Eat a normal, well-balanced diet. Avoid arthritis diet fads, which are common. Lose weight if you are obese, as obesity stresses the joints.

FUTURE CONSIDERATIONS FOR THE AGING ADULT

POSSIBLE COMPLICATIONS—Impaired vision; permanent deformity and crippling. This may develop rapidly, especially contractures (muscle shortening) or degeneration of the muscles around an inflamed joint.

PROBABLE OUTCOME
- The disease may be mild or severe. It is presently incurable, but with an early diagnosis it is possible to relieve the pain, prevent disability and lead an active life for a normal lifespan.
- Conservative treatment relieves the symptoms in 1 year in 75% of patients. About 5% to 10% are eventually disabled despite treatment.

PREVENTING RECURRENCE—There are no specific preventive measures.

CALL YOUR DOCTOR IF

- You have symptoms of rheumatoid arthritis.
- Any of the following occurs during treatment: Fever; symptoms in previously unaffected joints.
- New, unexplained symptoms develop. The drugs used in treatment may produce side effects.

ASBESTOSIS

BASIC INFORMATION FOR OLDER ADULTS

DESCRIPTION—Asbestosis is an inflammation of the lung due to breathing asbestos particles. This is not contagious. It may lead to lung cancer. Body parts involved: The lungs.

SPECIAL CONSIDERATIONS FOR AGING
- In the lungs, the transfer of carbon dioxide and oxygen to the bloodstream becomes less efficient.
- The vital capacity of the lungs decreases.

SIGNS & SYMPTOMS
Early symptoms:
- Shortness of breath.
- A cough that produces little or no sputum.
- A general ill feeling.

Late symptoms:
- Fitful sleep.
- Appetite loss.
- Chest pain.
- Hoarseness.
- Coughing blood.
- Symptoms of congestive heart failure.
- Bluish nails.

CAUSES & RISK FACTORS—Asbestosis is caused by many years of exposure to small particles of asbestos at home, at work or from a nearby asbestos plant. It may take 20 years after exposure for the disease to develop. The risk increases with:
- Poor nutrition.
- Smoking.
- Excessive alcohol consumption.

DOCTOR'S TREATMENT & DIAGNOSTIC TESTS
- Medical history and physical exam.
- X-rays of the chest.
- Pulmonary function tests.
- Self-care instructions focused on the older patient.

HOME TREATMENT BY SELF OR CARE-GIVER

GENERAL INSTRUCTIONS—The following measures may relieve the symptoms and protect against recurrent lung infections:
- Obtain medical treatment for any respiratory infection, including the common cold.
- Consider moving to a warm, dry climate if you have advanced disease.
- Practice bronchial drainage. Your physician will provide instructions.
- Use a cool-mist humidifier to loosen bronchial secretions so they can be coughed up easily.

MEDICATION (ADJUSTED FOR AGING)
- Your doctor may prescribe:
  Antibiotics for infections.

Bronchodilators (inhaled or oral) with inhalation therapy (supervised at first by an inhalation therapist) to open bronchial tubes to the maximum.
- For minor discomfort, you may use non-prescriptions drugs such as acetaminophen or aspirin.
- *Note:* Adverse reactions and side effects may be more frequent and severe in older persons. Remind your doctor of any medicines you already take.

ACTIVITY FOR OLDER PATIENTS
- Rest in bed with infections. You may read or watch TV.
- After treatment, resume normal activity as soon as your symptoms improve.
- See Appendix 20 regarding physical fitness for the active older adult.

FOOD & BEVERAGE
- No special diet is required.
- See Appendix 1 regarding good nutrition for people over 50.

FUTURE CONSIDERATIONS FOR THE AGING ADULT

POSSIBLE COMPLICATIONS
- Tuberculosis (late stages of silicosis).
- Heart failure due to lung disease.
- Lung collapse.
- Pleurisy.
- Lung cancer.

PROBABLE OUTCOME—This condition is currently considered incurable. However, the symptoms can be relieved or controlled. Scientific research into causes and treatment continues, so there is hope for increasingly effective treatment and a cure.

PREVENTING RECURRENCE
- During exposure to asbestos, wear a protective mask or a hood with an external air supply.
- Follow recommended industrial procedures to suppress asbestos dust.
- Don't smoke.
- Participate in a regular physical exercise program to maintain good cardiopulmonary fitness.

CALL YOUR DOCTOR IF

- You have symptoms of asbestosis.
- Any of the following occurs during treatment:
  A temperature spike of 101F (38.3C) or more.
  Increased chest pain or breathlessness.
  Blood in the sputum.
  Continuing weight loss.
- New, unexplained symptoms develop. The drugs used in treatment may produce side effects.

ASTHMA

BASIC INFORMATION FOR OLDER ADULTS

DESCRIPTION—Asthma is a chronic disorder with recurrent attacks of wheezing and shortness of breath. Body parts involved: The lungs, bronchi and bronchioles.

SPECIAL CONSIDERATIONS FOR AGING
- Unlikely to begin beyond age 45, but may start at any age.
- Stress from any emotional cause—fear, worry, anxiety, sadness, loneliness or anger—affects all aspects of any illness or disorder.

SIGNS & SYMPTOMS
Typical symptoms include:
- Chest tightness and shortness of breath; often a sense of suffocation.
- Wheezing upon breathing out.
- Coughing, especially at night, with little or no sputum.
- Rapid, shallow breathing that is easier when sitting up.
- Breathing difficulty with tightening neck muscles.

Symptoms of an acute attack include:
- Bluish skin.
- Exhaustion.
- Grunting respiration.
- Inability to speak.
- Mental changes, including restlessness or confusion.

CAUSES & RISK FACTORS—Caused by a spasm of the air passages (the bronchi and bronchioles), followed by swelling of the passages and thickening of the lung secretions (sputum). This decreases or closes off the air flow to the lungs. These changes are caused by allergens such as pollen, dust, fungus spores, feathers, animal dander, molds and some drugs and foods; lung inflammation and infections such as bronchitis; air irritants such as smoke and odors; exercise or excitement; and stress. The risk increases with other allergic conditions such as eczema or hay fever; a family history of asthma or allergies; exposure to air pollutants; smoking; the use of some drugs such as aspirin; and night-time.

DOCTOR'S TREATMENT & DIAGNOSTIC TESTS
- Medical history and physical exam.
- Chest x-rays.
- Laboratory blood studies and a pulmonary function test.
- Allergy testing, usually with skin tests.
- Self-care instructions focused on the older patient.
- Emergency room care and hospitalization for severe attacks.
- Psychotherapy or counseling if the asthma is stress-related.

HOME TREATMENT BY SELF OR CARE-GIVER

GENERAL INSTRUCTIONS
- Eliminate allergens and irritants at home and at work if possible.
- Keep regular medications with you at all times. Ask your doctor about having emergency drugs available.
- Sit upright during attacks.
- Practice deep breathing each morning to loosen accumulated lung secretions.

MEDICATION (ADJUSTED FOR AGING)—Your doctor may prescribe:
- Expectorants to loosen the sputum.
- Bronchodilators to open the air passages.
- Intravenous cortisone drugs (for emergencies only) to decrease the body's allergic response.
- Cortisone drugs by nebulizer, which have fewer adverse reactions than oral forms.
- Cromolyn sodium by nebulizer. This is a preventive drug.

ACTIVITY FOR OLDER PATIENTS—Stay active, but avoid sudden bursts of exercise. If an attack follows heavy exercise, sit and rest. Sip warm water. Treatment with bronchodilators often prevents exercise-caused asthma.

FOOD & BEVERAGE—No special diet is required, but avoid foods to which you are sensitive. Drink at least 3 quarts of liquid daily to keep secretions loose.

FUTURE CONSIDERATIONS FOR THE AGING ADULT

POSSIBLE COMPLICATIONS—Respiratory failure; pneumothorax; lung infection; COPD (see Glossary) from recurrent attacks.

PROBABLE OUTCOME—The symptoms can be controlled with treatment and strict adherence to prevention measures. Without treatment, severe attacks can be fatal.

PREVENTING RECURRENCE
- Avoid known allergens and air pollutants.
- Take prescribed preventive medicines regularly. Don't omit them when you feel well.
- See appendix 13 for suggestions to reduce stress.

CALL YOUR DOCTOR IF

- You have symptoms of asthma.
- You have an asthma attack that doesn't respond to treatment. *This is an emergency!*
- New, unexplained symptoms develop. The drugs used in treatment may produce side effects.

ILLNESSES & DISORDERS

ATELECTASIS

BASIC INFORMATION FOR OLDER ADULTS

DESCRIPTION—Atelectasis is the collapse of part or all of one lung, preventing the normal absorption of oxygen. Body parts involved: The lungs.

SPECIAL CONSIDERATIONS FOR AGING—
The vital capacity of the lungs decreases.

SIGNS & SYMPTOMS
Sudden, major collapse:
- Chest pain.
- Shortness of breath; rapid breathing.
- Shock (severe weakness, paleness of skin and rapid heartbeat).
- Dizziness.

Gradual collapse:
- A cough.
- Fever.
- No other symptoms.

CAUSES & RISK FACTORS—Caused by the obstruction of small or large air passages in the lungs by enlarged lymph glands in the chest; thick mucus plugs from an infection or another disease; tumors in the air passages; tumors on the blood vessels outside the air passages, causing pressure on the airways; inhaled objects, such as peanuts; prolonged chest or abdominal surgery with general anesthetic; chest injury or fractured ribs; and surgery on any part of the body. The risk increases with aging; smoking; any illness that has lowered your resistance or weakened you; chronic obstructive lung disease, including emphysema and bronchiectasis; and the use of drugs that depress alertness or consciousness, such as sedatives, barbiturates, tranquilizers or alcohol.

DOCTOR'S TREATMENT & DIAGNOSTIC TESTS
- Medical history and physical exam.
- Laboratory studies to measure oxygen and carbon dioxide in the blood.
- X-rays of the chest.
- Surgery to remove tumors.
- Bronchoscopy (see Glossary) to remove a foreign object or a mucus plug.
- Self-care instructions focused on the older patient.

HOME TREATMENT BY SELF OR CARE-GIVER

GENERAL INSTRUCTIONS
- Cooperate with requests to turn, cough and breathe deeply after surgery. Hold a pillow tightly against surgical incisions during the coughing exercises.
- Stop smoking.

- Learn to perform postural drainage (see Glossary) after hospitalization. An inhalation therapist, nurse or doctor can demonstrate the technique.

MEDICATION (ADJUSTED FOR AGING)
- Your doctor may prescribe:
  Antibiotics to fight infection that inevitably accompanies atelectasis.
  Pain relievers for minor pain.
- Don't take sedatives. They may contribute to a recurrence.
- *Note:* Adverse reactions and side effects may be more frequent and severe in older persons. Remind your doctor of any medicines you already take.

ACTIVITY FOR OLDER PATIENTS
- Resume your normal activities as soon as your symptoms improve.
- See Appendix 20 regarding physical fitness for the active older adult.

FOOD & BEVERAGE
- No special diet is required, but drink at least 8 glasses of water or other fluid daily to thin lung secretions.
- See Appendix 1 regarding good nutrition for people over 50.

FUTURE CONSIDERATIONS FOR THE AGING ADULT

POSSIBLE COMPLICATIONS
- Pneumonia; small lung abscess.
- Permanent lung scars and collapsed lung tissue.

PROBABLE OUTCOME—If atelectasis is caused by a mucus plug or inhaled foreign object, it is curable when the plug or object is removed. If it is caused by a tumor, the outcome depends on the nature of the tumor.

PREVENTING RECURRENCE
- Force yourself to cough and breath deeply every 1 to 2 hours after surgery with general anesthesia. Also change position often in bed if possible.
- Increase fluid intake during lung illness or after surgery—by mouth or intravenously—to keep lung secretions loose.

CALL YOUR DOCTOR IF

- You have symptoms of atelectasis.
- Any of the following occurs during treatment:
  Distended abdomen.
  Sudden shortness of breath.
  Blue fingernails and lips.
  Temperature spikes to 102F (38.9C) or higher.

ATHEROSCLEROSIS
(Hardening of the Arteries)

BASIC INFORMATION FOR OLDER ADULTS

DESCRIPTION—Atherosclerosis is a thickening of the inner lining of the arteries (the blood vessels that carry oxygen and other nutrients from the heart to other body parts). Atherosclerosis may lead to kidney damage, decreased circulation to the brain and extremities and coronary artery disease. Atherosclerosis is a major cause of strokes and heart attacks. Body parts involved: All arterial blood vessels in the body.

SPECIAL CONSIDERATIONS FOR AGING
- The large blood vessels become thicker and less elastic.
- Stress from any emotional cause—fear, worry, anxiety, sadness, loneliness or anger—affects all aspects of any illness or disorder.

SIGNS & SYMPTOMS—Symptoms are often absent until atherosclerosis reaches advanced stages. The symptoms depend on what part of the body has a decreased blood flow and the extent of disease. Common symptoms include:
- Muscle cramps if atherosclerosis involves vessels in the legs.
- Angina pectoris or heart attack if it involves blood vessels to the heart.
- Stroke or transient ischemic attack if it involves vessels to the neck and brain.
- Headache.

CAUSES & RISK FACTORS—Caused by patches of fatty tissue that damage the artery walls. These patches often collect at artery junctions. This collection may begin in early adulthood. At these points, the inner lining of the artery may trap fatty substances that circulate in the blood. As these fatty deposits accumulate, they reduce the blood vessel's elasticity and narrow the passageway, interfering with blood flow. The risk increases with stress; diabetes mellitus; high blood pressure; obesity; smoking; a sedentary lifestyle; poor nutrition, especially too much salt, saturated fat and cholesterol in the diet; and a family history of atherosclerosis.

DOCTOR'S TREATMENT & DIAGNOSTIC TESTS
- Medical history and physical exam.
- Laboratory studies, including an ECG (see Glossary), exercise tolerance test, blood studies of cholesterol and high-density lipoproteins (see Glossary) and blood sugar tests.
- X-rays of the chest and blood vessels.
- MRI and CT (see Glossary).
- Self-care instructions focused on the older patient.
- Psychotherapy or counseling to help you learn to cope with stress.

HOME TREATMENT BY SELF OR CARE-GIVER

GENERAL INSTRUCTIONS
- Follow instructions under Preventing Recurrence.
- Atherosclerosis is a complicated, serious disorder. This page can cover only the main points of diagnosis and treatment. Your doctor, nurse or librarian can provide sources of supplemental information.

MEDICATION (ADJUSTED FOR AGING)
- Recent studies show that lowering cholesterol levels in persons with high levels can increase life expectancy. If you have symptoms of a disorder caused by atherosclerosis—and diet and exercise fail to reduce cholesterol—your doctor may prescribe antihyperlipidemic drugs.
- *Note:* Adverse reactions and side effects may be more frequent and severe in older persons. Remind your doctor of any medicines you already take.

ACTIVITY FOR OLDER PATIENTS
- No restrictions are necessary.
- See Appendix 20 regarding physical fitness for the active older adult.

FOOD & BEVERAGE
- Eat a diet that is low in fat, low in salt and high in fiber.
- See Appendix 1 regarding good nutrition for people over 50.

FUTURE CONSIDERATIONS FOR THE AGING ADULT

POSSIBLE COMPLICATIONS—Heart attack; stroke; kidney disease; loss of vision.

PROBABLE OUTCOME—This condition is currently considered incurable. However, the symptoms can be controlled and progress of the disease can be slowed with treatment. Complications are eventually fatal. Research into causes and treatment continues, so there is hope for increasingly effective treatment and a cure.

PREVENTING RECURRENCE
- Don't smoke; exercise regularly.
- Follow the suggestions under Food & Beverage.
- Reduce stress to a manageable level when possible.
- If you have diabetes or high blood pressure, adhere strictly to your treatment program.

☎ CALL YOUR DOCTOR IF

You have high risk factors for atherosclerosis and want to become involved in a prevention program.

ILLNESSES & DISORDERS

189

ATHLETE'S FOOT
(Tinea Pedis; Ringworm of the Feet)

BASIC INFORMATION FOR OLDER ADULTS

DESCRIPTION—Athlete's foot is a common, contagious fungus infection of the skin on the feet. Body parts involved: The feet, especially the soles and the skin between the toes (usually the 4th and 5th toes).

SPECIAL CONSIDERATIONS FOR AGING
- The immune system becomes less effective, opening the way for viral, bacterial and other infections; malignancies; immune disorders; and allergies.
- Wound healing is less efficient.
- Skin permeability is increased.

SIGNS & SYMPTOMS
- Moist, soft, gray-white or red scales on the feet, especially between the toes.
- Dead skin between the toes.
- Itching in inflamed areas.
- Damp, musty foot odor.
- Small blisters on the feet (sometimes).

CAUSES & RISK FACTORS—Athlete's foot is caused by a trichophyton fungus infection. The risk increases with:
- Infrequent washing of the feet.
- Infrequent changes of shoes or socks.
- The use of locker rooms and public showers.
- Hot, humid weather.

DOCTOR'S TREATMENT & DIAGNOSTIC TESTS
- Medical history and physical exam.
- Laboratory culture and microscopic examination of scales.
- Self-care instructions focused on the older patient.

HOME TREATMENT BY SELF OR CARE-GIVER

GENERAL INSTRUCTIONS
- Remove scales and material between the toes daily.
- Keep the affected area cool and dry. Go barefoot, wear dry cotton socks or wear sandals during treatment.

MEDICATION (ADJUSTED FOR AGING)
- Use non-prescription antifungal powders, creams or ointments after each bath.
- For severe cases, your doctor may prescribe oral or more potent topical antifungal medications.

- *Note:* Adverse reactions and side effects may be more frequent and severe in older persons. Remind your doctor of any medicines you already take.

ACTIVITY FOR OLDER PATIENTS
- No restrictions are necessary.
- See Appendix 20 regarding physical fitness for the active older adult.

FOOD & BEVERAGE
- No special diet is required.
- See Appendix 1 regarding good nutrition for people over 50.

FUTURE CONSIDERATIONS FOR THE AGING ADULT

POSSIBLE COMPLICATIONS
- Secondary bacterial infection in the affected area.
- Id reaction (see Glossary) on the hands and face (rare).

PROBABLE OUTCOME—Usually curable in 3 weeks with treatment, but recurrence is common.

PREVENTING RECURRENCE
- Soak your feet daily in warm water and Epsom salts. Dry them thoroughly, and dust them with talc.
- Go barefoot when possible.
- Change shoes and socks daily.
- Wear socks made of cotton, wool or other natural, absorbent fibers. Avoid synthetics.
- Disinfect shower floors.

CALL YOUR DOCTOR IF

- You have severe symptoms of athlete's foot that persist despite self-treatment.
- You develop a fever or the infection seems to be spreading.

ATRIAL FIBRILLATION

BASIC INFORMATION FOR OLDER ADULTS

DESCRIPTION—Atrial fibrillation is a completely irregular heartbeat rhythm. Fibrillation means a quivering of heart muscle fibers. Body parts involved: The heart muscles; the atrium (also called the auricle), a chamber of the heart that connects to the left ventricle (the main chamber); the heart's electrical conduction system.

SPECIAL CONSIDERATIONS FOR AGING
- Heart muscle mass becomes thicker, but not stronger.
- The threshold for developing rhythm disturbances is lower.
- A sedentary life-style becomes more common.

SIGNS & SYMPTOMS
- No symptoms (sometimes).
- Continuously irregular heartbeat in which no 2 beats are of equal strength or duration. You may perceive them as ''flip- flops.''
- Weakness, dizziness or faintness (sometimes).
- Chest pain (sometimes).

CAUSES & RISK FACTORS—Causes include rheumatic heart disease caused by rheumatic fever; diseases of the mitral valve; atherosclerosis of the coronary arteries, with or without a previous heart attack; hyperthyroidism; congestive heart failure. The risk increases with stress; recent heart surgery; electrolyte disturbances, especially low potassium; pulmonary embolism; excessive use of some drugs, such as thyroid hormones, caffeine and others; smoking; excessive alcohol consumption; obesity; and hypertension.

DOCTOR'S TREATMENT & DIAGNOSTIC TESTS
- Medical history and physical exam.
- ECG (see Glossary).
- Blood studies to measure the levels of drugs used in treatment.
- Self-care instructions focused on the older patient.
- Hospitalization, sometimes with electric shock (electrocardioversion), which may restore normal rhythm.

HOME TREATMENT BY SELF OR CARE-GIVER

GENERAL INSTRUCTIONS
- Have family members and friends learn cardiopulmonary resuscitation (CPR) in case you have cardiac arrest.
- Don't smoke, use mind-altering drugs or drink more than 1 or 2 alcoholic drinks—if any—a day.
- Learn to check your own pulse for rate (beats per minute), rhythm (regular or irregular) and strength. Call your doctor if these change.

- See Appendix 13 for suggestions to minimize stress.

MEDICATION (ADJUSTED FOR AGING)
- Your doctor may prescribe:
  Heart medications such as digitalis, quinidine, calcium channel blockers or beta-adrenergic blockers to regulate the heartbeat.
  Anticoagulants to prevent blood clots.
- *Note:* Adverse reactions and side effects may be more frequent and severe in older persons. Remind your doctor of any medicines you already take.

ACTIVITY FOR OLDER PATIENTS
- Resume your normal activities slowly. Consult your doctor before resuming sexual relations or any other strenuous or exciting activity.
- See Appendix 20 regarding physical fitness for the active older adult.

FOOD & BEVERAGE
- Lose weight if you are obese, but don't use appetite suppressants. These may worsen rhythm disturbances. A reducing diet appears in Appendix 10.
- The underlying heart condition may require a low-salt or low-fat diet (see Appendices 8 and 9) and potassium supplements. See Appendix 1 regarding good nutrition for people over 50.

FUTURE CONSIDERATIONS FOR THE AGING ADULT

POSSIBLE COMPLICATIONS
- Acute pulmonary edema; arterial thrombosis or embolus; congestive heart failure.
- Other heartbeat irregularities that may trigger cardiac arrest.

PROBABLE OUTCOME—A normal heartbeat rhythm can be restored with electrocardio-version in about 50% of patients. In the other 50%, some symptoms can be controlled with medication. Those whose rhythm is restored to normal have a longer life expectancy, greater strength and more energy than those who have continuing atrial fibrillation.

PREVENTING RECURRENCE—Avoid the risk factors for atherosclerosis and coronary artery disease.

CALL YOUR DOCTOR IF

- You have symptoms of atrial fibrillation.
- Any of the following occurs during treatment:
  A change in the heart's rate, rhythm or strength.
  Chest pain, sweating and weakness.
  Shortness of breath with swollen feet and ankles.
  Pain in the calf of the leg while walking.
- New, unexplained symptoms develop. Drugs used in treatment may produce side effects.

BALDNESS
(Alopecia Areata)

BASIC INFORMATION FOR OLDER ADULTS

DESCRIPTION—Baldness is sudden hair loss in circular patches on the scalp. Hair loss is not accompanied by other visible evidence of scalp disease. This is not contagious. Body parts involved: The hair, scalp, eyebrows, eyelashes, beard, genital area and underarms (sometimes).

SPECIAL CONSIDERATIONS FOR AGING
- The hair bulb follicles are reduced in number.
- Wound healing is impaired.
- The skin produces a reduced quantity of vitamin D.
- The immune system is less efficient.

SIGNS & SYMPTOMS
- Sudden hair loss in sharply defined oval or circular patches. In rare cases, body hair loss may be total.
- No pain.
- No itch.
- Denuded site becomes white.

CAUSES & RISK FACTORS—The cause is unknown, but heredity and emotional factors, such as anxiety, may contribute to hair loss. The autoimmune system may also be involved. The risk can increase with:
- Stress and anxiety.
- A family history of baldness.
- Scalp infection.
- Any major surgery.
- Prolonged illness.
- High fever.
- Chemotherapy.

DOCTOR'S TREATMENT & DIAGNOSTIC TESTS
- Medical history and physical exam.
- Self-care instructions focused on the older patient.

HOME TREATMENT BY SELF OR CARE-GIVER

GENERAL INSTRUCTIONS
- Consider wearing a hairpiece or wig during the acute phase.
- Continue to bathe and shampoo as usual.
- Don't tug on normal hair close to areas of hair loss.

MEDICATION (ADJUSTED FOR AGING)
- Your doctor may prescribe a topical steroid. Apply it once or twice a day unless directed otherwise. Apply immediately after bathing or shampooing for better spreading and penetration. For the scalp and groin, use only low-potency steroid products without fluorine. In special cases, your doctor may inject steroids into affected areas and prescribe oral cortisone drugs for you to take on alternate days.
- A topical medication, minoxidil, may help.
- *Note:* Adverse reactions and side effects may be more frequent and severe in older persons. Remind your doctor of any medicines you already take.

ACTIVITY FOR OLDER PATIENTS
- No restrictions are necessary.
- See Appendix 20 regarding physical fitness for the active older adult.

FOOD & BEVERAGE
- No special diet is required.
- See Appendix 1 regarding good nutrition for people over 50.

FUTURE CONSIDERATIONS FOR THE AGING ADULT

POSSIBLE COMPLICATIONS
- Loss of all hair.
- Slow or incomplete regrowth.

PROBABLE OUTCOME—Usually curable, with spontaneous new growth in 18 months. Persons with a few small patches are generally cured completely. The disorder recurs in 25% of cases.

PREVENTING RECURRENCE—Cannot be prevented at present.

CALL YOUR DOCTOR IF

- You have symptoms of baldness.
- Any of the following occurs during treatment: Hair loss increases.
  Hair loss doesn't diminish in 4 weeks.
  Areas show signs of infection (redness, swelling, tenderness and warmth) after injections.

BALDNESS, PATTERN
(Male & Female)

BASIC INFORMATION FOR OLDER ADULTS

DESCRIPTION—Pattern baldness is gradual, painless hair loss that occurs in a distinctive pattern as a person ages. The earlier hair loss begins, the greater the eventual loss. Some persons have short periods of intense hair loss followed by long, stable periods. Body parts involved: The hair and scalp.

SPECIAL CONSIDERATIONS FOR AGING—The fatty layer of tissue under the skin becomes thinner.

SIGNS & SYMPTOMS
- In men, hair loss occurs on top of the head and in the temple areas of the scalp.
- In women, hair loss usually occurs only on top of the head.
- In both sexes, some scattered loss may also occur.

CAUSES & RISK FACTORS
Causes include:
- Genetic factors.
- Hormonal factors.
  Male hormones are an important factor in balding. Men who are castrated at a young age don't develop pattern baldness—regardless of genetic factors—unless they receive supplemental testosterone (a male hormone).
  Correspondingly, estrogen (a female hormone) may be protective in women, because hair loss rarely begins before menopause.
The risk increases with a a family history of pattern baldness. Hair loss that occurs after illness or pregnancy or as an adverse reaction to drugs is a different form of baldness.

DOCTOR'S TREATMENT & DIAGNOSTIC TESTS
- Medical history and physical exam if diagnosis is in doubt.
- Self-care instructions focused on the older patient.

HOME TREATMENT BY SELF OR CARE-GIVER

GENERAL INSTRUCTIONS
- Don't use medicated shampoos and ointments.
- If you cannot accept balding as part of aging, there are 2 options:
  Consider wearing a toupee or wig.

Consider a hair-transplant operation. This surgery may have complications, so discuss the advantages and disadvantages with your doctor before undergoing the procedure.

MEDICATION (ADJUSTED FOR AGING)
- Medicine is not necessary for this disorder. Your doctor may prescribe a topical form of minoxidil, which has proven helpful for a number of people.
- *Note:* Adverse reactions and side effects may be more frequent and severe in older persons. Remind your doctor of any medicines you already take.

ACTIVITY FOR OLDER PATIENTS
- No restrictions are necessary.
- See Appendix 20 regarding physical fitness for the active older adult.

FOOD & BEVERAGE
- No special diet is required.
- See Appendix 1 regarding good nutrition for people over 50.

FUTURE CONSIDERATIONS FOR THE AGING ADULT

POSSIBLE COMPLICATIONS—None.

PROBABLE OUTCOME—Incurable at present.

PREVENTING RECURRENCE—Cannot be prevented at present.

CALL YOUR DOCTOR IF

You want a medical referral for hair transplantation.

BAROTITIS MEDIA
(Barotrauma)

BASIC INFORMATION FOR OLDER ADULTS

DESCRIPTION—Barotitis media is damage to the middle ear caused by pressure changes. Body parts involved: The middle ear, the eustachian tube and the nerve endings in the ear.

SPECIAL CONSIDERATIONS FOR AGING—Hearing acuity diminishes.

SIGNS & SYMPTOMS
- Hearing loss (to varying degrees).
- A plugged feeling in the ear.
- Severe pain in the ears, over the cheekbones or in the forehead.
- Dizziness.
- Ringing noises in the ear.

CAUSES & RISK FACTORS—Caused by sudden increased pressure in the surrounding air, such as that which occurs in the rapid descent of an airplane or while scuba diving. In these activities, air moves from passages in the nose into the middle ear to maintain equal pressure on both sides of the eardrum. If the tube leading from the nose to the ear (the eustachian tube) doesn't function properly, the pressure in the middle ear is less than the pressure outside the ear. The negative pressure in the middle ear sucks the eardrum inward. Blood and mucus may later appear in the middle ear. This damage is more likely if you have a nose or throat infection when scuba diving or traveling by air. The risk increases with recent respiratory tract infection.

DOCTOR'S TREATMENT & DIAGNOSTIC TESTS
- Medical history and physical exam.
- Self-care instructions focused on the older patient.
- Surgery (sometimes) to open the eardrum and release fluid trapped in the middle ear. A plastic tube may be inserted through the surgically perforated eardrum to keep it open and equalize pressure. The tube falls out spontaneously in 9 to 12 months.

HOME TREATMENT BY SELF OR CARE-GIVER

GENERAL INSTRUCTIONS—If fluid drains from the ear, place a small piece of cotton in the outer ear canal to absorb it.

MEDICATION (ADJUSTED FOR AGING)
- Usually none is necessary.
- For minor discomfort, you may use non-prescription decongestants and pain relievers, such as acetaminophen.

- Your doctor may prescribe:
  Stronger prescription decongestant nasal sprays or tablets. Use for at least 2 weeks after damage.
  A steroid nasal spray.
  Antibiotics if infection is present.
- *Note:* Adverse reactions and side effects may be more frequent and severe in older persons. Remind your doctor of any medicines you already take.

ACTIVITY FOR OLDER PATIENTS
- Resume your normal activities as soon as your symptoms improve.
- See Appendix 20 regarding physical fitness for the active older adult.

FOOD & BEVERAGE
- No special diet is required.
- See Appendix 1 regarding good nutrition for people over 50.

FUTURE CONSIDERATIONS FOR THE AGING ADULT

POSSIBLE COMPLICATIONS—Without treatment, fluid may accumulate, become infected and rupture the eardrum. The rupture may affect nerve endings or scar the eardrum, causing permanent hearing loss.

PROBABLE OUTCOME—With treatment, most cases of barotitis media are reversible without permanent damage or hearing loss.

PREVENTING RECURRENCE
- Don't fly or scuba dive when you have an upper respiratory infection.
- If you must fly:
  Use non-prescription decongestant tablets or sprays. Follow package instructions.
  While ascending or descending, suck on hard candy or chew gum to force frequent swallowing.
  Take a moderate-sized breath, hold the nose and try to force air into the eustachian tube by gently puffing out the cheeks with the mouth closed.

CALL YOUR DOCTOR IF

- You have symptoms of barotitis media.
- Any of the following occurs during treatment:
  Severe headache.
  Fever.
  Severe pain.
  Dizziness.
- New, unexplained symptoms develop. The drugs used in treatment may produce side effects.

BELL'S PALSY

BASIC INFORMATION FOR OLDER ADULTS

DESCRIPTION—Bell's palsy, named after the physician who first described it, is paralysis on one side of the face. Body parts involved: The 7th cranial nerve and the facial muscles supplied by that nerve.

SPECIAL CONSIDERATIONS FOR AGING— Neurological diseases become more likely.

SIGNS & SYMPTOMS
- Sudden paralysis on one side of the face, including the muscles to the eyelid.
- Pain behind the ear on the affected side.
- Flat, expressionless features on one side of the face.
- Distorted smiles and frowns.
- Changes in taste, salivation or tear formation (sometimes).

CAUSES & RISK FACTORS—The cause is unknown. The paralysis is probably caused by a swelling of the facial nerve. The swelling may be caused by a virus, an autoimmune disease or a decrease in blood flow and pressure on the facial nerve as it passes through the temporal bone of the skull. The risk increases with face chilling.

DOCTOR'S TREATMENT & DIAGNOSTIC TESTS
- Medical history and physical exam.
- CT scan (see Glossary) to rule out other causes of pressure on the facial nerve.
- Self-care instructions focused on the older patient.
- Surgery (rare). Advancing age alone is not a deterrent.

HOME TREATMENT BY SELF OR CARE-GIVER

GENERAL INSTRUCTIONS
- If you have pain, apply heat to the painful area twice a day. Wring out a towel soaked in hot water and apply for 15 minutes. Cover or close the eye during heat treatments.
- If you cannot wink or close your eye well, buy a pair of wrap-around plastic bubble goggles. Wear them to protect your eye from dirt, dust and dryness. You may buy goggles from a sporting goods store or optician.
- At night, apply an eye patch to shut the lid so the eye stays moist and protected.
- As muscle strength returns, use facial massage and exercises. Massage the muscles of the forehead, cheek, lips and eyes using cream or oil. Exercise the weak muscles in front of a mirror. Open and close the eye, wink, smile and bare your teeth. Perform the massage and exercise for 15 or 20 minutes several times a day.

- Brush and floss your teeth more often to keep your mouth healthy.

MEDICATION (ADJUSTED FOR AGING)
- Your doctor may prescribe: Methylcellulose eye drops for comfort and protection of the exposed eye. Cortisone drugs for 2 weeks to reduce swelling and inflammation of the affected nerve.
- *Note:* Adverse reactions and side effects may be more frequent and severe in older persons. Remind your doctor of any medicines you already take.

ACTIVITY FOR OLDER PATIENTS
- Maintain your normal activities. Rest does not help Bell's palsy.
- See Appendix 20 regarding physical fitness for the active older adult.

FOOD & BEVERAGE
- A soft diet is often necessary.
- See Appendix 1 regarding good nutrition for people over 50.

FUTURE CONSIDERATIONS FOR THE AGING ADULT

POSSIBLE COMPLICATIONS—Eye irritation or injury because the eye does not close properly and is exposed to dust. If unprotected, the eye may develop ulcers on the cornea.

PROBABLE OUTCOME
- Bell's palsy is distressing, but it is not dangerous.
- The extent of nerve damage determines the extent of recovery. Improvement is gradual and recovery time varies, sometimes requiring many months.
- Patients with mild facial paralysis usually recover completely within several months. Patients with severe facial paralysis recover completely in 80% to 90% of cases.
- Surgery can sometimes improve facial appearance and muscle function in patients who do not recover fully.

PREVENTING RECURRENCE—Cannot be prevented at present.

CALL YOUR DOCTOR IF

- You have symptoms of Bell's palsy.
- Your eye becomes red or irritated despite treatment.
- You cannot prevent saliva from drooling from your mouth.
- Your pain worsens.
- You develop a fever.

BLADDER INFECTION
(Cystitis)

BASIC INFORMATION FOR OLDER ADULTS

DESCRIPTION—Cystitis is an inflammation or infection of the urinary bladder (the organ that stores urine from the kidneys) or the urethra (the tube through which urine travels from the bladder to the outside of the body). Body parts involved: The urinary bladder and the urethra.

SPECIAL CONSIDERATIONS FOR AGING
- Kidney function becomes less efficient.
- The blood flow to the kidneys decreases.

SIGNS & SYMPTOMS
- Burning and stinging on urination.
- Frequent urination, especially at night, although the amount of urine may be small.
- Increased urge to urinate.
- Pain in the lower part of the abdomen over the bladder.
- Low back pain.
- Blood in the urine; bad-smelling urine.
- Low-grade fever (under 101F).
- Painful sexual intercourse.
- Lack of urinary control (sometimes).

CAUSES & RISK FACTORS—Causes include increased sexual activity (in women, the cause is often aggravated by bruising of the urethra during intercourse); infection in other parts of the genitourinary system; stress; illness that has lowered resistance; excessive alcohol consumption; obstruction of urine in the urinary tract in men (usually partial obstruction caused by an enlarged or inflamed prostate gland); bacteria that reach the bladder from another part of the body through the bloodstream; bacteria that enter the urinary tract from the skin around the genitals and the anal area; injury to the urethra; the use of a urinary catheter to empty the bladder, such as following surgery.

DOCTOR'S TREATMENT & DIAGNOSTIC TESTS
- Medical history and physical exam.
- Urinalysis and careful urine collection for bacterial culture.
- Cystoscopy (see Glossary).
- Self-care instructions focused on the older patient.

HOME TREATMENT BY SELF OR CARE-GIVER

GENERAL INSTRUCTIONS—Carefully apply heat to the bladder area with a heat lamp or heating pad (set on low).

MEDICATION (ADJUSTED FOR AGING)—
Your doctor may prescribe:
- Antibiotics to fight the infection.
- Antispasmodics to relieve the pain.

ACTIVITY FOR OLDER PATIENTS
- Avoid sexual intercourse until you have been free of symptoms for 2 weeks to allow inflammation to subside.
- See Appendix 20 regarding physical fitness for the active older adult.

FOOD & BEVERAGE
- Drink 6 to 8 glasses of water daily.
- Avoid caffeine and alcohol during treatment.
- Drink cranberry juice to acidify urine. Some drugs are more effective with acid urine.

FUTURE CONSIDERATIONS FOR THE AGING ADULT

POSSIBLE COMPLICATIONS—Inadequate treatment can cause chronic urinary tract infections leading to kidney failure.

PROBABLE OUTCOME—Curable in 2 weeks with prompt medical treatment. Recurrence is common.

PREVENTING RECURRENCE.
- Drink a glass of water before sexual intercourse and urinate within 15 minutes after intercourse.
- Use a water-soluble lubricant during intercourse.
- Use female-superior or lateral positions in intercourse to protect the female urethra from injury.
- Take showers instead of tub baths.
- Request frequent urinalyses to monitor signs of infection.
- Drink 8 glasses of water every day.
- Avoid caffeine, which irritates the bladder.
- Avoid the use of catheters if possible.
- Obtain prompt medical treatment for urinary tract infections.
- Women: Do not douche. Clean the anal area thoroughly after bowel movements (wipe from the front to the rear rather than rear to front to avoid spreading fecal bacteria to the genital area).

CALL YOUR DOCTOR IF

- You have symptoms of cystitis.
- You have fever.
- Blood appears in the urine.
- Your discomfort and other symptoms don't decrease in 1 week.
- New, unexplained symptoms develop. The drugs used in treatment may produce side effects.
- Your symptoms recur after treatment.

BLADDER STONES, URINARY
(Calculi)

BASIC INFORMATION FOR OLDER ADULTS

DESCRIPTION—Bladder stones are small, solid particles that form within the bladder and are too large to pass in the urine through the urethra to the outside. Body parts involved: The bladder and urethra.

SPECIAL CONSIDERATIONS FOR AGING—Kidney function becomes less efficient.

SIGNS & SYMPTOMS
- Blood in the urine.
- Painful urination.
- A frequent urge to urinate, particularly at night, even though only small amounts of urine pass.
- A dull pain in the penis, scrotum, labia or back.

CAUSES & RISK FACTORS
Causes include:
- Reduced urine volume from dehydration.
- Increased excretion by the kidney of calcium, oxalate, urate, cystine, phosphate or xanthine.
- Reduction of normal protective substances that suppress stone formation (hereditary).

Risk factors include:
- Chronic bladder infection.
- Nerve injury that impairs bladder function.
- The long-term use of urinary catheters.
- A history of urinary stones.

DOCTOR'S TREATMENT & DIAGNOSTIC TESTS
- Medical history and physical exam.
- Laboratory studies such as blood chemistries, urinalysis, x-rays or a sonogram (ultrasound), and analysis of the composition of any stone that is passed.
- Surgery to remove the stone(s) (rare).
- Self-care instructions focused on the older patient.

HOME TREATMENT BY SELF OR CARE-GIVER

GENERAL INSTRUCTIONS—If you are waiting for the stone to pass, watch for it when you urinate. To trap it, urinate each time through a piece of gauze. The stone may pass without discomfort. When it passes, take it your doctor's office for analysis.

MEDICATION (ADJUSTED FOR AGING)
- Your doctor may prescribe:
  Narcotic pain relievers during the attack.
  Antibiotics if infection is present.
  Drugs to alkalize or acidify the urine after the attack, depending on the kind of stone.

- *Note:* Adverse reactions and side effects may be more frequent and severe in older persons. Remind your doctor of any medicines you already take.

ACTIVITY FOR OLDER PATIENTS
- If you know you have bladder stones, avoid situations in which a sudden, sharp pain might cause danger, such as climbing ladders.
- During a bladder-stone episode, stay as active as your strength allows. Don't go to bed. Activity may help the stone pass more easily.
- See Appendix 20 regarding physical fitness for the active older adult.

FOOD & BEVERAGE
- If the stone proves to be calcium or phosphorus, avoid milk and products made with milk, chocolate or nuts.
- If the stone is a phosphate, your doctor will prescribe an acid-ash diet to keep the urine slightly acid.
- If the stone is a urate or cystine stone, your doctor will prescribe an alkaline-ash diet to keep the urine slightly alkaline.
- For all types of stones, drink at least 13 glasses of fluid daily. Most of your fluid should be purified or distilled water. A small amount can be weak tea or other beverages.
- See Appendix 1 regarding good nutrition for people over 50.

FUTURE CONSIDERATIONS FOR THE AGING ADULT

POSSIBLE COMPLICATIONS
- Infection.
- Urinary blockage.

PROBABLE OUTCOME—Many bladder stones pass in the urine unassisted. Those that are too large to pass must be removed surgically or by shockwave treatment.

PREVENTING RECURRENCE
- Follow suggestions under Food & Beverage.
- Avoid activities that cause excessive sweating.

CALL YOUR DOCTOR IF

- You have symptoms of a bladder stone.
- You develop a fever or other symptoms of a bladder infection: stinging, burning on urination or a frequent urge to urinate.
- You develop new, unexplained symptoms during treatment. The drugs used in treatment may produce side effects.

BLADDER TUMOR

BASIC INFORMATION FOR OLDER ADULTS

DESCRIPTION—A bladder tumor is abnormal tissue growth in the bladder in which cell multiplication is uncontrolled. The tumor may be benign or malignant. Malignant bladder tumors usually don't spread to distant organs but may occasionally metastasize to the rectum, sigmoid colon, prostate gland or pelvic bones. Body parts involved: The bladder and (sometimes) the rectum, sigmoid colon, prostate gland or pelvic bones.

SPECIAL CONSIDERATIONS FOR AGING
- The immune system becomes less effective, opening the way for viral, bacterial and other infections; malignancies; immune disorders; and allergies.
- Usual signs and symptoms may be absent and be replaced by symptoms of confusion, dizziness, failure to thrive, falling, incontinence, increasing dementia, refusal to eat or drink, weight loss, depression, paranoia, hypo-chondriasis, psychosis or threats of suicide.
- Urinary incontinence becomes more frequent.
- Stress from any emotional cause—fear, worry, anxiety, sadness, loneliness or anger—affects all aspects of any illness or disorder.

SIGNS & SYMPTOMS
- Blood in the urine.
- Burning on urination.
- Increased frequency of urination, but passage of only small amounts of urine.
- Pain in the pelvic area.
- Unexplained weight loss.

CAUSES & RISK FACTORS—The cause is unknown. The risk increases with:
- Smoking.
- A family history of bladder tumors.
- Exposure to naphthylamines (dyes containing aniline) or chemicals used in the manufacture of rubber.

DOCTOR'S TREATMENT & DIAGNOSTIC TESTS
- Medical history and physical exam.
- Cystoscopy (see Glossary).
- X-rays of the bladder and urinary tract.
- Laboratory studies including urinalysis, cystoscopy and biopsy (see Glossary).
- Surgery to remove the tumor or possibly the bladder. If the tumor is malignant, anticancer drugs may be instilled in the bladder during surgery. The operation also may include a procedure to divert the urinary stream. Advancing age alone is not a deterrent.
- Radiation treatment.
- Treatment by diathermy (heat destruction) via cystoscope.
- Self-care instructions focused on the older patient.

HOME TREATMENT BY SELF OR CARE-GIVER

GENERAL INSTRUCTIONS
- Maintain as positive an attitude as possible during treatment.
- Treatment may cause side effects, but they are usually temporary.
- Your pain can be controlled. Don't hesitate to ask your doctor for pain medication.
- Fear may be your worst enemy.
- Call on family members and friends for whatever support and help you need.
- A bladder tumor is a complicated, serious disorder. This page can cover only the main points of diagnosis and treatment. Your doctor, nurse or librarian can provide sources of supplemental information.

MEDICATION (ADJUSTED FOR AGING)
- Your doctor may prescribe:
  Pain relievers.
  Oral anticancer drugs.
- *Note:* Adverse reactions and side effects may be more frequent and severe in older persons. Remind your doctor of any medicines you already take.

ACTIVITY FOR OLDER PATIENTS—After surgery or other treatment, resume your normal activities (including sex) as soon as possible.

FOOD & BEVERAGE
- No special diet is required.
- See Appendix 1 regarding good nutrition for people over 50.

FUTURE CONSIDERATIONS FOR THE AGING ADULT

POSSIBLE COMPLICATIONS
- Infection in the bladder or kidneys. The symptoms include back pain, fever and vomiting.
- Urinary obstruction.

PROBABLE OUTCOME—When diagnosed early, bladder cancer treatment is often successful, but recurrence is common and regular checkups are necessary. When the tumor has been present for a long time, the treatment outcome is poor.

PREVENTING RECURRENCE
- Avoid exposure to chemical or environmental hazards.
- Don't smoke.

CALL YOUR DOCTOR IF

- You have symptoms of a bladder tumor.
- New, unexplained symptoms develop. The drugs used in treatment may produce side effects.

BLADDER OR URETHRA INJURY

BASIC INFORMATION FOR OLDER ADULTS

DESCRIPTION—This disorder is characterized by damage to the urinary bladder (the organ that stores urine from the kidneys) or the urethra (the tube through which urine travels from the bladder to the outside of the body). Body parts involved: The urinary bladder and the urethra.

SPECIAL CONSIDERATIONS FOR AGING—Kidney function becomes less efficient.

SIGNS & SYMPTOMS
- Severe abdominal pain, boring in nature.
- Shock (sweating; faintness; nausea; panting; rapid pulse; pale, cold moist skin).
- Painful urination or inability to urinate.
- Bloody discharge from the urethra.
- Bloody urine.

CAUSES & RISK FACTORS—Usually caused by a pelvic bone fracture that punctures the bladder or urethra. The risk increases with:
- Excessive alcohol consumption.
- Accident-proneness.
- Hazardous occupations.
- Hazardous driving conditions.

DOCTOR'S TREATMENT & DIAGNOSTIC TESTS
- Medical history and physical exam.
- Laboratory urine studies.
- X-rays of the urinary tract.
- Emergency care; hospitalization.
- Surgery to repair a punctured bladder (usually). A damaged urethra may heal without surgery.
- Self-care instructions focused on the older patient.

HOME TREATMENT BY SELF OR CARE-GIVER

GENERAL INSTRUCTIONS—No specific instructions except those under other headings.

MEDICATION (ADJUSTED FOR AGING)
- Your doctor may prescribe antibiotics to prevent infection.
- *Note:* Adverse reactions and side effects may be more frequent and severe in older persons. Remind your doctor of any medicines you already take.

ACTIVITY FOR OLDER PATIENTS
- Stay as active as your strength allows. Allow 1 month for recovery. Don't return to work or resume sexual relations until healing is complete.
- See Appendix 20 regarding physical fitness for the active older adult.

FOOD & BEVERAGE
- No special diet is required.
- Drink 6 to 8 glasses of fluid daily.
- Don't drink alcohol.
- See Appendix 1 regarding good nutrition for people over 50.

FUTURE CONSIDERATIONS FOR THE AGING ADULT

POSSIBLE COMPLICATIONS
- Internal bleeding.
- Urine leakage into the abdomen, causing abdominal inflammation or infection.
- Recurrent infections from scars in the urethra that narrow the urinary passage.

PROBABLE OUTCOME—A punctured bladder or urethra requires emergency hospital treatment and surgery.

PREVENTING RECURRENCE—Protect yourself from injury whenever possible. Buckle your automobile seat belt and shoulder harness to minimize internal injury in case of accident. Don't drink and drive.

CALL YOUR DOCTOR IF

- You have any symptoms of bladder or urethra injury.
- You develop fever and chills during or after treatment.
- New, unexplained symptoms develop. The drugs used in treatment may produce side effects.

BLOOD PRESSURE, TOO HIGH
(Hypertension)

BASIC INFORMATION FOR OLDER ADULTS

DESCRIPTION—High blood pressure is an increase in the force against the arteries (blood vessels) as blood circulates through them. High blood pressure is sometimes called "the silent killer" because it often has no symptoms in the early stages. Body parts involved: The heart and blood vessels; the kidneys and eyes (advanced stages).

SPECIAL CONSIDERATIONS FOR AGING
- Many medical disorders in older people that once were thought to be "normal" consequences of aging are frequently diseases that can be treated.
- 50% of people over 60 have x-ray evidence of narrowing of the coronary arteries, yet only 50% of those people have symptoms.
- Stress from any emotional cause—fear, worry, anxiety, sadness, loneliness or anger—affects all aspects of any illness or disorder.

SIGNS & SYMPTOMS—Usually there are no symptoms unless the disease is severe. Following are the symptoms of a hypertensive crisis:
- Headache; drowsiness; confusion.
- Numbness and tingling in the hands and feet.
- Coughing up blood; nosebleeds.
- Severe shortness of breath.
- Seizures.

CAUSES & RISK FACTORS—The cause is usually unknown. A small number of cases result from:
- Chronic kidney disease.
- Severe narrowing of the aorta (the major artery of the heart).
- Tumors of some endocrine glands.
- Hardening of the arteries.
Risk factors include:
- Obesity; smoking; stress.
- Alcoholism.
- A diet that is high in salt or saturated fat.
- A sedentary lifestyle.
- Genetic factors. Hypertension is most common among blacks.
- A family history of hypertension, stroke, heart attack or kidney failure.
- The use of cortisone-like drugs, some immunosuppressant drugs and some appetite suppressants or decongestants.

DOCTOR'S TREATMENT & DIAGNOSTIC TESTS
- Medical history and physical exam.
- Laboratory studies such as blood studies of kidney function, urinalysis and ECG (see Glossary).
- X-rays of the chest and kidneys.
- Self-care instructions focused on the older patient.

HOME TREATMENT BY SELF OR CARE-GIVER

GENERAL INSTRUCTIONS
- Consider lifestyle changes and learn to reduce stress. See Appendix 13.
- Learn to take your own blood pressure. Your doctor or nurse can teach you.
- Go on a reducing diet if you are overweight.

MEDICATION (ADJUSTED FOR AGING)
- Many antihypertensive medications can reduce blood pressure. Your doctor will prescribe the type appropriate for you. Don't stop taking it without consulting your doctor.
- Don't take non-prescription cold and sinus remedies. These contain chemicals, such as ephedrine and pseudoephedrine, that raise blood pressure.
- *Note:* Adverse reactions and side effects may be more frequent and severe in older persons. Remind your doctor of any medicines you already take.

ACTIVITY FOR OLDER PATIENTS
- Exercise at least 3 times a week. This helps reduce stress and maintain normal body weight; it may also lower blood pressure.
- See Appendix 20 regarding physical fitness for the active older adult.

FOOD & BEVERAGE
- Consume a low-salt diet (see Appendix 9).
- Reduce if you are overweight (see Appendix 10).
- Reduce or discontinue alcohol consumption.

FUTURE CONSIDERATIONS FOR THE AGING ADULT

POSSIBLE COMPLICATIONS
- Stroke: heart attack; kidney failure.
- Congestive heart failure and pulmonary edema.
- Blindness caused by ruptured blood vessels.

PROBABLE OUTCOME—With treatment, complications are preventable (except for possible side effects of drugs). Life expectancy is near normal. Without treatment, life expectancy is reduced because of the likelihood of heart attack or stroke.

PREVENTING RECURRENCE—Essential high blood pressure (from unknown causes) cannot be prevented at present. If you have a family history of high blood pressure, obtain frequent blood pressure checks. If high blood pressure is detected early, treatment that includes diet, exercise, stress management and medication can usually prevent complications.

CALL YOUR DOCTOR IF

- You have symptoms of a hypertensive crisis.
- You have chest pain.

BLOOD TRANSFUSION REACTION

BASIC INFORMATION FOR OLDER ADULTS

DESCRIPTION—Blood transfusion reaction is a set of symptoms triggered by a blood transfusion. Body parts involved: The blood, blood vessels, kidneys, heart, skin, central nervous system, and lungs. (THIS IS AN EMERGENCY; SEEK MEDICAL CARE IMMEDIATELY!)

SPECIAL CONSIDERATIONS FOR AGING
- Kidney function becomes less efficient.
- Signs and symptoms may differ significantly from those listed below.

SIGNS & SYMPTOMS
Less serious:
- Chills and fever.
- Backache or other aches and pains.
- Hives and itching.

More serious:
- Blood cell destruction (hemolysis) causing shortness of breath, severe headache, chest or back pain and blood in the urine.

CAUSES & RISK FACTORS—Caused by receiving a transfusion of blood that is a different blood type from one's own. This may be due to errors in matching or the use of incompletely matched blood in an emergency. The risk increases with:
- Receiving a blood transfusion in an emergency situation when the careful typing and matching of blood must be bypassed.
- Receiving a blood transfusion from a donor who carries an infection.

DOCTOR'S TREATMENT & DIAGNOSTIC TESTS
- Medical history and physical exam.
- Laboratory blood tests to recheck blood compatibility and detect complications.
- Hospitalization. Patients receiving transfusions are usually in a hospital or outpatient surgical facility and reactions can be treated when they occur.
- Self-care instructions focused on the older patient.

HOME TREATMENT BY SELF OR CARE-GIVER

GENERAL INSTRUCTIONS—Stay awake and alert during a blood transfusion if possible so you can notify medical personnel immediately if symptoms occur.

MEDICATION (ADJUSTED FOR AGING)
- Your doctor may prescribe:
  Antihistamines to decrease hives and itching.
  Cortisone drugs to decrease the likelihood of acute kidney failure.
  Antihypertensives if blood pressure rises too high or hypertensives such as ephedrine or epinephrine if blood pressure drops too low.
- *Note:* Adverse reactions and side effects may be more frequent and severe in older persons. Remind your doctor of any medicines you already take.

ACTIVITY FOR OLDER PATIENTS
- Resume your normal activities as soon as your symptoms improve after transfusion.
- See Appendix 20 regarding physical fitness for the active older adult.

FOOD & BEVERAGE
- No special diet is required.
- See Appendix 1 regarding good nutrition for people over 50.

FUTURE CONSIDERATIONS FOR THE AGING ADULT

POSSIBLE COMPLICATIONS
- Acute kidney failure.
- Anaphylaxis.
- Congestive heart failure from overly rapid transfusion.
- Hypothermia from blood that is too cold.

PROBABLE OUTCOME—Most reactions clear gradually after the transfusion is halted. A few reactions are fatal.

PREVENTING RECURRENCE
- Blood bank and hospital personnel have received instructions in safety procedures to prevent reactions except in situations that are uncontrollable (see Causes).
- The use of diphenhydramine (an antihistamine) and acetaminophen prior to transfusion may prevent minor reactions.
- If surgery is planned at least 1 month in advance, your own blood may be drawn and stored for use during surgery if necessary. Transfusion with your own blood is least likely to produce a reaction.

CALL YOUR DOCTOR IF

You have symptoms of a blood transfusion reaction during or after a transfusion. Call immediately. *This is an emergency!*

BOILS
(Furuncles)

BASIC INFORMATION FOR OLDER ADULTS

DESCRIPTION—Boils are painful, deep bacterial infections of hair follicles. They are common and are contagious. Body parts involved: The skin and hair follicles.

SPECIAL CONSIDERATIONS FOR AGING
- The immune system becomes less effective, opening the way for viral, bacterial and other infections; malignancies; immune disorders; and allergies.
- The fatty layer of tissue under the skin becomes thinner.

SIGNS & SYMPTOMS
- A domed nodule that is painful, tender and red and has pus on the surface. A boil can appear suddenly and ripen in 24 hours. Boils are usually 1-1/2cm to 3cm in diameter; some are larger.
- Fever (rare).
- Swelling of the closest lymph glands.

CAUSES & RISK FACTORS—Boils are caused by an infection, usually from staphylococcus bacteria, that begins in the hair follicle and bores into the skin's deeper layers. The risk increases with:
- Poor nutrition.
- Illness that has lowered resistance.
- Diabetes mellitus.
- The use of immunosuppressive drugs.

DOCTOR'S TREATMENT & DIAGNOSTIC TESTS
- Medical history and physical exam.
- Laboratory culture of the pus to identify the germ.
- Self-care instructions focused on the older patient.
- For a large and painful boil, treatment may include incision and drainage of the boil.

HOME TREATMENT BY SELF OR CARE-GIVER

GENERAL INSTRUCTIONS
- Relieve the pain with gentle heat from warm-water soaks (see Glossary), a heating pad, a hot water bottle or a lamp close to the skin. Use 3 or 4 times daily for 20 minutes.
- Prevent the spread of boils by using clean towels only once or using paper towels and discarding them.
- Take showers instead of baths.

MEDICATION (ADJUSTED FOR AGING)
- Your doctor may prescribe antibiotics.
- Don't use non-prescription antibiotic creams or ointments on the boil's surface. They are ineffective.
- *Note:* Adverse reactions and side effects may be more frequent and severe in older persons. Remind your doctor of any medicines you already take.

ACTIVITY FOR OLDER PATIENTS
- Decrease activity until the boil heals. Avoid sweating.
- See Appendix 20 regarding physical fitness for the active older adult.

FOOD & BEVERAGE
- No special diet is required.
- See Appendix 1 regarding good nutrition for people over 50.

FUTURE CONSIDERATIONS FOR THE AGING ADULT

POSSIBLE COMPLICATIONS—The infection may enter the bloodstream and spread to other body parts.

PROBABLE OUTCOME—Without treatment, a boil will heal in 10 to 20 days. With treatment, the boil should heal in less time, the symptoms will be less severe and new boils should not appear. The pus that drains when a boil opens spontaneously may contaminate nearby skin, causing new boils.

PREVENTING RECURRENCE—Keep the skin clean.

CALL YOUR DOCTOR IF

- Any of the following occurs during treatment: Your symptoms don't improve in 3 to 4 days despite treatment.
  New boils appear.
  You develop a fever.
  Other family members develop boils.
- New, unexplained symptoms develop. The drugs used in treatment may produce side effects.

BRAIN OR EPIDURAL ABSCESS

BASIC INFORMATION FOR OLDER ADULTS

DESCRIPTION—A brain or epidural abscess is a collection of pus caused by a bacterial infection in the brain or the outermost of 3 membranes that cover the brain and spinal cord. Body parts involved: The brain, meninges (membranes that cover the brain) and skull. **(THIS IS AN EMERGENCY; SEEK MEDICAL CARE IMMEDIATELY!)**

SPECIAL CONSIDERATIONS FOR AGING
- Characteristic signs and symptoms of many disorders are frequently changed or absent.
- Many diseases become more common with age and all may present themselves in unusual ways.
- Usual signs and symptoms may be absent and be replaced by symptoms of confusion, dizziness, failure to thrive, falling, incontinence, increasing dementia, refusal to eat or drink, weight loss, depression, paranoia, hypochondriasis, psychosis or threats of suicide.
- The immune system becomes less effective, opening the way for viral, bacterial and other infections; malignancies; immune disorders; and allergies.

SIGNS & SYMPTOMS—The following symptoms usually appear gradually over several hours. They resemble the symptoms of a brain tumor or stroke:
- Pain in the back if the infection is in the covering of the spinal cord.
- Headache and drowsiness.
- Nausea and vomiting.
- Weakness, numbness or paralysis of one side of the body.
- Irregular gait; convulsions; fever.
- Confusion or delirium; difficulty in speaking.

CAUSES & RISK FACTORS—The primary source of a bacterial infection that causes a brain or epidural abscess often cannot be found. These 3 sources are the most common:
- An infection that spreads from an infected skull, such as osteomyelitis, mastoiditis or sinusitis.
- An infection that is introduced by a skull injury.
- An infection that spreads through the bloodstream from other infected organs, such as the lungs, skin or heart valves.

The risk increases with:
- Head injury.
- Illness that has lowered resistance, especially diabetes mellitus.
- Recent infection, especially around the nose, eyes and face.

DOCTOR'S TREATMENT & DIAGNOSTIC TESTS
- Medical history and physical exam.
- Laboratory studies of blood and spinal fluid.
- EEG, CT scan or MRI of the brain (see Glossary for all).
- X-rays of the skull.
- Surgery to drain pus.
- Self-care instructions focused on the older patient.

HOME TREATMENT BY SELF OR CARE-GIVER

GENERAL INSTRUCTIONS
- No specific instructions except those under other headings.
- A brain or epidural abscess is a complicated, serious disorder. This page can cover only the main points of diagnosis and treatment. Your doctor, nurse or librarian can provide sources of supplemental information.

MEDICATION (ADJUSTED FOR AGING)
- Your doctor may prescribe: Antibiotics for 4 to 6 weeks to fight infection. Anticonvulsants to prevent seizures.
- *Note:* Adverse reactions and side effects may be more frequent and severe in older persons. Remind your doctor of any medicines you already take.

ACTIVITY FOR OLDER PATIENTS
- While in the hospital, you will need bed rest. After a 2- to 3-week recovery, you should be as active as your strength and feeling of well-being allow.
- See Appendix 20 regarding physical fitness for the active older adult.

FOOD & BEVERAGE
- Eat a normal, well-balanced diet. Vitamin and mineral supplements should not be necessary unless you show evidence of deficiency or cannot eat normally.
- See Appendix 1 regarding good nutrition for people over 50.

FUTURE CONSIDERATIONS FOR THE AGING ADULT

POSSIBLE COMPLICATIONS—Seizures, coma and death without treatment.

PROBABLE OUTCOME—Usually curable with antibiotic treatment and surgery to drain pus.

PREVENTING RECURRENCE—Consult your doctor for treatment of any infection in your body—especially one around the nose or face—to prevent its spread.

CALL YOUR DOCTOR IF

- You have any symptoms of a brain or epidural abscess. *This is an emergency!*
- Your fever rises to 101F (38.3C) or higher.
- New, unexplained symptoms develop. The drugs used in treatment may produce side effects.

BRAIN INFECTION, VIRAL
(Viral or Aseptic Encephalitis; Acute Viral Encephalitis; Aseptic Encephalitis)

BASIC INFORMATION FOR OLDER ADULTS

DESCRIPTION—A viral brain infection is an acute inflammation of the brain caused by a contagious viral infection. Body parts involved: The brain and sometimes the meninges (the membranes that cover the brain).

SPECIAL CONSIDERATIONS FOR AGING
- The immune system becomes less effective, opening the way for viral, bacterial and other infections; malignancies; immune disorders; and allergies.
- Decreased nutrition increases the risk of infections.
- Side effects of medication and adverse reactions are more frequent and worse.

SIGNS & SYMPTOMS
Mild cases:
- No symptoms (sometimes).
- Fever; a general ill feeling.

Severe cases:
- Vomiting; headache; stiff neck.
- Pupils of different sizes.
- Unconsciousness.
- Personality changes; seizures.
- Occasional weakness or paralysis of an arm or leg.
- Double vision.
- Speech impairment.
- Hearing loss.
- Drowsiness that progresses to coma.
- Sensitivity to light.

CAUSES & RISK FACTORS
Causes include:
- Viruses that cause other illnesses, including polio, herpes, measles, mumps, chickenpox, infectious mononucleosis, infectious hepatitis, German measles, smallpox, coxsackie virus, echovirus diseases, Eastern and Western equine virus and the human immuno-deficiency virus (HIV).
- Viruses carried by mosquitoes or other insects.
- Lead poisoning.
- Vaccine reactions.
- Leukemia.

Risk factors include:
- Illness that has lowered resistance.
- Crowded or unsanitary living conditions.

DOCTOR'S TREATMENT & DIAGNOSTIC TESTS
- Medical history and physical exam.
- Laboratory studies of blood and cerebrospinal fluid.
- CT scan, EEG (see Glossary for both).
- Hospitalization (worst cases only).
- After diagnosis or hospitalization, self-care instructions focused on the older patient.

HOME TREATMENT BY SELF OR CARE-GIVER

GENERAL INSTRUCTIONS—No specific instructions except those under other headings.

MEDICATION (ADJUSTED FOR AGING)
- Antibiotics are not helpful with viral diseases such as this.
- Your doctor may prescribe:
  Antiviral drugs.
  Cortisone drugs to suppress inflammation (rare).
  Anticonvulsants.
- *Note:* Adverse reactions and side effects may be more frequent and severe in older persons. Remind your doctor of any medicines you already take.

ACTIVITY FOR OLDER PATIENTS—You will need bed rest in a darkened room. After a 2- to 3-week recovery, you should be as active as your strength and feeling of well-being allow.

FOOD & BEVERAGE
- No special diet is required.
- See Appendix 1 regarding good nutrition for people over 50.

FUTURE CONSIDERATIONS FOR THE AGING ADULT

POSSIBLE COMPLICATIONS—A small percentage of patients suffer permanent brain damage that impairs mental or muscle functions.

PROBABLE OUTCOME—Mild viral encephalitis is common and may go unnoticed. Severe cases usually require hospitalization. Unless the attack is severe, you can expect full recovery within 2 to 3 weeks.

PREVENTING RECURRENCE
- Avoid contact with anyone who has a viral brain infection.
- Consult your doctor for treatment of any infection in your body—especially those mentioned as causes—to attempt to prevent the spread of infection.

CALL YOUR DOCTOR IF

- You have any symptoms of a viral brain infection.
- You develop a fever.
- New, unexplained symptoms develop. The drugs used in treatment may produce side effects.

BRAIN TUMOR

BASIC INFORMATION FOR OLDER ADULTS

DESCRIPTION—A brain tumor is an abnormal growth in the brain that may be benign or malignant. A non-malignant brain tumor may cause as much disability as a malignant tumor unless it is treated properly. Brain tumors affect people in all age groups, but they are more common in older adults. Body parts involved: The brain and central nervous system.

SPECIAL CONSIDERATIONS FOR AGING
- The immune system becomes less effective, opening the way for viral, bacterial and other infections; malignancies; immune disorders; and allergies.
- Signs and symptoms may vary from the usual ones as listed.

SIGNS & SYMPTOMS
- Headaches that worsen when lying down.
- Vomiting with nausea or sudden vomiting without nausea.
- Vision disturbances, including double vision.
- Weakness in one side of the body.
- Lack of balance; dizziness.
- Loss of the sense of smell.
- Memory loss.
- Personality changes.
- Seizures.

CAUSES & RISK FACTORS—Some tumors begin in the brain (primary tumors), but most brain tumors have spread from the primary sites of other cancers—especially those of the breast, lungs, intestines or skin (malignant melanoma). The symptoms are caused by increasing pressure in the skull as the tumor enlarges. Risk factors are related to those for cancers of other body parts that spread to the brain, including:
- Poor nutrition, especially a low-fiber diet (intestinal cancer).
- Smoking (lung cancer).
- Excessive alcohol consumption (liver cancer).
- Excessive exposure to the sun (malignant melanoma).
- Previous cancer at any other site in the body.

DOCTOR'S TREATMENT & DIAGNOSTIC TESTS
- X-rays of the skull, bones, lungs and gastrointestinal tract.
- Laboratory studies of the blood and cerebrospinal fluid.
- CT scan, EEG and MRI exams (see Glossary for all).
- Surgery to remove the tumor if possible.

HOME TREATMENT BY SELF OR CARE-GIVER

MEDICATION (ADJUSTED FOR AGING)
- Your doctor may prescribe:
  Cortisone to diminish the swelling of the brain tissue.
  Anticonvulsant drugs to control seizures.
  Pain relievers.
  Anticancer drugs (chemotherapy).
- *Note:* Adverse reactions and side effects may be more frequent and severe in older persons. Remind your doctor of any medicines you already take.

ACTIVITY FOR OLDER PATIENTS
- Remain as active as your strength allows.
- See Appendix 20 regarding physical fitness for the active older adult.

FOOD & BEVERAGE
- No special diet is required.
- See Appendix 1 regarding good nutrition for people over 50.

FUTURE CONSIDERATIONS FOR THE AGING ADULT

POSSIBLE COMPLICATIONS—Adverse reactions to the medications used in treatment.

PROBABLE OUTCOME—Disability and death if the tumor is inoperable because of its size or location.

PREVENTING RECURRENCE—No general rules or suggestions possible.

CALL YOUR DOCTOR IF

- You have symptoms of a brain tumor.
- New, unexplained symptoms develop. The drugs used in treatment may produce side effects.

ILLNESSES & DISORDERS

BASIC INFORMATION FOR OLDER ADULTS

DESCRIPTION—Breast cancer is a malignant growth of breast tissue. Body parts involved: The nipple or tissue of the breast. Breast cancer spreads to nearby lymph glands, the lungs, pleura, bone (especially the skull), pelvis and liver.

SPECIAL CONSIDERATIONS FOR AGING
- Stress from any emotional cause—fear, worry, anxiety, sadness, loneliness or anger—affects all aspects of any illness or disorder.
- The immune system becomes less effective, opening the way for viral, bacterial and other infections; malignancies; immune disorders; and allergies.

SIGNS & SYMPTOMS—There are no symptoms in the early stages, but pre-symptom stages can be detected by mammogram. When symptoms finally occur, they include:
- Swelling or a lump in the breast.
- Vague discomfort in the breast without true pain.
- Retraction of the nipple.
- Distorted breast contour.
- Dimpled or pitted skin in the breast.
- Enlarged nodes under the arm (late).
- Bloody discharge from the nipple (rare).

CAUSES & RISK FACTORS—The cause is unknown. The risk increases with:
- Being over 50.
- Not having had children or conceiving in the late fertile years.
- A family history of breast cancer.
- Previous benign tumors of the breast (fibrocystic disease).

DOCTOR'S TREATMENT & DIAGNOSTIC TESTS
- Medical history and physical exam.
- X-rays of the breast and bones.
- Laboratory blood studies of hormones.
- Biopsy (see Glossary).
- Self-care instructions focused on the older patient.
- Surgery to remove the lump or the breast, lymph glands and lymphatic channels and muscles under the breast (sometimes). Advancing age alone is not a deterrent.
- Radiation therapy (sometimes).
- Hormonal or chemotherapy (sometimes).
- Substantial differences exist. You may benefit from a second opinion.

HOME TREATMENT BY SELF OR CARE-GIVER

GENERAL INSTRUCTIONS
- For an explanation of breast cancer surgery and postoperative care, see Mastectomy in the Surgeries section.
- Maintain as positive an attitude as possible during treatment.

- Treatment may cause side effects, but they are usually temporary.
- Your pain can be controlled. Don't hesitate to ask your doctor for pain medication.
- Fear may be your worst enemy.
- Call on family members and friends for whatever support and help you need.

MEDICATION (ADJUSTED FOR AGING)
- For minor discomfort during treatment, you may use non-prescription drugs such as acetaminophen or aspirin.
- Your doctor may prescribe:
  Pain relievers; cortisone drugs.
  Anticancer drugs, such as fluorouracil, cyclophosphamide, methotrexate, chlorambucil, vincristine, doxorubicin or melphalan.
  Hormones (male and female).

ACTIVITY FOR OLDER PATIENTS—After surgery, resume your normal activities gradually. Exercise for rehabilitation following surgery will depend on how much tissue has been removed and your general physical condition.

FOOD & BEVERAGE—No special diet is required. See Appendix 1 regarding good nutrition for people over 50.

FUTURE CONSIDERATIONS FOR THE AGING ADULT

POSSIBLE COMPLICATIONS
- Spread to vital organs if not treated early.
- Adverse reactions to anticancer drugs.

PROBABLE OUTCOME—Most breast cancer is curable if diagnosed and treated early. The 10-year survival rate among all women with breast cancer is less than 50%.

PREVENTING RECURRENCE
- Examine your breasts monthly for signs of cancer (see Appendix 14).
- Visit your doctor regularly for a professional examination.
- Obtain a baseline mammogram (see Glossary) between ages 35 and 40. Have mammograms every year thereafter if you have risk factors mentioned above.
- Eat a well-balanced diet that is low in fat.
- If you are pregnant, consider breast-feeding your baby. Women who have breast-fed have a lower incidence of breast cancer.

CALL YOUR DOCTOR IF

- You discover a lump or other change in the breast.
- Any of the following occurs after surgery: Nausea or vomiting; fever or swelling in the arm; pain that is not controlled by medication.
- New, unexplained symptoms develop. The drugs used in treatment may produce side effects.

BASIC INFORMATION FOR OLDER ADULTS

DESCRIPTION—Acute bronchitis is an inflammation of the air passages of the lungs. Body parts involved: The trachea, bronchi and bronchioles.

SPECIAL CONSIDERATIONS FOR AGING
- The immune system becomes less effective, opening the way for viral, bacterial and other infections; malignancies; immune disorders; and allergies.
- Decreased nutrition increases the risk of infections.
- Characteristic signs and symptoms of many disorders are frequently changed or absent.

SIGNS & SYMPTOMS
- A cough that produces little or no sputum initially, but does later on.
- A low fever (usually less than 101F or 38.3C).
- Burning chest discomfort or a feeling of pressure behind the breastbone.
- Wheezing or uncomfortable breathing (sometimes).

CAUSES & RISK FACTORS
Causes include:
- Infection from one of many respiratory viruses. Most cases of acute bronchitis begin with a cold virus in the nose and throat that spreads to the airways. A secondary bacterial infection is common.
- Lung inflammation from breathing air that contains irritants such as chemical fumes (ammonia), acid fumes, dust or smoke.

The risk increases with:
- Chronic obstructive pulmonary disease (COPD).
- Smoking.
- Cold, humid weather.
- Poor nutrition.
- Recent illness that has lowered resistance.

DOCTOR'S TREATMENT & DIAGNOSTIC TESTS
- Medical history and physical exam.
- Laboratory blood counts to detect complicating infections and cultures of sputum and blood to identify the bacteria.
- X-rays of the chest (for complications only).
- If you are in good overall health, self-care instructions focused on the older patient.

HOME TREATMENT BY SELF OR CARE-GIVER

GENERAL INSTRUCTIONS
- If you are a smoker, don't smoke during your illness. This delays recovery and makes complications more likely.
- Increase air moisture. Take frequent hot showers. Use a cool-mist humidifier beside your bed.

MEDICATION (ADJUSTED FOR AGING)
- For minor discomfort, you may use: Acetaminophen to reduce fever. Non-prescription cough suppressants. Use these only if your cough is non-productive (without sputum). It may be dangerous to stop a cough entirely as this traps excess mucus and irritants in the bronchial tubes, leading to pneumonia and poor oxygen exchange in the lungs.
- Your doctor may prescribe: Antibiotics to fight bacterial infections. Expectorants to thin mucus so it can be coughed up more easily. Cough suppressants.
- *Note:* Adverse reactions and side effects may be more frequent and severe in older persons. Remind your doctor of any medicines you already take.

ACTIVITY FOR OLDER PATIENTS
- Rest in bed until your temperature returns to normal. Then resume normal activity gradually as the symptoms improve.
- See Appendix 20 regarding physical fitness for the active older adult.

FOOD & BEVERAGE
- No special diet is required. Drink at least 8 to 10 glasses of fluid each day to help thin the mucus secretions so they can be coughed up more easily.
- See Appendix 1 regarding good nutrition for people over 50.

FUTURE CONSIDERATIONS FOR THE AGING ADULT

POSSIBLE COMPLICATIONS
- Bacterial lung infection (various kinds of pneumonia).
- Chronic bronchitis from recurrent episodes of acute bronchitis.

PROBABLE OUTCOME—Usually curable with treatment in 1 week. Cases with complications are usually curable in 2 weeks with medication.

PREVENTING RECURRENCE—Avoid close contact with persons who have bronchitis.

CALL YOUR DOCTOR IF

- You have symptoms of bronchitis.
- Any of the following occurs during the illness: High fever and chills. Chest pain. Thickened, discolored or blood-streaked sputum. Shortness of breath, even when the body is at rest. Vomiting.

BRONCHITIS, CHRONIC

BASIC INFORMATION FOR OLDER ADULTS

DESCRIPTION—Chronic bronchitis is the chronic inflammation and degeneration of the bronchial tubes, with or without active infection. Sputum is coughed up on most days for 3 months during 2 consecutive years. Body parts involved: The bronchial tubes (bronchi).

SPECIAL CONSIDERATIONS FOR AGING
- The immune system becomes less effective, opening the way for viral, bacterial and other infections; malignancies; immune disorders; and allergies.
- Characteristic signs and symptoms of many disorders are frequently changed or absent.

SIGNS & SYMPTOMS
- Frequent cough or coughing spasms.
- Shortness of breath; chest pain (rare).
- Sputum that is thick and difficult to cough up. Sputum production varies according to whether infection is present.
- Barrel chest (in the late stages).

CAUSES & RISK FACTORS—Caused by repeated irritation or infection in the bronchial tubes that makes them thicken, narrow and lose their elasticity. Underlying irritants include allergens, air pollution and tobacco smoke. The risk increases with:
- Smoking (the greatest risk factor).
- Any lung illness that has lowered resistance.
- A family history of tuberculosis or another disease of the respiratory tract.
- Exposure to air pollutants.
- Poor nutrition; obesity.
- Crowded living conditions.

DOCTOR'S TREATMENT & DIAGNOSTIC TESTS
- Medical history and physical exam.
- Laboratory studies of sputum, blood and pulmonary function; x-rays of the chest.
- Self-care instructions focused on the older patient.
- Many lung and heart disorders cause symptoms identical to those of chronic bronchitis. Your doctor must exclude these possibilities to make a diagnosis.

HOME TREATMENT BY SELF OR CARE-GIVER

GENERAL INSTRUCTIONS
- Stop smoking.
- If you work or live in an area with heavy air pollution, do everything you can to avoid or reduce it. Consider changing jobs and installing air conditioning with a filter and humidity control in your home.
- Avoid sudden temperature changes or exposure to cold, wet weather.
- Avoid talking loudly, laughing loudly, crying and exertion if these trigger coughing episodes.

- Practice bronchial drainage and deep-breathing techniques. Your physician will provide instructions.
- Sleep with 5-inch blocks under the foot of your bed.

MEDICATION (ADJUSTED FOR AGING)
- Don't take cough suppressants; they make chronic bronchitis worse.
- Your doctor may prescribe:
  Antibiotics to fight chronic or recurrent infection.
  Expectorants to loosen secretions.
  Bronchodilators to open bronchial tubes.
  Oxygen from an oxygen cylinder.

ACTIVITY FOR OLDER PATIENTS
- No restrictions are necessary. Remain as active as possible.
- See Appendix 20 regarding physical fitness for the active older adult.

FOOD & BEVERAGE
- No special diet is required. Increase your fluid intake to 8 to 10 glasses a day.
- See Appendix 1 regarding good nutrition for people over 50.

FUTURE CONSIDERATIONS FOR THE AGING ADULT

POSSIBLE COMPLICATIONS
- Recurrent pneumonia.
- Chronic obstructive pulmonary disease (COPD). COPD is incurable. It is characterized by purple lips and nails and congestive heart failure.

PROBABLE OUTCOME—Chronic bronchitis is usually curable with treatment if you are a non-smoker and don't have an underlying chronic disease, such as congestive heart failure, bronchiectasis or tuberculosis. Chronic bronchitis usually reduces life expectancy if you smoke and don't stop or if you have an underlying chronic disease.

PREVENTING RECURRENCE
- Don't smoke. This is the most reversible risk.
- Avoid irritating fumes in the environment.
- Obtain prompt medical treatment for respiratory infections.

CALL YOUR DOCTOR IF

- You have symptoms of chronic bronchitis.
- You develop a fever.
- Blood appears in the sputum.
- Your chest pain increases.
- Shortness of breath occurs even when you are resting or not coughing.
- The sputum thickens despite efforts to thin it.
- Vomiting occurs.

BUERGER'S DISEASE
(Thromboangiitis Obliterans)

BASIC INFORMATION FOR OLDER ADULTS

DESCRIPTION—Buerger's disease is a blockage of the small and medium arteries—usually in the legs and feet—due to the inflammation of the blood vessels. This causes clot formation. Cigarette smoking is a very important factor in developing this disease. It is extremely rare among non-smokers. Body parts involved: The arteries (and sometimes the veins) in the extremities.

SPECIAL CONSIDERATIONS FOR AGING
- The immune system becomes less efficient.
- The large and small arteries are thicker and less elastic.

SIGNS & SYMPTOMS
- Intermittent pain in the instep or the leg when exercising. The pain improves with rest.
- Pain, blueness, heat and tingling in the legs when they are exposed to cold.
- Painful ulcers on the toes and fingertips (sometimes).

CAUSES & RISK FACTORS—The cause is unknown, but the disease is probably triggered by nicotine. Cigarette smoking causes blood vessel spasms leading to the obstruction of the essential blood vessels in the extremities. The risk increases with:
- Collagen disease or atherosclerosis.
- Stress.
- Cold weather.
- A family history of Buerger's disease.

DOCTOR'S TREATMENT & DIAGNOSTIC TESTS
- Medical history and physical exam.
- Laboratory studies such as Doppler ultrasonography and arteriography (see Glossary for both).
- Self-care instructions focused on the older patient.
- Surgery (sympathectomy) to cut sympathetic nerves to the area (sometimes).

HOME TREATMENT BY SELF OR CARE-GIVER

GENERAL INSTRUCTIONS
- Other measures are rarely successful if smoking continues, so stop smoking.
- Avoid exposure to the cold. Wear warm footwear and gloves.
- Clip your nails carefully to avoid injuring the skin.
- Wear well-fitting shoes and cotton or wool socks. Don't wear socks made of synthetic material.
- Insert soft padding in your shoes to protect your feet.
- Don't go barefoot outdoors.
- Consult a podiatrist or have a visiting nurse see you regularly for foot and hand care.

MEDICATION (ADJUSTED FOR AGING)
- Your doctor may prescribe vasodilator drugs, but they are generally useless if you continue smoking.
- *Note:* Adverse reactions and side effects may be more frequent and severe in older persons. Remind your doctor of any medicines you already take.

ACTIVITY FOR OLDER PATIENTS
- Avoid cold weather, but stay active. Begin a conditioning program to become as physically fit as possible.
- See Appendix 20 regarding physical fitness for the active older adult.

FOOD & BEVERAGE
- No special diet is required.
- See Appendix 1 regarding good nutrition for people over 50.

FUTURE CONSIDERATIONS FOR THE AGING ADULT

POSSIBLE COMPLICATIONS—Gangrene in the foot or leg caused by a loss of blood supply. This may result in amputation.

PROBABLE OUTCOME—This condition is currently considered incurable. The symptoms can be controlled for a while, but the disease causes increasing disability—especially if amputation is necessary. Life expectancy is reduced. Scientific research into causes and treatment continues, so there is hope for increasingly effective treatment and a cure.

PREVENTING RECURRENCE
- Don't smoke.
- Avoid exposure to the cold. This also causes blood vessels to constrict and deprives extremities of a normal blood supply.

CALL YOUR DOCTOR IF

- You have symptoms of Buerger's disease.
- Uncontrollable pain begins.
- Ulcers develop on your toes or feet.

BUNION
(Hallux Valgus)

BASIC INFORMATION FOR OLDER ADULTS

DESCRIPTION—A bunion is an inflammation, swelling and protrusion of the base or side of the great (big) toe. Bunions may be congenital or hereditary. Body part involved: The great toe.

SPECIAL CONSIDERATIONS FOR AGING
- Long years of foot abuse with ill-fitting shoes.
- Bone strength decreases.
- Years of weight bearing cause wear and tear on the bones, joints and ligaments.

SIGNS & SYMPTOMS
- An inward-turned great toe that may overlap the second—and sometimes the third—toe.
- Thickened skin over the bony protrusion at the base of the great toe.
- Fluid accumulation under the thickened skin (sometimes).
- Foot pain and stiffness.

CAUSES & RISK FACTORS
Causes include:
- Arthritis.
- Narrow-toed, high-heeled shoes that compress the toes together.

The risk increases with a a family history of foot abnormalities.

DOCTOR'S TREATMENT & DIAGNOSTIC TESTS
- Medical history and physical exam.
- X-rays of the foot.
- In the early stages, self-care instructions focused on the older patient. This may prevent a bunion from worsening.
- Surgery to remove the bunion and correct the position of the bones.

HOME TREATMENT BY SELF OR CARE-GIVER

GENERAL INSTRUCTIONS
- Before bedtime, separate the great toe from the others with a foam rubber pad.
- Wear a thick, ring-shaped adhesive pad around and over the bunion when you are wearing shoes.
- Use arch supports to relieve pressure on the bunion. These are available in shoe repair shops.
- Make a cutout in your shoe where the pressure is greatest.
- Consider custom-made or specially molded shoes.

MEDICATION (ADJUSTED FOR AGING)
- Medicine usually is not necessary for this disorder unless infection develops.
- *Note:* Adverse reactions and side effects may be more frequent and severe in older persons. Remind your doctor of any medicines you already take.

ACTIVITY FOR OLDER PATIENTS
- If surgery is necessary, resume your normal activities gradually afterward. Walk on your heels until the surgical site heals. Elevate the foot of the bed to reduce swelling.
- See Appendix 20 regarding physical fitness for the active older adult.

FOOD & BEVERAGE
- No special diet is required.
- See Appendix 1 regarding good nutrition for people over 50.

FUTURE CONSIDERATIONS FOR THE AGING ADULT

POSSIBLE COMPLICATIONS
- Infection of the bunion, especially in persons with diabetes mellitus.
- Inflammation and arthritic changes in other joints caused by walking difficulty, which places abnormal stress on the foot, hip and spine.

PROBABLE OUTCOME—Usually curable with treatment and preventive measures to guard against recurrence.

PREVENTING RECURRENCE
- Exercise daily to keep the muscles of the feet and legs in good condition.
- Wear wide-toed shoes that fit well. Don't wear high heels or shoes without room for the toes in their normal positions.

CALL YOUR DOCTOR IF

- You have a bunion that is interfering with normal activities.
- Signs of infection, such as fever, heat, tenderness or pain, develop after treatment or surgery.

BURN

BASIC INFORMATION FOR OLDER ADULTS

DESCRIPTION—A burn is an injury to the skin, and sometimes other organs, due to contact with heat, radiation, electricity, fire or chemicals. Body parts involved: The skin, the underlying tissue and the respiratory system (sometimes).

SPECIAL CONSIDERATIONS FOR AGING
- The skin becomes thinner, so burns are more likely to be serious.
- The fatty layer of tissue under the skin becomes thinner.

SIGNS & SYMPTOMS
Burns are of 3 types:
- 1st-degree burns—Limited to the upper skin layer. They produce redness, tenderness, pain, swelling and slight fever.
- 2nd-degree burns—Affect deeper skin layers. The symptoms are more severe and include blisters.
- 3rd-degree burns—Involve all skin layers. The skin is white (it appears cooked) and there may be no pain in the initial stages.

2nd- and 3rd-degree burns over 10% of the skin surface will cause shock (rapid pulse, low blood pressure, cold sweat and paleness).

CAUSES & RISK FACTORS
Causes include:
- A rise in the temperature of the skin from heat sources such as fire, steam or electricity.
- Tissue injury caused by chemicals or radiation, including sunlight.

The risk increases with:
- Stress, carelessness, smoking in bed or excessive alcohol consumption, all of which make accidents more likely.
- Occupations involving exposure to heat or radiation, such as firefighting, police work or defense plant work.

DOCTOR'S TREATMENT & DIAGNOSTIC TESTS
- Medical history and physical exam.
- Laboratory blood and urine tests and studies of kidney and liver function (for severe burns).
- For most 1st-degree burns, self-care instructions focused on the older patient.
- Hospitalization for all large 3rd-degree burns and some 2nd-degree burns (special burn centers exist for the worst cases).
- Surgery to graft skin over 3rd-degree burns.

HOME TREATMENT BY SELF OR CARE-GIVER

GENERAL INSTRUCTIONS—For severe burns, seek emergency care. For less severe burns:
- Apply non-prescription body lotion to cool 1st-degree burns.
- Immerse small 2nd- or 3rd-degree burn areas in cold water for 10 minutes to reduce the pain and swelling.
- Keep the burn area clean. Soak in a tub or use lukewarm compresses once a day. You may add 2 tablespoons of powdered detergent to the tub to help soak off crusting areas. Use plain water for compresses.
- Prop the burn area higher than the rest of the body if possible.
- You may use dressings on the burn.

MEDICATION (ADJUSTED FOR AGING)
- To treat minor burns, you may use non-prescription antibiotic ointments, topical anesthetics and aspirin.
- To treat severe burns, your doctor may prescribe pain relievers, antibiotics and tetanus booster shots.

ACTIVITY FOR OLDER PATIENTS—Depends on the location and extent of the burn. Ask your doctor.

FOOD & BEVERAGE—No special diet is required for minor burns. More severe burns require intravenous feeding.

FUTURE CONSIDERATIONS FOR THE AGING ADULT

POSSIBLE COMPLICATIONS
- Infection at the burn site; permanent scarring.
- Pneumonia
- Shock due to the loss of fluids and electrolytes (with severe burns).
- Vision impairment if the eyes are injured.
- Tetanus and other infections.

PROBABLE OUTCOME—Most persons recover if the extent of burns (including 3rd-degree burns) is limited to 50% of the body surface. For less severe burns, skin usually repairs itself in 1 to 3 weeks.

PREVENTING RECURRENCE
- Wear sun-screen lotions outdoors.
- Fireproof your home. Install smoke alarms, plan emergency exits and have regular fire drills.
- Wear protective gear and observe safety precautions around heat or radiation.
- Don't touch uncovered electric wires.
- Discard extension cords with a pronged plug on one end and a bulb socket on the other. These are hazardous.

CALL YOUR DOCTOR IF

- You have a 2nd- or 3rd-degree burn or a 1st-degree burn that covers a large area.
- Any of the following occurs during treatment: There is no healing in 6 days.
  You experience chills and fever or increased pain, redness, swelling or pus in the burn area.

BURSITIS

BASIC INFORMATION FOR OLDER ADULTS

DESCRIPTION—Bursitis is an inflammation of a soft sac (bursa) containing lubricating liquid that protects a joint. Body parts involved: The bursas, especially near the shoulders, elbows, knees, pelvis, hips or Achilles' tendons.

SPECIAL CONSIDERATIONS FOR AGING
- Muscle tone decreases.
- Muscle bulk and power decrease.
- Characteristic signs and symptoms of many disorders are frequently changed or absent.

SIGNS & SYMPTOMS
- Pain, tenderness and limited movement in the affected area.
- When the shoulder is involved, radiation of the pain into the neck, arm and fingertips.
- Severe pain with movement of the arm or other affected joint.
- Fever (sometimes).

CAUSES & RISK FACTORS—Causes and risk factors are frequently unknown, but could be:
- Injury to a joint.
- Overuse of a joint (such as prolonged kneeling).
- Strenuous, unaccustomed exercise.
- Calcium deposits in a tendon with degeneration of the tendon.
- Acute or chronic infection.
- Arthritis.
- Gout.

DOCTOR'S TREATMENT & DIAGNOSTIC TESTS
- Medical history and physical exam.
- X-rays of the affected area.
- Injections of medicines and pain relievers into the affected area.
- Self-care instructions focused on the older patient.

HOME TREATMENT BY SELF OR CARE-GIVER

GENERAL INSTRUCTIONS
- Apply ice packs to the affected area during a flare-up or after receiving injections into the joint.
- After the acute stage, many doctors recommend continued ice treatment until the inflammation subsides. Others recommend heat. If you use heat, take hot showers, use a heat lamp, apply hot compresses or a heating pad or rub in deep-heating ointment.

MEDICATION (ADJUSTED FOR AGING)
- Your doctor may prescribe:
  Non-steroidal anti-inflammatory drugs.
  Cortisone injections into the bursa to reduce inflammation.
  Pain relievers.
- *Note:* Adverse reactions and side effects may be more frequent and severe in older persons. Remind your doctor of any medicines you already take.

ACTIVITY FOR OLDER PATIENTS
- Rest the inflamed area as much as possible. If you must resume normal activity immediately, wear a sling or use crutches until the pain becomes more bearable. To prevent a frozen joint (especially in the shoulder), begin normal, slow joint movement as soon as possible.
- See Appendix 20 regarding physical fitness for the active older adult.

FOOD & BEVERAGE
- No special diet is required.
- See Appendix 1 regarding good nutrition for people over 50.

FUTURE CONSIDERATIONS FOR THE AGING ADULT

POSSIBLE COMPLICATIONS—Frozen joint or permanent limitation of a joint's mobility.

PROBABLE OUTCOME—This is a common—but not serious—problem. The symptoms usually subside in 7 to 14 days with treatment.

PREVENTING RECURRENCE—Avoid injuries whenever possible. Wear seat belts in autos and protective gear for contact sports.

CALL YOUR DOCTOR IF

- You have symptoms of bursitis.
- The pain increases despite treatment.
- New, unexplained symptoms develop. The drugs used in treatment may produce side effects.

CALCIUM, TOO LITTLE
(Hypocalcemia)

BASIC INFORMATION FOR OLDER ADULTS

DESCRIPTION—Calcium is a mineral component of blood that helps regulate the heartbeat, transmit nerve impulses, contract the muscles and form bone and teeth. Too much *or* too little can cause serious—sometimes life-threatening—medical problems. Body parts involved: The membranes of all body cells; the muscles and bones; and the parathyroid glands and parathyroid hormones (which regulate the absorption and utilization of calcium).

SPECIAL CONSIDERATIONS FOR AGING—Decreased appetite means good nutrition becomes less likely.

SIGNS & SYMPTOMS
- Muscle spasms, twitching or cramps.
- Numbness and tingling in the arms, legs, hands and feet.
- Seizures.
- Irregular heartbeat.
- High blood pressure.

CAUSES & RISK FACTORS
Causes include:
- Underactive parathyroid glands from disease or damage during neck surgery.
- Inadequate dietary intake of calcium and vitamin D.
- Lack of adequate sunshine.
- Malabsorption of calcium from the gastrointestinal tract (usually for unknown reasons).
- Severe burns or infections.
- Pancreatitis.
- Kidney failure.
- Decreased blood levels of magnesium.

Risk factors include:
- The use of certain drugs, including thiazide diuretics and calcium channel blockers.
- Excessive alcohol consumption leading to poor nutrition.
- Chronic kidney disease.
- Inactivity or prolonged bed rest for any reason.

DOCTOR'S TREATMENT & DIAGNOSTIC TESTS
- Medical history and physical exam.
- Laboratory blood studies of calcium levels.
- ECG (see Glossary).
- X-rays of the bones.
- Self-care instructions focused on the older patient.

HOME TREATMENT BY SELF OR CARE-GIVER

GENERAL INSTRUCTIONS—The underlying cause must be corrected before you can follow a treatment program to prevent a recurrence.

MEDICATION (ADJUSTED FOR AGING)
- Your doctor may prescribe intravenous calcium gluconate or calcium carbonate for too little calcium.
- *Note:* Adverse reactions and side effects may be more frequent and severe in older persons. Remind your doctor of any medicines you already take.

ACTIVITY FOR OLDER PATIENTS
- After treatment, resume your normal activities as the symptoms improve.
- See Appendix 20 regarding physical fitness for the active older adult.

FOOD & BEVERAGE
- For a slightly low calcium level, take calcium supplements and vitamin D. Increase your intake of protein, milk and milk products.
- See Appendix 1 regarding good nutrition for people over 50.

FUTURE CONSIDERATIONS FOR THE AGING ADULT

POSSIBLE COMPLICATIONS
- Cardiac arrest.
- Fractures of weak bones.

PROBABLE OUTCOME—Unless calcium imbalance is caused by cancer, most cases are curable with treatment in 1 week.

PREVENTING RECURRENCE
- Eat a normal, balanced diet.
- Don't drink more than 1 or 2 alcoholic drinks—if any—a day.
- Don't use non-prescription antacids on a regular basis except under medical supervision.

CALL YOUR DOCTOR IF

Your symptoms recur after treatment.

ILLNESSES & DISORDERS

213

CALCIUM, TOO MUCH
(Hypercalcemia)

BASIC INFORMATION FOR OLDER ADULTS

DESCRIPTION—Calcium is a mineral component of blood that helps regulate the heartbeat, transmit nerve impulses, contract the muscles and form bone and teeth. Too much *or* too little can cause serious—sometimes life-threatening—medical problems. Body parts involved: The membranes of all body cells; the muscles and bones; and the parathyroid glands and parathyroid hormones (which regulate the absorption and utilization of calcium).

SPECIAL CONSIDERATIONS FOR AGING—Decreased appetite means good nutrition becomes less likely.

SIGNS & SYMPTOMS
- Lethargy.
- Appetite loss.
- Vomiting and diarrhea.
- Dehydration and thirst.
- Irregular heartbeat.
- Low blood pressure.
- Depression; delirium; confusion.
- Seizures or coma (in the worst cases only).

CAUSES & RISK FACTORS
Causes include:
- Overactive parathyroid glands.
- Multiple fractures and prolonged bed rest.
- Multiple myeloma.
- Tumors—benign *or* malignant—that destroy bone.

Risk factors include:
- Improper diet, especially overconsumption of milk products or non-prescription antacids that contain calcium.
- Repeated transfusions with citrated blood.
- Chronic kidney disease.
- Inactivity or prolonged bed rest for any reason.

DOCTOR'S TREATMENT & DIAGNOSTIC TESTS
- Medical history and physical exam.
- Laboratory blood studies of calcium levels.
- ECG (see Glossary).
- X-rays of the bones.
- Self-care instructions focused on the older patient.
- Hospitalization (sometimes).

HOME TREATMENT BY SELF OR CARE-GIVER

GENERAL INSTRUCTIONS—The underlying cause must be corrected before you can follow a treatment program to prevent a recurrence.

MEDICATION (ADJUSTED FOR AGING)
- Your doctor may prescribe intravenous saline solution and loop diuretics (furosemide and ethacrynic acid) for too much calcium.
- *Note:* Adverse reactions and side effects may be more frequent and severe in older persons. Remind your doctor of any medicines you already take.

ACTIVITY FOR OLDER PATIENTS
- After treatment, resume your normal activities as the symptoms improve.
- See Appendix 20 regarding physical fitness for the active older adult.

FOOD & BEVERAGE
- For a slightly high calcium level, restrict your consumption of dairy products and calcium-containing antacids.
- See Appendix 1 regarding good nutrition for people over 50.

FUTURE CONSIDERATIONS FOR THE AGING ADULT

POSSIBLE COMPLICATIONS
- Kidney stones.
- Peptic ulcer

PROBABLE OUTCOME—Unless the calcium imbalance is caused by cancer, most cases are curable with treatment in 1 week.

PREVENTING RECURRENCE
- Eat a normal, balanced diet.
- Don't drink more than 1 or 2 alcoholic drinks—if any—a day.
- Don't use non-prescription antacids on a regular basis except under medical supervision.

CALL YOUR DOCTOR IF
- You have symptoms of a calcium imbalance.
- Your symptoms recur after treatment.

CANKER SORES
(Aphthous Ulcers)

 ## BASIC INFORMATION FOR OLDER ADULTS

DESCRIPTION—Canker sores are painful ulcers that occur in the lining of the mouth. The ulcers are not cancerous, but they may be contagious. They may be confused with herpes infections. Body parts involved: The mouth and adjacent areas.

SPECIAL CONSIDERATIONS FOR AGING
- The immune system becomes less effective, opening the way for viral, bacterial and other infections; malignancies; immune disorders; and allergies.
- Many diseases become more common with age, and all may present themselves in unusual ways.
- Stress from any emotional cause—fear, worry, anxiety, sadness, loneliness or anger—affects all aspects of any illness or disorder.

SIGNS & SYMPTOMS—Mouth ulcers with the following characteristics:
- The ulcers are small, very painful, shallow and covered with a gray membrane. Borders are surrounded by an intense red halo.
- The ulcers appear on lips, gums, inner cheeks, tongue, palate and throat. 2 or 3 ulcers usually appear during an attack, but 10 to 15 ulcers are not uncommon.
- The ulcers may be so painful during the first 2 or 3 days that they interfere with eating or speaking.
- The ulcers are preceded by tingling or burning for 24 hours (sometimes).

CAUSES & RISK FACTORS—The cause is unknown, but the most likely causes include:
- Emotional or physical stress or anxiety.
- Injury to the mouth lining caused by rough dentures, hot food, toothbrushing or dental work.
- Irritation from foods such as chocolate, citrus, acidic foods (such as vinegar or pickles), salted nuts or potato chips.
- Virus infection.
Risk can increase with recent dental treatment.

DOCTOR'S TREATMENT & DIAGNOSTIC TESTS
- Medical history and physical exam.
- Laboratory culture of the sores to distinguish them from the sores of a herpes infection or to detect secondary bacterial infections.
- Self-care instructions focused on the older patient.

 ## HOME TREATMENT BY SELF OR CARE-GIVER

GENERAL INSTRUCTIONS
- Rinse your mouth 3 or more times a day with a salt solution (1/2 teaspoon salt to 8 oz. water).
- Clean the sores frequently with 2% hydrogen peroxide on a cotton applicator.

- If a canker sore is caused by a rough tooth, braces or dentures, consult your dentist. The sore won't heal until the cause is eliminated.

MEDICATION (ADJUSTED FOR AGING)
- Your doctor may prescribe:
Topical anesthetics to relieve the pain.
Antibiotics, such as tetracycline, to fight infection. Tetracycline is effective if the liquid form is held in the mouth for 2 to 5 minutes to coat the ulcers before swallowing. If started early, it prevents pain.
A protective dental paste with a steroid derivative. If it is applied as soon as the ulcer begins, this prevents pain.
- Keep the medicine prescribed by your doctor for the first attack. Use it immediately at the sign of a recurrent attack. The sooner treatment starts, the milder the attack.

ACTIVITY FOR OLDER PATIENTS—No restrictions are necessary.

FOOD & BEVERAGE—No restrictions are necessary, except to avoid foods that aggravate the ulcers. Drink as many fluids and eat as well-balanced a diet as possible while healing. To minimize the pain, sip liquids through straws. The foods that cause the least pain are milk, liquid gelatin, yogurt, ice cream and custard.

 ## FUTURE CONSIDERATIONS FOR THE AGING ADULT

POSSIBLE COMPLICATIONS—Dehydration in severe cases where eating and drinking are limited.

PROBABLE OUTCOME—Most ulcers heal without scarring in 2 weeks. Recurrent attacks are common. They vary from a single lesion 2 or 3 times a year to an uninterrupted succession of multiple lesions.

PREVENTING RECURRENCE
- Brush your teeth at least twice a day and floss regularly to keep your mouth clean and healthy.
- Avoid stress if possible. See Appendix 13.
- Avoid intimate contact with infected persons.
- Observe if canker sores develop after eating specific foods. Don't eat foods that seem to trigger attacks.

 ## CALL YOUR DOCTOR IF

- Temperature rises to 102F (38.9C) or higher.
- Ulcers don't improve in 3 days despite treatment.
- The pain is unbearable and isn't relieved by treatment.

CARCINOID SYNDROME

BASIC INFORMATION FOR OLDER ADULTS

DESCRIPTION—Carcinoid syndrome is a group of symptoms caused by malignant tumors (carcinoids). Carcinoids secrete serotonin, histamine, prostaglandins and hormones—powerful chemicals that cause carcinoid symptoms. Body parts involved: Primary tumors appear in the appendix, ileum, rectum, ovaries or stomach. The malignancy may spread and cause symptoms that affect the skin, blood vessels, kidneys, gastrointestinal tract, liver, heart and lungs.

SPECIAL CONSIDERATIONS FOR AGING
- The immune system becomes less effective, opening the way for viral, bacterial and other infections; malignancies; immune disorders; and allergies.
- Usual signs and symptoms may be absent and be replaced by symptoms of confusion, dizziness, failure to thrive, falling, incontinence, increasing dementia, refusal to eat or drink, weight loss, depression, paranoia, hypochondriasis, psychosis or threats of suicide.
- Stress from any emotional cause—fear, worry, anxiety, sadness, loneliness or anger—affects all aspects of any illness or disorder.

SIGNS & SYMPTOMS—Carcinoids are slow-growing and many persons with these tumors have no symptoms. The primary tumor may cause intestinal obstruction, which is characterized by painful cramps in the middle of the abdomen, vomiting, abdominal swelling and weight loss. In a few cases, carcinoid cells spread to other body parts and produce secondary, hormone-producing (serotonin) tumors. The symptoms of these secondary tumors may be triggered by heavy exercise or by the consumption of alcohol, bananas, tomatoes, plums, avocados, pineapple or walnuts. These symptoms include:
- Flushed skin on the head and neck.
- Watery eyes; unexplained weight loss.
- Diarrhea with abdominal cramps.
- Respiratory symptoms similar to those of asthma.
- Congestive heart failure; irregular heartbeat.
- Nausea and vomiting; low blood pressure.

CAUSES & RISK FACTORS—The causes are unknown. The risk factors include obesity, smoking and excessive alcohol consumption.

DOCTOR'S TREATMENT & DIAGNOSTIC TESTS
- Medical history and physical exam.
- Laboratory urine studies of levels of 5-hydroxyindoleacetic acid and serotonin.
- X-rays of the abdominal organs.
- Sigmoidoscopy and CT scan (see Glossary for both) of the colon; biopsy (see Glossary).
- Surgery to remove the tumors (sometimes).
- Self-care instructions focused on the older patient.

HOME TREATMENT BY SELF OR CARE-GIVER

GENERAL INSTRUCTIONS
- Maintain as positive an attitude as possible during treatment.
- Treatment may cause side effects, but they are usually temporary.
- Your pain can be controlled. Don't hesitate to ask your doctor for pain medication.
- Fear may be your worst enemy.
- Call on family members and friends for whatever support and help you need.

MEDICATION (ADJUSTED FOR AGING)
- For minor diarrhea, you may use non-prescription antidiarrheal medicines.
- Your doctor may prescribe:
  Anticancer drugs to kill malignant cells.
  Methyldopa to prevent formation of serotonin tumors.
  Phenothiazines to prevent flushed skin.
  Cortisone drugs to reduce inflammation anywhere in the body.

ACTIVITY FOR OLDER PATIENTS—Resume your normal activities as soon as your symptoms improve, but avoid strenuous exercise.

FOOD & BEVERAGE
- Include at least 2 protein servings a day.
- Take niacin supplements if recommended by your physician.
- Avoid foods that trigger the symptoms of secondary tumors.
- Don't drink alcohol.
- See Appendix 1 regarding good nutrition for people over 50.

FUTURE CONSIDERATIONS FOR THE AGING ADULT

POSSIBLE COMPLICATIONS—Malignancy may spread to other body parts.

PROBABLE OUTCOME—This condition is currently considered incurable.
However, the symptoms can be relieved or controlled and survival is possible for 10 to 20 years. Scientific research into causes and treatment continues, so there is hope for increasingly effective treatment and a cure.

PREVENTING RECURRENCE—Cannot be prevented at present.

CALL YOUR DOCTOR IF

- You have symptoms of carcinoid syndrome.
- The symptoms become disabling despite treatment.
- New, unexplained symptoms develop. The drugs used in treatment may produce side effects.

CARDIAC ARREST
(Sudden Death Syndrome)

BASIC INFORMATION FOR OLDER ADULTS

DESCRIPTION—Cardiac arrest is the total loss of the heart's pumping action. Delaying treatment for only 3 to 5 minutes may cause death or permanent brain damage. Body part involved: The heart. (THIS IS AN EMERGENCY; SEEK MEDICAL CARE IMMEDIATELY!)

SPECIAL CONSIDERATIONS FOR AGING
- 50% of people over 60 have x-ray evidence of narrowing of the coronary arteries, yet only 50% of those people have symptoms.
- Coronary artery disease is prevalent.

SIGNS & SYMPTOMS
- Brief dizziness, followed by fainting and unconsciousness.
- Bluish-white skin and dilated pupils.
- No pulse or breathing; seizures.
- Loss of bowel and bladder control (sometimes).

Simple fainting may resemble cardiac arrest, but pulse and breathing continue.

CAUSES & RISK FACTORS
Causes include:
- Heartbeat irregularities; heart attack (myocardial infarction; atherosclerotic heart disease).
- Lack of blood circulation and profound shock caused by a hemorrhage or overwhelming infection; loss of oxygen from drowning, choking or anesthesia.
- Major changes in the blood's electrolyte composition, as with a potassium or fluid imbalance.
- Electrical shock; drug overdose; hypothermia.

Risk factors include:
- Stress; diabetes mellitus.
- The use of drugs such as digitalis; diuretics; and adrenalin or any drug that raises blood pressure in a heart patient, including cold capsules, decongestant tablets and nasal sprays.
- The use of drugs of abuse, especially cocaine.

DOCTOR'S TREATMENT & DIAGNOSTIC TESTS
- Continuation of CPR begun at the scene (see General Instructions).
- Medical history and physical exam; lab tests.
- Hospitalization for observation for serious delayed reactions; after treatment, self-care instructions focused on the older patient.

HOME TREATMENT BY SELF OR CARE-GIVER

GENERAL INSTRUCTIONS
- If the victim is unconscious and *not* breathing, yell for help. Don't leave the victim. Begin mouth-to-mouth breathing immediately.

- If there is no heartbeat, give external cardiac massage. Don't stop CPR until help arrives.
- Have someone call 0 (operator) or 911 (emergency) for an ambulance or medical help.
- Administer oxygen, if available, after CPR has restored a heartbeat.
- The victim should be taken to the nearest hospital for intensive care—even if the victim has regained consciousness. Complications or death may occur 24 to 48 hours after the incident due to heart rhythm disturbances or damage to the central nervous system.
- Remain with a recovering patient to provide support and reassurance.

MEDICATION (ADJUSTED FOR AGING)—The doctor may later prescribe medications to treat the underlying cause of the cardiac arrest.

ACTIVITY FOR OLDER PATIENTS—After recovery, resume your normal activities gradually. Sexual relations may be resumed only after medical clearance from the doctor.

FOOD & BEVERAGE—Don't give fluid or foods to anyone with signs of cardiac arrest. He or she could choke.

FUTURE CONSIDERATIONS FOR THE AGING ADULT

POSSIBLE COMPLICATIONS—Death or permanent brain damage if heart action cannot be resumed in 3 to 5 minutes; mistaking a faint or other causes of unconsciousness for cardiac arrest.

PROBABLE OUTCOME—Bystanders skilled in recognizing cardiac arrest and performing CPR can often restore a heartbeat. The final outcome, however, depends on the underlying cause of the cardiac arrest.

PREVENTING RECURRENCE
- Obtain immediate medical treatment for any conditions listed as Causes. Refer to the appropriate chart in the Illnesses section.
- If you have heart disease, learn all you can about *all* the drugs you take, including non-prescription drugs.
- Encourage family members and friends to learn CPR. Call your local Red Cross or hospital for information.
- If you have heart trouble or are at risk, wear a Medic Alert bracelet or pendant (see Glossary).

CALL YOUR DOCTOR IF

- You see someone who appears to be experiencing cardiac arrest. Call for help immediately. *This is an emergency!* See General Instructions for additional emergency information.
- Signs of infection (fever, cough, muscle aches and fatigue) appear after apparent recovery.

BASIC INFORMATION FOR OLDER ADULTS

DESCRIPTION—Cardiomyopathy is an inflammatory disorder of the heart muscle. The heart muscle is weakened and cannot pump blood efficiently. Body parts involved: The heart muscle is the first body part involved, but decreasing heart function eventually affects the lungs, liver and circulatory system.

SPECIAL CONSIDERATIONS FOR AGING
- Characteristic signs and symptoms of many disorders are frequently changed or absent.
- Usual signs and symptoms may be absent and be replaced by symptoms of confusion, dizziness, failure to thrive, falling, incontinence, increasing dementia, refusal to eat or drink, weight loss, depression, paranoia, hypochondriasis, psychosis or threats of suicide.

SIGNS & SYMPTOMS—If cardiomyopathy is extensive enough to cause congestive heart failure, the following symptoms may occur:
- Irregular or rapid heartbeat.
- Shortness of breath with activity.
- Swelling of the feet and ankles.
- Fatigue.
- A cough with frothy, bloody sputum.
- Appetite loss.
- Loss of sex drive.
- Chest pain.

CAUSES & RISK FACTORS
Causes include:
- Virus infection.
- Nutritional deficiency, especially of vitamin B-1 (thiamine).
- Mineral deficiency, especially of potassium.
- Fat tissue replacing replacing muscle fibers in the heart.
- Amyloid deposits (see Glossary) due to other disorders.
- Tuberous sclerosis (see Glossary).
- Hemochromatosis (see Glossary).
- Severe anemia.
- Friedreich's ataxia (see Glossary).
- Stress.
- Terminal stage of coronary artery disease.
The risk increases with:
- Obesity.
- Smoking.
- Alcoholism.
- A family history of coronary artery disease or cardiomyopathy.
- The use of certain drugs, such as diuretics.

DOCTOR'S TREATMENT & DIAGNOSTIC TESTS
- Medical history and physical exam.
- ECG (see Glossary).
- X-rays of the heart and lungs.
- Biopsy of the heart muscle.
- Self-care instructions focused on the older patient.

HOME TREATMENT BY SELF OR CARE-GIVER

GENERAL INSTRUCTIONS—Weigh daily before breakfast and record the weight. Report any marked weight change to your doctor. This may indicate excess fluid accumulation.

MEDICATION (ADJUSTED FOR AGING)
- Your doctor may prescribe:
  Digitalis to improve heart function.
  Diuretics to decrease fluid retention.
  Vitamins or potassium supplements (if the disorder is caused by a deficiency).
- *Note:* Adverse reactions and side effects may be more frequent and severe in older persons. Remind your doctor of any medicines you already take.

ACTIVITY FOR OLDER PATIENTS—After treatment:
- Resume your normal activities gradually.
- Resume sexual relations when your sense of well-being allows and the symptoms are controlled.
- See Appendix 20 regarding physical fitness for the active older adult.

FOOD & BEVERAGE
- Low-salt diet (see Appendix 9).
- See Appendix 1 regarding good nutrition for people over 50.

FUTURE CONSIDERATIONS FOR THE AGING ADULT

POSSIBLE COMPLICATIONS—Congestive heart failure.

PROBABLE OUTCOME
- If the underlying disorder can be corrected, cardiomyopathy may be curable.
- If the underlying cause can't be corrected, cardiomyopathy is incurable. Some patients are candidates for a heart transplant.

PREVENTING RECURRENCE
- Don't drink alcoholic beverages.
- Eat a well-balanced diet.
- See Coronary Artery Disease in this section for prevention.

CALL YOUR DOCTOR IF

- You have symptoms of cardiomyopathy or the symptoms recur after treatment.
- You have chest pain.
- New, unexplained symptoms develop. The drugs used in treatment may produce side effects.

CARPAL TUNNEL SYNDROME

BASIC INFORMATION FOR OLDER ADULTS

DESCRIPTION—Carpal tunnel syndrome is a nerve disorder in the hand that causes pain and loss of feeling, especially in the thumb and the first 3 fingers. Body parts involved: The median nerve at the wrist joint; the blood vessels, nerves and tendons of the hand.

SPECIAL CONSIDERATIONS FOR AGING
- Joint disorders become more likely.
- Neurological diseases become more likely.
- Stress from any emotional cause—fear, worry, anxiety, sadness, loneliness or anger—affects all aspects of any illness or disorder.

SIGNS & SYMPTOMS
- Tingling or numbness in part of the hands.
- Sharp pains that shoot from the wrist up the arm, especially at night.
- Burning sensations in the fingers.
- Morning stiffness or cramping of hands.
- Thumb weakness.
- Frequent dropping of objects.
- Inability to make a fist.
- Shiny, dry skin on the hand.

CAUSES & RISK FACTORS—Caused by pressure on the median nerve due to swollen, inflamed or scarred tissue. The sources of pressure include:
- Inflammation of the tendon sheaths, frequently from arthritis.
- Fracture of the forearm.
- Sprain or dislocation of the wrist.

The risk increases with:
- Diabetes mellitus.
- Hypothyroidism.
- Menopause.
- Raynaud's disease.
- Work that requires strong hand action or continuous wrist action.

DOCTOR'S TREATMENT & DIAGNOSTIC TESTS
- Medical history and physical exam.
- Electromyograms (see Glossary).
- X-rays of the hand and wrist.
- Self-care instructions focused on the older patient.
- Surgery to free the pinched nerve.

HOME TREATMENT BY SELF OR CARE-GIVER

GENERAL INSTRUCTIONS
- You can decrease the discomfort by shaking your hands or dangling your arms. If you awaken at night with pain in your hand, hang it over the side of the bed, rub it or shake it.
- Consult your doctor about wearing a splint on the affected wrist at night.

MEDICATION (ADJUSTED FOR AGING)
- Your doctor may prescribe:
  Diuretics to decrease fluid retention that causes swollen tissue.
  Anti-inflammatory drugs to reduce inflammation.
  Cortisone injections at the wrist to reduce inflammation.
  Vitamin B-6 tablets or injections of vitamin B-12 may help. Consult your doctor.
- *Note:* Adverse reactions and side effects may be more frequent and severe in older persons. Remind your doctor of any medicines you already take.

ACTIVITY FOR OLDER PATIENTS
- Stay as active as your strength allows. If surgery has been necessary, allow 4 weeks for recovery. Exercises may be prescribed for the hand.
- See Appendix 20 regarding physical fitness for the active older adult.

FOOD & BEVERAGE
- Eat a normal, well-balanced diet that is low in sodium (see Appendix 9).
- See Appendix 1 regarding good nutrition for people over 50.

FUTURE CONSIDERATIONS FOR THE AGING ADULT

POSSIBLE COMPLICATIONS—Permanent numbness and a weak thumb or fingers in the affected hand.

PROBABLE OUTCOME—Usually curable—sometimes spontaneously, sometimes with surgery. Surgery is usually needed if muscle wasting or nerve changes have developed.

PREVENTING RECURRENCE—Cannot be prevented at present.

CALL YOUR DOCTOR IF

The symptoms of carpal tunnel syndrome don't disappear in 2 weeks.

CATARACT

BASIC INFORMATION FOR OLDER ADULTS

DESCRIPTION—A cataract is a clouding of the lens of the eye. The lens is a clear, flexible structure near the front of the eyeball. It helps to keep vision in focus and screens and refracts light rays. The lens has no blood supply. It is nourished by the vitreous humour (the watery protein substance that surrounds it). If hardening of the arteries prevents the proper nourishment of the vitreous humor—as often occurs in aging—the lens also loses its nourishment. The lens may then become less transparent and flexible and form cataracts. Cataracts may form in one or both eyes. If they form in both eyes, their growth rates may be very different. Cataracts are not cancerous. Body parts involved: The lens(es) of the eye(s).

SPECIAL CONSIDERATIONS FOR AGING—
Aging is the major risk factor, probably because there is cumulative damage to lens proteins with reduced solubility.

SIGNS & SYMPTOMS
- Blurred vision that may be worse in bright light. The blurring may first become apparent to one while driving at night, when lights seem to scatter or have halos.
- Double vision (occasionally).
- An opaque, milky white pupil (in the advanced stages only).
- Color perception changes.
- Near vision may have improved recently.

CAUSES & RISK FACTORS
- Natural aging.
- Injury to the eye.
- Illnesses associated with high blood sugar, such as diabetes mellitus.
- Inflammation, such as uveitis (see Glossary).
- Drugs, especially cortisone and its derivatives.
- Exposure to x-rays, microwaves and infrared radiation.

DOCTOR'S TREATMENT & DIAGNOSTIC TESTS
- Medical history and physical exam.
- Ophthalmologist's treatment.
- Surgery to remove the lens. Advancing age alone is not a deterrent.
- Self-care instructions focused on the older patient.

HOME TREATMENT BY SELF OR CARE-GIVER

GENERAL INSTRUCTIONS
- For a description of cataract surgery and postoperative care, see Cataract Removal in the Surgeries section. Special eyeglasses or contact lenses will be needed after surgery.
- Cataracts are a complicated, serious disorder. This page can cover only the main points of diagnosis and treatment. Your doctor, nurse or librarian can provide sources of supplemental information.

MEDICATION (ADJUSTED FOR AGING)
- Medicine is usually not necessary for this disorder.
- *Note:* Adverse reactions and side effects may be more frequent and severe in older persons. Remind your doctor of any medicines you already take.

ACTIVITY FOR OLDER PATIENTS
- No restrictions are necessary, except don't drive at night if your vision is poor.
- See Appendix 20 regarding physical fitness for the active older adult.

FOOD & BEVERAGE
- No special diet is required.
- See Appendix 1 regarding good nutrition for people over 50.

FUTURE CONSIDERATIONS FOR THE AGING ADULT

POSSIBLE COMPLICATIONS
- Loss of vision.
- Postoperative complications, including rupture of the eye, adhesions, infections and retinal detachment.

PROBABLE OUTCOME—Usually curable with surgery. Some cataracts never impair vision enough to require surgery. During the time cataracts are forming, frequent eyeglass changes may help vision.

PREVENTING RECURRENCE
- The use of cortisone drugs or any others that affect the eye lens should be monitored carefully by a doctor.
- Eye disorders which may cause cataract formation, such as iritis and uveitis, should receive prompt medical treatment.

CALL YOUR DOCTOR IF

You have symptoms of cataracts.

CELLULITIS
(Erysipelas)

BASIC INFORMATION FOR OLDER ADULTS

DESCRIPTION—Cellulitis is a non-contagious infection of the connective tissue beneath the skin that can affect the skin anywhere on the body, but it is most likely on the face or the lower legs. Erysipelas is the name of a severe cellulitis of the face. Body part involved: The connective tissue beneath the skin.

SPECIAL CONSIDERATIONS FOR AGING
- The skin becomes more permeable to bacteria, oil and water.
- The responsiveness of the skin's immune system decreases.
- The fatty layer of tissue under the skin becomes thinner.

SIGNS & SYMPTOMS
- Sudden tenderness, swelling and redness in an area of the skin. The area of cellulitis is initially 5cm to 20cm in diameter, and it grows rapidly in the first 24 hours. A thin red line often extends from the middle of the cellulitis toward the heart. Cellulitis does not develop into a boil.
- Fever, sometimes accompanied by chills and sweats.
- A general ill feeling.
- Swollen lymph glands nearest the cellulitis (sometimes).

CAUSES & RISK FACTORS—Cellulitis is caused by an infection from staphylococcus or streptococcus bacteria. Risk increases with:
- The use of immunosuppressive or cortisone drugs.
- Chronic illness, such as diabetes mellitus, or a recent infection that has lowered resistance.
- Any injury that breaks the skin.
- Poor nutrition.
- Venous ulcers (varicose ulcers; see Glossary)

DOCTOR'S TREATMENT & DIAGNOSTIC TESTS
- Medical history and physical exam.
- Laboratory blood culture if blood poisoning is suspected.
- Self-care instructions focused on the older patient.

HOME TREATMENT BY SELF OR CARE-GIVER

GENERAL INSTRUCTIONS—Use warm water soaks (see Appendix 18) to hasten healing and relieve the pain and inflammation.

MEDICATION (ADJUSTED FOR AGING)
- Your doctor may prescribe an antibiotic to fight infection. Finish the prescribed dose, even if the symptoms disappear quickly.
- *Note:* Adverse reactions and side effects may be more frequent and severe in older persons. Remind your doctor of any medicines you already take.

ACTIVITY FOR OLDER PATIENTS
- Rest in bed until the fever disappears and the other symptoms improve, then resume your normal activities.
- See Appendix 20 regarding physical fitness for the active older adult.

FOOD & BEVERAGE
- No special diet is required. Vitamin C supplements (250mg to 500mg daily) may hasten healing.
- See Appendix 1 regarding good nutrition for people over 50.

FUTURE CONSIDERATIONS FOR THE AGING ADULT

POSSIBLE COMPLICATIONS
- Blood poisoning if bacteria enter the bloodstream.
- Brain infection or meningitis if cellulitis occurs on the central part of the face.

PROBABLE OUTCOME—Usually curable in 7 to 10 days with treatment unless the patient has a chronic disease or is receiving immuno-suppressive treatment. In that case, cellulitis may lead to blood poisoning and become life threatening.

PREVENTING RECURRENCE
- Avoid skin damage. Use protective clothing or gear if you participate in strenuous work or sports.
- Keep the skin clean.

CALL YOUR DOCTOR IF

- You have symptoms of cellulitis, especially on the face.
- Any of the following occurs during treatment:
  Fever.
  Headache or vomiting.
  Drowsiness and lethargy.
  Blistering over the area of cellulitis.
  Red streaks that continue to extend despite treatment.
- New, unexplained symptoms develop. The drugs used in treatment may produce side effects.

ILLNESSES & DISORDERS

CERVICAL EROSION

BASIC INFORMATION FOR OLDER ADULTS

DESCRIPTION—Cervical erosion is a condition in which the lining of the uterus spreads to cover the tip of the cervix. This abnormally placed tissue is more likely to become inflamed or infected. It is not cancerous. Body parts involved: The cervix and the lining of the uterus.

SPECIAL CONSIDERATIONS FOR AGING
- Decreased hormone production (estrogen is a classic example).
- Estrogen production by the ovaries drops to zero at menopause, leading to disabling consequences in many women.
- Side effects of medication and adverse reactions are more frequent and worse.
- Repair from injury or disease is complete and effective, but recovery takes longer in older people.

SIGNS & SYMPTOMS
- No symptoms (usually).
- Increased mucus discharge from the vagina (sometimes).
- Unexplained vaginal bleeding (sometimes).

CAUSES & RISK FACTORS—The cause is usually unknown. Risk factors include:
- Stress.
- Repeated vaginal infections.
- Obesity.

DOCTOR'S TREATMENT & DIAGNOSTIC TESTS
- Medical history and physical exam, including pelvic examination.
- Pap smear (see Glossary).
- Minor surgery to cauterize or freeze the abnormal tissue (if a Pap smear is normal). Surgery is often done without anesthesia in the doctor's office or an outpatient surgical facility.
- Conization of the cervix (see Glossary) or hysterectomy (see the Surgeries section) if a Pap smear is not normal.
- Self-care instructions focused on the older patient.

HOME TREATMENT BY SELF OR CARE-GIVER

GENERAL INSTRUCTIONS
- Don't douche unless instructed to by your doctor.
- Obtain medical treatment for any vaginal infection you may also have.

MEDICATION (ADJUSTED FOR AGING)
- Your doctor may prescribe oral antibiotics or topical antibiotics to apply to the cervix.
- *Note:* Adverse reactions and side effects may be more frequent and severe in older persons. Remind your doctor of any medicines you already take.

ACTIVITY FOR OLDER PATIENTS
- After treatment (except following a hysterectomy), you may resume your normal activities and sexual relations immediately.
- See Appendix 20 regarding physical fitness for the active older adult.

FOOD & BEVERAGE
- No special diet is required.
- See Appendix 1 regarding good nutrition for people over 50.

FUTURE CONSIDERATIONS FOR THE AGING ADULT

POSSIBLE COMPLICATIONS—Occasionally precedes cancer of the cervix.

PROBABLE OUTCOME—The disorder is usually curable with treatment. Allow 3 months for the cervix to return completely to normal. Cervical erosion frequently recurs.

PREVENTING RECURRENCE—Cannot be prevented at present.

CALL YOUR DOCTOR IF

- You have symptoms of cervical erosion.
- Any of the following occurs after treatment: Increased discharge.
  Pain with intercourse or bleeding afterward.
- New, unexplained symptoms develop. The drugs used in treatment may produce side effects.

CERVICAL POLYPS

BASIC INFORMATION FOR OLDER ADULTS

DESCRIPTION—Cervical polyps are small, fragile, bulbous growths on stalks protruding through the cervix from the lining inside the uterus. They may be single or numerous. Body parts involved: The endometrium (the thin membrane lining the uterus) and the cervix (the lower third of the uterus, which opens into the vagina).

SPECIAL CONSIDERATIONS FOR AGING
- Decreased hormone production (estrogen is a classic example).
- Estrogen production by the ovaries drops to zero at menopause, leading to disabling consequences in many women.
- Side effects of medication and adverse reactions are more frequent and worse.
- Repair from injury or disease is complete and effective, but recovery takes longer in older people.

SIGNS & SYMPTOMS
- Unexpected spotting of blood.
- Spotting of blood after sexual intercourse or bowel movements.
- Vaginal discharge.

CAUSES & RISK FACTORS—Cervical polyps are caused by cervix inflammation due to infection, erosion or ulceration. They frequently accompany chronic infections in the vagina or cervix, although they are not contagious. The small growths are usually benign, but in very rare cases they represent early cancer of the cervix. The risk increases with:
- Diabetes mellitus.
- Recurrent vaginitis or cervicitis.

DOCTOR'S TREATMENT & DIAGNOSTIC TESTS
- Medical history and physical exam.
- Laboratory studies such as a Pap smear (see Glossary) and examination of the vaginal discharge.
- Self-care instructions focused on the older patient.
- Surgery to remove cervical polyps with a wire snare, electrocautery or liquid nitrogen. This can often be done in a simple office procedure. Your doctor may cauterize the cervix after removing the polyp to prevent regrowth of the same or another polyp. A polyp that accompanies cervicitis (inflammation or infection of the cervix) may require more extensive surgery. See Cervicitis in the Illnesses section.

HOME TREATMENT BY SELF OR CARE-GIVER

GENERAL INSTRUCTIONS
- Don't douche unless your doctor recommends it.
- Use small sanitary pads to protect your clothing from creams or suppositories.
- Keep creams or suppositories in the refrigerator.

MEDICATION (ADJUSTED FOR AGING)
- Your doctor may apply medication to the affected parts during office treatment. In addition, he or she may prescribe antibiotics by mouth or in vaginal suppositories or creams to fight infection.
- *Note:* Adverse reactions and side effects may be more frequent and severe in older persons. Remind your doctor of any medicines you already take.

ACTIVITY FOR OLDER PATIENTS
- No restrictions are necessary. Delay sexual relations until your doctor performs a follow-up pelvic exam and determines that healing is complete.
- See Appendix 20 regarding physical fitness for the active older adult.

FOOD & BEVERAGE—No special diet.

FUTURE CONSIDERATIONS FOR THE AGING ADULT

POSSIBLE COMPLICATIONS—None are expected, but in very rare instances cervical polyps may become malignant.

PROBABLE OUTCOME—Usually curable with surgery. You may feel brief, mild pain during the procedure and have mild to moderate cramps for several hours. Spotting of blood from the vagina may occur for 1 or 2 days.

PREVENTING RECURRENCE—To prevent vaginal or cervical infections that can precede cervical polyps:
- Wear cotton underpants or pantyhose with a cotton crotch to prevent accumulation of excessive heat and moisture, which can make you susceptible to vaginal and cervical infections.
- If you must take antibiotics for any reason, eat yogurt (with active yogurt cultures rather than pasteurized) or take acidophilus tablets (available from your pharmacy without prescription). This will reduce the chance that the antibiotics will allow the growth of infectious organisms in the cervix or vagina.
- Avoid contracting gonorrhea or other sexually transmitted diseases by having your sexual partner wear a condom during intercourse.

CALL YOUR DOCTOR IF

- You have symptoms of cervical polyps.
- Any of the following occurs after treatment: Discomfort persists longer than 1 week. Your symptoms recur. Unexplained vaginal bleeding or swelling develops.
- New, unexplained symptoms develop. The drugs used in treatment may produce side effects.

CERVICITIS

BASIC INFORMATION FOR OLDER ADULTS

DESCRIPTION—Cervicitis is an inflammation or infection of the cervix. There are 2 types, either of which may be contagious: Acute cervicitis, which is usually a bacterial or viral infection with specific symptoms; and chronic cervicitis, which is a long-term infection that may not have symptoms. Body parts involved: The cervix and the mucous membranes covering the cervix.

SPECIAL CONSIDERATIONS FOR AGING
- The immune system becomes less effective, opening the way for viral, bacterial and other infections; malignancies; immune disorders; and allergies.
- Decreased nutrition increases the risk of infections.
- Estrogen production by the ovaries drops to zero at menopause, leading to disabling consequences in many women.

SIGNS & SYMPTOMS
Acute cervicitis:
- Thick, yellow vaginal discharge.

Chronic cervicitis:
- Slight—sometimes unnoticeable—vaginal discharge.
- Backache.
- Discomfort with urination.
- Discomfort and bleeding with sexual intercourse.

Extensive chronic cervicitis:
- Profuse vaginal discharge.
- Spotting or bleeding after sexual intercourse.

CAUSES & RISK FACTORS—Acute cervicitis is usually caused by infection by one of many bacteria, including the one that causes gonorrhea or the herpes virus; chronic cervicitis is caused by repeated episodes of acute cervicitis or by one episode that is not treated long enough to heal completely. Risk factors include:
- Multiple sexual partners.
- Diabetes mellitus.
- Acute or recurrent vaginitis.

DOCTOR'S TREATMENT & DIAGNOSTIC TESTS
- Medical history and pelvic exam by a doctor.
- Laboratory studies such as a Pap smear (see Glossary) and culture of the discharge.
- Biopsy (see Glossary) of the cervix.
- Self-care instructions focused on the older patient.
- Destruction of abnormal cells with silver nitrate, cryosurgery, laser therapy or electrocautery (see Glossary for all).
- Surgery (hysterectomy) for widespread tissue destruction (rare). For more information, see Hysterectomy in the Surgeries section.

OTHER—If cervicitis is caused by a sexually transmitted infection, your sexual partner also needs treatment.

HOME TREATMENT BY SELF OR CARE-GIVER

GENERAL INSTRUCTIONS—Don't douche unless your doctor recommends it.

MEDICATION (ADJUSTED FOR AGING)—Your doctor may prescribe antiviral or antibiotic vaginal creams or suppositories to fight infection.

ACTIVITY FOR OLDER PATIENTS—No restrictions are necessary, except to avoid sexual relations until your doctor determines that the infection has healed.

FOOD & BEVERAGE—No special diet.

FUTURE CONSIDERATIONS FOR THE AGING ADULT

POSSIBLE COMPLICATIONS
- Cervical polyps.
- Pelvic inflammatory disease (PID).
- Malignant change in cervical cells (rare).

PROBABLE OUTCOME
- Mild cervicitis will heal without treatment.
- Acute cervicitis caused by venereal disease is contagious through sexual intercourse and is curable with medication.
- Most other cases of cervicitis can be cured with treatment in the doctor's office. All women with cervicitis need regular checkups until the condition heals.

PREVENTING RECURRENCE
- Wear cotton underpants or pantyhose with a cotton crotch. Avoid underpants made from non-ventilating materials. Synthetic materials hold in vaginal wetness and warmth, which may trigger vaginal or cervical infections.
- If you must take antibiotics for any reason, eat yogurt (with active yogurt cultures rather than pasteurized) or take acidophilus tablets (available from your pharmacy without prescription). This will reduce the chance that the antibiotics will allow the growth of infectious organisms in the cervix or vagina.
- Avoid contracting gonorrhea or other sexually transmitted diseases by having your sexual partner wear a condom during intercourse.

CALL YOUR DOCTOR IF

- You have symptoms of cervicitis.
- During treatment, discomfort persists longer than 1 week or symptoms worsen.
- Unexplained vaginal bleeding or swelling develops during or after treatment.
- New, unexplained symptoms develop. The drugs used in treatment may produce side effects.

BASIC INFORMATION FOR OLDER ADULTS

DESCRIPTION—Cancer of the cervix is a common but treatable and preventable cancer of the female reproductive system. Body parts involved: The cervix (the lower third of the uterus, which opens into the vagina).

SPECIAL CONSIDERATIONS FOR AGING
- Malignant diseases (especially in the colon, lung and breast) represent difficult-to-diagnose problems, but cancer of the cervix is relatively easy to detect.
- The immune system becomes less effective, opening the way for viral, bacterial and other infections; malignancies; immune disorders; and allergies.
- Malignant diseases progress more slowly.
- Stress from any emotional cause—fear, worry, anxiety, sadness, loneliness or anger—affects all aspects of any illness or disorder.

SIGNS & SYMPTOMS
In the early, easily treatable stages:
- No symptoms.
In the later stages:
- Unexplained vaginal bleeding.
- Persistent vaginal discharge.
- Pain and bleeding after intercourse.
In the final stages:
- Abdominal pain.
- Leaking of feces and urine through the vagina.
- Appetite and weight loss.
- Anemia.

CAUSES & RISK FACTORS—The cause is unknown. Risk factors include:
- Frequent sexual intercourse during the teen years.
- Multiple sex partners.
- Multiple pregnancies.
- Recurrent vaginal infections (bacterial or viral, including genital herpes and genital warts).
- Smoking.
- Sex partner with genital warts.

DOCTOR'S TREATMENT & DIAGNOSTIC TESTS
- Medical history and physical exam.
- Laboratory studies such as a Pap smear and biopsy (see Glossary).
- Surgical diagnostic procedures such as conization of the cervix (see Glossary).
- Surgery to remove the cancerous area. During the early stages, this may only involve a small area of the cervix. More advanced stages may require removal of the reproductive organs and other affected tissue. Advancing age alone is not a deterrent. For more information, see Hysterectomy in the Surgeries section.
- Chemotherapy and radiation therapy (advanced cancer).
- Following treatment, self-care instructions focused on the older patient.

HOME TREATMENT BY SELF OR CARE-GIVER

GENERAL INSTRUCTIONS
- Maintain as positive an attitude as possible during treatment.
- Treatment may cause side effects, but they are usually temporary.
- Your pain can be controlled. Don't hesitate to ask your doctor for pain medication.
- Fear may be your worst enemy.
- Call on family members and friends for whatever support and help you need.

MEDICATION (ADJUSTED FOR AGING)
- Medicine usually is not necessary for this disorder if it is diagnosed and treated early. If radical surgery and additional treatment are required, your doctor may prescribe:
  Anticancer drugs.
  Pain relievers.
- *Note:* Adverse reactions and side effects may be more frequent and severe in older persons. Remind your doctor of any medicines you already take.

ACTIVITY FOR OLDER PATIENTS—No restrictions are necessary.

FOOD & BEVERAGE
- No special diet is required.
- See Appendix 1 regarding good nutrition for people over 50.

FUTURE CONSIDERATIONS FOR THE AGING ADULT

POSSIBLE COMPLICATIONS—If cervical cancer is not treated early, it spreads beyond the uterus to other body parts and results in death.

PROBABLE OUTCOME—Usually curable if diagnosed before the tumor has spread.

PREVENTING RECURRENCE
- Avoid the risks listed above as much as possible.
- Obtain regular Pap smears (see Glossary). Regular pelvic examinations and Pap smears are very effective in detecting precancerous changes or cervical cancer in its symptom-free stage. Consult your doctor, Planned Parenthood or the public health department about how often to be examined. Many public agencies will perform a Pap smear at little or no cost to you.

CALL YOUR DOCTOR IF

- You have persistent vaginal bleeding or other symptoms of cervical cancer.
- You have not had a pelvic examination or Pap smear in the past year.

ILLNESSES & DISORDERS

CIRRHOSIS OF THE LIVER

BASIC INFORMATION FOR OLDER ADULTS

DESCRIPTION—Cirrhosis of the liver is a chronic scarring of the liver that leads to the loss of normal liver function. Body parts involved: The liver and its major blood vessels.

SPECIAL CONSIDERATIONS FOR AGING
- Disease in one organ system leads to problems in another system.
- The appetite becomes poorer.
- Stress from any emotional cause—fear, worry, anxiety, sadness, loneliness or anger—affects all aspects of any illness or disorder.
- Alcoholism is quite common in older people.

SIGNS & SYMPTOMS
Early stages:
- Fatigue; weakness.
- Poor appetite; nausea; weight loss.
- An enlarged liver.
- Red palms.

Late stages:
- Jaundice (yellow skin and eyes).
- Dark yellow or brown urine.
- Spider blood vessels of the skin (fine vessels which spread out from a central point).
- Hair loss.
- Breast enlargement in men.
- Fluid accumulation in the abdomen and legs.
- An enlarged spleen.
- Diarrhea; black or bloody stool.
- Bleeding and bruising.
- Mental confusion; coma.

CAUSES & RISK FACTORS—Cirrhosis means inflammation of the liver accompanied by the destruction of liver cells, cell regeneration and scarring. These may be preceded by prolonged excessive alcohol consumption, hepatitis, exposure to toxic chemicals or intestinal bypass surgery. The risk increases with:
- Poor nutrition.
- Hepatitis.
- Excessive alcohol consumption. Individuals vary widely in the amount and duration of alcohol consumption necessary to cause cirrhosis.
- Occupational exposure to chemicals that are toxic to the liver.

DOCTOR'S TREATMENT & DIAGNOSTIC TESTS
- Medical history and physical exam.
- Laboratory studies such as blood and urine tests of liver function.
- X-ray and/or biopsy of the liver.
- Self-care instructions focused on the older patient.
- Psychotherapy or counseling (for alcoholism).
- Surgery to relieve the pressure of the blood in the abdominal veins (rare and of limited benefit).

HOME TREATMENT BY SELF OR CARE-GIVER

GENERAL INSTRUCTIONS—If cirrhosis is caused by alcoholism, stop drinking. Ask for help from family members, friends and community agencies. For further information, see Alcoholism in the Illnesses section.

MEDICATION (ADJUSTED FOR AGING)—Your doctor may prescribe:
- Iron supplements for anemia resulting from hemorrhage or poor nutrition.
- Diuretics to reduce fluid retention.
- Antibiotics, such as neomycin, to reduce ammonia buildup.

ACTIVITY FOR OLDER PATIENTS—Resume your normal activities as soon as your symptoms improve.

FOOD & BEVERAGE
- In the early stages, eat a well-balanced diet that is high in carbohydrates, high in protein and low in salt (see Appendix 9). In the late stages you may need to reduce your protein intake.
- Vitamin and mineral supplements may be necessary.
- Don't drink alcohol.

FUTURE CONSIDERATIONS FOR THE AGING ADULT

POSSIBLE COMPLICATIONS
- Life-threatening hemorrhage, especially from the esophagus and stomach.
- Liver cancer.
- Body poisoning and coma from a buildup of ammonia and other body wastes.
- Sexual impotence.

PROBABLE OUTCOME—Cirrhosis can be arrested—no matter what the cause—if the underlying cause can be removed. Liver damage is irreversible, but the symptoms can be relieved or controlled. A nearly normal life is possible if cirrhosis is treated early and the treatment succeeds. If the underlying cause is not removed the liver scarring will continue, resulting in death from liver failure.

PREVENTING RECURRENCE
- Obtain treatment for alcoholism.
- Obtain prompt medical treatment for hepatitis.
- Survey your work environment for possible exposure to toxic chemicals.

CALL YOUR DOCTOR IF

- You have symptoms of cirrhosis.
- Any of the following occurs during treatment:
  Vomiting blood or passing a black stool.
  Mental confusion or coma.
  Fever or other signs of infection (redness, swelling, tenderness or pain).

COLD, COMMON

BASIC INFORMATION FOR OLDER ADULTS

DESCRIPTION—The common cold is a contagious viral infection of the upper respiratory passages. Body parts involved: The nose, throat, sinuses, ears, eustachian tubes, trachea, larynx and bronchial tubes.

SPECIAL CONSIDERATIONS FOR AGING
- The immune system becomes less effective, opening the way for viral, bacterial and other infections; malignancies; immune disorders; and allergies.
- Repair from injury or disease is complete and effective, but recovery takes longer in older people.
- The nasal mucous membrane becomes thinner and less elastic.
- Decreased nutrition increases the risk of infections.
- Signs and symptoms may differ significantly from those listed below.
- The total state of well-being in many older people makes them increasingly susceptible to infections and impairs their ability to prevent infections from spreading.
- Stress from any emotional cause—fear, worry, anxiety, sadness, loneliness or anger—affects all aspects of any illness or disorder.

SIGNS & SYMPTOMS
- Runny or stuffy nose. Nasal discharge is watery at first, then becomes thick and greenish yellow.
- Sore throat; hoarseness.
- A cough that produces little or no sputum.
- Low-grade fever; fatigue; chills.
- Watering eyes; appetite loss.
- Aching muscles and bones; headache.

CAUSES & RISK FACTORS—The common cold is caused by any of at least 200 viruses. Virus particles spread through the air or from person-to-person contact, especially hand shaking. Risk factors include:
- Stress; fatigue or overwork.
- Poor nutrition; smoking.
- Exposure to cold, wet weather.
- Crowded or unsanitary living conditions.

DOCTOR'S TREATMENT & DIAGNOSTIC TESTS
- Medical history and physical exam (sometimes).
- If a sore throat persists for 3 to 4 days, a laboratory throat culture to rule out bacterial infection with streptococcus or other germs.
- Self-care instructions focused on the older patient.

HOME TREATMENT BY SELF OR CARE-GIVER

GENERAL INSTRUCTIONS
- To relieve nasal congestion, use salt water drops (1/2 teaspoon of salt to 1 cup of warm water). Put 3 or 4 drops into each nostril several times a day.
- Use a cool-mist humidifier to increase the air moisture.

MEDICATION (ADJUSTED FOR AGING)
- No medicine, including antibiotics, can cure the common cold. To relieve the symptoms, you may use non-prescription drugs such as acetaminophen, decongestants, nose drops or sprays, cough remedies and throat lozenges.
- Vitamin C in large doses (up to 1000 mg a day) may shorten the cold's duration.
- *Note:* Adverse reactions and side effects may be more frequent and severe in older persons. Remind your doctor of any medicines you already take.

ACTIVITY FOR OLDER PATIENTS—Bed rest is not necessary, but avoid vigorous activity. Rest often.

FOOD & BEVERAGE
- Drink extra fluids, including water, fruit juice, tea and carbonated drinks. Avoid milk because it may thicken secretions in some persons.
- See Appendix 1 regarding good nutrition for people over 50.

FUTURE CONSIDERATIONS FOR THE AGING ADULT

POSSIBLE COMPLICATIONS—Bacterial infections of the ears, throat, sinuses or lungs.

PROBABLE OUTCOME—Spontaneous recovery in 7 to 14 days.

PREVENTING RECURRENCE
- To prevent spreading a cold to others, avoid unnecessary contact during the contagious phase (first 2 to 4 days).
- Wash your hands frequently, especially after blowing your nose or before handling food.
- Avoid risks listed above.

CALL YOUR DOCTOR IF

You cannot distinguish a common cold from the flu or any of the following occurs during the illness:
- Increased throat pain or white or yellow spots on the tonsils or other parts of the throat.
- Coughing episodes that last longer than intervals between coughing; cough that produces thick, yellow-green or gray sputum; cough that lasts longer than 7 days; or difficult or labored breathing between coughing bouts.
- Fever that lasts several days; shaking chills.
- Chest pain or shortness of breath.
- Earache or headache; skin rash.
- Pain in the teeth or over the sinuses.
- Unusual lethargy; irritability; delirium.
- Enlarged, tender glands in the neck.
- Dusky blue or gray lips, skin or nail beds.

ILLNESSES & DISORDERS

COLD SORES
(Fever Blisters; Herpes Simplex)

BASIC INFORMATION FOR OLDER ADULTS

DESCRIPTION—Cold sores represent a common, contagious virus infection (HSV 1; see Glossary). Cold sores are sometimes confused with impetigo. Body parts involved: The lips, gums and mouth area; the cornea (rare) or the genitals (occasionally).

SPECIAL CONSIDERATIONS FOR AGING
- The immune system becomes less effective, opening the way for viral, bacterial and other infections; malignancies; immune disorders; and allergies.
- Decreased nutrition increases the risk of infections.
- Mucous membranes become thinner and less elastic.

SIGNS & SYMPTOMS
- May be preceded by a tingling in the lips.
- Eruptions of very small, painful blisters—usually around the mouth, but sometimes on the genitals. The blisters are grouped together, and each is surrounded by a red ring. They fill with fluid, then dry up and disappear within a week.
- If the eye is infected, the symptoms include eye pain and redness, a feeling that something is in the eye, sensitivity to light and tearing.

CAUSES & RISK FACTORS—Cold sores are caused by infection with a herpes virus that invades the skin, often remaining for months or years before causing active inflammation. Most persons develop antibodies that control the virus unless risk factors (below) develop. The virus is transmitted by person-to-person contact or by contact with saliva, stools, urine or discharge from an infected eye. The blisters and ulcers are contagious until they heal, both in the first and in succeeding flare-ups. Risk factors include:
- Physical or emotional stress.
- Illness that has lowered resistance, including a cold, minor gastrointestinal upset or fever from any cause.
- Excessive exposure to the sun.
- Excessive exposure to cold wind (as while skiing).
- Dental treatment that stretches the mouth.
- The use of immunosuppressive drugs.

DOCTOR'S TREATMENT & DIAGNOSTIC TESTS
- Medical history and physical exam (sometimes); laboratory virus cultures (rare).
- Self-care instructions focused on the older patient.

HOME TREATMENT BY SELF OR CARE-GIVER

GENERAL INSTRUCTIONS
- Drink cool liquids or suck frozen juice bars to reduce discomfort.

- Apply an ice cube for 1 hour during the first 24 hours after a lesion appears. This may make it heal more quickly.
- Don't rub or scratch an infected eye.
- To prevent flare-ups, use zinc oxide or sunscreen preparations on your lips when you spend much time outdoors.

MEDICATION (ADJUSTED FOR AGING)
- Use acetaminophen or aspirin to relieve minor pain.
- Don't try to treat an infected eye—especially with cortisone ointments or drops—without consulting your doctor. Cortisone preparations promote growth of the herpes virus in the cornea.
- Your doctor may prescribe:
  Antiviral topical or oral medication.
  Antibiotic ointment if lesions become infected with bacteria.
  Topical medication for eye infections.

ACTIVITY FOR OLDER PATIENTS
- No restrictions are necessary, except to avoid close contact—especially kissing or oral sex—until the lesions heal.
- Avoid newborns or patients who are taking immunosuppressant drugs.

FOOD & BEVERAGE—No special diet.

FUTURE CONSIDERATIONS FOR THE AGING ADULT

POSSIBLE COMPLICATIONS
- Permanent vision impairment if herpes eye infections are untreated.
- Severe, widespread infection in patients with eczema.
- Meningitis or encephalitis (rare).

PROBABLE OUTCOME—Spontaneous recovery in a few days to a week, occasionally longer. Recurrence is common. The virus remains in the body for life, but it is usually dormant.

PREVENTING RECURRENCE
- Avoid physical contact with others who have active lesions.
- Wash your hands often during a flare-up to avoid spreading the virus.

CALL YOUR DOCTOR IF

Any of the following occurs with a cold sore:
- Signs of secondary bacterial infection, such as fever, pus instead of clear fluid in the lesions, headache and muscle aches.
- Eruption of lesions on the genitals similar to those around the mouth.
- New, unexplained symptoms. The drugs used in treatment may produce side effects.

COLITIS, ULCERATIVE
(Granulomatous Colitis)

BASIC INFORMATION FOR OLDER ADULTS

DESCRIPTION—Ulcerative colitis is a serious chronic inflammatory disease of the colon characterized by ulceration and episodes of bloody diarrhea. The ulcerated areas are inflamed and may form abscesses in the lining of the large intestine. Ulcerative colitis may be confused with some bacterial infections of the colon. Body parts involved: The rectum and large bowel.

SPECIAL CONSIDERATIONS FOR AGING
- Characteristic signs and symptoms of many disorders are frequently changed or absent.
- Usual signs and symptoms may be absent and be replaced by symptoms of confusion, dizziness, failure to thrive, falling, incontinence, increasing dementia, refusal to eat or drink, weight loss, depression, paranoia, hypochondriasis, psychosis or threats of suicide.
- The immune system becomes less effective, opening the way for viral, bacterial and other infections; malignancies; immune disorders; and allergies.
- Stress from any emotional cause—fear, worry, anxiety, sadness, loneliness or anger—affects all aspects of any illness or disorder.

SIGNS & SYMPTOMS
Early symptoms include:
- Pain in the left side of the abdomen that improves after bowel movements.
- Episodes of bloody diarrhea with mucus, alternating with symptom free intervals.

Symptoms during an acute attack include:
- Increased bloody diarrhea (up to 10 to 20 bowel movements a day).
- Severe cramps and pain around the rectum.
- Sweating; dehydration.
- Nausea; appetite and weight loss.
- A bloated abdomen.
- A fever as high as 104F (40C).
- A rapid heartbeat.

CAUSES & RISK FACTORS—The cause is unknown. The risk increases with stress, anxiety or depression; a family history of ulcerative colitis; and excessive alcohol consumption.

DOCTOR'S TREATMENT & DIAGNOSTIC TESTS
- Medical history and physical exam.
- Laboratory stool and blood studies.
- X-ray of the colon (barium enema).
- Sigmoidoscopy (see Glossary).
- Biopsy of the colon lining.
- Self-care instructions focused on the older patient.
- Psychological counseling.
- Surgery to remove the diseased colon (sometimes). For an explanation of this surgery and postoperative care, consult your doctor.
- Hospitalization during severe episodes.

HOME TREATMENT BY SELF OR CARE-GIVER

GENERAL INSTRUCTIONS
- To reduce cramps, apply a hot water bottle, warm moist towels or heating pad to the abdomen.
- Try to reduce stress. See Appendix 13.

MEDICATION (ADJUSTED FOR AGING)
- Don't use aspirin. It increases the risk of bleeding.
- Your doctor may prescribe:
  Antidiarrhea medication for minimal symptoms.
  Sulfa drugs, such as sulfasalazine, for moderate symptoms.
  Medicated enemas (usually with hydrocortisone).
  Cortisone drugs for severe disease.

ACTIVITY FOR OLDER PATIENTS—Bed rest may be necessary during acute attacks. However, resume normal activity as soon as your symptoms improve.

FOOD & BEVERAGE
- Don't drink alcohol.
- During early treatment, avoid milk and milk products.
- See Appendix 1 regarding good nutrition for people over 50.

FUTURE CONSIDERATIONS FOR THE AGING ADULT

POSSIBLE COMPLICATIONS
- Life-threatening blood loss, ulceration through the intestinal wall or peritonitis during acute attacks.
- Malnutrition, wasting of the body or chronic disability.
- Inflammation of the joints, eyes and skin.
- Colon cancer; the risk is greater in persons with ulcerative colitis.

PROBABLE OUTCOME—Often curable with medical treatment or surgery and counseling to reduce stress or depression or to control excessive alcohol consumption. If it is not curable, the symptoms can be controlled with treatment.

PREVENTING RECURRENCE—There are no specific preventive measures.

CALL YOUR DOCTOR IF

- You have symptoms of ulcerative colitis.
- Fever and chills develop.
- The frequency of bowel movements or bleeding increases.
- Your abdomen becomes distended.
- Jaundice (yellow eyes and skin) develops.
- Vomiting begins or the abdominal pain increases.

CONGESTIVE HEART FAILURE

BASIC INFORMATION FOR OLDER ADULTS

DESCRIPTION—Congestive heart failure is a complication of many serious diseases in which the heart loses its full pumping capacity. Blood backs up into other organs, especially the lungs and liver. Body parts involved: The heart, blood vessels, lungs, liver and extremities.

SPECIAL CONSIDERATIONS FOR AGING
- Older people have decreased reserve power for heart function.
- The total heart functions less efficiently— especially among smokers.
- The heart's muscle mass becomes thicker, but not stronger.

SIGNS & SYMPTOMS
- Shortness of breath, especially with exertion or when lying flat in bed.
- Fatigue, weakness or faintness.
- A cough (usually with sputum); wheezing.
- Swelling of the abdomen, legs and ankles.
- Rapid or irregular heartbeat.
- Low blood pressure; distended neck veins.
- An enlarged liver.

CAUSES & RISK FACTORS—Causes include high blood pressure; heart valve disease; heart attack; coronary artery disease; heartbeat irregularities; severe lung disease such as emphysema; congenital heart disease; cardiomyopathy; hyperthyroidism; severe anemia; heart tumor (rare); and infections complicating underlying heart disease. The risk increases with:
- Infections with high fever; smoking; obesity.
- Excessive alcohol consumption.
- The use of certain drugs, such as beta-adrenergic blockers or excessive digitalis.
- A diet that is high in fat and salt.

DOCTOR'S TREATMENT & DIAGNOSTIC TESTS
- Medical history and physical exam.
- Laboratory blood studies and urinalysis.
- X-rays of the heart, lungs and blood vessels (angiography).
- ECG (see Glossary) and heart catheterization studies (occasionally).
- Radioactive studies of heart muscle efficiency.
- Echocardiogram (occasionally; see Glossary).
- Self-care instructions focused on the older patient.
- Surgery on the heart valves, coronary arteries or ventricular aneurysms (sometimes).
- Hospitalization (in severe cases).

HOME TREATMENT BY SELF OR CARE-GIVER

GENERAL INSTRUCTIONS
- Weigh daily and keep a record.
- Don't smoke.

MEDICATION (ADJUSTED FOR AGING)
- Your doctor may prescribe:
  Diuretics to decrease fluid retention and swelling. (The dosage may start off low and then increase.)
  Digitalis to strengthen and regulate the heartbeat.
  Antiarrhythmic drugs to stabilize the heartbeat.
  "Afterload" vasodilators to reduce blood pressure, even if it is normal.
  Potassium replacements if you take diuretics or digitalis.
- *Note:* Adverse reactions and side effects may be more frequent and severe in older persons. Remind your doctor of any medicines you already take.

ACTIVITY FOR OLDER PATIENTS—In the early stages, bed rest with the upper body elevated is as important as medication. Avoid unnecessary exertion (such as climbing stairs) until the condition is under control. Then consult your doctor about acceptable activity.

FOOD & BEVERAGE
- Achieve your ideal weight to reduce the heart's workload.
- Eat a low-salt, low-fat, high-fiber diet (see Appendices 8 and 9).
- Don't drink alcohol.

FUTURE CONSIDERATIONS FOR THE AGING ADULT

POSSIBLE COMPLICATIONS—Pulmonary edema.

PROBABLE OUTCOME—Life expectancy is reduced, but many forms are well controlled for a while with medication and sometimes surgery. The underlying cause may be treated. Other forms cause chronic illness. Any infection may worsen the condition.

PREVENTING RECURRENCE—If you have a condition that can lead to congestive heart failure, obtain medical care and adhere to your treatment program. Follow your dietary guidelines and don't drink alcohol or smoke.

CALL YOUR DOCTOR IF

- You have symptoms of congestive heart failure.
- Any of the following occurs during treatment:
  Symptoms of infection, such as fever, muscle aches, headache and dizziness.
  Worsening of the symptoms, especially rapid or irregular heartbeat or wheezing at night.
  Cough with increased sputum or blood.
  Weight gain of 3 or 4 pounds in 1 or 2 days.
- New, unexplained symptoms develop. The drugs used in treatment may produce side effects.

CONSTIPATION

BASIC INFORMATION FOR OLDER ADULTS

DESCRIPTION—Constipation is the passing of infrequent, difficult or uncomfortable bowel movements. Body part involved: The colon.

SPECIAL CONSIDERATIONS FOR AGING
- The total digestive system becomes more sluggish.
- The muscles of the abdomen and pelvic floor become weak.
- Stress from any emotional cause—fear, worry, anxiety, sadness, loneliness or anger—affects all aspects of any illness or disorder.

SIGNS & SYMPTOMS—People vary widely in bowel activity. Any of the following may be a sign of constipation:
- Infrequent bowel movements, sometimes accompanied by abdominal swelling.
- Hard feces; sensation of continuing fullness after a bowel movement.
- Straining during bowel movements.
- Pain or bleeding with bowel movements.

CAUSES & RISK FACTORS—Causes include inadequate fluid intake; insufficient fiber in the diet (fiber adds bulk, holds water and creates easily passed, soft feces); inactivity; depression; hypothyroidism; hypercalcemia; anal fissure; chronic kidney failure; back pain; the use of laxatives over a long period; colon or rectal cancer; irritable bowel syndrome; diverticular disease; travel; and the use of unfamiliar or unclean facilities. Risk factors include:
- Stress; illness requiring complete bed rest.
- The use of certain drugs, including belladonna, calcium channel blockers, beta-adrenergic blockers, tricyclic antidepressants, narcotics, atropine or aspirin.

DOCTOR'S TREATMENT & DIAGNOSTIC TESTS
- Medical history and physical exam. Tell your doctor of any major change in your bowel pattern that lasts longer than 1 week; it may be a sign of cancer.
- Laboratory tests of the blood and stool to detect internal bleeding.
- Sigmoidoscopy (rare; see Glossary).
- Self-care instructions focused on the older patient.

HOME TREATMENT BY SELF OR CARE-GIVER

GENERAL INSTRUCTIONS
- Set aside a regular time each day for bowel movements. The best time is often within 1 hour after breakfast. Don't try to hurry. Sit at least 10 minutes, whether or not a bowel movement occurs.
- Drinking hot water, tea or coffee may help stimulate the bowel.
- If constipation persists for 3 or 4 days, use a non-prescription, disposable enema for temporary relief. If you prefer not to use a commercial enema preparation, you may give yourself an enema as follows:
  Spread a bath mat on the bathroom floor or in the tub.
  Fill an enema bag with lukewarm water.
  Hang the enema bag no higher than 30 inches from the floor.
  Lie on your left side on the mat.
  Insert the nozzle gently into the rectum.
  Let the water flow in slowly, a little at a time.
  If it hurts, stop the water flow until the pain subsides, then start the flow again.
  Use the entire quart of water.
  Hold the fluid inside until you are uncomfortable.
  Then sit on the toilet for a bowel movement.

MEDICATION (ADJUSTED FOR AGING)—For *occasional* constipation, you may use stool softeners, mild non-prescription laxatives or enemas. Don't use laxatives or enemas regularly as this can cause dependency. Avoid harsh laxatives and cathartics, such as epsom salts.

ACTIVITY FOR OLDER PATIENTS—Exercise and good physical fitness help maintain healthy bowel patterns. See Appendix 20 for exercise suggestions.

FOOD & BEVERAGE
- Drink at least 8 glasses of water each day. Include bulk foods, such as bran and raw fruits and vegetables, in your diet. Avoid refined cereals and breads, pastries and sugar.
- See Appendix 1 regarding good nutrition for people over 50.

FUTURE CONSIDERATIONS FOR THE AGING ADULT

POSSIBLE COMPLICATIONS—Hemorrhoids; laxative dependency; hernia from excessive straining; uterine or rectal prolapse; spastic colitis; bowel obstruction.

PROBABLE OUTCOME—Usually curable with exercise, diet and adequate fluids.

PREVENTING RECURRENCE
- Eat a well-balanced, high-fiber diet.
- Exercise regularly.
- Drink at least 8 glasses of water a day.
- If your physical mobility is restricted, talk to your doctor about the ongoing use of laxatives or enemas.

CALL YOUR DOCTOR IF

- You have constipation that persists despite self-care—especially if the constipation represents a change in your normal bowel patterns.
- Constipation is accompanied by fever or severe abdominal pain.
- There is blood in your stools.

CORN OR CALLUS

BASIC INFORMATION FOR OLDER ADULTS

DESCRIPTION—A corn is a thickening (bump) of the outer skin layer, usually over a bony area such as a toe joint. A corn involves the toe joints and the skin between the toes. A callus is a painless thickening of skin caused by repeated pressure or irritation. It can occur on any part of the body, especially the hands, feet or knees, that endures repeated pressure or irritation. Body parts involved: Those mentioned above.

SPECIAL CONSIDERATIONS FOR AGING
- Years of weight bearing cause wear and tear on the bones, joints and ligaments.
- The bones become thinner.

SIGNS & SYMPTOMS
- Corn—A small, tender, painful raised bump on the side or over the joint of a toe. A corn is usually 3 mm to 10 mm in diameter and has a hard center.
- Callus—A rough, thickened area of skin that appears after repeated pressure or irritation.

CAUSES & RISK FACTORS—Corns and calluses form to protect a skin area from injury caused by repeated irritation (rubbing or squeezing). Pressure causes the cells in the irritated area to grow at a faster rate, leading to overgrowth. Risk factors include:
- Shoes that fit poorly.
- Occupations that involve pressure on the hands or knees, such as carpentry, writing, guitar playing or tile laying.

DOCTOR'S TREATMENT & DIAGNOSTIC TESTS
- Medical history and physical exam by a doctor of medicine or a podiatrist (sometimes).
- Self-care instructions focused on the older patient.

HOME TREATMENT BY SELF OR CARE-GIVER

GENERAL INSTRUCTIONS
- If you have diabetes or poor circulation, consider consulting a podiatrist for treatment.
- Remove the source of pressure if possible. Discard ill-fitting shoes.
- Use corn and callus pads to reduce pressure on irritated areas.
- Peel or rub the thickened area with a pumice stone to remove it. Don't cut it with a razor. Soak the area in warm water to soften it before peeling.

- Ask a shoe repairman to sew a metatarsal bar onto your shoe to use while a corn is healing.
- Avoid surgery. It does not remove the cause. Post-surgical scarring is painful and may complicate healing.

MEDICATION (ADJUSTED FOR AGING)
- After peeling the upper layers of the corn once or twice a day, apply ointment. Use a non-prescription 5% or 10% salicylic ointment. Cover with adhesive tape.
- Your doctor may inject a corn or callus with cortisone medicine to suppress any inflammation or pain.
- *Note:* Adverse reactions and side effects may be more frequent and severe in older persons. Remind your doctor of any medicines you already take.

ACTIVITY FOR OLDER PATIENTS
- Resume your normal activities as soon as your symptoms improve.
- See Appendix 20 regarding physical fitness for the active older adult.

FOOD & BEVERAGE
- No special diet is required.
- See Appendix 1 regarding good nutrition for people over 50.

FUTURE CONSIDERATIONS FOR THE AGING ADULT

POSSIBLE COMPLICATIONS—Back, hip, knee or ankle pain caused by a change in one's gait due to severe discomfort.

PROBABLE OUTCOME—Usually curable if the underlying cause can be removed. Allow 3 weeks for recovery. Recurrence is likely—even with treatment—if the cause is not removed.

PREVENTING RECURRENCE
- Don't wear shoes that fit poorly.
- Avoid activities that create constant pressure on specific skin areas.
- When possible, wear protective gear, such as gloves or knee pads.

CALL YOUR DOCTOR IF

- You have corns or calluses that persist despite self-treatment.
- Any signs of infection, such as redness, swelling, pain, heat or tenderness, develop around a corn or callus.

CORNEA, INFECTION OF
(Keratitis)

BASIC INFORMATION FOR OLDER ADULTS

DESCRIPTION—Infection of the cornea is an inflammation of the cornea (the clear central portion of the eye that covers the pupil). Body parts involved: The eye(s).

SPECIAL CONSIDERATIONS FOR AGING
- The immune system becomes less effective, opening the way for viral, bacterial and other infections; malignancies; immune disorders; and allergies.
- Characteristic signs and symptoms of many disorders are frequently changed or absent.
- Decreased nutrition increases the risk of infections.
- The amount of mucus in the eyes decreases.

SIGNS & SYMPTOMS
- Eye pain.
- Photophobia (sensitivity to light).
- Tears.

CAUSES & RISK FACTORS
Causes include:
- Bacterial, viral or fungal infections. The most common is herpes simplex virus Type I (HSV I; see Glossary).
- Drying of the eye caused by an eyelid disorder or insufficient tear formation.
- A foreign object in the eye.
- Intense light, such as from welding arcs or the reflection of intense sunlight from snow or water. (Symptoms may not appear for 24 hours after exposure.)
- Vitamin A deficiency (rare in normal diet).
- Allergy or sensitivity to eye cosmetics, air pollution, airborne particles (pollen, dust, mold or yeasts) and other allergens.

Risk factors include:
- Poor nutrition, especially insufficient vitamin A.
- Illness that has lowered resistance.
- Crowded or unsanitary living conditions.
- Viral infections elsewhere in the body, especially cold sores or genital herpes.

DOCTOR'S TREATMENT & DIAGNOSTIC TESTS
- Medical history and physical exam by an ophthalmologist.
- Laboratory culture of the discharge from the eye.
- Surgery to replace the cornea (in severe cases only). Advancing age alone is not a deterrent.
- Self-care instructions focused on the older patient.

HOME TREATMENT BY SELF OR CARE-GIVER

GENERAL INSTRUCTIONS—A temporary eye patch is often necessary. It may limit your ability to take care of yourself.

MEDICATION (ADJUSTED FOR AGING)
- Your ophthalmologist may prescribe: Antibiotic or antiviral eye drops and ointments.
  Artificial tears.
- Don't treat any eye inflammation without consulting your doctor. *Don't use non-prescription eye drops containing topical corticosteroids.* These may worsen the condition or cause eyeball perforation.

ACTIVITY FOR OLDER PATIENTS
- Eye patching will restrict activity. Resume your normal activities gradually.
- See Appendix 20 regarding physical fitness for the active older adult.

FOOD & BEVERAGE
- No special diet is required.
- See Appendix 1 regarding good nutrition for people over 50.

FUTURE CONSIDERATIONS FOR THE AGING ADULT

POSSIBLE COMPLICATIONS
- Glaucoma.
- Ulceration of the cornea.
- Permanent scarring in the eye.
- Vision loss.

PROBABLE OUTCOME—Depends on the cause. With early treatment, most types of cornea infection are curable.

PREVENTING RECURRENCE
- Wear protective glasses if your work involves eye hazards.
- Eat a well-balanced diet that contains sufficient vitamin A or take multiple vitamin supplements containing vitamin A.

CALL YOUR DOCTOR IF

- You have symptoms of cornea infection.
- Your vision diminishes in any way.

CORNEAL ABRASION AND ULCER

BASIC INFORMATION FOR OLDER ADULTS

DESCRIPTION—Corneal abrasion and ulcer is an open sore in the cornea (the clear central portion of the eye that covers the pupil). Body parts involved: The cornea (covering of the eye), conjunctiva (white of the eye), iris (colored part of the eye) and aqueous humor (fluid in the eyeball).

SPECIAL CONSIDERATIONS FOR AGING
- The immune system becomes less effective, opening the way for viral, bacterial and other infections; malignancies; immune disorders; and allergies.
- Repair from injury or disease is complete and effective, but recovery takes longer in older people.

SIGNS & SYMPTOMS
- Eye pain, usually severe.
- Sensitivity to bright light.
- Eyelid spasm.
- Tearing.
- Blurred vision.
- Redness in the white of the eye.

CAUSES & RISK FACTORS
Causes include:
- Ill-fitting contact lenses or prolonged use.
- Injury to the cornea or the embedding in the cornea of a foreign body, such as a small piece of steel, sand or glass. A bacterial infection—usually pneumococcal, streptococcal or staphylococcal—may follow the injury.
- Infection by the virus *herpes simplex,* which produces cold sores on the mouth.
- Infections of the eyelids and conjunctiva.
- Defective closure of the lid.

All the above infections are contagious from person to person or from one part of the body to another—especially finger-to-eye contact after touching cold sores on the mouth.

Risk factors include:
- Recent infection or eye injury.
- Smoking or other environmental eye irritants.

DOCTOR'S TREATMENT & DIAGNOSTIC TESTS
- Medical history and physical exam by an ophthalmologist.
- Laboratory studies to identify the bacterium, virus or fungus responsible for the infection and ulcer.
- Self-care instructions focused on the older patient.

HOME TREATMENT BY SELF OR CARE-GIVER

GENERAL INSTRUCTIONS
- Apply cool water compresses to the eye as often as they feel good.
- Patching the eye may decrease discomfort.

MEDICATION (ADJUSTED FOR AGING)
- Your doctor may prescribe antibiotic eye drops, ointments or oral antibiotics for bacterial infections. Your doctor will administer medication for viral and fungus infections.
- For minor pain, you may use non-prescription drugs such as acetaminophen.
- *Note:* Adverse reactions and side effects may be more frequent and severe in older persons. Remind your doctor of any medicines you already take.

ACTIVITY FOR OLDER PATIENTS
- After treatment, resume normal activity as soon as possible.
- See Appendix 20 regarding physical fitness for the active older adult.

FOOD & BEVERAGE
- No special diet is required.
- See Appendix 1 regarding good nutrition for people over 50.

FUTURE CONSIDERATIONS FOR THE AGING ADULT

POSSIBLE COMPLICATIONS—Neglected corneal ulcers may penetrate the cornea, allowing infection to enter the eyeball. This can cause permanent vision loss.

PROBABLE OUTCOME
- A corneal ulcer is a serious eye problem. It is usually curable in 2 to 3 weeks if treated by an ophthalmologist.
- If scars from previous corneal ulcers impair vision significantly, a corneal transplant (grafting a new cornea onto the eye) may make vision nearly normal.

PREVENTING RECURRENCE
- Wash your hands frequently.
- Avoid injury. Wear safety goggles to protect your eyes when they will be exposed to flying wood shavings or splinters or to bits of metal or stone.
- Don't touch your eyes if you have cold sores.

CALL YOUR DOCTOR IF

- You have symptoms of a corneal abrasion and ulcer.
- Any of the following occurs during treatment: Fever over 101F (38.3C).
  Pain that is not relieved by acetaminophen.
  Changed vision.
- New, unexplained symptoms develop. The drugs used in treatment may produce side effects.

CORONARY ARTERY DISEASE
(Coronary Atherosclerosis; Ischemic Heart Disease; Coronary Heart Disease)

BASIC INFORMATION FOR OLDER ADULTS

DESCRIPTION—Coronary artery disease is a hardening and narrowing of the coronary arteries, which provide blood to the heart. There are two main coronary arteries. When either or both narrow, they can no longer provide adequate oxygen for the heart. Body parts involved: The blood vessels to the heart.

SPECIAL CONSIDERATIONS FOR AGING
- Many diseases become more common with age, and all may present themselves in unusual ways.
- Coronary artery disease becomes notoriously difficult to diagnose with aging.
- 50% of people over 60 have x-ray evidence of narrowing of the coronary arteries, yet only 50% of those people have symptoms.
- Stress from any emotional cause—fear, worry, anxiety, sadness, loneliness or anger—affects all aspects of any illness or disorder.

SIGNS & SYMPTOMS
- Early stages: No symptoms (often).
- Later stages: Angina pectoris (discomfort or pain in the chest that is brought on by exercise and disappears with rest); heart attack.

CAUSES & RISK FACTORS—The causes are often unknown, except for association with the risk factors below. The arteries are narrowed due to hardening of the arteries, and blood clots frequently form and block the arteries. Risk factors include:
- Smoking; stress; obesity.
- A family history of coronary artery disease, diabetes, high blood pressure or atherosclerosis.
- Poor nutrition, especially too much fat in the diet; a previous heart attack or stroke.
- Fatigue or overwork; lack of exercise.

DOCTOR'S TREATMENT & DIAGNOSTIC TESTS
- Medical history and physical exam.
- Laboratory studies such as an ECG (see Glossary), exercise tolerance test and blood studies to measure the total fat, cholesterol and lipoproteins; x-rays of the chest.
- Coronary angiogram (cardiac catheterization).
- Self-care instructions after diagnosis to help you make necessary lifestyle changes.
- In severe cases, surgery to bypass the coronary arteries (see Coronary Artery Bypass Graft in the Surgeries section) or balloon angioplasty (see Glossary). Advancing age alone is not a deterrent. Although these procedures may decrease or eliminate the symptoms for a while, they do not control the underlying disease.
- A heart transplant can cure end-stage coronary artery disease when no simple procedures will help.

HOME TREATMENT BY SELF OR CARE-GIVER

GENERAL INSTRUCTIONS—Try to reduce as many risk factors as possible. Consider lifestyle changes (see Appendix 12).

MEDICATION (ADJUSTED FOR AGING)—Your doctor may prescribe:
- Nitroglycerin, anticoagulants, calcium channel blockers, ACE inhibitors or beta-adrenergic blockers for angina pectoris and blood vessel spasms.
- Vasodilator drugs to increase the blood supply to the heart muscle.

ACTIVITY FOR OLDER PATIENTS
- Engage in a program of moderate, daily physical exercise (see Appendix 20).
- Consult your doctor about sexual activity.

FOOD & BEVERAGE—Eat a low-fat, low-salt diet (see Appendices 8 and 9).

FUTURE CONSIDERATIONS FOR THE AGING ADULT

POSSIBLE COMPLICATIONS—Life-threatening myocardial infarction (death of the cells of the heart muscle from inadequate blood supply).

PROBABLE OUTCOME—This condition is currently considered incurable. However, the symptoms can usually be relieved or controlled. Treatment can prolong your life and improve its quality.

PREVENTING RECURRENCE
- Don't smoke; exercise regularly.
- Eat a low-fat, low-salt, high-fiber diet.
- Take one aspirin a day (consult your doctor).
- Reduce stress to a manageable level when possible (see Appendix 13).
- If you have diabetes or hypertension, adhere strictly to the treatment schedule, including diet restrictions.

CALL YOUR DOCTOR IF

- You develop deep chest discomfort (aching or pressure) that radiates to the jaw, left arm or back. Call immediately. *This may be an emergency!*
- You sweat and feel short of breath.
- You have high risk factors and wish to become involved in a program of prevention.
- After exertion, you develop chest, neck or jaw pain that goes away with rest.

CREEPING ERUPTIONS
(Larva Migrans, Cutaneous)

BASIC INFORMATION FOR OLDER ADULTS

DESCRIPTION—Creeping eruptions is a skin infestation of hookworm or roundworm larvae. These parasites usually infect dogs and cats. Body parts involved: The areas of the skin that come in contact with the ground, usually the feet, legs or buttocks.

SPECIAL CONSIDERATIONS FOR AGING
- The skin becomes thinner.
- The skin produces less vitamin D, so supplemental oral vitamin D may be needed.
- The responsiveness of the skin's immune system decreases.

SIGNS & SYMPTOMS—A skin rash or small blisters progressing to thin, raised lines on the skin leading from the parasite's entry point. The random lines create tunnel-like lesions that lengthen up to 1cm a day. Most persons have several tracks simultaneously, each of a different length and pattern.

CAUSES & RISK FACTORS—Caused by an infestation of the larvae of hookworms and roundworms found in the intestinal tracts of dogs and cats. Risk factors include:
- Contact with warm, moist sand in which cats or dogs have defecated.
- Work that requires crawling in confined spaces and contact with infected soil, as when plumbers work under houses.

DOCTOR'S TREATMENT & DIAGNOSTIC TESTS
- Medical history and physical exam.
- Self-care instructions focused on the older patient.

HOME TREATMENT BY SELF OR CARE-GIVER

GENERAL INSTRUCTIONS—No specific instructions except those listed under other headings.

MEDICATION (ADJUSTED FOR AGING)
- Your doctor may prescribe:
  Topical thiabendazole for local application in a 2% solution with dimethyl sulfoxide (DMSO). Follow the instructions carefully. Apply it to the end of the track (farthest from the point of entry).
  Oral thiabendazole for serious infestations by many larvae. This form causes adverse reactions and side effects.

- *Note:* Adverse reactions and side effects may be more frequent and severe in older persons. Remind your doctor of any medicines you already take.

ACTIVITY FOR OLDER PATIENTS
- No restrictions are necessary.
- See Appendix 20 regarding physical fitness for the active older adult.

FOOD & BEVERAGE
- No special diet is required.
- See Appendix 1 regarding good nutrition for people over 50.

FUTURE CONSIDERATIONS FOR THE AGING ADULT

POSSIBLE COMPLICATIONS—Secondary bacterial infection of the affected skin.

PROBABLE OUTCOME—Usually curable in 1 to 2 weeks with treatment.

PREVENTING RECURRENCE
- Handle cat litter carefully. Avoid touching the soil.
- Avoid contact with soil used by cats and dogs for elimination.
- Have pets treated for worms.

CALL YOUR DOCTOR IF

- You have symptoms of creeping eruptions.
- The skin lesions develop pus, indicating secondary infection.
- You take oral thiabendazole and new, unexplained symptoms develop.

CROHN'S DISEASE
(Regional Ileitis; Granulomatous Ileitis or Ileocolitis; Regional Enteritis)

BASIC INFORMATION FOR OLDER ADULTS

DESCRIPTION—Crohn's disease is an inflammatory disease of the ileum, the lower part of the small intestine. Body parts involved: The ileum, colon and other parts of the gastro-intestinal tract; regional lymph nodes; and the mesentery (outside covering of the intestines).

SPECIAL CONSIDERATIONS FOR AGING
- The digestive system becomes more sluggish.
- The immune system becomes less effective, opening the way for viral, bacterial and other infections; malignancies; immune disorders; and allergies.
- The total state of well-being in many older people makes them increasingly susceptible to infections and impairs their ability to prevent infections from spreading.

SIGNS & SYMPTOMS
- Cramping abdominal pain, especially after eating. The pain is sometimes in the right lower abdomen, mimicking appendicitis.
- Nausea and diarrhea; a general ill feeling; fever.
- Appetite and weight loss.
- Abdominal tenderness; an abdominal mass that can be felt; bloody stools (sometimes).

CAUSES & RISK FACTORS—The cause is unknown. Risk factors include:
- A medical history of food allergies.
- A family history of Crohn's disease.

DOCTOR'S TREATMENT & DIAGNOSTIC TESTS
- Medical history and physical exam.
- Laboratory blood studies.
- Surgical diagnostic procedures such as sigmoidoscopy or colonoscopy (see Glossary for both).
- X-rays of the colon and small intestine.
- Biopsy.
- Self-care instructions focused on the older patient.
- Surgery (ileostomy) to resect the inflamed area (sometimes). Although non-surgical treatment is preferred, advancing age alone is not a deterrent.

HOME TREATMENT BY SELF OR CARE-GIVER

GENERAL INSTRUCTIONS
- Use heat to relieve the pain. Apply a heating pad or warm compresses to the abdomen. If abdominal cramps are continuous or severe, notify your doctor.
- Check your stool daily for signs of bleeding. Take any suspicious specimens, such as a black-colored stool, to your doctor's office for analysis. Carry the specimen in a closed glass jar or styrofoam cup.

MEDICATION (ADJUSTED FOR AGING)—
Your doctor may prescribe:
- Pain relievers.
- Antidiarrhea medication.
- Vitamin supplements.
- Anti-inflammatory drugs and immuno-suppressant medication.
- Antibiotics to fight infections.

ACTIVITY FOR OLDER PATIENTS
- During acute attacks, rest in bed or a chair. Get up only to go to the bathroom, to bathe or to eat.
- During periods between attacks, rest often during the day and sleep up to 10 hours a night.

FOOD & BEVERAGE
- Eat a low-residue, high-protein, high-carbohydrate diet that is high in vitamins and minerals. Meats, potatoes and their substitutes are the mainstays of the diet. Consult a dietician for advice.
- If you have possible food allergies, omit milk, wheat, eggs, nuts and other suspected foods. Omit each one—especially milk—for 3 or 4 days, then try it again.

FUTURE CONSIDERATIONS FOR THE AGING ADULT

POSSIBLE COMPLICATIONS
- Intestinal obstruction; bleeding and anemia.
- A fistula between the bowel and the bladder.
- Perirectal abscess; kidney disorders.
- Perforation of the inflamed bowel.
- Increased susceptibility to cancer of the ileum.
- Joint pain and inflammation; eye inflammation.
- Malabsorption of nutrients; vitamin B-12 deficiency.

PROBABLE OUTCOME—Attacks usually begin in patients in their early 20s and may continue for years. In about 5 to 20% of the cases, the disease starts after age 60. Intervals between attacks vary from every few months to every few years. Occasionally symptoms appear once or twice, then disappear. If you and your doctor decide that your condition requires surgery, it can improve your condition and delay progress of the disease for many years. However, despite surgery, recurrences are quite possible.

PREVENTING RECURRENCE—Cannot be prevented at present.

CALL YOUR DOCTOR IF

- You have symptoms of Crohn's disease.
- You have black, tarry stools or blood in the stool.
- Your abdomen swells.
- Your temperature rises to 101F (38.3C) or higher.

CRYPTOCOCCOSIS
(Torulosis)

BASIC INFORMATION FOR OLDER ADULTS

DESCRIPTION—Cryptococcosis is a fungal disease that usually begins in the lung and may spread to other body parts. It is much more serious when there are underlying illnesses or risk factors. Body parts involved: The lungs, central nervous system, kidneys, bones and skin.

SPECIAL CONSIDERATIONS FOR AGING
- The immune system becomes less effective, opening the way for viral, bacterial and other infections; malignancies; immune disorders; and allergies.
- Usual signs and symptoms may be absent and be replaced by symptoms of confusion, dizziness, failure to thrive, falling, incontinence, increasing dementia, refusal to eat or drink, weight loss, depression, paranoia, hypochondriasis, psychosis or threats of suicide.
- The total state of well-being in many older people makes them increasingly susceptible to infections and impairs their ability to prevent infections from spreading.

SIGNS & SYMPTOMS
- Severe headache; stiff neck; fever.
- Blurred vision; drowsiness.
- Protein in the urine.
- Mental disturbances, such as confusion, depression, agitation or inappropriate speech or dress.
- A cough.

CAUSES & RISK FACTORS—Cryptococcosis is caused by infection from the fungus *cryptococcus neoformans* (also called *filobasidiella neoformans*). The fungus is acquired by breathing air that contains spores of this organism, which comes from soil. The serious, progressive, systemic form of this fungus disease is most apt to occur in persons who are seriously ill with other diseases or who are receiving immunosuppressive treatment. The risk factors include:
- Geographic location (the disease is most common in the southeastern U.S.).
- The use of cortisone, immunosuppressive or antimetabolite drugs.
- Illness that has lowered resistance—especially Hodgkin's disease—or others, including uremia, diabetes, chronic lung disease, tuberculosis, leukemia or severe burns.

DOCTOR'S TREATMENT & DIAGNOSTIC TESTS
- Medical history and physical exam.
- Laboratory studies of the cerebrospinal fluid, blood and urine.
- X-rays of the chest and bones.
- Lung biopsy and bronchoscopy.
- Hospitalization for intensive care in severe cases.

- After diagnosis and hospitalization, self-care instructions focused on the older patient.

HOME TREATMENT BY SELF OR CARE-GIVER

GENERAL INSTRUCTIONS
- It is usually not necessary to isolate persons with cryptococcosis.
- Weigh daily and keep a weight chart. Report changes of 3 pounds or more (up or down) to your doctor.

MEDICATION (ADJUSTED FOR AGING)—If the disease remains confined to the lungs, no medication may be needed. If complications arise, your doctor may prescribe potent antifungal drugs. These are effective for skin, bone or kidney involvement and life-saving for cryptococcal meningitis. Treatment with these drugs requires hospitalization.

ACTIVITY FOR OLDER PATIENTS—If you have a mild form of the disease that does not require strong antifungal medication, rest in bed until the cough and fever disappear.

FOOD & BEVERAGE
- No special diet is required.
- See Appendix 1 regarding good nutrition for people over 50.

FUTURE CONSIDERATIONS FOR THE AGING ADULT

POSSIBLE COMPLICATIONS—This fungus can cause severe, debilitating illness. In rare cases, the fungi spread from the lungs throughout the body, causing skin ulcers and bone, kidney and brain infections.

PROBABLE OUTCOME—Usually curable if the infection remains confined to the lung or if treatment with potent antifungal medicines is successful against complications.

PREVENTING RECURRENCE—Obtain medical treatment for any of the serious illnesses listed as risks. Relapse may occur.

CALL YOUR DOCTOR IF

- You have symptoms of cryptococcosis, especially a severe headache or stiff neck.
- Any of the following occurs during treatment:
  Weight loss.
  Fever of 101F (38.3C) taken orally.
  Diarrhea that cannot be controlled.
  Severe headache and stiff neck.
- New, unexplained symptoms develop. The drugs used in treatment may produce side effects.

CUSHING'S SYNDROME

BASIC INFORMATION FOR OLDER ADULTS

DESCRIPTION—Cushing's syndrome is an endocrine disorder caused by excessive adrenal hormones. Body parts involved: The adrenal glands (located over the kidneys) and pituitary gland (at the base of the brain).

SPECIAL CONSIDERATIONS FOR AGING
- Usual signs and symptoms may be absent and be replaced by symptoms of confusion, dizziness, failure to thrive, falling, incontinence, increasing dementia, refusal to eat or drink, weight loss, depression, paranoia, hypochondriasis, psychosis or threats of suicide.
- The immune system becomes less effective, opening the way for viral, bacterial and other infections; malignancies; immune disorders; and allergies.

SIGNS & SYMPTOMS
- Round face and puffy eyes.
- Ruddy red complexion.
- Growth of facial hair in women.
- Fat accumulation over the upper back and trunk, accompanied by purple "stretch marks."
- High blood pressure.
- Mental and emotional changes, including psychosis.
- Enlarged clitoris in women.
- Diabetes mellitus; peptic ulcers; osteoporosis.
- Low resistance to infection.
- Insomnia.
- Thin, easily bruised skin.

CAUSES & RISK FACTORS—The signs and symptoms result from the overproduction of the cortisone-like hormone produced by the adrenal glands. This may result from:
- A tumor in the adrenal glands.
- A pituitary tumor, causing production of excessive ACTH (adrenocorticotropic hormone), which the pituitary gland produces to stimulate the adrenal glands to secrete hormones.
- The prolonged use of cortisone drugs.

The risk increases with the prolonged use of ACTH to treat pituitary cancer.

DOCTOR'S TREATMENT & DIAGNOSTIC TESTS
- Study of pictures taken before symptoms began, which are helpful in noting changes in appearance.
- Medical history and physical exam.
- Laboratory blood and urine studies of white blood cell counts, pituitary and adrenal gland function and hormone levels.
- CT scans of the pituitary and adrenal glands.
- Consultation with an endocrinologist.
- Surgery (sometimes) to remove ACTH-producing tumors from the pituitary or to remove adrenal gland tumors. Advancing age alone is not a deterrent.
- Hospitalization for high-voltage radiation treatment of the pituitary gland (sometimes).
- Self-care instructions focused on the older patient.

HOME TREATMENT BY SELF OR CARE-GIVER

GENERAL INSTRUCTIONS
- Learn all you can about this condition and its treatment. You must often monitor your own reactions to medications. Discontinuing drugs suddenly is dangerous.
- Wear a Medic Alert bracelet or pendant (see Glossary).
- Protect yourself from fractures. Accident-proof your home. Wear seat belts in autos.

MEDICATION (ADJUSTED FOR AGING)—Your doctor may prescribe:
- Drugs such as aminoglutethimide or mitotane to suppress adrenal gland function.
- Cortisone drugs if adrenal glands must be removed surgically.
- Drugs to replace pituitary hormones (sometimes).
- Antihypertensive drugs to lower blood pressure.
- Calcium supplements to treat osteoporosis.

ACTIVITY FOR OLDER PATIENTS—No restrictions are necessary. Energy will increase once treatment begins.

FOOD & BEVERAGE—Consult your doctor about possible salt restriction.

FUTURE CONSIDERATIONS FOR THE AGING ADULT

POSSIBLE COMPLICATIONS—Bone fractures due to osteoporosis; pituitary tumor if adrenal glands are removed (rare).

PROBABLE OUTCOME
- If caused by an adrenal gland tumor, the disorder is curable with the surgical removal of the tumor or glands. Lifelong, carefully monitored drug therapy is essential if the glands are removed.
- If caused by a pituitary tumor, the disorder is curable with the surgical removal or radiation of the tumor, but tumors may recur.
- If caused by the prolonged use of cortisone drugs or ACTH, the condition may improve if these are withdrawn *gradually under medical supervision.*

PREVENTING RECURRENCE—If the use of ACTH or cortisone is necessary for other disorders, such as asthma, arthritis, kidney disease or Addison's disease, take the lowest dose possible for the shortest time. Consult your doctor.

CALL YOUR DOCTOR IF

- You have symptoms of Cushing's syndrome.
- You have signs of infection, such as fever, chills, muscle aches, headache and dizziness.

DANDRUFF
(Seborrheic Dermatitis)

BASIC INFORMATION FOR OLDER ADULTS

DESCRIPTION—A form of seborrheic dermatitis, dandruff is a skin condition characterized by greasy or dry white scales. It is not contagious. Body parts involved: The skin of the scalp, eyebrows, forehead and face; the folds around the nose and behind the ears; the external ear canals; the skin of the trunk, especially over the breastbone (sternum); or in skin folds.

SPECIAL CONSIDERATIONS FOR AGING
- The skin becomes thinner.
- The skin becomes dryer and rougher.

SIGNS & SYMPTOMS—Flaking, white scales over reddish patches on the skin. The scales anchor to hair shafts. They may itch, but they are usually painless unless complicated by infection.

CAUSES & RISK FACTORS—The cause is unknown. The risk increases with:
- Stress.
- Hot, humid weather or cold, dry weather.
- Infrequent shampoos.
- Oily skin.
- Other skin disorders, such as acne rosacea, acne or psoriasis.
- Obesity.
- Parkinson's disease.
- The use of drying lotions that contain alcohol.

DOCTOR'S TREATMENT & DIAGNOSTIC TESTS
- Medical history and physical exam.
- Self-care instructions focused on the older patient.

HOME TREATMENT BY SELF OR CARE-GIVER

GENERAL INSTRUCTIONS
- Shampoo vigorously and as often as once a day. The shampoo you use is not as important as the way you scrub your scalp. Loosen scales with your fingernails while shampooing and leave shampoo on at least 5 minutes.
- If shampooing is inconvenient or not physically possible, apply a topical steroid lotion.

MEDICATION (ADJUSTED FOR AGING)
- For minor dandruff, you may use non-prescription dandruff shampoos and lubricating skin lotion.
- For severe problems, your doctor may prescribe:
  Shampoos that contain coal tar or scalp creams that contain cortisone. To apply medication to the scalp, part the hair a few strands at a time and rub the ointment or lotion vigorously into the scalp.
  Topical steroids for other affected parts.
- *Note:* Adverse reactions and side effects may be more frequent and severe in older persons. Remind your doctor of any medicines you already take.

ACTIVITY FOR OLDER PATIENTS
- No restrictions are necessary. Outdoor activities in summer may help.
- See Appendix 20 regarding physical fitness for the active older adult.

FOOD & BEVERAGE
- No special diet is required. Avoid foods that seem to worsen your condition.
- See Appendix 1 regarding good nutrition for people over 50.

FUTURE CONSIDERATIONS FOR THE AGING ADULT

POSSIBLE COMPLICATIONS
- Embarrassment and social discomfort.
- Secondary bacterial infection in affected areas.

PROBABLE OUTCOME—This is a chronic condition, but it is often characterized by long periods of inactivity. During active phases, the symptoms can be controlled with treatment.

PREVENTING RECURRENCE—Cannot be prevented. To minimize severity or frequency of flare-ups:
- Shampoo frequently.
- Dry skin folds thoroughly after bathing.
- Wear loose, ventilated clothing.

CALL YOUR DOCTOR IF

- You have symptoms of dandruff that don't respond to self-care.
- Patches of dandruff ooze, form crusts or drain pus.

DEHYDRATION

BASIC INFORMATION FOR OLDER ADULTS

DESCRIPTION—Dehydration means loss of water and essential body salts. Body parts involved: The blood, gastrointestinal tract and kidneys.

SPECIAL CONSIDERATIONS FOR AGING
- This is one of the diseases common in older people.
- Signs and symptoms may differ significantly from those listed below.
- Repair from injury or disease is complete and effective, but recovery takes longer in older people.

SIGNS & SYMPTOMS
- Dry mouth and lips.
- Decreased or absent urination.
- Sunken eyes.
- Dry, wrinkled skin with poor resilience.
- Confusion; coma.
- Low blood pressure.
- Severe thirst.
- Increase in heart rate and breathing.
- Lightheadedness.

CAUSES & RISK FACTORS
Causes include:
- Persistent vomiting or diarrhea from any cause.
- Persistent high fever.
- Heavy sweating.
- The use of drugs that deplete fluids and electrolytes, such as diuretics.
- Overexposure to the sun or heat.
Risk factors include:
- Recent illness with high fever.
- Diabetes mellitus.
- Chronic kidney disease.

DOCTOR'S TREATMENT & DIAGNOSTIC TESTS
- Medical history and physical exam.
- Laboratory blood studies, including blood counts and electrolyte measurement (see Glossary).
- Self-care instructions focused on the older patient.
- Hospitalization to receive intravenous fluids (severe or prolonged illness only).

HOME TREATMENT BY SELF OR CARE-GIVER

GENERAL INSTRUCTIONS
- Weigh daily on an accurate home scale and record the weight so you can be aware of fluid loss.
- If you have vomiting or diarrhea, keep a record of the number of episodes so you can estimate your fluid loss.

- For minor dehydration, take frequent small amounts of clear liquids. Large amounts may trigger vomiting.
- Drink electrolyte solutions. A solution of 1 pint water, 1 teaspoon sugar and 1/2 teaspoon salt may be adequate.

MEDICATION (ADJUSTED FOR AGING)
- Your doctor may prescribe intravenous fluids to replace lost water.
- *Note:* Adverse reactions and side effects may be more frequent and severe in older persons. Remind your doctor of any medicines you already take.

ACTIVITY FOR OLDER PATIENTS
- Rest in bed until you recover. You may read or watch TV.
- See Appendix 20 regarding physical fitness for the active older adult.

FOOD & BEVERAGE
- Depends on the underlying disorder. Salty foods decrease the effect of dehydration.
- See Appendix 1 regarding good nutrition for people over 50.

FUTURE CONSIDERATIONS FOR THE AGING ADULT

POSSIBLE COMPLICATIONS—Blood pressure drop, shock and death from prolonged, severe dehydration.

PROBABLE OUTCOME—Curable with control of the underlying cause and replacement of necessary fluids.

PREVENTING RECURRENCE
- Obtain medical treatment for underlying causes of dehydration.
- If you are vomiting or have diarrhea, take small amounts of liquid with non-prescription electrolyte supplements or drinks every 30 to 60 minutes.
- If you use diuretics, weigh daily. Report to your doctor a weight loss of more than 3 pounds in 1 day or 5 pounds in 1 week.
- Form a habit of drinking at least 8 glasses of water or other fluid daily.

CALL YOUR DOCTOR IF

You have symptoms of dehydration.

DEMENTIA
(Chronic Brain Syndrome)

BASIC INFORMATION FOR OLDER ADULTS

DESCRIPTION—Dementia is a mental impairment caused by a variety of diseases that produce permanent brain deterioration. Body part involved: The brain.

SPECIAL CONSIDERATIONS FOR AGING
- Nerve cell loss begins at age 20 to 40 and continues throughout life. Cells in the brain and other parts of the central nervous system cannot reproduce or replace themselves after injury or disease.
- The blood vessels nourishing the brain are less healthy. They become thicker and lose their elasticity.
- Behavior changes may occur with relatively minor illnesses, such as anemia, because of reduced oxygen to the brain.

SIGNS & SYMPTOMS
- Forgetfulness, especially of recent events.
- Unpredictable, sometimes violent, behavior.
- Confusion.
- Loss of interest in normal activities.
- Disorientation, especially at night.
- Poor personal hygiene and appearance.
- Depression.
- Poor judgment.
- Staggering gait.
- Incoherent speech.

CAUSES & RISK FACTORS—Dementia involves the degeneration and loss of the gray matter from the brain. The causes include: Alzheimer's disease; inadequate blood supply to the brain due to blood clots, hypertension or hardening of the arteries; alcoholism; chronic infection, such as lung disease; chronic poisoning from industrial chemicals, such as mercury; an inherited condition, such as Huntington's chorea; brain injury from any cause; some endocrine conditions, such as diabetes or hypothyroidism; brain tumor; Parkinson's disease. The risk increases with:
- Chemical or environmental exposure to heavy metals.
- Excessive alcohol consumption.
- The use of cocaine, LSD or mescaline or glue sniffing.
- A family history of Alzheimer's disease.

DOCTOR'S TREATMENT & DIAGNOSTIC TESTS
- Medical history and physical exam.
- Laboratory blood studies.
- X-rays of the head and other body parts.
- EEG, CT scan or MRI (see Glossary).
- Neurological examination to detect curable conditions.
- Psychotherapy or counseling for family members.
- Care-giver instructions.
- Nursing home care if the disorder is too advanced for home care.

HOME TREATMENT BY SELF OR CARE-GIVER

GENERAL INSTRUCTIONS
- Family members can notice early behavior changes and seek prompt medical care; provide simple reminders, such as a clock, daily calendar or name tag; minimize changes in daily routine and environment; encourage social activities and contacts; treat the person with respect and kindness; and provide a protected, non-judgmental environment when the patient cannot provide self-care.
- When home care is no longer possible, find a good extended-care facility; visit the patient often—even if he or she doesn't seem to recognize you.
- Care-givers will need help to avoid "burn-out."

MEDICATION (ADJUSTED FOR AGING)—The doctor may prescribe medication appropriate to treat the underlying condition.

ACTIVITY FOR OLDER PATIENTS—Encourage as much activity as possible.

FOOD & BEVERAGE—Provide a well-balanced diet.

FUTURE CONSIDERATIONS FOR THE AGING ADULT

POSSIBLE COMPLICATIONS
- Infections, falls, injuries and poor nutrition. These occur because the ill person cannot care for himself or herself.
- Misdiagnosis. Some curable conditions, such as pernicious anemia, hypothyroidism, chronic drug toxicity and subdural hematoma, have symptoms that mimic dementia.

PROBABLE OUTCOME—This condition is currently considered incurable. Medicine may prevent the condition from worsening, but it cannot restore lost brain function.

PREVENTING RECURRENCE
- Obtain early medical treatment for underlying causes, such as hypertension, alcoholism, diabetes and hypothyroidism.
- Protect yourself from head injury. Wear seat belts in vehicles. Wear protective head gear for riding bicycles, motorcycles and participating in contact sports. Don't drive after drinking or using mind-altering drugs.
- Survey your workplace for chemical hazards and protect yourself from exposure.
- To prevent atherosclerosis, don't smoke, eat a diet low in fat (see Appendix 8), exercise regularly (see Appendix 20) and reduce stress.

CALL YOUR DOCTOR IF

You observe symptoms of dementia in a family member.

BASIC INFORMATION FOR OLDER ADULTS

DESCRIPTION—Dentures are false teeth—either full or partial appliances. In some cases, they may cause pain or other disorders. However, problems usually don't arise if dentures fit well, look natural, feel good and are cared for properly. Body parts involved: The gums and temporomandibular joints.

SPECIAL CONSIDERATIONS FOR AGING
- Repair from injury or disease is complete and effective, but recovery takes longer in older people.
- Aging may contribute to poor nutrition, which in turn complicates denture problems.

SIGNS & SYMPTOMS
- Pain with your dentures in place.
- Inflamed or dark red gums that bleed easily.
- Possible hard pads at pressure points (dental granulomas).

CAUSES & RISK FACTORS
Causes include:
- Pressure on mouth tissues from the dentures.
- Jawbone deterioration.
The risk increases with poor nutrition.

DOCTOR'S TREATMENT & DIAGNOSTIC TESTS
- Medical history and physical exam by a dentist.
- Self-care instructions focused on the older patient.

HOME TREATMENT BY SELF OR CARE-GIVER

GENERAL INSTRUCTIONS
- You may want to eat a soft diet until the pain subsides.
- Practice speaking aloud to gain muscle control and tone so your speech is normal. Speak slowly at first until you feel at ease.
- Remove your dentures at night to rest your gums. Store dentures in a glass of water mixed with denture cleanser so they will not dry out and warp.
- Clean and massage your gums regularly with a finger, cloth or brush.
- Clean your dentures daily. Use a stiff brush and regular toothpaste to clean your dentures as you would natural teeth. Tartar accumulates on dentures as on natural teeth.
- Clean the dentures over a basin of water to cushion a fall if you should drop them.
- If stubborn stains appear, place the dentures in a glass of water mixed with 1 teaspoon of chlorine bleach. (Don't use bleach if your dentures contain metal. The chemical may damage the metal.)

- If you have a partial denture, clean your natural teeth and gums thoroughly, especially around the base of the teeth.

MEDICATION (ADJUSTED FOR AGING)
- Your doctor may prescribe antifungal medicine if you develop thrush.
- *Note:* Adverse reactions and side effects may be more frequent and severe in older persons. Remind your doctor of any medicines you already take.

ACTIVITY FOR OLDER PATIENTS
- No restrictions are necessary.
- See Appendix 20 regarding physical fitness for the active older adult.

FOOD & BEVERAGE
- No special diet is required if dentures fit properly.
- See Appendix 1 regarding good nutrition for people over 50.

FUTURE CONSIDERATIONS FOR THE AGING ADULT

POSSIBLE COMPLICATIONS
- Susceptibility to fungus infection (thrush), especially with the use of antibiotics.
- Protruding jaw and sunken cheeks after many years of wearing dentures.
- Trapped food particles in partial dentures.

PROBABLE OUTCOME—Artificial teeth are not as efficient as natural teeth, and an adjustment period is necessary. Most people adapt well to dentures, but some persons never adjust to them completely. Problems can usually be treated.

PREVENTING RECURRENCE—Consult your dentist regularly for checkups.

☎ CALL YOUR DOCTOR IF

- Your dentures won't stay in place when you smile, laugh or talk.
- Sore spots develop on your gums. These are common and can be treated easily and quickly by your dentist.
- White spots develop in your mouth which become irritated when you try to brush them away.
- Your dentures break. Save all the pieces for your dentist. Your dentist can usually repair dentures quickly. Don't try to repair them yourself.

ILLNESSES & DISORDERS

DEPRESSION

BASIC INFORMATION FOR OLDER ADULTS

DESCRIPTION—Depression is manifested as a feeling of continuing sadness, despondency or hopelessness. Body part involved: The central nervous system.

SPECIAL CONSIDERATIONS FOR AGING
- Usual signs and symptoms may be absent and be replaced by symptoms of confusion, dizziness, increasing dementia, refusal to eat or drink, weight loss, depression, paranoia, hypochondriasis, psychosis or threats of suicide.
- Nerve cells in aging people are especially susceptible to the action of drugs, particularly mind-altering drugs such as narcotics, alcohol, sleep inducers, pain killers, antihistamines, muscle relaxants, antinausea medications and others.

SIGNS & SYMPTOMS
- Loss of interest in life; boredom.
- Listlessness; fatigue; social isolation.
- Insomnia; excessive or disturbed sleeping.
- Appetite loss or overeating; constipation.
- Loss of sex drive.
- Difficulty concentrating or making decisions.
- Unexplained crying bouts.
- Intense guilt feelings over minor or imaginary misdeeds.
- Irritability, anxiety or agitation.
- Various pains, such as headache or chest pain, without evidence of disease.
- Thoughts of death or suicide.

CAUSES & RISK FACTORS—Causes include failure in one's occupation, marriage or other relationships; the death or loss of a loved one; the loss of something important (such as a job, home or investments); a job change or a move to a new area; surgery, such as mastectomy; major illness or disability; passing from one life stage to another, such as menopause or retirement; the use of some drugs, such as reserpine, beta-adrenergic blockers or benzodiazepines; withdrawal from mood-altering drugs, such as narcotics, amphetamines or caffeine; and some diseases, including diabetes mellitus, cancer of the pancreas and hormonal abnormalities. Risk factors include:
- Unexpressed anger or other emotions.
- A compulsive, rigid, perfectionistic or highly dependent personality.
- A family history of depression; alcoholism.
- Being institutionalized; isolation and inactivity.

DOCTOR'S TREATMENT & DIAGNOSTIC TESTS
- Medical history and physical exam (sometimes by a psychiatrist).
- Psychological testing.
- For mild depression, self-care instructions focused on the older patient.
- Psychotherapy or counseling.
- Hospitalization for severe depression.
- Electroconvulsive therapy (rarely) for severe depression.

HOME TREATMENT BY SELF OR CARE-GIVER

GENERAL INSTRUCTIONS
- Join a support group. Contact social agencies or churches for help.
- Call your local suicide-prevention hotline if you feel suicidal.
- Join a senior citizens' center or attend a day-care program.

MEDICATION (ADJUSTED FOR AGING)—
Your doctor may prescribe:
- Antidepressant drugs (often tricyclics) to accompany therapy.
- Lithium for mania alternating with the depression.

ACTIVITY FOR OLDER PATIENTS
- No restrictions are necessary. Maintain your daily activities and interests—even if you don't feel like it.
- Attend social functions, concerts, athletic events, plays and movies.
- Keep in touch with friends and loved ones.
- Engage in regular exercise (see Appendix 20). This helps relieve depression.

FOOD & BEVERAGE—Eat a normal, well-balanced diet—even if you have no appetite. Vitamin and mineral supplements may be necessary.

FUTURE CONSIDERATIONS FOR THE AGING ADULT

POSSIBLE COMPLICATIONS
- Suicide. Warning signs include withdrawal from family and friends; neglect of personal appearance; mention of wanting "to end it all" or being "a burden to others"; evidence of a suicide plan, such as buying or cleaning a gun; sudden cheerfulness after despondency.
- Hallucinations or psychotic behavior.
- Manic behavior, characterized by inappropriate overactivity and comic or irresponsible behavior.

PROBABLE OUTCOME—Spontaneous recovery in many cases, but professional help can shorten the duration and help you learn to cope in the future. Recurrence is common. The recovery rate is high despite one's pessimism while depressed.

PREVENTING RECURRENCE—Maintain good communication with your family and friends.

CALL YOUR DOCTOR IF

- You have symptoms of depression.
- You feel suicidal or hopeless.

DERMATITIS, ALLERGIC
(Eczema, Atopic)

BASIC INFORMATION FOR OLDER ADULTS

DESCRIPTION—Allergic dermatitis is a chronic inflammatory disease of the skin that is often associated with other allergic disorders that affect the respiratory system, such as asthma or hay fever. Body part involved: The skin.

SPECIAL CONSIDERATIONS FOR AGING
- The skin becomes thinner.
- The immune system becomes less effective, opening the way for viral, bacterial and other infections; malignancies; immune disorders; and allergies.
- Stress from any emotional cause—fear, worry, anxiety, sadness, loneliness or anger—affects all aspects of any illness or disorder.

SIGNS & SYMPTOMS
- Itching rash in areas where heat and moisture are retained, such as the creases of the elbows, knees, neck, face, hands, feet, groin, genitals and around the anus.
- Dry, thickened skin in affected areas.
- Uncontrolled scratching (frequently unconscious).
- Chronic fatigue from loss of sleep due to severe itching.

CAUSES & RISK FACTORS—The cause of atopic dermatitis is unknown, but it is probably inherited and is probably related to immune system deficiency. Risk factors include:
- Hay fever or asthma.
- Food allergy.
- A family history of atopic dermatitis or other allergic disorders.
- Stress. The rash and itching increase during stressful periods.
- The use of immunosuppressive drugs.

DOCTOR'S TREATMENT & DIAGNOSTIC TESTS
- Laboratory blood studies and patch tests to identify allergies.
- Self-care instructions focused on the older patient.

HOME TREATMENT BY SELF OR CARE-GIVER

GENERAL INSTRUCTIONS
- Use cool-water soaks (see Appendix 18) for crusting, oozing lesions. These decrease itching and remove crusts.
- Bathe in cool water with cleansing agents other than soap.
- Wear loose-fitting, cotton clothing; avoid wool and synthetics.
- Don't allow yourself to be vaccinated against smallpox. It can cause a life-threatening reaction.
- Avoid fabric softeners and anti-static laundry products.
- Use petroleum- or lanolin-based ointments after bathing.
- Reduce stress in your life if possible. See Appendix 13 for suggestions.

MEDICATION (ADJUSTED FOR AGING)
- To relieve minor itching, use non-prescription topical steroids or coal tar preparations.
- For severe itching, your doctor may prescribe: More potent topical steroids.
  Oral cortisone drugs (rarely and for short periods only).
  Antihistamines or mild tranquilizers.
  Lubricating ointments for the hands.
  Antibiotics (sometimes) to fight secondary infections.
- *Note:* Adverse reactions and side effects may be more frequent and severe in older persons. Remind your doctor of any medicines you already take.

ACTIVITY FOR OLDER PATIENTS
- No restrictions are necessary except to keep cool. Avoid prolonged exposure to heat.
- See Appendix 20 regarding physical fitness for the active older adult.

FOOD & BEVERAGE
- An allergy diet (see Appendix 6) may be necessary if food allergy is suspected.
- See Appendix 1 regarding good nutrition for people over 50.

FUTURE CONSIDERATIONS FOR THE AGING ADULT

POSSIBLE COMPLICATIONS
- Secondary bacterial infection in the affected area.
- Increased susceptibility to adverse drug reactions.
- Decreased resistance to fungal and viral infections.
- Permanent scarring from scratching.

PROBABLE OUTCOME—Unpredictable. Flare-ups and remissions may occur throughout life.

PREVENTING RECURRENCE—Cannot be prevented at present.

CALL YOUR DOCTOR IF
- You have symptoms of allergic dermatitis.
- You develop a fever or uncontrolled itching during a flare-up.

DERMATITIS, CONTACT
(Housewives' Eczema)

BASIC INFORMATION FOR OLDER ADULTS

DESCRIPTION—Contact dermatitis, a skin inflammation caused by contact with an irritating substance, is not contagious. Body part involved: The skin, especially that of the hands, feet and groin.

SPECIAL CONSIDERATIONS FOR AGING
- The skin becomes thinner.
- The immune system becomes less effective, opening the way for viral, bacterial and other infections; malignancies; immune disorders; and allergies.

SIGNS & SYMPTOMS
- Itching (sometimes).
- Slight redness.
- Cracks and fissures in the skin.
- Bright red, weeping areas (severe cases).

CAUSES & RISK FACTORS
Causes include:
- Contact with irritants, such as sprays, acids, topical medications or solvents. The irritant removes the fatty layer of the skin. This causes dehydration and shrinking of the surface cells.
- Some metals in jewelry.
- Poison ivy.
- Cosmetics.

Risk factors include:
- Constant exposure to hot water, detergents or other irritants that change the moisture content of the skin.
- Burns from hot water or sunburn.

DOCTOR'S TREATMENT & DIAGNOSTIC TESTS
- Medical history and physical exam.
- Self-care instructions focused on the older patient.

HOME TREATMENT BY SELF OR CARE-GIVER

GENERAL INSTRUCTIONS
- Avoid the chemical or material causing the skin irritation.
- Use bath oil or glycerin-based soap instead of soap for bathing.
- Pat skin dry rather than rubbing it.
- Reduce water temperature to lukewarm for bathing or other uses.
- Use only cream, lotion or ointment prescribed for the condition. Other commercial products may aggravate the condition. Apply ointment or cream to hands 6 or 7 times a day. For other body parts, lubricate twice a day, especially after bathing.

- Minimize the use of solvents and wear heavy-duty, cotton-lined vinyl gloves to prevent contact with irritating substances such as water; soap; detergent; metal scouring pads; scouring powder; paint; paint thinner; turpentine; and polish for cars, floors, shoes, furniture or metal.
- Dry the insides of gloves after use. Discard gloves if they develop a hole.
- Wear gloves when you peel or squeeze lemons, oranges, grapefruit, tomatoes or potatoes.
- Wear leather or heavy-duty fabric gloves for housework or gardening.
- Use a dishwashing machine to wash dishes or ask someone else to do it.
- Remove rings before doing housework or washing hands.

MEDICATION (ADJUSTED FOR AGING)
- Your doctor may prescribe topical creams, ointments or lotions. These may include steroid preparations to reduce inflammation or lubricants to preserve moisture.
- *Note:* Adverse reactions and side effects may be more frequent and severe in older persons. Remind your doctor of any medicines you already take.

ACTIVITY FOR OLDER PATIENTS
- Resume your normal activities gradually as irritation subsides.
- See Appendix 20 regarding physical fitness for the active older adult.

FOOD & BEVERAGE
- No special diet is required.
- See Appendix 1 regarding good nutrition for people over 50.

FUTURE CONSIDERATIONS FOR THE AGING ADULT

POSSIBLE COMPLICATIONS—Pain and disfigurement of the hands from constant lesions.

PROBABLE OUTCOME—The symptoms can be controlled with treatment and avoidance of the irritant. Recurrence is common, so treatment may be necessary for years.

PREVENTING RECURRENCE
- Avoid contact with any irritant which has caused dermatitis in the past.
- Protect skin from sunburn and other burns.

CALL YOUR DOCTOR IF

- You develop a fever.
- Signs of infection (swelling, tenderness, redness or warmth) develop at the site of irritation.
- Treatment does not relieve the symptoms in 1 week.

DIABETES MELLITUS, INSULIN-DEPENDENT
(Type I Diabetes)

BASIC INFORMATION FOR OLDER ADULTS

DESCRIPTION—Diabetes mellitus is a chronic disease characterized by the body's inability to produce enough insulin to process carbohydrates, fat and protein efficiently. Treatment requires injections of insulin. Insulin-dependent diabetes is often called *ketosis-prone diabetes* if it begins in adulthood and *juvenile diabetes* if it begins in childhood. Body parts involved: The islet cells of the pancreas that produce insulin and all body cells that need insulin to convert food into chemicals the body can use.

SPECIAL CONSIDERATIONS FOR AGING
- *Non*-insulin-dependent diabetes mellitus is more common in older people than this type.
- Stress from any emotional cause—fear, worry, anxiety, sadness, loneliness or anger—affects all aspects of any illness or disorder.

SIGNS & SYMPTOMS
- Fatigue; excessive thirst; frequent urination.
- Increased appetite *and* weight loss.
- Itching around the genitals.
- Increased susceptibility to infections, especially urinary tract infections and yeast infections of the skin, mouth or vagina.
- Deterioration of vision (advanced stages).
- Loss of energy and easy fatiguability.

CAUSES & RISK FACTORS—Causes include insufficient production of insulin by the islet cells of the pancreas for unknown reasons; interference with the use of insulin in the body cells for unknown reasons; and virus infection of the pancreas. Risk factors include a family history of diabetes mellitus. It often skips one generation.

DOCTOR'S TREATMENT & DIAGNOSTIC TESTS
- Medical history and physical exam.
- Laboratory urine and blood studies to measure glucose, cholesterol and insulin.
- Self-care instructions focused on the older patient.
- Hospitalization for severe complications.
- Surgery for treatment of some complications, such as failing eyesight, gangrene or coronary artery disease. Age alone is not a deterrent.
- Regular foot care by a podiatrist and regular eye examination by a specialist.

HOME TREATMENT BY SELF OR CARE-GIVER

GENERAL INSTRUCTIONS
- Learn all you can about controlling diabetes and recognizing the signs and symptoms of ketoacidosis (very high blood sugar) or hypoglycemia (very low blood sugar); see Call Your Doctor If below. Learn the techniques of home monitoring of blood sugar.
- Keep a vial of glucagon available at all times to use if hypoglycemia occurs.
- Learn to give yourself insulin injections. They will be necessary every day for life.
- Wear a Medic Alert bracelet or pendant (see Glossary).
- Seek medical treatment for any infection.
- Join a diabetic patient-support group.

MEDICATION (ADJUSTED FOR AGING)—Your doctor will prescribe insulin by injection. The dosage must be individualized and occasionally adjusted.

ACTIVITY FOR OLDER PATIENTS
- Regular daily exercise is an important part of controlling diabetes. Consult your doctor.
- If insulin-dependent diabetes is poorly controlled, avoid activities such as climbing a ladder or working in high places.

FOOD & BEVERAGE—A special diet will be prescribed by your doctor.

FUTURE CONSIDERATIONS FOR THE AGING ADULT

POSSIBLE COMPLICATIONS
- Cardiovascular disease, especially stroke, atherosclerosis and coronary artery disease.
- Kidney failure; blindness.
- Peripheral vascular disease, with gangrene in the legs and feet and sexual impotence in men.
- Life-threatening hypoglycemia (low blood sugar) if too much insulin is used.
- Life-threatening ketoacidosis (very high blood sugar) with breakdown of body cells.

PROBABLE OUTCOME—This disease is presently considered incurable, but the symptoms and progress of the disease can be controlled with rigid adherence to a treatment program. Life expectancy is somewhat reduced, but many with diabetes have a nearly normal life span.

PREVENTING RECURRENCE—Cannot be prevented.

CALL YOUR DOCTOR IF

- You have symptoms of diabetes mellitus.
- Any of the following occurs during treatment:
  Inability to think clearly, weakness, sweating, paleness, rapid heartbeat, seizures or coma (may indicate hypoglycemia).
  Fruity odor on the breath, changes in breathing pattern or stupor (may indicate ketoacidosis).
  Several days of illness or weakness.
  Numbness, tingling or pain in the feet or hands.
  Chest pain.

DIABETES MELLITUS, NON-INSULIN-DEPENDENT
(Type II Diabetes)

BASIC INFORMATION FOR OLDER ADULTS

DESCRIPTION—This type of diabetes is a disease characterized by the body's inability to produce enough insulin to process carbohydrates, fat and protein efficiently. Often called *maturity-onset diabetes,* non-insulin-dependent diabetes mellitus is most prevalent among obese adults. Body parts involved: The islet cells of the pancreas that produce insulin and all body cells that need insulin to convert food into chemicals the body can use.

SPECIAL CONSIDERATIONS FOR AGING
- This form of diabetes is more common in older people than the form that requires insulin injections for treatment.
- Stress from any emotional cause—fear, worry, anxiety, sadness, loneliness or anger—affects all aspects of any illness or disorder.

SIGNS & SYMPTOMS
- Overweight; increased appetite.
- Fatigue and loss of energy.
- Excessive thirst; frequent urination.
- Decreased resistance to infection, especially urinary tract infections and yeast infections of the skin, mouth or vagina.

CAUSES & RISK FACTORS—Causes include: Insufficient production of insulin by the pancreas to sustain normal function of body cells; interference with insulin's utilization in the cells of the body for unknown reasons. Risk factors include:
- Obesity; stress.
- The use of certain drugs, including thiazide diuretics and cortisone or phenytoin.
- A family history of diabetes mellitus.

DOCTOR'S TREATMENT & DIAGNOSTIC TESTS
- Medical history and physical exam.
- Laboratory urine and blood studies to measure glucose, cholesterol and insulin levels.
- Self-care instructions focused on the older patient.
- Surgery for treatment of some complications, such as gangrene or heart disease. Advancing age alone is not a deterrent.

HOME TREATMENT BY SELF OR CARE-GIVER

GENERAL INSTRUCTIONS
- Learn to test your urine for glucose (sugar).
- Learn all you can about controlling diabetes and recognizing the signs and symptoms of complications.
- Wear a Medic Alert pendant or bracelet (see Glossary).

- Lose weight to a normal level and maintain your ideal weight.
- Obtain prompt medical treatment for any infection or injury.

MEDICATION (ADJUSTED FOR AGING)—Your doctor may prescribe oral medicines to reduce blood sugar (hypoglycemics). These are not always necessary. They can often be discontinued when body weight becomes normal.

ACTIVITY FOR OLDER PATIENTS
- Regular daily exercise is an important part of controlling diabetes. Consult your doctor.
- See Appendix 20 regarding physical fitness for the active older adult.

FOOD & BEVERAGE—A special diet will be necessary to reduce your weight, limit your consumption of refined carbohydrates, balance unrefined carbohydrates with protein and fat and increase your consumption of plant fiber. Your doctor will provide instructions.

FUTURE CONSIDERATIONS FOR THE AGING ADULT

POSSIBLE COMPLICATIONS
- Cardiovascular disease, especially atherosclerosis, stroke and coronary artery disease.
- Vision impairment.
- Peripheral vascular disease, with gangrene in the legs and feet and sexual impotence in men (sometimes).
- Hypoglycemia if oral hypoglycemic medication is used (rare).

PROBABLE OUTCOME—This form of diabetes can often be controlled with weight loss. Good control decreases the chance of complications. In some cases, it progresses to insulin-dependent diabetes, a more serious form.

PREVENTING RECURRENCE—Control your weight to avoid becoming obese.

CALL YOUR DOCTOR IF

- You have symptoms of diabetes mellitus.
- Any of the following occurs during treatment: Inability to think clearly, weakness, sweating, paleness, rapid heartbeat, seizures or coma (may indicate hypoglycemia). Numbness, tingling or pain in your feet or hands. Infection that does not improve in 3 days. Chest pain. Worsening of your original symptoms despite adherence to treatment.

DIARRHEA, ACUTE

BASIC INFORMATION FOR OLDER ADULTS

DESCRIPTION—Acute diarrhea is the passage of many loose, watery or unformed bowel movements. This is a symptom, not a disease. Body parts involved: The colon and small intestine.

SPECIAL CONSIDERATIONS FOR AGING
- Decreased nutrition increases the risk of infections.
- The immune system becomes less effective, opening the way for viral, bacterial and other infections; malignancies; immune disorders; and allergies.
- Repair from injury or disease is complete and effective, but recovery takes longer in older people.
- Stress from any emotional cause—fear, worry, anxiety, sadness, loneliness or anger—affects all aspects of any illness or disorder.

SIGNS & SYMPTOMS
- Cramping abdominal pain.
- Loose, watery or unformed bowel movements.
- Lack of bowel control (sometimes).
- Fever (sometimes).

CAUSES & RISK FACTORS
Causes include:
- Emotional upsets or acute stress.
- Food poisoning.
- Infections (viral, parasitic or bacterial).
- Regional enteritis.
- Malabsorption syndromes.
- Disease or tumor of the pancreas (malignant or benign).
- Diverticulitis.
- Foods such as prunes or beans.
- Excessive alcohol consumption.
- The use of drugs such as laxatives, antacids, antibiotics, quinine or anticancer drugs.
- Food allergy.
- Radiation treatments for cancer.

Risk factors include:
- Stress.
- Recent illness.
- Excessive alcohol consumption.
- Crowded or unsanitary living conditions.
- Travel to other countries.

DOCTOR'S TREATMENT & DIAGNOSTIC TESTS
- Medical history and physical exam if the symptoms persist longer than 2 to 3 days.
- Laboratory stool studies (for prolonged diarrhea).
- Self-care instructions focused on the older patient.

OTHER—Everyone is likely to have bouts of diarrhea occasionally from insignificant causes which disappear and leave no lasting effects. Most cases of acute diarrhea last a short time, and a search for the cause may not be necessary.

HOME TREATMENT BY SELF OR CARE-GIVER

GENERAL INSTRUCTIONS
- If cramps are present, place hot compresses or a hot water bottle on the abdomen.
- Maintain fluid intake.
- Replace lost fluid and electrolytes (salts) by drinking water with added salt and sugar (1 teaspoon salt and 4 teaspoons sugar in 1 quart of water).

MEDICATION (ADJUSTED FOR AGING)
- For minor discomfort, you may use non-prescription drugs.
- *Note:* Adverse reactions and side effects may be more frequent and severe in older persons. Remind your doctor of any medicines you already take.

ACTIVITY FOR OLDER PATIENTS
- Decrease activity until diarrhea stops.
- See Appendix 20 regarding physical fitness for the active older adult.

FOOD & BEVERAGE
- If diarrhea is accompanied by nausea, suck ice chips only.
- If you are not nauseated, drink small amounts of clear liquid such as herbal tea, ginger ale, broth or gelatin until diarrhea stops.
- After your symptoms disappear, eat soft foods such as cooked cereal, rice, eggs, custard, baked potato and yogurt for 1 or 2 days.
- Resume a normal diet 2 or 3 days after the diarrhea stops. Avoid fruit, alcohol and highly seasoned foods for several more days.
- See Appendix 1 regarding good nutrition for people over 50.

FUTURE CONSIDERATIONS FOR THE AGING ADULT

POSSIBLE COMPLICATIONS—Dehydration if diarrhea is prolonged.

PROBABLE OUTCOME—Spontaneous recovery in 24 to 48 hours.

PREVENTING RECURRENCE—If diarrhea is recurrent and a cause can be identified, treatment or avoidance of the cause should prevent recurrence.

CALL YOUR DOCTOR IF

- Diarrhea lasts more than 48 hours.
- Mucus, blood or worms appear in the stool.
- Fever rises to 101F (38.3C) or higher.
- Severe pain develops in the abdomen or rectum.
- Dehydration develops. Signs include dry mouth, wrinkled skin, excessive thirst, and little or no urination.

DIC
(Disseminated Intravascular Coagulation;
Defibrinogenation Syndrome; Coagulopathy)

 **BASIC INFORMATION
FOR OLDER ADULTS**

DESCRIPTION—DIC is a serious disruption of blood-clotting mechanisms resulting in hemorrhaging or internal bleeding. This disorder is a complication of an underlying disorder. Body parts involved: The blood vessels and the blood in all parts of the body. (THIS IS AN EMERGENCY; SEEK MEDICAL CARE IMMEDIATELY!)

SPECIAL CONSIDERATIONS FOR AGING
- The immune system becomes less effective, opening the way for viral, bacterial and other infections; malignancies; immune disorders; and allergies.
- Stress from social isolation increases the risk of infection.
- Usual signs and symptoms may be absent and be replaced by symptoms of confusion, dizziness, failure to thrive, falling, incontinence, increasing dementia, refusal to eat or drink, weight loss, depression, paranoia, hypochondriasis, psychosis or threats of suicide.

SIGNS & SYMPTOMS
- Bleeding and hemorrhaging from any or several body parts. The bleeding may be heavy. Common signs of bleeding include: Bloody vomit or red or black stools. Vaginal bleeding. Red or cloudy urine. Unexplained bruising.
- Severe abdominal or back pain caused by bleeding into body organs.
- Convulsions (rare).
- Coma (rare).

CAUSES & RISK FACTORS—DIC is caused by a depletion of the blood-clotting components, which causes widespread bleeding. This condition can be the result of:
- Widespread or major infection.
- Widespread cancer.
- Some kinds of surgery.
- Widespread tissue destruction, as with extensive burns.
- Poisonous snakebite.
- Transfusion of mismatched blood.
Risk factors include:
- Poor nutrition.
- Illness that has lowered resistance.

**DOCTOR'S TREATMENT
& DIAGNOSTIC TESTS**
- Medical history and physical exam.
- Laboratory blood tests, especially of the blood-clotting mechanism.
- Hospitalization.

- Surgery to correct the underlying disorder (sometimes).
- After treatment, self-care instructions focused on the older patient.

 **HOME TREATMENT BY
SELF OR CARE-GIVER**

GENERAL INSTRUCTIONS
- Patients with this condition are often desperately ill and require intensive hospital care. Family members can help by maintaining a positive, hopeful attitude.
- During recovery, don't scrub or take scabs off sores. This may trigger new bleeding.

MEDICATION (ADJUSTED FOR AGING)
- Your doctor may prescribe: Blood transfusions or blood component infusions. Heparin (an anticoagulant administered by injection).
- *Note:* Adverse reactions and side effects may be more frequent and severe in older persons. Remind your doctor of any medicines you already take.

ACTIVITY FOR OLDER PATIENTS
- Rest in bed until your doctor approves a return to normal activity. You may read or watch TV.
- See Appendix 20 regarding physical fitness for the active older adult.

FOOD & BEVERAGE
- No special diet is required.
- See Appendix 1 regarding good nutrition for people over 50.

 **FUTURE CONSIDERATIONS
FOR THE AGING ADULT**

POSSIBLE COMPLICATIONS
- Kidney failure.
- Brain damage with seizures or coma.
- Shock.
- Death.

PROBABLE OUTCOME—Depends on the severity. If the underlying cause of DIC is treated promptly, full recovery is likely.

PREVENTING RECURRENCE—Obtain prompt medical treatment for the underlying causes.

 CALL YOUR DOCTOR IF

- You have symptoms of DIC. *This is an emergency!*
- Any bleeding recurs or the abdomen swells rapidly during treatment.

DIPHTHERIA

BASIC INFORMATION FOR OLDER ADULTS

DESCRIPTION—Diphtheria is a highly contagious throat infection. Body parts involved: The throat, heart and central nervous system. (THIS IS AN EMERGENCY; SEEK MEDICAL CARE IMMEDIATELY!)

SPECIAL CONSIDERATIONS FOR AGING
- Stress from social isolation increases the risk of infection.
- The immune system becomes less effective, opening the way for viral, bacterial and other infections; malignancies; immune disorders; and allergies.
- Decreased nutrition increases the risk of infections.

SIGNS & SYMPTOMS
Early stages:
- Sore throat.
- Low-grade fever.
- Swollen neck glands.
- Yellow spots or sores on the skin (sometimes).
Late stages:
- Airway obstruction and breathing difficulty.
- Shock (characterized by low blood pressure, rapid heartbeat, paleness, cold skin, sweating, and an anxious appearance).

CAUSES & RISK FACTORS—Diphtheria is caused by a bacterial germ, *corynebacterium diphtheriae,* that infects the throat and sometimes the skin. The incubation period is 5 to 9 days following exposure. The germ produces poisons that spread to the heart, central nervous system and other organs. Risk factors include:
- Poor nutrition.
- An outbreak in the community.
- Crowded or unsanitary living conditions.
- Lack of up-to-date immunizations.
- Visiting developing countries of the world without being immunized.

DOCTOR'S TREATMENT & DIAGNOSTIC TESTS
- Medical history and physical exam.
- Laboratory studies such as throat culture and blood counts.
- Hospitalization.

OTHER—Notify the local health department of any case of diphtheria. Anyone having contact with the patient must be examined and treated.

HOME TREATMENT BY SELF OR CARE-GIVER

GENERAL INSTRUCTIONS
- Quarantine the patient until fully recovered. Protect susceptible individuals (the non-immunized, very young or elderly) from exposure.
- Dispose of all secretions (from the nose and mouth) and excretions (urine and feces) in an acceptable manner. Call the local health department for instructions.

MEDICATION (ADJUSTED FOR AGING)
- Your doctor may prescribe:
  Diphtheria antitoxin to neutralize the diphtheria toxin.
  Antibiotics to fight remaining diphtheria germs.
- *Note:* Adverse reactions and side effects may be more frequent and severe in older persons. Remind your doctor of any medicines you already take.

ACTIVITY FOR OLDER PATIENTS
- You will need prolonged bed rest (2 to 3 months or until fully recovered), especially if the heart is involved. You may watch TV or read.
- See Appendix 20 regarding physical fitness for the active older adult.

FOOD & BEVERAGE
- No special diet is required.
- See Appendix 1 regarding good nutrition for people over 50.

FUTURE CONSIDERATIONS FOR THE AGING ADULT

POSSIBLE COMPLICATIONS
- Heart inflammation and heart failure.
- Suffocation if the throat structure completely closes.
- Nerve inflammation.
- Misdiagnosis as a less serious infection, resulting in dangerous delay of treatment.

PROBABLE OUTCOME—Usually curable in 1 week, followed by slow recovery for several weeks. A delay in treatment may result in death or long-term heart disease.

PREVENTING RECURRENCE
- Be immunized with diphtheria vaccine. See Appendix 16 for an immunization schedule.
- Improve your nutrition and standard of living.

CALL YOUR DOCTOR IF

- You have symptoms of diphtheria or observe them in someone else. *This is an emergency!*
- Anyone in your family is exposed to diphtheria.
- Your immunizations are not current.
- Any of the following occurs during treatment: Temperature spikes to 102F (38.9C). Increasing breathing difficulty. Increasing shortness of breath. Confusion.

DISK, RUPTURED
(Herniated Disk; Slipped Disk)

BASIC INFORMATION FOR OLDER ADULTS

DESCRIPTION—A ruptured disk is a sudden or gradual break in the supportive ligaments surrounding one of the spinal disks (cushions which separate the bony spinal vertebrae). Body parts involved: The disks of the neck or lower spine are the most common sites.

SPECIAL CONSIDERATIONS FOR AGING
- Years of weight bearing cause wear and tear on the bones, joints and ligaments.
- The bones become thinner.
- Stress from any emotional cause—fear, worry, anxiety, sadness, loneliness or anger—affects all aspects of any illness or disorder.

SIGNS & SYMPTOMS
Ruptures in the lower back:
- Severe pain in the lower back or the back of one leg, buttock or foot (sciatica). The pain usually affects one side and worsens with movement, coughing, sneezing, lifting or straining.
- Weakness, numbness or muscular wasting of the affected leg.

Ruptures in the neck:
- Pain in the neck, shoulder or down one arm. The pain worsens with movement.
- Weakness, numbness or muscular wasting of the affected arm.

CAUSES & RISK FACTORS—A ruptured disk is characterized by the weakening and rupture of the disk material, creating pressure on nearby spinal nerves. Causes include sudden injury or chronic stress, such as from constant lifting or obesity. Risk factors include:
- Heavy lifting.
- Poor physical condition.

DOCTOR'S TREATMENT & DIAGNOSTIC TESTS
- Medical history and physical exam.
- X-rays of the neck or lower spine, including myelogram (see Glossary).
- CT scan (see Glossary).
- Self-care instructions focused on the older patient.
- Traction at home or in the hospital (sometimes).
- Surgery (usually called laminectomy) to relieve the pressure on the nerves if bed rest does not relieve the symptoms.
- New procedures are simpler than laminectomy, but not always successful.
- Rehabilitation to strengthen the muscles.
- Psychotherapy or counseling to help you learn coping methods for enduring pain and frustration.

HOME TREATMENT BY SELF OR CARE-GIVER

GENERAL INSTRUCTIONS
- Apply ice packs to the painful area during the first 72 hours and occasionally thereafter if they provide relief. Alternately, try to relieve the pain with a heat lamp, hot showers or baths or warm compresses.
- Don't allow an untrained person to do any back manipulation.
- See Appendix 15 for back care suggestions.

MEDICATION (ADJUSTED FOR AGING)
- For minor discomfort, you may use non-prescription drugs such as aspirin.
- Your doctor may prescribe:
  Pain relievers.
  Muscle relaxants, such as diazepam or methocarbamol.
  Non-steroidal anti-inflammatory drugs to reduce inflammation around the rupture.
  Laxatives or stool softeners to prevent constipation.

ACTIVITY FOR OLDER PATIENTS—Rest in bed at least 2 weeks during the acute phase. You may read or watch TV. Slowly resume your normal activities, including sexual relations, when the symptoms improve. Follow the rehabilitation plan your doctor prescribes.

FOOD & BEVERAGE—No special diet is required. Increase consumption of dietary fiber and drink at least 8 glasses of fluid a day to prevent constipation or fecal impaction.

FUTURE CONSIDERATIONS FOR THE AGING ADULT

POSSIBLE COMPLICATIONS—Loss of bladder and bowel function; paralysis; muscle wasting and weakness.

PROBABLE OUTCOME—Spontaneous recovery in many cases. Try at least 2 weeks in bed before considering other therapy unless complications occur. When necessary, a ruptured disk is curable with surgery.

PREVENTING RECURRENCE
- Practice proper posture when lifting.
- Exercise regularly to maintain muscle tone.

CALL YOUR DOCTOR IF

- You have symptoms of a ruptured disk.
- Any of the following occurs during treatment: Increased pain or weakness in the extremities. Loss of bladder or bowel control.
- New, unexplained symptoms develop. The drugs used in treatment may produce side effects.

DIVERTICULAR DISEASE
(Diverticulosis; Diverticulitis)

BASIC INFORMATION FOR OLDER ADULTS

DESCRIPTION—Diverticulosis is the presence of small, saclike swellings (diverticulae) in the wall of the colon. Diverticulae may be present without any symptoms. Diverticulitis is the inflammation of the diverticulae. It is not contagious or cancerous. Body part involved: The left side of the large intestine.

SPECIAL CONSIDERATIONS FOR AGING
- The immune system becomes less effective, opening the way for viral, bacterial and other infections; malignancies; immune disorders; and allergies.
- Decreased nutrition increases the risk of infections.
- The total digestive system becomes sluggish.

SIGNS & SYMPTOMS
Symptoms of diverticulosis:
- Mild cramping, bloated feeling or tenderness in the left side of the abdomen that is relieved by passing gas or moving the bowels.
- Occasional bright red blood in the stool. Non-infected diverticulae sometimes bleed.
- Constipation or diarrhea (sometimes).
- No symptoms (usually).

Symptoms of diverticulitis:
- Intermittent cramping, abdominal pain that becomes constant. The pain may be disabling from the onset or may not become disabling for several days.
- Fever.
- Nausea.
- Tenderness over the affected area of the colon.

CAUSES & RISK FACTORS—The cause is unknown, but the tendency is inherited. Recent evidence suggests that the highly refined, low-residue diet common in the U.S. and other developed countries may contribute to the formation of diverticulae. Pressure builds up inside the sigmoid colon as a result of spasms due to lack of dietary bulk. The inner lining eventually pushes through to form the small pouches. Risk factors include:
- An improper diet that lacks fiber.
- A family history of diverticulosis.
- Coronary artery disease or gallbladder disease.
- Obesity.

DOCTOR'S TREATMENT & DIAGNOSTIC TESTS
- Medical history and physical exam.
- X-rays of the lower intestinal tract (barium enema).
- Sigmoidoscopy (see Glossary).
- Self-care instructions focused on the older patient.
- Hospitalization (for complications only).
- Surgery to remove part of the colon if the diverticulae become infected or bleed significantly.

HOME TREATMENT BY SELF OR CARE-GIVER

GENERAL INSTRUCTIONS
- Try to have a bowel movement at about the same time each day. Allow at least 10 minutes and don't strain.
- Check your stool daily for bleeding. If the stool is black, remove it from the toilet and take it to your doctor's office for analysis.
- To relieve mild pain and spasms, apply warm compresses to the abdomen.

MEDICATION (ADJUSTED FOR AGING)
- Your doctor may prescribe:
  Antibiotics if the diverticulae are infected. Antispasmodic drugs to relieve the symptoms. Bulk-producing laxatives if you are unable to eat a high-fiber diet. Don't take laxatives unless they are prescribed.
- *Note:* Adverse reactions and side effects may be more frequent and severe in older persons. Remind your doctor of any medicines you already take.

ACTIVITY FOR OLDER PATIENTS
- If you have fever or severe pain, stay in bed. Resume your normal activity as soon as your symptoms improve.
- See Appendix 20 regarding physical fitness for the active older adult.

FOOD & BEVERAGE—Eat a well-balanced diet that is high in fiber, low in salt and low in fat (see Appendices 1, 8 and 9).

FUTURE CONSIDERATIONS FOR THE AGING ADULT

POSSIBLE COMPLICATIONS—If the diverticulae become infected, they may bleed profusely or perforate (erode through the intestinal wall) and cause peritonitis. Both of these complications are medical and surgical emergencies.

PROBABLE OUTCOME—Diverticulosis is dangerous only if the diverticulae become infected or bleed. Diverticulitis is curable with surgery.

PREVENTING RECURRENCE—Cannot be prevented at present, but the risk can be reduced by:
- Eating a diet that is high in fiber throughout life.
- Maintaining good cardiovascular fitness. This disease may be related to blood vessel disorders.

CALL YOUR DOCTOR IF

- You develop a fever.
- Severe pain continues despite treatment.
- Blood appears in the stool.
- Vomiting or abdominal swelling occurs.

DROWNING, NEAR

BASIC INFORMATION FOR OLDER ADULTS

DESCRIPTION—Near drowning refers to the immediate aftereffects of prolonged submersion under water. Body parts involved: The lungs, blood and heart. (THIS IS AN EMERGENCY; SEEK MEDICAL CARE IMMEDIATELY!)

SPECIAL CONSIDERATIONS FOR AGING
- In the lungs, the transfer of carbon dioxide and oxygen to the bloodstream becomes less efficient.
- The chest muscles used for breathing become weaker.

SIGNS & SYMPTOMS
- Confusion or unconsciousness.
- Little or no breathing or heartbeat.
- Bluish-white paleness.

CAUSES & RISK FACTORS
Submersion under water causes either:
- Spasm of the larynx (the tube from the throat to the lungs). After rescue, this spasm prevents oxygen from reaching the lungs.
- Water in the lungs resulting in life-threatening changes in the circulating blood.
Risk factors include:
- Excessive alcohol consumption.
- Accidents—especially head injuries—while swimming.
- Suicidal tendencies.

DOCTOR'S TREATMENT & DIAGNOSTIC TESTS
- Continuation of cardiopulmonary resuscitation (CPR) begun at the scene (see General Instructions).
- Medical history and physical exam.
- Laboratory blood tests.
- Hospitalization for observation for serious delayed reactions.
- After treatment, self-care instructions focused on the older patient.

HOME TREATMENT BY SELF OR CARE-GIVER

GENERAL INSTRUCTIONS
- If the victim is unconscious and *not* breathing, yell for help. Don't leave the victim. Begin mouth-to-mouth breathing immediately.
- If there is no heartbeat, give external cardiac massage.
- Have someone call 0 (operator) or 911 (emergency) for an ambulance or medical help.
- Don't stop CPR until help arrives.
- Administer oxygen, if available, after CPR has restored a heartbeat. (Emergency oxygen may be available in welders' shops.)
- The victim should be taken to the nearest hospital for intensive care—even if the victim has regained consciousness. Complications or death may occur 24 to 48 hours after the accident due to heart rhythm disturbances or damage to the central nervous system.
- Remain with a recovering patient to provide support and reassurance. Near drowning is a traumatic experience.

MEDICATION (ADJUSTED FOR AGING)
- The doctor may prescribe:
  Oxygen.
  Cortisone drugs to prevent or treat lung inflammation.
  Antibiotics to prevent lung infection.
  Bronchodilators to enable oxygen to enter the lungs.
- *Note:* Adverse reactions and side effects may be more frequent and severe in older persons. Remind your doctor of any medicines you already take.

ACTIVITY FOR OLDER PATIENTS
- You need complete bed rest until activity is permitted by your doctor.
- See Appendix 20 regarding physical fitness for the active older adult.

FOOD & BEVERAGE
- Intravenous nutrients will be given if you are unconscious upon hospitalization. After recovery, no special diet is necessary.
- See Appendix 1 regarding good nutrition for people over 50.

FUTURE CONSIDERATIONS FOR THE AGING ADULT

POSSIBLE COMPLICATIONS—Pulmonary edema (body fluid in the lungs); permanent brain damage; heart irregularities, including cardiac arrest and death; lung infection.

PROBABLE OUTCOME—Depends on the length of time under water. With early rescue and treatment, full recovery is possible. Special body mechanisms may permit full recovery from near drowning in icy water even after prolonged immersion.

PREVENTING RECURRENCE
- Learn cardiopulmonary resuscitation (CPR).
- Encourage all family members—including infants—to learn to swim. Swimming can be learned at any age.
- Install a fence around your home swimming pool.
- Never swim alone.
- Don't drink alcohol and swim.

CALL YOUR DOCTOR IF

- Someone appears to have drowned. Call for emergency help immediately. *This is an emergency!* See General Instructions for additional emergency information.
- Signs of infection (fever, cough, muscle aches and fatigue) appear after apparent recovery.

DRUG ABUSE & ADDICTION

BASIC INFORMATION FOR OLDER ADULTS

DESCRIPTION—Drug abuse and addiction is a compulsive and destructive use of mind-altering substances despite adverse medical, psychological and social consequences. Body parts involved: The central nervous system, liver, kidneys and blood. (See Appendix 21 for the safe use of medications.)

SPECIAL CONSIDERATIONS FOR AGING
- Usual signs and symptoms may be absent and be replaced by symptoms of confusion, dizziness, failure to thrive, falling, incontinence, increasing dementia, refusal to eat or drink, weight loss, depression, paranoia, hypochondriasis, psychosis or threats of suicide.
- Alcoholism may be particularly difficult to diagnose in elderly patients.

SIGNS & SYMPTOMS—Depend on the substance of abuse. Most produce:
- A temporary pleasant mood alteration.
- Relief from anxiety; feelings of self-confidence.
- Increased sensitivity to sights and sounds.
- Altered activity levels—either stupor and sleeplike states *or* frenzies.
- Unpleasant or painful symptoms when the abused substance is withdrawn.

CAUSES & RISK FACTORS—Substances of abuse may produce addiction (a physiological need) or dependence (a psychological need). The most common substances of abuse include nicotine; caffeine; alcohol; amphetamines; barbiturates; cocaine; marijuana; opiates, including codeine, heroin, methadone, morphine and opium; psychedelic drugs, including PCP ("angel dust"), mescaline and LSD; and volatile substances, such as glue, solvents and paints. Risk factors include illness that requires prescription pain relievers or tranquilizers; a family history of drug abuse; genetic factors (some persons may be more susceptible to addiction than others); excessive alcohol consumption; fatigue or overwork; poverty; and psychological problems, including depression, dependency or poor self-esteem.

DOCTOR'S TREATMENT & DIAGNOSTIC TESTS
- Medical history and physical exam.
- Laboratory blood tests.
- Observations of family members or others.
- Psychotherapy or counseling.
- Hospitalization for drug withdrawal symptoms.
- Group withdrawal programs.

HOME TREATMENT BY SELF OR CARE-GIVER

GENERAL INSTRUCTIONS
- Admit you have a problem.
- Seek professional help.

- Be open and honest with your family and good friends and ask for their help.
- Avoid friends who tempt you to resume your habit.
- Join self-help groups.

MEDICATION (ADJUSTED FOR AGING)—
Your doctor may prescribe:
- Disulfiram (Antabuse) for alcoholism. This drug produces severe illness when alcohol is consumed.
- Methadone for narcotic abuse. This drug is a less potent narcotic used to decrease the severity of physical withdrawal symptoms.
- Gradual withdrawal from any prescription medicines you are addicted to.

ACTIVITY FOR OLDER PATIENTS
- No restrictions are necessary. Exercise regularly and vigorously.
- See Appendix 20 regarding physical fitness for the active older adult.

FOOD & BEVERAGE—Eat a normal, well-balanced diet that is high in protein. Vitamin supplements may be necessary if you suffer from malnutrition.

FUTURE CONSIDERATIONS FOR THE AGING ADULT

POSSIBLE COMPLICATIONS
- Sexually transmitted diseases, which are more likely among addicts.
- Severe infections, such as endocarditis, hepatitis or blood poisoning, from intravenous injections with non-sterile needles.
- Malnutrition.
- Accidental injury to oneself or others while in a drug-induced state.
- Loss of job or family.
- Irreversible damage to body organs.
- Death caused by overdose.

PROBABLE OUTCOME—Curable with strong motivation, good medical care and support from family members and friends.

PREVENTING RECURRENCE
- Don't socialize with persons who use drugs.
- Seek counseling for mental health problems, such as depression or chronic anxiety, before they lead to drug problems.
- Develop wholesome interests and activities.
- After surgery, illness or injury, discontinue the use of prescription pain relievers and tranquilizers as soon as possible. Don't use more than you need.

CALL YOUR DOCTOR IF

- You abuse or are addicted to drugs and want help.
- New, unexplained symptoms develop. Drugs used in treatment may produce side effects.

BASIC INFORMATION FOR OLDER ADULTS

DESCRIPTION—Drug hypersensitivity refers to a variety of allergic responses caused by medication. These are not inherited or contagious. Body parts involved: The skin, blood vessels and lungs.

SPECIAL CONSIDERATIONS FOR AGING—
Unusual and unexpected reactions to drugs and medications are more likely.

SIGNS & SYMPTOMS
Usual signs and symptoms include:
- Rash, itching or hives.
- Jaundice (yellow skin and eyes).
- Flushed skin.
- Facial swelling.
- Anxiety.
- Serum sickness (fever, rash, joint pain and nerve damage).
- Anaphylaxis (wheezing and breathing difficulty). For signs and symptoms, see Anaphylaxis in the Illnesses section.
- Various blood disorders, such as hemolytic anemia.
- Peripheral neuropathy (nerve damage).
- Vasculitis (blood vessel inflammation).

The following reactions to medications are usually *not* the result of allergies:
- Vomiting or diarrhea.
- Fever.
- Photosensitivity (a skin reaction to sunlight).

CAUSES & RISK FACTORS—Medications are materials that are foreign to the body. When a medication is injected—or, less often, when one is taken orally—the body develops antibodies to the medication. Subsequent exposure to the medication causes an allergic reaction in the body. Risk factors include:
- The use of almost any drugs, but especially the following:
  Penicillin and cephalosporin antibiotics.
  Sulfa drugs.
  Animal serums
  Vaccines.
  Local anesthetics.
  Allergy extracts.
  Iodine-containing compounds, such as those used in some x-rays.
- The injection of medications, especially in high doses.
- A medical history of other allergies such as hay fever, asthma or eczema.
- Current infectious illness (probably because infection increases the functioning of the immune system).

DOCTOR'S TREATMENT & DIAGNOSTIC TESTS
- Medical history and physical exam.
- Self-care instructions focused on the older patient.

HOME TREATMENT BY SELF OR CARE-GIVER

GENERAL INSTRUCTIONS
- See the Emergency First Aid section for the treatment of anaphylaxis.
- Wear a Medic Alert pendant or bracelet (see Glossary) if you have drug hypersensitivity.
- Keep an anaphylaxis kit at home, on your person, nearby at work and in your car for emergency use if anyone in the family has had a severe drug reaction. Ask your doctor how to obtain one.

MEDICATION (ADJUSTED FOR AGING)
- Your doctor may prescribe:
  Cortisone drugs to decrease the inflammatory reaction.
  Antihistamines to decrease the body's allergic response.
- *Note:* Adverse reactions and side effects may be more frequent and severe in older persons. Remind your doctor of any medicines you already take.

ACTIVITY FOR OLDER PATIENTS
- Resume your normal activities as soon as your symptoms improve.
- See Appendix 20 regarding physical fitness for the active older adult.

FOOD & BEVERAGE
- No special diet is required.
- See Appendix 1 regarding good nutrition for people over 50.

FUTURE CONSIDERATIONS FOR THE AGING ADULT

POSSIBLE COMPLICATIONS
- Death from severe anaphylaxis reactions.
- Disability for many months from serum sickness.

PROBABLE OUTCOME—Most reactions disappear once the medication is permanently discontinued.

PREVENTING RECURRENCE
- Tell your doctor about any drug reactions you have had.
- Learn the name of any medication you are given. If it causes a reaction, you must avoid it in the future.
- Don't take any medication—including non-prescription drugs—unless it is necessary.

CALL YOUR DOCTOR IF

You have symptoms of drug hypersensitivity or observe them in someone else.

DUMPING SYNDROME

BASIC INFORMATION FOR OLDER ADULTS

DESCRIPTION—Dumping syndrome includes a group of symptoms that are a complication of the surgical removal of all or part of the stomach. Most patients experience the problem to a minor degree for 1 to 6 months after surgery. It becomes a serious problem in 1% or 2% of patients. The symptoms are of 2 types—early dumping syndrome and late dumping syndrome. The symptoms of the first begin a few minutes to 45 minutes after every meal. The symptoms of the second begin 2 to 3 hours after eating. Most persons experience late dumping syndrome; one person does not have both forms. Body parts involved: The gastro-intestinal system and the cardiovascular system.

SPECIAL CONSIDERATIONS FOR AGING
- The total digestive system becomes sluggish.
- The esophageal muscles decrease in strength with aging.
- Stress from any emotional cause—fear, worry, anxiety, sadness, loneliness or anger—affects all aspects of any illness or disorder.

SIGNS & SYMPTOMS
Early dumping syndrome:
- Weakness and fainting.
- Sweating; dizziness; vomiting.
- Irregular or rapid heartbeat.
- Decreased blood pressure.
- Flushing of the skin.
- Shortness of breath.
- Explosive diarrhea and abdominal cramps.

Late dumping syndrome:
- Sweating, anxiety and tremors.
- Exhaustion and faintness.
- Decreased blood pressure.
- Headache.

CAUSES & RISK FACTORS
Causes include:
- Early dumping syndrome—Rapid entry of food and fluids directly into the small intestine, producing decreased blood pressure and increased blood flow to the intestines.
- Late dumping syndrome—Low blood sugar caused by excessive insulin production in response to the sudden dumping of food and fluids into the intestine.

The larger the amount of stomach removed, the greater the risk of severe dumping syndrome.

DOCTOR'S TREATMENT & DIAGNOSTIC TESTS
- Medical history and physical exam.
- Laboratory studies of blood sugar levels.
- After diagnosis, self-care instructions focused on the older patient.

HOME TREATMENT BY SELF OR CARE-GIVER

GENERAL INSTRUCTIONS
- Early dumping syndrome—Lie down for 45 minutes until the symptoms pass.
- Late dumping syndrome—Eat small amounts of sugar candy or drink sweetened orange juice.

MEDICATION (ADJUSTED FOR AGING)
- Your doctor may prescribe:
  Anticholinergics to block the dumping syndrome reflex.
  Pectin to reduce the severity of diarrhea.
  Vitamin and mineral supplements to compensate for poor absorption.
- *Note:* Adverse reactions and side effects may be more frequent and severe in older persons. Remind your doctor of any medicines you already take.

ACTIVITY FOR OLDER PATIENTS
- Between symptoms—No restrictions.
- With symptoms—Rest until the symptoms pass.

FOOD & BEVERAGE
- Early dumping syndrome—Diet control is the most important treatment. Eat a diet that is low in sugar and other simple carbohydrates. Increase fat and protein consumption. Eat 6 small, evenly spaced meals a day. Take meals dry, without water or beverages, and drink fluids only between meals.
- Late dumping syndrome—Avoid refined sugar and foods containing sugar.
- See Appendix 1 regarding good nutrition for people over 50.

FUTURE CONSIDERATIONS FOR THE AGING ADULT

POSSIBLE COMPLICATIONS—Malnutrition and weight loss; anxiety.

PROBABLE OUTCOME—Spontaneous recovery for most patients. Early dumping syndrome usually lasts 3 to 4 months. Late dumping syndrome usually lasts 1 year, but it may persist for many years.

PREVENTING RECURRENCE—Some degree of dumping syndrome cannot be prevented, but the number of recurrences and their severity can be minimized with dietary changes (see Food & Beverage).

CALL YOUR DOCTOR IF

- You have symptoms of dumping syndrome that are not relieved by the measures outlined above.
- You vomit blood; have black, tarry stools; or have other signs of gastrointestinal bleeding.
- New, unexplained symptoms develop. The drugs used in treatment may produce side effects.

DYSENTERY, BACILLARY
(Shigellosis)

BASIC INFORMATION FOR OLDER ADULTS

DESCRIPTION—Bacillary dysentery is a bacterial infection of the surface layers of the intestinal tract. This is contagious with close personal contact and occurs in epidemics. It has a 1- to 4-day incubation period. Body parts involved: The lower small intestine (ileum) and the large intestine (colon).

SPECIAL CONSIDERATIONS FOR AGING
- Stress from social isolation increases the risk ofinfection.
- The immune system becomes less effective, opening the way for viral, bacterial and other infections; malignancies; immune disorders; and allergies.
- Usual signs and symptoms may be absent and be replaced by symptoms of confusion, dizziness, failure to thrive, falling, incontinence, increasing dementia, refusal to eat or drink, weight loss, depression, paranoia, hypochondriasis, psychosis or threats of suicide.

SIGNS & SYMPTOMS
- Abdominal cramps; fever.
- Diarrhea (up to 20 or 30 watery bowel movements in 1 day).
- Blood, mucus or pus in the stool.
- Nausea or vomiting; muscle aches or pain.
- A white blood cell count that is lower than normal at the onset (sometimes).

CAUSES & RISK FACTORS—The cause is *shigella bacillus,* a bacterium that invades the lining of the colon. It spreads from person to person, usually from contaminated hands to the mouth, contaminated food or drinking water. Risk factors include:
- Travel to foreign countries.
- Crowded or unsanitary living conditions.

DOCTOR'S TREATMENT & DIAGNOSTIC TESTS
- Medical history and physical exam.
- Laboratory stool culture.
- Self-care instructions focused on the older patient.
- Hospitalization of persons who are severely ill. Hospital care will include isolation and giving intravenous fluid supplements.

HOME TREATMENT BY SELF OR CARE-GIVER

GENERAL INSTRUCTIONS
- Isolate the patient from others.
- Use warm compresses or a hot water bottle wrapped in a towel on the abdomen to relieve the pain.
- Maintain fluid intake. For instructions, see Dehydration in the Illnesses section.

MEDICATION (ADJUSTED FOR AGING)
- Your doctor may prescribe antibiotics.
- Don't use paregoric preparations or other antidiarrhea drugs unless your doctor prescribes them. These may prolong the illness. If used, discontinue them as soon as possible.

ACTIVITY FOR OLDER PATIENTS—Bed rest is necessary, except for trips to the bathroom, until fever, diarrhea and other symptoms have been gone for at least 3 days. Exercise your legs regularly in bed. Resume your normal activities slowly.

FOOD & BEVERAGE
- Consume a liquid or soft diet until the diarrhea stops, then return to normal diet.
- See Appendix 1 regarding good nutrition for people over 50.

FUTURE CONSIDERATIONS FOR THE AGING ADULT

POSSIBLE COMPLICATIONS
- Dangerous dehydration.
- In rare cases, the bacteria may enter the bloodstream from the digestive tract and infect other body organs, such as the kidneys, gallbladder, liver or heart, and the joints. This may cause shock and death.

PROBABLE OUTCOME—Usually curable in 7 days with treatment. Most shigella infections are mild and don't require drastic treatment. However, in a severe attack excessive dehydration can be fatal if treatment is unsuccessful.

PREVENTING RECURRENCE
- Wash your hands after bowel movements and before handling food.
- Isolate anyone with symptoms of bacillary dysentery.
- Immerse soiled clothes and bedclothes in covered buckets of soap and water until they can be boiled.

CALL YOUR DOCTOR IF

- You have symptoms of bacillary dysentery.
- Any of the following occurs during treatment:
  A fever of 102F (38.9C) or more.
  A sore throat, headache or earache.
  Shortness of breath or a severe cough.
  Traces of blood in the sputum.
  Severe abdominal pain or abdominal swelling.
  Rectal bleeding.
  Pain in the calf or leg.
  Swollen joints.
  Signs of dehydration (lethargy, sunken eyes, rapid weight loss or dry skin).

EAR INFECTION, MIDDLE
(Otitis Media)

BASIC INFORMATION FOR OLDER ADULTS

DESCRIPTION—Otitis media is an infection in the middle ear. This is not contagious from person to person, but the respiratory infection causing it may be infectious. Body parts involved: The middle ear, where nerves and small bones connect to the eardrum on one side and the eustachian tube on the other side.

SPECIAL CONSIDERATIONS FOR AGING
- Some degree of hearing loss occurs.
- The immune system becomes less effective, opening the way for viral, bacterial and other infections; malignancies; immune disorders; and allergies.

SIGNS & SYMPTOMS
- Irritability.
- Pain in the ear, either sharp or aching.
- A feeling of fullness in the ear.
- Hearing loss.
- Fever.
- Discharge or leakage from the ear.
- Diarrhea; vomiting (sometimes).

CAUSES & RISK FACTORS
Causes include:
- Bacterial or viral infections that spread to the middle ear by way of the eustachian tube. These are usually upper respiratory virus infections in the nose or throat.
- Sinus and eustachian tube blockage caused by nasal allergies or enlarged adenoids.
- A ruptured eardrum.

Risk factors include:
- A recent illness, such as a respiratory infection, that has lowered resistance.
- Crowded or unsanitary living conditions.
- Genetic factors. Some American Indians—especially the Navajo—seem more susceptible.
- High altitude.
- Cold climate.

DOCTOR'S TREATMENT & DIAGNOSTIC TESTS
- Medical history and physical exam.
- X-ray or CT scan (sometimes; see Glossary for both).
- After diagnosis, self-care instructions focused on the older patient.
- Surgery to insert plastic tubes through the eardrum to drain pus or fluid from the middle ear (rare).

HOME TREATMENT BY SELF OR CARE-GIVER

GENERAL INSTRUCTIONS—Apply warm compresses to the areas around the ears to relieve the pain.

MEDICATION (ADJUSTED FOR AGING)
- Use ear drops to relieve the pain. You may use non-prescription drops or those prescribed for a previous infection. They will not cure the infection.
- Use non-prescription decongestant or antihistaminic nasal sprays or drops to help open the eustachian tube and relieve pressure in the middle ear.
- Use non-prescriptions drugs such as acetaminophen to reduce the pain and fever.
- Your doctor may prescribe antibiotics if the infection appears to be bacterial rather than viral. Finish the medication. The infection may remain active for several days after the symptoms disappear.
- *Note:* Adverse reactions and side effects may be more frequent and severe in older persons. Remind your doctor of any medicines you already take.

ACTIVITY FOR OLDER PATIENTS—Rest in bed or reduce activity until the fever and pain subside, then resume your normal activities.

FOOD & BEVERAGE—No special diet.

FUTURE CONSIDERATIONS FOR THE AGING ADULT

POSSIBLE COMPLICATIONS
- Eardrum rupture.
- Hearing impairment—usually temporary, but sometimes permanent.
- Mastoiditis (rare).
- Meningitis (rare).

PROBABLE OUTCOME—Usually curable with treatment.

PREVENTING RECURRENCE—If you have an ear infection followed by a hearing loss or enlarged adenoids, ask your doctor about using a steroid nasal spray, preventive antibiotics, antihistamines or decongestants during future respiratory infections. This may prevent fluid accumulation.

CALL YOUR DOCTOR IF

- You have symptoms of a middle ear infection.
- Any of the following occurs during treatment:
  Fever.
  Severe headache.
  Earache that persists longer than 2 days despite treatment.
  Swelling around the ear.
  Convulsions.
  Twitching of the face muscles.
  Dizziness.

EAR INFECTION, OUTER
(Otitis Externa; Swimmer's Ear)

BASIC INFORMATION FOR OLDER ADULTS

DESCRIPTION—Otitis externa is an inflammation or infection of the ear canal that extends from the eardrum to the outside of the ear. Body part involved: The skin of the ear canal.

SPECIAL CONSIDERATIONS FOR AGING
- The immune system becomes less effective, opening the way for viral, bacterial and other infections; malignancies; immune disorders; and allergies.
- Usual signs and symptoms may be absent and be replaced by symptoms of confusion, dizziness, failure to thrive, falling, incontinence, increasing dementia, refusal to eat or drink, weight loss, depression, paranoia, hypochondriasis, psychosis or threats of suicide.
- Decreased nutrition increases the risk of infections.

SIGNS & SYMPTOMS
- Ear pain that worsens when the earlobe is pulled; slight fever (sometimes).
- Discharge of pus from the ear.
- Temporary hearing loss in the affected ear.

CAUSES & RISK FACTORS
Causes by a bacterium or fungus that has infected the delicate skin lining of the ear canal. Infection may develop because of:
- Swimming in dirty, polluted water.
- Excessive swimming in chlorinated pools. Chlorinated water dries out the ear canal, allowing bacteria or fungi to enter the skin.
- Excessive moisture from any cause.
- Irritation from swabs; metal objects such as bobby pins; or ear plugs, especially if they are left in a long time.
- Inadequate production of protective earwax.

Risk factors include:
- Previous ear infections.
- Skin allergies.
- Diabetes mellitus or other disorders that predispose one to infection.

DOCTOR'S TREATMENT & DIAGNOSTIC TESTS
- Medical history and physical exam.
- X-ray, CT scan or MRI (see Glossary for all).
- Self-care instructions focused on the older patient.
- Severe cases may require treatment by an ear, nose and throat specialist.

HOME TREATMENT BY SELF OR CARE-GIVER

GENERAL INSTRUCTIONS
- Your doctor will probably cleanse the ear canal and insert a cotton wick. The wick allows medication to reach all infected parts.

Moisten the wick with medication every hour for the first 24 hours. Continue to use drops according to your doctor's instructions after the wick is removed. Clean the tip of the dropper with alcohol after each use. Don't let other persons use the medicine.
- After you have had otitis externa, keep the prescription ear drops on hand. If the ear canals get wet for any reason, such as swimming or shampooing, put drops in both ears at bedtime.

MEDICATION (ADJUSTED FOR AGING)
- You may use non-prescription drugs such as acetaminophen or aspirin for minor pain.
- Your doctor may prescribe:
  Ear drops that contain antibiotics and cortisone drugs to control inflammation and fight infection.
  Oral antibiotics for severe infection.
  Codeine or narcotics for a short time to relieve severe pain.

ACTIVITY FOR OLDER PATIENTS
- Resume your normal activities as soon as your symptoms improve.
- Avoid getting water in your ears for 3 weeks after all the symptoms disappear. Any moisture—even from showering or washing your hair—can trigger a recurrence.

FOOD & BEVERAGE—No special diet.

FUTURE CONSIDERATIONS FOR THE AGING ADULT

POSSIBLE COMPLICATIONS
- Severe pain.
- A chronic inflammation that is difficult to cure.
- A boil in the ear canal.
- Cellulitis (a deep tissue infection). See Cellulitis in the Illnesses section.

PROBABLE OUTCOME—Usually curable with treatment in 7 to 10 days.

PREVENTING RECURRENCE
- Don't clean your ears with any object or chemical.
- Don't use ear plugs, alcohol in the ears, lamb's wool or anything else to keep your ears dry. These are not only useless; they may be harmful.

CALL YOUR DOCTOR IF

- You have symptoms of otitis externa.
- Any of the following occurs during treatment:
  The pain persists despite treatment.
  You feel your ears need cleaning. But remember that a small amount of earwax helps protect against infection.

EARDRUM, RUPTURED
(Tympanic Membrane Perforation)

BASIC INFORMATION FOR OLDER ADULTS

DESCRIPTION—A ruptured eardrum occurs with the perforation of the thin membrane (the tympanic membrane) that separates the inner ear from the outer ear. Body parts involved: The eardrum (tympanic membrane) and the middle ear.

SPECIAL CONSIDERATIONS FOR AGING—
Some degree of hearing loss occurs.

SIGNS & SYMPTOMS
- Sudden pain in the ear.
- Partial hearing loss.
- Bleeding or discharge from the ear. The discharge may resemble pus within 24 to 48 hours after rupture.
- Ringing in the ear.
- Dizziness.

CAUSES & RISK FACTORS
Causes include:
- Perforation of the eardrum when a sharp object is inserted into the ear, such as a cotton swab to clean the ear or relieve an itch, an unseen twig on a tree or hot slag from an industrial site.
- Sudden inward pressure in the ear, such as from a slap, a swimming or diving accident or a nearby explosion.
- Sudden outward pressure or suction, such as from a kiss over the ear.
- Severe middle ear infection.
Risk factors include:
- Recent middle ear infection.
- Head injury.

DOCTOR'S TREATMENT & DIAGNOSTIC TESTS
- Medical history and physical exam. When the eardrum ruptures, the contents of the middle ear (primarily bones) can be seen with a special instrument called an otoscope. A healthy eardrum is almost transparent.
- Self-care instructions focused on the older patient.
- Microsurgery to repair the perforation (rare).

HOME TREATMENT BY SELF OR CARE-GIVER

GENERAL INSTRUCTIONS
- Don't blow your nose if possible. If you must, blow gently.
- Keep the ear canal dry. Don't swim, take showers or get caught in the rain. Insert a wisp of cotton in the ear canal to keep moisture out of it when bathing.

MEDICATION (ADJUSTED FOR AGING)
- Your doctor may prescribe:
  Antibiotics to prevent or treat infections.
  Sedatives or tranquilizers to reduce apprehension.
  Pain relievers. For minor pain, you may use non-prescription drugs such as acetaminophen.
- *Note:* Adverse reactions and side effects may be more frequent and severe in older persons. Remind your doctor of any medicines you already take.

ACTIVITY FOR OLDER PATIENTS
- Resume your normal activities as soon as your symptoms improve.
- See Appendix 20 regarding physical fitness for the active older adult.

FOOD & BEVERAGE
- No special diet is required.
- See Appendix 1 regarding good nutrition for people over 50.

FUTURE CONSIDERATIONS FOR THE AGING ADULT

POSSIBLE COMPLICATIONS
- Ear infection with fever, vomiting and diarrhea.
- Significant blood loss (rare).
- Meningitis.
- Mastoiditis (see Glossary).
- Permanent hearing loss (rare).

PROBABLE OUTCOME—If the ruptured eardrum does not become infected, it will usually repair itself in 2 months. If it becomes infected, the infection is curable with treatment and hearing is usually not affected permanently.

PREVENTING RECURRENCE
- Don't put any object into the ear canal.
- Avoid injuries that may cause a rupture (see Causes).
- Obtain prompt medical treatment for middle ear infections.

CALL YOUR DOCTOR IF

- You have symptoms of a ruptured eardrum, especially a pus-like discharge.
- Any of the following occurs during treatment:
  Fever.
  Pain that persists despite treatment.
  Dizziness that continues longer than 12 to 24 hours.
- New, unexplained symptoms develop. The drugs used in treatment may produce side effects.

ILLNESSES & DISORDERS

EARWAX BLOCKAGE
(Cerumen Impaction)

BASIC INFORMATION FOR OLDER ADULTS

DESCRIPTION—Cerumen impaction is the blockage of the external ear canal due to an overproduction of earwax. Wax is produced by the ears to protect the canal leading from the eardrum to the outside of the ear. Body part involved: The external ear canal of one or both ears.

SPECIAL CONSIDERATIONS FOR AGING
- The hearing becomes impaired. The high tones go first.
- Characteristic signs and symptoms of many disorders are frequently changed or absent.

SIGNS & SYMPTOMS
- Decreased hearing.
- Ear pain.
- Plugged feeling in the ear.
- Ringing in the ear.

CAUSES & RISK FACTORS
Earwax blockage is caused by the overproduction of wax by glands in the external ear canal. Risk factors include:
- Exposure to dust or debris.
- A family history of overproduction of earwax.

DOCTOR'S TREATMENT & DIAGNOSTIC TESTS
- Medical history and physical exam.
- Self-care instructions focused on the older patient. Sometimes wax can be removed easily at home with ear drops and irrigation of the ear canal.
- If the wax is difficult to dislodge, your doctor can remove it.

HOME TREATMENT BY SELF OR CARE-GIVER

GENERAL INSTRUCTIONS—To remove earwax at home:
- *Caution:* If you have a perforated eardrum, don't try to remove earwax yourself. See your doctor.
- Buy non-prescription wax-softening ear drops.
- Lie down with the affected ear toward the ceiling.
- Pull the top of the ear gently up and back toward the back of the head.
- Instill the ear drops; use the amount given in the package directions.
- Leave the drops in the ear for 20 minutes. Continue to lie down if possible. Plug the ear with cotton.
- Sit up, leaning a little toward the affected side.
- Use a soft rubber bulb syringe to irrigate the ear canal gently with plain warm water or equal parts warm water and hydrogen peroxide.
- Repeat irrigations until the ear feels clear. If the ear doesn't clear, consult your doctor.
- Don't try to remove wax with a stick or cotton swab. You may damage the eardrum or cause infection in the ear canal.

MEDICATION (ADJUSTED FOR AGING)
- For minor pain, you may use non-prescription drugs such as acetaminophen.
- After treatment, your doctor may prescribe wax-softening ear drops to use when needed.
- *Note:* Adverse reactions and side effects may be more frequent and severe in older persons. Remind your doctor of any medicines you already take.

ACTIVITY FOR OLDER PATIENTS
- No restrictions are necessary.
- See Appendix 20 regarding physical fitness for the active older adult.

FOOD & BEVERAGE
- No special diet is required.
- See Appendix 1 regarding good nutrition for people over 50.

FUTURE CONSIDERATIONS FOR THE AGING ADULT

POSSIBLE COMPLICATIONS
- Ear infection.
- Eardrum damage.

PROBABLE OUTCOME—Earwax can be removed, but stubborn cases require patience.

PREVENTING RECURRENCE—Avoid areas where the air is dusty or filled with debris. This stimulates the overproduction of earwax.

CALL YOUR DOCTOR IF

- You have symptoms of an earwax blockage that do not clear despite the treatment described above.
- Fever and ear pain accompany an earwax blockage. Do *not* irrigate the ear in this case.

ECZEMA, NUMMULAR
(Xerotic Eczema)

BASIC INFORMATION FOR OLDER ADULTS

DESCRIPTION—Nummular eczema is severely chapped skin that becomes cracked, fissured and inflamed. The disorder is most common in winter. It is not contagious. Body part involved: The skin anywhere on the body, but most commonly on the legs.

SPECIAL CONSIDERATIONS FOR AGING
- The responsiveness of the skin's immune system decreases.
- Decreased nutrition, common among chronically ill older people, increases the risk of any disease or disorder.

SIGNS & SYMPTOMS—Lesions with the following characteristics:
- The lesions are round plaques (flat-topped patches) 2cm to 5cm in diameter. The plaques are sometimes piled like flat discs on top of each other. They usually have very definite borders.
- The plaques itch, burn and sting.
- Redness is most pronounced within the cracks and fissures that crisscross the surfaces of the plaques.
- The plaques usually don't weep or become crusty.

CAUSES & RISK FACTORS
Causes include:
- Insufficient oil on the skin's surface, which allows evaporation of water through the skin. The cells of the skin shrink so much that islands of cells begin to separate, causing cracks and fissures.
- Excessive bathing or rubbing of the skin, which causes the oil in the skin to decrease.

The risk increases in an environment with low humidity, especially in homes heated with hot-air fans in the winter.

DOCTOR'S TREATMENT & DIAGNOSTIC TESTS
- Medical history and physical exam.
- Phototherapy (see Glossary) to treat the symptoms if other treatments fail.
- Self-care instructions focused on the older patient.

HOME TREATMENT BY SELF OR CARE-GIVER

GENERAL INSTRUCTIONS
- See instructions under Preventing Recurrence.
- Use hand cream 4 to 8 times per day on the hands and twice daily on the trunk and extremities. When possible, apply it immediately after bathing—while the skin is wet—to trap additional moisture before evaporation occurs. Bath oils probably don't help.

MEDICATION (ADJUSTED FOR AGING)
- For minor discomfort, you may use non-prescription skin lubricants, such as petroleum jelly, mineral oil or cold cream.
- For serious discomfort, your doctor may prescribe topical cortisone creams or lotions.
- *Note:* Adverse reactions and side effects may be more frequent and severe in older persons. Remind your doctor of any medicines you already take.

ACTIVITY FOR OLDER PATIENTS
- No restrictions are necessary.
- See Appendix 20 regarding physical fitness for the active older adult.

FOOD & BEVERAGE
- No special diet is required.
- See Appendix 1 regarding good nutrition for people over 50.

FUTURE CONSIDERATIONS FOR THE AGING ADULT

POSSIBLE COMPLICATIONS—Secondary bacterial infection in the affected area.

PROBABLE OUTCOME—Usually curable with treatment, but recurrence is common unless environmental conditions can be controlled.

PREVENTING RECURRENCE—Reduce water loss from the skin by:
- Bathing less frequently and using cool water.
- Using soap sparingly.
- Patting the skin dry rather than rubbing it.
- Applying skin lubricants to dry skin before chapped areas become inflamed.
- Using humidifiers in rooms with very dry air.

CALL YOUR DOCTOR IF

- You have severely chapped skin and self-care does not relieve the symptoms in 1 week.
- Chapped skin becomes inflamed.

ILLNESSES & DISORDERS

ELECTRIC SHOCK

BASIC INFORMATION FOR OLDER ADULTS

DESCRIPTION—Electric shock is an injury caused by electricity passing through the body. Body parts involved: The total body in many cases. (THIS IS AN EMERGENCY; SEEK MEDICAL CARE IMMEDIATELY!)

SPECIAL CONSIDERATIONS FOR AGING
- Characteristic signs and symptoms of many disorders are frequently changed or absent.
- Injured tissues repair more slowly.

SIGNS & SYMPTOMS—Depend on where the current enters the body and the kind of electrical current. Following are the most common:
- Burns at points of contact. The burns are often deep.
- Heart damage, including cardiac arrest.
- Severe muscle spasms that may cause fractures.
- Breathing paralysis.
- Unconsciousness.

CAUSES & RISK FACTORS—Electric shock can result from contact with electricity from downed power lines, exposed appliance wires, faulty electrical equipment, lightning strikes or other electrical sources. Risk factors include:
- Standing on wet ground or under a tree during an electrical storm.
- Mishandling electrical equipment.
- Occupations that involve electrical machinery or lines.

DOCTOR'S TREATMENT & DIAGNOSTIC TESTS
- Emergency cardiopulmonary resuscitation (CPR) at the time of injury if the victim is unconscious and not breathing; see General Instructions.
- Diagnosis is usually obvious from the circumstances.
- Self-care instructions focused on the older patient (for minor burns only).
- Hospitalization.

HOME TREATMENT BY SELF OR CARE-GIVER

GENERAL INSTRUCTIONS
- If the victim is touching live electrical wires, shut off the power or remove the wires with a non-metal object before giving aid. Don't electrocute yourself trying to help someone else.
- If the victim is unconscious and not breathing: Yell for help. Don't leave the victim. Begin mouth-to-mouth breathing immediately. If there is no heartbeat, give external cardiac massage. Have someone call 0 (operator) or 911 (emergency) for an ambulance or medical help. Don't stop cardiopulmonary resuscitation (CPR) until help arrives.

- If multiple persons are struck, give CPR first to victims who are not moving (those who are moving are likely to recover).

MEDICATION (ADJUSTED FOR AGING)
- Medicine usually is not necessary for electric shock.
- *Note:* Adverse reactions and side effects may be more frequent and severe in older persons. Remind your doctor of any medicines you already take.

ACTIVITY FOR OLDER PATIENTS
- No restrictions are necessary if the shock is mild. If the shock is severe, you may resume your normal activities gradually as your injuries heal.
- See Appendix 20 regarding physical fitness for the active older adult.

FOOD & BEVERAGE
- No special diet is required following electric shock.
- See Appendix 1 regarding good nutrition for people over 50.

FUTURE CONSIDERATIONS FOR THE AGING ADULT

POSSIBLE COMPLICATIONS
- Pneumonia.
- Permanent brain damage.
- Severe burns of the skin and underlying muscle.
- Death from heart damage.

PROBABLE OUTCOME—Depends on the extent of injury. Full recovery is likely if major brain or heart damage does not occur.

PREVENTING RECURRENCE
- Inspect your house, especially the kitchen, bathroom and workshop, for hazards. Use grounded plugs wherever possible.
- Don't use hair dryers or radios in the bathroom where they can fall into a tub or sink.
- Use safety plugs in empty electrical outlets to prevent grandchildren from inserting metal objects.
- Don't try to repair electrical equipment unless you know how.
- Wear protective gloves and clothing for work that involves exposure to electricity.
- Replace worn cords or wiring at home or work.
- Use ground-fault electrical interrupters when possible.
- Go indoors during electrical storms. Lightning may strike several miles away from actual rainfall.

CALL YOUR DOCTOR IF

- You or someone around you receives an electric shock severe enough to cause injury. *This is an emergency!*
- Any of the following occurs during convalescence: Irregular heartbeat. Fever. Cough with sputum.

EMPHYSEMA

BASIC INFORMATION FOR OLDER ADULTS

DESCRIPTION—Emphysema is a chronic lung condition in which the microscopic sacs in the lungs (the alveoli) become overstretched, destroying the elasticity of the fibers that open and close the air sacs during breathing. Body parts involved: The alveoli.

SPECIAL CONSIDERATIONS FOR AGING
- In the lungs, the transfer of carbon dioxide and oxygen to the bloodstream becomes less efficient.
- The vital capacity of the lungs decreases.
- Obstruction of the airways becomes more common, especially among people who have smoked tobacco for many years.
- Stress from any emotional cause—fear, worry, anxiety, sadness, loneliness or anger—affects all aspects of any illness or disorder.

SIGNS & SYMPTOMS
- No symptoms in the early stages (often).
- Shortness of breath that increases in severity over several years.
- Wheezing; coughing that produces scant sputum.
- Occasional recurrent infections of the lungs or bronchial tubes; a barrel-shaped chest.
- Swelling in the legs and feet (edema).

CAUSES & RISK FACTORS—The basic cause is unknown. Causative factors include many years of cigarette smoking; air pollution; inflammation of the air sacs in the lungs; and an inherited alpha$_1$-antitrypsin deficiency. Risk factors include smoking; occupations that require forced breathing, such as glass blowing or playing a wind instrument; repeated lung infections that decrease the function of lung tissue; and allergies or a family history of allergies.

DOCTOR'S TREATMENT & DIAGNOSTIC TESTS
- Medical history and physical exam.
- Laboratory studies such as blood tests and spirometry (see Glossary); x-rays of the chest.
- Self-care instructions focused on the older patient.
- Hospitalization for complications.

HOME TREATMENT BY SELF OR CARE-GIVER

GENERAL INSTRUCTIONS
- Don't smoke; avoid breathing irritants.
- If you work in an area with severe air pollution, do all you can to decrease your exposure. Change jobs if necessary.
- Install air conditioning with a filter and humidity control in your home.
- Treat any accompanying allergies to minimize aggravation of emphysema.
- Avoid sudden temperature or humidity changes, loud talking, laughing, crying or exertion if these trigger coughing episodes.
- Floss and brush your teeth regularly to reduce the chance of oral infection.
- Elevate the foot of your bed with 4- or 5-inch blocks. This helps prevent mucus from accumulating in the lower parts of the lungs.
- Learn and practice breathing exercises. Ask your doctor for instructions.
- Supplemental oxygen may be required. Follow instructions from your doctor and equipment supplier.

MEDICATION (ADJUSTED FOR AGING)
- Your doctor may prescribe:
  Antibiotics to fight or prevent secondary infections.
  Bronchodilators to relax spasms of the bronchial tubes.
- Arrange for immunizations against influenza and pneumonia.

ACTIVITY FOR OLDER PATIENTS—Activity will be limited, but stay as active as your strength allows.

FOOD & BEVERAGE
- Drink at least 8 glasses of fluid a day. This thins lung secretions so they can be coughed up more easily.
- Your doctor may recommend a salt-restricted diet to help reduce the fluid in the body. See Appendix 9.

FUTURE CONSIDERATIONS FOR THE AGING ADULT

POSSIBLE COMPLICATIONS—Susceptibility to lung infections; chronic obstructive pulmonary disease (COPD); respiratory failure; congestive heart failure.

PROBABLE OUTCOME—Emphysema is incurable, but the symptoms can be controlled to retard the progress and severity of the disease. Although emphysema reduces life expectancy, many persons live many years with it. Without treatment, complications can be fatal.

PREVENTING RECURRENCE
- Don't smoke; avoid places with polluted air.
- Exercise moderately in fresh, clean air.
- Prevent flu and pneumonia with immunizations.
- Avoid persons with respiratory infections.
- Obtain antibiotic treatment for lung infections.

CALL YOUR DOCTOR IF

- You have symptoms of emphysema.
- Any of the following occurs after diagnosis:
  Fever.
  Blood in the sputum.
  Increased shortness of breath or shortness of breath without coughing or when at rest.
  Chest pain.
  Sputum that increases, thickens or changes color despite treatment.

ILLNESSES & DISORDERS

BASIC INFORMATION FOR OLDER ADULTS

DESCRIPTION—Empyema is an accumulation of pus between layers of infected pleura (thin membranes that cover the lungs). Body parts involved: The lungs and pleura.

SPECIAL CONSIDERATIONS FOR AGING
- Characteristic signs and symptoms of many disorders are frequently changed or absent.
- The immune system becomes less effective, opening the way for viral, bacterial and other infections; malignancies; immune disorders; and allergies.
- Decreased nutrition increases the risk of infections.

SIGNS & SYMPTOMS
- Chest pain. The pain varies from vague discomfort to a stabbing pain. It is often worse with coughing or breathing. It may extend to the lower chest wall or abdomen.
- Rapid, shallow breathing.
- Chills.
- Fever.
- Extreme fatigue.
- Bad breath.
- Weight loss.

CAUSES & RISK FACTORS
Empyema is a complication of:
- Lung or chest infections, such as pneumonia, tuberculosis or lung abscess.
- Collapsed lung or chest injury.
- Malignancy in other parts of the body.
- Collagen vascular disease, such as systemic lupus erythematosus.
- Infection in another part of the body that has spread to the chest.
- Congestive heart failure.
- Kidney disorders.
- Liver disorders.

Risk factors include:
- Poor nutrition.
- Recent illness.
- Smoking.
- Fatigue or overwork.
- Wet, cold climates.
- Crowded or unsanitary living conditions.

DOCTOR'S TREATMENT & DIAGNOSTIC TESTS
- Medical history and physical exam.
- Laboratory culture of pus from the empyema cavity.
- X-rays of the chest.
- Self-care instructions focused on the older patient.
- Hospitalization.
- Surgery to drain the pus (sometimes).

HOME TREATMENT BY SELF OR CARE-GIVER

GENERAL INSTRUCTIONS
- To reduce the chest pain, wrap the entire chest *loosely* with 2 or 3 non-adhesive, 6-inch elastic bandages or use a rib belt.
- Use a cool-mist humidifier to loosen bronchial secretions so they may be coughed up more easily.
- Practice these breathing exercises:
  Purse your lips and breathe forcefully against resistance (as if blowing out a candle) 10 times. Repeat every hour.
  Take 10 deep breaths every hour.
- Don't smoke.

MEDICATION (ADJUSTED FOR AGING)
- Your doctor may prescribe antibiotics to fight infection. The type of antibiotic will depend on the type of germ responsible and sensitivity studies (see Glossary).
- For minor pain, you may use non-prescription drugs such as acetaminophen.

ACTIVITY FOR OLDER PATIENTS—Reduce your activity level until the pain and fever are gone. Gradually return to your normal activity level. Allow 2 months for recovery.

FOOD & BEVERAGE—No special diet is required. Take vitamin supplements, and increase your fluid intake.

FUTURE CONSIDERATIONS FOR THE AGING ADULT

POSSIBLE COMPLICATIONS
- Meningitis.
- Pericarditis.
- Endocarditis.
- Brain abscess.

PROBABLE OUTCOME—Successful treatment depends on discovery and treatment of the underlying disorder. Draining the pus from the infected space hastens healing. High doses of antibiotics are needed and hospitalization is usually required.

PREVENTING RECURRENCE—Obtain medical treatment for any serious disorder or infection that may cause empyema.

CALL YOUR DOCTOR IF

- You have symptoms of empyema.
- Any of the following occurs during treatment:
  A fever develops.
  The pain increases.
  Your breathlessness worsens.
  The cough becomes dry and non-productive.
  Your fingernails or toenails turn blue or dark.
  Blood appears in the sputum.

ENDOMETRIAL HYPERPLASIA
(Adenomatous Hyperplasia of the Uterus; Adenomyosis; Adenomatosis)

BASIC INFORMATION FOR OLDER ADULTS

DESCRIPTION—Endometrial hyperplasia is an overgrowth of tissue in the endometrium (the inner lining of the uterus). This is not cancerous. Body parts involved: The uterus and the endometrium.

SPECIAL CONSIDERATIONS FOR AGING
- Repair from injury or disease is complete and effective, but recovery takes longer in older people.
- Characteristic signs and symptoms of many disorders are frequently changed or absent.

SIGNS & SYMPTOMS—Bleeding after menopause.

CAUSES & RISK FACTORS—The cause is excessive estrogen (a female hormone) that is produced by the body or results from the use of hormone-containing medications. Endometrial hyperplasia rarely occurs in women who had normal menstrual cycles prior to menopause. The risk increases with estrogen replacement therapy after menopause. If you were diagnosed when you were younger, menopause may relieve your symptoms.

DOCTOR'S TREATMENT & DIAGNOSTIC TESTS
- Medical history and physical exam.
- Laboratory tests such as blood tests of hormone levels and a Pap smear (see Glossary).
- D&C (dilatation and curettage; see Glossary) to obtain tissue for microscopic examination to rule out malignancy.
- Hysterectomy (surgery to remove the uterus) sometimes. Advancing age alone is not a deterrent.
- Self-care instructions focused on the older patient.

HOME TREATMENT BY SELF OR CARE-GIVER

GENERAL INSTRUCTIONS
- Try to reduce psychological stress that can complicate your illness and delay your recovery. If you can't resolve the stress, ask for help from family, friends or competent counselors.
- Use heat to relieve the pain. Place warm compresses or a hot water bottle on your abdomen or back.
- Take frequent warm baths to relax muscles and relieve discomfort. Sit in a tub of warm water for 10 to 15 minutes.
- Don't douche unless your doctor recommends it.

- For an explanation of the surgery and postoperative care, see Hysterectomy in the Surgeries section.

MEDICATION (ADJUSTED FOR AGING)
- If the D&C does not relieve the symptoms and you don't want a hysterectomy, your doctor will probably prescribe progesterone, a female hormone.
- Avoid aspirin, as it may increase bleeding.
- Acetaminophen may be used for pain if necessary.
- *Note:* Adverse reactions and side effects may be more frequent and severe in older persons. Remind your doctor of any medicines you already take.

ACTIVITY FOR OLDER PATIENTS
- No restrictions are necessary unless you have surgery. Then resume your activities gradually. Ask your doctor about resuming sexual relations following surgery or D&C. Don't hesitate to discuss this. It is an important part of your life.
- See Appendix 20 regarding physical fitness for the active older adult.

FOOD & BEVERAGE
- No special diet is required.
- See Appendix 1 regarding good nutrition for people over 50.

FUTURE CONSIDERATIONS FOR THE AGING ADULT

POSSIBLE COMPLICATIONS
- Perforation of the uterus and peritonitis as a complication of surgery (rare).
- Excessive, uncontrollable bleeding.

PROBABLE OUTCOME—Often curable with D&C or hysterectomy. If a woman chooses not to have surgery, hormone therapy usually controls the symptoms.

PREVENTING RECURRENCE—There are no specific preventive measures.

CALL YOUR DOCTOR IF

- You have symptoms of endometrial hyperplasia.
- The following symptoms occur during hormone treatment or after surgery or D&C:
  Excessive bleeding (saturating more than 1 pad or tampon every hour).
  Signs of infection, such as fever, general ill feeling, headache, dizziness or muscle aches.
- New, unexplained symptoms develop. Hormones used in treatment may produce side effects.

EPIDIDYMITIS

BASIC INFORMATION FOR OLDER ADULTS

DESCRIPTION—Epididymitis is an inflammation and infection of the epididymis, an oblong structure attached to the upper part of each testicle. Body parts involved: The testicles and the epididymes.

SPECIAL CONSIDERATIONS FOR AGING
- The immune system becomes less effective, opening the way for viral, bacterial and other infections; malignancies; immune disorders; and allergies.
- Injured tissues repair more slowly.
- Decreased nutrition increases the risk of infections.

SIGNS & SYMPTOMS
- An enlarged, hardened, painful testicle.
- Fever.
- Tender scrotal contents.
- Tenderness of the second testicle (sometimes).
- Acute urethritis (often).

CAUSES & RISK FACTORS
Usually epididymitis is a complication of a bacterial infection elsewhere in the body, such as:
- Gonococcal infection of the urethra.
- Prostate infection.
- Bladder or kidney infection.

Epididymitis may also complicate an infection of the scrotum or be caused by scrotal injury. The risk increases with:
- Recent illness, especially acute or chronic prostatitis, urethritis or urinary tract infection.
- Prostatectomy, cystoscopy (see Glossary) or the use of a urethral catheter.

DOCTOR'S TREATMENT & DIAGNOSTIC TESTS
- Medical history and physical exam.
- Laboratory studies such as urinalysis and culture of prostate secretions to identify the germ responsible.
- Self-care instructions focused on the older patient.

HOME TREATMENT BY SELF OR CARE-GIVER

GENERAL INSTRUCTIONS
- Support the weight of the scrotum and tender testicles. Roll a soft bath towel and place it between your legs under the inflamed area.
- Apply an ice bag, warm compresses or a hot water bottle to the inflamed parts. Use whichever relieves the pain best.
- Wear an athletic supporter or two pairs of athletic briefs when you resume normal activity.

MEDICATION (ADJUSTED FOR AGING)
- Your doctor may prescribe:
  Antibiotics to fight infection.
  Pain relievers.
  Stool softeners.
  Hormones to decrease sexual tension if necessary.
- *Note:* Adverse reactions and side effects may be more frequent and severe in older persons. Remind your doctor of any medicines you already take.

ACTIVITY FOR OLDER PATIENTS
- Rest in bed until the fever, pain and swelling improve. Don't engage in sexual intercourse. If sexual desire and erections become a problem, consult your doctor for medication. Wait at least 1 month after *all* symptoms disappear before resuming sexual relations.
- Slowly resume normal activities.
- See Appendix 20 regarding physical fitness for the active older adult.

FOOD & BEVERAGE
- Don't drink alcohol, tea, coffee or carbonated beverages. These irritate the urinary system.
- Eat natural laxative foods such as prunes, fresh fruit, whole-grain cereals and nuts to prevent constipation.
- See Appendix 1 regarding good nutrition for people over 50.

FUTURE CONSIDERATIONS FOR THE AGING ADULT

POSSIBLE COMPLICATIONS
- Constipation (sometimes) because bowel movements aggravate the pain.
- Sterility or narrowing and blockage of the urethra if the epididymitis involves both testicles. This requires surgery.

PROBABLE OUTCOME—Usually curable with treatment.

PREVENTING RECURRENCE
- Use rubber condoms during intercourse to protect yourself from venereal disease. Don't engage in sexual activity with persons who have venereal disease.
- Avoid urethral catheters if possible.

CALL YOUR DOCTOR IF

- You have symptoms of epididymitis.
- The pain is not relieved by the measures outlined above.
- You develop a fever.
- You become constipated.
- Your symptoms don't improve within 4 days after treatment begins.

ESOPHAGEAL REFLUX
(Hiatal Hernia)

BASIC INFORMATION FOR OLDER ADULTS

DESCRIPTION—Esophageal reflux is a weakness or opening in the diaphragm (the muscle that separates the chest cavity from the abdominal cavity). Part of the stomach protrudes upwards into the chest. Body parts involved: The esophagus, stomach and diaphragm.

SPECIAL CONSIDERATIONS FOR AGING
- The esophageal muscles decrease in strength.
- Stress from any emotional cause—fear, worry, anxiety, sadness, loneliness or anger—affects all aspects of any illness or disorder.

SIGNS & SYMPTOMS—Often no symptoms are felt. When there are symptoms, they usually develop within 1 hour or more after eating and include:
- "Heartburn" (a burning sensation in the area of the heart and behind the breastbone). Heartburn may be confused with heart attack symptoms.
- Belching; gastric reflux.
- Swallowing difficulty (rare).

CAUSES & RISK FACTORS—Causes include congenital weakness in the muscular ring of the diaphragm through which the esophagus passes and empties into the stomach and an abdominal injury that causes pressure that tears a hole in the diaphragm. Either can allow gastric (stomach) acid to flow backward from the stomach into the esophagus, irritating the esophagus. The hernia weakens the sphincter that controls the opening between the stomach and the esophagus. The stomach may even protrude into the lower chest. Lying flat or abdominal pressure (such as straining) may push the stomach upward. Risk factors include:
- Chronic constipation and straining during bowel movements.
- Obesity; smoking.
- Constant straining or lifting with tightening of the abdominal muscles.

DOCTOR'S TREATMENT & DIAGNOSTIC TESTS
- Medical history and physical exam.
- X-rays of the esophagus and stomach.
- Gastroscopy with a flexible gastroscope (see Glossary); biopsy (rare).
- Self-care instructions focused on the older patient.
- Surgery to close the weakness in the diaphragm and keep the stomach in its natural place (rare).

HOME TREATMENT BY SELF OR CARE-GIVER

GENERAL INSTRUCTIONS
- Raise the head of your bed 4 to 6 inches. This allows gravity to keep stomach acid away from the hernia.
- Avoid large meals. Eat 4 or 5 small meals a day instead. Don't eat anything for at least 2 hours before bedtime.
- Don't lie down or bend over immediately following a meal.
- Lose weight if you are overweight. A reducing diet appears in Appendix 10.
- Don't smoke.
- Don't wear tight pantyhose, girdles, belts or pants.
- Don't strain during bowel movements, urination or lifting.

MEDICATION (ADJUSTED FOR AGING)—Your doctor may prescribe:
- Antacids. These are most effective for some persons when they take them 1 hour before meals and at bedtime. Others find them more helpful 1 to 2 hours after meals and at bedtime. Try both ways to find the best schedule for you.
- Stool softeners.
- Drugs which hasten gastric emptying.

ACTIVITY FOR OLDER PATIENTS—No restrictions are necessary.

FOOD & BEVERAGE
- Avoid alcoholic beverages, caffeine-containing beverages (coffee, tea, cocoa and cola drinks) and any other food, juice or spice that aggravates your symptoms. Eat slowly.
- See Appendix 1 regarding good nutrition for people over 50.

FUTURE CONSIDERATIONS FOR THE AGING ADULT

POSSIBLE COMPLICATIONS
- Bleeding from the esophagus. This can be excessive, leading to shock.
- Misdiagnosis as a heart attack.

PROBABLE OUTCOME—The symptoms can usually be controlled with the suggestions listed above. If they cannot be controlled and it appears that the irritation of the esophagus is causing scarring and ulceration, the condition can be corrected with surgery.

PREVENTING RECURRENCE—There are no specific preventive measures.

CALL YOUR DOCTOR IF

- You have symptoms of a esophageal reflux, especially the sensation that food stops beneath your breastbone. Call immediately if you experience pain accompanied by shortness of breath, sweating or nausea.
- You vomit blood or have recurrent vomiting.
- Your temperature rises over 100F (37.8C).
- Your symptoms don't improve with treatment in 1 month.

ESOPHAGEAL STRICTURE OR CORROSIVE ESOPHAGITIS

 ## BASIC INFORMATION FOR OLDER ADULTS

DESCRIPTION—Esophageal stricture is a narrowing of the esophagus (the tube connecting the mouth to the stomach) caused by inflammation. The narrowing interferes with swallowing. Corrosive esophagitis is narrowing of the esophagus caused by chemical damage. Body part involved: The esophagus.

SPECIAL CONSIDERATIONS FOR AGING
- The esophageal muscles decrease in strength with aging.
- Characteristic signs and symptoms of many disorders are frequently changed or absent.
- The total digestive system becomes sluggish.

SIGNS & SYMPTOMS
- Sudden or gradual decrease in the ability to swallow. Gradual swallowing difficulty affects solid foods first, then liquids.
- Pain in the mouth and chest after eating.
- Increased salivation.
- Rapid breathing.
- Vomiting, sometimes with mucus or blood. Cancer of the esophagus often causes similar symptoms.
- Gastric reflux during sleep.

CAUSES & RISK FACTORS—Caused by scarring of the esophagus following inflammation or damage due to:
- Chronic heartburn or a hiatal hernia.
- Prolonged use of feeding tubes.
- Accidental swallowing of lye or other corrosive chemicals. *This is an emergency!*
- Deliberate swallowing of lye or other corrosive chemicals by a suicidal person.
- Bulimia.

The risk increases with the careless storage of corrosive chemicals, such as lye, kerosene, harsh detergent or bleach.

DOCTOR'S TREATMENT & DIAGNOSTIC TESTS
- Medical history and physical exam.
- Surgical diagnostic procedures such as endoscopy (see Glossary).
- X-rays of the esophagus (barium swallow).
- Hospitalization for supportive care and intravenous nutrition.
- Surgery to remove the stricture if other measures fail. Advancing age alone is not a deterrent.
- Periodic dilatation of the esophagus.
- Psychotherapy or counseling for suicidal persons.
- Self-care instructions focused on the older patient.

 ## HOME TREATMENT BY SELF OR CARE-GIVER

GENERAL INSTRUCTIONS—The stricture must be stretched regularly (about once a month) with a large, heavy dilator. Your doctor will provide specific instructions. The dilator is an inflatable bag that is swallowed and monitored fluoroscopically. The stricture will eventually return if regular treatments are not continued.

MEDICATION (ADJUSTED FOR AGING)
- Your doctor may prescribe:
  Cortisone drugs to reduce inflammation and diminish the possibility of scarring.
  Antibiotics to prevent infection.
  A drug to relax the smooth muscles, which should be taken prior to meals.
- *Note:* Adverse reactions and side effects may be more frequent and severe in older persons. Remind your doctor of any medicines you already take.

ACTIVITY FOR OLDER PATIENTS
- Resume your normal activities gradually.
- See Appendix 20 regarding physical fitness for the active older adult.

FOOD & BEVERAGE
- Eat a soft or liquid diet (see Appendix 11) after treatment until normal swallowing is possible. Avoid spicy foods that irritate the esophagus.
- Don't drink alcohol.
- See Appendix 1 regarding good nutrition for people over 50.

 ## FUTURE CONSIDERATIONS FOR THE AGING ADULT

POSSIBLE COMPLICATIONS
- Malnutrition from an inability to eat normally.
- Perforation of the damaged esophagus. This may be life-threatening.

PROBABLE OUTCOME—Usually curable with treatment. Normal swallowing can be maintained with regular treatment to stretch the stricture.

PREVENTING RECURRENCE
- Store all chemicals where they can't be mistaken for other substances.
- Avoid the prolonged use of feeding tubes.

 ## CALL YOUR DOCTOR IF

- You have symptoms of esophageal stricture or corrosive esophagitis.
- Any of the following occurs during treatment:
  Chest pain.
  Fever.
  Inability to speak.
  Feeling of air bubbles under the skin of the chest.

BASIC INFORMATION FOR OLDER ADULTS

DESCRIPTION—Esophagus cancer is a growth of tissue in the esophagus (the tube connecting the mouth to the stomach) in which cells multiply in an uncontrolled fashion. Cancer that begins in the esophagus (primary) usually occurs in the lower third of the esophagus where it passes through the chest. Body parts involved: The esophagus.

SPECIAL CONSIDERATIONS FOR AGING
- Malignant diseases are less likely to spread rapidly
- Usual signs and symptoms may be absent and be replaced by symptoms of confusion, dizziness, failure to thrive, falling, incontinence, increasing dementia, refusal to eat or drink, weight loss, depression, paranoia, hypochondriasis, psychosis or threats of suicide.
- Side effects of medication and adverse reactions are more frequent and worse.
- Stress from any emotional cause—fear, worry, anxiety, sadness, loneliness or anger—affects all aspects of any illness or disorder.

SIGNS & SYMPTOMS
- Swallowing difficulty or pain.
- Rapid weight loss.
- Regurgitation of bloody mucus.
- Respiratory infections

CAUSES & RISK FACTORS—The cause is unknown. Most esophagus cancers are primary (begin in the esophagus), but some spread from other body parts. It is not inherited. Risk factors include:
- Smoking.
- Excessive alcohol consumption.
- Previous head and neck tumors.
- Celiac disease.

DOCTOR'S TREATMENT & DIAGNOSTIC TESTS
- Medical history and physical exam.
- Biopsy (see Glossary) of the tumor.
- X-ray of the upper intestinal tract.
- Surgery to remove the cancer. Advancing age alone is not a deterrent.
- Radiation treatment (sometimes).
- Self-care instructions focused on the older patient.

HOME TREATMENT BY SELF OR CARE-GIVER

GENERAL INSTRUCTIONS
- Maintain as positive an attitude as possible during treatment.
- Treatment may cause side effects, but they are usually temporary.

- Your pain can be controlled. Don't hesitate to ask your doctor for pain medication.
- Fear may be your worst enemy.
- Call on family members and friends for whatever support and help you need.
- Esophagus cancer is a complicated, serious disorder. This page can cover only the main points of diagnosis and treatment. Your doctor, nurse or librarian can provide sources of supplemental information.

MEDICATION (ADJUSTED FOR AGING)
- Your doctor may prescribe:
  Medicine to relieve the pain.
  Tranquilizers to reduce anxiety.
  Anticancer drugs (chemotherapy) sometimes.
- *Note:* Adverse reactions and side effects may be more frequent and severe in older persons. Remind your doctor of any medicines you already take.

ACTIVITY FOR OLDER PATIENTS
- Remain as active as possible.
- See Appendix 20 regarding physical fitness for the active older adult.

FOOD & BEVERAGE—Your doctor may prescribe a special diet, depending on the treatment chosen.

FUTURE CONSIDERATIONS FOR THE AGING ADULT

POSSIBLE COMPLICATIONS—If treatment doesn't begin immediately, esophagus cancer spreads rapidly to the lungs and liver.

PROBABLE OUTCOME—This condition is currently considered incurable. Early diagnosis and aggressive treatment offer the only chance of survival. In any case, the symptoms can be relieved or controlled. Medical literature cites a few instances of unexplained recovery. Scientific research into causes and treatment continues, so there is hope for increasingly effective treatment and a cure.

PREVENTING RECURRENCE
- Don't smoke.
- Don't drink.
- Obtain medical treatment for any gastrointestinal disorder that lasts longer than 5 days.

CALL YOUR DOCTOR IF

- You have symptoms of cancer of the esophagus, especially difficulty swallowing.
- The pain becomes intolerable despite treatment.
- New, unexplained symptoms develop. The drugs used in treatment may produce side effects.

EXTRADURAL HEMORRHAGE
(Epidural Hemorrhage)

BASIC INFORMATION FOR OLDER ADULTS

DESCRIPTION—An extradural hemorrhage is bleeding between the skull and the outermost of 3 membranes that cover the brain (meninges). It may be confused with meningitis. Body parts involved: The skull, meninges and brain. (THIS IS AN EMERGENCY; SEEK MEDICAL CARE IMMEDIATELY!)

SPECIAL CONSIDERATIONS FOR AGING
- Characteristic signs and symptoms of many disorders are frequently changed or absent.
- The blood vessels are less elastic and more fragile.

SIGNS & SYMPTOMS—These symptoms develop within 24 to 96 hours after a head injury:
- A headache that steadily worsens.
- Drowsiness or unconsciousness.
- Nausea or vomiting.
- Inability to move the arms and legs.
- A change in the sizes of the eye pupils.
- Seizures.

CAUSES & RISK FACTORS—Head injury is the cause of extradural hemorrhage. Risk factors include:
- The use of anticoagulant drugs.
- Bleeding disorders, such as hemophilia, ideopathic thrombocytopenic purpura (ITT) or aplastic anemia.
- Injuries. These occur more often after excessive alcohol consumption or the use of mind-altering drugs.

DOCTOR'S TREATMENT & DIAGNOSTIC TESTS
- Medical history and physical exam.
- Laboratory studies of the blood and cerebrospinal fluid.
- Hospital diagnostic tests such as x-rays of the head, arteriography, radioscopic scan and CT scan (see Glossary for all).
- Surgery to stop the bleeding and remove blood clots.
- Self-care instructions focused on the older patient.

HOME TREATMENT BY SELF OR CARE-GIVER

GENERAL INSTRUCTIONS—No specific instructions except those under other headings.

MEDICATION (ADJUSTED FOR AGING)
- Your doctor may prescribe cortisone drugs to reduce the swelling inside the skull.
- *Note:* Adverse reactions and side effects may be more frequent and severe in older persons. Remind your doctor of any medicines you already take.

ACTIVITY FOR OLDER PATIENTS
- Stay as active as your strength allows. Work and exercise moderately. Rest when you tire. If speech or muscle control has been damaged, you may need physical therapy or speech therapy.
- See Appendix 20 regarding physical fitness for the active older adult.

FOOD & BEVERAGE
- Eat a normal, well-balanced diet. Vitamin and mineral supplements should not be necessary unless you cannot eat normally.
- See Appendix 1 regarding good nutrition for people over 50.

FUTURE CONSIDERATIONS FOR THE AGING ADULT

POSSIBLE COMPLICATIONS—Fatal compression of the brain if the bleeding lasts longer than 24 hours.

PROBABLE OUTCOME—Quick diagnosis and prompt surgery usually bring complete recovery.

PREVENTING RECURRENCE
- Get medical advice when head injuries occur.
- Avoid head injury in the following ways:
  Use seat belts in cars.
  Wear protective head gear during contact sports or while riding a bicycle or motorcycle.
  Don't drive after drinking alcohol or using mind-altering drugs.

CALL YOUR DOCTOR IF

- You have had a head injury—even if it seems minor—and you develop any symptoms of extradural hemorrhage. *This is an emergency!*
- Any of the following occurs during treatment:
  You develop a fever.
  The surgical wound becomes red, swollen or tender.
  Your headache worsens.

BASIC INFORMATION FOR OLDER ADULTS

DESCRIPTION—This disorder is characterized by the embedding of a small speck of metal, wood, stone, sand, paint or other foreign material in the eye, usually involving the conjunctiva (outer eye covering). Body parts involved: The eye and the conjunctiva. **(THIS IS AN EMERGENCY; SEEK MEDICAL CARE IMMEDIATELY!)**

SPECIAL CONSIDERATIONS FOR AGING
- Repair from injury or disease is complete and effective, but recovery takes longer in older people.
- Characteristic signs and symptoms of many disorders are frequently changed or absent.

SIGNS & SYMPTOMS
- Severe pain, irritation and redness in the eye.
- The presence of a foreign body that is visible with the naked eye (usually). Sometimes the foreign body is very small, trapped under the eyelid and invisible except with medical examination.
- A scratchy feeling with blinking.
- The symptoms may improve with the foreign body still present.

CAUSES & RISK FACTORS—The cause is accidental. Risk factors include:
- Windy weather.
- Occupations, hobbies or activities, such as carpentry or grinding, in which fine particles of wood or other materials fly loose in the air.

DOCTOR'S TREATMENT & DIAGNOSTIC TESTS
- Emergency room care (sometimes).
- Medical history and physical exam. This may include staining the eye with a harmless substance (fluorescein) to outline the object and examine the eye through a magnifying lens.
- Self-care instructions focused on the older patient.

HOME TREATMENT BY SELF OR CARE-GIVER

GENERAL INSTRUCTIONS
- Ask someone else to drive you to the doctor's office. Don't try to drive yourself.
- Don't rub the eye.
- Keep the eye closed if possible until you are examined.
- Wear an eye patch to keep the eye closed or wear dark glasses for 24 hours after removal of the foreign body to protect your eye from bright light.

- Use moist compresses to relieve discomfort after removal. Prepare them by folding a clean cloth in several layers. Dip it in warm water, wring it out slightly and apply it to the eye. Dip the compress often to keep it moist. Apply the compress for 1 hour, rest 1 hour and then repeat.

MEDICATION (ADJUSTED FOR AGING)
- Your doctor may prescribe:
  Antibiotic eye drops or ointment to prevent infection.
  Pain relievers.
  Local anesthetic eye drops.
- *Note:* Adverse reactions and side effects may be more frequent and severe in older persons. Remind your doctor of any medicines you already take.

ACTIVITY FOR OLDER PATIENTS
- Resume your normal activities gradually after removal of the foreign body and the patch if one is applied.
- See Appendix 20 regarding physical fitness for the active older adult.

FOOD & BEVERAGE
- No special diet is required.
- See Appendix 1 regarding good nutrition for people over 50.

FUTURE CONSIDERATIONS FOR THE AGING ADULT

POSSIBLE COMPLICATIONS
- Infection, especially if the foreign body is not removed completely.
- Severe, permanent vision damage caused by the penetration of deeper eye layers.

PROBABLE OUTCOME—Most objects can be removed simply under local anesthesia in a doctor's office or emergency room.

PREVENTING RECURRENCE—Wear protective eye coverings if your occupation or hobby involves the risk of eye injury.

CALL YOUR DOCTOR IF

- You have a foreign body in your eye. *This is an emergency!*
- Any of the following occurs after removal:
  The pain increases or does not disappear in 2 days.
  You develop a fever.
  Your vision changes.

EYE INJURIES
(Contusions or Lacerations of the Eye)

BASIC INFORMATION FOR OLDER ADULTS

DESCRIPTION—Eye injuries include blunt injuries (contusions) or cuts (lacerations). Body parts involved: The eyeball, eyelid, bones around the eyeball (eye socket) and muscles attached to the eyeball. (THIS IS AN EMERGENCY; SEEK MEDICAL CARE IMMEDIATELY!)

SPECIAL CONSIDERATIONS FOR AGING
- Repair from injury or disease is complete and effective, but recovery takes longer in older people.
- Side effects of medication and adverse reactions are more frequent and worse.

SIGNS & SYMPTOMS
- Swelling, redness, tenderness, pain, bleeding or bruising ("black eye") in or around the eye.
- Change in ability to see clearly.

CAUSES & RISK FACTORS
Caused by a blunt or sharp blow or cut to the eye or surrounding structures. Risk factors include:
- Fights. Fights are more likely with alcohol consumption or in hostile environments that foster aggression.
- Occupations or hobbies that expose the eye to injury, such as athletics, carpentry or steel construction work.

DOCTOR'S TREATMENT & DIAGNOSTIC TESTS
- Medical history and physical exam.
- X-rays of bone surrounding the eye.
- Treatment may include suturing a laceration.
- Hospitalization if bleeding occurs in the eye.
- Self-care instructions focused on the older patient.

HOME TREATMENT BY SELF OR CARE-GIVER

GENERAL INSTRUCTIONS
- Protect your eyes from bright light or sunlight by wearing dark glasses temporarily.
- Use ice packs or warm moist compresses to relieve the discomfort. Prepare a compress by folding a clean cloth in several layers. Dip it in warm water, wring it out slightly and apply it to the eye. Dip the compress often to keep it moist. Apply the compress for an hour, rest an hour and repeat.
- Sleep with your head elevated with 2 pillows until the symptoms subside.

MEDICATION (ADJUSTED FOR AGING)
- Your doctor may prescribe:
  Antibiotic eye drops or ointments to prevent infection.
  Pain relievers.
  Eye drops to dilate the eye pupil and rest the eye muscles (sometimes).
- *Note:* Adverse reactions and side effects may be more frequent and severe in older persons. Remind your doctor of any medicines you already take.

ACTIVITY FOR OLDER PATIENTS
- Resume your normal activities gradually after treatment.
- See Appendix 20 regarding physical fitness for the active older adult.

FOOD & BEVERAGE
- No special diet is required.
- See Appendix 1 regarding good nutrition for people over 50.

FUTURE CONSIDERATIONS FOR THE AGING ADULT

POSSIBLE COMPLICATIONS
- Permanent vision loss.
- Infection.

PROBABLE OUTCOME—Usually curable with treatment to prevent infection and suture of lacerations in and around the eye. Sutures are usually removed in about 7 days. Allow 2 weeks for complete healing.

PREVENTING RECURRENCE—Wear protective eye coverings if possible during any exposure to eye injury.

CALL YOUR DOCTOR IF

- You have a cut or other injury to your eye. *This is an emergency!*
- Any of the following occurs after eye injury:
  Fever.
  Severe eye pain that persists despite treatment.
  Vision changes.

EYE TUMOR

BASIC INFORMATION FOR OLDER ADULTS

DESCRIPTION—An eye tumor is a growth in the eye in which cell multiplication is uncontrolled and progressive. Eye tumors are of 3 types: retinoblastoma, malignant melanoma and a secondary tumor that has spread from another part of the body. An eye tumor usually involves one eye. Retinoblastoma invades both eyes in 25% of cases. Body parts involved: The eyes.

SPECIAL CONSIDERATIONS FOR AGING
- Malignant diseases are less likely to spread rapidly.
- Pupil size becomes smaller.

SIGNS & SYMPTOMS
The following are characteristic of all 3 types of eye tumors:
- Possibly no signs in the early stages except occasionally a whitish light reflection in the pupil.
- Gradual loss of vision.
- Bulging eyes (sometimes).

Retinoblastoma may have the following additional signs:
- Crossed eyes.
- A tumor that is visible through the pupil.

CAUSES & RISK FACTORS
- Melanoma and secondary tumors—Unknown.
- Retinoblastoma—Inherited tendency. The risk is greater if there is a a family history of retinoblastoma.

DOCTOR'S TREATMENT & DIAGNOSTIC TESTS
- Medical history and physical exam.
- Echography (see Glossary).
- Fluorescein dye tests (see Glossary) to outline the blood vessels in the eye.
- X-rays of the skull.
- Self-care instructions focused on the older patient.
- One of the following:
  Surgery to remove the tumor.
  Radiation therapy.
  Cryotherapy (see Glossary).
  Treatment with laser beams.

HOME TREATMENT BY SELF OR CARE-GIVER

GENERAL INSTRUCTIONS
- The surgeon will provide instructions for postoperative care.
- Maintain as positive an attitude as possible during treatment.
- Treatment may cause side effects, but they are usually temporary.
- Your pain can be controlled. Don't hesitate to ask your doctor for pain medication.
- Fear may be your worst enemy.
- Call on family members and friends for whatever support and help you need.
- An eye tumor is a complicated, serious disorder. This page can cover only the main points of diagnosis and treatment. Your doctor, nurse or librarian can provide sources of supplemental information.

MEDICATION (ADJUSTED FOR AGING)
- Your doctor may prescribe:
  Pain relievers.
  Anticancer drugs (chemotherapy).
- *Note:* Adverse reactions and side effects may be more frequent and severe in older persons. Remind your doctor of any medicines you already take.

ACTIVITY FOR OLDER PATIENTS
- After treatment, resume your normal activities as soon as possible.
- See Appendix 20 regarding physical fitness for the active older adult.

FOOD & BEVERAGE
- No special diet is required.
- See Appendix 1 regarding good nutrition for people over 50.

FUTURE CONSIDERATIONS FOR THE AGING ADULT

POSSIBLE COMPLICATIONS
- Spread to other parts of the body.
- Partial or complete loss of vision.

PROBABLE OUTCOME—Some eye tumors are curable in 6 months with medical treatment. Other eye tumors are considered incurable. A fatal spread to other body parts usually occurs rapidly. However, medical literature cites a few instances of unexplained recovery. Scientific research into causes and treatment continues, so there is hope for increasingly effective treatment and a cure.

PREVENTING RECURRENCE—Cannot be prevented at present.

CALL YOUR DOCTOR IF

- You have symptoms of an eye tumor.
- Your pain becomes intolerable during treatment.
- New, unexplained symptoms develop that may indicate the malignancy has spread to other body parts.

EYELID, DROOPING
(Ptosis)

BASIC INFORMATION FOR OLDER ADULTS

DESCRIPTION—Ptosis is the drooping of the upper eyelid, partially or completely covering the eye. Body parts involved: The upper eyelid and the eye.

SPECIAL CONSIDERATIONS FOR AGING—Muscle bulk and power decrease.

SIGNS & SYMPTOMS—Drooping of one or both eyelids, accompanied by poor blinking reflexes. The extent of the droop may vary at different times of the day.

CAUSES & RISK FACTORS—Ptosis may accompany other problems, including:
- Paralysis of the nerve fibers to the eyelids.
- Myasthenia gravis.
- Muscular dystrophy.
- Diabetes.
- Brain tumor.
- Head or eyelid injury.
- Tumor in the upper lobe of a lung.
The risk increases with a family history of ptosis.

DOCTOR'S TREATMENT & DIAGNOSTIC TESTS
- Medical history and physical exam.
- X-rays of various body regions to look for the underlying cause.
- Self-care instructions focused on the older patient.
- Some ophthalmologists recommend keeping the lid raised with a support that is part of eyeglasses.
- Surgery to strengthen the muscles of the eyelid (sometimes). Advancing age alone is not a deterrent.

HOME TREATMENT BY SELF OR CARE-GIVER

GENERAL INSTRUCTIONS
- Keep the eye moist with non-prescription artificial tears.
- Wear safety goggles to protect the eyes from injury when you are exposed to dust or flying debris.

MEDICATION (ADJUSTED FOR AGING)
- Medicine usually is not necessary for ptosis, but it may be necessary for the underlying disorder.
- *Note:* Adverse reactions and side effects may be more frequent and severe in older persons. Remind your doctor of any medicines you already take.

ACTIVITY FOR OLDER PATIENTS
- No restrictions are necessary.
- See Appendix 20 regarding physical fitness for the active older adult.

FOOD & BEVERAGE
- No special diet is required.
- See Appendix 1 regarding good nutrition for people over 50.

FUTURE CONSIDERATIONS FOR THE AGING ADULT

POSSIBLE COMPLICATIONS
- Permanent disfigurement.
- Irritation and infection in the eye caused by poor blinking reflexes and continuous contact between the eyelid and eye surface.
- Visual disturbance.

PROBABLE OUTCOME—Sometimes curable if the underlying cause can be corrected by surgery or medication.

PREVENTING RECURRENCE—There are no specific preventive measures.

CALL YOUR DOCTOR IF

- You have symptoms of ptosis.
- Ptosis worsens or vision is affected.

EYELID EDGE, INFECTION OF
(Blepharitis)

BASIC INFORMATION FOR OLDER ADULTS

DESCRIPTION—Blepharitis is an inflammation of the eyelid edges. Body parts involved: The eyelids, eyelashes, meibomian glands (which lubricate the lids) and conjunctiva (whites of the eyes).

SPECIAL CONSIDERATIONS FOR AGING
- The immune system becomes less effective, opening the way for viral, bacterial and other infections; malignancies; immune disorders; and allergies.
- The eyes develop increased sensitivity to glare.

SIGNS & SYMPTOMS
- Redness and greasy scales on the edges of one or both eyelids.
- Eyelashes that fall out.
- Small ulcers on the eyelid. If the lid edges ulcerate, crusts will form. If the crusts are removed, the lids will bleed.
- Irritation of the eye if flakes from the lid fall into the eye.
- A feeling that something is in the eye. This includes itching, burning, redness, swelling of the lid, sensitivity to bright light and tearing.
- Discharge from the lids, which glues the lashes together during sleep.

CAUSES & RISK FACTORS
Causes include:
- Bacterial infection, usually staphylococcal, of the eyelash follicles and the meibomian glands.
- Allergic reaction (for less serious inflammations only).
- Body lice (rare).

The risk increases with:
- A medical history of seborrheic dermatitis or eczema of the scalp and other body parts.
- Exposure to chemical or environmental irritants.
- Crowded or unsanitary living conditions.
- Poor nutrition.

DOCTOR'S TREATMENT & DIAGNOSTIC TESTS
- Medical history and physical exam.
- Laboratory culture of the discharge from the lids.
- Self-care instructions focused on the older patient.
- If blepharitis is caused by lice, your doctor will remove them with tweezers or medication.

HOME TREATMENT BY SELF OR CARE-GIVER

GENERAL INSTRUCTIONS
- Use warm-water soaks (see Appendix 18) to reduce inflammation and hasten healing. Apply the soaks for 20 minutes, then rest at least 1 hour. Repeat as often as needed.
- Remove the scales from the lids each day.
- Don't wear eye makeup until the inflammation subsides.
- Use baby shampoo or a washcloth to gently wash your eyelashes once a day.

MEDICATION (ADJUSTED FOR AGING)
- Your doctor may prescribe antibiotic ointment or eyedrops, which may contain cortisone drugs.
- *Note:* Adverse reactions and side effects may be more frequent and severe in older persons. Remind your doctor of any medicines you already take.

ACTIVITY FOR OLDER PATIENTS
- No restrictions are necessary.
- See Appendix 20 regarding physical fitness for the active older adult.

FOOD & BEVERAGE
- No special diet is required.
- See Appendix 1 regarding good nutrition for people over 50.

FUTURE CONSIDERATIONS FOR THE AGING ADULT

POSSIBLE COMPLICATIONS
- Loss of eyelashes.
- Ulceration of the cornea (the covering of the eye).
- Scarred eyelids.

PROBABLE OUTCOME—Blepharitis is stubbornly resistant to treatment, but it is sometimes curable in 8 to 12 months. Recurrence is common.

PREVENTING RECURRENCE
- Wash your hands often, and dry them with clean towels.
- Avoid environments that contain dust or other irritating substances.
- Use hypoallergenic eye makeup.

CALL YOUR DOCTOR IF

- You have symptoms of blepharitis.
- You have pain in the *eye*.
- Your vision changes.
- New, unexplained symptoms develop. The drugs used in treatment may produce side effects.

EYELID, INFLAMMATION OF
(Chalazion)

BASIC INFORMATION FOR OLDER ADULTS

DESCRIPTION—Chalazion is an inflammation of the eyelid that manifests itself as a mass on the eyelid resulting from the chronic inflammation of a meibomian gland (a gland which lubricates the lid). Body part involved: The eyelid.

SPECIAL CONSIDERATIONS FOR AGING
- The appetite generally becomes poorer.
- The immune system becomes less effective, opening the way for viral, bacterial and other infections; malignancies; immune disorders; and allergies.
- Repair from injury or disease is complete and effective, but recovery takes longer in older people.

SIGNS & SYMPTOMS—A painless swelling on the eyelid, which at first may resemble a sty. The eyelid may swell, and the eye may feel irritated. After a few days these early symptoms disappear, leaving a painless, slow-growing, firm lump in the eyelid. The skin over the lump can be moved loosely.

CAUSES & RISK FACTORS—An inflammation of the eyelid is caused by the blockage of a duct leading to the surface of the eyelid from the meibomian gland. The blockage may be due to an infection (usually staphylococcal) around the duct opening. The risk increases with:
- Stress.
- Fatigue or overwork.
- The use of eye cosmetics.
- Poor nutrition.

DOCTOR'S TREATMENT & DIAGNOSTIC TESTS
- Medical history and physical exam.
- Laboratory culture of the discharge.
- Self-care instructions focused on the older patient.
- Surgical removal under local anesthesia in the doctor's office if the chalazion does not heal spontaneously in 6 weeks.

HOME TREATMENT BY SELF OR CARE-GIVER

GENERAL INSTRUCTIONS—Use warm-water soaks (see Appendix 18) to reduce the inflammation and hasten healing. Apply the soaks for 20 minutes, then rest at least 1 hour. Repeat as often as needed.

MEDICATION (ADJUSTED FOR AGING)
- Your doctor may prescribe:
  Topical antibiotic ointments or creams such as erythromycin or bacitracin. Apply a thin layer of medication to the lid edges 3 or 4 times daily. A heavy layer wastes medicine and is no more beneficial than a thin layer. Antibiotic eye drops to prevent the spread of infection to other parts of the eye. Oral antibiotics or antibiotic injections usually are not needed.
- *Note:* Adverse reactions and side effects may be more frequent and severe in older persons. Remind your doctor of any medicines you already take.

ACTIVITY FOR OLDER PATIENTS
- No restrictions are necessary.
- See Appendix 20 regarding physical fitness for the active older adult.

FOOD & BEVERAGE
- No special diet is required.
- See Appendix 1 regarding good nutrition for people over 50.

FUTURE CONSIDERATIONS FOR THE AGING ADULT

POSSIBLE COMPLICATIONS—The eyelid infection may become chronic and spread to other glands in the eye.

PROBABLE OUTCOME—The inflammation may heal spontaneously. If not, it is usually curable with surgical removal.

PREVENTING RECURRENCE
- Wash your hands often, and dry them with clean towels.
- Avoid environments that contain dust or other irritating substances.
- Eat a normal, well-balanced diet.

CALL YOUR DOCTOR IF

- You have symptoms of eyelid inflammation that last longer than 2 weeks.
- You have pain in the *eye*.
- Your vision changes.
- New, unexplained symptoms develop. The drugs used in treatment may produce side effects.

EYELID, INWARD-TURNING
(Entropion)

 BASIC INFORMATION FOR OLDER ADULTS

DESCRIPTION—Entropion is a disorder of the lower eyelid (usually) in which it curls inward toward the eye. Body parts involved: One or both eyelids and the eye(s).

SPECIAL CONSIDERATIONS FOR AGING
- Characteristic signs and symptoms of many disorders are frequently changed or absent.
- The immune system becomes less effective, opening the way for viral, bacterial and other infections; malignancies; immune disorders; and allergies.
- Repair from injury or disease is complete and effective, but recovery takes longer in older people.

SIGNS & SYMPTOMS—Inflammation of the eye (swelling, redness, pain and excessive tears) caused when the inward-turning eyelid and its lashes rub against the cornea.

CAUSES & RISK FACTORS—Several different factors may cause an eyelid to turn inward:
- Relaxation of the eyelid's supporting tissue, coupled with the inward pull of the eyelid muscles.
- Chronic eye inflammation (including allergy), creating scar tissue in the eyelid.

The risk increases with aging.

DOCTOR'S TREATMENT & DIAGNOSTIC TESTS
- Medical history and physical exam.
- Self-care instructions focused on the older patient.
- Your doctor may attach a small strip of adhesive tape to the lower lid as a temporary measure before surgery.
- Minor surgery (usually) to correct the condition.

 HOME TREATMENT BY SELF OR CARE-GIVER

GENERAL INSTRUCTIONS
- Apply warm compresses to the eyelid several times a day to relieve inflammation and discomfort. To prepare the compresses:
  Pour warm water in a clean bowl.
  Soak a clean cloth in the water. Wring it out almost dry.
  Apply the warm, moist cloth to the closed eye for 10 to 15 minutes.
  Remoisten the cloth frequently.
- Wear protective glasses or goggles if you are exposed to wind or pollutants.

MEDICATION (ADJUSTED FOR AGING)
- Your doctor may prescribe:
  Artificial tears until surgery can be performed.
  Antibiotics if infection is present.
- *Note:* Adverse reactions and side effects may be more frequent and severe in older persons. Remind your doctor of any medicines you already take.

ACTIVITY FOR OLDER PATIENTS
- No restrictions are necessary.
- See Appendix 20 regarding physical fitness for the active older adult.

FOOD & BEVERAGE
- No special diet is required.
- See Appendix 1 regarding good nutrition for people over 50.

 FUTURE CONSIDERATIONS FOR THE AGING ADULT

POSSIBLE COMPLICATIONS—Ulceration of the cornea due to irritation by the eyelash and eyelid.

PROBABLE OUTCOME—Usually curable with surgery.

PREVENTING RECURRENCE—Obtain prompt medical attention for any eye infection.

 CALL YOUR DOCTOR IF

- You have symptoms of an inward-turning eyelid.
- Any of the following occurs after surgery:
  Eye pain, redness and photosensitivity.
  Your vision changes in any way.

EYELID, OUTWARD-TURNING
(Ectropion)

 BASIC INFORMATION FOR OLDER ADULTS

DESCRIPTION—Ectropion is a disorder of the lower eyelid in which it weakens and turns outward (inside out). Body parts involved: One or both eyelids and the eye(s).

SPECIAL CONSIDERATIONS FOR AGING
- Characteristic signs and symptoms of many disorders are frequently changed or absent.
- Disease in one organ system leads to problems in another system.
- Repair from injury or disease is complete and effective, but recovery takes longer in older people.

SIGNS & SYMPTOMS
- An outward turning of the lower eyelid, causing an unattractive facial appearance.
- Inflammation (pain, redness and swelling) in the affected eyelid.
- Inadequate eye lubrication caused by lubricating tears running down the cheek instead of into the eye.

CAUSES & RISK FACTORS
Causes include:
- Weakening of the muscles and tissues that normally support the lid against the eye.
- Paralysis of the nerve that supplies the eyelid muscles.
- Contraction of scar tissue from previous wounds or burns.
The risk increases with age.

DOCTOR'S TREATMENT & DIAGNOSTIC TESTS
- Medical history and physical exam.
- Minor surgery to restore normal tension to the eyelid.
- Self-care instructions focused on the older patient.

 HOME TREATMENT BY SELF OR CARE-GIVER

GENERAL INSTRUCTIONS
- Apply warm compresses to the eyelids several times a day to relieve inflammation and discomfort. To prepare the compresses: Pour warm water in a clean bowl. Soak a clean cloth in the water. Wring it out almost dry. Apply the warm, moist cloth to the closed eye for 10 to 15 minutes. Remoisten the cloth frequently.
- Wear protective glasses or goggles if you are exposed to wind or pollutants.

MEDICATION (ADJUSTED FOR AGING)
- Your doctor may prescribe: Artificial tears until surgery can be performed. Antibiotics if infection is present.
- *Note:* Adverse reactions and side effects may be more frequent and severe in older persons. Remind your doctor of any medicines you already take.

ACTIVITY FOR OLDER PATIENTS
- No restrictions are necessary.
- See Appendix 20 regarding physical fitness for the active older adult.

FOOD & BEVERAGE
- No special diet is required.
- See Appendix 1 regarding good nutrition for people over 50.

 FUTURE CONSIDERATIONS FOR THE AGING ADULT

POSSIBLE COMPLICATIONS—Damage to the cornea caused by dryness.

PROBABLE OUTCOME—Usually curable with surgery.

PREVENTING RECURRENCE—Cannot be prevented at present.

 CALL YOUR DOCTOR IF

- You have symptoms of an outward-turning eyelid.
- Any of the following occurs after surgery: Eye pain, redness and photosensitivity. Your vision changes in any way.

EYES, BULGING
(Exophthalmos; Proptosis)

 BASIC INFORMATION FOR OLDER ADULTS

DESCRIPTION—Exophthalmos is a protrusion or bulging of one or both eyes. Body parts involved: The eye(s).

SPECIAL CONSIDERATIONS FOR AGING
- The detection of thyroid disease frequently represents a diagnostic enigma in the elderly.
- There is less efficient response to physical stress (fright and flight) due to the decreased responsiveness of the adrenal glands.
- Stress from any emotional cause—fear, worry, anxiety, sadness, loneliness or anger—affects all aspects of any illness or disorder.

SIGNS & SYMPTOMS
- Bulging of the eyes, which creates a staring or frightened look.
- Double vision.
- Blurred vision.
- Pain (sometimes).
- Infrequent blinking (sometimes).

CAUSES & RISK FACTORS—Caused by a swelling of the tissue behind the eye, which could be due to:
- An overactive thyroid gland (the most common cause).
- Infection or tumor in the supportive tissues behind the eye.
- Aneurysm, blood clot or hemorrhage in the veins or arteries behind the eye.
- Injury to the eye or face.

The risk factors are unknown.

DOCTOR'S TREATMENT & DIAGNOSTIC TESTS
- Biopsy (see Glossary) of the tissue behind the eyes.
- Blood tests of thyroid function.
- Radioactive studies of thyroid function.
- X-rays of the head.
- CT scan (see Glossary).
- Surgery to:
  Remove a tumor, blood clot or aneurysm. Return the eyes to their normal positions if necessary after the underlying cause is corrected. Advancing age alone is not a deterrent.
- Self-care instructions focused on the older patient.

 HOME TREATMENT BY SELF OR CARE-GIVER

GENERAL INSTRUCTIONS
- If the disorder is caused by injury, see a doctor immediately.
- If your vision is affected, don't drive or engage in dangerous activity.
- If your eyelids don't blink properly, wear goggles to protect them from wind or dust.

MEDICATION (ADJUSTED FOR AGING)
- If your lids don't blink properly, use non-prescription lubricating eye drops.
- Your doctor may prescribe drugs to treat the underlying cause, such as:
  Antithyroid drugs for hyperthyroidism.
  Antibiotics to fight infection.
  Cortisone drugs to reduce inflammation.
- *Note:* Adverse reactions and side effects may be more frequent and severe in older persons. Remind your doctor of any medicines you already take.

ACTIVITY FOR OLDER PATIENTS
- No restrictions are necessary.
- See Appendix 20 regarding physical fitness for the active older adult.

FOOD & BEVERAGE
- No special diet is required.
- See Appendix 1 regarding good nutrition for people over 50.

 FUTURE CONSIDERATIONS FOR THE AGING ADULT

POSSIBLE COMPLICATIONS—Injury to the eye and impaired vision.

PROBABLE OUTCOME—Spontaneous recovery in most cases after the underlying cause is treated. If not, surgery can often correct any remaining protrusion.

PREVENTING RECURRENCE—Obtain prompt medical treatment for the underlying disorder.

 CALL YOUR DOCTOR IF

- You have symptoms of bulging eyes.
- Your symptoms don't improve within 5 days after treatment begins.
- New, unexplained symptoms develop. The drugs used in treatment may produce side effects.

FACIAL BONES, FRACTURE OF

BASIC INFORMATION FOR OLDER ADULTS

DESCRIPTION—The fracture of facial bones means that there are broken bones in the face. Body parts involved: The facial nerves, blood vessels, skin and bones. The facial bones include those of the upper jaw (maxilla), lower jaw (mandible), cheek (zygoma), area around the eyes (orbital) and nose. For more information about fractures of the nose, see Nose Fracture in the Illnesses section.

SPECIAL CONSIDERATIONS FOR AGING
- The total weight and density of bone decrease.
- Muscle bulk and power decrease.
- Repair from injury or disease is complete and effective, but recovery takes longer in older people.

SIGNS & SYMPTOMS—The following apply to the site of injury:
- Swelling.
- Tenderness, crepitation (a crackly feeling upon touching) or pain.
- Redness that becomes multicolored soon after injury.
- Loss of sensation in the lips and nose from nerve damage.
- Double or blurred vision.

CAUSES & RISK FACTORS—Caused by injury, especially from auto or bicycle accidents, sports injuries and fist fights. The risk increases with:
- Excessive alcohol consumption.
- A hostile, aggressive personality.
- Participation in contact sports.

DOCTOR'S TREATMENT & DIAGNOSTIC TESTS
- Medical history and physical exam.
- Laboratory blood studies to measure blood loss.
- X-rays of the skull and facial bones.
- Consultation with a plastic surgeon, oral surgeon, ophthalmologist or ear, nose and throat specialist.
- Surgery to realign fractured bones and reconstruct normal facial contours.
- Self-care instructions focused on the older patient.

HOME TREATMENT BY SELF OR CARE-GIVER

GENERAL INSTRUCTIONS
- Don't exercise to the point where you must pant for breath. Breathing may be difficult for a while.
- Protect your face from pressure. Sleep on your back.
- Don't blow your nose hard or use makeup until healing is complete.
- If your jaws are wired, learn how to release them quickly in case of emergency, such as severe coughing or vomiting.

MEDICATION (ADJUSTED FOR AGING)
- Your doctor may prescribe:
  Pain relievers.
  Antibiotics to fight infection if necessary.
- *Note:* Adverse reactions and side effects may be more frequent and severe in older persons. Remind your doctor of any medicines you already take.

ACTIVITY FOR OLDER PATIENTS
- Rest quietly for about 2 days, then resume your normal activities as your strength returns.
- See Appendix 20 regarding physical fitness for the active older adult.

FOOD & BEVERAGE—Eat a high-protein liquid diet (see Appendix 7) for several days. If your jaw is wired, the liquid diet will be necessary for up to 8 weeks. Add soft solid foods when you can. Take vitamin and mineral supplements to hasten healing.

FUTURE CONSIDERATIONS FOR THE AGING ADULT

POSSIBLE COMPLICATIONS
- Infection in the injured area.
- Permanent disfigurement.

PROBABLE OUTCOME
- Surgery usually produces good cosmetic results and a return to normal function. It should be done as soon as possible after injury.
- Teeth that have been knocked out can sometimes be replanted.
- A broken jaw is corrected by securing the teeth with wire or plastic splints so the jaw heals in its proper position. Speech will be changed while the wires are in place, but it should return to normal when they are removed. Normal vision should return if the eye is not injured. Allow about 6 weeks for recovery.

PREVENTING RECURRENCE—Avoid injury whenever possible. Wear protective headgear for contact sports or when riding motorcycles or bicycles. Use auto seat belts. Don't drive after drinking or using mind-altering drugs.

CALL YOUR DOCTOR IF

- You have a facial bone fracture.
- Any of the following occurs during treatment:
  Fever.
  Impaired vision.
  Severe headache.
  Loss of sensation in face.
  Intolerable pain.
  Illness of any kind during healing.
  Loosening of wires or splints.
- New, unexplained symptoms develop. The drugs used in treatment may produce side effects.

FAINTING
(Syncope)

BASIC INFORMATION FOR OLDER ADULTS

DESCRIPTION—Fainting is sudden, temporary loss of consciousness. Body parts involved: The circulatory system (heart and blood vessels) and the brain.

SPECIAL CONSIDERATIONS FOR AGING—Blood pressure drop is much more common upon standing following sitting or lying down.

SIGNS & SYMPTOMS
- Sudden lightheadedness.
- General weakness, then falling.
- Blurred vision (sometimes).
- Nausea (sometimes).
- Paleness and sweating.
- Rapid heartbeat and rapid breathing. If heartbeat or breathing is not present, this may be cardiac arrest rather than fainting.

CAUSES & RISK FACTORS—Fainting occurs with a sudden decrease in blood flow to the brain. This may be caused by:
- Heartbeat abnormalities (a heartbeat that is too fast, too slow or irregular).
- Prolonged straining, such as from severe coughing or attempted bowel movements when constipated.
- Sudden emotional stress or fear.
- Heart diseases that limit the amount of blood the heart pumps.
- Getting out of bed or a chair suddenly (orthostatic hypotension).
- Acute pain; epilepsy; low blood sugar.
- Heart attack (rare).

The risk increases with:
- Stress; heart disease.
- Excessive use of alcohol.
- The use of certain drugs, such as heart medications that slow the heartbeat. These include digitalis, beta-adrenergic blockers and other antihypertensive drugs.
- Hot, humid weather; being in a stuffy room.

DOCTOR'S TREATMENT & DIAGNOSTIC TESTS
- Care and observation of your symptoms by bystanders.
- If the fainting is caused by other conditions (see Causes), medical history and physical exam.
- After you have regained consciousness, self-care instructions focused on the older patient.

HOME TREATMENT BY SELF OR CARE-GIVER

GENERAL INSTRUCTIONS
- If someone faints and is *not* breathing:
  Yell for help. Don't leave the victim.
  Begin mouth-to-mouth breathing immediately.

If there is no heartbeat, give external cardiac massage.
Have someone call 0 (operator) or 911 (emergency) for an ambulance or medical help. Don't stop CPR until help arrives.
- If someone faints, *is* breathing and has a pulse, leave the person on the ground and elevate both legs. This helps return blood to the heart.
- If you feel faint, sit down immediately and bend over or lie down.
- If you are subject to frequent fainting spells, avoid activities in which fainting may endanger your life, such as climbing to high places, driving vehicles or operating dangerous machinery.

MEDICATION (ADJUSTED FOR AGING)
- Medication usually is not necessary for fainting. Medication may be necessary for underlying disorders.
- *Note:* Adverse reactions and side effects may be more frequent and severe in older persons. Remind your doctor of any medicines you already take.

ACTIVITY FOR OLDER PATIENTS—Resume your normal activities as soon as you regain consciousness.

FOOD & BEVERAGE—No special diet is required unless fainting episodes are caused by low blood sugar. If so, eat 5 or 6 small meals a day. The meals should be high in protein, high in complex carbohydrates and low in simple carbohydrates (sugar). Drink adequate fluids and avoid alcohol.

FUTURE CONSIDERATIONS FOR THE AGING ADULT

POSSIBLE COMPLICATIONS
- Injury while fainting.
- Mistaking cardiac arrest for fainting.

PROBABLE OUTCOME—Simple fainting disappears in 1 or 2 minutes.

PREVENTING RECURRENCE
- Avoid sudden changes in physical activity.
- If fainting episodes are caused by medication, consult your doctor about changing drugs.

CALL YOUR DOCTOR IF

- You see someone who has fainted and who is not breathing and has no pulse. Call for help immediately. *This is an emergency!* See General Instructions for additional emergency information.
- Someone faints and does not regain consciousness quickly.
- Fainting is a symptom of another condition (see Causes).

FARMER'S LUNG

BASIC INFORMATION FOR OLDER ADULTS

DESCRIPTION—Farmer's lung is an inflammation of the lung due to the inhalation of fungus germs from moldy hay or grain. This is an allergic response and is not contagious or cancerous. Body parts involved: The lungs.

SPECIAL CONSIDERATIONS FOR AGING
- The immune system becomes less effective, opening the way for viral, bacterial and other infections; malignancies; immune disorders; and allergies.
- Stress from social isolation increases the risk of infection.
- Decreased nutrition, common among chronically ill older people, increases the risk of any disease or disorder.

SIGNS & SYMPTOMS—In persons who are sensitive to the fungus, the following appear 4 to 8 hours after exposure to hay. They usually diminish in a few hours, but may last up to 2 weeks:
- Breathlessness (sometimes with wheezing).
- Dry cough.
- Chest pain.
- Chills and fever.
- Headache and muscle aches.

The following occur with repeated episodes over many years. All these are similar to emphysema and chronic obstructive pulmonary disease (COPD) from any cause.
- Increasing shortness of breath with wheezing on exertion.
- A cough with sputum.
- Fatigue.
- Weight loss.

CAUSES & RISK FACTORS—Caused by an allergy to the fungus in moldy hay called *micropolyspora faeni* or *thermoactinomyces vulgaris*. The time it takes to develop the allergy varies from person to person. The risk increases with:
- A family history of allergy.
- Smoking.

DOCTOR'S TREATMENT & DIAGNOSTIC TESTS
- Medical history and physical exam.
- Laboratory studies of lung function and blood.
- X-rays of the chest.
- Self-care instructions focused on the older patient.

HOME TREATMENT BY SELF OR CARE-GIVER

GENERAL INSTRUCTIONS
- Avoid exposure to moldy hay or grain.
- Obtain medical treatment for any respiratory infection, including the common cold.

MEDICATION (ADJUSTED FOR AGING)
- For minor discomfort, you may use non-prescription drugs such as:
  Cough preparations to loosen the secretions.
  Acetaminophen for the pain.
- For serious symptoms, your doctor may prescribe:
  Cortisone drugs to suppress the inflammatory response.
  Antibiotics to fight any secondary infections.
- *Note:* Adverse reactions and side effects may be more frequent and severe in older persons. Remind your doctor of any medicines you already take.

ACTIVITY FOR OLDER PATIENTS
- Resume your normal activities as soon as your symptoms improve.
- See Appendix 20 regarding physical fitness for the active older adult.

FOOD & BEVERAGE
- No special diet is required.
- See Appendix 1 regarding good nutrition for people over 50.

FUTURE CONSIDERATIONS FOR THE AGING ADULT

POSSIBLE COMPLICATIONS—Continued exposure can lead to chronic obstructive pulmonary disease (COPD) or respiratory failure.

PROBABLE OUTCOME—Usually curable—even in late stages of the disease—if exposure can be avoided.

PREVENTING RECURRENCE
- Avoid exposure to the fungus. If you cannot avoid exposure, wear a mask or hood during exposure.
- Don't smoke.
- Treat hay in silos with chemicals that prevent the growth of fungus spores.

CALL YOUR DOCTOR IF

- You have symptoms of farmer's lung.
- Any of the following occurs during or after treatment:
  Your temperature spikes to over 101F (38.3C).
  The chest pain increases.
  Your breathlessness worsens.
  Blood appears in the sputum.
  You experience unexplained weight loss.
- New, unexplained symptoms develop. The drugs used in treatment may produce side effects.

FECAL IMPACTION

BASIC INFORMATION FOR OLDER ADULTS

DESCRIPTION—Fecal impaction is a severe form of acute constipation in which a large mass of feces cannot be passed. Fecal impaction is not a serious condition, but it complicates other illnesses. Body parts involved: The lower colon and the rectum.

SPECIAL CONSIDERATIONS FOR AGING
- Colon motility decreases.
- Characteristic signs and symptoms of many disorders are frequently changed or absent.
- Daily fluid and fiber intake usually decreases.

SIGNS & SYMPTOMS
- Absence of normal bowel movements.
- A sense of fullness in the rectum with inability to pass a stool.
- Lack of urinary control.
- A firm mass in the lower left abdomen (sometimes).
- Pain or cramps (sometimes). Impaction often develops slowly without discomfort.
- Thin, watery discharge from the rectum.

CAUSES & RISK FACTORS
Causes include:
- Rectal disorders that make normal bowel movements uncomfortable, such as painful hemorrhoids or anal fissure.
- Rectal or colon tumors.
- Barium that is swallowed for x-rays of the intestinal tract.
- Loss of nerve supply to the colon or rectum, as with a spinal cord injury.
- Insufficient fiber and liquid in the diet.
The risk increases with:
- Bed rest for any condition, such as a recent heart attack, surgery or fracture.
- Back disorders with nerve pressure.
- Decreased fluid and fiber intake.
- The chronic or long-term use of laxatives.
- The use of some drugs, such as narcotic pain killers, antiparkinsonism drugs, atropine, phenothiazines or tricyclic antidepressants.

DOCTOR'S TREATMENT & DIAGNOSTIC TESTS
- Medical history and physical exam, including a rectal exam, by a doctor.
- Treatment involving the removal of the feces manually or by enema (sometimes).
- Self-care instructions focused on the older patient.

HOME TREATMENT BY SELF OR CARE-GIVER

GENERAL INSTRUCTIONS
- If your doctor prescribes it, use an oil-retention enema before and after manual removal of the impaction. Follow the instructions on the package.
- For suggestions on improving your bowel habits, see Constipation in the Illnesses section.

MEDICATION (ADJUSTED FOR AGING)
- After removal of the impaction, your doctor may prescribe laxatives or stool softeners.
- *Note:* Adverse reactions and side effects may be more frequent and severe in older persons. Remind your doctor of any medicines you already take.

ACTIVITY FOR OLDER PATIENTS
- No restrictions are necessary. Be as active as possible. Good physical fitness improves bowel function.
- See Appendix 20 regarding physical fitness for the active older adult.

FOOD & BEVERAGE
- Eat a normal, well-balanced diet with adequate fiber (see Appendix 1).
- Drink at least 8 glasses of fluid each day.

FUTURE CONSIDERATIONS FOR THE AGING ADULT

POSSIBLE COMPLICATIONS
- Persons who have had a recent (within 1 week) heart attack may suffer fatal rupture of the heart muscle while straining to pass a fecal impaction.
- Rectal prolapse (protrusion outside the body).
- Aggravation of hemorrhoids.

PROBABLE OUTCOME—Usually curable with treatment, but recurrence is common unless the underlying cause is removed.

PREVENTING RECURRENCE
- If you are confined to bed, drink extra fluids and increase your consumption of dietary fiber.
- If simple constipation develops, use a mild laxative, such as milk of magnesia, a stool softener or an enema.

CALL YOUR DOCTOR IF

- You have symptoms of a fecal impaction.
- Your normal bowel pattern changes.
- You cannot pass feces while under treatment for other conditions.

ILLNESSES & DISORDERS

FEVER OF UNDETERMINED ORIGIN (FUO)

BASIC INFORMATION FOR OLDER ADULTS

DESCRIPTION—FUO is a prolonged (3 weeks or more) temperature above 101F for which no cause is evident. Body parts involved: Any body organ or system may be the source of a fever-producing condition.

SPECIAL CONSIDERATIONS FOR AGING
- The immune system becomes less effective, opening the way for viral, bacterial and other infections; malignancies; immune disorders; and allergies.
- Decreased nutrition increases the risk of infections.
- Decreased nutrition, common among chronically ill older people, increases the risk of any disease or disorder.

SIGNS & SYMPTOMS—Fever (measured rectally) for at least 2 weeks. The fever may be intermittent.

CAUSES & RISK FACTORS
Causes include:
- Infections.
- Collagen or autoimmune diseases.
- Tumors and cancer, especially kidney cancer and leukemia.
- Self-induced in some psychologically unstable persons.
- Dehydration.

The risk increases with:
- Poor nutrition.
- Illness that has lowered resistance.
- Chemical or environmental exposure to polluted water or air.
- Travel in areas with unsanitary conditions.
- Exposure to others with contagious diseases.

DOCTOR'S TREATMENT & DIAGNOSTIC TESTS
- Maintenance of an accurate daily temperature chart.
- Medical history and physical exam. Because fever may be the first evidence of a serious condition in an early stage, your doctor may recommend thorough diagnostic testing.
- Laboratory studies such as blood studies and a urine culture (see Glossary).
- X-rays of the chest.
- Self-care instructions focused on the older patient.

HOME TREATMENT BY SELF OR CARE-GIVER

GENERAL INSTRUCTIONS—Until the fever's cause has been diagnosed, keep a daily temperature chart. Rectal temperatures are most accurate.

MEDICATION (ADJUSTED FOR AGING)
- For minor discomfort, you may use non-prescription drugs such as acetaminophen.
- Until the underlying cause is determined, your doctor may withhold prescription drugs to avoid masking the symptoms of the underlying disorder. Occasionally, in critically ill patients awaiting results of laboratory studies, the doctor may recommend a therapeutic trial of antibiotics or other drugs.
- *Note:* Adverse reactions and side effects may be more frequent and severe in older persons. Remind your doctor of any medicines you already take.

ACTIVITY FOR OLDER PATIENTS
- Be as active as you can be.
- Get plenty of bed rest.
- See Appendix 20 regarding physical fitness for the active older adult.

FOOD & BEVERAGE
- No special diet is required.
- See Appendix 1 regarding good nutrition for people over 50.

FUTURE CONSIDERATIONS FOR THE AGING ADULT

POSSIBLE COMPLICATIONS—Depend on the underlying condition causing the fever.

PROBABLE OUTCOME—Spontaneous recovery in about 10% of cases. In other cases, the outcome depends on successful detection and treatment of the underlying disorder.

PREVENTING RECURRENCE—There are no specific preventive measures.

CALL YOUR DOCTOR IF

- You have an unexplained fever that lasts longer than 24 hours.
- New symptoms develop. They may provide a clue about the underlying cause of the fever.

FIBROCYSTIC BREAST DISEASE
(Chronic Cystic Mastitis)

BASIC INFORMATION FOR OLDER ADULTS

DESCRIPTION—Fibrocystic breast disease is a disorder of the female breast characterized by non-malignant lumps. Body parts involved: The breasts.

SPECIAL CONSIDERATIONS FOR AGING
- Many body changes occur as a result of estrogen deficiency beginning at menopause. These include vaginal dryness, shortening and narrowing of the vagina, greater susceptibility to vaginal infections, frequent bladder infections, reductions in the size of the clitoris and increased facial hair. Changes in other systems of the body may lead to a greater tendency to osteoporosis, hardening of the arteries and other disorders.
- Fat decreases in tissue just below the skin.

SIGNS & SYMPTOMS—Lumps in the breasts with the following characteristics:
- The lumps are usually on both sides. Solitary lumps may occur, but multiple lumps are common.
- The lumps offer resistance when pressed with the fingertips, and they may be tender.
- The lumps may be accompanied by generalized breast pain.
- The lumps are of different sizes. When the lumps are relatively large and near the surface, they can be moved freely within the breast.
- Lumps deep within the breast may be indistinguishable from breast cancer.

CAUSES & RISK FACTORS—The cause is unknown, but it is probably related to estrogen and other hormones produced by the ovaries. Preliminary studies indicate that smoking cigarettes is associated with a higher incidence and greater extent of fibrocystic breast disease.

DOCTOR'S TREATMENT & DIAGNOSTIC TESTS
- Medical history and physical exam.
- Mammogram (see Glossary).
- Surgical diagnostic procedures such as biopsy or cyst aspiration (see Glossary).
- Self-care instructions focused on the older patient.

HOME TREATMENT BY SELF OR CARE-GIVER

GENERAL INSTRUCTIONS
- Examine your breasts carefully each month (see Appendix 14). Report any changes in lumps that have been previously diagnosed to your doctor.
- Visit your doctor at least every 6 months for a breast exam or other studies, especially if you have a a family history of cancer.

MEDICATION (ADJUSTED FOR AGING)
- To decrease the size of lumps or inhibit the formation of new lumps, your doctor may prescribe:
  Vitamin E.
  Female hormones.
- *Note:* Adverse reactions and side effects may be more frequent and severe in older persons. Remind your doctor of any medicines you already take.

ACTIVITY FOR OLDER PATIENTS
- No restrictions are necessary.
- See Appendix 20 regarding physical fitness for the active older adult.

FOOD & BEVERAGE
- No special diet is required, but avoid smoking, caffeine, chocolate and cola drinks.
- See Appendix 1 regarding good nutrition for people over 50.

FUTURE CONSIDERATIONS FOR THE AGING ADULT

POSSIBLE COMPLICATIONS—Misdiagnosis. Some lumps appear to be benign, but are cancerous. Diagnostic studies, including biopsy, are often necessary to rule out malignancy.

PROBABLE OUTCOME
- Women with fibrocystic breast disease continue to have breast lumps that appear and dissolve; some remain permanently. The disorder is presently incurable, but it does not jeopardize health.
- Some cysts can be aspirated in a doctor's office, causing the lump to disappear. If the lump does not disappear completely after aspiration, it may be cancerous and should be diagnosed by biopsy and microscopic analysis.

PREVENTING RECURRENCE—Until research is conclusive, avoid smoking.

CALL YOUR DOCTOR IF

- You have undiagnosed lumps in a breast.
- You detect a change in a lump or new lumps appear.
- Nipple discharge appears.
- You have not had a breast exam in 2 years.
- New, unexplained symptoms develop. Hormones used in treatment may produce side effects.

FIBROID TUMORS OF THE UTERUS
(Myomas; Leiomyomas)

 BASIC INFORMATION FOR OLDER ADULTS

DESCRIPTION—Fibroid tumors of the uterus are abnormal growths of cells in the muscular wall of the uterus (myometrium). The term "fibroids" is misleading. The cells are not fibrous; they are composed of abnormal muscle cells. Uterine fibroids are almost always benign (not cancerous). Body parts involved: The uterus and the cervix (sometimes).

SPECIAL CONSIDERATIONS FOR AGING
- Fibroids usually, but not always, decrease in size after menopause.
- Stress from any emotional cause—fear, worry, anxiety, sadness, loneliness or anger—affects all aspects of any illness or disorder.

SIGNS & SYMPTOMS
- No symptoms (often).
- Bleeding after menopause.
- Painful sexual intercourse or bleeding after intercourse.
- Anemia (weakness, fatigue and paleness).
- Feelings of pressure on the urinary bladder or rectum.
- Increased vaginal discharge (rare).

CAUSES & RISK FACTORS—The cause is
unknown; however, fibroids may be hereditary. Some studies indicate that women with fibroids may have higher levels of the human growth hormone. The risk increases with genetic factors. Fibroid tumors are 3 to 5 times more common in black women than in Caucasian women.

DOCTOR'S TREATMENT & DIAGNOSTIC TESTS
- Medical history and physical exam.
- Laboratory studies such as sonography, laparoscopy or hysterosalpingogram (see Glossary for all).
- Self-care instructions focused on the older patient.
- Hospitalization if surgery is necessary. Fibroids are generally removed surgically if they cause excessive bleeding or become malignant.

 HOME TREATMENT BY SELF OR CARE-GIVER

GENERAL INSTRUCTIONS
- If your doctor recommends surgery, ask for a full explanation and discussion before making a decision.
- Record the dates of bleeding and the number of pads or tampons you use each day.

MEDICATION (ADJUSTED FOR AGING)
- Your doctor may prescribe iron supplements if you are anemic from excessive blood loss.
- *Note:* Adverse reactions and side effects may be more frequent and severe in older persons. Remind your doctor of any medicines you already take.

ACTIVITY FOR OLDER PATIENTS
- No restrictions are necessary.
- See Appendix 20 regarding physical fitness for the active older adult.

FOOD & BEVERAGE
- No special diet is required.
- See Appendix 1 regarding good nutrition for people over 50.

 FUTURE CONSIDERATIONS FOR THE AGING ADULT

POSSIBLE COMPLICATIONS—Malignant change in the fibroid tumor (occurs in fewer than 0.5% of cases). This rare complication is usually signaled by very rapid growth.

PROBABLE OUTCOME
- These tumors usually decrease in size without treatment after menopause.
- Fibroids can often be removed surgically without removing the entire uterus.

PREVENTING RECURRENCE—Cannot be prevented at present.

 CALL YOUR DOCTOR IF

- You have symptoms of a fibroid tumor.
- A fibroid tumor has been diagnosed and the symptoms become more severe.
- You saturate a pad or tampon more often than once an hour.

FIBROSITIS
(Fibromyositis or Fibromyalgia)

BASIC INFORMATION FOR OLDER ADULTS

DESCRIPTION—Fibrositis is an inflammation of the muscles, muscle sheaths and connective tissue layers of the tendons, muscles, bones and joints. Body parts involved: The muscular areas of the low back, neck, shoulders, chest, arms, hips and thighs.

SPECIAL CONSIDERATIONS FOR AGING
- The immune system becomes less effective, opening the way for viral, bacterial and other infections; malignancies; immune disorders; and allergies.
- The percentage of muscle tissue decreases.

SIGNS & SYMPTOMS
- Stiffness and weakness.
- Sudden, painful muscle spasms ("charley horses") that worsen with activity.
- Nodules or localized areas that are tender to the touch (trigger points).
- Painful muscle areas.
- Fatigue.
- Difficulty remaining asleep.

CAUSES & RISK FACTORS—The cause is unknown. Risk factors include:
- Stress.
- Muscle injury.
- Exposure to dampness or cold.
- A medical history of disorders that produce joint inflammation, such as rheumatoid arthritis or polyarteritis.
- Viral infections.
- Poor nutrition.
- Fatigue or overwork.
- Poor posture.
- Starting a vigorous exercise program.

DOCTOR'S TREATMENT & DIAGNOSTIC TESTS
- Medical history and physical exam.
- Laboratory blood studies to measure inflammation and tests to rule out rheumatoid arthritis or polymyalgia. There is no specific test for fibromyositis.
- Self-care instructions focused on the older patient.

HOME TREATMENT BY SELF OR CARE-GIVER

GENERAL INSTRUCTIONS
- Heat relieves the pain. Take hot showers (let the water beat on painful areas), whirlpool or plain tub baths in hot water. Use warm compresses.
- Have someone gently massage painful areas.

MEDICATION (ADJUSTED FOR AGING)
- For minor discomfort, you may use non-prescription drugs such as aspirin, acetaminophen or ibuprofen.
- Your doctor may prescribe: Cortisone injections into "trigger points." Non-steroidal anti-inflammatory drugs.
- *Note:* Adverse reactions and side effects may be more frequent and severe in older persons. Remind your doctor of any medicines you already take.

ACTIVITY FOR OLDER PATIENTS
- Stay as active as possible, even when you are in pain.
- Have your doctor recommend an appropriate exercise program. Start exercising slowly.
- See Appendix 20 regarding physical fitness for the active older adult.

FOOD & BEVERAGE
- No special diet is required.
- See Appendix 1 regarding good nutrition for people over 50.

FUTURE CONSIDERATIONS FOR THE AGING ADULT

POSSIBLE COMPLICATIONS
- Muscle atrophy; disability.
- The abuse of pain-killing medications.

PROBABLE OUTCOME—Spontaneous recovery in some persons. Other persons may have flare-ups and remissions indefinitely. The disease is uncomfortable, but not life-threatening. The symptoms can be controlled with treatment.

PREVENTING RECURRENCE—Avoid risk factors when possible.

CALL YOUR DOCTOR IF

- You have symptoms of fibrositis that last more than 2 or 3 days.
- New, unexplained symptoms develop. The drugs used in treatment may produce side effects.

BASIC INFORMATION FOR OLDER ADULTS

DESCRIPTION—This disorder is an imbalance in the mixture of water and salts (electrolytes) needed for normal body function. Necessary salts include sodium, potassium, calcium, bicarbonate and phosphate. Body parts involved: The total body. All body parts—even hard bone—are bathed in a precise blend of water and natural salts.

SPECIAL CONSIDERATIONS FOR AGING
- Daily fluid intake usually decreases with aging.
- Total body water decreases.
- The percentage of muscle tissue decreases.
- Side effects of medication and adverse reactions are more frequent and worse.

SIGNS & SYMPTOMS—Depend on whether water or salts are out of proportion. The following may indicate either:
- Dry mouth.
- Wrinkled skin.
- Increased, decreased or absent urination.
- Fatigue.
- Puffy legs, hands, face or abdomen.
- Lung congestion.
- Weakness and confusion.
- Heartbeat irregularities.
- Lightheadedness.

CAUSES & RISK FACTORS
- Fluids and salts may be *lost* by vomiting; diarrhea; heavy perspiration; some medications, such as diuretics; and the use of nasogastric tubes during hospitalization.
- Fluid and salts may *accumulate* from congestive heart failure; excessive intravenous fluids; acute or chronic kidney failure; diabetes insipidus; adrenal disease; chronic lung disease; and the use of cortisone drugs, female hormones or sodium bicarbonate.

The risk increases with fever; diarrhea and/or vomiting; kidney disease; diabetes mellitus; heart disease; unusual or extreme diets; anorexia nervosa or bulimia; alcoholism; and the use of diuretics and other medicines.

DOCTOR'S TREATMENT & DIAGNOSTIC TESTS
- Medical history and physical exam.
- Laboratory studies of the urine, stool, blood and electrolytes—especially sodium, chloride and potassium.
- Radioactive studies of total body water.
- After diagnosis of a minor imbalance, self-care instructions focused on the older patient.
- For a serious imbalance, hospitalization to receive intravenous fluids and treatment, including treatment of the underlying cause.

HOME TREATMENT BY SELF OR CARE-GIVER

GENERAL INSTRUCTIONS
- Keep a fluid-balance record during serious illnesses at home. Record the liquids you take in each day (use a measuring cup to estimate). Measure and record how much urine you pass each day. Ask your doctor if he wants a specimen for testing.
- Weigh yourself daily on an accurate home scale. Any sudden weight increase or decrease may indicate fluid changes.

MEDICATION (ADJUSTED FOR AGING)
- For fluid loss, your doctor may prescribe: Salt-containing drinks to make at home. Intravenous fluids during hospitalization.
- For fluid accumulation and sodium overload, your doctor may prescribe diuretics and potassium supplements.
- *Note:* Adverse reactions and side effects may be more frequent and severe in older persons. Remind your doctor of any medicines you already take.

ACTIVITY FOR OLDER PATIENTS—Rest in bed until your strength returns.

FOOD & BEVERAGE
- For a serious fluid imbalance, your doctor may withhold solid food until the fluid balance returns to normal.
- See Appendix 1 regarding good nutrition for people over 50.

FUTURE CONSIDERATIONS FOR THE AGING ADULT

POSSIBLE COMPLICATIONS—Heartbeat irregularities; cardiac arrest and death.

PROBABLE OUTCOME—Usually curable in 24 to 48 hours with early treatment, depending on the underlying cause.

PREVENTING RECURRENCE
- For vomiting or diarrhea, take small amounts of clear liquids, such as fruit juice, sodas, tea or gelatin water every 30 minutes. A replacement solution of 1 pint water, 1 teaspoon sugar and 1/2 teaspoon salt may help (mix carefully).
- Use commercial replacement solutions.
- During serious illness, keep a fluid-balance record (see General Instructions).

CALL YOUR DOCTOR IF

- You have symptoms of a fluid and electrolyte imbalance or dehydration.
- Your weight increases or decreases 4 or more pounds in 1 day.

FOLLICULITIS, BACTERIAL

BASIC INFORMATION FOR OLDER ADULTS

DESCRIPTION—Bacterial folliculitis is a superficial or deep bacterial irritation and infection of the hair follicles of the skin. This is contagious. Body part involved: The skin anywhere on the body, but usually that of the exposed areas of the arms, legs and neck and the beard area of the face.

SPECIAL CONSIDERATIONS FOR AGING
- The immune system becomes less effective, opening the way for viral, bacterial and other infections; malignancies; immune disorders; and allergies.
- The fatty layer of tissue under the skin becomes thinner.
- The sweat glands produce less sweat.
- Signs and symptoms may differ significantly from those listed below.

SIGNS & SYMPTOMS—Pustules (small white blisters with pus inside) with the following characteristics:
- The pustules are yellow-white and surrounded by narrow red rings.
- The pustules are 1mm to 2mm in size; there may be few or many.
- The pustules discharge a blood-stained pus of dead cells.
- Some pustules are pierced by hairs; others may be adjacent to hair follicles.

CAUSES & RISK FACTORS
Causes include:
- Infection of the hair follicles with staphylococcus bacteria, usually after minor skin injury. The infection is spread to other parts of the body by the fingernails, frequently from staphylococcus in the nose.
- Infection with *pseudomonas* bacteria following the use of contaminated hot tubs or spas. This is rare but increasing.

Risk factors include:
- Contact with an infected person.
- Recent illness, such as a nose infection.
- Diabetes.
- Eczema or dermatitis.
- Crowded or unsanitary living conditions.
- Inflammation or chronic skin abrasion (such as from tight clothing or chronic rubbing).

DOCTOR'S TREATMENT & DIAGNOSTIC TESTS
- Medical history and physical exam.
- Laboratory culture of the discharge from the pustule (rare).
- Self-care instructions focused on the older patient.

HOME TREATMENT BY SELF OR CARE-GIVER

GENERAL INSTRUCTIONS
- Don't scratch the pustules. The germs that cause them can be transferred from under the fingernails to other parts of the body.
- Use warm-water soaks (see Appendix 18) to relieve the itching and hasten healing.
- Shower frequently in preference to taking tub baths.
- Wash the clothing worn next to your skin in boiling water.

MEDICATION (ADJUSTED FOR AGING)
- If there are only a few pustules, you may use non-prescription topical antibiotics such as bacitracin, mycitracin or neomycin. Apply and gently massage a small amount into the affected areas 3 or 4 times a day. Use only the small amount needed for coverage; larger quantities don't help.
- If there are many pustules, your doctor may prescribe injections or oral antibiotics, such as erythromycin or dicloxacillin, to fight infection.

ACTIVITY FOR OLDER PATIENTS—Resume your normal activities as soon as your symptoms improve.

FOOD & BEVERAGE—No special diet.

FUTURE CONSIDERATIONS FOR THE AGING ADULT

POSSIBLE COMPLICATIONS—The infection may enter the bloodstream and spread to other body parts.

PROBABLE OUTCOME
- Without treatment, boils or deep skin infections may develop.
- Without treatment, an individual pustule heals in 7 days. But as some heal, new ones appear.
- Treatment will shorten the course of the infection. Healing should be complete in 2 weeks. However, recurrence is common.

PREVENTING RECURRENCE
- Keep skin clean. Scrub skin twice daily with an antibacterial soap. Use separate towels and washcloths.
- Avoid hot, humid environments, which foster bacterial growth.

CALL YOUR DOCTOR IF

- The pustules spread despite treatment.
- You develop a fever.
- Your ankles swell.
- You develop a boil or signs of spreading infection.
- The symptoms of bacterial folliculitis recur after treatment.

FOLLICULITIS, FUNGAL

BASIC INFORMATION FOR OLDER ADULTS

DESCRIPTION—Fungal folliculitis is a superficial or deep fungal irritation and infection of the hair follicles of the skin. It is contagious and may resemble a herpes infection. Body parts involved: The skin on the hands, arms, legs, face and scalp.

SPECIAL CONSIDERATIONS FOR AGING
- The immune system becomes less effective, opening the way for viral, bacterial and other infections; malignancies; immune disorders; and allergies.
- The fatty layer of tissue under the skin becomes thinner.
- The sweat glands produce less sweat.
- Signs and symptoms may differ significantly from those listed below.

SIGNS & SYMPTOMS—Plaques (patches or flat areas) with clearly defined borders and pustules (small, white blisters with pus inside) on top. The pustules are 1mm to 2mm in diameter and frequently appear in clusters.

CAUSES & RISK FACTORS—Caused by a fungus infection that produces a small abscess next to the hair follicle. Risk factors include:
- Illness that has lowered resistance.
- Diabetes.
- Eczema or dermatitis.
- Exposure to heat and high humidity.
- Drugs that suppress the immune system (immunosuppressants).

DOCTOR'S TREATMENT & DIAGNOSTIC TESTS
- Medical history and physical exam.
- Laboratory culture of the pustule.
- Self-care instructions focused on the older patient.

HOME TREATMENT BY SELF OR CARE-GIVER

GENERAL INSTRUCTIONS
- Avoid injury to the skin.
- Women should use depilatory creams instead of razors.
- Men should not shave during treatment until lesions on the face heal.

MEDICATION (ADJUSTED FOR AGING)
- Your doctor may prescribe griseofulvin (an oral antifungal medication) and topical antifungal agents. Follow the directions on the label. These medications may cause side effects or adverse reactions. The side effects usually disappear when your body adjusts to the drug or the drug is discontinued.
- *Note:* Adverse reactions and side effects may be more frequent and severe in older persons. Remind your doctor of any medicines you already take.

ACTIVITY FOR OLDER PATIENTS
- No restrictions are necessary.
- See Appendix 20 regarding physical fitness for the active older adult.

FOOD & BEVERAGE
- No special diet is required.
- See Appendix 1 regarding good nutrition for people over 50.

FUTURE CONSIDERATIONS FOR THE AGING ADULT

POSSIBLE COMPLICATIONS—Bacterial folliculitis and fungal folliculitis are difficult to differentiate. Fungal folliculitis may be misdiagnosed and treated with steroid creams, which aggravate the disorder.

PROBABLE OUTCOME—Usually curable in 6 weeks with treatment.

PREVENTING RECURRENCE
- Protect your skin as much as possible from minor injury.
- Avoid hot, humid environments.

CALL YOUR DOCTOR IF

- You have symptoms of fungal folliculitis.
- Any of the following occurs during treatment: Signs of spreading infection (redness, swelling, warmth and pain). Fever over 101F (38.3C).
- New, unexplained symptoms develop. The drugs used in treatment may produce side effects.

FRACTURES, BONE

BASIC INFORMATION FOR OLDER ADULTS

DESCRIPTION—A bone fracture is a complete or incomplete break in a bone. This is a serious problem in older people and seems to trigger disorders in many other body systems. The following are different types of fractures:

- Complete fracture—The broken bone is completely separated.
- Incomplete (greenstick) fracture—The broken bone is not completely separated.
- Comminuted fracture—There are more than 2 bone fragments at the fracture site.
- Open (compound) fracture—The fractured bone has broken the skin.
- Closed fracture (including stress fracture)—The fractured bone has not broken the skin.
- Compression fracture—The break occurs due to extreme pressure on the bone.
- Impacted fracture—The broken ends have been driven into each other.
- Avulsion fracture—Force has been applied to a strong tendon, causing it to pull on and break off a portion of bone.
- Pathologic fracture—A break occurs due to minor injury in bone that has been weakened or destroyed by disease.

Body parts involved: The bones and surrounding areas.

SPECIAL CONSIDERATIONS FOR AGING
- The bones become thinner.
- Bone strength decreases.
- Muscle bulk and power decrease.

SIGNS & SYMPTOMS
- Pain and swelling at the fracture site.
- Tenderness close to the fracture.
- Paleness and deformity (sometimes).
- Loss of pulse below the fracture, usually in an extremity. *This is an emergency!*
- Numbness, tingling or paralysis below the fracture (rare). *This is an emergency!*
- Bleeding or bruising at the site.
- Weakness and inability to bear weight.

CAUSES & RISK FACTORS—Caused by injury. The risk increases with osteoporosis, falls, tumors of the bone or bone marrow and reckless behavior that increases the chance of an injury or auto accident.

DOCTOR'S TREATMENT & DIAGNOSTIC TESTS
- Medical history and physical exam.
- Laboratory studies to determine blood loss.
- X-rays of injured parts; CT scan; bone scan.
- Almost all fractures require immobilization with casts or splints.
- Hospitalization for anesthesia and treatment of severe fractures.
- Surgery if the fracture must be repaired with rods, plates or screws.
- Physical therapy for rehabilitation.
- Self-care instructions focused on the older patient.

HOME TREATMENT BY SELF OR CARE-GIVER

GENERAL INSTRUCTIONS
- Seek emergency first aid care.
- See additional information regarding fractures and the care of casts in Appendix 17.

MEDICATION (ADJUSTED FOR AGING)—Your doctor may prescribe pain relievers; muscle relaxants.

ACTIVITY FOR OLDER PATIENTS
- There may be special exercises to maintain muscle tone. Consult your doctor.
- Resume your normal activities as soon as your symptoms improve.

FOOD & BEVERAGE—No special diet is required. Take vitamin C and zinc supplements to promote bone healing.

FUTURE CONSIDERATIONS FOR THE AGING ADULT

POSSIBLE COMPLICATIONS
- Failure to heal (non-union); shock.
- Travel of a fat embolus (clump of fat cells) from the injury site to the lungs or brain.
- Obstruction of nearby arteries.
- Compartment syndrome (swelling of an injured muscle within a confined compartment surrounded by an unyielding envelope of tissue or a cast).

PROBABLE OUTCOME—Usually curable with skillful first aid and aftercare. The broken bone should be manipulated, realigned and immobilized as soon as possible. Realignment is much more difficult after 6 hours. Healing time varies. Recovery is complete when there is no bone motion at the fracture site and x-rays show complete healing.

PREVENTING RECURRENCE
- Don't drive after drinking alcohol or using mind-altering drugs.
- Wear protective gear for sports.
- Use your auto seat belt or harness.
- If you have osteoporosis, adhere to your treatment program and avoid situations in which injury is likely.

CALL YOUR DOCTOR IF

- You have symptoms of a bone fracture.
- Any of the following occurs after immobilization or surgery *(report any of these signs to your doctor immediately!)*:
  Swelling above or below the fracture site.
  Severe, persistent pain.
  Blue or gray skin below the fracture site, especially under the nails.
  Numbness or loss of feeling below the fracture site.

FROSTBITE

BASIC INFORMATION FOR OLDER ADULTS

DESCRIPTION—Frostbite is temporary or permanent tissue damage from exposure to subfreezing temperature. Body parts involved: The arms and legs (especially the fingers and toes); the face (especially the nose and ears).

SPECIAL CONSIDERATIONS FOR AGING
- Characteristic signs and symptoms of many disorders are frequently changed or absent.
- The skin becomes thinner.
- There is less efficient response to physical stress (fright and flight) due to the decreased responsiveness of the adrenal glands.
- The temperature regulation mechanism (the thalamus) becomes less efficient.

SIGNS & SYMPTOMS
During exposure:
- Gradual numbness, hardness and paleness in the affected area.

Upon rewarming:
- Pain and tingling or burning (sometimes severe) in the affected area, with color change from white to red, then purple.
- Blisters (in severe cases).
- Shivering; slurred speech; memory loss.

CAUSES & RISK FACTORS—Caused by the formation of ice crystals in the skin and blood vessels leading to tissue injury or tissue death, depending on the temperature and the length of exposure. Risk factors include:
- Diabetes mellitus; peripheral neuropathy.
- Blood vessel disease such as Raynaud's phenomenon.
- Smoking; excessive alcohol consumption.
- Windy weather, which increases the chill factor.

DOCTOR'S TREATMENT & DIAGNOSTIC TESTS
- Medical history and physical exam.
- X-rays of damaged areas.
- Self-care until medical help is available.
- Hospitalization (sometimes).
- Surgery to remove permanently damaged (gangrenous) tissue (sometimes).

HOME TREATMENT BY SELF OR CARE-GIVER

GENERAL INSTRUCTIONS—The following instructions apply to emergency care until medical care is available:
- Treat hypothermia first. See Hypothermia in the Illnesses section.
- Upon reaching shelter, remove the clothing from the frostbitten parts.
- *Never* massage damaged tissue.

- Immerse the affected parts in warm water (about 100F or 37.8C). Use a thermometer if one is available. Higher temperatures may cause further injury.
- Drink warm fluids with a high sugar content if available.
- Don't smoke.
- After rewarming, cover the affected areas with soft cloth bandages.
- Don't use the affected limbs until you have medical attention. If your feet are involved, don't walk.
- Maintain body-to-body contact with any companion.

MEDICATION (ADJUSTED FOR AGING)
- Your doctor may prescribe:
  Analgesics, including narcotics, to relieve severe pain. Don't use strong pain killers longer than 4 to 7 days.
  Antibiotics to fight infection.
- You may use non-prescriptions drugs such as acetaminophen for minor pain.

ACTIVITY FOR OLDER PATIENTS—Resume your normal activities after treatment.

FOOD & BEVERAGE—No special diet.

FUTURE CONSIDERATIONS FOR THE AGING ADULT

POSSIBLE COMPLICATIONS
- Amputation of dead or infected tissue, especially fingers, toes, the nose or ears, following severe exposure.
- Cardiac arrest if frostbite is accompanied by total body hypothermia.

PROBABLE OUTCOME—For mild cases, full recovery is possible with treatment. Severe cases usually require amputation of the affected part.

PREVENTING RECURRENCE
- Anticipate sudden temperature changes and carry a jacket, gloves, socks, hat and scarf.
- Don't drink or smoke prior to anticipated exposure.
- Continue to move your arms and legs.

CALL YOUR DOCTOR IF

- You have symptoms of frostbite or observe them in someone else.
- Any of the following occurs during treatment: Increased pain, swelling, redness or drainage at the site of injury.
  Fever, muscle aches, dizziness or a general ill feeling.
- New, unexplained symptoms develop. The drugs used in treatment may produce side effects.

GALLBLADDER, INFECTION OF
(Cholecystitis or Cholangitis)

BASIC INFORMATION FOR OLDER ADULTS

DESCRIPTION—An infection of the gallbladder involves the gallbladder (cholecystitis) or the ducts that drain bile from the gallbladder to the small intestine (cholangitis). It may be confused with hepatitis, pancreatitis or duodenal ulcer. Body parts involved: The gallbladder (located under the liver) and the bile ducts in the liver leading to the gallbladder.

SPECIAL CONSIDERATIONS FOR AGING
- The immune system becomes less effective, opening the way for viral, bacterial and other infections; malignancies; immune disorders; and allergies.
- Gallbladder function becomes sluggish.

SIGNS & SYMPTOMS
- Cramping pain in the upper right side of the abdomen. Pain may also occur in the chest (imitating a heart attack), in the upper back or in the right shoulder. These symptoms frequently follow a meal that is rich in fats.
- Tenderness in the upper abdomen.
- Nausea and vomiting.
- Belching.
- Slight fever. If high fever and chills occur, a bacterial infection is present.
- Jaundice (sometimes).
- Pale stools (sometimes).
- Skin itching (sometimes).

CAUSES & RISK FACTORS—Caused by an inflammation or a bacterial infection, which are usually caused by gallstone formation and the blockage of bile ducts. The risk increases with:
- A diet that is high in fat.
- Gallstones, whether or not they have caused symptoms.
- Chronic or acute pancreatitis.
- Coronary artery disease.
- A family history of gallbladder disease.

DOCTOR'S TREATMENT & DIAGNOSTIC TESTS
- Medical history and physical exam.
- Laboratory blood studies.
- X-rays of the gallbladder.
- Ultrasonography (see Glossary) of the gallbladder and the bile ducts.
- Radioisotope studies (see Glossary) of the liver and pancreas.
- Destruction of gallstones by lithotripsy (sometimes; see Glossary).
- Surgery to remove an infected gallbladder and gallstones. Gallstone surgery is rarely an emergency.
- Hospitalization (usually).
- Following treatment, self-care instructions focused on the older patient.

HOME TREATMENT BY SELF OR CARE-GIVER

GENERAL INSTRUCTIONS—After an acute attack, consider having elective surgery to prevent a future emergency.

MEDICATION (ADJUSTED FOR AGING)
- Don't medicate yourself with non-prescription pain relievers during an attack. These may mask the symptoms of a bacterial infection, allowing it to worsen and delaying treatment.
- Your doctor may prescribe analgesics, including narcotics, to relieve the pain.

ACTIVITY FOR OLDER PATIENTS—Rest in bed until the symptoms disappear or recovery from surgery is complete. While in bed, move your legs often to reduce the likelihood of deep-vein blood clotting. You may read or watch TV.

FOOD & BEVERAGE
- Because of nausea and vomiting, intravenous fluids are usually necessary during attacks. Begin taking clear liquids or a non-fat diet as soon as you can tolerate solid foods.
- See Appendix 1 regarding good nutrition for people over 50.

FUTURE CONSIDERATIONS FOR THE AGING ADULT

POSSIBLE COMPLICATIONS
- Gallbladder rupture and peritonitis.
- Gallbladder abscess.
- Misdiagnosis as a heart attack.

PROBABLE OUTCOME—The symptoms of some mild attacks subside spontaneously in 1 to 4 days if no complications develop. Most episodes require hospitalization and treatment. Recurrences are common. Attacks will cease with surgery to remove the gallbladder.

PREVENTING RECURRENCE
- Avoid any food that gives you indigestion.
- Have surgery to remove gallstones, even if they cause no symptoms.

CALL YOUR DOCTOR IF

- You have symptoms of a gallbladder infection. If the symptoms are accompanied by shortness of breath, sweating and nausea, *call immediately!*
- Any of the following occurs during an attack:
  Fever.
  Jaundice.
  Recurrent vomiting.
  Intolerable pain.

GALLSTONES
(Cholelithiasis)

BASIC INFORMATION FOR OLDER ADULTS

DESCRIPTION—Gallstones are stones in the gallbladder (the organ under the liver that stores bile). Most gallstones are composed primarily of cholesterol and are not cancerous. An estimated 25% of people over 50 will develop gallstones. Body parts involved: The gallbladder and the bile ducts.

SPECIAL CONSIDERATIONS FOR AGING
- The immune system becomes less effective, opening the way for viral, bacterial and other infections; malignancies; immune disorders; and allergies.
- Gallbladder function becomes sluggish.
- Nutrition frequently becomes suboptimal.

SIGNS & SYMPTOMS
- Colicky pain in the upper right abdomen or between the shoulder blades.
- Nausea and vomiting.
- Bloating or belching.
- Intolerance of fatty foods (indigestion, bloating and belching).
- Jaundice.
- No symptoms in about 40% of cases.

CAUSES & RISK FACTORS—The cause is unknown, but the most common theories are:
- Failure of the gallbladder to empty competently.
- Alterations in the bile mucus.
- Increased bilirubin (see Glossary) concentration in the bile.
- Infection in the tubes that carry bile out of the liver.

Risk factors include:
- Recent illness, such as coronary artery disease, cirrhosis of the liver or a disorder of the small intestine.
- A family history of gallstones.
- Genetic factors. Some ethnic groups are more susceptible. For example, about 70% of American Indians have gallstones.
- Obesity.
- Excessive alcohol consumption.

DOCTOR'S TREATMENT & DIAGNOSTIC TESTS
- Medical history and physical exam.
- Laboratory studies such as blood count, blood chemistry, CT scan (see Glossary) and ultrasound (see Glossary).
- X-rays of the gallbladder.
- Self-care instructions focused on the older patient.
- Surgery to remove the gallbladder and stones in the bile ducts. Advancing age alone is not a deterrent. For more information, see Gallbladder Removal in the Surgeries section.
- Shockwave treatment (lithotripsy).

- An experimental procedure in which a tube is inserted into the gallbladder and a solution that dissolves cholesterol is flushed through.

HOME TREATMENT BY SELF OR CARE-GIVER

GENERAL INSTRUCTIONS
- If you know you have gallstones and experience pain in the upper right abdomen, apply heat to the area. If the pain worsens or continues more than 3 hours, call your doctor.
- Surgery for gallstones that cause no symptoms is controversial. You and your doctor should discuss the benefits and risks before making a decision.

MEDICATION (ADJUSTED FOR AGING)
- For minor discomfort, you may use non-prescription drugs such as acetaminophen.
- Your doctor may prescribe oral medication to try to dissolve the stones. This treatment is still experimental.
- *Note:* Adverse reactions and side effects may be more frequent and severe in older persons. Remind your doctor of any medicines you already take.

ACTIVITY FOR OLDER PATIENTS
- No restrictions are necessary, except to rest during attacks of gallbladder colic.
- See Appendix 20 regarding physical fitness for the active older adult.

FOOD & BEVERAGE
- During an attack sip water occasionally, but don't eat.
- At other times, eat a low-fat diet (see Appendix 8).

FUTURE CONSIDERATIONS FOR THE AGING ADULT

POSSIBLE COMPLICATIONS—Infection or rupture of the gallbladder.

PROBABLE OUTCOME—Many persons with gallstones have no symptoms. For those who do, the disorder is curable with surgery.

PREVENTING RECURRENCE
- There are no specific preventive measures, except a low-fat diet (see Appendix 8).
- After an initial attack, a second attack is more likely to occur within 2 years.

CALL YOUR DOCTOR IF

- You have symptoms of gallstones.
- You develop a fever.

GANGRENE

BASIC INFORMATION FOR OLDER ADULTS

DESCRIPTION—Gangrene is dead tissue, usually due to the loss of the blood supply to the tissue, which develops when a wound becomes infected or tissue is destroyed by an accident. Body parts involved: Any body part, but the most common are the toes, feet, legs, fingers, hands and arms. The most dangerous are the abdominal organs.

SPECIAL CONSIDERATIONS FOR AGING
- The immune system becomes less effective, opening the way for viral, bacterial and other infections; malignancies; immune disorders; and allergies.
- Decreased nutrition, common among chronically ill older people, increases the risk of any disease or disorder.
- Older people are more likely to have multiple disorders.

SIGNS & SYMPTOMS
- Black skin with dead underlying muscle and bone.
- Crepitation of the skin. This feels like air bubbles under the skin.
- Swelling.
- Pain or loss of sensation in the affected area.
- Bad-smelling discharge from ulcers in dead tissues.
- A fever up to 101F (38.3C).

CAUSES & RISK FACTORS—Gangrene occurs when the blood flow to a body part is blocked or severely reduced. Blood flow may be interrupted by infection with *clostridia perfringens* germs that enter the body through a wound or cut; tissue injury caused by accidents, surgery or deep puncture wounds; a crushing injury that cuts off the blood supply; a blood clot in an artery; hardening of the arteries; and prolonged frostbite. Risk factors include:
- Diabetes mellitus.
- Smoking, which impairs blood circulation.
- Excessive alcohol consumption, which interferes with blood vessel function.

DOCTOR'S TREATMENT & DIAGNOSTIC TESTS
- Medical history and physical exam.
- Cultures from the gangrene site or blood.
- X-rays of any suspicious area to detect gas in the tissues.
- During convalescence, self-care instructions focused on the older patient.
- Tetanus immunization.
- Time in a hyperbaric chamber (a depressurization chamber) to halt the progress of gangrene.
- Surgery to remove dead tissue, sometimes by amputation.
- Physical therapy if amputation is necessary.

HOME TREATMENT BY SELF OR CARE-GIVER

GENERAL INSTRUCTIONS—After surgery or intensive hospital care:
- Don't smoke!
- Wear sterile gloves to change your dressings.
- Place any materials that touch ulcerated areas in double plastic bags and destroy them.
- Have whirlpool treatments and massages to increase circulation.

MEDICATION (ADJUSTED FOR AGING)— Your doctor may prescribe:
- Antibiotics—usually intravenously in the early stages—to fight infection.
- Pain relievers.
- Anticoagulants to prevent blood clotting.

ACTIVITY FOR OLDER PATIENTS—Rest in bed until the gangrene stops progressing and healing begins. Then resume activity gradually. Move your legs frequently while you are in bed to prevent blood clots in the deep veins.

FOOD & BEVERAGE
- Eat a high-protein, high-calorie diet while your body is repairing damaged tissue.
- Take vitamin and mineral supplements, including zinc. Ask your doctor for advice.
- Drink adequate fluids (6 to 8 glasses daily).

FUTURE CONSIDERATIONS FOR THE AGING ADULT

POSSIBLE COMPLICATIONS
- Blood poisoning; shock.
- DIC (disseminated intravascular coagulation), a blood-clotting disorder.
- Limb amputation to prevent death.

PROBABLE OUTCOME—Usually curable in the early stages with antibiotic treatment and surgery to remove dead tissue. Without treatment, gangrene may lead to fatal infection.

PREVENTING RECURRENCE
- If you have diabetes, adhere closely to your treatment program to control diabetes. Examine your feet often for signs of unhealthy tissue. Keep your nails trimmed. Wear comfortable, well-fitting shoes.
- If you have hardening of the arteries, see Atherosclerosis in the Illnesses section for preventive measures.
- Consult your doctor for signs of infection (warmth, swelling, redness, pain or tenderness) in a skin injury.

☎ CALL YOUR DOCTOR IF

- You have symptoms of gangrene.
- You have persistent pain despite medication and treatment.
- Fever develops during convalescence.

GENITAL ITCHING
(Pruritus Vulvae)

BASIC INFORMATION FOR OLDER ADULTS

DESCRIPTION—Pruritus vulvae is an acute or chronic disorder of the skin around the vulva (the vaginal lips) that is common in women over 45. This disorder is characterized by severe itching. It is not contagious. Body parts involved: The vulva and the surrounding skin.

SPECIAL CONSIDERATIONS FOR AGING
- The skin becomes dryer and rougher.
- The skin becomes thinner.
- Many body changes occur as a result of estrogen deficiency beginning at menopause. These include vaginal dryness, shortening and narrowing of the vagina, greater susceptibility to vaginal infections, frequent bladder infections, reductions in the size of the clitoris and increased facial hair. Changes in other systems of the body may lead to a greater tendency to osteoporosis, hardening of the arteries and other disorders.
- Stress from any emotional cause—fear, worry, anxiety, sadness, loneliness or anger—affects all aspects of any illness or disorder.

SIGNS & SYMPTOMS
- Intense itching, sensitivity and irritation in the genital area. The skin may be dry.
- A thin, white vaginal discharge (sometimes).
- Discomfort during sexual intercourse.

CAUSES & RISK FACTORS—Causes include skin disease, such as psoriasis or lichen planus; systemic disease, such as diabetes; atrophy and dryness caused by estrogen deficiency; skin reaction to irritants, such as toilet tissue, soap, douches, deodorants, powders, perfumes and fabric; systemic allergies, including food allergies; and disorders of the vagina, such as vaginitis. Risk factors include:
- Stress.
- Hot, humid weather.
- Diabetes mellitus.
- Lack of urinary control.

DOCTOR'S TREATMENT & DIAGNOSTIC TESTS
- Medical history and physical exam.
- Self-care instructions focused on the older patient.
- Doctor's treatment if self-care isn't effective in 2 weeks.

HOME TREATMENT BY SELF OR CARE-GIVER

GENERAL INSTRUCTIONS
- Follow the suggestions under Preventing Recurrence.
- Keep the area as dry and cool as possible. Wear loose clothing.
- Don't scratch the itchy area. Scratching will aggravate the soreness and irritation.

- Wash the genital area with water and unscented soap only once a day.
- Use a lubricant, such as a lubricating jelly or baby oil, during intercourse.
- After urinating or having a bowel movement, clean the genital area gently with absorbent cotton or antiseptic wipes. Wipe from front to back (vagina to anus). Use petroleum jelly to help relieve the symptoms.
- Don't douche or use talcum powder.
- Pouring a glass of warm water over genital area when urinating will lessen the burning sensation.

MEDICATION (ADJUSTED FOR AGING)
- You may use low-potency, non-prescription steroid creams or ointments. If these are not effective, your doctor may prescribe:
  More potent steroid creams or lotions to reduce the inflammation. These require 24 to 36 hours to provide relief.
  Ointments that contain hormones.
  Benzodiazepines or antihistamines at night to ensure rest.
- *Note:* Adverse reactions and side effects may be more frequent and severe in older persons. Remind your doctor of any medicines you already take.

ACTIVITY FOR OLDER PATIENTS—Avoid overexertion, heat and excessive sweating.

FOOD & BEVERAGE—No special diet is required, but avoid foods to which you may be allergic.

FUTURE CONSIDERATIONS FOR THE AGING ADULT

POSSIBLE COMPLICATIONS—Secondary bacterial infection of the inflamed skin.

PROBABLE OUTCOME—Home treatment usually provides relief in 4 to 7 days. If medical treatment becomes necessary, allow 2 weeks for recovery.

PREVENTING RECURRENCE
- Wear cotton rather than nylon underpants.
- Avoid contact with the irritants listed above.
- Obtain medical treatment for underlying causes.

CALL YOUR DOCTOR IF

- You have symptoms of genital itching.
- Your symptoms don't improve in 2 weeks despite treatment.
- Scratching leads to skin infection.
- New, unexplained symptoms develop. The drugs used in treatment may produce side effects.

BASIC INFORMATION FOR OLDER ADULTS

DESCRIPTION—Giardiasis is a bowel infection caused by a parasite found in contaminated food or water. Body part involved: The gastrointestinal tract, especially the small bowel.

SPECIAL CONSIDERATIONS FOR AGING
- The immune system becomes less effective, opening the way for viral, bacterial and other infections; malignancies; immune disorders; and allergies.
- Colon motility decreases.

SIGNS & SYMPTOMS
- Sudden diarrhea and abdominal cramping. Some persons have only mild diarrhea and indigestion.
- Loose, bulky, bad-smelling stools.
- A slight fever (uncommon).

CAUSES & RISK FACTORS—Caused by infestation by a microscopic parasite, *giardia lamblia*. Giardia parasites enter the body through food or water and multiply in the small intestine. Local inflammation, causing diarrhea and other symptoms, occurs in 1 or 2 days to 3 weeks. Risk factors include:
- Crowded or unsanitary living conditions, especially a substandard water supply and poor sanitation system.
- Institutional living.
- Drinking stream water while camping.
- Previous stomach surgery. Stomach acid normally provides some protection against this infection.
- Oral-anal sexual practices.

DOCTOR'S TREATMENT & DIAGNOSTIC TESTS
- Medical history and physical exam. Tell your doctor if you have been traveling or camping in the previous month.
- Laboratory stool studies to detect parasites. May need to be repeated if early studies are negative.
- Self-care instructions focused on the older patient.

HOME TREATMENT BY SELF OR CARE-GIVER

GENERAL INSTRUCTIONS
- Prevention is the best treatment. Be cautious when you are away from normal water supplies.
- Practice careful personal hygiene if you have diarrhea or are around those who do.

MEDICATION (ADJUSTED FOR AGING)
- Don't use non-prescription drugs for gastrointestinal problems. These can mask symptoms.
- Your doctor may prescribe an antiparasite drug, metronidazole, which is very effective. Alcohol interacts with metronidazole to cause abdominal cramps and nausea, so don't drink alcohol during treatment.
- Since stool examinations are frequently false positive, your doctor may treat on the basis of clinical history and examination.
- *Note:* Adverse reactions and side effects may be more frequent and severe in older persons. Remind your doctor of any medicines you already take.

ACTIVITY FOR OLDER PATIENTS
- No restrictions are necessary.
- See Appendix 20 regarding physical fitness for the active older adult.

FOOD & BEVERAGE
- Maintain an adequate fluid intake (at least 8 glasses of water or liquid a day).
- See Appendix 1 regarding good nutrition for people over 50.

FUTURE CONSIDERATIONS FOR THE AGING ADULT

POSSIBLE COMPLICATIONS
- Chronic bowel inflammation.
- Malabsorption and weight loss.
- Dehydration.

PROBABLE OUTCOME—Spontaneous recovery in about 1 month for most persons. Medication hastens recovery.

PREVENTING RECURRENCE
- Boil water that is not known to be safe or treat it with commercial chemical purifiers.
- Avoid uncooked foods that may have been rinsed in contaminated water.
- Wash your hands often, especially before meals, to avoid catching the infection from other persons.

CALL YOUR DOCTOR IF

- You have symptoms of giardiasis.
- New, unexplained symptoms develop. The drugs used in treatment may produce side effects.

BASIC INFORMATION FOR OLDER ADULTS

DESCRIPTION—Acute glaucoma is a condition of the eye in which the fluid that normally drains into and out of the eye is suddenly obstructed. The obstruction causes severe pain and loss of vision. Body parts involved: The eye(s). **(THIS IS AN EMERGENCY; SEEK MEDICAL CARE IMMEDIATELY!)**

SPECIAL CONSIDERATIONS FOR AGING
- This medical problem is much more likely to occur in older persons.
- The pupil size becomes smaller.
- Stress from any emotional cause—fear, worry, anxiety, sadness, loneliness or anger—affects all aspects of any illness or disorder.

SIGNS & SYMPTOMS
- Severe, throbbing eye pain and headache.
- Redness in the eye.
- Blurred vision or halos around lights.
- A tender, firm eyeball.
- A dilated, fixed pupil.
- A swollen upper eyelid.
- Vomiting and weakness (due to severe eye pain).

CAUSES & RISK FACTORS—The cause is unknown. Risk factors include:
- A family history of glaucoma or farsightedness.
- Emotional upsets.
- Smoking.

DOCTOR'S TREATMENT & DIAGNOSTIC TESTS
- Medical history and physical exam.
- Laboratory studies such as tonometry (measurement of the pressure within the eyeball).
- Hospitalization during the attack until the pressure in the eye decreases.
- Surgery (iridectomy with a laser beam) to prevent further attacks—if other treatment is unsuccessful.
- Self-care instructions focused on the older patient.

HOME TREATMENT BY SELF OR CARE-GIVER

GENERAL INSTRUCTIONS
- Avoid emotional upset, which raises pressure in the eye.
- Don't smoke. Tobacco constricts the blood vessels, reducing the blood supply to the eye.

- Acute glaucoma is a complicated, serious disorder. This page can cover only the main points of diagnosis and treatment. Your doctor, nurse or librarian can provide sources of supplemental information.

MEDICATION (ADJUSTED FOR AGING)
- Your doctor may prescribe:
  Eye drops to lower the pressure inside the eye. Follow the instructions and schedule carefully, even if the symptoms subside or the eye drops are occasionally uncomfortable.
  Diuretics to decrease the fluid pressure in the eye.
  Pain relievers.
- *Note:* Adverse reactions and side effects may be more frequent and severe in older persons. Remind your doctor of any medicines you already take.

ACTIVITY FOR OLDER PATIENTS
- After treatment, resume your normal activities gradually, but avoid fatigue. Resume sexual relations when the eye pressure is under control.
- See Appendix 20 regarding physical fitness for the active older adult.

FOOD & BEVERAGE—Eat a low-salt diet (see Appendix 9).

FUTURE CONSIDERATIONS FOR THE AGING ADULT

POSSIBLE COMPLICATIONS—Total blindness in the affected eye if treatment is delayed or unsuccessful.

PROBABLE OUTCOME—The symptoms can be controlled if treatment begins quickly.

PREVENTING RECURRENCE—Consult your doctor regularly for checkups to detect glaucoma before symptoms begin. If you are over 40, have the pressure inside the eye checked at least once a year. The test is simple and painless.

CALL YOUR DOCTOR IF

- You have symptoms of acute glaucoma. *This is an emergency!*
- New, unexplained symptoms develop. The drugs used in treatment may produce side effects.

GLAUCOMA, CHRONIC
(Open-Angle Glaucoma)

BASIC INFORMATION FOR OLDER ADULTS

DESCRIPTION—Chronic glaucoma is a condition of the eye in which the fluid that normally drains into and out of the eye is gradually obstructed. This causes loss of vision. Chronic glaucoma—unlike acute glaucoma—usually causes no pain. Body parts involved: The eye(s).

SPECIAL CONSIDERATIONS FOR AGING
- This medical problem is much more likely to occur in older persons.
- The pupil size becomes smaller.
- Stress from any emotional cause—fear, worry, anxiety, sadness, loneliness or anger—affects all aspects of any illness or disorder.

SIGNS & SYMPTOMS
Early stages:
- Loss of peripheral vision in small areas.
- Blurred vision on one side toward the nose.

Later stages:
- Larger areas of vision loss, usually in both eyes.

Late stages:
- A hard eyeball.
- Halos around lights.
- Blind spots.
- Poor night vision.

CAUSES & RISK FACTORS—The symptoms are caused by pressure in the eyeball that damages the fibers in the optic nerve. Glaucoma is probably hereditary, but it may be suspected in any person who requires frequent lens changes, has mild headaches or vague visual disturbances or sees halos around electric lights or whose vision does not adapt well from light to dark. Risk factors include:
- A family history of acute or chronic glaucoma.
- Emotional stress.
- Smoking.

DOCTOR'S TREATMENT & DIAGNOSTIC TESTS
- Medical history and physical exam.
- Laboratory studies such as tonometry (measurement of the pressure within the eyeball).
- Self-care instructions focused on the older patient.
- Surgery (if other treatment is unsuccessful or unfeasible).

HOME TREATMENT BY SELF OR CARE-GIVER

GENERAL INSTRUCTIONS
- Avoid emotional upheavals and fatigue, which increase pressure in the eye.
- Don't smoke. Tobacco constricts the blood vessels, restricting the blood supply to the eye.

- Chronic glaucoma is a complicated, serious disorder. This page can cover only the main points of diagnosis and treatment. Your doctor, nurse or librarian can provide sources of supplemental information.

MEDICATION (ADJUSTED FOR AGING)
- Your doctor may prescribe:
  Eye drops to lower the pressure inside the eye. Follow the instructions and schedule carefully, even if the symptoms subside or eye drops are occasionally uncomfortable. Use the drops 4 to 5 times daily.
  Diuretics to reduce excess fluid.
- *Note:* Adverse reactions and side effects may be more frequent and severe in older persons. Remind your doctor of any medicines you already take.

ACTIVITY FOR OLDER PATIENTS
- Resume your normal activities gradually.
- See Appendix 20 regarding physical fitness for the active older adult.

FOOD & BEVERAGE—Eat a low-salt diet (see Appendix 9).

FUTURE CONSIDERATIONS FOR THE AGING ADULT

POSSIBLE COMPLICATIONS—Loss of vision before other symptoms begin.

PROBABLE OUTCOME—The symptoms can usually be controlled with treatment. Glaucoma treatment is lifelong. Vision is usually not impaired permanently if glaucoma is treated.

PREVENTING RECURRENCE
- Make sure that the tension in the eyeball is measured with every eye examination (at least once a year after age 40).
- Tell your doctor of any changes in your ability to see.

CALL YOUR DOCTOR IF

- You have symptoms of chronic glaucoma.
- Medicine in the eye becomes intolerable.
- Any sign of eye infection develops, such as fever.
- Pain begins in the eye.
- Redness occurs in the eye.
- Your vision changes suddenly.

GLOMERULONEPHRITIS
(Post-Infectious, Acute or Chronic Glomerulonephritis)

BASIC INFORMATION FOR OLDER ADULTS

DESCRIPTION—Glomerulonephritis is an inflammation of the glomeruli (the small, round filters in the kidneys). Damaged glomeruli cannot effectively filter waste products from the bloodstream. Body parts involved: The kidneys.

SPECIAL CONSIDERATIONS FOR AGING
- The blood flow to the kidneys decreases.
- The immune system becomes less effective, opening the way for viral, bacterial and other infections; malignancies; immune disorders; and allergies.

SIGNS & SYMPTOMS—Mild glomerulonephritis produces no symptoms. Diagnosis is possible only with urine studies. Severe glomerulonephritis produces the following:
- Smoky or slightly red urine.
- A general ill feeling.
- Drowsiness.
- Nausea or vomiting.
- Headaches.
- Fever (sometimes).
- Appetite loss.
- Decreased urination.
- Fluid accumulation in the body, especially puffy eyes and ankles.
- Shortness of breath.
- High blood pressure.
- Protein in the urine.
- Disturbed vision.

CAUSES & RISK FACTORS—Acute glomerulonephritis follows a streptococcal infection. The most common infection sites are the throat and the skin. Kidney symptoms usually begin 2 or 3 weeks after the strep infection. Chronic glomerulonephritis is rare and may have different causes than acute glomerulonephritis. The risk increases with:
- Exposure to people in public places where strep infections can be transmitted.
- Autoimmune disorders.
- Lupus erythematosus (one of the connective tissue diseases).

DOCTOR'S TREATMENT & DIAGNOSTIC TESTS
- Medical history and physical exam.
- Laboratory studies such as blood counts, repeated urinalyses to determine the presence of protein or other abnormal elements and streptococcal antibody titer (a sophisticated blood study).
- Kidney function tests and biopsy of a small portion of kidney tissue.
- Self-care instructions focused on the older patient.
- Hospitalization (in severe cases).

HOME TREATMENT BY SELF OR CARE-GIVER

GENERAL INSTRUCTIONS
- Record your temperature 3 times a day.
- Collect and record the amount of urine passed in each 24-hour period. Occasionally some of this collection should be analyzed in the doctor's office.

MEDICATION (ADJUSTED FOR AGING)—
Your doctor may prescribe:
- Cortisone or cytotoxic drugs if the illness is severe.
- Diuretics to increase urination.
- Antihypertensives if high blood pressure accompanies the illness.
- Iron and vitamin supplements if anemia develops.

ACTIVITY FOR OLDER PATIENTS
- Stay in bed, except to go to the bathroom, until all signs of illness have passed. This may be several weeks or months. Bed rest ensures an adequate blood flow to the kidneys; blood flow is best when lying down.
- Resume your normal activities after recovery. Your doctor will determine when all signs and symptoms have disappeared.

FOOD & BEVERAGE
- As long as your kidneys function properly, you may eat a normal, well-balanced diet. Greatly decrease the sodium in your diet.
- Your doctor may prescribe a special diet to reduce the load on the kidneys.

FUTURE CONSIDERATIONS FOR THE AGING ADULT

POSSIBLE COMPLICATIONS—Kidney failure, which may require dialysis or other dramatic treatment.

PROBABLE OUTCOME—The symptoms subside in 2 weeks to several months.

PREVENTING RECURRENCE
- Avoid exposure to people with strep infection.
- Consult your doctor for antibiotic treatment of any infection that may be strep.

CALL YOUR DOCTOR IF

- You have symptoms of glomerulonephritis.
- Any of the following occur during treatment:
  Severe headache or convulsion.
  Failure to pass at least 22 ounces of urine in a 24-hour period.
  Fever.
  Skin rash.
  Increased fluid retention.
  Increased nausea, vomiting or diarrhea.

GONORRHEA

BASIC INFORMATION FOR OLDER ADULTS

DESCRIPTION—Gonorrhea is an infectious disease of the reproductive organs that is sexually transmitted (a venereal disease). Body parts involved: Males—the urethra; females—the urethra and reproductive system; both sexes—the rectum, throat, joints and eyes (sometimes).

SPECIAL CONSIDERATIONS FOR AGING
- The immune system becomes less effective, opening the way for viral, bacterial and other infections; malignancies; immune disorders; and allergies.
- Characteristic signs and symptoms of many disorders are frequently changed or absent.
- Disease in one organ system leads to problems in another system.

SIGNS & SYMPTOMS
- Burning urination.
- Thick green-yellow discharge from the penis or vagina.
- Little or no fever.
- Pain or tenderness with sexual intercourse (sometimes).
- Rectal discomfort and discharge (sometimes).
- Joint pain.
- A rash, especially on the palms.
- Mild sore throat (sometimes).

Females often have few or no symptoms. Males usually have more pronounced symptoms.

CAUSES & RISK FACTORS—Caused by an infection from gonococcus bacteria that grow well on delicate, moist tissue. The bacteria are usually transmitted sexually, but some cases are of unknown origin. Sexual activity involving the rectum or the mouth may transmit infection to those areas if either partner is infected. Risk factors include:
- Many sexual partners, whether heterosexual or homosexual.
- Rape.

DOCTOR'S TREATMENT & DIAGNOSTIC TESTS
- Medical history and physical exam.
- Blood studies.
- Laboratory culture and microscopic analysis of the discharge from the vagina, urethra, rectum or throat.
- Hospitalization for complications.

OTHER—This condition must be reported to the local health department to prevent its spread. Your cooperation is important, and your confidentiality will be maintained.

HOME TREATMENT BY SELF OR CARE-GIVER

GENERAL INSTRUCTIONS
- Use separate linens and disposable eating utensils during treatment.
- Wash your hands frequently, especially after urination and bowel movements.
- Don't touch your eyes with your hands.
- Inform all sexual contacts so they can seek treatment and avoid infecting others. They may have the disease even if symptoms aren't apparent.

MEDICATION (ADJUSTED FOR AGING)
- Your doctor will prescribe antibiotics to fight the infection.
- You may take non-prescriptions drugs such as acetaminophen or aspirin to reduce the discomfort—but not in place of antibiotics. Home remedies or folk medicine treatments are ineffective.

ACTIVITY FOR OLDER PATIENTS—No restrictions are necessary, except don't resume sexual activity until a follow-up culture shows the infection is cured.

FOOD & BEVERAGE—No special diet is required. Reduce your consumption of caffeine and alcohol during treatment. These irritate the urethra.

FUTURE CONSIDERATIONS FOR THE AGING ADULT

POSSIBLE COMPLICATIONS
- Gonococcal eye infection.
- Blood poisoning (gonococcal septicemia).
- Infectious arthritis.
- Pelvic inflammatory disease (PID).
- Epididymitis.
- Endocarditis.
- Sexual impotence in men if untreated (sometimes).

PROBABLE OUTCOME—Usually curable in 1 to 2 weeks with treatment.

PREVENTING RECURRENCE
- Avoid sexual partners whose health practices and status are uncertain.
- Use a rubber condom during sexual intercourse.
- Women should never use someone else's douche equipment.

CALL YOUR DOCTOR IF

- You have symptoms of gonorrhea.
- You develop chills, fever, abdominal pain, swelling of the testicles, genital sores or joint pain either before or during treatment.
- New, unexplained symptoms develop. The drugs used in treatment may produce side effects.

GOUT

BASIC INFORMATION FOR OLDER ADULTS

DESCRIPTION—Gout is characterized by recurrent attacks of joint inflammation caused by deposits of uric acid crystals in the joints. Body parts involved: The joints, especially the base of the big toe. Gout may also involve the elbow, knee, hand, foot, ankle, arm or shoulder.

SPECIAL CONSIDERATIONS FOR AGING
- Years of weight bearing cause wear and tear on the bones, joints and ligaments.
- Characteristic signs and symptoms of many disorders are frequently changed or absent.

SIGNS & SYMPTOMS
- Sudden onset of severe pain in the inflamed joint, usually at the base of the big toe or in the larger joints.
- The involved joints are red, hot, swollen and very tender. The skin over the joint is red and shiny.
- Fever (sometimes).

CAUSES & RISK FACTORS
Causes include:
- Genetic transmission.
- A high level of uric acid in the blood due to increased production of uric acid or decreased elimination of uric acid by the kidneys.
- The use of diuretic drugs (water pills) such as furosemide and hydrochlorothiazide.
- The use of some antibiotics.
- Some blood diseases, such as polycythemia and leukemia.

Risk factors include:
- A family history of gout.
- The use of drugs such as diuretics or antibiotics.

DOCTOR'S TREATMENT & DIAGNOSTIC TESTS
- Laboratory studies to determine blood levels of uric acid.
- Therapeutic trials with antigout medications.
- Self-care instructions focused on the older patient.

OTHER—The excessive consumption of rich food and alcohol does not cause gout, as was once believed, but it may trigger attacks.

HOME TREATMENT BY SELF OR CARE-GIVER

GENERAL INSTRUCTIONS
- Use warm or cold compresses on painful joints.
- Keep the weight of bedclothes off any painful joint by making a frame that raises the sheets off the feet.

MEDICATION (ADJUSTED FOR AGING)
- Your doctor may prescribe:
  Pain relievers.
  Non-steroidal anti-inflammatory drugs to control the inflammation in painful joints.
  Lifelong medication, such as allopurinol to decrease uric acid production or probenecid to increase the excretion of uric acid from the kidneys.
  These medications have significant side effects and adverse reactions. Obtain as much information as possible regarding their use.
- *Note:* Adverse reactions and side effects may be more frequent and severe in older persons. Remind your doctor of any medicines you already take.

ACTIVITY FOR OLDER PATIENTS—Acute attacks will end sooner with complete rest.

FOOD & BEVERAGE
- Don't eat liver, sweetbreads, kidneys or sardines.
- Drink 8 to 10 glasses of water daily.
- Don't drink alcoholic beverages.

FUTURE CONSIDERATIONS FOR THE AGING ADULT

POSSIBLE COMPLICATIONS—If untreated, may cause:
- Crippled, deformed joints.
- Kidney stones.
- Inflammation of the bones, ligaments and tendons.

PROBABLE OUTCOME—The first attack may last a few days, but recurrent attacks are common without treatment to reduce the uric acid level in the blood. The symptoms can be eliminated with treatment.

PREVENTING RECURRENCE—Cannot be prevented at present. Recurrent attacks can usually be prevented with medication.

CALL YOUR DOCTOR IF

- You have symptoms of gout.
- Any of the following occurs during treatment:
  Fever of 101F (38.3C) or higher.
  Skin rash, sore throat, red tongue or bleeding gums.
  Marked swelling of the feet or abrupt weight increase.
  Diarrhea or vomiting.
- The symptoms are not relieved in 3 days despite treatment.
- New, unexplained symptoms develop that may indicate an adverse reaction of the drug or interactions between drugs.

GUILLAIN-BARRE SYNDROME
(Infectious Polyneuropathy;
Acute Idiopathic Polyneuritis)

BASIC INFORMATION FOR OLDER ADULTS

DESCRIPTION—Guillain-Barré syndrome is an inflammatory condition of the nerves that causes rapid weakness and loss of sensation. Body part involved: The central nervous system. (THIS IS AN EMERGENCY; SEEK MEDICAL CARE IMMEDIATELY!)

SPECIAL CONSIDERATIONS FOR AGING
- The immune system becomes less effective, opening the way for viral, bacterial and other infections; malignancies; immune disorders; and allergies.
- Characteristic signs and symptoms of many disorders are frequently changed or absent.
- Repair from injury or disease is complete and effective, but recovery takes longer in older people.
- Decreased nutrition, common among chronically ill older people, increases the risk of any disease or disorder.

SIGNS & SYMPTOMS
Early stages:
- Muscle weakness in the hands and feet, arms and legs, abdomen and chest. The weakness spreads within 72 hours; it may create life-threatening breathing difficulty.
- Shock (weakness, faintness, cold hands and feet, rapid heartbeat and sweating).
Later stages:
- Complete paralysis (sometimes) for weeks or months.

CAUSES & RISK FACTORS—The cause is unknown, but this syndrome may be an autoimmune disorder. It sometimes follows an immunization or minor surgery. Risk factors include:
- Recent surgery.
- Recent immunization.
- Recent illness, such as a minor respiratory infection, gastroenteritis, Hodgkin's disease or lupus erythematosus.

DOCTOR'S TREATMENT & DIAGNOSTIC TESTS
- Medical history and physical exam.
- Laboratory study of spinal fluid.
- Hospitalization.
- Use of a respirator if the muscles used for respiration become greatly weakened.
- Self-care instructions focused on the older patient.

HOME TREATMENT BY SELF OR CARE-GIVER

GENERAL INSTRUCTIONS
- Remain mentally and socially active during recovery.
- Cough to rid your lungs of mucus.
- Guillain-Barré syndrome is a complicated, serious disorder. This page can cover only the main points of diagnosis and treatment. Your doctor, nurse or librarian can provide sources of supplemental information.

MEDICATION (ADJUSTED FOR AGING)
- Your doctor may prescribe:
  Laxatives to prevent constipation.
  Cortisone drugs, although they are not always effective.
- *Note:* Adverse reactions and side effects may be more frequent and severe in older persons. Remind your doctor of any medicines you already take.

ACTIVITY FOR OLDER PATIENTS—Remain as active as your muscle strength permits. Have a family member or visiting nurse passively move and stretch your muscles. Slowly return to normal activity.

FOOD & BEVERAGE—No special diet is required. Drink at least 8 glasses of fluid a day to prevent constipation.

FUTURE CONSIDERATIONS FOR THE AGING ADULT

POSSIBLE COMPLICATIONS
- Paralysis of eyelid muscles, resulting in eye damage.
- Thrombophlebitis.
- Pneumonia; respiratory failure.
- Pressure sores if you are immobilized.
- Constipation or fecal impaction.

PROBABLE OUTCOME—Complete recovery without residual effects in most cases. Some persons recover in 15 to 20 days, while others require a year or more. Many mechanical devices help you maintain mobility until you recover.

PREVENTING RECURRENCE—Cannot be prevented at present.

CALL YOUR DOCTOR IF

- You have symptoms of Guillain-Barré syndrome. *This is an emergency!*
- Any of the following occurs during treatment:
  Fever.
  Breathing difficulty.
  Sores on the skin.
  Vision changes.
  Swollen or tender calves.
  Constipation.
- New, unexplained symptoms develop. The drugs used in treatment may produce side effects.

GUM INFECTION
(Gingivitis)

BASIC INFORMATION FOR OLDER ADULTS

DESCRIPTION—Gingivitis is an inflammation or infection of the gums. Body parts involved: The gum tissues around the teeth.

SPECIAL CONSIDERATIONS FOR AGING
- The immune system becomes less effective, opening the way for viral, bacterial and other infections; malignancies; immune disorders; and allergies.
- Older people frequently drink an inadequate amount of water.
- Disease in one organ system leads to problems in another system.

SIGNS & SYMPTOMS
- Gums that are swollen, tender, red and soft around the teeth.
- Gums that bleed easily.
- Bad breath.
- Fever (rarely).
- No pain.

CAUSES & RISK FACTORS—Causes include poor nutrition, especially vitamin deficiencies that cause diseases such as scurvy or pellagra; plaque (food particles, germs and mucus at the base of the teeth); blood disorders, including leukemia; adverse reactions to drugs, such as anticonvulsants (primarily phenytoin and barbiturates); exposure to lead and bismuth; and injury to the gums. Risk factors include diabetes; poor nutrition, especially vitamin deficiency; infections; careless flossing of the teeth or brushing too vigorously.

DOCTOR'S TREATMENT & DIAGNOSTIC TESTS
- Medical history and physical exam by a doctor or dentist.
- Laboratory culture of the plaque to identify the bacteria responsible for the infection.
- Self-care instructions focused on the older patient.
- Surgery to remove the infected gum tissue if other treatment fails. Advancing age alone is not a deterrent.

HOME TREATMENT BY SELF OR CARE-GIVER

GENERAL INSTRUCTIONS
- Brush your teeth properly. Scrub clear, sticky plaque off the teeth daily with a soft toothbrush. Place the brush at the gum line and gently rotate it, pointing the bristles toward the gum. Brush one section of teeth at a time. A soft brush is less likely to damage the teeth and gums than a hard brush.
- Floss your teeth at least once a day. Use waxed or unwaxed dental floss. Wind most of it around the middle finger of each hand. Use the index fingers as guides to force the floss between the teeth gently. Gently clean adjacent tooth surfaces with a back-and-forth, sawing motion at the gum line. Floss between all lower teeth. Loosen the floss and place it on the tops of the thumbs. Floss between all upper teeth, using the thumbs as guides.
- Use a fluoride toothpaste.
- Make regular appointments with your dentist for cleaning of the teeth and the treatment of cavities.

MEDICATION (ADJUSTED FOR AGING)—Your doctor or dentist may prescribe:
- Antibiotics to fight infection.
- Fluoride mouthwash.
- Vitamins if you have a deficiency.

ACTIVITY FOR OLDER PATIENTS—No restrictions are necessary.

FOOD & BEVERAGE—No special diet is required. Avoid candy, sweet drinks or sweet snacks. Sugar stimulates the production of acid, which attacks normal teeth. The best desserts are fruit and cheese rather than ice cream or other high-sugar desserts.

FUTURE CONSIDERATIONS FOR THE AGING ADULT

POSSIBLE COMPLICATIONS
- Periodontitis (advanced gum disease).
- Trench mouth.
- Extensive involvement may require painful, prolonged gum surgery.

PROBABLE OUTCOME—Usually curable in 1 to 2 weeks with treatment.

PREVENTING RECURRENCE
- Practice good oral hygiene (see General Instructions) to prevent the formation of plaque.
- Have regular dental checkups twice a year.
- Eat a well-balanced diet. Take vitamin supplements if you cannot eat well-balanced meals.

CALL YOUR DOCTOR IF

- You have symptoms of a gum infection.
- Any of the following occurs during treatment:
  The bleeding increases.
  The pain becomes intolerable.
  Your temperature rises to 101F (38.3C) or higher.
  Your neck or face becomes swollen.
  Swallowing becomes difficult.
- New, unexplained symptoms develop. The drugs used in treatment may produce side effects.

HEAD INJURY

BASIC INFORMATION FOR OLDER ADULTS

DESCRIPTION—This disorder involves an injury to the head, with or without unconsciousness or other visible signs. Body part involved: The head.

SPECIAL CONSIDERATIONS FOR AGING
- Characteristic signs and symptoms of many disorders are frequently changed or absent.
- Falling is one of the universal risks of becoming older.

SIGNS & SYMPTOMS—Depend on the extent of injury. The presence or absence of swelling at the injury site is not related to the seriousness of injury. Signs and symptoms include any or all of the following:
- Drowsiness or confusion.
- Vomiting and nausea.
- Blurred vision.
- Pupils of different sizes.
- Loss of consciousness, either temporarily or for long periods.
- Amnesia or memory lapses.
- Irritability.
- Headache.
- Bleeding of the scalp if the skin is broken.

CAUSES & RISK FACTORS—Caused by injury. The worst injuries usually result from motor vehicle accidents. Risk factors include:
- Excessive alcohol consumption.
- Contact sports, especially football or boxing.
- Seizure disorders.
- Falls.

DOCTOR'S TREATMENT & DIAGNOSTIC TESTS
- Medical history and physical exam.
- Laboratory studies of the blood and cerebrospinal fluid.
- X-rays of the skull and neck.
- CT scan (see Glossary) of the head.
- Care-giver instructions focused on the older patient.
- Hospitalization for observation if the signs and symptoms are severe.

HOME TREATMENT BY SELF OR CARE-GIVER

GENERAL INSTRUCTIONS
- The extent of injury can be determined only with careful examination and observation. After a doctor's examination, the injured person may be sent home, but a responsible person must stay with the person and watch for serious symptoms. The first 24 hours after injury are critical, although serious aftereffects can appear later.
- If you are watching the patient, awaken him or her every 2 hours for 24 hours or as recommended by your doctor. Report to the doctor immediately if you can't awaken or arouse the person.

Also report any of the following:
Vomiting.
Inability to move arms and legs equally well on both sides.
Temperature above 100F (37.8C).
Stiff neck.
Pupils of unequal sizes or shapes.
Convulsions.
Noticeable restlessness.
Severe headache that persists longer than 4 hours after injury.
Confusion.

MEDICATION (ADJUSTED FOR AGING)
- Don't give *any* medicine—including non-prescription acetaminophen or aspirin—until the diagnosis is certain.
- *Note:* Adverse reactions and side effects may be more frequent and severe in older persons. Remind your doctor of any medicines you already take.

ACTIVITY FOR OLDER PATIENTS
- The patient should rest in bed until the doctor determines that the danger is over. Normal activity may then be resumed as the symptoms improve.
- See Appendix 20 regarding physical fitness for the active older adult.

FOOD & BEVERAGE
- Consume a full liquid diet (see Appendix 7) until the danger passes.
- See Appendix 1 regarding good nutrition for people over 50.

FUTURE CONSIDERATIONS FOR THE AGING ADULT

POSSIBLE COMPLICATIONS
Bleeding under the skull (subdural hemorrhage and hematoma); bleeding into the brain.

PROBABLE OUTCOME
- Usually curable with early recognition of danger signs and medical treatment. Complications can be life-threatening or cause permanent disability.
- Severe head injuries sometimes take several years for recovery.

PREVENTING RECURRENCE
- Don't drive after drinking or using mind-altering drugs.
- Wear protective headgear for contact sports and cycling.
- Use your auto seat belt or shoulder harness.

CALL YOUR DOCTOR IF

You have symptoms of a head injury or observe them in someone else.

BASIC INFORMATION FOR OLDER ADULTS

DESCRIPTION—A migraine headache is an intense, incapacitating headache, accompanied by other symptoms, that occurs repeatedly in some persons. Body parts involved: The blood vessels leading to the scalp and brain.

SPECIAL CONSIDERATIONS FOR AGING
- The blood vessels nourishing the brain are less healthy. They become thicker and lose their elasticity.
- Characteristic signs and symptoms of many disorders are frequently changed or absent.
- Stress from any emotional cause—fear, worry, anxiety, sadness, loneliness or anger—affects all aspects of any illness or disorder.

SIGNS & SYMPTOMS—The nature of migraine attacks varies between persons and from time to time in the same person. The symptoms of a classic migraine attack appear in the following sequence:
- Inability to see clearly, followed by seeing bright spots and zig-zag patterns. Visual disturbances may last several minutes or several hours, but they disappear once the headache begins.
- A dull, boring pain in the temple that spreads to the entire side of the head. The pain becomes intense and throbbing.
- Nausea and vomiting.

In other types of migraine attack, the above symptoms (vision disturbances, headache or vomiting) may be absent, or other symptoms may be present. Some persons become pale with bloodshot eyes and a runny nose or eyes.

CAUSES & RISK FACTORS—Caused by the constriction, then dilation and inflammation of the blood vessels that go to the scalp and brain. Vision disturbances occur when the blood vessels narrow. The headache begins when they widen again. Attacks may be triggered by:
- Tension. Emotional problems are probably the most common reason for migraine attacks, but headaches don't necessarily coincide with emotional upset. They often occur on weekends when stress is decreased.
- Fatigue.
- The consumption of alcohol or certain foods.

Risk factors include:
- Stress; a family history of migraines.
- Smoking; excessive alcohol consumption.
- The use of many prescription and non-prescription drugs.
- Bright lights, loud noises or strong smells.

DOCTOR'S TREATMENT & DIAGNOSTIC TESTS
- Medical history and physical exam.
- Laboratory blood studies.
- CT scan (see Glossary) of the head.
- Self-care instructions focused on the older patient.

HOME TREATMENT BY SELF OR CARE-GIVER

GENERAL INSTRUCTIONS—At the first sign of a migraine attack:
- Apply a cold cloth or ice pack to your head or splash your face with cold water.
- Take pain relievers, such as aspirin or acetaminophen.
- Lie down in a quiet, dark room for several hours. Relax if possible. Listen to music, sleep or meditate.
- Don't read.

MEDICATION (ADJUSTED FOR AGING)
- Your doctor may prescribe:
  Antihistamines to expand the blood vessels.
  Antiemetics to decrease the nausea and vomiting.
  Vasoconstrictors to narrow the blood vessels.
  Pain relievers.
  Beta-adrenergic or calcium channel blockers or tricyclic antidepressants to prevent attacks if headaches are so frequent or severe that you can't function normally. These medications may have undesirable side effects and may not help everyone.
- *Note:* Adverse reactions and side effects may be more frequent and severe in older persons. Remind your doctor of any medicines you already take.

ACTIVITY FOR OLDER PATIENTS—Rest during attacks. Between attacks, exercise to achieve maximum fitness (see Appendix 20).

FOOD & BEVERAGE—Because some attacks are caused by foods, such as cheese or chocolate, keep a record of what you ate before each attack. Avoid foods that seem to trigger migraine attacks. Otherwise, no special diet is necessary.

FUTURE CONSIDERATIONS FOR THE AGING ADULT

POSSIBLE COMPLICATIONS—None are expected.

PROBABLE OUTCOME—The symptoms can be controlled with treatment.

PREVENTING RECURRENCE
- See Appendix 13 for suggestions to reduce stress.
- 1 aspirin a day may prevent migraine attacks in adults. Ask your doctor for advice.
- The use of the drug propranolol prevents attacks in some persons.

CALL YOUR DOCTOR IF

- You have a migraine attack that persists longer than 24 hours despite treatment.
- Frequent migraine attacks interfere with your life.

BASIC INFORMATION FOR OLDER ADULTS

DESCRIPTION—Simple tension or vascular headaches are of 3 types:
- Headaches from muscle strain in the scalp, neck and face.
- Headaches from constricted blood vessels in the head that cause pressure on the walls of the blood vessels.
- Headaches from dilated blood vessels in the brain.

Body parts involved: The sensory nerves in the skin, scalp, blood vessels and muscles of the head.

SPECIAL CONSIDERATIONS FOR AGING
- The blood vessels nourishing the brain are less healthy. They become thicker and lose their elasticity.
- Characteristic signs and symptoms of many disorders are frequently changed or absent.
- Stress from any emotional cause—fear, worry, anxiety, sadness, loneliness or anger—affects all aspects of any illness or disorder.

SIGNS & SYMPTOMS—Any of the following:
- Moderate pain in the front or back of the head accompanied by tight muscles in the neck or scalp.
- Constant pain over the temples, accompanied by the feeling that a vise is over the back of the head.
- Throbbing pain all over the head.
- Nausea and vomiting (sometimes).

CAUSES & RISK FACTORS—Causes include tension, which strains the muscles of the neck, scalp, face and jaw; sleep disturbances; excessive eating or irregular meals; physically exhausting work; anxiety or depression; eye strain, including that from sun glare; the use of drugs or alcohol; low blood sugar; allergic reactions; toothache; or ear infection. Risk factors include:
- Stress, either mental or physical.
- Environments that are noisy, stuffy, hot or poorly lit or have irritating odors.
- Exposure to or consumption of nitrites, sulfites, monosodium glutamate or other food additives.

DOCTOR'S TREATMENT & DIAGNOSTIC TESTS
- Medical history and physical exam.
- Laboratory studies such as a CT scan or MRI (see Glossary) for unrelenting pain.
- Self-care instructions focused on the older patient.
- Biofeedback training or counseling for chronic headaches caused by stress.

HOME TREATMENT BY SELF OR CARE-GIVER

GENERAL INSTRUCTIONS
- If possible, stop what you are doing and try to relax.
- Massage your shoulders, neck, jaw and scalp.
- Take a hot bath or shower.
- Lie down. Place a warm or cold cloth, whichever feels better, over the aching area.

MEDICATION (ADJUSTED FOR AGING)
- You may take acetaminophen or aspirin to relieve the pain.
- *Note:* Adverse reactions and side effects may be more frequent and severe in older persons. Remind your doctor of any medicines you already take.

ACTIVITY FOR OLDER PATIENTS—Rest in a quiet room during an attack.

FOOD & BEVERAGE
- Most persons feel better if they don't eat, unless the headache is from low blood sugar.
- Don't drink alcohol.

FUTURE CONSIDERATIONS FOR THE AGING ADULT

POSSIBLE COMPLICATIONS—None are expected for a simple headache.

PROBABLE OUTCOME—Most tension or vascular headaches can be relieved with simple treatment.

PREVENTING RECURRENCE
- Get enough sleep—an average of 8 hours for men and 7 hours for women.
- Don't skip meals, especially breakfast.
- Don't overeat.
- Exercise regularly (see Appendix 20) to reduce tension and improve circulation.
- Drink alcohol moderately—no more than 1 or 2 drinks a day if at all.
- Don't smoke cigarettes and avoid smoky environments.
- Don't use mood-altering, mind-altering, stimulant or sedative drugs.
- Avoid foods that contain nitrites or other additives to which you are sensitive.

CALL YOUR DOCTOR IF

You have a headache and any of the following:
- A fever.
- A recent head injury.
- Drowsiness.
- Nausea or vomiting.
- Pain in one eye.
- Blurred vision.
- High blood pressure.
- Pain and tenderness around the eyes and cheekbones that worsens when you lean forward.
- Vision disturbances and vomiting prior to the headache.
- Persistent headache pain that lasts longer than 24 hours without other symptoms.
- You suspect a prescription or non-prescription drug caused the headache.

HEARING IMPAIRMENT OR LOSS
(Deafness)

BASIC INFORMATION FOR OLDER ADULTS

DESCRIPTION—This disorder is characterized by a decreased ability or complete inability to hear. Classifications include:
- Conductive loss, in which the bones of the middle ear degenerate and don't transmit sound waves. See Otosclerosis in this section.
- Sensorineural loss, in which the 8th cranial nerve (the acoustic nerve) is damaged, often for unknown reasons.
- Mixed loss, involving both conductive and sensorineural disabilities.

Body parts involved: The bones of the middle ear that conduct sound (conductive and mixed loss); the branches of the 8th cranial nerve that transmit sound to the brain (sensorineural and mixed loss).

SPECIAL CONSIDERATIONS FOR AGING
- Hearing loss. The high tones go first.
- The loss of nerve cells begins between ages 20 and 40 and continues throughout life. The cells in the brain and other parts of the central nervous system cannot reproduce or replace themselves.
- Coordination and balance become impaired.

SIGNS & SYMPTOMS
- Difficulty in discriminating (listening selectively) to environmental sounds.
- Ringing in the ears; dizziness.
- Difficulty in understanding the speech of others, especially with distracting background noise.

CAUSES & RISK FACTORS—Causes include a congenital disorder that is transmitted as a dominant or recessive genetic trait; chronic middle ear infections or the spread of infection to the inner ear; earwax blocking the ear canal; blood vessel disorders, including hypertension; head injury; brain tumor; a blood clot that travels to the acoustic nerve; multiple sclerosis; syphilis; blood coagulation disorders; and prolonged exposure to sound levels of 85 decibels or above. Risk factors include:
- A family history of congenital or acquired deafness; Meniere's disease.
- The use of drugs such as aminoglycosides, non-steroidal anti-inflammatories, bumetanide, capreomycin, cisplatin, erythromycins, gentamicin, minocylcine, rancomycin, strep- tomycin, tobramycin, quinine, furosemide, ethacrynic acid or heavy doses of aspirin.
- Occupations or hobbies involving high noise levels.

DOCTOR'S TREATMENT & DIAGNOSTIC TESTS
- Medical history and physical exam.
- Laboratory studies such as blood studies, audiogram, Weber test, and Rinne test (see Glossary for all).

- Surgery for conductive-type deafness (sometimes).
- Speech therapy and rehabilitation if necessary.
- Self-care instructions focused on the older patient.

HOME TREATMENT BY SELF OR CARE-GIVER

GENERAL INSTRUCTIONS
- Contact local rehabilitation facilities to learn sign language and lip reading.
- Learn to use and wear a hearing aid if one is prescribed.
- Consult your phone company about special audio equipment for your phone.
- Resist the temptation to withdraw socially because of your hearing difficulty. Isolation will increase your communication problems and will make adjustment more difficult.
- Devices are available to assist you in hearing sounds from TV and radio while allowing family members to listen at normal levels.
- Special portable devices to amplify sound can be used in concert halls, movies or large meetings.

MEDICATION (ADJUSTED FOR AGING)—Medicine usually is not necessary for this disorder.

ACTIVITY FOR OLDER PATIENTS—No restrictions are necessary.

FOOD & BEVERAGE—No special diet.

FUTURE CONSIDERATIONS FOR THE AGING ADULT

POSSIBLE COMPLICATIONS—Permanent deafness.

PROBABLE OUTCOME—Some conductive hearing loss is curable with surgery. Hearing loss caused by prolonged exposure to loud noise sometimes disappears when the noise is eliminated. Other types of hearing loss are usually permanent.

PREVENTING RECURRENCE
- Avoid prolonged use or overdosage of drugs that cause hearing loss.
- Obtain medical treatment for underlying disorders that cause hearing loss.
- Avoid prolonged exposure to loud noise. If exposure is unavoidable, protect your ears with ear plugs.

CALL YOUR DOCTOR IF

You suspect you have a hearing loss, especially if you must often ask others to repeat themselves or family members frequently ask you if your hearing is all right.

HEART ATTACK
(Myocardial Infarction)

BASIC INFORMATION FOR OLDER ADULTS

DESCRIPTION—A heart attack is the death of cells of the heart muscle due to the reduction or obstruction of the blood flow through the coronary arteries. Body parts involved: The coronary arteries, heart muscle and platelets and clotting factors in the blood. (THIS IS AN EMERGENCY; SEEK MEDICAL CARE IMMEDIATELY!)

SPECIAL CONSIDERATIONS FOR AGING
- Characteristic signs and symptoms of many disorders are frequently changed or absent.
- The coronary arteries nourishing the heart become thicker and lose their elasticity.
- Stress from any emotional cause affects all aspects of any illness or disorder.

SIGNS & SYMPTOMS
- Chest pain or a "heavy, squeezing or crushing" feeling in the chest.
- Sweating; cold, clammy skin.
- Pain that radiates from the midchest over the breastbone to the jaw, neck, either arm, the area between the shoulder blades or the upper abdomen (sometimes).
- A feeling of impending doom.
- Shortness of breath; nausea and vomiting.

CAUSES & RISK FACTORS—Caused by a partial or complete blockage of the coronary arteries. The symptoms are often triggered by an emotional crisis, a heavy meal or heavy exercise. Risk factors include:
- Smoking; obesity; stress; high blood cholesterol levels or low HDL cholesterol (see Glossary).
- High blood pressure; diabetes mellitus.
- A diet that is high in fat, refined sugar and salt.
- A family history of coronary artery disease.
- A sedentary lifestyle; fatigue or overwork.
- Exercise in heat or cold and wind.

DOCTOR'S TREATMENT & DIAGNOSTIC TESTS
- Continuation of cardiopulmonary resuscitation (CPR) if it was necessary (see General Instructions).
- Medical history and physical exam.
- Laboratory blood studies; ECG (see Glossary).
- Radioactive technetium 99 scan (see Glossary).
- Hospitalization.
- Surgery (pacemaker insertion, angioplasty or coronary artery bypass graft). For further information see the Surgeries section.
- Following treatment, self-care instructions.

HOME TREATMENT BY SELF OR CARE-GIVER

GENERAL INSTRUCTIONS
- If you think you are experiencing a heart attack, call your doctor or call 0 (operator) or 911 (emergency) for help.
- If a heart attack victim is unconscious and *not* breathing:
Yell for help. Don't leave the victim.
Begin mouth-to-mouth breathing immediately.
If there is no heartbeat, give external cardiac massage. Don't stop CPR until help arrives.
Have someone call 0 or 911 for help.

MEDICATION (ADJUSTED FOR AGING)—Your doctor may prescribe pain relievers; antiarrhythmic and antianginal drugs, such as beta-adrenergic blockers or calcium channel blockers, to stabilize an irregular heartbeat; anticoagulants to prevent blood clots; nitroglycerin to widen the arteries and increase the blood supply to the heart; digitalis to strengthen the contractions of the heart muscle and stabilize the heartbeat.

ACTIVITY FOR OLDER PATIENTS—Resume your normal activities gradually during recovery. Consult your doctor before resuming sexual relations. Enroll in a cardiac rehabilitation program if available.

FOOD & BEVERAGE—Eat a low-fat, low-salt, high-fiber diet (see Appendices 8 and 9).

FUTURE CONSIDERATIONS FOR THE AGING ADULT

POSSIBLE COMPLICATIONS—Irregular heart rhythms; shock; pericarditis; congestive heart failure; pleural effusion (see Glossary); deep-vein thrombosis; pulmonary embolism; rupture of the heart septum or wall; ventricular aneurysm (see Glossary).

PROBABLE OUTCOME—With immediate emergency care and hospitalization in a coronary care unit, most persons recover from a first heart attack. Treatment delay is often fatal. Survivors should allow 4 to 8 weeks for recovery.

PREVENTING RECURRENCE
- Follow the suggestions for the prevention of hardening of the arteries under Atherosclerosis in the Illnesses section. Ask your doctor about taking one aspirin daily.
- Have family members learn CPR.

CALL YOUR DOCTOR IF

- You have symptoms of a heart attack. *This is an emergency!*
- You see someone who appears to be experiencing a heart attack. See General Instructions.
- Any of the following occurs during recovery: Chest pain that is not relieved by prescribed medication; shortness of breath or cough while at rest; nausea, vomiting or diarrhea; fever; or bleeding from the gums or other sites.

HEART BLOCK
(Atrioventricular Block)

BASIC INFORMATION FOR OLDER ADULTS

DESCRIPTION—Heart block is a persistent disruption (either mild or major) in the transmission of electrical signals between the heart's upper and lower chambers. The contractions of the atria (the upper heart chambers) lose synchronization with those of the ventricles (the lower heart chambers). The heartbeat is no longer regulated normally to quicken under exertion or stress and to slow down at other times. Body parts involved: The electrical transmission system of the heart that coordinates the contractions of the heart muscle cells. The heart's natural pacemaker initiates the electrical system.

SPECIAL CONSIDERATIONS FOR AGING
- The coronary arteries nourishing the heart are less healthy. They become thicker and lose their elasticity.
- Unusual and unexpected reactions to drugs and medications are more likely.
- Characteristic signs and symptoms of many disorders are frequently changed or absent.

SIGNS & SYMPTOMS
- No symptoms (sometimes) for less severe forms.
- Slow, irregular heartbeat.
- Dizziness.
- Sudden loss of consciousness.
- Convulsions (sometimes).

CAUSES & RISK FACTORS
Causes include:
- Coronary artery disease, a sign of atherosclerosis (hardening of the arteries). However, in many cases there is no history of heart disease.
- Congenital heart abnormalities.
- Excessive digitalis and some other medications.
Risk factors include:
- Stress.
- An improper diet that is high in fat and salt.
- Obesity; smoking; diabetes mellitus.
- Heart disease, including atherosclerosis, congestive heart failure or heart valve disease.
- High blood pressure.
- A previous electrolyte imbalance.
- The use of some drugs, such as digitalis, quinidine or beta-adrenergic blockers.
- Sick sinus syndrome (see Glossary).

DOCTOR'S TREATMENT & DIAGNOSTIC TESTS
- Medical history and physical exam.
- ECG (see Glossary).
- Monitoring by a Holter monitor, a 12- or 24-hour continuous ECG monitor (see Glossary).
- Self-care instructions focused on the older patient.
- Surgery to implant an artificial pacemaker (sometimes). Advancing age alone is not a deterrent.

HOME TREATMENT BY SELF OR CARE-GIVER

GENERAL INSTRUCTIONS
- Wear a Medic Alert bracelet or pendant (see Glossary) in case you suddenly lose consciousness.
- Don't smoke.

MEDICATION (ADJUSTED FOR AGING)
- There are no medications that cure heart block, but there are some that make it worse. Don't take medications to relieve allergies or nasal congestion, including antihistamines, or any stimulant, including caffeine, cocaine or marijuana.
- *Note:* Adverse reactions and side effects may be more frequent and severe in older persons. Remind your doctor of any medicines you already take.

ACTIVITY FOR OLDER PATIENTS
- Don't think of yourself as an invalid. Unless your doctor advises against it, mild exercise is helpful and not to be feared. Begin a regular exercise program—walking is ideal—and increase the amount daily.
- See Appendix 20 regarding physical fitness for the active older adult.

FOOD & BEVERAGE
- Lose weight if you are overweight. A reducing diet appears in Appendix 10. Don't use amphetamines or other appetite suppressants to curb your appetite.
- Avoid the excessive use of alcoholic beverages. Alcohol depresses the heartbeat.
- Avoid caffeine in all forms—coffee, tea, cocoa, cola drinks and chocolate.

FUTURE CONSIDERATIONS FOR THE AGING ADULT

POSSIBLE COMPLICATIONS—Uncontrolled slow, rapid or irregular heartbeat and cardiac arrest.

PROBABLE OUTCOME—The symptoms can be controlled with surgery to implant a pacemaker.

PREVENTING RECURRENCE
- Obtain medical treatment for any underlying disease.
- Don't smoke.
- Exercise regularly (see Appendix 20).
- Eat a diet that is low in fat (see Appendix 8) and low in salt (see Appendix 9).

CALL YOUR DOCTOR IF

- You have symptoms of heart block, especially an episode with loss of consciousness.
- After diagnosis, stress increases in your life.

HEART LINING INFECTION
(Endocarditis; Bacterial Endocarditis; Infective Endocarditis)

BASIC INFORMATION FOR OLDER ADULTS

DESCRIPTION—Endocarditis is a non-contagious infection of the valves or lining of the heart. Body parts involved: The heart muscle, heart valves and endocardium (lining of the heart chambers and valves).

SPECIAL CONSIDERATIONS FOR AGING
- The immune system becomes less effective, opening the way for viral, bacterial and other infections; malignancies; immune disorders; and allergies.
- The total heart functions less efficiently—especially among smokers.
- Older people have decreased heart function reserves.

SIGNS & SYMPTOMS
Early symptoms:
- Fatigue and weakness; weight loss.
- Intermittent fever, chills and excessive sweating, especially at night.
- Vague aches and pains; heart murmur.
Late symptoms:
- Severe chills and high fever.
- Shortness of breath on exertion.
- Swelling of the feet, legs and abdomen.
- Rapid or irregular heartbeat.

CAUSES & RISK FACTORS—Caused by bacteria or fungi that enter the blood and infect the valves and heart lining of persons with damaged hearts (see risks below). The bacteria or fungi further damage the heart valves, muscles and linings. The risk of heart valve damage increases with:
- Rheumatic fever; congenital heart disease.
- Open heart surgery; major dental treatment.
- Genitourinary procedures (see Glossary).
The risk of a heart lining infection following heart valve damage increases with:
- Injections of contaminated materials into the bloodstream, such as self-administered intravenous drugs.
- Excessive alcohol consumption.
- The use of immunosuppressive drugs.
- Artificial heart valves.

DOCTOR'S TREATMENT & DIAGNOSTIC TESTS
- Medical history and physical exam.
- Laboratory blood counts and blood cultures.
- ECG (see Glossary).
- X-rays of the heart and lungs, including an echocardiogram and angiogram (see Glossary).
- Ultrasound.
- Hospitalization.
- After the acute illness, selfcare instructions focused on the older patient.

HOME TREATMENT BY SELF OR CARE-GIVER

GENERAL INSTRUCTIONS
- If you have damaged heart valves, tell any doctor or dentist who treats you.
- Once you have had a heart lining infection, stay under a doctor's care to prevent a relapse.

MEDICATION (ADJUSTED FOR AGING)—Your doctor may prescribe antibiotics to fight infection. Antibiotic treatment is often intravenous.

ACTIVITY FOR OLDER PATIENTS
- Rest in bed until you are fully recovered. While in bed, flex your legs often to prevent clots from forming in deep veins.
- Resume your normal activities, including sexual relations, when your strength allows.

FOOD & BEVERAGE—No special diet unless you have an underlying heart disorder. In that case, follow a low-salt diet (see Appendix 9).

FUTURE CONSIDERATIONS FOR THE AGING ADULT

POSSIBLE COMPLICATIONS—Blood clots that may travel to the brain, kidneys or abdominal organs, causing infections, abscesses, stroke or heart rhythm disturbances (atrial fibrillation is most common).

PROBABLE OUTCOME—Usually curable with early diagnosis and treatment, but recovery may take weeks. If treatment is delayed, heart function deteriorates, resulting in congestive heart failure and death.

PREVENTING RECURRENCE—If you have heart valve damage or a heart murmur:
- Request antibiotics prior to medical procedures that may introduce bacteria into the blood. These include dental work and surgery of the urinary or gastrointestinal tract.
- Don't drink more than 1 or 2—if any—alcoholic drinks in 1 day.
- Don't use illicit drugs such as heroin or cocaine.

CALL YOUR DOCTOR IF

- You have symptoms of a heart lining infection.
- Any of the following occurs during or after treatment:
  Weight gain without diet changes.
  Blood in the urine.
  Chest pain.
  Sudden weakness or numbness in the muscles of the face, trunk or limbs.

HEART RHYTHM IRREGULARITY
(Arrhythmia)

BASIC INFORMATION FOR OLDER ADULTS

DESCRIPTION—Arrhythmia is an abnormality in the rhythm of the heartbeat. Body parts involved: The heart and the nerves that transmit impulses to coordinate the contractions of the heart muscle.

SPECIAL CONSIDERATIONS FOR AGING
- 50% of people over 60 have x-ray evidence of narrowing of the coronary arteries, yet only 50% of those people have symptoms.
- Unusual and unexpected reactions to drugs and medications are more likely.
- Characteristic signs and symptoms of many disorders are frequently changed or absent.
- Stress from any emotional cause affects all aspects of any illness or disorder.

SIGNS & SYMPTOMS
- Awareness of one's own heartbeat, including whether it skips; is always fast, slow or irregular; or suddenly changes rhythm.
- Shortness of breath.
- Sudden faintness or weakness.
- No symptoms (frequently).

CAUSES & RISK FACTORS—Causes include heart diseases such as rheumatic fever, congenital heart disease, cardiomyopathy, previous heart attack or heart muscle inflammation; endocrine disorders, especially thyroid and adrenal gland diseases; fluid and electrolyte imbalance, especially too little or too much potassium; side effects of certain drugs, especially digitalis, beta-adrenergic blockers, stimulants and diuretics; overdose of certain drugs, including antidepressants, marijuana and cocaine; and postoperative effects following chest or heart surgery. Risk factors include:
- Stress; hypertension; smoking.
- Chronic kidney disease.
- The use of certain drugs, such as caffeine, alcohol, amphetamines and many non-prescription cough and cold remedies.
- Fatigue, overwork or sleep deprivation.

DOCTOR'S TREATMENT & DIAGNOSTIC TESTS
- Medical history and physical exam.
- Laboratory blood studies.
- ECG and 24-hour Holter monitoring (see Glossary for both); x-rays of the heart, including echocardiogram (see Glossary).
- Psychotherapy or counseling if stress is a major factor.
- DC cardioversion (see Glossary) in a hospital or outpatient surgical facility.
- Surgery to correct some heart problems (coronary artery bypass, replacement of the damaged valve or insertion of a pacemaker). Advancing age alone is not a deterrent.
- Self-care instructions focused on the older patient.

HOME TREATMENT BY SELF OR CARE-GIVER

GENERAL INSTRUCTIONS
- Consider lifestyle changes. See Appendix 13.
- Wear a Medic Alert bracelet or pendant (see Glossary) with the name of your condition.
- A few arrhythmias are fatal unless cardiopulmonary resuscitation (CPR) is performed immediately. Take a course to learn CPR, especially if someone in your home or neighborhood has heart disease.

MEDICATION (ADJUSTED FOR AGING)
- Your doctor may prescribe antiarrhythmic medications. You may need to try several to find the most effective one.
- *Note:* Adverse reactions and side effects may be more frequent and severe in older persons. Remind your doctor of any medicines you already take.

ACTIVITY FOR OLDER PATIENTS—Resume most normal activities as soon as your symptoms improve. Consult your doctor about exercise.

FOOD & BEVERAGE
- Some heart medicines require extra potassium, found mostly in citrus fruits, bananas, dried apricots or peaches, raisins, lentils and whole-grain cereals. Ask your doctor if you need to eat more of these.
- Don't eat or drink caffeine-containing foods or beverages, such as coffee, tea, cola or chocolate.
- See Appendix 1 regarding good nutrition for people over 50.

FUTURE CONSIDERATIONS FOR THE AGING ADULT

POSSIBLE COMPLICATIONS—Fainting; congestive heart failure; death from prolonged (more than 3 to 6 minutes) cardiac arrest.

PROBABLE OUTCOME—Most rhythm disturbances can be controlled with treatment. Very occasional irregular heartbeats are harmless and require no treatment.

PREVENTING RECURRENCE—If you have any disorders listed as causes or risks, follow your treatment program carefully to control the disease. If medication is part of your treatment, consult your doctor about having blood levels monitored and electrolytes measured periodically.

CALL YOUR DOCTOR IF

- You have symptoms of heart rhythm irregularity.
- New, unexplained symptoms develop. The drugs used in treatment may produce side effects.

HEART VALVE DISEASE
(Valvular Heart Disease)

BASIC INFORMATION FOR OLDER ADULTS

DESCRIPTION—Heart valve disease is a complication of diseases that distort or destroy the valves of the heart. Body parts involved: The heart valves (the aortic, mitral, tricuspid and pulmonic valves).

SPECIAL CONSIDERATIONS FOR AGING
- 50% of people over 60 have x-ray evidence of narrowing of the coronary arteries, yet only 50% of those people have symptoms.
- The coronary arteries nourishing the heart are less healthy. They become thicker and lose their elasticity.
- The heart rate does not increase to the expected degree in response to stress.

SIGNS & SYMPTOMS
- No symptoms (sometimes).
- Fatigue and weakness; chest pain.
- Dizziness or fainting.
- Shortness of breath; lung congestion.
- Heart rhythm irregularities.
- Heart murmurs (abnormal heart sounds heard by the doctor through a stethoscope).
- Abnormal blood pressure (high or low).

CAUSES & RISK FACTORS—The heart has 4 valves. The mitral and tricuspid valves (the main heart valves) control blood flow into the ventricles. The aortic and pulmonic valves control blood flow out of the heart. Heart valve disease can be either narrowed valves, which obstruct the blood flow (stenosis), or widened or scarred valves, which allow blood to leak backward into the heart (insufficiency). The disorder may be inherited or may be caused by any of the following:
- Rheumatic fever.
- A complication of strep throat.
- Atherosclerosis; high blood pressure.
- Congenital heart defects; endocarditis.
- Syphilis (rare).
Risk factors include:
- A family history of heart valve disease.
- Fatigue or overwork.
- The use of self-injected IV drugs, which are a major risk.

DOCTOR'S TREATMENT & DIAGNOSTIC TESTS
- Medical history and physical exam.
- Laboratory blood tests.
- ECG (see Glossary).
- Heart catheterization (see Glossary).
- X-rays of the heart, lungs and blood flow (angiography).
- Self-care instructions focused on the older patient.
- Hospitalization.
- Surgery to replace or open defective valves (sometimes). Advancing age alone is not a deterrent.

HOME TREATMENT BY SELF OR CARE-GIVER

GENERAL INSTRUCTIONS—Tell any doctor, dentist or anesthesiologist who treats you that you have heart valve disease. Remind those involved, even if you think they know the details of your medical history.

MEDICATION (ADJUSTED FOR AGING)
- Your doctor may prescribe:
  Antibiotics to treat or prevent bacterial infection of abnormal heart valves.
  Antiarrhythmic drugs to stabilize heartbeat irregularities.
  Digitalis medication to strengthen or regulate the heartbeat.
- *Note:* Adverse reactions and side effects may be more frequent and severe in older persons. Remind your doctor of any medicines you already take.

ACTIVITY FOR OLDER PATIENTS—Get as much exercise as you can tolerate. No restrictions are necessary are necessary with some forms of heart valve disease. Have your doctor recommend an exercise program.

FOOD & BEVERAGE—Eat a low-fat, low-salt diet (see Appendices 8 and 9).

FUTURE CONSIDERATIONS FOR THE AGING ADULT

POSSIBLE COMPLICATIONS—Infection of the valves; congestive heart failure.

PROBABLE OUTCOME—Depends on the underlying condition. Many complications of valvular disease can be controlled with medication or cured with surgery.

PREVENTING RECURRENCE
- Obtain medical treatment for diseases that cause heart valve damage, such as high blood pressure, endocarditis and syphilis.
- Take antibiotics for streptococcal infections to prevent rheumatic fever.
- If you have a a family history of congenital heart disease, obtain genetic counseling before starting a family.

CALL YOUR DOCTOR IF

- You have symptoms of heart valve disease.
- During treatment, you develop signs of infection, such as fever, chills, muscle aches, headache, fatigue and a general ill feeling.

HEARTBEAT, RAPID
(Tachycardia; Paroxysmal Tachycardia)

BASIC INFORMATION FOR OLDER ADULTS

DESCRIPTION—Tachycardia is a heartbeat that is much more rapid than usual and is not caused by overexertion. Tachycardia ranges from 150 to 300 beats per minute. A person with no heart disease may exercise and raise the heartbeat to 160 or more. This is normal and is not a medical problem. Body parts involved: The heart muscle and the electrical system of the heart.

SPECIAL CONSIDERATIONS FOR AGING
- Unusual and unexpected reactions to drugs and medications are more likely.
- 50% of people over 60 have x-ray evidence of narrowing of the coronary arteries, yet only 50% of those people have symptoms.
- The coronary arteries nourishing the heart are less healthy; they become thicker and lose their elasticity.
- Stress from any emotional cause—fear, worry, anxiety, sadness, loneliness or anger—affects all aspects of any illness or disorder.

SIGNS & SYMPTOMS
- Heart pounding or palpitations. The pulse at the wrist or neck will be 100 to 180 beats per minute, which is much faster than normal.
- Faintness or a feeling of impending death.
- Chest pain; involuntary cough; breathlessness.

CAUSES & RISK FACTORS—The cause is unknown. This condition usually occurs in young persons with no evidence of disease, but it may also occur in older patients who have coronary artery disease. Risk factors include:
- Heart disease or chronic lung disease.
- Stress, fatigue or overwork; smoking.
- The use of some drugs, such as caffeine, ephedrine or other sympathomimetic drugs.
- Fever.
- Hyperthyroidism.

DOCTOR'S TREATMENT & DIAGNOSTIC TESTS
- Medical history and physical exam.
- ECG (see Glossary).
- Self-care instructions focused on the older patient.
- Hospitalization if the attack persists despite treatment.
- DC electrocardioversion, a controlled electric shock (rarely necessary).

HOME TREATMENT BY SELF OR CARE-GIVER

GENERAL INSTRUCTIONS—The following sometimes reduce heartbeat:
- Hold your breath briefly.
- Pinch the skin on your arm enough to cause pain.
- Bathe your face in cold water, submerge your head briefly in a sink of cool water or take a cool shower and let the water beat on your head.
- Hold your nostrils closed and blow gently through the nose, making the eardrums pop.
- Massage the carotid area in the neck, *if you have been taught to do this safely.* Ask your doctor for instructions.

MEDICATION (ADJUSTED FOR AGING)
- For repeated attacks, your doctor may prescribe medications to control your heart rhythm. These include digitalis, quinidine, calcium channel blockers, procainamide and beta-adrenergic blockers.
- *Note:* Adverse reactions and side effects may be more frequent and severe in older persons. Remind your doctor of any medicines you already take.

ACTIVITY FOR OLDER PATIENTS
- Lie down during an attack until your heartbeat returns to normal, then resume your activities.
- Between attacks, exercise regularly with your doctor's approval; physical fitness helps prevent tachycardia.
- See Appendix 20 regarding physical fitness for the active older adult.

FOOD & BEVERAGE
- No special diet is required.
- See Appendix 1 regarding good nutrition for people over 50.

FUTURE CONSIDERATIONS FOR THE AGING ADULT

POSSIBLE COMPLICATIONS—Uninterrupted tachycardia can lead to life-threatening congestive heart failure, heart attack or cardiac arrest.

PROBABLE OUTCOME—Rapid heartbeat can usually be controlled with treatment.

PREVENTING RECURRENCE
- Don't smoke.
- Reduce stress if possible. See Appendix 13.
- Avoid decongestants, appetite suppressants and excessive coffee, cola and other stimulants with or without caffeine.

CALL YOUR DOCTOR IF

- You have an episode of rapid, irregular heartbeat that does not end in 4 or 5 minutes.
- You develop shortness of breath.
- You have chest pain.

HEARTBURN

BASIC INFORMATION FOR OLDER ADULTS

DESCRIPTION—Heartburn is discomfort in the upper digestive tract. Heartburn is a symptom—not a disease—and has nothing to do with the heart. Body parts involved: The stomach and esophagus.

SPECIAL CONSIDERATIONS FOR AGING
- Stress from any emotional cause affects all aspects of any illness or disorder.
- The esophageal muscles decrease in strength with aging.
- Older people frequently drink an inadequate amount of water.

SIGNS & SYMPTOMS—The following signs are worse at night:
- Belching or slight regurgitation of the stomach's contents into the mouth, producing an acid taste; vomiting (rarely).
- A heavy, burning or uncomfortable sensation in the chest.
- Swallowing difficulty.
- Mild abdominal pain.

CAUSES & RISK FACTORS
Causes include:
- Hiatal hernia (part of stomach protruding into the chest); ulcers of the esophagus.
- Irritation of the lower esophagus caused by stomach acid spilling into the esophagus.
- Weakness or malfunction of the sphincter muscle between the esophagus and the stomach.

Risk factors include:
- Stress and excessive air swallowing.
- Improper diet; obesity.
- Smoking; excessive alcohol consumption.
- The use of drugs such as aspirin, arthritis medicine or cortisone.

DOCTOR'S TREATMENT & DIAGNOSTIC TESTS
- Medical history and physical exam.
- Laboratory studies such as blood studies and an ECG (see Glossary) to exclude the chance of heart disease; esophagoscopy (see Glossary).
- X-rays of the upper digestive tract.
- Self-care instructions focused on the older patient.
- Hospitalization for special studies or surgery (rarely).

HOME TREATMENT BY SELF OR CARE-GIVER

GENERAL INSTRUCTIONS
- Elevate the head of the bed 4 to 6 inches with blocks.
- Eat small, frequent meals.
- Don't smoke.
- Lose weight if you are overweight.
- Don't bend over, lie down or exercise immediately after eating.
- Don't wear tight pantyhose, girdles, belts or pants.

MEDICATION (ADJUSTED FOR AGING)
- For minor discomfort, you may use non-prescription liquid antacids. These preparations coat the inside of the esophagus and neutralize stomach acid. Follow the instructions on the bottle. The usual dose is 1 tablespoon taken 1 hour after meals and at bedtime.
- *Note:* Adverse reactions and side effects may be more frequent and severe in older persons. Remind your doctor of any medicines you already take.

ACTIVITY FOR OLDER PATIENTS—Resume your normal activities as soon as the symptoms subside.

FOOD & BEVERAGE
- Avoid foods and beverages that stimulate the secretion of heavy stomach acid, such as spicy dishes, coffee, acid fruit juice or alcohol. Avoid chocolate and reduce your consumption of fatty foods, cabbage and beans.
- Eat frequent small meals.
- See Appendix 1 regarding good nutrition for people over 50.

FUTURE CONSIDERATIONS FOR THE AGING ADULT

POSSIBLE COMPLICATIONS
- Misdiagnosis as a heart attack, which produces symptoms similar to those of heartburn.
- If heartburn is caused by a large hiatal hernia, surgery may be necessary to repair the hernia.
- If heartburn is caused by ulcers in the esophagus, surgery may be necessary to remove scar tissue. Scar tissue forms with repeated ulceration and healing and may interfere with swallowing.

PROBABLE OUTCOME—The symptoms can be controlled with treatment, but recurrence is common.

PREVENTING RECURRENCE
- Consider lifestyle changes (see Appendix 12).
- Avoid eating before going to bed.
- Don't take a nap after eating. Lying down may worsen the problem.

CALL YOUR DOCTOR IF

- Swallowing becomes more difficult.
- You regurgitate blood when you have heartburn.
- The heartburn continues despite self-care.
- The following symptoms accompany the heartburn:
  Shortness of breath.
  Sweating.
  Pain in the jaw, neck and arm.
  Nausea.

HEATSTROKE OR HEAT EXHAUSTION
(Sunstroke or Heat Prostration)

 BASIC INFORMATION FOR OLDER ADULTS

DESCRIPTION—Heatstroke and heat exhaustion are disorders caused by prolonged exposure to hot temperatures, limited fluid intake or failure of the temperature regulation mechanisms in the brain. Body parts involved: The total body. (THIS IS AN EMERGENCY; SEEK MEDICAL CARE IMMEDIATELY!)

SPECIAL CONSIDERATIONS FOR AGING
- Older people tolerate temperature extremes poorly.
- Stress from any emotional cause—fear, worry, anxiety, sadness, loneliness or anger—affects all aspects of any illness or disorder.
- Decreased nutrition, common among chronically ill older people, increases the risk of any disease or disorder.

SIGNS & SYMPTOMS
Heatstroke:
- Sudden dizziness, weakness, faintness and headache.
- Skin that is hot and dry without sweating.
- High body temperature.
- Rapid heartbeat.
- Muscle cramps.

Heat exhaustion:
- Skin that is cool and moist.
- Pale or gray skin color.
- Slow pulse.
- Confusion; thirst; weakness.
- Muscle cramps.
- Low or normal body temperature.
- Dark yellow or orange urine.
- Nausea or vomiting.

CAUSES & RISK FACTORS—Heatstroke is caused by a failure of the body's heat-regulating mechanisms, leading to a heat buildup in the body. The failure may be a result of general effects of aging; alcoholism; chronic illness; diabetes; blood vessel disease. Heat exhaustion is caused by a loss of body fluids and salt from sweating and failure to drink enough replacement fluid. Risk factors of both conditions include:
- Sweating and inadequate fluid intake.
- Recent illness involving fluid loss from vomiting or diarrhea.
- Hot, humid weather.
- Working in a hot environment.

DOCTOR'S TREATMENT & DIAGNOSTIC TESTS
- Medical history and physical exam.
- Laboratory studies of blood and urine to measure electrolyte levels.
- After diagnosis of mild cases, self-care instructions focused on the older patient.
- Hospitalization to lower body temperature and provide intravenous replacement fluids.

 HOME TREATMENT BY SELF OR CARE-GIVER

GENERAL INSTRUCTIONS
- If someone with symptoms is very hot and *not sweating:*
  Cool the person rapidly. Use a cold-water bath or wrap the person in wet sheets. Arrange for transportation to the nearest hospital. *This is an emergency!*
- If someone is faint *but sweating:*
  Give the person liquids (water, soft drinks or fruit juice). Don't give salt pills. Arrange for transportation to the hospital, except in mild cases. Call your doctor for advice.

MEDICATION (ADJUSTED FOR AGING)
- Medicine usually is not necessary for these disorders. Don't take salt tablets.
- *Note:* Adverse reactions and side effects may be more frequent and severe in older persons. Remind your doctor of any medicines you already take.

ACTIVITY FOR OLDER PATIENTS
- Activity may be resumed as soon as your symptoms improve.
- See Appendix 20 regarding physical fitness for the active older adult.

FOOD & BEVERAGE
- No special diet is required.
- See Appendix 1 regarding good nutrition for people over 50.

 FUTURE CONSIDERATIONS FOR THE AGING ADULT

POSSIBLE COMPLICATIONS
- Shock.
- Brain damage caused by prolonged high body temperature (106F or 41.1C).

PROBABLE OUTCOME—Prompt treatment usually brings full recovery in 1 to 2 days.

PREVENTING RECURRENCE
- Wear light, loose-fitting clothing in hot weather.
- Drink water often; don't wait until you're thirsty.
- Drink extra water if you sweat heavily. If urine output decreases, increase your water intake.
- If you become overheated, improve your ventilation. Open a window or use a fan or air conditioner. This promotes sweat evaporation, which cools the skin.

 CALL YOUR DOCTOR IF

You have symptoms of heatstroke or heat exhaustion or observe them in someone else. Call immediately. *This is an emergency!*

HEEL SPUR
(Calcaneal Spur)

 BASIC INFORMATION FOR OLDER ADULTS

DESCRIPTION—A heel spur is a hard, bony growth in the tissue of the heel that causes pain and difficulty walking. Body parts involved: The heel, including the calcaneus (the major bone in the heel).

SPECIAL CONSIDERATIONS FOR AGING
- Characteristic signs and symptoms of many disorders are frequently changed or absent.
- Disease in one organ system leads to problems in another system.

SIGNS & SYMPTOMS—Pain and tenderness in the sole of the foot under the heel bone.

CAUSES & RISK FACTORS—Caused by stress or injury to the heel tissues, which causes inflammation and calcification c. the ligaments in the foot. Risk factors include:
- Prolonged standing.
- Running or jogging. The condition is less likely with vigorous walking.
- Obesity.

DOCTOR'S TREATMENT & DIAGNOSTIC TESTS
- Medical history and physical exam by a doctor or podiatrist.
- X-rays of the heel.
- Self-care instructions focused on the older patient.
- Surgery to remove the spur (rare).
- Ultrasound therapy or hydrotherapy.

 HOME TREATMENT BY SELF OR CARE-GIVER

GENERAL INSTRUCTIONS—Place a heel cup or felt insert in your shoe to relieve the pressure on your heel.

MEDICATION (ADJUSTED FOR AGING)
- To relieve minor pain, you may use non-prescriptions drugs such as acetaminophen or aspirin.
- Your doctor may:
  Inject steroids into the inflamed area to reduce inflammation.
  Prescribe oral non-steroidal anti-inflammatory drugs.
- *Note:* Adverse reactions and side effects may be more frequent and severe in older persons. Remind your doctor of any medicines you already take.

ACTIVITY FOR OLDER PATIENTS
- Stay off your feet as much as possible, especially at the beginning of treatment.
- See Appendix 20 regarding physical fitness for the active older adult.

FOOD & BEVERAGE
- No special diet is required, unless you are overweight. If so, lose weight to reduce the stress on your feet. A reducing diet appears in Appendix 10.
- See Appendix 1 regarding good nutrition for people over 50.

 FUTURE CONSIDERATIONS FOR THE AGING ADULT

POSSIBLE COMPLICATIONS—Lower back or knee disorders caused by constant limping.

PROBABLE OUTCOME—Usually curable with conservative treatment. If not, heel spurs are sometimes curable with surgery.

PREVENTING RECURRENCE
- Avoid activities that put constant strain on the foot.
- Wear a shoe with a rubber or felt heel cushion.

 CALL YOUR DOCTOR IF

- You have symptoms of a heel spur.
- Your pain or disability persists despite treatment.

HEMATOMA

BASIC INFORMATION FOR OLDER ADULTS

DESCRIPTION—A hematoma is a collection of pooled blood in any part of the body under the skin within a relatively constricted area. Hematomas probably accompany all serious contusions of the body, but they are sometimes difficult to diagnose because of the large muscle masses. Body parts involved: All body parts, including the soft tissues (nerves, tendons, ligaments, muscles and blood vessels) surrounding the hematoma.

SPECIAL CONSIDERATIONS FOR AGING
- Repair from injury or disease is complete and effective, but recovery takes longer.
- Muscle bulk and power decrease.

SIGNS & SYMPTOMS
- Swelling at the injury site; tenderness.
- Fluctuance (a feeling of tenseness to the touch, like pushing on an overinflated balloon).
- Redness that progresses through several color changes—purple, green-yellow and yellow—before it completely heals.

CAUSES & RISK FACTORS—Caused by direct injury, usually with a blunt object. Bleeding into tissues causes the surrounding tissue to be pushed away. The risk increases with:
- Contact sports.
- A medical history of any bleeding disorder such as hemophilia.
- Poor nutrition, including vitamin deficiency.
- The use of anticoagulants or aspirin.

DOCTOR'S TREATMENT & DIAGNOSTIC TESTS
- Medical history and physical exam for all except minor injuries.
- Doctor's care unless the hematoma is very small.
- X-rays of the injured area to assess the injury and to rule out the possibility of an underlying bone fracture. The total extent of the injury may not be apparent for 48 to 72 hours following injury.
- Needle aspiration of blood from the hematoma if it is accessible. At the same time, hyaluronidase (an enzyme) can be injected into the hematoma space to hasten the absorption of blood.
- Self-care for minor hematomas or for serious hematomas during the rehabilitation phase.
- Physical therapy following serious hematomas.

HOME TREATMENT BY SELF OR CARE-GIVER

GENERAL INSTRUCTIONS
- Use instructions for RICE, the first letters of *rest, ice, compression* and *elevation*. See Appendix 37 for details.
- Continue ice massage 3 or 4 times a day for 15 minutes at a time. Fill a large styrofoam cup with water and freeze. Tear a small amount of foam

from the top so the ice protrudes. Massage firmly over the injured area in a circle about the size of a softball.
- Don't put heavy pressure on the hematoma. You may trigger the bleeding again.

MEDICATION (ADJUSTED FOR AGING)
- For minor discomfort, you may use: Nonprescription medicines such as acetaminophen or ibuprofen. Topical liniments and ointments.
- Your doctor may prescribe stronger medicine for pain if needed.

ACTIVITY FOR OLDER PATIENTS
- Begin activities slowly and stop exercise as soon as pain begins. Increase your activity level as your healing progresses. To prevent a delay in healing, protect the area of the hematoma from excessive motion soon after injury. Motion breaks down the clot and causes irritation leading to possible scar formation, calcification and restricted movement after healing.
- Begin daily rehabilitation exercises when supportive wrapping is no longer needed. Use gentle ice massage for 10 minutes prior to exercise.

FOOD & BEVERAGE
- During recovery, eat a well-balanced diet that includes protein, such as meat, fish, poultry, cheese, milk and eggs. Increase fiber and fluid intake to prevent constipation that may result from decreased activity.
- Maintain a moderate to low-fat diet (120 to 130 grams of fat per day).

FUTURE CONSIDERATIONS FOR THE AGING ADULT

POSSIBLE COMPLICATIONS
- Infection introduced either through a break in the skin at the time of injury or during aspiration of the hematoma.
- Prolonged healing time if activity is resumed too soon.
- Calcification of the blood remaining in the hematoma if the blood is not completely removed or absorbed.

PROBABLE OUTCOME—The average healing time is 2 weeks to 2 months unless the blood is removed with aspiration. The healing time is much less with this treatment.

PREVENTING RECURRENCE—Apply an ice compress quickly after even minor injury.

CALL YOUR DOCTOR IF
- You have signs of a hematoma that doesn't begin to improve in 1 or 2 days.
- The skin is broken and signs of infection (drainage, increasing pain, fever, headache, muscle aches, dizziness or a general ill feeling) occur.

HEMIPLEGIA

BASIC INFORMATION FOR OLDER ADULTS

DESCRIPTION—Hemiplegia is the partial or complete paralysis of one side of the body. Body parts involved: The brain or spinal cord. (ACUTE ONSET OF THIS CONDITION IS AN EMERGENCY; SEEK MEDICAL HELP IMMEDIATELY!)

SPECIAL CONSIDERATIONS FOR AGING
- Stress from any emotional cause—fear, worry, anxiety, sadness, loneliness or anger—affects all aspects of any illness or disorder.
- Neurological diseases become more likely.
- The blood vessels nourishing the brain become thicker and lose their elasticity.

SIGNS & SYMPTOMS—Because of the anatomy of the brain and spinal cord, injury to one side of the brain affects the opposite side of the body. The following signs and symptoms vary greatly between individuals:
- Weakness or paralysis of the arm and leg on the affected side.
- Difficulty speaking, understanding or recognizing words.
- Altered or lost sensation on the affected side.
- Difficulty with self-feeding.
- Urinary incontinence.
- Blurred, double or decreased vision.

CAUSES & RISK FACTORS—Caused by brain injury in an area that controls one side of the body. Injury may result from stroke (the most common), which may be caused by bleeding in the brain or by a blood clot or other obstruction of a blood vessel to the brain; brain tumor or hemorrhage; head injury; multiple sclerosis; or encephalitis (brain inflammation). Risk factors include:
- Hypertension; diabetes.
- Bleeding disorders.

DOCTOR'S TREATMENT & DIAGNOSTIC TESTS
- Medical history and physical exam.
- Laboratory studies of blood, urine and cerebrospinal fluid; ECG (see Glossary).
- X-rays of the brain and neck.
- Hospitalization.
- Psychotherapy or counseling to help you overcome depression and learn to cope with disability.
- Physical therapy.
- Long-term nursing home care (sometimes).
- Care-giver instructions.

HOME TREATMENT BY SELF OR CARE-GIVER

GENERAL INSTRUCTIONS
- Ask family members and friends for support and obtain professional help in readjusting your life.
- Sleep on an egg-crate foam mattress or a waterbed to prevent pressure sores.

MEDICATION (ADJUSTED FOR AGING)
- No medication can repair damaged brain tissue, but your doctor may prescribe: Medications to control hypertension, diabetes or other underlying disorders. Anticoagulants to prevent blood clot formation if a stroke resulting from a clot caused the paralysis.
- *Note:* Adverse reactions and side effects may be more frequent and severe in older persons. Remind your doctor of any medicines you already take.

ACTIVITY FOR OLDER PATIENTS
- Resume your normal activities gradually. With rehabilitation you can compensate for or restore many lost functions.
- Use passive exercise for paralyzed or partially paralyzed muscles to prevent contractures. A physical therapist can provide instructions.

FOOD & BEVERAGE
- No special diet is required for hemiplegia, but diabetes or hypertension may require special diets. Consult your doctor.
- See Appendix 1 regarding good nutrition for people over 50.

FUTURE CONSIDERATIONS FOR THE AGING ADULT

POSSIBLE COMPLICATIONS—Pressure sores; shortening of the muscles (contractures); slow deterioration of the musculoskeletal system.

PROBABLE OUTCOME—Depends on the extent of injury. Brain tissue does not repair itself, but other parts of the brain can take over lost functions.

PREVENTING RECURRENCE
- Obtain medical treatment to control hypertension or diabetes.
- Protect yourself from head injury: Use seat belts in cars. Wear protective headgear during contact sports or while riding a bicycle or motorcycle. Don't drink alcohol or use mind-altering drugs and drive.

CALL YOUR DOCTOR IF

- You have symptoms of hemiplegia. *This is an emergency!*
- Any of the following occurs during treatment: Signs of infection, such as fever, muscle aches, chills and headache. Difficulty in emptying the bladder.
- New, unexplained symptoms develop. The drugs used in treatment may produce side effects.

HEMORRHOIDS
(Piles)

BASIC INFORMATION FOR OLDER ADULTS

DESCRIPTION—Hemorrhoids are dilated (varicose) veins of the rectum or anus. Body parts involved: The veins under the rectal or anal membrane.

SPECIAL CONSIDERATIONS FOR AGING
- The blood vessels throughout the body are less healthy. They become thicker and lose their elasticity.
- Constipation is more common in older people.
- The intake of water and other fluids is frequently inadequate.

SIGNS & SYMPTOMS
- Rectal bleeding. Bright red blood may appear as streaks on toilet paper adhering to fecal residue, or it may appear as a slow trickle for a short while following bowel movements.
- Pain, itching or mucus discharge after bowel movements.
- A lump that can be felt in the anus.
- A sensation that the rectum has not emptied completely after a bowel movement (large hemorrhoids only).

CAUSES & RISK FACTORS
Causes include:
- Repeated pressure in the anal or rectal veins—usually caused by straining during bowel movements.
- Abdominal or rectal tumors—either benign or malignant.

Risk factors include:
- A diet that lacks fiber; constipation.
- Prolonged sitting.
- Obesity.

DOCTOR'S TREATMENT & DIAGNOSTIC TESTS
- Medical history and physical exam.
- Anoscopy (see Glossary) or sigmoidoscopy (see Glossary).
- X-rays of the lower intestinal tract.
- Self-care instructions focused on the older patient.
- Surgery to remove the hemorrhoids (sometimes).

HOME TREATMENT BY SELF OR CARE-GIVER

GENERAL INSTRUCTIONS
- Straining during bowel movements increases the pain. Never strain to push a stool out.
- Lift feet on a low footstool to aid bowel movement.
- Clean the anal area gently with soft, moist paper after each bowel movement.

- To relieve the pain, sit in 8 to 10 inches of hot water for 10 to 20 minutes several times a day.
- To reduce the pain and swelling of a blood clot or protruding hemorrhoid, stay in bed for 1 day and apply ice packs to the anal area.

MEDICATION (ADJUSTED FOR AGING)
- For minor pain, you may use non-prescription drugs that contain zinc oxide or low-strength steroids.
- Your doctor may prescribe a stool softener or bulk laxative, such as psyllium seed.
- *Note:* Adverse reactions and side effects may be more frequent and severe in older persons. Remind your doctor of any medicines you already take.

ACTIVITY FOR OLDER PATIENTS
- No restrictions are necessary. Bowel function improves with good physical conditioning.
- See Appendix 20 regarding physical fitness for the active older adult.

FOOD & BEVERAGE
- To prevent constipation, eat a well-balanced diet that contains many high-fiber foods such as fresh fruit, bran muffins, beans, vegetables and whole-grain cereals.
- See Appendix 1 regarding good nutrition for people over 50.

FUTURE CONSIDERATIONS FOR THE AGING ADULT

POSSIBLE COMPLICATIONS
- Iron-deficiency anemia if the blood loss is significant.
- Severe pain caused by a blood clot in a hemorrhoid.
- Infection or ulceration of a hemorrhoid.

PROBABLE OUTCOME—Completely curable with surgery.

PREVENTING RECURRENCE
- Don't try to hurry bowel movements.
- Lose weight if you are overweight.

CALL YOUR DOCTOR IF

- A hard lump develops where a hemorrhoid has been.
- Hemorrhoids cause severe pain that isn't relieved by the treatment described above.
- Rectal bleeding is excessive (more than a trace or streak on toilet paper or stool).

HEPATITIS, ACUTE VIRAL

BASIC INFORMATION FOR OLDER ADULTS

DESCRIPTION—Acute viral hepatitis is an inflammation of the liver caused by a virus. Body part involved: The liver.

SPECIAL CONSIDERATIONS FOR AGING
- The immune system becomes less effective, opening the way for viral, bacterial and other infections; malignancies; immune disorders; and allergies.
- The total state of wellbeing in many older people makes them increasingly susceptible to infections and impairs their ability to prevent infections from spreading.
- Decreased nutrition increases the risk of infections.

SIGNS & SYMPTOMS
Early stages:
- Flu-like symptoms, such as fever, fatigue, nausea, vomiting, diarrhea and loss of appetite.

Several days later:
- Jaundice (yellow eyes and skin) caused by a buildup of bile in the blood.
- Dark urine from bile spilling over into the urine.
- Light, "clay-colored" or whitish stools.

CAUSES & RISK FACTORS—Caused by any of 3 different but related viruses that may infect the liver:
- Type A—Usually enters the body through water or food, especially raw shellfish that has been contaminated by sewage or through close personal contact such as sharing food or kissing.
- Type B—Usually enters the body through blood transfusions contaminated with the virus or through injections with non-sterile needles or syringes.
- Type Non-A, Non-B—Usually enters the body through contaminated blood transfusions.

Risk factors include:
- Travel to areas with poor sanitation.
- Oral-anal sexual practices.
- The use of intravenous, mind-altering drugs.
- Alcoholism.
- Blood transfusions.
- Working in a hospital.
- Working or participating in a day-care center or residential programs for retarded persons.
- Kidney dialysis treatment.
- Poor nutrition.
- Illness that has lowered resistance.

DOCTOR'S TREATMENT & DIAGNOSTIC TESTS
- Medical history and physical exam.
- Laboratory blood tests to identify the infection (Type A and Type B) and study liver function.
- Urinalysis.
- After diagnosis of mild cases, self-care instructions focused on the older patient.
- Hospitalization in severe cases to prevent dehydration.

HOME TREATMENT BY SELF OR CARE-GIVER

GENERAL INSTRUCTIONS
- Most persons with hepatitis can be cared for at home without undue risk. Strict isolation is not necessary, but the infected person should have separate eating and drinking utensils or use disposable ones.
- If you have hepatitis or are caring for someone with it, wash your hands carefully and often, especially after bowel movements.

MEDICATION (ADJUSTED FOR AGING)—Your doctor may prescribe cortisone drugs for severe cases to reduce liver inflammation.

ACTIVITY FOR OLDER PATIENTS—Bed rest is necessary until jaundice disappears and appetite returns. People differ widely in the rate at which they can return to normal activity.

FOOD & BEVERAGE
- Despite poor appetite, eating small, well-balanced meals helps promote recovery. Drink at least 8 glasses of water each day. *Don't drink alcohol.*
- See Appendix 1 regarding good nutrition.

FUTURE CONSIDERATIONS FOR THE AGING ADULT

POSSIBLE COMPLICATIONS—Liver failure in severe cases.

PROBABLE OUTCOME—Jaundice and other symptoms peak and then gradually disappear over 3 to 16 weeks. Most people in good general health recover fully in 1 to 4 months. A small percentage (1% to 2%) may proceed to chronic hepatitis. Recovery from viral hepatitis usually provides permanent immunity against it.

PREVENTING RECURRENCE
- Avoid the risk factors listed above.
- If you are exposed to someone with hepatitis, consult your doctor about receiving gamma globulin injections to prevent or decrease the risk of hepatitis.
- If you are in a high-risk group, such as hospital workers, dentists, dental workers or male homosexuals, consult your doctor about being vaccinated for Type B hepatitis. Vaccines are not available for the other forms of hepatitis.

CALL YOUR DOCTOR IF

- You have symptoms of hepatitis or have been exposed to someone who has it.
- Any of the following occurs during treatment:
  Increasing loss of appetite.
  Excessive drowsiness or mental confusion.
  Vomiting, diarrhea or abdominal pain.
  Deepening jaundice.
  Skin rash or itching.

HEPATOMA
(Malignant Liver Tumor; Hepatocellular Carcinoma)

 BASIC INFORMATION FOR OLDER ADULTS

DESCRIPTION—Hepatoma is a malignant tumor that begins in the liver—i.e., a primary tumor as opposed to cancer that has spread from another site. Body part involved: The liver.

SPECIAL CONSIDERATIONS FOR AGING
- The immune system becomes less effective, opening the way for viral, bacterial and other infections; malignancies; immune disorders; and allergies.
- Decreased nutrition, common among chronically ill older people, increases the risk of any disease or disorder.

SIGNS & SYMPTOMS
- A hard mass in the right upper abdomen.
- Unexplained weight loss and appetite loss.
- Jaundice (yellow skin and eyes; rare).
- Abdominal discomfort that resembles a pulled muscle.
- Low blood sugar (weakness, sweating, hunger, tremor and headache).
- Fever.
- Fluid in the abdomen; enlarged spleen.
- A bleeding tendency in the gastrointestinal tract and other sites.
- Decreased mental function (sometimes).

CAUSES & RISK FACTORS
Causes include:
- Pre-existing cirrhosis of the liver. 50% of persons with hepatoma have cirrhosis.
- Possibly a slow virus.
Risk factors include:
- A medical history of hepatitis; alcoholism.
- Birth control pills.
- Anabolic steroids used by some athletes to build muscles.
- Geographic locations. This condition is especially common in South Africa and Southeast Asia.

DOCTOR'S TREATMENT & DIAGNOSTIC TESTS
- Medical history and physical exam.
- Laboratory blood studies of liver function and hepatitis B antigen.
- CT scan (see Glossary) of the liver and ultrasound.
- X-rays of the abdomen, including angiography (see Glossary) of liver blood vessels.
- Liver biopsy.
- Surgery to remove the tumor if possible. Only 25% can be removed successfully. Advancing age alone is not a deterrent. Liver transplants have been successful in a few patients.
- Psychotherapy or counseling to help you cope with an incurable illness.
- Self-care instructions focused on the older patient.

 HOME TREATMENT BY SELF OR CARE-GIVER

GENERAL INSTRUCTIONS
- No specific instructions except those listed under other headings.
- Hepatoma is a complicated, serious disorder. This page can cover only the main points of diagnosis and treatment. Your doctor, nurse or librarian can provide sources of supplemental information.

MEDICATION (ADJUSTED FOR AGING)
- For minor discomfort, you may use non-prescription drugs such as acetaminophen. Your doctor may prescribe pain relievers if necessary.
- Anticancer drugs have produced disappointing results so far.
- *Note:* Adverse reactions and side effects may be more frequent and severe in older persons. Remind your doctor of any medicines you already take.

ACTIVITY FOR OLDER PATIENTS
- Stay as active as your strength allows.
- See Appendix 20 regarding physical fitness for the active older adult.

FOOD & BEVERAGE
- No special diet is required. Don't drink alcohol.
- See Appendix 1 regarding good nutrition for people over 50.

 FUTURE CONSIDERATIONS FOR THE AGING ADULT

POSSIBLE COMPLICATIONS
- Liver failure.
- Spread to other organs, especially the lungs, adrenal glands and bones.

PROBABLE OUTCOME--This condition is currently considered incurable. Only a small number of patients survive 5 years following surgery. However, the symptoms can be relieved or controlled, and medical literature cites a few instances of unexplained recovery. Scientific research into causes and treatment continues, so there is hope for increasingly effective treatment and a cure.

PREVENTING RECURRENCE
- Don't drink more than 1 or 2 alcoholic drinks—if any—a day.
- Immunization against hepatitis B may be helpful.

 CALL YOUR DOCTOR IF

- You have symptoms of hepatoma.
- You develop signs of bleeding, especially from the gastrointestinal tract. Signs include bloody vomit or vomit that contains black material resembling coffee grounds, blood in the stool or black, tarry stools.

HERNIA

BASIC INFORMATION FOR OLDER ADULTS

DESCRIPTION—A hernia is the protrusion of an internal organ through a weakness or abnormal opening in the muscle around it. The most common types include inguinal hernia, femoral hernia, incisional hernia, umbilical hernia and hiatal hernia (see Esophageal Reflux in the Illnesses section). Body parts involved:
- Inguinal or femoral—The connective tissue in the groin.
- Incisional—The muscles at the site of a previous surgery.
- Umbilical—The muscles around the navel.
- Hiatal—The diaphragm and esophagus.

SPECIAL CONSIDERATIONS FOR AGING
- Repair from injury or disease is complete and effective, but recovery takes longer in older people.
- Percent of strong muscle tissue decreases.

SIGNS & SYMPTOMS
- A protrusion that usually returns to normal position with gentle pressure or by lying down.
- Mild discomfort or pain at the site of the protrusion (sometimes).
- Scrotal swelling, with or without pain.
- Severe pain when the hernia bulges out and can't be replaced.

CAUSES & RISK FACTORS—Caused by a weakness in connective tissue or a muscle wall. This may be present from birth or acquired later in life. Incisional hernias result from previous surgery. Risk factors include:
- Chronic cough.
- Obesity.
- Straining, as with chronic constipation.
- Lifting a heavy object.

DOCTOR'S TREATMENT & DIAGNOSTIC TESTS
- Medical history and physical exam.
- Laboratory blood studies.
- X-rays of the abdomen.
- Surgery to repair the opening caused by the weakened muscle or connective tissue. Advancing age alone is not a deterrent.
- Self-care instructions focused on the older patient.

HOME TREATMENT BY SELF OR CARE-GIVER

GENERAL INSTRUCTIONS
- For an explanation of surgery to repair an inguinal hernia and postoperative care, see Hernia Repair, Inguinal, in the Surgeries section.

- Whenever you lie down prior to surgery, push your hernia gently into place if it protrudes visibly.
- Don't wear a hernia truss. It injures or weakens tissues, making surgery difficult or impossible.

MEDICATION (ADJUSTED FOR AGING)
- For minor discomfort, you may use non-prescription drugs such as acetaminophen.
- *Note:* Adverse reactions and side effects may be more frequent and severe in older persons. Remind your doctor of any medicines you already take.

ACTIVITY FOR OLDER PATIENTS
- Avoid lifting heavy objects.
- See Appendix 20 regarding physical fitness for the active older adult.

FOOD & BEVERAGE
- Adjust your diet to avoid constipation.
- See Appendix 1 regarding good nutrition for people over 50.

FUTURE CONSIDERATIONS FOR THE AGING ADULT

POSSIBLE COMPLICATIONS—If an abdominal hernia becomes strangulated (loses its blood supply), the protruding part may cause intestinal obstruction with fever, severe pain, vomiting and shock.

PROBABLE OUTCOME—Hernias are usually curable with surgery.

PREVENTING RECURRENCE
- A weak area may not herniate until it ruptures with heavy lifting or straining. If you must lift something, lift properly. Bend your knees, lift the object and rise using your leg muscles. Keep the object close to your body. Don't strain or hold your breath. Don't lift by bending from the waist and lifting using your back muscles.
- If constipation is a problem, see Constipation in the Illnesses section for treatment.
- If you have a chronic cough, seek appropriate medical care.
- Strengthen your abdominal muscles by appropriate exercise (ask your doctor).

CALL YOUR DOCTOR IF

You have symptoms of a hernia. If you have fever or severe pain, call immediately!

HERPES, GENITAL

BASIC INFORMATION FOR OLDER ADULTS

DESCRIPTION—Genital herpes is a virus infection of the genitals or the skin around the rectum or buttocks. It is usually (but not always) transmitted by sexual contact (intercourse or oral sex). Genital herpes may increase the risk of cervical cancer. Body parts involved: The penis; vagina; cervix; thighs; buttocks (sometimes).

SPECIAL CONSIDERATIONS FOR AGING
- The immune system becomes less effective, opening the way for infections.
- Decreased nutrition increases the risk of any disease or disorder.
- Characteristic signs and symptoms of many disorders are frequently changed or absent.
- Stress from any emotional cause affects all aspects of any illness or disorder.

SIGNS & SYMPTOMS
- Painful blisters, preceded by itching and irritation, on the vaginal lips or the penis. In women, the blisters may extend into the vagina to the cervix and urethra. After a few days, the blisters rupture and leave painful, shallow ulcers which last 1 to 3 weeks.
- Difficult, painful urination.
- Enlarged lymph glands.
- Fever and a general ill feeling.

CAUSES & RISK FACTORS—Caused by *herpes simplex* virus, Type 2 (HSV-2; see Glossary). (*Herpes simplex virus*, Type 1 (HSV-1) causes common cold sores, which appear around the mouth.) Genital herpes is transmitted from someone who has active herpes lesions, usually (but not always) by sexual contact. The lesions may be on the genitals, hands, lips or mouth (including Type 1 virus). The virus lies dormant inside infected cells until conditions for multiplication are right; then the infected cells grow. Risk factors include:
- Serious illness that has lowered resistance.
- The use of immunosuppressive or anticancer drugs; a rundown condition.
- Stress, which increases susceptibility to a primary infection or a recurrence. Stress may lead to the diminished efficiency of the immune responses that usually suppress the growth of the virus.

DOCTOR'S TREATMENT & DIAGNOSTIC TESTS
- Medical history and physical exam.
- Self-care instructions focused on the older patient.

HOME TREATMENT BY SELF OR CARE-GIVER

GENERAL INSTRUCTIONS
- Take warm baths to which a tablespoon of salt is added.
- There are no particular instructions for men.

- Women should wear cotton underpants or pantyhose with a cotton crotch—not underpants made from non-ventilating materials.
- Women should not douche unless told to by a doctor.
- To reduce the pain during urination, women may urinate in a bath or shower, through a tubular device such as a toilet paper roll or a plastic cup with the end cut out or while pouring a glass of warm water over the vaginal area.

MEDICATION (ADJUSTED FOR AGING)—Your doctor may prescribe an antiviral drug, such as acyclovir, in oral or topical form. This new drug reduces the intensity and duration of the first attack. It does not prevent recurrent attacks.

ACTIVITY FOR OLDER PATIENTS
- Reduce your normal activities until your fever diminishes and you feel well.
- Don't resume sexual relations until the symptoms have disappeared.

FOOD & BEVERAGE—No special diet.

FUTURE CONSIDERATIONS FOR THE AGING ADULT

POSSIBLE COMPLICATIONS
- Generalized and serious disease in persons who must take anticancer drugs or immunosuppressive drugs.
- Secondary bacterial infection.
- The virus may have a part in the development of cervical cancer. Women who have had herpes should get a Pap smear at least once a year.

PROBABLE OUTCOME
- Genital herpes is currently considered incurable, but the symptoms can be relieved with treatment.
- During symptom-free periods, the virus returns to its dormant state. Your symptoms recur when the virus is reactivated. Recurrent symptoms are not new infections.
- The discomfort varies from person to person and from time to time in the same person. The first herpes infection is much more uncomfortable than following ones.

PREVENTING RECURRENCE
- Avoid sexual intercourse if either partner has blisters or sores; avoid oral sex with a partner who has cold sores on the mouth.
- Use a rubber condom during intercourse if either sex partner has inactive genital herpes.

CALL YOUR DOCTOR IF

- You have symptoms of genital herpes.
- The symptoms worsen or don't improve in 1 week despite treatment.
- Unusual vaginal bleeding or swelling occurs.
- The fever returns during treatment or you become generally ill.
- The symptoms recur after treatment.

HERPETIC WHITLOW

BASIC INFORMATION FOR OLDER ADULTS

DESCRIPTION—Herpetic whitlow is an inflammation of the skin folds around the nails caused by a contagious herpes virus. Body parts involved: The bed of a fingernail (most likely) or toenail.

SPECIAL CONSIDERATIONS FOR AGING
- Characteristic signs and symptoms of many disorders are frequently changed or absent.
- The immune system becomes less effective, opening the way for viral, bacterial and other infections; malignancies; immune disorders; and allergies.
- Decreased nutrition increases the risk of infections.

SIGNS & SYMPTOMS
- Sudden pain around the nail.
- Redness, swelling and warmth around the nail.
- Swelling of the lymph glands nearby, such as in the elbow or armpit if a fingernail is affected.
- Groupings of tiny blisters that are barely visible around the nail.

CAUSES & RISK FACTORS—Caused by the *herpes hominus* virus, Type 1 or Type 2. Herpetic whitlow is often transmitted to the fingers from cold sores (*herpes simplex*) on the mouth. Risk factors include:
- Occupational exposure to constant wetness, such that experienced by dishwashers or maintenance personnel.
- Occupational exposure to herpes infection, such as that experienced by nurses, dentists or dental assistants who provide mouth care.

DOCTOR'S TREATMENT & DIAGNOSTIC TESTS
- Medical history and physical exam.
- Laboratory culture of discharge from the infected area.
- Self-care instructions focused on the older patient.
- Minor surgical procedure if the infection is severe.

HOME TREATMENT BY SELF OR CARE-GIVER

GENERAL INSTRUCTIONS
- Protect your hands and feet to prevent further injury or spread of the infection to others. Wear heavy-duty vinyl gloves to avoid contact with irritating substances such as water, soap, detergent, metal scrubbing pads, scouring pads, scouring powder and other chemicals. Wear shoes or sandals in public showers or outdoors.
- Don't touch other persons until the inflammation clears.

MEDICATION (ADJUSTED FOR AGING)
- Your doctor may prescribe: Topical steroid preparations to reduce the inflammation. They include creams, ointments and lotions. Apply the topical steroid only once or twice a day unless directed otherwise. Apply immediately after bathing for better spreading and penetration. Oral or topical antiviral medications.
- *Note:* Adverse reactions and side effects may be more frequent and severe in older persons. Remind your doctor of any medicines you already take.

ACTIVITY FOR OLDER PATIENTS
- No restrictions are necessary.
- See Appendix 20 regarding physical fitness for the active older adult.

FOOD & BEVERAGE
- No special diet is required.
- See Appendix 1 regarding good nutrition for people over 50.

FUTURE CONSIDERATIONS FOR THE AGING ADULT

POSSIBLE COMPLICATIONS
- Spread of the herpes infection to other body parts, such as the lips or genitals.
- Osteomyelitis, a bacterial infection of the bone and bone marrow (rare).

PROBABLE OUTCOME—The first episode is usually curable in 2 months with treatment. However, recurrent attacks are common.

PREVENTING RECURRENCE
- Avoid exposure to people who have active herpes infections.
- Keep your hands and feet warm and dry.

CALL YOUR DOCTOR IF

- You have symptoms of herpetic whitlow.
- Your temperature rises over 101F (38.3C).
- Your symptoms don't improve in 3 days despite treatment.
- Herpes lesions appear elsewhere on the body.

ILLNESSES & DISORDERS

HICCUPS
(Hiccoughs; Singultus)

BASIC INFORMATION FOR OLDER ADULTS

DESCRIPTION—Hiccups are repeated involuntary spasmodic contractions of the diaphragm. Hiccups are a symptom—not a disease. Body parts involved: The diaphragm (the big muscle that separates the chest from the abdomen) and the phrenic nerve (the nerve that connects the diaphragm to the brain).

SPECIAL CONSIDERATIONS FOR AGING—Characteristic signs and symptoms of many disorders are frequently changed or absent. For example, hiccups may be the only early sign of appendicitis.

SIGNS & SYMPTOMS—A sharp, quick sound produced from the vocal cords by a spasm of the diaphragm. The spasm closes the muscles in the back of the throat during inhalation.

CAUSES & RISK FACTORS—Caused by the irritation of the nerves from the brain that control the breathing muscles, especially the diaphragm. The cause of short hiccup episodes is usually unknown. Prolonged or recurrent hiccup episodes may be caused by:
- Swallowing hot or irritating substances.
- Diseases of the pleura (thin membrane layers that cover the lungs).
- Pneumonia.
- Uremia.
- Alcoholism.
- The use of certain prescription or non-prescription drugs.
- Disorders of the stomach, esophagus, bowel or pancreas.
- Bladder irritation.
- Hepatitis.
- The spread of cancer from another part of the body to the liver or part of the pleura.
- Recent surgery, especially abdominal surgery.
- Emotional causes.

Risk factors include:
- An illness that has diminished your health.
- Recent abdominal surgery.
- The use of drugs, especially those that irritate the stomach.

DOCTOR'S TREATMENT & DIAGNOSTIC TESTS
- Medical history and physical exam.
- Self-care instructions focused on the older patient.
- Surgery to cut the phrenic nerve (for severe, prolonged cases only).

HOME TREATMENT BY SELF OR CARE-GIVER

GENERAL INSTRUCTIONS—These instructions are for short hiccup episodes. Prolonged hiccups require medical care.
- Hold your breath and count to 10.
- Breathe into a paper bag, then ihale the air in the bag. Don't use a plastic bag because it may cling to your nostrils.
- Insert your thumb between your teeth and your upper lip; press the upper lip with your index finger just below the right nostril.
- Drink a glass of water rapidly.
- Swallow dry bread or crushed ice.
- Pull gently on your tongue.
- Close your eyelids and apply gentle pressure to your eyeballs.
- Swallow a teaspoon of dry sugar.

MEDICATION (ADJUSTED FOR AGING)
- For prolonged or recurrent hiccups, your doctor may prescribe a mild tranquilizer or sedative.
- *Note:* Adverse reactions and side effects may be more frequent and severe in older persons. Remind your doctor of any medicines you already take.

ACTIVITY FOR OLDER PATIENTS
- No restrictions are necessary.
- See Appendix 20 regarding physical fitness for the active older adult.

FOOD & BEVERAGE
- No special diet is required.
- See Appendix 1 regarding good nutrition for people over 50.

FUTURE CONSIDERATIONS FOR THE AGING ADULT

POSSIBLE COMPLICATIONS—None unless the hiccups are prolonged, which may indicate serious disease.

PROBABLE OUTCOME—Short hiccup episodes usually don't indicate disease. They will subside with the treatment discussed below. Continued hiccups can be debilitating and require medical attention to determine the cause.

PREVENTING RECURRENCE—Cannot be prevented at present.

CALL YOUR DOCTOR IF

- The hiccups persist longer than 8 hours.
- You suspect a prescription drug may be causing the hiccups.

HIP FRACTURE

BASIC INFORMATION FOR OLDER ADULTS

DESCRIPTION—A hip fracture is a complete or partial break in the femur, the major bone in the hip joint. Body parts involved: The femur, including the muscles and tendons that attach the head of the femur to the acetabulum (hip socket in the bony pelvis).

SPECIAL CONSIDERATIONS FOR AGING
- For many reasons, older people are less likely to maintain a good level of physical conditioning.
- Muscle bulk and power decrease.
- The bones become thinner.
- Many body changes occur as a result of estrogen deficiency beginning at menopause. These include a greater tendency to osteoporosis, hardening of the arteries and other disorders.

SIGNS & SYMPTOMS
- Intolerable pain when trying to walk.
- Swelling, tenderness and bruising in the hip area.
- Deformed hip appearance.

CAUSES & RISK FACTORS
Caused by injury, especially falls. Risk factors include:
- Activities that increase the risk of injury.
- Osteoporosis, especially post-menopausal osteoporosis.
- Bone cancer.
- Multiple medications which may reduce alertness.
- Osteogenesis imperfecta (see Glossary).
- Calcium imbalance.
- Poor nutrition, especially insufficient calcium and protein.

DOCTOR'S TREATMENT & DIAGNOSTIC TESTS
- Medical history and physical exam.
- X-rays and bone scans of the hip.
- Surgery to reattach broken fragments, usually by screwing them together with a metal or plastic fixation device.
- Physical therapy and rehabilitation.

HOME TREATMENT BY SELF OR CARE-GIVER

GENERAL INSTRUCTIONS
- Self-care is not appropriate; surgery is the only treatment. The surgeon reattaches the fractured bone parts and secures them with surgical steel pins. Unlike most fractures, hip fractures usually don't require casts.
- After surgery, bathe and shower as usual. You may wash the incision gently with mild unscented soap. Wound dressings are optional.
- Heat relieves the pain of the incision. Use a heat lamp or a towel in warm water and wrung out.

MEDICATION (ADJUSTED FOR AGING)—
Your doctor may prescribe:
- Pain relievers.
- Antibiotics to fight infection if necessary.
- Stool softeners to prevent constipation.

ACTIVITY FOR OLDER PATIENTS
- After awakening from anesthesia, move the unaffected leg often to decrease the possibility of deep-vein blood clots. Most surgeons urge patients to get up and move about as soon as possible. Resume your normal activities gradually as healing progresses.
- You will probably use a walker at first, then progress to a cane after 6 to 12 weeks. A rehabilitation program is mandatory for full recovery.

FOOD & BEVERAGE
- Consume clear liquids for the 1st day after surgery, then no special diet. Ask your doctor if you should take calcium supplements.
- See Appendix 1 regarding good nutrition for people over 50.

FUTURE CONSIDERATIONS FOR THE AGING ADULT

POSSIBLE COMPLICATIONS
- Infection of the surgical wound.
- Nerve and blood vessel damage at the fracture site.
- Accompanying dislocation.
- Inadequate blood supply to the injured area, causing tissue death of the bone.
- Poor healing (non-union) of the fracture.
- Blood clots due to bed confinement and restricted activity.

PROBABLE OUTCOME—Usually curable with surgery and rehabilitation.

PREVENTING RECURRENCE
- Ensure an adequate calcium intake (1000mg to 1500mg a day) with milk and milk products or calcium supplements.
- Protect yourself against falls, especially in the home.
- Women should consult a doctor about taking estrogen after menopause begins.

CALL YOUR DOCTOR IF

- You have symptoms of a hip fracture. Call immediately if you have numbness or loss of feeling below the fracture site. *This is an emergency!*
- Any of the following occurs after surgery: Swelling above or below the fracture site. Chills, fever, muscle aches or headache. Increased pain, swelling, redness or discharge at the surgical site. Constipation.

BASIC INFORMATION FOR OLDER ADULTS

DESCRIPTION—Histoplasmosis is a fungus infection that is confined mostly to people who live in the eastern and midwestern parts of the U.S. Most cases are minor and go undiagnosed. Body parts involved: The lungs; central nervous system; gastrointestinal system; eyes.

SPECIAL CONSIDERATIONS FOR AGING
- The immune system becomes less effective, opening the way for viral, bacterial and other infections; malignancies; immune disorders; and allergies.
- Decreased nutrition increases the risk of infections.
- Characteristic signs and symptoms of many disorders are frequently changed or absent.

SIGNS & SYMPTOMS
- Persistent cough and other symptoms similar to those of a cold.
- Loss of appetite, diarrhea and weight loss.
- Fever; headache.
- Irritability.
- Paleness.
- Abdominal swelling.
- Breathing difficulty (rare).
- Some vision changes (seeing flashing spots in the peripheral visual fields).

CAUSES & RISK FACTORS—Caused by infection by the fungus *histoplasma capsulatum*. People become infected by breathing dust that contains fungus spores. The fungus is found in soil contaminated by the feces of birds and bats that carry the fungus. The contaminated soil is most often in pigeon lofts, barns, chicken houses, damp areas under bridges, along streams and in caves. The risk increases with:
- Recent severe illness, especially uremia, diabetes mellitus, chronic lung disease, cancer or severe burns.
- Geographic location. This disease occurs most often on the western slopes of the Appalachians and in the Mississippi, Missouri and Ohio River valleys.
- The use of immunosuppressive, anticancer or cortisone drugs.

DOCTOR'S TREATMENT & DIAGNOSTIC TESTS
- Medical history and physical exam.
- Laboratory studies such as a sputum culture, blood studies and skin tests.
- Self-care instructions focused on the older patient.
- Hospitalization for complications.

HOME TREATMENT BY SELF OR CARE-GIVER

GENERAL INSTRUCTIONS
- Isolation is not necessary. The disease is not transmitted from person to person.

- Use a cool-mist humidifier with pure water and no medicine in it to increase the air moisture. This helps thin lung secretions so they can be coughed up more easily.
- Don't smoke.
- Weigh daily and keep a record. Report any changes (up or down) to your doctor.

MEDICATION (ADJUSTED FOR AGING)
- For severe cases, your doctor may prescribe antifungal drugs that must be given intravenously in a hospital.
- Don't suppress the cough with cough medicine if it produces sputum. It is ridding the lungs of mucus. If the cough is painful and non-productive, consult your doctor about a prescription cough suppressant.
- You may use non-prescription drugs such as acetaminophen or aspirin to relieve the pain.
- *Note:* Adverse reactions and side effects may be more frequent and severe in older persons. Remind your doctor of any medicines you already take.

ACTIVITY FOR OLDER PATIENTS
- Stay in bed until the fever, pain and shortness of breath have been gone for at least 48 hours. Then resume your normal activities gradually. Many people are fatigued and weak after recovery. Don't expect too much too soon.
- See Appendix 20 regarding physical fitness for the active older adult.

FOOD & BEVERAGE
- No special diet is required.
- See Appendix 1 regarding good nutrition for people over 50.

FUTURE CONSIDERATIONS FOR THE AGING ADULT

POSSIBLE COMPLICATIONS—Spread of the infection to the heart, spleen, adrenal glands and meninges (the membranes that cover the brain). This is rare, but it can be fatal.

PROBABLE OUTCOME—Usually curable—even with complications—with intensive care and 10 to 12 weeks of treatment with antifungal drugs. Most people only feel tired or "bad" for several weeks.

PREVENTING RECURRENCE—Avoid areas where the soil is likely to be infected with histoplasma spores.

CALL YOUR DOCTOR IF

- You have symptoms of histoplasmosis.
- Any of the following occurs during treatment:
  Weight loss continues.
  Fever rises to 101F (38.3C) orally.
  Diarrhea is uncontrollable.
  Severe headache and stiff neck begin.

HIVES
(Urticaria; Giant Urticaria)

BASIC INFORMATION FOR OLDER ADULTS

DESCRIPTION—Hives is an allergic disorder characterized by skin changes with raised areas, redness and itching. Body parts involved: The skin anywhere on the body, including the scalp, lips, palms and soles.

SPECIAL CONSIDERATIONS FOR AGING
- The immune system becomes less effective, opening the way for infections and allergies.
- Decreased nutrition, common among chronically ill older people, increases the risk of any disease or disorder.
- Unusual and unexpected reactions to drugs and medications are more likely.
- Stress from any emotional cause affects all aspects of any illness or disorder.

SIGNS & SYMPTOMS—Itchy skin papules (small, raised bumps) with the following characteristics:
- They swell and produce pink or red lesions called wheals. The wheals have clearly defined edges and flat tops. They measure 1cm to 5cm in diameter.
- Wheals join together quickly and form large, flat plaques (larger areas of raised, skin-colored lesions).
- Wheals and plaques change shape, resolve and reappear in minutes or hours. This rapid change is unique to hives.

CAUSES & RISK FACTORS—Hives is characterized by the release of histamines, sometimes for unknown reasons. The most common causes are medications (nearly every drug causes hives in some persons); insect bites; viral infections; autoimmune disease; dysproteinemias; exposure to cold, heat, water or sunlight; cancer, especially leukemia; exposure to animals, especially cats; eating eggs, fruits, nuts and shellfish; and food dyes and preservatives (possibly). Risk factors include stress; other allergies or a a family history of allergies.

DOCTOR'S TREATMENT & DIAGNOSTIC TESTS
- Medical history and physical exam.
- Allergy skin tests and desensitization injections.
- Self-care instructions focused on the older patient.
- Emergency room care for life-threatening reactions.

HOME TREATMENT BY SELF OR CARE-GIVER

GENERAL INSTRUCTIONS
- Don't take drugs (including aspirin, laxatives, sedatives, vitamins, antacids, pain killers or cough syrups) that have not been prescribed for you.
- Don't wear tight underwear or foundation garments. Any skin irritation may trigger new outbreaks.

- Don't take hot baths or showers.
- Apply cold-water compresses or soaks (see Appendix 18) to relieve the itching.

MEDICATION (ADJUSTED FOR AGING)
- You may try applying calamine lotion to relieve the itching.
- Your doctor may prescribe: Antihistamines, ephedrine, terbutaline or cortisone drugs to relieve itching and rash. Sedatives or tranquilizers for anxiety. Epinephrine by injection to treat severe symptoms.
- *Note:* Adverse reactions and side effects may be more frequent and severe in older persons. Remind your doctor of any medicines you already take.

ACTIVITY FOR OLDER PATIENTS—Decrease your activities until several days after the hives disappear. Avoid getting hot, sweaty or excited.

FOOD & BEVERAGE
- If foods are suspected as a cause, keep a food diary to help identify the offending food.
- Avoid alcohol and coffee or other caffeine-containing beverages. These may trigger outbreaks.

FUTURE CONSIDERATIONS FOR THE AGING ADULT

POSSIBLE COMPLICATIONS—Swelling of the larynx and inability to breathe; hives may be the first sign of life-threatening anaphylaxis. If so, they will be followed by itching, runny nose, wheezing, paleness, cold sweats and low blood pressure. Without prompt treatment, coma and cardiac arrest can occur.

PROBABLE OUTCOME—Depends on the cause. If caused by a medication or acute viral infection, hives usually disappears within hours or days. Some cases become chronic and last for months or years. Most eventually go into spontaneous remission—even if the cause is not identified.

PREVENTING RECURRENCE
- If you have had hives and identified the cause, avoid the source.
- Keep an anaphylaxis kit if you experience severe reactions.

CALL YOUR DOCTOR IF

- Any of the following occurs during an episode of hives. If so, *this is an emergency*: Swollen lips. Shortness of breath or wheezing. A tight or constricted feeling in the throat.
- New, unexplained symptoms develop. The drugs used in treatment may produce side effects.

ILLNESSES & DISORDERS

HODGKIN'S DISEASE

BASIC INFORMATION FOR OLDER ADULTS

DESCRIPTION—A form of lymphoma, Hodgkin's disease is a malignant tumor of the lymph glands. Body parts involved: The lymphocytes (white blood cells), lymph glands (glands which check infection and produce immune substances) and spleen (a large lymph gland).

SPECIAL CONSIDERATIONS FOR AGING
- The immune system becomes less effective, opening the way for viral, bacterial and other infections; malignancies; immune disorders; and allergies.
- Malignant diseases are less likely to spread rapidly.
- Older patients become less able to tolerate maximal x-ray and chemotherapy treatments.
- Stress from any emotional cause—fear, worry, anxiety, sadness, loneliness or anger—affects all aspects of any illness or disorder.

SIGNS & SYMPTOMS
- Itching all over the body.
- Swollen, rubbery, non-tender distinct lymph glands anywhere in the body—but most commonly in the armpit or groin.
- Intermittent fever and night sweats.
- Pain in the diseased area after drinking alcohol.
- Weight loss.
- Jaundice (yellow skin and eyes).
- A general ill feeling.
- Anemia.
- Bleeding from the gastrointestinal tract.

CAUSES & RISK FACTORS—The cause is unknown, but research suggests a virus infection may be a factor or that the Epstein-Barr virus may be involved. Risk factors include:
- Autoimmune diseases.
- Immunodeficiencies.

DOCTOR'S TREATMENT & DIAGNOSTIC TESTS
- Medical history and physical exam.
- Laboratory studies of blood and bone marrow.
- Lymphangiogram (see Glossary).
- Biopsy (see Glossary) of lymph nodes or other body parts.
- X-rays or CT scans (see Glossary) of various body parts that may be involved.
- Hospitalization for short periods to confirm diagnosis and for treatment.
- Surgery to discover the extent of disease. Advancing age alone is not a deterrent.
- Radiation therapy.
- Self-care instructions focused on the older patient.

HOME TREATMENT BY SELF OR CARE-GIVER

GENERAL INSTRUCTIONS
- Maintain as positive an attitude as possible during treatment.

- Treatment may cause side effects, but they are usually temporary.
- Your pain can be controlled. Don't hesitate to ask your doctor for pain medication.
- Fear may be your worst enemy.
- Call on family members and friends for whatever support and help you need.
- Hodgkin's disease is a complicated, serious disorder. This page can cover only the main points of diagnosis and treatment. Your doctor, nurse or librarian can provide sources of supplemental information.

MEDICATION (ADJUSTED FOR AGING)
- Your doctor may prescribe anticancer drugs (chemotherapy). Medication may cause side effects or adverse reactions in some people. New symptoms may be caused by the medicine, the original disorder or a new illness. Side effects caused by medicine usually disappear when the body adjusts to the drug or when the drug is discontinued.
- *Note:* Adverse reactions and side effects may be more frequent and severe in older persons. Remind your doctor of any medicines you already take.

ACTIVITY FOR OLDER PATIENTS
- Remain as active as your strength allows.
- See Appendix 20 regarding physical fitness for the active older adult.

FOOD & BEVERAGE
- No special diet is required.
- See Appendix 1 regarding good nutrition for people over 50.

FUTURE CONSIDERATIONS FOR THE AGING ADULT

POSSIBLE COMPLICATIONS—Spread of the malignancy to other parts of the body.

PROBABLE OUTCOME—Usually curable with radiation therapy and anticancer drugs if diagnosed and treated early. With treatment, the 10-year survival rate is about 70%. The potential for cure varies according to the cell type discovered from biopsy of the lymph nodes and the spread of the disease prior to treatment.

PREVENTING RECURRENCE—There are no specific preventive measures.

CALL YOUR DOCTOR IF

- You have symptoms of Hodgkin's disease.
- Any of the following occurs during treatment:
  Fever.
  Signs of infection (redness, swelling, pain or tenderness) anywhere in the body.
  Swelling of the feet and ankles.
  Discomfort when urinating or decreased urination in 1 day.
- You think your medicine is causing symptoms.

HYDROCEPHALUS, NORMAL-PRESSURE

BASIC INFORMATION FOR OLDER ADULTS

DESCRIPTION—Normal-pressure hydrocephalus is a dilatation of the brain ventricles (the chambers in the brain filled with cerebrospinal fluid). In this type of hydrocephalus, the fluid is not under increased pressure. Body part involved: The brain.

SPECIAL CONSIDERATIONS FOR AGING—Normal-pressure hydrocephalus is one of the few human disorders that occurs only among the elderly population.

SIGNS & SYMPTOMS
- Dementia, characterized by confusion, depression, paranoia, memory impairment (variable), anxiety, slow disintegration of the personality and intellect, impaired insight and judgment, restricted interests, rigid outlook, difficulty in conceptual thinking, poverty of thought, diminished initiative, easy distractibility, speech disturbances and "night walking."
- Incontinence.
- Unsteadiness and hesitation when walking.

CAUSES & RISK FACTORS
Causes include:
- Previous surface inflammation of the brain caused by bleeding (subarachnoid hemorrhage).
- Infection or head injury.
Stress may hasten the symptoms of dementia.

DOCTOR'S TREATMENT & DIAGNOSTIC TESTS
- Medical history and physical exam.
- Laboratory blood studies and urinalysis.
- PET scan; CT scan; EEG (see Glossary for all).
- Radioactive studies with a gamma emissions camera.
- Follow-up outpatient visits to monitor your progress and adjustment to treatment.
- Hospitalization for surgery to shunt cerebrospinal fluid away from ventricles in the brain.

OTHER—Normal-pressure hydrocephalus is an enormously complicated problem with long-lasting implications for patients and all family members. Seek as much knowledge as you can and request help from community social services.

HOME TREATMENT BY SELF OR CARE-GIVER

GENERAL INSTRUCTIONS—Follow a neurosurgeon's instructions, plus the following:
- Keep the patient's room reasonably bright.
- Keep drug or alcohol use to a minimum.
- Provide radio and/or television.
- Make explanations simple and concise.
- Display large calendars and clocks.

MEDICATION (ADJUSTED FOR AGING)
- The doctor may prescribe haloperidol if needed to calm the patient.
- *Note:* Adverse reactions and side effects may be more frequent and severe in older persons. Remind your doctor of any medicines the patient already takes.

ACTIVITY FOR OLDER PATIENTS—Care-givers should:
- Encourage socialization.
- Encourage the continuation of performable tasks.

FOOD & BEVERAGE
- No special diet is required.
- See Appendix 1 regarding good nutrition for people over 50.

FUTURE CONSIDERATIONS FOR THE AGING ADULT

POSSIBLE COMPLICATIONS—Further mental deterioration.

PROBABLE OUTCOME—Surgery (shunting of the cerebrospinal fluid) frequently improves the symptoms.

PREVENTING RECURRENCE—There are no proven preventive measures.

CALL YOUR DOCTOR IF

- Symptoms of normal-pressure hydrocephalus occur.
- New, unexplained symptoms develop. Medicine used in treatment may produce side effects.
- You wish referral to any number of community social services designed to help patients with mental illness.

HYPERVENTILATION SYNDROME
(Panic Attack)

BASIC INFORMATION FOR OLDER ADULTS

DESCRIPTION—With hyperventilation syndrome breathing is so fast that the carbon dioxide level in the blood is decreased, temporarily upsetting the normal blood chemistry. Body parts involved: The central nervous system; lungs; skin; hands; feet.

SPECIAL CONSIDERATIONS FOR AGING
- Characteristic signs and symptoms of many disorders are frequently changed or absent.
- Stress from any emotional cause—fear, worry, anxiety, sadness, loneliness or anger—affects all aspects of any illness or disorder.

SIGNS & SYMPTOMS
- Rapid breathing.
- Numbness and tingling around the mouth, hands and feet.
- Weakness or faintness.
- Muscle spasms or contractions in the hands and feet.
- Fainting (occasionally).

CAUSES & RISK FACTORS—Caused by a change in the normal ratio of acid to other elements in the blood due to breathing out too much carbon dioxide. This leads to alkalosis, an increase in blood alkalinity. Hyperventilation can accompany fever, disease of the heart and lungs or severe injury. If disease or injury is not present, hyperventilation is caused by anxiety. Risk factors include:
- Stress.
- Feelings of guilt.
- Fatigue or overwork.
- Illness.
- Smoking.
- Excessive alcohol consumption.

DOCTOR'S TREATMENT & DIAGNOSTIC TESTS
- Medical history and physical exam.
- Self-care instructions focused on the older patient.
- Psychotherapy or counseling if the hyperventilation occurs often and is caused by anxiety.

HOME TREATMENT BY SELF OR CARE-GIVER

GENERAL INSTRUCTIONS—During an attack, following the instructions below will increase the amount of carbon dioxide in the blood and relieve the symptoms.
- Cover your mouth and nose completely with a paper bag, then breathe slowly into the bag and rebreathe the air. The air in the bag contains additional carbon dioxide.
- Breathe slowly in and out of the bag at least 10 times.
- Put the bag aside and breathe normally a few minutes.
- Repeat the process until the symptoms diminish or disappear.
- If the symptoms return, repeat the process as often as needed.

MEDICATION (ADJUSTED FOR AGING)—Medicine usually is not necessary for this disorder.

ACTIVITY FOR OLDER PATIENTS
- After treatment, resume normal activity as soon as possible.
- See Appendix 20 regarding physical fitness for the active older adult.

FOOD & BEVERAGE
- No special diet is required.
- See Appendix 1 regarding good nutrition for people over 50.

FUTURE CONSIDERATIONS FOR THE AGING ADULT

POSSIBLE COMPLICATIONS
- Seizures.
- Fainting.

PROBABLE OUTCOME
- The symptoms can be controlled if you follow the instructions listed.
- If hyperventilation is caused by a disease, it will stop when the disease is cured.
- Recurrent attacks caused by anxiety should stop if the underlying stress can be eliminated.

PREVENTING RECURRENCE
- Avoid anxiety-producing situations.
- See Appendix 13 for suggestions to reduce stress.

CALL YOUR DOCTOR IF

- You have symptoms of hyperventilation that don't diminish with self-treatment.
- Any of the following occurs during an attack:
  Fainting.
  Seizure.
  Sudden fever.

HYPOCHONDRIASIS

BASIC INFORMATION FOR OLDER ADULTS

DESCRIPTION—Hypochondriasis is anxiety that accompanies a person's conviction that he or she has a serious or fatal disease despite evidence to the contrary from medical examinations and tests. Body part involved: The brain.

SPECIAL CONSIDERATIONS FOR AGING
- Many medical disorders in older people that were once thought to be "normal" consequences of aging are frequently diseases that can be treated.
- Usual signs and symptoms may be absent and be replaced by symptoms of confusion, dizziness, failure to thrive, falling, incontinence, increasing dementia, refusal to eat or drink, weight loss, depression, paranoia, hypochondriasis, psychosis or threats of suicide.

SIGNS & SYMPTOMS
- Anxiety and persistent reports of symptoms involving any body part. Concern about heart disease or cancer is common.
- The abuse of prescription and nonprescription drugs.
- The symptoms may change, but the person's belief that a serious condition exists does not. Frequently reported symptoms include insomnia, sexual dysfunction and gastrointestinal discomfort, such as bloating, belching and cramps.
- Afflicted patients continuously seek medical advice and tests as well as medications.

CAUSES & RISK FACTORS
Causes include:
- Overly protective parents in childhood.
- Lack of social outlets and contacts.
- Guilt feelings and an imagined need for punishment.
- An extreme need for attention.
Risk factors include:
- Stress.
- Major life changes, such as a divorce, job change, marriage, move, loss of a valued person or object, menopause or retirement.
- Depression.
- Psychosis.
- Other psychological disorders.

DOCTOR'S TREATMENT & DIAGNOSTIC TESTS
- Medical history and physical exam. After a thorough medical evaluation, repeat testing should be avoided.
- Psychotherapy or counseling for specific psychological problems. It usually won't help the hypochrondriasis.
- Biofeedback for pain problems.
- Self-care instructions focused on the older patient.

HOME TREATMENT BY SELF OR CARE-GIVER

GENERAL INSTRUCTIONS—Persons with hypochondriasis are often difficult to live with because of their constant worry and demands for attention. Realize that the person really suffers and try to be supportive. Reward positive behavior that is not related to physical complaints. Don't encourage the "sick role."

MEDICATION (ADJUSTED FOR AGING)
- Medicine usually is not necessary for this disorder. Your doctor may prescribe mild tranquilizers or antidepressants for a short time while therapy is being arranged.
- *Note:* Adverse reactions and side effects may be more frequent and severe in older persons. Remind your doctor of any medicines you already take.

ACTIVITY FOR OLDER PATIENTS
- Embark on a program that will lead to an acceptable degree of physical fitness. Exercise daily.
- See Appendix 20 regarding physical fitness for the active older adult.

FOOD & BEVERAGE
- Learn as much as possible about good nutrition and adhere to these teachings.
- See Appendix 1 regarding good nutrition for people over 50.

FUTURE CONSIDERATIONS FOR THE AGING ADULT

POSSIBLE COMPLICATIONS
- Wasting money on unnecessary—and sometimes dangerous—medical care.
- Insisting on unnecessary surgical procedures or medications.
- Failure of a doctor to take the symptoms of real disease seriously when they do develop.

PROBABLE OUTCOME—Generally resistant to treatment. Most patients with hypochondriasis maintain a lifelong belief that they have a serious disease and they change doctors frequently.

PREVENTING RECURRENCE—In childhood, don't reward illness by giving a child special privileges and undue attention for being sick. Provide adequate love and support during healthy periods.

CALL YOUR DOCTOR IF

- You have symptoms of hypochondriasis and want professional help to overcome the problem.
- New, unexplained symptoms develop. Tranquilizers used in treatment may produce side effects or dependence.

ILLNESSES & DISORDERS

BASIC INFORMATION FOR OLDER ADULTS

DESCRIPTION—This form of hypoglycemia constitutes low blood sugar in a patient who is taking medication, such as insulin or oral anti-diabetic drugs, for diabetes. Body parts involved: The brain at first, but this quickly involves all body cells. (THIS IS AN EMERGENCY; SEEK MEDICAL CARE IMMEDIATELY!)

SPECIAL CONSIDERATIONS FOR AGING—Usual signs and symptoms may be absent and be replaced by symptoms of confusion, dizziness, failure to thrive, falling, incontinence, increasing dementia, refusal to eat or drink, weight loss, depression, paranoia, hypochondriasis, psychosis or threats of suicide.

SIGNS & SYMPTOMS

Mild hypoglycemic reaction:
- Excessive hunger; weakness; nervousness.
- Emotional instability; difficulty concentrating.
- Sweating; headache.

Moderate hypoglycemic reaction:
- Increased weakness; excessive sweating; cold, clammy skin; pounding heartbeat.
- Numbness around the mouth or fingers.
- Memory loss; increasing confusion.
- Double vision; staring expression.
- Difficulty walking.

Severe hypoglycemic reaction:
- Muscle twitching; lack of urinary control.
- Unconsciousness; convulsions.

CAUSES & RISK FACTORS—Caused by too much insulin or oral antidiabetic drug or not enough food for the condition your body is in. Factors which affect this include more exercise than usual; irregular meals, skipped meals or partial meals; loose bowel movements, diarrhea or vomiting of the last meal; infection; anger or excitement. Risk factors include:
- Stress; illness with fever.
- Smoking, which decreases blood sugar.
- The use of other drugs which may also reduce blood sugar, such as diuretics, caffeine or alcohol.
- A disorder of the liver or pancreas.

DOCTOR'S TREATMENT & DIAGNOSTIC TESTS
- Medical history and physical exam.
- Laboratory studies of blood sugar.
- Self-care instructions focused on the older patient.

HOME TREATMENT BY SELF OR CARE-GIVER

GENERAL INSTRUCTIONS
- Wear a Medic Alert bracelet or pendant (see Glossary).
- For a mild hypoglycemic reaction, drink 1/2 cup of orange juice or a non-dietetic soft drink or eat 1/2 candy bar, 6 or 7 hard candies or 2 teaspoons of honey, syrup or sugar. Repeat if necessary in 10 to 15 minutes.
- For a moderate hypoglycemic reaction, eat or drink something sugary as above, but follow it with a carbohydrate that is absorbed more slowly, such as a banana, apple, cereal, bread or crackers.
- For a severe hypoglycemic reaction in which the person is disoriented, give a small drink of fruit juice or smear syrup inside the mouth. If the person is unconscious (and you are trained to do so), inject glucagon (1/2 to 1cc) deeply into a muscle and at right angles to the big muscle in the arm or leg. After the person regains consciousness, give sweet foods as above. Prop the person in a sitting position as soon as possible. Call the doctor.

MEDICATION (ADJUSTED FOR AGING)
- Always carry hard candy. Your doctor may prescribe glucagon to have available for emergencies.
- *Note:* Adverse reactions and side effects may be more frequent and severe in older persons. Remind your doctor of any medicines you already take.

ACTIVITY FOR OLDER PATIENTS
- After treatment, resume normal activity as soon as possible.
- See Appendix 20 regarding physical fitness for the active older adult.

FOOD & BEVERAGE
- Ask your doctor if your basic diet plan needs to be changed.
- See Appendix 1 regarding good nutrition for people over 50.

FUTURE CONSIDERATIONS FOR THE AGING ADULT

POSSIBLE COMPLICATIONS—Repeated attacks can cause permanent brain damage.

PROBABLE OUTCOME—This disorder is curable in 10 to 15 minutes if glucose can be given orally or by injection.

PREVENTING RECURRENCE
- Follow diet, exercise and medication instructions for diabetics carefully.
- Keep hard candy available for early symptoms.
- Request glucagon and an injection kit from your doctor.

CALL YOUR DOCTOR IF

- You have diabetes, take medication and have symptoms of hypoglycemia—especially severe symptoms. *This is an emergency!*
- The symptoms don't disappear with the treatment above.
- Hypoglycemic reactions occur frequently.

HYPOGLYCEMIA, FUNCTIONAL

BASIC INFORMATION FOR OLDER ADULTS

DESCRIPTION—Functional hypoglycemia is low blood sugar caused by the excessive production of insulin by the pancreas. This is not a disease. It is often misdiagnosed when the diagnosis is based on symptoms alone. Body parts involved: The pancreas at first, but eventually all body cells.

SPECIAL CONSIDERATIONS FOR AGING
- Usual signs and symptoms may be absent and be replaced by symptoms of confusion, dizziness, failure to thrive, falling, incontinence, increasing dementia, refusal to eat or drink, weight loss, depression, paranoia, hypochondriasis, psychosis or threats of suicide.
- Stress from any emotional cause—fear, worry, anxiety, sadness, loneliness or anger—affects all aspects of any illness or disorder.

SIGNS & SYMPTOMS—The following vary greatly among people in frequency and severity:
- Weakness or faintness.
- Sweating.
- Excessive hunger.
- Nervousness and trembling hands.
- Heartbeat irregularities.
- Headache.
- Confusion.
- Personality changes.
- Loss of consciousness.
- Seizures (sometimes).

CAUSES & RISK FACTORS—Functional hypoglycemia probably results when the pancreas produce too much insulin in response to sugars and other carbohydrates, heavy exercise or unknown causes. The following drugs decrease blood sugar levels in some persons: tobacco, caffeine, alcohol, aspirin, sulfonurea medications, phenformin, haloperidol, propoxyphene and chlorpromazine. Some doctors believe functional hypoglycemia may be the first indication that diabetes mellitus is developing. Risk factors include:
- Stress.
- Improper diet.
- Smoking.
- The use of drugs such as those listed above.
- Fatigue or overwork.
- Stomach surgery.
- High fevers.

DOCTOR'S TREATMENT & DIAGNOSTIC TESTS
- Medical history and physical exam.
- Laboratory studies such as blood sugar and glucose tolerance tests.

- Self-care instructions focused on the older patient.
- Psychotherapy or counseling to help you learn to cope with stress.

HOME TREATMENT BY SELF OR CARE-GIVER

GENERAL INSTRUCTIONS
- Consider lifestyle changes. See Appendix 13.
- Carry glucose tablets, sugar lumps or candy.
- Let friends know about the symptoms. If you become disoriented, they can provide something sweet.
- Talk to your doctor about discontinuing drugs that may cause the problem.

MEDICATION (ADJUSTED FOR AGING)—Medicine usually is not necessary for this disorder.

ACTIVITY FOR OLDER PATIENTS
- No restrictions are necessary.
- See Appendix 20 regarding physical fitness for the active older adult.

FOOD & BEVERAGE
- Eat 5 or 6 small meals a day that are low in simple carbohydrates, moderate in fats and high in protein. Don't skip meals. Between-meal snacks should include protein, such as chicken, eggs, cheese or skim milk, rather than carbohydrates. Avoid highly concentrated sweets, such as candy.
- See Appendix 1 regarding good nutrition for people over 50.

FUTURE CONSIDERATIONS FOR THE AGING ADULT

POSSIBLE COMPLICATIONS—Repeated attacks can cause personality changes.

PROBABLE OUTCOME—The symptoms can be controlled with treatment.

PREVENTING RECURRENCE
- Follow instructions under Food & Beverage. Don't skip meals.
- Avoid stress.
- Don't smoke.
- Don't drink alcohol.

☎ CALL YOUR DOCTOR IF

You have symptoms of functional hypoglycemia.

ID REACTION
(Autoeczematization; Autosensitization)

BASIC INFORMATION FOR OLDER ADULTS

DESCRIPTION—An id reaction is an allergic response to a skin disorder of the feet, groin or other area that is producing an itching rash somewhere else in the body. Body parts involved: The parts with the original disorder (the groin, ears, hands, or feet) and the parts with the allergic response (the hands, feet, arms, legs or trunk).

SPECIAL CONSIDERATIONS FOR AGING
- The number of autoantibodies (see Glossary) increases.
- The immune system becomes less effective, opening the way for viral, bacterial and other infections; malignancies; immune disorders; and allergies.

SIGNS & SYMPTOMS
- Itching (often severe).
- Vesicles (small, fluid-filled blisters) of varying sizes on the skin.

CAUSES & RISK FACTORS—The cause is unknown. An id reaction may be a disorder of the body's immunological response to the original ailment. It occurs most often with some forms of dermatitis, outer ear infections and eczema of the hand or foot. Risk factors include:
- A recent skin rash anywhere.
- Stress.
- A medical history of allergies.

DOCTOR'S TREATMENT & DIAGNOSTIC TESTS
- Medical history and physical exam.
- Laboratory culture of the original skin disorder.
- Self-care instructions focused on the older patient.

HOME TREATMENT BY SELF OR CARE-GIVER

GENERAL INSTRUCTIONS
- Treat the original skin disorder until it heals completely to prevent a recurrence of the id reaction. For instructions, consult your doctor or refer to the disorder in this book.
- Minimize stress if possible. (See Appendix 13.)

MEDICATION (ADJUSTED FOR AGING)
- Your doctor may prescribe topical or oral cortisone drugs. Oral steroids quickly control the id reaction, but slow the healing of the underlying disorder.
- *Note:* Adverse reactions and side effects may be more frequent and severe in older persons. Remind your doctor of any medicines you already take.

ACTIVITY FOR OLDER PATIENTS
- No restrictions are necessary.
- See Appendix 20 regarding physical fitness for the active older adult.

FOOD & BEVERAGE
- No special diet is required.
- See Appendix 1 regarding good nutrition for people over 50.

FUTURE CONSIDERATIONS FOR THE AGING ADULT

POSSIBLE COMPLICATIONS—Adverse reaction to the medication used in treatment.

PROBABLE OUTCOME—Usually curable in 2 weeks. Recurrence is rapid if treatment is discontinued before the id reaction and the original disorder are completely gone.

PREVENTING RECURRENCE—Treat all skin disorders thoroughly until they disappear.

CALL YOUR DOCTOR IF

- You have symptoms of an id reaction.
- Any of the following occurs during treatment: A fever higher than 101F (38.3C). Heat, redness, pain or tenderness in any of the lesions. This indicates infection.
- New, unexplained symptoms develop. The drugs used in treatment may produce side effects.

IDIOPATHIC HYPERTROPHIC SUBAORTIC STENOSIS
(IHSS)

BASIC INFORMATION FOR OLDER ADULTS

DESCRIPTION—Idiopathic hypertrophic subaortic stenosis is a chronic heart condition that produces an enlarged heart muscle, restricting the amount of blood the heart pumps. Body part involved: The heart.

SPECIAL CONSIDERATIONS FOR AGING
- 50% of people over 60 have x-ray evidence of narrowing of the coronary arteries, yet only 50% of those people have symptoms.
- The coronary arteries nourishing the heart are less healthy. They become thicker and lose their elasticity.
- The total heart functions less efficiently—especially among smokers.

SIGNS & SYMPTOMS
- Chest pain (angina pectoris).
- Heart rhythm irregularity.
- Fainting.
- Shortness of breath.
- Swollen feet and ankles.
- Distended neck veins.
- Heart failure.
- Heart murmur (see Glossary).

CAUSES & RISK FACTORS—Causes include a thickening of the left chamber (ventricle) of the heart for unknown reasons. This obstructs the flow of blood and the heart may be unable to pump enough blood during exertion. In some cases, this condition is inherited as a dominant genetic trait. The risk increases with a family history of IHSS.

DOCTOR'S TREATMENT & DIAGNOSTIC TESTS
- Medical history and physical exam.
- Laboratory studies such as cardiac catheterization (see Glossary) to measure the blood flow through the heart's chambers.
- X-rays of the heart.
- ECG and echocardiogram (see Glossary for both) of the heart.
- Treatment may include consultation with a cardiologist.
- Surgery to reduce the obstruction if medication does not control the problem. Advancing age alone is not a deterrent.
- DC electrocardioversion (electric shock to the heart) to treat life-threatening heartbeat irregularities and improve heart output.
- Self-care instructions focused on the older patient.

HOME TREATMENT BY SELF OR CARE-GIVER

GENERAL INSTRUCTIONS
- Stay under close medical supervision.
- Wear a Medic Alert bracelet or pendant (see Glossary).
- Family members, close friends and business acquaintances should learn cardiopulmonary resuscitation (CPR) in case cardiac arrest occurs.

MEDICATION (ADJUSTED FOR AGING)
- Your doctor may prescribe beta-adrenergic blockers or calcium channel blockers to prevent heartbeat irregularities.
- Don't use nitroglycerin for angina pain. It dilates the arteries, which may be harmful.
- If digitalis is prescribed for you, discuss the risks with your doctor. It may trigger heartbeat irregularities.
- *Note:* Adverse reactions and side effects may be more frequent and severe in older persons. Remind your doctor of any medicines you already take.

ACTIVITY FOR OLDER PATIENTS—Your doctor should guide you about how much physical activity is ideal. Your ability to increase activity is dependent on your response to therapy. Don't regard yourself as an invalid.

FOOD & BEVERAGE—A low-salt diet (see Appendix 9) may be necessary if you have fluid accumulation (a possible sign of congestive heart failure).

FUTURE CONSIDERATIONS FOR THE AGING ADULT

POSSIBLE COMPLICATIONS
- Fatal heartbeat irregularity.
- Bacterial infection of the heart valve.

PROBABLE OUTCOME—Usually curable with medication or surgery.

PREVENTING RECURRENCE—If you have a a family history of IHSS, obtain genetic counseling before starting a family.

CALL YOUR DOCTOR IF

- You have symptoms of IHSS or your symptoms worsen during treatment.
- New, unexplained symptoms develop. The drugs used in treatment may produce side effects.

IMMUNODEFICIENCY DISEASE

BASIC INFORMATION FOR OLDER ADULTS

DESCRIPTION—Immunodeficiency disease is a defect in the body's immune system. A healthy immune system protects the body against germs (bacteria, viruses and fungi), cancer (partial protection) and any foreign material that enters the body. When the system fails, the body becomes susceptible to infection and cancer. Similar but unrelated disorders are caused by acquired immune deficiency syndrome (AIDS). Also similar is the immunosuppression some people develop due to potent drugs that are used to treat several disorders. Body parts involved: The immune system (the blood, bone marrow, lymph tissue, liver, spleen and thymus gland).

SPECIAL CONSIDERATIONS FOR AGING
- Decreased nutrition, common among chronically ill older people, increases the risk of any disease or disorder.
- The number of autoantibodies (see Glossary) increases.
- The immune system becomes less effective, opening the way for viral, bacterial and other infections; malignancies; immune disorders; and allergies.
- Stress from any emotional cause—fear, worry, anxiety, sadness, loneliness or anger—affects all aspects of any illness or disorder.

SIGNS & SYMPTOMS—Recurrent, severe infections and illnesses. The most common include:
- Ear or respiratory infections, such as otitis media and pneumonia.
- Yeast infections, especially candidiasis.
- Cancer, especially leukemia and lymphoma.
- Bleeding disorders; eczema.
- Meningitis or encephalitis.

CAUSES & RISK FACTORS
Causes include:
- Congenital defects that involve an incomplete or absent immune system.
- Surgical removal of the spleen before age 2.
- The use of immunosuppressive drugs.
- Radiation treatment.
- Some cancers, such as Hodgkin's disease.
- Hypogammaglobulinemia (see Glossary).
- Viral infections.
Risk factors include:
- Poor nutrition.
- A family history of immunodeficiency disease.

DOCTOR'S TREATMENT & DIAGNOSTIC TESTS
- Medical history and physical exam.
- Laboratory blood studies of antibodies; a microscopic examination of blood and tissue cells and skin tests.
- X-rays of the thymus gland.
- Radioactive studies of immune function.
- Surgery to transplant bone marrow or the thymus gland (occasionally).

- Hospitalization for the treatment of serious infection.
- Self-care instructions focused on the older patient.

HOME TREATMENT BY SELF OR CARE-GIVER

GENERAL INSTRUCTIONS
- Avoid exposure to persons with contagious illnesses.
- Don't take *any* type of vaccine without medical advice.
- Follow all instructions carefully if you must take cortisone or immunosuppressive drugs that have been prescribed for you without getting a second medical opinion.

MEDICATION (ADJUSTED FOR AGING)
- Your doctor may prescribe:
  Antibiotics to fight infections.
  Injections of antibodies.
  Transfusions of blood components.
  Injections of gamma globulin (sometimes).
- *Note:* Adverse reactions and side effects may be more frequent and severe in older persons. Remind your doctor of any medicines you already take.

ACTIVITY FOR OLDER PATIENTS—Bed rest
is usually necessary during acute illnesses. Otherwise, there are no restrictions on your activity.

FOOD & BEVERAGE—No special diet.

FUTURE CONSIDERATIONS FOR THE AGING ADULT

POSSIBLE COMPLICATIONS
- Uncontrolled bacterial, viral or fungal infections that don't respond to treatment.
- Cancer.
- Infectious arthritis.

PROBABLE OUTCOME—Severe forms of
immunodeficiency are usually fatal. Minor forms can be treated successfully.

PREVENTING RECURRENCE
- Maintain good nutrition.
- Practice safe sex.

CALL YOUR DOCTOR IF

- You have symptoms of immunodeficiency disease.
- After diagnosis you have signs of infection, such as:
  Chills; fever; muscle aches.
  Headache; dizziness.
  A cough with thick, discolored or blood-streaked sputum.

IMPOTENCE, MALE SEXUAL
(Erectile Dysfunction)

BASIC INFORMATION FOR OLDER ADULTS

DESCRIPTION—Male sexual impotence is the inability to have or maintain an erection of the penis that is necessary for satisfactory sexual intercourse. Body parts involved: The male reproductive system; the central nervous system.

SPECIAL CONSIDERATIONS FOR AGING
- Men require a longer penile erection time.
- Sexual response gradually slows—especially in males.
- The level of testosterone (the male sex hormone) is lower.
- There are changes in the circulatory system.
- Stress from any emotional cause affects all aspects of any illness or disorder.

SIGNS & SYMPTOMS—Absent penile erections or erections that are too weak, brief or painful for sexual intercourse.

CAUSES & RISK FACTORS—About 50% of cases have psychological causes. These include:
- Guilt feelings; psychological disorders, including depression, anxiety and psychosis.
- A poor relationship with one's sexual partner.
- Lack of sexual information, including an understanding of the emotional aspects of sexuality and information about female anatomy and physiology.
- Concern about sexual performance.
Physiological causes include:
- Temporary fatigue; diabetes mellitus.
- Atherosclerosis (hardening of the arteries).
- The use of some antihypertensive medications.
- Disorders of the central nervous system, such as spinal cord injury, multiple sclerosis, stroke or syphilis.
- Endocrine disorders that involve the pituitary, thyroid, adrenal or sexual glands.
- Alcoholism; drug abuse, especially of marijuana, cocaine, narcotics, tranquilizers, sedatives, hypnotics and hallucinogenics.
- Decreased circulation to the penis from any cause.
Risk factors include:
- Stress; excessive alcohol consumption.
- Recent illness that has lowered strength.
- Recent major surgery, especially cardiovascular or prostate surgery.
- The use of drugs—including necessary prescription drugs and illicit drugs.

DOCTOR'S TREATMENT & DIAGNOSTIC TESTS
- Medical history and physical exam.
- Laboratory blood studies of hormone levels.
- Self-care instructions focused on the older patient.
- Psychotherapy or counseling from a qualified professional sex therapist.
- Sleep studies to measure night-time erections (sometimes).

- Surgery to implant an inflatable or non-inflatable penile prosthesis (sometimes).

HOME TREATMENT BY SELF OR CARE-GIVER

GENERAL INSTRUCTIONS
- An experimental therapy is the use of papaverine injections into the penis. Discuss this possibility with your doctor.
- See Appendix 13 for suggestions to reduce stress and improve your overall health.

MEDICATION (ADJUSTED FOR AGING)
- Medication is not helpful for impotence caused by psychological factors. Be wary of persons who offer cures with shots or pills.
- Medication may be prescribed to treat the underlying medical condition.
- If you suspect that a medication is causing impotence, consult your doctor about changing your prescription or dosage.

ACTIVITY FOR OLDER PATIENTS—No restrictions are necessary. Resume sexual relations when potency returns or surgery heals.

FOOD & BEVERAGE—Eat a well-balanced diet and take vitamin and mineral supplements.

FUTURE CONSIDERATIONS FOR THE AGING ADULT

POSSIBLE COMPLICATIONS
- Depression and loss of self-esteem.
- Marital problems or the breakdown of close personal relationships.

PROBABLE OUTCOME
- Spontaneous recovery or recovery after brief counseling in many cases with psychological origins.
- For other cases with physical origins, treatment and improvement of the underlying disorder may improve sexual performance.

PREVENTING RECURRENCE
- Maintain good communication with your partner. Don't be hesitant about discussing the problem, exploring your needs and asking for help. Your partner's understanding is critical to solving the problem.
- Don't drink more than 1 or 2 alcoholic drinks—if any—a day. Don't use other drugs that can be abused.
- If you have diabetes, adhere closely to your treatment program.

CALL YOUR DOCTOR IF

You have symptoms of impotence, especially if you take medications or have any of the disorders listed as causes.

BASIC INFORMATION FOR OLDER ADULTS

DESCRIPTION—Functional incontinence is a type of incontinence that occurs infrequently or represents a failure to comprehend the need to urinate. Body parts involved: The urinary bladder and urethra.

SPECIAL CONSIDERATIONS FOR AGING
- Many body changes occur as a result of estrogen deficiency beginning at menopause. These include vaginal dryness, shortening and narrowing of the vagina, greater susceptibility to vaginal infections, frequent bladder infections, reductions in the size of the clitoris and increased facial hair. Changes in other systems of the body may lead to a greater tendency to osteoporosis, hardening of the arteries and other disorders.
- Urinary incontinence becomes more frequent.
- Stress from any emotional cause—fear, worry, anxiety, sadness, loneliness or anger—affects all aspects of any illness or disorder.

SIGNS & SYMPTOMS
- Forgetting to urinate.
- Urinating at inappropriate times or places.
- Occasional problems in getting to the toilet in time.

CAUSES & RISK FACTORS
- Medications that induce incontinence.
- Urinary tract infection.
- Vaginal infection.
- Stool (fecal) impaction.
- Diabetes.

DOCTOR'S TREATMENT & DIAGNOSTIC TESTS
- Medical history and physical exam.
- Urinalysis to determine if a urinary tract infection is causing the symptoms.
- Self-care instructions focused on the older patient.

HOME TREATMENT BY SELF OR CARE-GIVER

GENERAL INSTRUCTIONS
- Learn to recognize, control and develop the muscles of the pelvic floor. These are the ones you use to interrupt urination in mid-stream. The following exercises (Kegel exercises) strengthen these muscles so you can control or relax them completely:
  To identify which muscles are involved, alternately start and stop urinating when using the toilet.
  Practice tightening and releasing these muscles while sitting, standing, walking, driving, watching TV or listening to music. For a while, you may experience some pelvic pain.

Tighten the muscles a small amount at a time, "like an elevator going up to the 10th floor." Then release very slowly, "one floor at a time."
Tighten the muscles from front to back, including the anus, as in the previous exercise.
Practice these exercises every morning, afternoon and evening. Start with 5 each time and gradually work up to 20 or 30 each time.
- Following treatment of the underlying cause, it may be necessary to rely on external devices or superabsorbent pads. Your doctor will recommend the best method for you.
- Specially trained nurses or therapists will help you learn how to cope with the problem.

MEDICATION (ADJUSTED FOR AGING)
- Medicine usually is not necessary for this disorder, but your doctor may prescribe antibiotics if you have a complicating urinary tract infection.
- *Note:* Adverse reactions and side effects may be more frequent and severe in older persons. Remind your doctor of any medicines you already take.

ACTIVITY FOR OLDER PATIENTS—No restrictions are necessary.

FOOD & BEVERAGE
- Lose weight if you are obese. A reducing diet appears in Appendix 10.
- Fluid intake may be adjusted by your doctor.

FUTURE CONSIDERATIONS FOR THE AGING ADULT

POSSIBLE COMPLICATIONS
- Urinary tract infections.
- Social isolation due to concern about embarrassment.

PROBABLE OUTCOME—Likely to continue unless the underlying causes can be treated.

PREVENTING RECURRENCE
- Eat a normal, well-balanced diet and exercise regularly to build and maintain muscle strength.
- Learn and practice Kegel exercises (see General Instructions) before the symptoms of functional incontinence begin.

CALL YOUR DOCTOR IF

- You have symptoms of functional incontinence.
- Any sign of infection develops, such as fever, pain on urination, frequent urination or a general ill feeling.

INCONTINENCE, OVERFLOW
(Paradoxic Incontinence)

BASIC INFORMATION FOR OLDER ADULTS

DESCRIPTION—Overflow incontinence is characterized by a constant dribble of urine due to an inability to empty the bladder normally. Body parts involved: The urinary bladder and urethra.

SPECIAL CONSIDERATIONS FOR AGING
- In women, many body changes occur as a result of estrogen deficiency beginning at menopause. These include vaginal dryness, greater susceptibility to vaginal infections and frequent bladder infections. Changes in other systems of the body may lead to a greater tendency to other disorders.
- In men, one of the normal changes of aging is the gradual enlargement of the prostate, which can lead to incontinence and other urinary tract problems.
- Urinary incontinence becomes more frequent.
- Stress from any emotional cause affects all aspects of any illness or disorder.

SIGNS & SYMPTOMS
—Unintentional loss of urine with lifting, sneezing, singing, coughing, laughing, or straining to have a bowel movement.

CAUSES & RISK FACTORS
- Stretching of the bladder (from retaining urine too long).
- The use of some drugs (e.g., tranquilizers).
- Prostate gland obstruction in men.

DOCTOR'S TREATMENT & DIAGNOSTIC TESTS
- Medical history and physical exam.
- Urinalysis to determine if a urinary tract infection is causing the symptoms.
- Self-care instructions focused on the older patient.
- Surgery to tighten relaxed or damaged muscles that support the bladder.
- Prostatectomy to remove the prostate in men with indications for surgery.
- Balloon urethra dilatation.
- Intermittent catheterization under sterile conditions.

HOME TREATMENT BY SELF OR CARE-GIVER

GENERAL INSTRUCTIONS
- Learn to recognize, control and develop the muscles of the pelvic floor. These are the ones you use to interrupt urination in midstream. The following exercises (Kegel exercises) strengthen these muscles so you can control or relax them completely:
  To identify which muscles are involved, alternately start and stop urinating when using the toilet.
  Practice tightening and releasing these muscles while sitting, standing, walking, driving, watching TV or listening to music. For a

while, you may experience some pelvic pain. Tighten the muscles a small amount at a time, "like an elevator going up to the 10th floor." Then release very slowly, "one floor at a time." Tighten the muscles from front to back, including the anus, as in the previous exercise. Practice these exercises every morning, afternoon and evening. Start with 5 each time and gradually work up to 20 or 30 each time.
- Wear absorbent underpants or super-absorbent pads.
- Use a planned schedule for emptying the bladder.
- Keep a daily diary of fluid intake and urination frequency. This will help you assess your progress.

MEDICATION (ADJUSTED FOR AGING)—
Your doctor may prescribe:
- Bethanechol, prazosin and others drugs.
- Antibiotics if you have a complicating urinary tract infection.
- A pessary (support device) made of rubber or other material to fit inside the vagina to support the uterus and the lower muscular layer of the bladder.

ACTIVITY FOR OLDER PATIENTS
—No restrictions are necessary.

FOOD & BEVERAGE
- Lose weight if you are obese. A reducing diet appears in Appendix 10.
- Your fluid intake may be adjusted by your doctor.

FUTURE CONSIDERATIONS FOR THE AGING ADULT

POSSIBLE COMPLICATIONS—Complete loss of urinary control requiring surgery; urinary tract infections; social isolation due to concern about embarrassment.

PROBABLE OUTCOME—If the overflow incontinence is not severe enough to require surgery, exercise can improve the muscle function. If it is severe, it can be helped with surgery.

PREVENTING RECURRENCE
- Eat a normal, well-balanced diet and exercise regularly to build muscle strength.
- Learn and practice Kegel exercises (see General Instructions) before the symptoms of overflow incontinence begin.

CALL YOUR DOCTOR IF

- You have symptoms of overflow incontinence.
- Any sign of infection develops, such as fever, pain on urination, frequent urination or a general ill feeling.
- The symptoms don't improve after 3 months of Kegel exercises or the symptoms become intolerable and you wish to consider surgery.

ILLNESSES & DISORDERS

BASIC INFORMATION FOR OLDER ADULTS

DESCRIPTION—Stress incontinence is an involuntary loss of urine that accompanies any action that suddenly increases the pressure in the abdomen. It affects women more often than men. Body parts involved: The urinary bladder and urethra.

SPECIAL CONSIDERATIONS FOR AGING
- Many body changes occur as a result of estrogen deficiency beginning at menopause. These include vaginal dryness, greater susceptibility to vaginal infections and frequent bladder infections. Changes in other systems of the body may lead to a greater tendency to other disorders.
- Urinary incontinence becomes more frequent.
- Stress from any emotional cause affects all aspects of any illness or disorder.

SIGNS & SYMPTOMS—Unintentional loss of urine with lifting, sneezing, singing, coughing, laughing, or straining to have a bowel movement.

CAUSES & RISK FACTORS—Caused by the shortening of the urethra and loss of the normal muscular support for the bladder and the floor of the pelvis. These changes occur during pregnancy and after childbirth, particularly repeated childbirth. They may also occur as a natural consequence of aging. Risk factors include:
- Repeated childbirth; obesity.
- Chronic lung disease with a cough.
- Surgery that may traumatize the urethra.
- Injury of the urethra from any cause.

DOCTOR'S TREATMENT & DIAGNOSTIC TESTS
- Medical history and physical exam.
- Urinalysis to determine if a urinary tract infection is causing the symptoms.
- Provocative stress test (see Glossary).
- Self-care instructions focused on the older patient.
- Surgery to tighten relaxed or damaged muscles that support the bladder.
- Implant of an artificial urinary sphincter in some cases.

HOME TREATMENT BY SELF OR CARE-GIVER

GENERAL INSTRUCTIONS
- Learn to recognize, control and develop the muscles of the pelvic floor. These are the ones you use to interrupt urination in mid-stream. The following exercises (Kegel exercises) strengthen these muscles so you can control or relax them completely:
To identify which muscles are involved, alternately start and stop urinating when using the toilet.
Practice tightening and releasing these muscles while sitting, standing, walking, driving, watching TV or listening to music. For a

while, you may experience some pelvic pain. Tighten the muscles a small amount at a time, "like an elevator going up to the 10th floor." Then release very slowly, "one floor at a time." Tighten the muscles from front to back, including the anus, as in the previous exercise. Practice these exercises every morning, afternoon and evening. Start with 5 each time and gradually work up to 20 or 30 each time.
- Wear absorbent underpants or super-absorbent pads.
- Use a planned schedule for emptying your bladder.
- Keep a daily diary of fluid intake and urination frequency. This will help assess progress.

MEDICATION (ADJUSTED FOR AGING)—Medicine usually is not necessary for this disorder, but your doctor may prescribe:
- Antibiotics if you have a complicating urinary tract infection.
- A pessary (support device) made of rubber or other material to fit inside the vagina to support the uterus and the lower muscular layer of the bladder.

ACTIVITY FOR OLDER PATIENTS—No restrictions are necessary.

FOOD & BEVERAGE
- Lose weight if you are obese. A reducing diet appears in Appendix 10.
- Your fluid intake may be adjusted by your doctor.

FUTURE CONSIDERATIONS FOR THE AGING ADULT

POSSIBLE COMPLICATIONS—Complete loss of urinary control requiring surgery; urinary tract infections; social isolation due to concern about embarrassment.

PROBABLE OUTCOME—If the stress incontinence is not severe enough to require surgery, exercise can improve the muscle function. If it is severe, it can be helped with surgery.

PREVENTING RECURRENCE
- Eat a normal, well-balanced diet and exercise regularly to build and maintain muscle strength.
- Learn and practice Kegel exercises (see General Instructions) before the symptoms of stress incontinence begin.

CALL YOUR DOCTOR IF

- You have symptoms of stress incontinence.
- Any sign of infection develops, such as fever, pain on urination, frequent urination or a general ill feeling.
- The symptoms don't improve after 3 months of Kegel exercises or the symptoms become intolerable and you wish to consider surgery.

BASIC INFORMATION FOR OLDER ADULTS

DESCRIPTION—Urge incontinence is an inability to control the bladder once the urge to urinate occurs. It affects women more often than men. Body parts involved: The urinary bladder and urethra.

SPECIAL CONSIDERATIONS FOR AGING
- Many body changes occur as a result of estrogen deficiency beginning at menopause. These include vaginal dryness, greater susceptibility to vaginal infections and frequent bladder infections. Changes in other systems of the body may lead to a greater tendency to other disorders.
- Urinary incontinence becomes more frequent.
- Stress from any emotional cause affects all aspects of any illness or disorder.

SIGNS & SYMPTOMS—An involuntary loss of urine almost immediately after feeling a slight urge to urinate. The volume of lost urine may range from a few drops to complete bladder emptying.

CAUSES & RISK FACTORS—Caused by overactive muscles that make the bladder contract and empty. Urge incontinence is usually associated with other urinary problems. Risk factors include:
- Obesity.
- Surgery that may traumatize the urethra.
- Injury of the urethra from any cause.

DOCTOR'S TREATMENT & DIAGNOSTIC TESTS
- Medical history and physical exam.
- Urinalysis to determine if a urinary tract infection is causing the symptoms.
- Self-care instructions focused on the older patient.
- Surgery to tighten relaxed or damaged muscles that support the bladder.

HOME TREATMENT BY SELF OR CARE-GIVER

GENERAL INSTRUCTIONS
- Learn to recognize, control and develop the muscles of the pelvic floor. These are the ones you use to interrupt urination in midstream. The following exercises (Kegel exercises) strengthen these muscles so you can control or relax them completely:
  To identify which muscles are involved, alternately start and stop urinating when using the toilet. Practice tightening and releasing these muscles while sitting, standing, walking, driving, watching TV or listening to music. For a while, you may experience some pelvic pain. Tighten the muscles a small amount at a time, "like an elevator going up to the 10th floor." Then release very slowly, "one floor at a time." Tighten the muscles from front to back, including the anus, as in the previous exercise.

Practice these exercises every morning, afternoon and evening. Start with 5 each time and gradually work up to 20 or 30 each time.
- Wear absorbent underpants or super-absorbent pads.
- Use a planned schedule for emptying the bladder.
- Keep a daily diary of fluid intake and urination frequency. This will help you assess your progress.
- Use a bedside commode or urinal and bedpan if necessary.

MEDICATION (ADJUSTED FOR AGING)—Your doctor may prescribe:
- Oxybutynin chloride, propantheline, dicyclomine or imipramine.
- Antibiotics if you have a complicating urinary tract infection.
- A pessary (support device) made of rubber or other material to fit inside the vagina to support the uterus and the lower muscular layer of the bladder.

ACTIVITY FOR OLDER PATIENTS—No restrictions are necessary.

FOOD & BEVERAGE
- Lose weight if you are obese. A reducing diet appears in Appendix 10.
- Your fluid intake may be adjusted by your doctor.

FUTURE CONSIDERATIONS FOR THE AGING ADULT

POSSIBLE COMPLICATIONS—Urinary tract infections; social isolation due to concern about embarrassment.

PROBABLE OUTCOME—There are several different forms of treatment available, some still experimental. If the first treatment techniques don't work, discuss alternatives with your doctor.

PREVENTING RECURRENCE
- Eat a normal, well-balanced diet and exercise regularly to build and maintain muscle strength.
- Learn and practice Kegel exercises (see General Instructions) before the symptoms of stress incontinence begin.

☎ CALL YOUR DOCTOR IF

- You have symptoms of urge incontinence.
- Any sign of infection develops, such as fever, pain on urination, frequent urination or a general ill feeling.
- The symptoms don't improve after 3 months of Kegel exercises and medicines or the symptoms become intolerable and you wish to consider surgery.
- New, unexplained symptoms develop. The drugs used in treatment may produce side effects.

INDIGESTION
(Dyspepsia)

BASIC INFORMATION FOR OLDER ADULTS

DESCRIPTION—Indigestion is vague chest or abdominal discomfort—with no apparent organic cause—that occurs during or soon after eating or drinking. Body parts involved: The stomach; esophagus; small intestine.

SPECIAL CONSIDERATIONS FOR AGING
- The esophageal muscles decrease in strength with aging.
- The appetite becomes poorer.
- Stress from any emotional cause affects all aspects of any illness or disorder.

SIGNS & SYMPTOMS
- Mild nausea; heartburn.
- Upper abdominal pain; gas or belching.
- Bloated or full feeling; acid taste.

CAUSES & RISK FACTORS—The symptoms seem to be related to eating, drinking or swallowing air while talking or chewing gum. They occur most often with emotional upset while eating; excessive smoking; constipation; eating improperly cooked food; eating food with a high fat content; poor digestion of gas-forming foods such as beans, cucumbers, cabbage, turnips and onions; food allergy; or overindulgence in alcohol. Risk factors include:
- Stress; fatigue or overwork.
- Smoking; excessive alcohol consumption.
- The use of drugs that may irritate the stomach.
- Peptic ulcers, gallstones or an inflamed esophagus.

DOCTOR'S TREATMENT & DIAGNOSTIC TESTS
- Medical history and physical exam.
- X-rays of the upper digestive tract.
- Gastroscopy (see Glossary).
- Self-care instructions focused on the older patient.

OTHER—Persistent symptoms can indicate disease in the digestive tract or other body parts. Occasionally symptoms occur in patients with no apparent disease. This indicates an abnormal function in a normal part of the body.

HOME TREATMENT BY SELF OR CARE-GIVER

GENERAL INSTRUCTIONS—Treatment and prevention are similar:
- Allow time for leisurely meals. Chew your food carefully and thoroughly. Avoid conflicts during meals.
- Don't smoke immediately before a meal.
- Avoid excitement or exercise immediately after a meal.
- Drinking milk may relieve the symptoms.
- Avoid situations than make you swallow air, such as chewing gum.
- Observe episodes of indigestion for changes in symptoms. If their character, timing, frequency or severity changes, a more serious disorder may be responsible. These include heartburn from irritation of the lower esophagus, gallbladder infection, ulcers or stomach cancer. See separate headings in the Illnesses section for each.

MEDICATION (ADJUSTED FOR AGING)
- For minor discomfort, you may use non-prescription antacids.
- For serious discomfort, your doctor may prescribe H_2 blockers, antispasmodics or tranquilizers to relieve tension.

ACTIVITY FOR OLDER PATIENTS—No restrictions are necessary.

FOOD & BEVERAGE
- No special diet is required. Avoid foods—especially those listed under Causes—if they produce discomfort.
- See Appendix 1 regarding good nutrition for people over 50.

FUTURE CONSIDERATIONS FOR THE AGING ADULT

POSSIBLE COMPLICATIONS—Indigestion may mimic signs of a heart attack or serious disease of the esophagus or stomach, causing the serious disorder to be ignored.

PROBABLE OUTCOME—The symptoms can be controlled with treatment, but recurrence is likely.

PREVENTING RECURRENCE
- Avoid foods you don't digest well.
- Don't smoke.
- Don't eat fast; relax after meals.
- Avoid emotional situations during meals.

CALL YOUR DOCTOR IF

- The pattern of symptoms changes markedly.
- You develop the following:
  Vomiting, weight loss or appetite loss.
  Black, tarry stools or vomiting of blood.
  Fever.
  Severe pain in the upper right abdomen.
  Discomfort that continues unrelated to meals, eating or chewing gum.
- Indigestion is accompanied by:
  Shortness of breath.
  Sweating.
  Pain radiating to the jaw, neck or arm.

INFLUENZA
(Flu; Grippe)

BASIC INFORMATION FOR OLDER ADULTS

DESCRIPTION—Flu is a common, contagious respiratory infection caused by a virus. The incubation time after exposure is 24 to 48 hours. Body parts involved: The upper respiratory system.

SPECIAL CONSIDERATIONS FOR AGING
- The immune system becomes less effective, opening the way for viral, bacterial and other infections; malignancies; immune disorders; and allergies.
- Characteristic signs and symptoms of many disorders are frequently changed or absent.
- Stress from social isolation increases the risk of infection.

SIGNS & SYMPTOMS
- Chills and moderate to high fever.
- Muscle aches, including backache.
- A cough, usually with little or no sputum.
- Sore throat; hoarseness; runny nose.
- Headache; fatigue.
- Loss of appetite; chest pain.

CAUSES & RISK FACTORS—Caused by infection from viruses of the myxovirus class. There are 3 main types—A, B and C. Types A and B may alter to produce new strains. The viruses are spread by personal contact. Risk factors include:
- Stress; fatigue or overwork; poor nutrition.
- A recent illness that has lowered resistance.
- Chronic illness, especially chronic lung disease.

DOCTOR'S TREATMENT & DIAGNOSTIC TESTS
- Medical history and physical exam.
- Laboratory studies such as blood tests and sputum culture (only for complications).
- X-rays of the chest.
- Self-care instructions focused on the older patient.

HOME TREATMENT BY SELF OR CARE-GIVER

GENERAL INSTRUCTIONS
- To relieve nasal congestion, use salt-water drops (1 teaspoon of salt to 1 quart of water).
- To relieve a sore throat, gargle often with warm or cold double-strength tea.
- Use a cool-mist humidifier to increase the air moisture. This thins lung secretions so they can be coughed up more easily. Don't put medicine in the humidifier; it does not help.
- To avoid spreading germs to others, wash your hands frequently—especially after blowing your nose or before handling food.
- Rest in bed until your fever is gone.

MEDICATION (ADJUSTED FOR AGING)
- For minor discomfort, you may use non-prescription drugs such as acetaminophen, cough syrups, nasal sprays or decongestants.
- Your doctor may prescribe:
  An antiviral drug, amantadine, for seriously ill persons or for those at greatest risk from complications.
  Antibiotics to combat any complicating bacterial infection.

ACTIVITY FOR OLDER PATIENTS
- Rest is the best medicine. If you are in good general health, rest helps your body fight the virus.
- Gradually resume your normal activities.

FOOD & BEVERAGE—No special diet is required. If you have a high fever, drink extra fluids—at least 8 glasses of water a day. Extra fluids, including fruit juice, tea and carbonated drinks, also help thin lung secretions. Avoid milk because it thickens secretions in some persons.

FUTURE CONSIDERATIONS FOR THE AGING ADULT

POSSIBLE COMPLICATIONS—Bacterial infections, including middle ear infections, bronchitis or pneumonia. These can be especially dangerous for chronically ill persons or those over age 65.

PROBABLE OUTCOME—Spontaneous recovery in 7 to 14 days if no complications occur. If complications arise, treatment with antibiotics is usually necessary and recovery may take 3 to 6 weeks.

PREVENTING RECURRENCE
- Avoid the risk factors listed above.
- Have a yearly influenza vaccine injection, particularly if you are over age 65 or have chronic heart or lung disease. A vaccine protects against only a few—not all—types of flu.
- Avoid unnecessary contact with persons who have upper respiratory infections during the flu season (winter).

CALL YOUR DOCTOR IF

- You have symptoms of influenza.
- Any of the following occurs during treatment:
  Increased fever or cough.
  Blood in the sputum.
  Earache.
  Shortness of breath or chest pain.
  A thick discharge from the nose, sinuses or ears.
  Sinus pain.
  Neck pain or stiffness.
- New, unexplained symptoms develop. The drugs used in treatment may produce side effects.

INSECT BITES & STINGS

BASIC INFORMATION FOR OLDER ADULTS

DESCRIPTION—Insect bites or stings cause skin eruptions and other symptoms. The victim often doesn't remember being bitten or stung. Body parts involved: The skin on any part of the body; the lymph glands in the neck, armpit, groin or elbow.

SPECIAL CONSIDERATIONS FOR AGING
- Decreased nutrition, common among chronically ill older people, increases the risk of any disease or disorder.
- The immune system becomes less effective, opening the way for viral, bacterial and other infections; malignancies; immune disorders; and allergies.

SIGNS & SYMPTOMS—Red lumps in the skin. The lumps usually appear within minutes after the bite or sting, but some don't appear for 6 to 12 hours. Skin reactions fall into 2 categories:
- A toxic reaction with pain, such as from bee stings.
- A toxic reaction with itching due to the body's release of histamine at the bite site, such as from mosquitoes.

CAUSES & RISK FACTORS—Caused by bites or stings from mosquitoes, fleas, chiggers, bedbugs, ants, spiders, bees and other insects. The risk increases with:
- Being in an area with a heavy insect infestation.
- Warm weather in spring and summer.
- Travel in tropical countries.

DOCTOR'S TREATMENT & DIAGNOSTIC TESTS
- Medical history and physical exam.
- Self-care instructions focused on the older patient.

HOME TREATMENT BY SELF OR CARE-GIVER

GENERAL INSTRUCTIONS
- Wash the area with soap and water. Use calamine lotion to relieve itching.
- Avoid scratching.
- Use immersion or wrapped soaks (see Appendix 18) to relieve the itching and hasten healing. Warm-water soaks are usually more soothing for pain or inflammation. Cool-water soaks feel better for itching.
- If you have experienced anaphylaxis (a severe allergic reaction) following an insect bite, ask your doctor for an anaphylaxis kit to treat it in the future.

MEDICATION (ADJUSTED FOR AGING)
- For minor discomfort, you may use: Non-prescription oral antihistamines to decrease the itching.
  Non-prescription topical steroid preparations to reduce the inflammation and itching. Use them according to the label directions. On your face and groin, use only low-potency steroid products without fluorine.
- For serious symptoms, your doctor may: Prescribe stronger topical steroids or oral steroids if the reaction is severe.
  Inject epinephrine or cortisone to prevent or diminish the symptoms of anaphylaxis.
- For bee, wasp, yellowjacket or hornet stings, rub a paste of meat tenderizer and water into the site.
- For ant bites, rub the site with ammonia; repeat as often as necessary.
- For black widow spider or scorpion bites, capture the insect and seek medical attention.
- For tick and mite bites, apply a petroleum product until the insect withdraws.

ACTIVITY FOR OLDER PATIENTS—No restrictions are necessary.

FOOD & BEVERAGE—No special diet.

FUTURE CONSIDERATIONS FOR THE AGING ADULT

POSSIBLE COMPLICATIONS
- A secondary bacterial infection at the site of the bite. This may cause swollen lymph glands in the neck, armpit, groin or elbow.
- Anaphylaxis (for hypersensitive persons). See Anaphylaxis in the Illnesses section.

PROBABLE OUTCOME—Most troublesome symptoms disappear in 2 to 3 days, but scratching may prolong the symptoms for several weeks. Treatment helps, but it doesn't cure quickly.

PREVENTING RECURRENCE
- After identifying the cause, remove it if possible. Treat animals for fleas and ticks, and exterminate insects in the house or kennel.
- If you cannot avoid exposure, apply insect repellents with diethyltoluamide (DEET).
- Recent evidence indicates that B vitamins may be deterrents to insect bites.

CALL YOUR DOCTOR IF

- You have symptoms of anaphylaxis. *This is an emergency!*
- Self-care does not relieve the symptoms or the symptoms don't improve after 2 to 3 days of medical treatment.
- A bitten area becomes red, swollen, warm and tender, indicating infection.
- Your temperature rises to 101F (38.3C).

BASIC INFORMATION FOR OLDER ADULTS

DESCRIPTION—Insomnia means sleep disturbance—either difficulty falling asleep or difficulty remaining asleep. Difficulty in sleeping occurs in about 1 of 3 adults. Body parts involved: The central nervous system; other body parts involved depend on the cause.

SPECIAL CONSIDERATIONS FOR AGING
- The brain shrinks in volume. The older the person, the more the shrinkage.
- Neurological diseases become more likely.
- Nerve cells in aging people are especially susceptible to the action of drugs, particularly mind-altering drugs such as narcotics, alcohol, sleep inducers, pain killers, antihistamines, muscle relaxants and others.
- Stress from any emotional cause affects all aspects of any illness or disorder.

SIGNS & SYMPTOMS
- Restlessness when trying to fall asleep.
- Brief sleep followed by wakefulness.
- Normal sleep until very early in the morning (3 or 4 a.m.), then wakefulness, often with frightening thoughts.
- Periods of sleeplessness that alternate with periods of excessive sleep or sleepiness at inconvenient times.
- Daytime fatigue; irritability.

CAUSES & RISK FACTORS—Causes include:
- Depression. This is usually characterized by early-morning wakefulness.
- Overactivity of the thyroid gland.
- Anxiety caused by stress.
- Sexual problems, such as impotence or lack of a sex partner.
- A noisy environment (including a snoring partner).
- Allergies and early-morning wheezing.
- Heart or lung conditions that cause shortness of breath when lying down.
- Painful disorders, such as fibromyositis or arthritis.
- Urinary or gastrointestinal problems that require urination or bowel movements during the night.
- The consumption of stimulants, such as coffee, tea or cola drinks.
- The use of some medications, including dextro-amphetamines, cortisone drugs or decongestants.
- Daytime napping; erratic work hours.
- A new environment or location; jet lag.
- Lack of physical exercise; alcoholism.
- Drug abuse, including the overuse of sleep-inducing drugs.
- Withdrawal from addictive substances or some prescription or over-the-counter drugs.
- A misconception about how much sleep is needed.
The risk increases with stress, obesity or smoking.

DOCTOR'S TREATMENT & DIAGNOSTIC TESTS
- Medical history and physical exam.
- Laboratory thyroid studies; EEG (see Glossary).
- Tests in a sleep-study laboratory.

- Self-care instructions focused on the older patient.
- Psychotherapy or counseling if the cause is psychological.

FUTURE CONSIDERATIONS FOR THE AGING ADULT

GENERAL INSTRUCTIONS
- Seek ways to minimize stress. See Appendix 13.
- Obtain medical treatment for any underlying medical disorder.
- Don't use stimulants for several hours before bedtime.
- Relax in a warm bath before bedtime.
- Maintain a log of your sleep patterns. You may be getting more sleep than you thought.
- Establish a regular time for going to bed and getting up.

MEDICATION (ADJUSTED FOR AGING)
- Your doctor may prescribe sleep-inducing drugs for a short time if temporary insomnia is interfering with your daily activities; you have a medical disorder that regularly disturbs your sleep; you need to establish regular sleep patterns.
- The long-term use of sleep inducers may be counter-productive or addictive. Don't use sleeping pills given to you by friends and don't take non-prescription sleeping pills.

ACTIVITY FOR OLDER PATIENTS
- Exercise regularly (see Appendix 20) to create healthy fatigue, but not within 2 hours of going to bed.
- Have sexual relations if they are fulfilling and satisfying before going to sleep.
- Keep active during the day. Avoid naps.

FOOD & BEVERAGE—No special diet is required, but don't eat within 3 hours of bedtime if indigestion has previously disturbed your sleep. Drinking a glass of warm milk before bedtime may help.

FUTURE CONSIDERATIONS FOR THE AGING ADULT

POSSIBLE COMPLICATIONS—Impaired relationships; poor work performance; lower resistance to disease; injury from falling asleep around machinery or while driving.

PROBABLE OUTCOME—Most persons can establish good sleep patterns if the underlying cause of insomnia is treated or eliminated.

PREVENTING RECURRENCE—Establish a life-style that fosters healthy sleep patterns (see General Instructions). If you are unable to sleep, get up and do something. Avoid lengthy daytime napping.

CALL YOUR DOCTOR IF

- You have insomnia.
- New, unexplained symptoms develop. The drugs used in treatment may produce side effects.

INTESTINAL OBSTRUCTION

BASIC INFORMATION FOR OLDER ADULTS

DESCRIPTION—Intestinal obstruction is the partial or complete blockage of the intestines. Body parts involved: The small and large intestines. (THIS IS AN EMERGENCY; SEEK MEDICAL CARE IMMEDIATELY!)

SPECIAL CONSIDERATIONS FOR AGING
- The total digestive system become sluggish.
- Usual signs and symptoms may be absent and be replaced by symptoms of confusion, dizziness, failure to thrive, falling, incontinence, increasing dementia, refusal to eat or drink, weight loss, depression, paranoia, hypochondriasis, psychosis or threats of suicide.

SIGNS & SYMPTOMS
- Abdominal pain and cramps.
- Nausea and vomiting. In the advanced stages, the vomit resembles feces.
- Weakness, dizziness or fainting.
- Little or no urine due to fluid loss.
- Audible noises from the abdomen in the early stages. Later *no* sounds are audible.
- Abdominal bloating, swelling and gas.
- Fever (sometimes).
- Diarrhea (with a partial obstruction only).
- Rectal bleeding (sometimes).
- Inability to pass gas or stool.

CAUSES & RISK FACTORS
Causes include:
- Paralytic ileus—i.e., the muscle contractions of the intestine stop.
- Adhesions (constricting bands of fibrous tissue that result from previous surgery).
- Intestinal hernias.
- Intestinal inflammation or tumors—either benign or cancerous.
- Tumors in adjacent organs that cause pressure on the intestines.
- Foreign objects inside the intestines (swallowed objects or parasites such as worms).
- A twisted bowel (volvulus; see Glossary).
- Severe constipation (fecal impaction).
The risk increases with previous abdominal surgery.

DOCTOR'S TREATMENT & DIAGNOSTIC TESTS
- Medical history and physical exam.
- Laboratory blood studies to measure fluids and electrolytes and to detect bleeding or infection.
- X-rays of the intestinal tract and abdomen (upper and lower GI series).
- The removal of gas and intestinal contents through a flexible tube inserted in the throat (usually in a hospital).
- Surgery to remove the obstruction (usually). Advancing age alone is not a deterrent.
- Hospitalization for diagnosis and replacement of lost fluids prior to surgery.
- Self-care instructions focused on the older patient.

HOME TREATMENT BY SELF OR CARE-GIVER

GENERAL INSTRUCTIONS
- Intestinal obstruction usually develops rapidly into an emergency. Home remedies are of no value and some—such as enemas or laxatives—may be harmful.
- Intestinal obstruction is a complicated, serious disorder. This page can cover only the main points of diagnosis and treatment. Your doctor, nurse or librarian can provide sources of supplemental information.

MEDICATION (ADJUSTED FOR AGING)
- Medication is not helpful for intestinal obstruction. However, your doctor may prescribe medication appropriate for the underlying disorder.
- *Note:* Adverse reactions and side effects may be more frequent and severe in older persons. Remind your doctor of any medicines you already take.

ACTIVITY FOR OLDER PATIENTS—Rest in bed until the obstruction is corrected. If surgery is necessary, resume your normal activities gradually.

FOOD & BEVERAGE
- Don't eat or drink anything until the obstruction is corrected. You will probably receive intravenous nourishment until then.
- See Appendix 1 regarding good nutrition for people over 50.

FUTURE CONSIDERATIONS FOR THE AGING ADULT

POSSIBLE COMPLICATIONS—Dehydration and shock; bowel gangrene; peritonitis; a tumor in the colon.

PROBABLE OUTCOME
- Surgery can usually correct the obstruction, but it may not correct the underlying cause, such as cancer.
- Without treatment, complications can be fatal.

PREVENTING RECURRENCE
- Eat a diet that is high in fiber and drink at least 6 to 8 glasses of liquid a day to avoid constipation or fecal impaction.
- Obtain prompt medical treatment to repair a hernia.
- See your doctor if your bowel habits change significantly for longer than 7 days. This may be an early symptom of bowel cancer.

CALL YOUR DOCTOR IF

- Your bowel habits change.
- You have early symptoms of intestinal obstruction.

IRIS, INFLAMMATION AND INFECTION OF
(Iritis; Uveitis)

BASIC INFORMATION FOR OLDER ADULTS

DESCRIPTION—Iritis is an inflammation of parts of the eye, mainly the iris (the ring of colored tissue around the pupil of the eye). It may sometimes be confused with pinkeye (conjunctivitis). Body parts involved: The eye(s).

SPECIAL CONSIDERATIONS FOR AGING
- The immune system becomes less effective, opening the way for viral, bacterial and other infections; malignancies; immune disorders; and allergies.
- Visual acuity decreases.
- The pupils become smaller.

SIGNS & SYMPTOMS
Acute iritis of sudden onset:
- Severe eye pain.
- Photophobia (sensitivity to light).
- Eye redness.
- A smaller pupil in the affected eye (sometimes).
- Tears.
- Blurred vision.

Iritis of gradual onset:
- Eye pain.
- Photophobia.
- Floating spots in the field of vision.
- Blurred vision.

CAUSES & RISK FACTORS
Causes include:
- An infection that spreads to the eye from other body parts. Common infections include:
  Toxoplasmosis.
  Tuberculosis.
  Histoplasmosis.
  Syphilis.
  Sarcoidosis.
  Viruses.
- Injury to the eye.
- An autoimmune reaction (possibly).
- Unknown in many cases.

Risk factors include:
- Rheumatoid arthritis.
- Ulcerative colitis.

DOCTOR'S TREATMENT & DIAGNOSTIC TESTS
- Medical history and physical exam by an ophthalmologist.
- Self-care instructions focused on the older patient.

HOME TREATMENT BY SELF OR CARE-GIVER

GENERAL INSTRUCTIONS—Wear dark glasses—even indoors—until treatment is complete.

MEDICATION (ADJUSTED FOR AGING)
- Your ophthalmologist may prescribe: Eye drops (mydriatics) that dilate the pupil and prevent scarring. You may need to use eye drops for a long time. Ask your doctor how to instill them in the eye correctly. Oral cortisone drugs or cortisone eye drops to reduce inflammation. Discuss the side effects of cortisone drugs with your doctor.
- *Note:* Adverse reactions and side effects may be more frequent and severe in older persons. Remind your doctor of any medicines you already take.

ACTIVITY FOR OLDER PATIENTS
- Rest in bed until the symptoms subside. Allow 1 to 2 weeks.
- See Appendix 20 regarding physical fitness for the active older adult.

FOOD & BEVERAGE
- No special diet is required.
- See Appendix 1 regarding good nutrition for people over 50.

FUTURE CONSIDERATIONS FOR THE AGING ADULT

POSSIBLE COMPLICATIONS
- Glaucoma.
- Cataracts.
- Permanent partial vision loss.

PROBABLE OUTCOME—Your vision can usually be preserved with prompt treatment.

PREVENTING RECURRENCE—Cannot be prevented at present.

CALL YOUR DOCTOR IF

- You have symptoms of iritis—either sudden or gradual. Call immediately.
- Your vision changes in any way.
- New, unexplained symptoms develop. The drugs used in treatment may produce side effects.

JAW DISLOCATION
(Temporomandibular Joint Dislocation)

 BASIC INFORMATION FOR OLDER ADULTS

DESCRIPTION—The temporomandibular joints connect the lower jaw (mandible) to the skull. They are just forward of the ears. With jaw dislocation, one cannot close the mouth because the head of the mandible (the condyle) slides backward into a depression in the skull. Body part involved: The jaw.

SPECIAL CONSIDERATIONS FOR AGING
- Muscle bulk and power decrease.
- Bone strength decreases.

SIGNS & SYMPTOMS
- Inability to close the mouth.
- Pain and swelling in the jaw.
- Bleeding under the skin of the jaw.
- Obvious asymmetry of the face.
- Numbness of the chin and lower lip (sometimes).
- Drooling.
- Difficulty speaking.

CAUSES & RISK FACTORS
Causes include:
- Injury from an auto accident.
- Physical violence.
- Some persons dislocate their mandibles with little provocation, as with yawning, yelling, biting large pieces of food or opening the mouth very wide for any reason.
The risk increases with injuries most often associated with:
- Accident-proneness.
- A violent lifestyle.
- Excessive alcohol consumption or the use of mind-altering drugs.
- Non-use of seat belts.

DOCTOR'S TREATMENT & DIAGNOSTIC TESTS—The muscles tighten and the pain increases within 15 to 30 minutes after dislocation, so a dislocated jaw should be treated quickly. Treatment usually involves the following:
- Medical history and physical exam.
- X-rays of the jaw.
- After diagnosis and treatment, self-care instructions focused on the older patient.
- Surgery to stabilize the joint for recurring dislocations (rare).

 HOME TREATMENT BY SELF OR CARE-GIVER

GENERAL INSTRUCTIONS
- Make sure an injured person with a fractured or dislocated jaw has no breathing obstruction. If there is an obstruction, seek emergency help immediately.

- If your jaw is injured, don't panic. Stay calm. Go to the nearest dental office or emergency facility for help.
- Don't try to talk with a dislocated jaw. Write messages instead. Don't try to push or force your mouth closed. Your mouth cannot close normally until the dislocation is corrected.

MEDICATION (ADJUSTED FOR AGING)
- Your doctor may prescribe:
  Pain relievers.
  Muscle relaxants.
- *Note:* Adverse reactions and side effects may be more frequent and severe in older persons. Remind your doctor of any medicines you already take.

ACTIVITY FOR OLDER PATIENTS
- Rest in bed with your head turned to one side. You may read or watch TV. Resume your normal activities in 2 to 3 days. Allow 6 weeks for the muscles and tendons attached to the joint to heal.
- See Appendix 20 regarding physical fitness for the active older adult.

FOOD & BEVERAGE—A liquid diet (see Appendix 7) may be necessary for up to 4 weeks. Start with clear liquids, then graduate to a full liquid diet, including blenderized foods, milkshakes and juices. Don't chew solid foods without your doctor's or dentist's permission.

 FUTURE CONSIDERATIONS FOR THE AGING ADULT

POSSIBLE COMPLICATIONS—Obstruction of the airway and inhalation of mucus and blood into the lungs, leading to pneumonia. This occurs most often with dislocation and fracture.

PROBABLE OUTCOME—Usually curable with treatment.

PREVENTING RECURRENCE
- Avoid opening your mouth widely if possible when you yawn, bite large pieces of food, yell or scream during excitement, call out loudly or sing.
- Use seat belts in vehicles.
- Don't drive after drinking alcohol or using mind-altering drugs.

 CALL YOUR DOCTOR IF

- You have symptoms of a dislocated jaw.
- Your pain is intolerable.

JOINT DISLOCATION OR SUBLUXATION

BASIC INFORMATION FOR OLDER ADULTS

DESCRIPTION—Joint dislocation means injury to a joint so that the adjoining bones no longer touch each other. Subluxation is a minor dislocation; the joint surfaces still touch, but not in normal relation to each other. Body parts involved: The bones in joints, especially the jaw, shoulder, knee and spine.

SPECIAL CONSIDERATIONS FOR AGING
- Years of weight bearing cause wear and tear on the bones, joints and ligaments.
- For many reasons, older people are less likely to maintain a good level of physical conditioning.

SIGNS & SYMPTOMS
- Sudden joint pain, swelling or deformity after an injury.
- Limited or absent movement around a joint.

CAUSES & RISK FACTORS
Causes include:
- An injury that stretches or tears the ligaments that surround a joint and hold the bones together.
- Shallow or abnormally formed joint surfaces (congenital).
- Rheumatoid arthritis or other diseases of the ligaments and tissues around a joint.

Risk factors include:
- Rheumatoid arthritis.
- A family history of congenital hip dislocation.
- Repeated injury to a joint.

DOCTOR'S TREATMENT & DIAGNOSTIC TESTS
- Medical history and physical exam.
- X-rays of the joint and adjacent bones.
- Treatment may include manipulating the joint to reposition the bones.
- Self-care instructions focused on the older patient.
- Surgery to restore the joint to its normal position (sometimes). Recurring dislocation may require surgical reconstruction or replacement of the joint. Advancing age alone is not a deterrent.

HOME TREATMENT BY SELF OR CARE-GIVER

GENERAL INSTRUCTIONS—Immediately after injury:
- Apply ice packs to the involved joint to prevent swelling.
- Use a splint or sling to prevent movement while transporting the injured person to the doctor.
- Don't allow an untrained person to attempt to manipulate the joint back into place.

- If your doctor puts a cast on the joint, see Appendix 17.

MEDICATION (ADJUSTED FOR AGING)
- Your doctor may prescribe:
  General anesthesia or muscle relaxants to make joint manipulation possible.
  Acetaminophen or aspirin to relieve moderate pain.
  Narcotic pain relievers for severe pain.
- *Note:* Adverse reactions and side effects may be more frequent and severe in older persons. Remind your doctor of any medicines you already take.

ACTIVITY FOR OLDER PATIENTS
- Resume your normal activities gradually after treatment. Follow the rehabilitation program your doctor prescribes.
- See Appendix 20 regarding physical fitness for the active older adult.

FOOD & BEVERAGE
- Drink only water before manipulation or surgery to correct the dislocation. Solid food makes general anesthesia more hazardous.
- See Appendix 1 regarding good nutrition for people over 50.

FUTURE CONSIDERATIONS FOR THE AGING ADULT

POSSIBLE COMPLICATIONS—Damage to nearby nerves or major blood vessels, causing numbness, coldness and paleness.

PROBABLE OUTCOME—Usually curable with prompt treatment. After the dislocation has been corrected, the joint may require immobilization with a cast or sling for 2 to 8 weeks.

PREVENTING RECURRENCE—If you are involved in heavy work or strenuous sports, learn to protect the involved joints. Use protective devices, such as wrapped elastic bandages, tape wraps, knee or shoulder pads and special support stockings.

CALL YOUR DOCTOR IF

- You have difficulty moving a joint after injury.
- Any extremity becomes numb, pale or cold after injury. *This is an emergency!*
- Dislocations occur repeatedly that you can ''pop'' back into normal position.

BASIC INFORMATION FOR OLDER ADULTS

DESCRIPTION—Actinic keratosis is a small area of sun-damaged skin that is precancerous. Body parts involved: The skin of exposed areas, especially the scalp, face, ears, lips, arms and hands.

SPECIAL CONSIDERATIONS FOR AGING
- The fatty layer of tissue under the skin becomes thinner.
- The skin becomes more permeable to bacteria, oil and water.
- The skin becomes less elastic.

SIGNS & SYMPTOMS—Brownish or reddish scaly patches on exposed areas of skin. The patches are painless.

CAUSES & RISK FACTORS—Caused by prolonged exposure to the sun's radiation. Risk factors include:
- Outdoor occupations such as farming.
- Outdoor sports.
- Light complexion.

DOCTOR'S TREATMENT & DIAGNOSTIC TESTS
- Medical history and physical exam.
- Self-care instructions focused on the older patient.
- Skin biopsy.

HOME TREATMENT BY SELF OR CARE-GIVER

GENERAL INSTRUCTIONS—After diagnosis:
- Minimize direct exposure to the sun.
- See your doctor for checkups every 6 months to ensure early detection and treatment of skin cancers.

MEDICATION (ADJUSTED FOR AGING)
- Your doctor may use:
  Liquid nitrogen to freeze the affected tissue.
  Applications of 5-fluorouacil to the affected area. This causes uncomfortable inflammation, but it is very effective.
  Vitamin A, which is still experimental.
- *Note:* Adverse reactions and side effects may be more frequent and severe in older persons. Remind your doctor of any medicines you already take.

ACTIVITY FOR OLDER PATIENTS
- No restrictions are necessary.
- See Appendix 20 regarding physical fitness for the active older adult.

FOOD & BEVERAGE
- No special diet is required.
- See Appendix 1 regarding good nutrition for people over 50.

FUTURE CONSIDERATIONS FOR THE AGING ADULT

POSSIBLE COMPLICATIONS
- Skin damage.
- Skin cancer (including malignant melanoma, basal-cell carcinoma and squamous-cell carcinoma).

PROBABLE OUTCOME—An individual keratosis will disappear with treatment, but new lesions are likely to recur. If neglected, actinic keratosis can lead to skin cancer.

PREVENTING RECURRENCE—Protect yourself against direct exposure to the sun. When outdoors, wear a hat and protective clothing. Use sunscreen lotions and creams with SPF ratings of 15 or more.

CALL YOUR DOCTOR IF

You have signs of actinic keratosis. Even though this causes no symptoms, it is precancerous.

KERATOSIS, SEBORRHEIC

BASIC INFORMATION FOR OLDER ADULTS

DESCRIPTION—Seborrheic keratosis is a non-contagious, inflammatory, scaling disease of the skin often called seborrheic warts. Body parts involved: The chest, back, face and arms.

SPECIAL CONSIDERATIONS FOR AGING
- The sweat glands produce less sweat.
- The skin produces less vitamin D, so supplemental oral vitamin D may be needed.
- The fatty layer of tissue under the skin becomes thinner.

SIGNS & SYMPTOMS—Papules (small, raised bumps) with the following characteristics:
- The papules are flat-topped with well-defined borders.
- Young papules are relatively flat and light brown. More advanced papules are dark brown or black.
- The papules are wider than they are tall, and they appear to be "stuck on."
- The papules measure 5mm to 20mm in diameter. They are distributed on the chest, back, face and arms.
- The papules don't itch or hurt.
- There may be only 1 or 2 papules or there may be up to 100.

CAUSES & RISK FACTORS—The cause is unknown. Risk factors include:
- A family history of the disorder.
- Excessive exposure to the sun.
- Other skin injury.

DOCTOR'S TREATMENT & DIAGNOSTIC TESTS
- Medical history and physical exam.
- Biopsy (see Glossary).
- Self-care instructions focused on the older patient.
- Diagnosis to rule out skin cancer.
- Removal of the lesions if they are unsightly, are irritated by clothing or interfere with grooming. Removal methods include cryo-surgery, chemocautery, light electrosurgery or shave biopsy (see Glossary for all).

HOME TREATMENT BY SELF OR CARE-GIVER

GENERAL INSTRUCTIONS—After removal, a blister (sometimes with blood) will develop at the treatment site. The top of the blister will come off spontaneously in about 2 weeks. You should have little or no scarring. Wash and use makeup or cosmetics as usual. If clothing irritates the blister, cover it with a small adhesive bandage.

MEDICATION (ADJUSTED FOR AGING)—Medicine is usually not necessary for this disorder.

ACTIVITY FOR OLDER PATIENTS
- No restrictions are necessary.
- See Appendix 20 regarding physical fitness for the active older adult.

FOOD & BEVERAGE
- No special diet is required.
- See Appendix 1 regarding good nutrition for people over 50.

FUTURE CONSIDERATIONS FOR THE AGING ADULT

POSSIBLE COMPLICATIONS—Seborrheic keratoses on the edges of the eyelids may require special treatment.

PROBABLE OUTCOME—The number of lesions increases with time. Each lesion is permanent unless removed. Seborrheic keratoses are harmless and require no treatment, but most people want them removed.

PREVENTING RECURRENCE—There are no specific preventive measures.

CALL YOUR DOCTOR IF

- You have symptoms of seborrheic keratosis.
- You want unsightly seborrheic keratoses removed.
- Treated areas become infected, as evidenced by pain, tenderness, redness, swelling or heat.
- Any lesion changes color or bleeds.

KIDNEY CANCER

BASIC INFORMATION FOR OLDER ADULTS

DESCRIPTION—Kidney cancer is an uncontrolled growth of malignant cells in the kidney. The cancer may begin in the kidney (primary) or spread to the kidney from other sites (secondary). Body parts involved: One or both kidneys.

SPECIAL CONSIDERATIONS FOR AGING
- Malignant diseases (especially in the colon, lung and breast) represent difficult-to-diagnose problems.
- Characteristic signs and symptoms of many disorders are frequently changed or absent.
- Stress from any emotional cause—fear, worry, anxiety, sadness, loneliness or anger—affects all aspects of any illness or disorder.

SIGNS & SYMPTOMS
- Blood in the urine.
- Pain in the flank (the lower back on either side of the spine).
- Unexplained fever, usually low.
- A swelling or mass in the abdomen.
- Hypertension (sometimes).
- Weight loss.

CAUSES & RISK FACTORS—The causes and risk factors are unknown.

DOCTOR'S TREATMENT & DIAGNOSTIC TESTS
- Medical history and physical exam.
- Laboratory studies of the blood and urine to measure kidney function.
- X-rays of the kidneys, associated blood vessels and surrounding tissue.
- CT scan of the abdomen.
- Renal angiography.
- Surgery to remove the affected kidney. Advancing age alone is not a deterrent.
- Postoperative radiation treatment if the cancer has spread. Otherwise, radiation is usually not helpful.
- After surgery, self-care instructions focused on the older patient.

HOME TREATMENT BY SELF OR CARE-GIVER

GENERAL INSTRUCTIONS
- Maintain as positive an attitude as possible during treatment.
- Treatment may cause side effects, but they are usually temporary.
- Your pain can be controlled. Don't hesitate to ask your doctor for pain medication.
- Fear may be your worst enemy.
- Call on family members and friends for whatever support and help you need.

- Kidney cancer is a complicated, serious disorder. This page can cover only the main points of diagnosis and treatment. Your doctor, nurse or librarian can provide sources of supplemental information.

MEDICATION (ADJUSTED FOR AGING)
- Your doctor may prescribe pain relievers and anticancer drugs (chemotherapy).
- *Note:* Adverse reactions and side effects may be more frequent and severe in older persons. Remind your doctor of any medicines you already take.

ACTIVITY FOR OLDER PATIENTS
- No restrictions are necessary.
- See Appendix 20 regarding physical fitness for the active older adult.

FOOD & BEVERAGE
- No special diet is required.
- See Appendix 1 regarding good nutrition for people over 50.

FUTURE CONSIDERATIONS FOR THE AGING ADULT

POSSIBLE COMPLICATIONS—Spread of the cancer (metastasis) to nearby tissues or through the bloodstream to the lungs, bone, liver or lymph glands.

PROBABLE OUTCOME—Depends on how early the kidney cancer is discovered. The 5-year survival rate is 50% to 60% if the cancer is diagnosed and treated before it spreads from the kidney. Survival for 5 years is unlikely if the cancer is discovered after it spreads. However, medical literature cites instances of unexplained recovery.

PREVENTING RECURRENCE—Cannot be prevented at present. Seek early medical care if you have urinary symptoms, pain or unexplained fever.

CALL YOUR DOCTOR IF

You have symptoms of kidney cancer.

KIDNEY FAILURE, ACUTE

BASIC INFORMATION FOR OLDER ADULTS

DESCRIPTION—Acute kidney failure is the sudden failure of the kidneys to function. This condition usually has a short, relatively severe course, but often it is curable. Body parts involved: The kidneys. (THIS IS AN EMERGENCY; SEEK MEDICAL CARE IMMEDIATELY!)

SPECIAL CONSIDERATIONS FOR AGING
- Characteristic signs and symptoms of many disorders are frequently changed or absent.
- The blood flow to the kidneys decreases.
- Kidney function becomes less efficient.
- The prostate gland atrophies.

SIGNS & SYMPTOMS
Early stages:
- Little or no urine output.

Later stages:
- Nausea, vomiting, diarrhea and appetite loss.
- Mental changes, including irritability, drowsiness, stupor or coma; convulsions.
- Severe itching; high or low blood pressure.
- Unexplained bruising, bleeding spots under the skin or spontaneous bleeding.
- Pale skin and weak pulse.
- The symptoms of the underlying cause (see below) will also be present.

CAUSES & RISK FACTORS—Conditions in the kidney or in other areas of the body can cause the kidneys to stop functioning. This leads to a buildup of waste products in the blood and tissues. Underlying conditions include shock with very low blood pressure; blood poisoning (septicemia); congestive heart failure; fluid and electrolyte imbalance; reaction to a blood transfusion; a severe accident with extensive muscle injury; acute glomerulonephritis; multiple myeloma; obstruction of the blood vessels that supply the kidneys; kidney stones that obstruct both ureters or the urethra; severe bleeding or burns; prostate enlargement; the use of certain medications, including anticancer drugs, kanamycin, amphotericin B, anticonvulsants or excessive vitamin D; and overdose of many poisons or drugs, especially mind-altering drugs. Risk factors include:
- Having just one kidney.
- Recent surgery; accidents with severe injuries.
- A medical history of conditions affecting the kidneys, such as diabetes or gout.

DOCTOR'S TREATMENT & DIAGNOSTIC TESTS
- Medical history and physical exam.
- Laboratory blood counts and blood and urine tests that measure kidney function and fluid and electrolyte balance; ECG (see Glossary).
- Needle biopsy (see Glossary) of the kidneys.
- X-rays of the abdomen, kidneys, ureters and bladder to detect kidney stones.
- Surgery if the cause can be corrected by surgery. Advancing age alone is not a deterrent.
- Hospitalization for fluid and electrolyte therapy, blood transfusion and kidney dialysis (sometimes).
- Temporary dialysis (sometimes) until kidney function returns.
- Self-care instructions focused on the older patient.

HOME TREATMENT BY SELF OR CARE-GIVER

GENERAL INSTRUCTIONS—No specific instructions except those listed under other headings.

MEDICATION (ADJUSTED FOR AGING)
- Your doctor may prescribe:
  Medications appropriate to control the underlying condition.
  Antibiotics if infection develops.
  Reduced dosages of other medicines you currently take.
- *Note:* Adverse reactions and side effects may be more frequent and severe in older persons. Remind your doctor of any medicines you already take.

ACTIVITY FOR OLDER PATIENTS
- Rest in bed until the condition is cured. Then resume your normal activities as soon as your symptoms improve.
- See Appendix 20 regarding physical fitness for the active older adult.

FOOD & BEVERAGE
- Food and water intake is rigorously controlled to prevent fluid and electrolyte imbalance and to minimize the buildup of body wastes.
- Your doctor will provide you with a diet plan to meet your special, individual needs.

FUTURE CONSIDERATIONS FOR THE AGING ADULT

POSSIBLE COMPLICATIONS—Congestive heart failure; increased risk of infections; chronic kidney failure; lifelong dialysis.

PROBABLE OUTCOME—If the underlying condition can be controlled and the kidney failure can be treated promptly, complete recovery is likely. If not, the disorder can lead to chronic kidney failure. Kidney transplant is possible if chronic failure develops.

PREVENTING RECURRENCE—There are no specific preventive measures. Avoid the causes and risk factors listed above when possible.

CALL YOUR DOCTOR IF

- You have symptoms of kidney failure. *This is an emergency!*
- Any of the following occurs during treatment:
  Chills, fever, headache or muscle aches.
  Shortness or breath.
  Unexpected bleeding from any body opening.

KIDNEY FAILURE, CHRONIC
(Uremia)

BASIC INFORMATION FOR OLDER ADULTS

DESCRIPTION—Chronic kidney failure is the inability of the kidneys to eliminate the body's nitrogen waste products. It usually develops gradually. Body parts involved: The kidneys, which eventually affect all body systems.

SPECIAL CONSIDERATIONS FOR AGING
- Characteristic signs and symptoms of many disorders are frequently changed or absent.
- The blood flow to the kidneys decreases.
- Kidney function becomes less efficient.
- The prostate gland atrophies.
- Stress from any emotional cause affects all aspects of any illness or disorder.

SIGNS & SYMPTOMS—Few symptoms or none until 60% to 75% of kidney filtration fails. Then 1 or more of the following:
- Listlessness, mental confusion and drowsiness.
- High blood pressure; shortness of breath.
- Bad breath; bleeding gums and mouth ulcers.
- Abdominal pain; itching skin.
- Numbness, tingling and burning in the legs and feet; muscle cramps.
- Decreased sex drive.
- Anemia, paleness and fatigue; unusual bleeding.
- Muscle and bone pain. Bones break easily.

CAUSES & RISK FACTORS—Causes include collagen diseases, such as systemic lupus erythematosus; chronic glomerulonephritis; chronic abnormalities, such as polycystic kidney disease; kidney damage due to diabetes mellitus; urinary tract obstruction; overdose of many drugs and chemicals, especially phenacetin or streptomycin; and blood vessel diseases, such as hardening of the arteries in or leading to the kidney. The risk increases with the use of mind-altering drugs.

DOCTOR'S TREATMENT & DIAGNOSTIC TESTS
- Medical history and physical exam.
- Laboratory blood counts and blood and urine tests that measure kidney function and fluid and electrolyte balance; ECG (see Glossary).
- Needle biopsy (see Glossary) of kidneys.
- X-rays of the abdomen, kidneys, ureters and bladder to detect kidney stones.
- Kidney transplant if possible.
- Kidney dialysis (see Glossary) if available.
- Hospitalization for complications and care in the final stages.
- Self-care instructions focused on the older patient.

HOME TREATMENT BY SELF OR CARE-GIVER

GENERAL INSTRUCTIONS
- To decrease the itching, add 1 cup of oatmeal to your daily bath. Use skin moisturizers on itching areas.
- Brush your teeth and use mouthwash often to minimize gum and mouth problems.
- Weigh daily and keep a record. Report any change of 3 pounds (up or down) to your doctor.
- Measure the fluids you drink and the urine you pass each day. Keep a record and take it with you on doctor visits. You should pass about 2500cc or more of urine a day. If you pass less, decrease your fluid intake so intake does not exceed output by more than 800cc a day. For example, if you pass 2000cc in 24 hours, don't drink more than 2800cc in the next 24 hours.

MEDICATION (ADJUSTED FOR AGING)
- Your doctor may prescribe:
  Diuretics to reduce fluid accumulation.
  Iron and folic acid supplements for anemia.
  Stool softeners to prevent constipation.
  Digitalis for congestive heart failure.
  Adjustments to dosage and schedule for any medicines you currently take.
- *Note:* Adverse reactions and side effects may be more frequent and severe in older persons. Remind your doctor of any medicines you already take.

ACTIVITY FOR OLDER PATIENTS—Reduce your activity. Don't become overheated or fatigued. Sleep more at night and rest during the day. If you are confined to bed, flex your legs often to reduce the chance of blood clots in the leg veins.

FOOD & BEVERAGE
- Eat a low-salt, low-potassium, low-protein diet with added fiber. Eat frequent small, high-calorie meals.
- Your doctor will provide you with a diet plan to meet your individual needs.

FUTURE CONSIDERATIONS FOR THE AGING ADULT

POSSIBLE COMPLICATIONS—Pericarditis; myocarditis; pneumonia; pancreatitis; hormone deficiencies; fluid and electrolyte imbalance; gastrointestinal ulcers.

PROBABLE OUTCOME—Kidney transplants can cure some younger patients. Otherwise, kidney failure is a condition that worsens gradually, although a near-normal lifespan is possible if the condition stabilizes. Kidney dialysis can improve your life and prolong it for several years.

PREVENTING RECURRENCE—Obtain treatment for underlying diseases *before* uremia results.

CALL YOUR DOCTOR IF

- You have symptoms of uremia.
- Any of the following occurs during treatment:
  Fever; vomiting or diarrhea.
  Urine output of less than 2000cc.
  Severe headache; convulsions.

KIDNEY INFECTION, ACUTE
(Acute Pyelonephritis)

BASIC INFORMATION FOR OLDER ADULTS

DESCRIPTION—Acute pyelonephritis is a non-contagious bacterial infection of the kidney with rapidly developing severe symptoms. Acute kidney infections are less common among older adults than chronic kidney infections. Body parts involved: The kidneys; the urinary tract.

SPECIAL CONSIDERATIONS FOR AGING
- The immune system becomes less effective, opening the way for viral, bacterial and other infections; malignancies; immune disorders; and allergies.
- Decreased nutrition increases the risk of infections.
- Older people frequently drink inadequate amounts of water.

SIGNS & SYMPTOMS—Sudden onset of:
- Fever and shaking chills; marked fatigue.
- Burning, frequent urination; abdominal pain.
- Cloudy urine or blood in the urine.
- Aching (sometimes severe) in one or both sides of the lower back.

CAUSES & RISK FACTORS—Caused by bacteria (most commonly *escherichia coli*) invading one or both kidneys. The infection may begin in the bladder. The most common sources of bacterial infection are:
- Vigorous sexual activity in women, which allows bacteria to enter the urethra and bladder.
- Infections elsewhere in the body that travel to the kidneys through the bloodstream or lymph glands.
- Blockage or abnormality of the urinary system, caused by stones, obstructions, bladder dysfunction from nerve diseases, tumors or congenital abnormalities.
- Catheters, tubes or surgical procedures used for other medical conditions.

Risk factors include:
- Diabetes mellitus.
- Chronic infection or a tumor of the urinary bladder.
- Infrequent emptying of the urinary bladder.
- Paralysis from a spinal cord injury or tumor.
- Childhood renal infections.
- The past use of any drug containing phenacetin.

DOCTOR'S TREATMENT & DIAGNOSTIC TESTS
- Medical history and physical exam.
- Urinalysis, blood tests and urine culture (see Glossary).
- Self-care instructions focused on the older patient.

OTHER—Acute kidney infections in males of any age may indicate a serious underlying disease, such as a tumor, obstruction or prostate disorder. Consult your doctor even if the symptoms disappear spontaneously.

HOME TREATMENT BY SELF OR CARE-GIVER

GENERAL INSTRUCTIONS—To collect urine for urinalysis or culture:
- Females—Clean the vaginal area with warm, soapy water; sponge dry. Spread the vaginal lips with one hand and urinate briefly into the toilet bowl. Then urinate into the container.
- Males—Pull back the foreskin of the penis if you are not circumcised. Clean the end of the penis with soapy water. Urinate briefly into the toilet bowl, then into the container.

MEDICATION (ADJUSTED FOR AGING)—Your doctor may prescribe:
- Oral antibiotics. Take all the antibiotics prescribed, even if the symptoms disappear.
- Antibiotics (intravenous or by injection) if oral antibiotics don't cure the infection.
- Urinary analgesics to relieve the pain.

ACTIVITY FOR OLDER PATIENTS—Rest in bed until your high fever and discomfort subside. Don't resume sexual relations until the fever or urinary symptoms have cleared.

FOOD & BEVERAGE—No special diet. Drink at least 2 quarts of liquid daily; include cranberry juice or vitamin C to acidify the urine.

FUTURE CONSIDERATIONS FOR THE AGING ADULT

POSSIBLE COMPLICATIONS—Chronic kidney infection; hypertension.

PROBABLE OUTCOME—Usually curable in about 3 weeks with treatment. Make a return visit to your doctor to ensure a complete cure.

PREVENTING RECURRENCE—There are no specific preventive measures for males. For females:
- After bowel movements, always wipe from the vaginal area toward the rectum.
- Avoid prolonged moistness around the urethra, such as that caused by nylon underpants or wet swimsuits.
- Avoid sexual positions that irritate or hurt the urethra or bladder; urinate within 15 minutes after sexual intercourse.

CALL YOUR DOCTOR IF

- You have symptoms of a kidney infection.
- Any of the following occurs during treatment: The symptoms and fever persist after 48 hours of antibiotic treatment. Occasionally a different antibiotic is needed.
  The symptoms return (especially if accompanied by fever) after antibiotic treatment.
- New, unexplained symptoms develop. Drugs used in treatment may produce side effects.

KIDNEY INFECTION, CHRONIC
(Chronic Pyelonephritis)

BASIC INFORMATION FOR OLDER ADULTS

DESCRIPTION—Chronic kidney infection is an infection of the kidneys that develops slowly and lasts for months or years, leading to scarring and the eventual loss of kidney function. Body parts involved: The kidneys.

SPECIAL CONSIDERATIONS FOR AGING
- The immune system becomes less effective, opening the way for viral, bacterial and other infections; malignancies; immune disorders; and allergies.
- Decreased nutrition increases the risk of infections.
- Older people frequently drink inadequate amounts of water.

SIGNS & SYMPTOMS—Usually produces no signs or symptoms, unlike acute kidney infection. The following occur if chronic kidney failure develops:
- Anemia.
- Weakness.
- Loss of appetite.
- Hypertension.
- Pain in one or both sides of the lower back.
- Protein and blood in the urine.

CAUSES & RISK FACTORS—Caused by frequent acute bacterial kidney infections. Risk factors include:
- A history of diabetes mellitus.
- Urinary obstruction, such as stones or tumors.
- The long-term use of catheters.

DOCTOR'S TREATMENT & DIAGNOSTIC TESTS
- Medical history and physical exam.
- Laboratory blood studies of kidney function, urinalysis and urine culture (see Glossary).
- X-rays of the kidneys.
- Self-care instructions focused on the older patient.
- Surgery to relieve obstruction in the urinary tract if one exists.

HOME TREATMENT BY SELF OR CARE-GIVER

GENERAL INSTRUCTIONS—Follow your treatment plan carefully. This may not be easy for an illness that causes few symptoms in the early stages.

MEDICATION (ADJUSTED FOR AGING)
- Your doctor may prescribe:
  Antibiotics for months or years.
  Drugs to keep the urine slightly acid.
- *Note:* Adverse reactions and side effects may be more frequent and severe in older persons. Remind your doctor of any medicines you already take.

ACTIVITY FOR OLDER PATIENTS
- No restrictions are necessary.
- See Appendix 20 regarding physical fitness for the active older adult.

FOOD & BEVERAGE
- No special diet is required. Drink 2 quarts of liquid daily; include cranberry juice to acidify the urine.
- See Appendix 1 regarding good nutrition for people over 50.

FUTURE CONSIDERATIONS FOR THE AGING ADULT

POSSIBLE COMPLICATIONS—Kidney-caused hypertension; chronic kidney failure.

PROBABLE OUTCOME
- The symptoms can be controlled with treatment. If only one kidney is chronically infected and antibiotic treatment is unsuccessful, surgical removal of the affected kidney may prevent complications.
- If chronic kidney failure develops in both kidneys, a kidney transplant or kidney dialysis (see Glossary) can be life-saving.

PREVENTING RECURRENCE
- Obtain prompt medical treatment for acute kidney infections, including 2 or more weeks of antibiotic treatment. Don't discontinue the prescribed medication even if the symptoms disappear after a few days of treatment.
- Obtain treatment for any abnormality of the urinary tract that causes infection.

CALL YOUR DOCTOR IF

- You have symptoms of chronic kidney failure.
- You have symptoms of an acute kidney infection, such as urgent, frequent or burning urination; fever and chills; fatigue; cloudy urine.

KIDNEY, POLYCYSTIC

BASIC INFORMATION FOR OLDER ADULTS

DESCRIPTION—Polycystic kidney is an inherited kidney disorder in which cysts develop in the kidneys. The cysts enlarge the kidneys and reduce their function. This condition is not cancerous. Most cases show no symptoms until adulthood. Then the symptoms progress slowly for up to 20 years. Body parts involved: The kidneys.

SPECIAL CONSIDERATIONS FOR AGING—Characteristic signs and symptoms of many disorders are frequently changed or absent.

SIGNS & SYMPTOMS
Early stages:
- Blood in the urine that may be visible only by microscopic examination.
- Repeated kidney infections.
- A mass in the abdomen.
- Hypertension.
- No symptoms (frequently) until the cysts replace so much normal kidney structure that kidney failure occurs.

Late stages (kidney failure):
- Pain in the lower back.
- Frequent urination.
- Increasing fatigue and weakness.
- Headache.
- Bad breath.
- Nausea, vomiting or diarrhea.
- Fluid retention, especially swelling around the ankles or eyes.
- Shortness of breath.
- Chest pain.
- Itching skin.

CAUSES & RISK FACTORS—This disease is inherited; the cause is unknown. The risk increases with a family history of polycystic kidney disease.

DOCTOR'S TREATMENT & DIAGNOSTIC TESTS
- Medical history and physical exam.
- X-rays and ultrasonography of kidneys and other parts of the urinary tract.
- Self-care instructions focused on the older patient.
- Surgery to perform a kidney transplant. Advancing age alone is not a deterrent.
- Hospitalization for dialysis.

HOME TREATMENT BY SELF OR CARE-GIVER

GENERAL INSTRUCTIONS
- There is no specific treatment for polycystic kidney disease. The treatment described below applies primarily to patients with polycystic disease who have chronic kidney failure or other complications such as high blood pressure.
- Dialysis and transplants are the best long-range treatments.

MEDICATION (ADJUSTED FOR AGING)
- Without complications, medicine is usually not necessary for this disorder.
- If necessary, your doctor may prescribe antibiotics for infection or antihypertensives to control high blood pressure. Most drugs are excreted by the kidneys. If you have chronic kidney failure and take prescription drugs, the dose may need adjustment because of this disorder.
- *Note:* Adverse reactions and side effects may be more frequent and severe in older persons. Remind your doctor of any medicines you already take.

ACTIVITY FOR OLDER PATIENTS
- Take short, frequent rest periods during the day. Otherwise, stay as active as your strength allows.
- See Appendix 20 regarding physical fitness for the active older adult.

FOOD & BEVERAGE
- Eat a low-salt, low-protein diet (see Appendix 9).
- Drink at least 8 glasses of fluid every day.
- Iron and multiple vitamin supplements may be necessary to ensure good nutrition because of the dietary restrictions. Your doctor may also prescribe calcium and vitamin D supplements to prevent the softening of the bones (osteoporosis).

FUTURE CONSIDERATIONS FOR THE AGING ADULT

POSSIBLE COMPLICATIONS—Urinary tract infections; chronic kidney failure.

PROBABLE OUTCOME—Polycystic kidney disease is currently considered incurable. Your doctor may slow the progressive kidney damage by treating complications as they arise. Scientific research into causes and treatment continues. This offers hope for increasingly effective treatment and eventual cure.

PREVENTING RECURRENCE—Cannot be prevented at present. If polycystic kidney disease runs in your family, consult your doctor for tests to discover if you have kidney cysts. Even if you feel well and don't have the disease, get regular checkups. If you have a family history of polycystic kidney disease, advise your children to seek genetic counseling before starting a family.

CALL YOUR DOCTOR IF

- You have symptoms of polycystic kidney.
- You have symptoms of kidney failure.
- You have fever or other signs of infection.
- Urination decreases.

KIDNEY STONES
(Renal Calculi; Urinary Calculi; Urinary Stones)

BASIC INFORMATION FOR OLDER ADULTS

DESCRIPTION—Kidney stones are small, solid particles that form in one or both kidneys and sometimes travel into the ureter. Stones vary from the size of a grain of sand to that of a golf ball, and there may be one or several. Body parts involved: The kidneys; ureters; bladder; urethra.

SPECIAL CONSIDERATIONS FOR AGING
- Older people frequently drink inadequate amounts of water.
- Suboptimal nutrition is more likely in older people.

SIGNS & SYMPTOMS
- Episodes of severe, colicky (intermittent) pain every few minutes. The pain usually appears first in the back, just below the ribs. Over several hours or days, the pain follows the stone's course through the ureter toward the groin. The pain stops when the stone passes.
- Frequent nausea; traces of blood in the urine. The urine may appear cloudy or dark.

CAUSES & RISK FACTORS—Causes include excessive calcium in the urine due to a disturbance in the parathyroid gland that upsets the calcium metabolism or the excessive intake of calcium or vitamin D; gout (in the case of uric acid stones); and the blockage of urine from any cause. Risk factors include:
- Decreased urine volume caused by dehydration or hot, dry weather.
- Improper diet (too much calcium).
- A family history of kidney stones.
- Hyperparathyroidism.
- Excessive alcohol consumption.
- Bed confinement for any reason.
- Reduced intestinal area due to surgery.
- Excessive use of sodium bicarbonate for stomach acidity (rare).

DOCTOR'S TREATMENT & DIAGNOSTIC TESTS
- Medical history and physical exam.
- Urinalysis and blood studies for calcium and phosphorus.
- X-rays of the urinary tract; monitoring of the stones using ultrasound scan (see Glossary).
- Self-care instructions focused on the older patient.
- Surgery, cystoscopy or lithotritor shockwave treatment to remove stones if they don't pass spontaneously. Advancing age alone is not a deterrent.

HOME TREATMENT BY SELF OR CARE-GIVER

GENERAL INSTRUCTIONS—Strain all urine through gauze to detect the passage of the stone. Take it to the doctor for analysis of its composition.

MEDICATION (ADJUSTED FOR AGING)—
Your doctor may prescribe:
- Pain relievers.
- Antispasmodics to relax the ureter muscles and help the stone pass.

ACTIVITY FOR OLDER PATIENTS
- If you know you have kidney stones, avoid situations in which a sudden pain might cause danger, such as climbing ladders or working on roofs or girders.
- During a kidney stone episode, stay as active as possible. Don't go to bed. Activity may help the stone pass.

FOOD & BEVERAGE
- If the stone proves to be composed of calcium or phosphorus, avoid products made with milk, chocolate and nuts.
- If the stone is a phosphate, your doctor will prescribe an acid-ash diet to keep the urine slightly acid.
- If the stone is a urate or cystine stone, your doctor will prescribe an alkaline-ash diet to keep the urine slightly alkaline.
- For all types of stones, drink at least 13 glasses of fluid daily. Most of the fluid should be purified water.

FUTURE CONSIDERATIONS FOR THE AGING ADULT

POSSIBLE COMPLICATIONS—Urinary tract infection; damage to the kidney, necessitating surgical removal.

PROBABLE OUTCOME—Large stones usually remain in the kidney without symptoms, although they damage the kidney. Small stones pass easily into the ureter through the urine. Stones that are big enough to pass—but not small enough to pass with ease—cause excruciating pain. These usually pass in a few days. If the stone stops and blocks the urine, it must be removed to prevent further kidney damage.

PREVENTING RECURRENCE
- Drink 3 quarts of fluid, mostly purified water, every day.
- Avoid milk and milk products if you have had a calcium or phosphorus kidney stone.
- Avoid excessive sweating.

CALL YOUR DOCTOR IF

- You have symptoms of a kidney stone.
- Your temperature rises to 101F (38.3C).
- You develop symptoms of a kidney infection: stinging and burning on urination or a frequent urge to urinate.
- New, unexplained symptoms develop. The drugs used in treatment may produce side effects.

BASIC INFORMATION FOR OLDER ADULTS

DESCRIPTION—This condition involves the bruising or tearing of the kidney or ureter. The kidneys filter waste materials from the bloodstream and produce urine. The ureters are the tubes that carry urine from the kidneys to the bladder. Body parts involved: The kidney; the ureter. (THIS IS AN EMERGENCY; SEEK MEDICAL CARE IMMEDIATELY!)

SPECIAL CONSIDERATIONS FOR AGING
- The percentage of muscle tissue decreases.
- The bones become thinner.

SIGNS & SYMPTOMS
- Pain or tenderness in the back, just below the ribs on the injured side.
- Fever (sometimes).
- Blood in the urine.

If you have severe pain with large amounts of blood in your urine, one or both kidneys may be seriously injured.

CAUSES & RISK FACTORS—Caused by a blow or penetrating wound to the side of the body under the ribs. Risk factors include:
- Excessive alcohol consumption.
- Accident-proneness.
- Hazardous occupations.
- Hazardous driving conditions.

DOCTOR'S TREATMENT & DIAGNOSTIC TESTS
- Medical history and physical exam.
- Laboratory urine studies.
- X-rays of the urinary tract.
- Hospitalization for shock or internal bleeding.
- Surgery to repair the ureter or remove the kidney if other treatment fails. Advancing age alone is not a deterrent.
- Self-care instructions focused on the older patient.

HOME TREATMENT BY SELF OR CARE-GIVER

GENERAL INSTRUCTIONS—No special instructions except those listed under other headings.

MEDICATION (ADJUSTED FOR AGING)
- Your doctor may prescribe:
  Pain relievers. Antibiotics to treat or protect against infection.
- *Note:* Adverse reactions and side effects may be more frequent and severe in older persons. Remind your doctor of any medicines you already take.

ACTIVITY FOR OLDER PATIENTS
- You will need bed rest for 1 to 2 weeks after the injury.
- After recovery, resume normal activities gradually.
- See Appendix 20 regarding physical fitness for the active older adult.

FOOD & BEVERAGE
- No special diet is required.
- Drink 6 to 8 glasses of fluid daily.
- Don't drink alcohol.
- See Appendix 1 regarding good nutrition for people over 50.

FUTURE CONSIDERATIONS FOR THE AGING ADULT

POSSIBLE COMPLICATIONS
- Internal bleeding.
- Shock (sweating; faintness; nausea; panting; rapid pulse; pale, cold, moist skin).
- Urine leakage into the abdomen, causing abdominal inflammation or infection.
- Scarring and narrowing of the injured ureter.

PROBABLE OUTCOME—Usually curable with time, bed rest and surgery or protection against infection. The surgery to remove an injured kidney (if it does not heal with other measures) is not complicated. After recovery, you can lead a normal life with one kidney.

PREVENTING RECURRENCE—Protect yourself from injury whenever possible. Buckle your automobile seat belt to minimize internal injury in case of accident. Don't drink and drive.

CALL YOUR DOCTOR IF

- You have any symptoms of kidney or ureter injury. *This is an emergency!*
- Your symptoms recur after treatment, especially blood in the urine.
- New, unexplained symptoms develop. The drugs used in treatment may produce side effects.

LABYRINTHITIS

BASIC INFORMATION FOR OLDER ADULTS

DESCRIPTION—Labyrinthitis is an inflammation of the semicircular canals in the inner ear. Body parts involved: The semicircular canals of the inner ear. These fluid-filled canals help maintain balance.

SPECIAL CONSIDERATIONS FOR AGING
- Nerve cell loss begins at age 20 to 40 and continues throughout life. Cells in the brain and other parts of the central nervous system cannot reproduce or replace themselves.
- Neurological diseases become more likely.

SIGNS & SYMPTOMS
- Extreme dizziness—especially with head movement—that begins gradually and peaks in 48 hours.
- Involuntary eye movement.
- Nausea and vomiting (sometimes).
- Loss of balance, especially falling toward the affected side.
- Temporary hearing loss (sometimes).

CAUSES & RISK FACTORS
Causes include:
- A virus infection (usually) in the inner ear.
- Bacterial infection in the inner ear.
- Spread of a chronic middle ear infection.
- Ingestion of toxic drugs.
- Allergy.
- Cholesteatoma (an accumulation of debris covered by skin in the outer ear canal).

Risk factors include:
- Stress.
- A recent viral illness, especially respiratory infection.
- A family history of allergies.
- Smoking.
- Excessive alcohol consumption.
- The use of some prescription or non-prescription drugs, especially aspirin.
- Fatigue or overwork.

DOCTOR'S TREATMENT & DIAGNOSTIC TESTS
- Medical history and physical exam.
- Laboratory culture of any discharge that leaks from the infected ear.
- Audiometry (see Glossary).
- Self-care instructions focused on the older patient.
- Surgery to remove cholesteatoma if necessary.

HOME TREATMENT BY SELF OR CARE-GIVER

GENERAL INSTRUCTIONS
- No specific instructions except those listed under other headings.

- Labyrinthitis is a complicated, serious disorder. This page can cover only the main points of diagnosis and treatment. Your doctor, nurse or librarian can provide sources of supplemental information.

MEDICATION (ADJUSTED FOR AGING)
- Your doctor may prescribe:
  Antinausea medications.
  Tranquilizers to reduce dizziness.
  Diuretics to decrease fluid accumulation in the inner ear.
  Antibiotics to fight bacterial infection.
- *Note:* Adverse reactions and side effects may be more frequent and severe in older persons. Remind your doctor of any medicines you already take.

ACTIVITY FOR OLDER PATIENTS
- Keep the head as still as possible. Rest in bed until dizziness subsides. Then resume your normal activities gradually. Avoid hazardous activities, such as driving, climbing or working around dangerous machinery, until 1 week after the symptoms disappear.
- See Appendix 20 regarding physical fitness for the active older adult.

FOOD & BEVERAGE
- No special diet is required, but decrease salt and fluid intake.
- See Appendix 1 regarding good nutrition for people over 50.

FUTURE CONSIDERATIONS FOR THE AGING ADULT

POSSIBLE COMPLICATIONS—Permanent hearing loss on the affected side (rare).

PROBABLE OUTCOME—Recovery—either spontaneous or with treatment—in 1 to 6 weeks.

PREVENTING RECURRENCE
- Obtain prompt medical treatment for ear infections.
- Don't take medication that has produced dizziness without consulting your doctor.

CALL YOUR DOCTOR IF

- You have symptoms of labyrinthitis.
- Any of the following occurs during treatment:
  Decreased hearing in either ear.
  Persistent vomiting.
  Convulsions.
  Fainting.
  Fever of 101F (38.3C) or higher.
- New, unexplained symptoms develop. The drugs used in treatment may produce side effects.

LACTOSE INTOLERANCE
(Milk Intolerance; Lactase Deficiency)

BASIC INFORMATION FOR OLDER ADULTS

DESCRIPTION—Lactose intolerance is difficulty digesting cow's milk. It occurs—with varying severity—in 75% of the black population, 90% of Orientals or American Indians and fewer than 20% of Caucasians of northwest European origin. It is not contagious or cancerous, and it occurs in varying degrees in almost all older adults. Body part involved: The digestive system.

SPECIAL CONSIDERATIONS FOR AGING
- The stomach produces less acid.
- Decreased nutrition, common among chronically ill older people, increases the risk of any disease or disorder.

SIGNS & SYMPTOMS
- Rumbling abdominal sounds, abdominal cramps and diarrhea.
- Gas and bloating.
- Nausea.
- Headaches.
- Diarrhea.

CAUSES & RISK FACTORS—Caused by a deficiency or absence of the enzyme lactase. Lactase is necessary to digest all milk except mother's milk. Without it, sugars in milk absorb fluid and cause diarrhea. Although some infants are born with the disorder, lactose intolerance usually develops in adulthood. The risk increases with:
- A family history of lactase deficiency.
- Intestinal diseases.

DOCTOR'S TREATMENT & DIAGNOSTIC TESTS
- Medical history and physical exam.
- Laboratory studies such as a stool exam and lactose tolerance test.
- X-rays of the lower intestinal tract.
- Therapeutic trial of a milk-free diet.
- Self-care instructions focused on the older patient.

HOME TREATMENT BY SELF OR CARE-GIVER

GENERAL INSTRUCTIONS—No special instructions except those listed under other headings.

MEDICATION (ADJUSTED FOR AGING)
- A supplement to neutralize lactose in milk. The enzyme lactase is available without a prescription to be added to milk and milk products.
- *Note:* Adverse reactions and side effects may be more frequent and severe in older persons. Remind your doctor of any medicines you already take.

ACTIVITY FOR OLDER PATIENTS
- No restrictions are necessary.
- See Appendix 20 regarding physical fitness for the active older adult.

FOOD & BEVERAGE
- Avoid milk and milk products, such as cheese and ice cream. Yogurt can be eaten.
- See Appendix 1 regarding good nutrition for people over 50.

FUTURE CONSIDERATIONS FOR THE AGING ADULT

POSSIBLE COMPLICATIONS
- Headaches.
- Diarrhea.

PROBABLE OUTCOME—This condition is currently considered incurable. However, the symptoms can be relieved or controlled with a diet that is free of milk and milk products. The symptoms worsen at times for unexplained reasons.

PREVENTING RECURRENCE—Cannot be prevented at present.

CALL YOUR DOCTOR IF

- You have symptoms of lactose intolerance.
- Temperature rises to 101F (38.3C) or higher.
- A milk-free diet doesn't relieve the symptoms.

ILLNESSES & DISORDERS

LARGE INTESTINE, CANCER OF
(Colon Cancer; Colorectal Cancer)

BASIC INFORMATION FOR OLDER ADULTS

DESCRIPTION—Cancer of the large intestine is an uncontrolled growth of malignant cells in the rectum or colon (large intestine). Body parts involved: The large intestine, including the cecum, ascending colon, transverse colon, descending colon and sigmoid colon; the rectum (50% of all colorectal cancers occur here).

SPECIAL CONSIDERATIONS FOR AGING
- Colon cancer is particularly difficult to diagnose in older persons.
- Malignant diseases are less likely to spread rapidly.
- The immune system becomes less effective, opening the way for viral, bacterial and other infections; malignancies; immune disorders; and allergies.
- Stress from any emotional cause—fear, worry, anxiety, sadness, loneliness or anger—affects all aspects of any illness or disorder.

SIGNS & SYMPTOMS
- No symptoms in the early stages (frequently).
- Bloody or black, tarry stools.
- Cramping abdominal pain.
- Feeling of fullness.
- Change in bowel habits, such as diarrhea, constipation or narrow-caliber stools.
- Unexplained weight loss.
- Pain in the rectum.
- Anemia.
- Loss of bowel control (sometimes).

CAUSES & RISK FACTORS—The cause is unknown. Risk factors include:
- Ulcerative colitis and some other chronic disorders of the gastrointestinal tract.
- Improper diet that is low in fiber and high in fat.
- Previous rectal polyps.
- A family history of rectal polyps or colorectal cancer.
- Chronic parasitic infections (schistosomiasis or amebiasis).

DOCTOR'S TREATMENT & DIAGNOSTIC TESTS
- Medical history and physical exam.
- Laboratory blood studies and stool tests.
- Sigmoidoscopy; colonoscopy (see Glossary for both).
- X-rays of the colon (barium enema) and kidney (intravenous pyelogram).
- Surgery to remove the tumor. It is sometimes necessary to divert the bowel through a surgical opening in the abdomen (colostomy). Advancing age alone is not a deterrent.
- Radiation treatment before and after surgery.
- Self-care instructions focused on the older patient.

HOME TREATMENT BY SELF OR CARE-GIVER

GENERAL INSTRUCTIONS
- If you have a colostomy, you will require special instructions for care of the opening. Consult your doctor. For an explanation of surgery and postoperative care, see Colostomy in the Surgeries section.
- Maintain as positive an attitude as possible during treatment.
- Treatment may cause side effects, but they are usually temporary.
- Your pain can be controlled. Don't hesitate to ask your doctor for pain medication.
- Fear may be your worst enemy.
- Call on family members and friends for whatever support and help you need.

MEDICATION (ADJUSTED FOR AGING)—
Your doctor may prescribe:
- Pain relievers.
- Medicine to regulate bowel movements.
- Anticancer drugs (chemotherapy), although they are usually not very effective.

ACTIVITY FOR OLDER PATIENTS
- Avoid sports or activities that might injure the stoma (surgical bowel opening).
- Resume your normal activities, including sexual relations, as soon as possible after surgery. A colostomy should not prevent intercourse.

FOOD & BEVERAGE—Eat a low-fat, high-fiber diet (see Appendices 1 and 8).

FUTURE CONSIDERATIONS FOR THE AGING ADULT

POSSIBLE COMPLICATIONS—Spread of the cancer to other body parts and death.

PROBABLE OUTCOME—Curable in 80% to 90% of cases with early surgery to remove the tumor.

PREVENTING RECURRENCE
- Eat a diet that is high in fiber and low in fat.
- Have annual physical examinations and request rectal and colon exams and tests for blood in the stool.
- If you have any of the risk factors listed above, buy from your pharmacy a kit for detection of blood in the stool. Check for bleeding every 2 months.

CALL YOUR DOCTOR IF

- You have symptoms of cancer of the large intestine, especially rectal bleeding or a significant change in bowel habits that lasts longer than 7 days.
- You develop anemia (fatigue, paleness and rapid heartbeat).

BASIC INFORMATION FOR OLDER ADULTS

DESCRIPTION—A polyp of the large intestine is a benign growth shaped like a grape on a stalk or lying flat against the inner lining of the large intestine. Polyps occur singly or in groups. They are more common than malignant tumors. Body parts involved: The large intestine, most often in the rectum and the sigmoid colon.

SPECIAL CONSIDERATIONS FOR AGING
- Polyps are particularly difficult to diagnose in older persons unless periodic sigmoidoscopy is part of your health-care routine.
- Malignant diseases are less likely to spread rapidly.
- The immune system becomes less effective, opening the way for viral, bacterial and other infections; malignancies; immune disorders; and allergies.

SIGNS & SYMPTOMS
- No symptoms (usually).
- Rectal bleeding (sometimes).
- Mucus discharge from the rectum (sometimes).

CAUSES & RISK FACTORS—The cause is unknown. The risk increases with a family history of intestinal polyps.

DOCTOR'S TREATMENT & DIAGNOSTIC TESTS
- Medical history and physical exam.
- Laboratory studies of blood and stool.
- Sigmoidoscopy; colonoscopy (see Glossary).
- Barium enema x-ray (see Glossary).
- Surgery or other procedure to remove polyps.
- Self-care instructions focused on the older patient.

HOME TREATMENT BY SELF OR CARE-GIVER

GENERAL INSTRUCTIONS
- Surgery to remove a polyp is usually done by inserting a proctoscope or sigmoidoscope into the anus. Polyps are snipped off or destroyed by electric cauterization. If a pathologist's report indicates that the polyp is malignant, the total excision of the polyp and surrounding tissue is necessary.
- For multiple polyps, a portion of the colon may be removed through an abdominal incision (laparotomy).

MEDICATION (ADJUSTED FOR AGING)—Medicine usually is not necessary for this disorder.

ACTIVITY FOR OLDER PATIENTS
- No restrictions are necessary.
- See Appendix 20 regarding physical fitness for the active older adult.

FOOD & BEVERAGE—Eat a diet that is high in fiber (see Appendix 1) and low in fat (see Appendix 8) to reduce the risk of malignant change.

FUTURE CONSIDERATIONS FOR THE AGING ADULT

POSSIBLE COMPLICATIONS—Malignant change in about 1% of polyps.

PROBABLE OUTCOME—Usually curable with surgery, although polyps may recur.

PREVENTING RECURRENCE—If you have had polyps in the past, you should have regular sigmoidoscopic (see Glossary) examinations—at least once a year or more, depending on your doctor's recommendation.

CALL YOUR DOCTOR IF

- You have bleeding or mucus discharge from the rectum.
- Other members of your family have had polyps or colorectal cancer. You should have periodic examinations.
- Any of the following occurs after surgery: Increased rectal bleeding. Fever, chills or aches. These may indicate an infection at the surgical site.

ILLNESSES & DISORDERS

BASIC INFORMATION FOR OLDER ADULTS

DESCRIPTION—Laryngitis is a minor inflammation of the larynx (the "voice box" that contains the vocal cords) and the surrounding tissues that causes temporary hoarseness. Body parts involved: The larynx; the upper part of the neck behind the Adam's apple.

SPECIAL CONSIDERATIONS FOR AGING
- The immune system becomes less effective, opening the way for viral, bacterial and other infections; malignancies; immune disorders; and allergies.
- Decreased nutrition, common among chronically ill older people, increases the risk of any disease or disorder.
- Characteristic signs and symptoms of many disorders are frequently changed or absent.
- Loss of salivary gland tissue and moisture in the larynx.
- Muscle atrophy.

SIGNS & SYMPTOMS
- Hoarseness or loss of voice.
- High, trembly, weak voice.
- Sore throat; tickling in the back of the throat.
- Sensation of a lump in the throat.
- Slight fever (sometimes).
- Swallowing difficulty (rare).

CAUSES & RISK FACTORS
Causes include:
- Viruses (common).
- Bacteria (rare).
- Allergies.
- Excessive use of the voice.
- Electrolyte balance disturbances, especially low potassium, that cause muscle weakness (sometimes).
- Tumors (rare).

Risk factors include:
- Exposure to irritants distributed by air conditioning systems, such as mold, pollen and pollutants.
- Extremely cold weather.
- Smoking.
- Excessive alcohol consumption.
- Recent respiratory illness, such as bronchitis or pneumonia.
- Decrease in breathing effort.

DOCTOR'S TREATMENT & DIAGNOSTIC TESTS
- Medical history and physical exam. Treatment by an ear, nose and throat specialist might be helpful for persistent cases.
- Self-care instructions focused on the older patient.

HOME TREATMENT BY SELF OR CARE-GIVER

GENERAL INSTRUCTIONS
- Don't use your voice. Whisper or write notes. For most cases, resting the voice for a few days is all that is needed.
- If breathing effort has decreased, a speech therapist may help.
- Use a cool-mist humidifier to increase air moisture and ease the constricted feeling in the throat. Warm, steamy showers also help.
- Use non-prescription lozenges or sugar-free hard candies to stimulate saliva flow.

MEDICATION (ADJUSTED FOR AGING)
- For minor discomfort, you may use non-prescriptions drugs such as acetaminophen, aspirin or cough syrup.
- Your doctor may prescribe antibiotics for bacterial infection.
- *Note:* Adverse reactions and side effects may be more frequent and severe in older persons. Remind your doctor of any medicines you already take.

ACTIVITY FOR OLDER PATIENTS
- Rest more frequently.
- See Appendix 20 regarding physical fitness for the active older adult.

FOOD & BEVERAGE
- No special diet is required.
- See Appendix 1 regarding good nutrition for people over 50.

FUTURE CONSIDERATIONS FOR THE AGING ADULT

POSSIBLE COMPLICATIONS—Total breathing obstruction if laryngitis is part of a serious infection of the respiratory system, such as epiglottitis.

PROBABLE OUTCOME—Spontaneous recovery for viral laryngitis in 10 to 14 days. Bacterial infections are usually curable in 7 to 10 days with antibiotic treatment.

PREVENTING RECURRENCE
- Avoid yelling or straining your voice.
- Treat respiratory infections carefully.

CALL YOUR DOCTOR IF

- You have hoarseness or other symptoms of laryngitis that last longer than 2 weeks. This may be an early sign of cancer.
- You feel very ill or have a high fever or breathing difficulty.

LARYNX CANCER
(Laryngeal Cancer)

BASIC INFORMATION FOR OLDER ADULTS

DESCRIPTION—Uncontrolled growth of malignant cells in the larynx (the "voice box" that contains the vocal cords) and the surrounding tissues. Body parts involved: The larynx; the upper part of the neck behind the Adam's apple.

SPECIAL CONSIDERATIONS FOR AGING
- The immune system becomes less effective, opening the way for viral, bacterial and other infections; malignancies; immune disorders; and allergies.
- Decreased nutrition, common among chronically ill older people, increases the risk of any disease or disorder.
- Malignant diseases are less likely to spread rapidly.
- Stress from any emotional cause—fear, worry, anxiety, sadness, loneliness or anger—affects all aspects of any illness or disorder.

SIGNS & SYMPTOMS
- Hoarseness that does not disappear after resting the voice.
- A "lump-in-the-throat" feeling.
- Painful or difficult swallowing.
- Hard, swollen lymph glands in the neck.

CAUSES & RISK FACTORS—Caused by smoking. Other causes are unknown. Risk factors include:
- Heavy smoking.
- Excessive alcohol consumption.
- Polyps of the vocal cords.
- Chronic inflammation of the vocal cords from any cause.

DOCTOR'S TREATMENT & DIAGNOSTIC TESTS
- Medical history and physical exam.
- Biopsy (see Glossary) of the vocal cords or other affected tissue.
- Treatment by an ear, nose and throat specialist.
- Hospitalization for radiation treatment.
- Surgery to remove the cancer and other involved tissue (sometimes). Advancing age alone is not a deterrent.
- Speech therapy to help you learn to speak without vocal cords if surgery is necessary.
- Self-care instructions focused on the older patient.

HOME TREATMENT BY SELF OR CARE-GIVER

GENERAL INSTRUCTIONS
- Be alert to hoarseness that persists beyond 2 weeks. Early diagnosis and treatment—as with other cancers—offer the best hope for complete cure.

- If your vocal cords are removed, join a support group for persons like you who have faced the same situation. This will help minimize your stress and help you adjust.
- Larynx cancer is a complicated, serious disorder. This page can cover only the main points of diagnosis and treatment. Your doctor, nurse or librarian can provide sources of supplemental information.
- Maintain as positive an attitude as possible during treatment.
- Treatment may cause side effects, but they are usually temporary.
- Your pain can be controlled. Don't hesitate to ask your doctor for pain medication.
- Fear may be your worst enemy.
- Call on family members and friends for whatever support and help you need.

MEDICATION (ADJUSTED FOR AGING)—
Medicine usually is not necessary for this disorder. Anticancer drugs (chemotherapy) are not often prescribed; radiation therapy is used instead.

ACTIVITY FOR OLDER PATIENTS
- Resume your normal activities gradually after treatment or surgery.
- See Appendix 20 regarding physical fitness for the active older adult.

FOOD & BEVERAGE—No special diet is required, unless surgery is performed. In that case, a liquid diet (see Appendix 7) is necessary until the affected area heals.

FUTURE CONSIDERATIONS FOR THE AGING ADULT

POSSIBLE COMPLICATIONS—Life-threatening spread of the cancer to other body parts.

PROBABLE OUTCOME—Often curable with early diagnosis and treatment. In the late stages, this condition is currently considered incurable. However, the symptoms can be relieved or controlled. Scientific research into causes and treatment continues, so there is hope for increasingly effective treatment and a cure.

PREVENTING RECURRENCE
- Stop smoking.
- Don't drink more than 1 or 2 alcoholic drinks—if any—a day.
- Don't abuse your voice.

CALL YOUR DOCTOR IF

You have symptoms of larynx cancer.

LEGIONNAIRE'S DISEASE
(Legionella Pneumophilia Bronchopneumonia)

BASIC INFORMATION FOR OLDER ADULTS

DESCRIPTION—Legionnaire's disease is a form of lung infection (bronchopneumonia) named after an epidemic that affected 182 people attending an American Legion convention in 1976. Body parts involved: The bronchial tubes and lungs.

SPECIAL CONSIDERATIONS FOR AGING
- The immune system becomes less effective, opening the way for viral, bacterial and other infections; malignancies; immune disorders; and allergies.
- Decreased nutrition, common among chronically ill older people, increases the risk of any disease or disorder.
- The total state of wellbeing in many older people makes them increasingly susceptible to infections and impairs their ability to prevent infections from spreading.
- More susceptibility to this particular disease.

SIGNS & SYMPTOMS
- A general ill feeling.
- Headache.
- Chills and fever up to 105F (40.6C).
- Muscle aches.
- A cough without sputum that progresses to one with gray or blood-streaked sputum.
- Nausea; vomiting; diarrhea.
- Disorientation.

CAUSES & RISK FACTORS—Caused by an infection from bacteria (*legionella pneumophilia*) that is not contagious between persons. The germ is transmitted through the air, and the incubation period after exposure is 2 to 10 days. In the 1976 epidemic, the germ was transmitted through the cooling and evaporating elements of a large central air conditioning system. The bacteria are also found in excavation sites and newly plowed soil. Risk factors include:
- Chronic, debilitating illness including diabetes mellitus, chronic kidney failure and emphysema.
- Smoking. This increases the risk 3 to 4 times.
- Excessive alcohol consumption.
- The use of immunosuppressive drugs, including cortisone and anticancer drugs.

DOCTOR'S TREATMENT & DIAGNOSTIC TESTS
- Medical history and physical exam.
- Laboratory blood studies and culture of sputum.
- Lung biopsy.
- Hospitalization for intensive care and oxygen (severe cases).
- For mild cases or during convalescence after hospitalization, self-care instructions focused on the older patient.

HOME TREATMENT BY SELF OR CARE-GIVER

GENERAL INSTRUCTIONS—The following apply to mild cases or to care after hospitalization:
- Use a cool-mist humidifier to increase air moisture and thin lung secretions so they can be coughed up more easily.
- Use a warm compress on the chest to relieve the chest pain.
- Practice deep breathing exercises as often as your strength allows.
- Avoid loud talking, laughing or singing. They may trigger excessive coughing.
- Keep warm. If you become chilled, the germ can become more virulent.

MEDICATION (ADJUSTED FOR AGING)
- Your doctor may prescribe antibiotics. Be sure to finish all prescribed medication.
- If the cough is painful and doesn't produce sputum, you may use non-prescription medicine to suppress it. If the cough produces sputum, don't suppress it.
- You may take aspirin or acetaminophen to reduce fever.

ACTIVITY FOR OLDER PATIENTS—Rest in bed until you are completely well. You may read or watch TV. Allow 2 to 4 weeks for recovery.

FOOD & BEVERAGE—No special diet.

FUTURE CONSIDERATIONS FOR THE AGING ADULT

POSSIBLE COMPLICATIONS—Shock or delirium; congestive heart failure; kidney failure; heart rhythm disturbances.

PROBABLE OUTCOME—Usually curable with prompt diagnosis and treatment. If untreated, 15% of cases are fatal.

PREVENTING RECURRENCE
- Have cooling and heating systems cleaned and inspected regularly. Change filters often.
- Don't smoke.
- Don't drink more than 1 or 2 alcoholic drinks—if any—a day.

CALL YOUR DOCTOR IF

- You have symptoms of Legionnaire's disease.
- Any of the following occurs during or after treatment:
  Temperature spike to 102F (38.9C).
  Severe chest pain despite treatment.
  Increased shortness of breath.
  Dark or bluish nails, lips or skin.
  Blood in the sputum.
- New, unexplained symptoms develop. Drugs used in treatment may produce side effects.

LEUKEMIA, ACUTE

BASIC INFORMATION FOR OLDER ADULTS

DESCRIPTION—Acute leukemia is a malignant overgrowth of white blood cells in the bone marrow or the tissues that are part of the lymphatic system (the lymph glands, spleen and liver). These excess cells accumulate and spill into the bloodstream, eventually involving other tissues. Common forms of leukemia include acute lymphocytic leukemia (ALL), which is especially prevalent in children; acute myelogenous leukemia (AML); and acute non-lymphocytic leukemia (ANLL). Body parts involved: The bone marrow and lymph tissue in the early stages, eventually all body tissues.

SPECIAL CONSIDERATIONS FOR AGING
- Malignant diseases are difficult to diagnose.
- The immune system becomes less effective, opening the way for viral, bacterial and other infections and malignancies.
- Older patients become less able to tolerate maximal x-ray and chemotherapy treatments.
- Decreased nutrition increases the risk of infections.
- Stress from any emotional cause affects all aspects of any illness or disorder.
- Signs and symptoms may differ significantly from those listed below.

SIGNS & SYMPTOMS
- Low fever; tiredness; a general ill feeling.
- Increasing paleness; anemia.
- Easy bruising and spontaneous bleeding (such as nosebleeds or bleeding from the gums or gastrointestinal tract).
- An enlarged spleen and abdominal pain.
- Susceptibility to infection, especially pneumonia.
- Mouth infections with ulcers and sores.
- Headache and lethargy if the meninges (membranes covering the brain) are affected.

CAUSES & RISK FACTORS—The cause is unknown, but there are many suspected predisposing factors—especially viruses and radiation. Risk factors include a family history of leukemia; excessive exposure to x-rays; being an identical twin of someone with leukemia; exposure to benzene and other toxic industrial chemicals; the use of cytotoxic or immunosuppressant drugs; and chronic bone marrow disorders.

DOCTOR'S TREATMENT & DIAGNOSTIC TESTS
- Medical history and physical exam.
- Laboratory studies of blood, bone marrow and cerebrospinal fluid.
- After diagnosis and treatment and during remission, self-care instructions.
- Hospitalization for treatment in the initial stage or for relapse.
- A bone marrow transplant, sometimes suggested for younger people, is not used for older adults.

HOME TREATMENT BY SELF OR CARE-GIVER

GENERAL INSTRUCTIONS
- Avoid ill persons and crowds to prevent dangerous exposure to infection.
- Rinse your mouth often with a warm salt-water solution to decrease the number of mouth ulcers. Use 1 tablespoon salt in 8 oz. water.
- Use a soft toothbrush to prevent gum abrasion.
- Maintain as positive an attitude as possible during treatment.
- Treatment may cause side effects, but they are usually temporary.
- Your pain can be controlled. Don't hesitate to ask your doctor for pain medication.
- Fear may be your worst enemy.
- Call on family members and friends for whatever support and help you need.

MEDICATION (ADJUSTED FOR AGING)—Your doctor may prescribe:
- Blood transfusions.
- Anticancer (chemotherapy) drugs.
- Cortisone drugs; pain relievers.
- Antibiotics to fight infection.
- Uricosuric drugs to increase the excretion of uric acid that may accumulate as a side effect of anticancer drugs.

ACTIVITY FOR OLDER PATIENTS—No restrictions are necessary during remissions. Bed rest is usually necessary during active phases.

FOOD & BEVERAGE—Drink extra fluids. Adults should drink 8 to 10 glasses of fluid daily. During chemotherapy, eat and drink high-calorie foods and beverages, such as milkshakes or eggnog.

FUTURE CONSIDERATIONS FOR THE AGING ADULT

POSSIBLE COMPLICATIONS—Hemorrhage; death from the destruction of the body's defenses against infection.

PROBABLE OUTCOME—Due to lack of tolerance for treatment, the long-term survival rate is poor. Relapses are likely.

PREVENTING RECURRENCE—Cannot be prevented. If you have a a family history of leukemia, have your children seek genetic counseling before starting a family.

CALL YOUR DOCTOR IF

- You have symptoms of leukemia.
- Any of the following occurs during active stages *or* remissions:
  Fever, chills, cough or sore throat; constipation. Abnormal bleeding. Apply pressure and ice while awaiting your doctor's return call.
- New, unexplained symptoms develop. The drugs used in treatment may produce side effects.

LEUKEMIA, CHRONIC LYMPHOCYTIC

BASIC INFORMATION FOR OLDER ADULTS

DESCRIPTION—Chronic lymphocytic leukemia is a very slow-growing cancer of the blood-forming organs. About a third of leukemia victims have this form. It is often discovered in a routine blood test for unrelated purposes. Body parts involved: The blood-forming organs (the bone marrow, lymph glands, liver and spleen).

SPECIAL CONSIDERATIONS FOR AGING
- This is one of the few diseases that is common only in the elderly.
- The immune system becomes less effective, opening the way for viral, bacterial and other infections and malignancies.
- Decreased nutrition increases the risk of any disease or disorder.
- Characteristic signs and symptoms of many disorders are frequently changed or absent.
- Stress from any emotional cause affects all aspects of any illness or disorder.

SIGNS & SYMPTOMS
In the early stages, the following appear gradually:
- Fatigue and general weakness.
- Mild to moderate anemia.
- Firm, enlarged lymph nodes.
- Unexplained weight loss.
- Enlarged liver and spleen.
- Susceptibility to infection.
- Skin nodules (sometimes).
- Low-grade fever and sweating at night.
In late stages, the following appear:
- Inability to resist bacterial, viral or fungal infections.
- Incapacitating weakness.

CAUSES & RISK FACTORS—The cause is unknown. Unlike some forms of leukemia, excessive exposure to radiation does *not* seem to be a factor. The risk increases with a family history of chronic lymphocytic leukemia or chronic viral infection.

DOCTOR'S TREATMENT & DIAGNOSTIC TESTS
- Medical history and physical exam.
- Laboratory studies of the blood and bone marrow.
- Chemotherapy.
- Self-care instructions focused on the older patient.
- Hospitalization for anticancer drugs and radiation treatment.
- Psychotherapy or counseling for the patient and family.

HOME TREATMENT BY SELF OR CARE-GIVER

GENERAL INSTRUCTIONS
- Be extra careful about avoiding illness:
  Wash your hands frequently.
  Don't become chilled.
  Avoid contact with all obviously ill people, especially children with infections.
- Avoid crowds during cold and flu seasons.
- Maintain as positive an attitude as possible during treatment.
- Treatment may cause side effects, but they are usually temporary.
- Your pain can be controlled. Don't hesitate to ask your doctor for pain medication.
- Fear may be your worst enemy.
- Call on family members and friends for whatever support and help you need.

MEDICATION (ADJUSTED FOR AGING)
- Many persons with this disorder require little treatment. Treatment plans are highly individualized.
- Your doctor may prescribe:
  Anticancer medications, including cortisone drugs.
  Antigout drugs.
- *Don't take aspirin* or any product containing aspirin. Aspirin increases the likelihood of bleeding.
- *Note:* Adverse reactions and side effects may be more frequent and severe in older persons. Remind your doctor of any medicines you already take.

ACTIVITY FOR OLDER PATIENTS—No restrictions are necessary.

FOOD & BEVERAGE
- No special diet is required. Eat as heartily as possible.
- See Appendix 1 regarding good nutrition for people over 50.

FUTURE CONSIDERATIONS FOR THE AGING ADULT

POSSIBLE COMPLICATIONS—Bleeding; severe anemia; infections; gout.

PROBABLE OUTCOME—This condition is currently considered incurable. However, the symptoms can be relieved or controlled. Many patients live for years with few or no symptoms, and medical literature cites a few instances of unexplained recovery. Scientific research into causes and treatment continues, so there is hope for increasingly effective treatment and a cure.

PREVENTING RECURRENCE—There are no specific preventive measures.

CALL YOUR DOCTOR IF

- You have symptoms of chronic lymphocytic leukemia.
- Any of the following occurs after diagnosis and treatment:
  Recurrence or worsening of the symptoms.
  Signs of infection, such as fever and chills.
  Black, tarry stools, bleeding gums or nosebleed.
- New, unexplained symptoms develop. The drugs used in treatment may produce side effects.

LEUKOPLAKIA

BASIC INFORMATION FOR OLDER ADULTS

DESCRIPTION—Leukoplakia is the thickening of an area of the delicate lining of the mouth, tongue or vulva (the lips around the opening of the vagina). This is not contagious, but it may be premalignant. Body parts involved: The inside of the cheek, floor of the mouth, tongue, palate or roof of the mouth; the vulva.

SPECIAL CONSIDERATIONS FOR AGING
- Many body changes occur as a result of estrogen deficiency beginning at menopause. These include vaginal dryness, shortening and narrowing of the vagina, greater susceptibility to vaginal infections, frequent bladder infections, reductions in the size of the clitoris and increased facial hair. Changes in other systems of the body may lead to a greater tendency to osteoporosis, hardening of the arteries and other disorders.
- Decreased nutrition, common among chronically ill older people, increases the risk of any disease or disorder.

SIGNS & SYMPTOMS
- A small white patch in the affected area. The patch feels firm, rough and stiff.
- Sensitivity to hot and spicy food.
- No symptoms in the early stages (sometimes).

CAUSES & RISK FACTORS—Some causes (such as that for leukoplakia of the vulva) are unknown; others include:
- Deficiency of vitamins A or B.
- Deficiency of male or female hormones.
- Chronic irritation in the mouth. The irritation may be from jagged teeth, ill-fitting dentures, hot or spicy food or the excessive consumption of alcohol or nicotine.

Risk factors include:
- The use of tobacco products, including cigarettes, chewing tobacco, snuff, pipes or cigars.
- Dentures.

DOCTOR'S TREATMENT & DIAGNOSTIC TESTS
- Medical history and physical exam by a doctor or dentist.
- Biopsy (see Glossary).
- Surgery to remove the lesions.
- Self-care instructions focused on the older patient.

HOME TREATMENT BY SELF OR CARE-GIVER

GENERAL INSTRUCTIONS—There are no instructions for vulvular leukoplakia. Following oral surgery or biopsy:
- If bleeding occurs, press cotton gauze gently for 5 minutes against the operation site.

- 24 hours after the operation, rinse the mouth with a warm salt-water solution. Use 1/2 teaspoon salt in 8 oz. warm water. Repeat every 1 or 2 hours.
- Brush and floss your teeth often and use antiseptic mouthwash during the healing process. A clean mouth heals faster.
- Return to the doctor or dentist for the removal of sutures 5 to 7 days after the operation. By then, the laboratory report may be complete.

MEDICATION (ADJUSTED FOR AGING)
- For minor pain, you may use non-prescription drugs such as acetaminophen.
- Your doctor may prescribe topical or oral forms of vitamin A (sometimes).
- *Note:* Adverse reactions and side effects may be more frequent and severe in older persons. Remind your doctor of any medicines you already take.

ACTIVITY FOR OLDER PATIENTS
- No restrictions are necessary.
- See Appendix 20 regarding physical fitness for the active older adult.

FOOD & BEVERAGE
- Consume a liquid or soft diet for 24 hours after oral surgery or biopsy; then no special diet is required.
- See Appendix 1 regarding good nutrition for people over 50.

FUTURE CONSIDERATIONS FOR THE AGING ADULT

POSSIBLE COMPLICATIONS—The lesion may become cancerous if untreated.

PROBABLE OUTCOME—Sometimes curable with surgery and removal of the source of irritation, such as tobacco.

PREVENTING RECURRENCE
- Don't smoke or use tobacco products.
- Inspect the mouth regularly if you wear dentures or smoke.
- Decrease your consumption of hot or highly seasoned foods if suspicious lesions develop.
- There is no known way to prevent vulvular leukoplakia.

CALL YOUR DOCTOR IF

- You have symptoms of leukoplakia.
- Any of the following occurs after surgery: Bleeding after 12 hours or more. Severe pain.

LICE
(Pediculosis; Head Lice; Body Lice; "Crabs")

BASIC INFORMATION FOR OLDER ADULTS

DESCRIPTION—Lice are tiny parasites that live on the body or in clothing and cause skin inflammation. Body parts involved: The skin—especially that of hairy areas anywhere, such as the scalp, eyebrows or genital area—and that in areas in which the clothing is in close contact with the skin, such as the shoulders, waist, genital area or buttocks.

SPECIAL CONSIDERATIONS FOR AGING
- Decreased nutrition increases the risk of any disease or disorder.
- Characteristic signs and symptoms of many disorders are frequently changed or absent.

SIGNS & SYMPTOMS
- Itching and scratching, sometimes intense and usually in hair-covered areas.
- Eggs ("nits") on hair shafts.
- Scalp inflammation and matted hair.
- Enlarged lymph glands at the back of the scalp or in the groin (sometimes).
- Red bite marks and hives.

CAUSES & RISK FACTORS—Caused by tiny (3mm to 4mm) parasites that bite through the skin to obtain nourishment (blood). The bites cause itching and inflammation. Some lice live on the skin, although they are difficult to see. Others live in clothing near the skin. The eggs of the lice (nits) adhere to hairs. Risk factors include:
- Crowded or unsanitary living conditions.
- A family history of lice.
- Sexual intercourse with an infected person.
- Contact with an infected person.
- Sharing hairbrushes or headwear.

DOCTOR'S TREATMENT & DIAGNOSTIC TESTS
- Your own observation of the symptoms. You may see nits (like tiny footballs) on the sides of hairs.
- Medical history and physical exam.
- Self-care instructions focused on the older patient.

HOME TREATMENT BY SELF OR CARE-GIVER

GENERAL INSTRUCTIONS—The following measures apply to all members of the household and to any sexual partners of household members:
- Use a medicated shampoo, cream or lotion prescribed by your doctor.
- Machine-wash *all* clothing and linen in hot water. Dry it in the dryer's hot-air cycle. Iron the clothing and linen if possible. Washing removes the lice, and ironing destroys the nits.
- If you don't have a washing machine, iron the clothes and linen or seal them for 10 days in a plastic bag to kill the lice and nits.
- Dry-clean non-washable items or seal them in a plastic bag for 10 days.

- Clothing can be disinfected with insecticide powder.
- Boil articles such as combs, curlers, hairbrushes and barrettes.
- The hair does not have to be shaved.

MEDICATION (ADJUSTED FOR AGING)
- Your doctor may prescribe anti-lice (pediculicide) cream, lotion or shampoo. Apply creams or lotions to infected body parts according to instructions. To use the shampoo:
  Wet your hair. Apply 1 tablespoon of shampoo. Lather for 4 minutes, working the lather well into the scalp.
  If shampoo gets in your eyes, wash it out immediately with water.
  Rinse your hair thoroughly and towel it dry. Don't use this towel again without laundering it. Comb your hair with a fine-toothed comb dipped in hot vinegar to remove the lice. The comb must run through the hair repeatedly from the scalp outward until the hair is completely free of nits. A single application of shampoo is effective in more than 90% of cases. Don't use it more frequently than recommended, because the shampoo may irritate the skin or be absorbed into the body.
  A repeat application may be necessary in 10 to 14 days.
- If the lice infect your eyelashes, they must be removed carefully by your doctor. The prescribed medications should *not* go into the eye or on the eyelashes. You may apply petroleum jelly to the eyelash follicles for 7 or 8 days after removal.

ACTIVITY FOR OLDER PATIENTS—No restrictions are necessary.

FOOD & BEVERAGE—No special diet.

FUTURE CONSIDERATIONS FOR THE AGING ADULT

POSSIBLE COMPLICATIONS—Infection at the site of deep scratching may cause diseases such as typhus (rare).

PROBABLE OUTCOME—Usually curable with medicated creams, lotions and shampoos. Allow 5 days after treatment for the symptoms to disappear. Lice often recur.

PREVENTING RECURRENCE
- Bathe and shampoo often.
- Avoid wearing the same clothing more than a day or two; change bed linens often.
- Don't share combs, brushes or hats with others.

CALL YOUR DOCTOR IF

You, your sexual partner or anyone in your household has symptoms of lice—or they recur.

LIPIDS, EXCESSIVE IN BLOOD
(Hyperlipidemia; High Cholesterol; Hypercholesterolemia; High Level of Fat in the Blood)

BASIC INFORMATION FOR OLDER ADULTS

DESCRIPTION—Hyperlipidemia is a disorder characterized by above-normal levels of fat in the blood. The different types indicate the level of the fat in the blood. Body parts involved: The blood and the arteries.

SPECIAL CONSIDERATIONS FOR AGING
- Characteristic signs and symptoms of many disorders are frequently changed or absent.
- Many medical disorders in older people that once were thought to be "normal" consequences of aging are frequently diseases that can be treated.

SIGNS & SYMPTOMS—Most of the types of hyperlipidemia produce similar symptoms, including:
- Yellowish nodules of fat in the skin beneath the eyes, elbows and knees and in the tendons.
- An enlarged spleen and liver (with some types).
- A whitish ring around the eye pupils (with some types).
- Abdominal pain.

CAUSES & RISK FACTORS—The blood contains a variety of fats (lipids) that join to blood proteins, forming lipoproteins. These include cholesterol, triglycerides and high-density lipoproteins (HDL). They provide energy and are "building blocks" for some tissues and hormones. In excess, they filter out of the blood and are deposited in blood vessels, tendons and other tissues, where they cause symptoms and disease. Risk factors include:
- An improper diet that is high in fat and cholesterol.
- A family history of hyperlipidemia.
- The use of estrogen for postmenopausal estrogen replacement therapy.
- Diabetes mellitus.
- Hypothyroidism.
- Nephrosis (a kidney disease).
- Alcoholism.
- Obesity.
- Lupus erythematosus.
- The use of cortisone-like drugs.

DOCTOR'S TREATMENT & DIAGNOSTIC TESTS
- Medical history and physical exam.
- Laboratory blood studies to measure blood lipids.
- Self-care instructions focused on the older patient.
- Surgery to remove fat deposits in the skin and tendons.

HOME TREATMENT BY SELF OR CARE-GIVER

GENERAL INSTRUCTIONS—See Appendix 13 for suggestions to reduce stress and improve health. Stress increases the risk of heart disease, a major complication of hyperlipidemia.

MEDICATION (ADJUSTED FOR AGING)
- Your doctor may prescribe:
  Medications to control blood lipids. Many new drugs of this type are now appearing on the market with variable and unpredictable results.
  Medications to treat underlying diseases, such as diabetes or thyroid conditions.
- *Note:* Adverse reactions and side effects may be more frequent and severe in older persons. Remind your doctor of any medicines you already take.

ACTIVITY FOR OLDER PATIENTS
- No restrictions are necessary unless the tendons are weakened by fat deposits.
- See Appendix 20 regarding physical fitness for the active older adult.

FOOD & BEVERAGE
- Eat a diet that is low in fat. See Appendix 8.
- Lose weight if you are overweight. See Appendix 10 for a reducing diet.
- Don't drink alcohol.

FUTURE CONSIDERATIONS FOR THE AGING ADULT

POSSIBLE COMPLICATIONS
- Heart attack.
- Stroke.
- Acute pancreatitis.

PROBABLE OUTCOME—Usually treatable or controllable with lifelong dietary control and medication.

PREVENTING RECURRENCE
- Eat a diet that is low in fat. See Appendix 8.
- If you have diabetes, adhere closely to your treatment program.

CALL YOUR DOCTOR IF

- You have symptoms or a family history of excessive lipids in the blood.
- New, unexplained symptoms develop. The drugs used in treatment may produce side effects.

LIPOMAS

BASIC INFORMATION FOR OLDER ADULTS

DESCRIPTION—Lipomas are benign tumors of fat tissue. Body parts involved: The trunk; neck; back; upper thighs; arms.

SPECIAL CONSIDERATIONS FOR AGING
- The responsiveness of the skin's immune system decreases.
- The fatty layer of tissue under the skin becomes thinner.

SIGNS & SYMPTOMS—Nodules under the skin with the following characteristics:
- The nodules are dome-shaped and about 2cm to 10cm in diameter. Some grow larger.
- The nodules feel "doughy," smooth and easily movable.
- Only one—or many—lipomas may occur at one time.
- The nodules cause no pain.

CAUSES & RISK FACTORS—The cause is unknown, but the tendency is probably inherited. Minor injury may trigger growth. The risk increases with a family history of lipomas.

DOCTOR'S TREATMENT & DIAGNOSTIC TESTS
- Medical history and physical exam.
- Surgery to remove the lipoma (sometimes). The surgery may be for cosmetic reasons.
- Self-care instructions focused on the older patient.

HOME TREATMENT BY SELF OR CARE-GIVER

GENERAL INSTRUCTIONS—After surgical removal:
- Apply rubbing alcohol to the scab twice a day.
- Apply an adhesive bandage to the scab during the day. Leave it uncovered at night.
- Wash the wound as usual. Dry gently and completely after bathing or swimming.
- If the scab cracks or oozes, apply non-prescription antibiotic ointment several times a day.
- Return to your doctor for removal of sutures in 5 to 10 days.

MEDICATION (ADJUSTED FOR AGING)—Medication usually is not necessary for this disorder.

ACTIVITY FOR OLDER PATIENTS
- After surgical removal, resume your normal activities gradually. Allow 1 month for complete healing.
- See Appendix 20 regarding physical fitness for the active older adult.

FOOD & BEVERAGE
- No special diet is required.
- See Appendix 1 regarding good nutrition for people over 50.

FUTURE CONSIDERATIONS FOR THE AGING ADULT

POSSIBLE COMPLICATIONS—Large lipomas may interfere with muscle function.

PROBABLE OUTCOME—These tumors are benign and require no treatment, but they may be removed if they are unsightly or interfere with muscle function. Surgical removal is usually done in a doctor's office.

PREVENTING RECURRENCE—Cannot be prevented at present. If you are obese, you can reduce the size of lipomas by losing weight.

CALL YOUR DOCTOR IF

Any of the following occurs after surgery:
- Fever.
- Bleeding which does not respond to moderate pressure.
- Signs of infection (warmth, swelling or redness) at the surgical site.

BASIC INFORMATION FOR OLDER ADULTS

DESCRIPTION—Liver cancer is an uncontrolled growth of malignant cells in the liver. Liver cancer may be primary, resulting from abnormal liver or bile duct cells. Or it may be secondary, spreading from another cancerous site, which is more common. The most common sources are cancers of the rectum, colon, lung, breast, pancreas, esophagus or skin (malignant melanoma). Body parts involved: The liver and the bile ducts.

SPECIAL CONSIDERATIONS FOR AGING

- The immune system becomes less effective, opening the way for viral, bacterial and other infections; malignancies; immune disorders; and allergies.
- Characteristic signs and symptoms of many disorders are frequently changed or absent.
- Malignant diseases are less likely to spread rapidly.
- Decreased nutrition, common among chronically ill older people, increases the risk of any disease or disorder.
- Stress from any emotional cause—fear, worry, anxiety, sadness, loneliness or anger—affects all aspects of any illness or disorder.

SIGNS & SYMPTOMS

- Loss of appetite and weight loss.
- A tender mass in the right upper abdomen.
- Pain in the upper abdomen.
- A low-grade fever, usually less than 101F (38.3C).
- Yellow eyes and skin (sometimes).
- A swollen abdomen from fluid retention (sometimes).
- Mental status changes, such as confusion or forgetfulness.

CAUSES & RISK FACTORS—The cause is unknown. The risk increases with:
- Cirrhosis of the liver.
- The use of anabolic steroids.
- Excessive alcohol consumption.
- A previous hepatitis B infection.
- Cancer at another site, such as the breast, which may spread to the liver.

DOCTOR'S TREATMENT & DIAGNOSTIC TESTS

- Medical history and physical exam.
- Laboratory blood studies.
- CT scan or ultrasound scan (see Glossary for both).
- X-rays of the chest.
- Liver biopsy.
- Angiogram (see Glossary).
- Self-care instructions focused on the older patient.
- Surgery to confirm the diagnosis. Advancing age alone is not a deterrent.
- Radiation therapy.
- Liver transplant. This procedure is available at a few medical centers in the U.S.

HOME TREATMENT BY SELF OR CARE-GIVER

GENERAL INSTRUCTIONS
- Liver cancer is a complicated, serious disorder. This page can cover only the main points of diagnosis and treatment. Your doctor, nurse or librarian can provide sources of supplemental information.
- Maintain as positive an attitude as possible during treatment.
- Treatment may cause side effects, but they are usually temporary.
- Your pain can be controlled. Don't hesitate to ask your doctor for pain medication.
- Fear may be your worst enemy.
- Call on family members and friends for whatever support and help you need.

MEDICATION (ADJUSTED FOR AGING)
- Your doctor may prescribe: Anticancer drugs (chemotherapy). Pain relievers.
- *Note:* Adverse reactions and side effects may be more frequent and severe in older persons. Remind your doctor of any medicines you already take.

ACTIVITY FOR OLDER PATIENTS—No restrictions are necessary. Stay as active as your strength allows.

FOOD & BEVERAGE—Eat a low-salt diet (see Appendix 9).

FUTURE CONSIDERATIONS FOR THE AGING ADULT

POSSIBLE COMPLICATIONS
- Sodium retention, leading to life-threatening fluid accumulation in the abdomen and lower body parts.
- Kidney failure; death from loss of liver function.

PROBABLE OUTCOME—This condition is currently considered incurable and fatal within a short time. However, the pain can be controlled. Treatment is usually attempted, although it is not likely to be successful. Scientific research into causes and treatment continues, so there is hope for increasingly effective treatment and a cure.

PREVENTING RECURRENCE—There are no specific preventive measures.

CALL YOUR DOCTOR IF

- You have symptoms of liver cancer, especially unexplained weight loss, a low fever or a mass in the abdomen.
- You develop a swollen abdomen during treatment.
- New, unexplained symptoms develop. The drugs used in treatment may produce side effects.

ILLNESSES & DISORDERS

LUNG ABSCESS

BASIC INFORMATION FOR OLDER ADULTS

DESCRIPTION—A lung abscess is an infected area of lung tissue surrounded by lung inflammation. The infected lung tissue dies and is replaced with pus. The infection is not contagious from person to person. Body parts involved: The lung(s).

SPECIAL CONSIDERATIONS FOR AGING
- The immune system becomes less effective, opening the way for viral, bacterial and other infections; malignancies; immune disorders; and allergies.
- Decreased nutrition, common among chronically ill older people, increases the risk of any disease or disorder.
- The total state of well-being in many older people makes them increasingly susceptible to infections and impairs their ability to prevent infections from spreading.
- The ability to clear mucus from the air passages decreases.
- The chest muscles become weaker.

SIGNS & SYMPTOMS
- A cough with sputum. The sputum is puslike, often blood-streaked and sometimes smells bad.
- Bad breath.
- Sweating.
- Fever to 101F (38.3C) or higher.
- Chills.
- Weight loss.
- Chest pain (sometimes).

CAUSES & RISK FACTORS—A lung abscess is usually a complication of pneumonia. It sometimes occurs when an unconscious or sedated person inhales infected material from the upper breathing passages. The patient may be unconscious from a head injury or an anesthetic (including dental anesthesia), intoxicated from alcohol or heavily sedated. Lung abscesses are generally caused by virulent bacteria, such as klebsiella, pseudomona, staphylococcus or beta-hemolytic streptococcus. Risk factors include:
- Recent illness, especially pneumonia that has been slow to heal.
- Alcoholism.
- Recent general anesthesia.
- Injury causing unconsciousness.

DOCTOR'S TREATMENT & DIAGNOSTIC TESTS
- Medical history and physical exam.
- Laboratory blood tests and a culture of pus from the abscess to determine what antibiotic to use.
- X-rays of the lung.
- Surgery (sometimes) to aspirate pus from the abscess or to remove the abscess and part of the lung if the abscess does not heal.
- Self-care instructions focused on the older patient.

HOME TREATMENT BY SELF OR CARE-GIVER

GENERAL INSTRUCTIONS
- Don't smoke; practice deep breathing exercises as often as possible.
- Learn postural drainage to help rid the lung of bronchial secretions. Lie on the bed on your stomach with your head and chest hanging over the edge. Force yourself to cough. Continue until you cannot raise any more sputum. Practice this twice a day for 5 to 10 minutes.

MEDICATION (ADJUSTED FOR AGING)—Your doctor may prescribe antibiotics for prolonged periods to fight infection and prevent a recurrence.

ACTIVITY FOR OLDER PATIENTS—No restrictions are necessary.

FOOD & BEVERAGE—No special diet. Increase your fluid intake to a minimum of 1 glass of fluid at least 8 times a day. By drinking extra liquids, the body is forced to eliminate part of the fluid through the lungs. This makes thick lung secretions thinner so they can be coughed up more easily.

FUTURE CONSIDERATIONS FOR THE AGING ADULT

POSSIBLE COMPLICATIONS
- Chronic abscess, leading to weight loss, anemia, bronchiectasis or chronic lung disease if the abscess does not respond well to antibiotic treatment.
- Rupture of the abscess, causing empyema or massive bleeding in the lung.
- Spread of the infection to other body parts, especially the brain.

PROBABLE OUTCOME—Usually curable with prolonged antibiotic treatment (up to 6 months).

PREVENTING RECURRENCE
- Obtain prompt medical treatment for respiratory infections, especially pneumonia.
- Keep the teeth and mouth in good condition to prevent oral infections that could result in a lung abscess.

CALL YOUR DOCTOR IF

- You have symptoms of a lung abscess.
- Any of the following occurs during treatment: Your rever rises to 101F (38.3C) or higher. The sputum thickens despite treatment. Postural drainage reveals a change in the color, amount or consistency of the sputum.
- Symptoms of a lung infection recur after treatment, especially a sputum-producing cough, fever or general ill feeling.
- New, unexplained symptoms develop. The drugs used in treatment may produce side effects.

LUNG CANCER
(Bronchogenic Carcinoma)

BASIC INFORMATION FOR OLDER ADULTS

DESCRIPTION—Lung cancer is a malignant tissue growth in the lung. Lung cancer is the leading cause of cancer deaths in men and the second most common cause in women. Body parts involved: The bronchial tubes and the lungs. The cancer spreads to the larynx, liver, brain, bones and kidneys.

SPECIAL CONSIDERATIONS FOR AGING
- The immune system becomes less effective, opening the way for viral, bacterial and other infections; malignancies; immune disorders; and allergies.
- Decreased nutrition increases the risk of any disease or disorder.
- Characteristic signs and symptoms of many disorders are frequently changed or absent.
- Weakening of chest muscles.
- Stress from any emotional cause affects all aspects of any illness or disorder.

SIGNS & SYMPTOMS
- Persistent cough; wheezing; chest pain.
- Sputum that may contain blood.
- Fatigue and weakness; weight loss.

CAUSES & RISK FACTORS—Causes include cigarette, cigar or pipe smoking; air pollution; and the spread of cancer from somewhere else in the body. Risk factors include:
- Smoking. A smoker is 22 times more likely to develop lung cancer than a non-smoker.
- Exposure to passive smoke may increase the risk.
- Environmental exposure to asbestos, uranium ore, nickel, chromates, bischloromethyl ether or air pollution.

DOCTOR'S TREATMENT & DIAGNOSTIC TESTS
- Medical history and physical exam.
- Laboratory studies of cells in the sputum and pleural fluid; x-rays of the lungs.
- Surgery for diagnosis (bronchoscopy), biopsy (see Glossary) or removal of cancerous lung tissue if cancer is still small. Advancing age alone is not a deterrent.
- About 2 weeks in an extended-care facility for physical therapy to regain lost lung function after surgery.
- Radiation treatment (sometimes).
- Self-care instructions focused on the older patient.

OTHER—Lung cancer causes more deaths than any other form of cancer. Its incidence is increasing. It is related almost exclusively to cigarette smoking.

HOME TREATMENT BY SELF OR CARE-GIVER

GENERAL INSTRUCTIONS
- Maintain as positive an attitude as possible during treatment.
- Treatment may cause side effects, but they are usually temporary.
- Your pain can be controlled. Don't hesitate to ask your doctor for pain medication.
- Fear may be your worst enemy.
- Call on family members and friends for whatever support and help you need.
- For an explanation of lung cancer surgery and post-operative care, see Lung Resection in the Surgeries section.

MEDICATION (ADJUSTED FOR AGING)
- For minor pain, you may use non-prescription drugs such as acetaminophen or aspirin.
- Your doctor may prescribe:
  Medication to reduce your pain, nausea or anxiety.
  Anticancer drugs (chemotherapy).

ACTIVITY FOR OLDER PATIENTS—After surgery, resume your normal activities gradually.

FOOD & BEVERAGE—No special diet.

FUTURE CONSIDERATIONS FOR THE AGING ADULT

POSSIBLE COMPLICATIONS
- Destructive spread to other body parts, including the brain.
- Lung collapse; fluid on the lung.
- Club-shaped fingers.

PROBABLE OUTCOME—Without surgery, this condition is currently considered incurable. Only 25% of tumors can be removed surgically. However, the symptoms can be relieved or controlled. The survival rate after 5 years is less than 10%.

PREVENTING RECURRENCE
- Avoid pollutants. Wear a protective mask if you work with pollutants.
- Don't smoke. Because tumors don't develop for a long time, smokers can quit at any time and greatly reduce the risk of developing lung cancer.
- Visit your doctor for regular health checkups that may include a chest x-ray if you are a heavy smoker.

CALL YOUR DOCTOR IF

- You have symptoms of lung cancer.
- Any of the following occurs after surgery or during drug treatment:
  Intolerable pain.
  Nausea or vomiting.
  Sleeplessness.
- New, unexplained symptoms develop. The drugs used in treatment may produce side effects.

LUNG DISEASE, CHRONIC
(Bronchiectasis)

BASIC INFORMATION FOR OLDER ADULTS

DESCRIPTION—Chronic lung disease occurs when the bronchial tubes become blocked and accumulate thick secretions. Frequent secondary infections occur. It is not contagious unless associated with tuberculosis. Body parts involved: The lungs and the bronchial tubes.

SPECIAL CONSIDERATIONS FOR AGING
- The immune system becomes less effective, opening the way for viral, bacterial and other infections; malignancies; immune disorders; and allergies.
- In the lungs, the transfer of carbon dioxide and oxygen to the blood becomes less efficient.
- Characteristic signs and symptoms of many disorders are frequently changed or absent.
- Decreased nutrition increases the risk of infections.

SIGNS & SYMPTOMS
- Frequent coughing with bad-smelling green or yellow sputum, sometimes flecked with blood.
- Repeated lung infections; shortness of breath.
- A general ill feeling; frequent fatigue.
- Anemia (frequently).

CAUSES & RISK FACTORS—Caused by damage to the small bronchial tubes, which may develop over years. Common sources of damage include:
- Repeated lung infections (pneumonia).
- Chronic bronchitis; allergies; smoke or dust.
- Inhalation of a foreign object.
- Tuberculosis; fungus infection; cystic fibrosis.

The risk increases with:
- Smoking.
- Poor nutrition; obesity; fatigue or overwork.
- A family history of tuberculosis.
- Exposure to allergens; cold, humid weather.

DOCTOR'S TREATMENT & DIAGNOSTIC TESTS
- Medical history and physical exam.
- X-rays of the lung, including a bronchogram (see Glossary).
- Sputum culture; bronchoscopy.
- Self-care instructions focused on the older patient.
- Surgery to remove isolated areas of damaged lung tissue (rare).

HOME TREATMENT BY SELF OR CARE-GIVER

GENERAL INSTRUCTIONS
- Don't smoke.
- Learn and practice postural drainage (see Glossary) twice a day.
- Sleep with 3- to 5-inch blocks under the foot of the bed to prevent mucus from collecting in the lower lobes of the lungs.

- If you work around heavy air pollution, do everything possible to limit your exposure—including changing jobs.
- Install air conditioning with a filter and humidity control in your home.
- Avoid sudden temperature changes.
- Avoid loud talking, loud laughing, crying, exertion or sudden temperature changes if these trigger coughing episodes.
- Keep the teeth and mouth in excellent condition.
- If you have an allergic background, avoid allergens.

MEDICATION (ADJUSTED FOR AGING)—Your doctor may prescribe:
- Antibiotics for 10 days every month if bacterial infections have caused bronchiectasis or triggered episodes of pneumonia or acute bronchitis.
- Bronchodilators to enlarge the airways.
- Expectorants to loosen secretions.

ACTIVITY FOR OLDER PATIENTS
- Remain as active as possible.
- See Appendix 20 regarding physical fitness for the active older adult.

FOOD & BEVERAGE—Increase your fluid intake. Drink a minimum of 8 glasses of fluid a day. This thins lung secretions so they can be coughed out more easily.

FUTURE CONSIDERATIONS FOR THE AGING ADULT

POSSIBLE COMPLICATIONS
- COPD (chronic obstructive pulmonary disease).
- Repeated pneumonia; destruction of lung tissue.

PROBABLE OUTCOME—With treatment, most patients with chronic lung disease can lead nearly normal lives without major disability.

PREVENTING RECURRENCE
- Don't ever smoke.
- Obtain medical treatment for lung infections.
- Avoid as many risks as possible.
- Get immunization against influenza and pneumonia.

CALL YOUR DOCTOR IF

- You have symptoms of chronic lung disease.
- After diagnosis, you have symptoms of a respiratory infection or bronchitis.
- You develop a fever.
- Blood appears in the sputum, the sputum thickens despite treatment or postural drainage reveals a change in the color, amount or character of the sputum.
- Your chest pain increases.
- Shortness of breath occurs without coughing or when you are at rest.

LUPUS ERYTHEMATOSUS, DISCOID

BASIC INFORMATION FOR OLDER ADULTS

DESCRIPTION—Discoid lupus erythematosus is a skin disorder. It is different from systemic lupus erythematosus, a disease of the connective tissue that affects many different organs. About 1 in 20 persons with discoid lupus progresses to systemic lupus. This disorder is characterized by remissions and flare-ups. Body parts involved: The skin of the face, scalp, ears, neck and arms.

SPECIAL CONSIDERATIONS FOR AGING
- The immune system becomes less effective, opening the way for viral, bacterial and other infections; malignancies; immune disorders; and allergies.
- Decreased nutrition, common among chronically ill older people, increases the risk of any disease or disorder.
- There is less efficient response to physical stress (fright and flight) due to the decreased responsiveness of the adrenal glands.

SIGNS & SYMPTOMS—Plaques (red, raised skin lesions) with the following characteristics:
- The plaques are 1cm to 4cm in diameter and have clearly defined borders.
- They may appear anywhere on the face, but the cheeks and jawline are the most common sites. Some people describe them as "butterfly" lesions when two lesions of unequal size appear on both sides of the nose.
- The plaques sometimes appear on the scalp with localized patches of hair loss.
- The plaques scar as they heal.

CAUSES & RISK FACTORS
- The cause is unknown, but is probably an autoimmune disorder.
- The risk increases with exposure to sunlight.

DOCTOR'S TREATMENT & DIAGNOSTIC TESTS
- Medical history and physical exam.
- Laboratory blood studies and biopsy of skin lesions to rule out systemic lupus erythematosus.
- Self-care instructions focused on the older patient.

HOME TREATMENT BY SELF OR CARE-GIVER

GENERAL INSTRUCTIONS
- Don't go outdoors between 10 a.m. and 2 p.m., when the sun's ultraviolet light is strongest. If you can't avoid exposure to bright sunlight, wear protective clothing and maximum-protection sun-screen products. Avoid fluorescent lighting if possible.
- See your doctor for regular checkups, even when you are in remission.

MEDICATION (ADJUSTED FOR AGING)
- Your doctor may prescribe:
  Injections of triamcinolone into lesions or hydroxychloroquine by mouth to shrink the lesions.
  Topical steroids (occasionally) to decrease the redness of the lesions.
- *Note:* Adverse reactions and side effects may be more frequent and severe in older persons. Remind your doctor of any medicines you already take.

ACTIVITY FOR OLDER PATIENTS
- No restrictions are necessary.
- See Appendix 20 regarding physical fitness for the active older adult.

FOOD & BEVERAGE
- No special diet is required.
- See Appendix 1 regarding good nutrition for people over 50.

FUTURE CONSIDERATIONS FOR THE AGING ADULT

POSSIBLE COMPLICATIONS
- Extensive scarring of the face.
- Systemic lupus erythematosus.

PROBABLE OUTCOME—This disorder is characterized by remissions and flare-ups. It runs its course in 10 to 20 years. 95% of patients (those who don't progress to systemic lupus) live a normal lifespan.

PREVENTING RECURRENCE—There are no specific preventive measures. Protection from sunlight decreases the severity.

CALL YOUR DOCTOR IF

- You have symptoms of discoid lupus erythematosus.
- Any of the following occurs during treatment: Lesions on the hands.
  Swelling, redness and pain in joints.
- New, unexplained symptoms develop. The drugs used in treatment may produce side effects.

LUPUS ERYTHEMATOSUS, SYSTEMIC

BASIC INFORMATION FOR OLDER ADULTS

DESCRIPTION—Systemic lupus erythematosus is an inflammatory disease of the connective tissue. Lupus is not inherited or cancerous. Body parts involved: The connective tissue (collagen). Many body systems are affected, including the joints, skin, kidneys, brain, heart and lungs.

SPECIAL CONSIDERATIONS FOR AGING
- The immune system becomes less effective, opening the way for viral, bacterial and other infections; malignancies; immune disorders; and allergies.
- Decreased nutrition, common among chronically ill older people, increases the risk of any disease or disorder.
- There is less efficient response to physical stress (fright and flight) due to the decreased responsiveness of the adrenal glands.

SIGNS & SYMPTOMS—Lupus symptoms frequently flare up and then subside. Episodes generally include fever and fatigue, plus any 4 of the following:
- A rash, usually on the cheeks.
- Ulcers in the mouth.
- Red palms and hands.
- Joint pain with redness, swelling and tenderness—but no deformity.
- Swelling of the face and legs.
- Shortness of breath.
- Rapid or irregular heartbeat.
- Chest pain.
- Hair loss.
- Swelling of the lymph glands.
- Protein in the urine.
- Increased sensitivity to the sun.
- Anemia.
- Mental changes, including psychosis.

CAUSES & RISK FACTORS—The cause is unknown, but lupus is probably an autoimmune disorder. In an autoimmune disorder, the body's immune system functions abnormally and attacks its own normal tissue—usually connective tissue. Risk factors include stress; the use of drugs such as hydralazine, procainamide, methyldopa and chlorpromazine; and genetic factors (the incidence is higher among blacks).

DOCTOR'S TREATMENT & DIAGNOSTIC TESTS
- Medical history and physical exam. Patients with vague, recurrent symptoms may require long-term observation before a final diagnosis can be made.
- Laboratory studies of antinuclear antibodies, blood count and sedimentation rate (see Glossary).
- Self-care instructions focused on the older patient.

HOME TREATMENT BY SELF OR CARE-GIVER

GENERAL INSTRUCTIONS
- Obtain prompt medical treatment for any infection.
- Don't take any immunizations or drugs without consulting your doctor. Immunizations and some drugs may cause relapses or worsen your current symptoms.
- Use sunscreen with a skin protection factor (SPF) of 15 or more.

MEDICATION (ADJUSTED FOR AGING)
- Your doctor may prescribe immunosuppressive, steroidal and non-steroidal anti-inflammatory drugs or anti-malarial drugs. These relieve the symptoms but don't cure the disease.
- *Note:* Adverse reactions and side effects may be more frequent and severe in older persons. Remind your doctor of any medicines you already take.

ACTIVITY FOR OLDER PATIENTS—Remain as active as possible.

FOOD & BEVERAGE—If your kidneys or heart are affected, restrict your salt intake. Otherwise, no special diet is necessary.

FUTURE CONSIDERATIONS FOR THE AGING ADULT

POSSIBLE COMPLICATIONS—Bacterial or viral pneumonia; impaired kidney function; pericarditis; seizures; hypertension.

PROBABLE OUTCOME—Lupus is currently considered incurable. The disease is characterized by remissions and relapses. Life expectancy is reduced, but the symptoms can be relieved or controlled for many years. Medical literature cites instances of unexplained recovery. Scientific research into causes and treatment continues, so there is hope for increasingly effective treatment and a cure.

PREVENTING RECURRENCE—Cannot be prevented at present.

CALL YOUR DOCTOR IF

- You have symptoms of systemic lupus erythematosus.
- Any of the following occurs after diagnosis:
  A fever of 101F (38.3C) or higher.
  Blood in the urine.
  Shortness of breath.
  Chest pain.
  A bloody stool.
  Severe abdominal pain.
  Any illness with fever.
- New, unexplained symptoms develop. The drugs used in treatment may produce side effects.

LYME DISEASE
(LD; Lyme Arthritis)

BASIC INFORMATION FOR OLDER ADULTS

DESCRIPTION—Lyme disease is an inflammatory disorder characterized by a skin rash that is followed in weeks to months by symptoms in the central nervous system, cardiovascular system and joints. The majority of people who get Lyme disease do not become seriously ill. It can be a self-limited illness that goes away without treatment. Body parts involved: The skin of the thighs, buttocks or underarms; the central nervous system; the heart and blood vessels; the large joints, especially in the knees.

SPECIAL CONSIDERATIONS FOR AGING
- The immune system becomes less effective, opening the way for viral, bacterial and other infections; malignancies; immune disorders; and allergies.
- Decreased nutrition increases the risk of infections.
- The total state of wellbeing in many older people makes them increasingly susceptible to infections and impairs their ability to prevent infections from spreading.

SIGNS & SYMPTOMS
First stage:
- A red papule (small, raised bump) on the skin of the thighs, buttocks or armpits that grows as large as 5cm.

Later stages—any or some of the following:
- Muscle aches and pains.
- Fatigue and lethargy.
- Chills and fever.
- Stiff neck with headache.
- Backache.
- Nausea and vomiting.
- Sore throat.
- Enlargement of the spleen and lymph glands.
- Migrating joint pain, eventually accompanied by redness and warmth.
- An enlarged heart and heart rhythm disturbances.

CAUSES & RISK FACTORS—Caused by a germ (a spirochete) that is transmitted by the bite of a tiny tick, *ixodes dammini*. Many patients report a tick bite at the site of the skin lesion 3 days to 3 weeks prior to the skin rash. The risk increases with exposure to areas where ticks are numerous, such as long grass or brush.

DOCTOR'S TREATMENT & DIAGNOSTIC TESTS
- Medical history and physical exam.
- Laboratory blood studies.
- Self-care instructions focused on the older patient.

HOME TREATMENT BY SELF OR CARE-GIVER

GENERAL INSTRUCTIONS
- Early treatment is important to prevent progression and irreversible neurological damage.

- Use crutches to keep weight off affected joints if necessary.
- Heat relieves the joint pain. Take warm baths, and use heat lamps or whirlpool treatments.

MEDICATION (ADJUSTED FOR AGING)
- Your doctor may prescribe:
  An antibiotic for at least 10 days.
  Non-steroidal anti-inflammatory drugs.
  Cortisone drugs to reduce the inflammatory response in the heart or the central nervous system.
- *Note:* Adverse reactions and side effects may be more frequent and severe in older persons. Remind your doctor of any medicines you already take.

ACTIVITY FOR OLDER PATIENTS
- Rest in bed until the symptoms of active inflammation subside. You may read or watch TV. Then resume normal activities gradually.
- See Appendix 20 regarding physical fitness for the active older adult.

FOOD & BEVERAGE
- No special diet is required.
- See Appendix 1 regarding good nutrition for people over 50.

FUTURE CONSIDERATIONS FOR THE AGING ADULT

POSSIBLE COMPLICATIONS
- Congestive heart failure.
- Permanent joint deformity.
- Permanent brain damage (rare).

PROBABLE OUTCOME—The skin rash is curable in some patients in 10 days with treatment, and this may prevent the development of other symptoms. If not, the symptoms in the joints, central nervous system and cardiovascular system usually subside slowly over 2 to 3 years. The symptoms often recur after several years—without another tick bite.

PREVENTING RECURRENCE
- Wear protective clothing with tight collars and cuffs when you may be exposed to ticks.
- Use effective insect repellents, such as 100% DEET, in areas with ticks.
- Have dogs and cats wear tick-repellant collars.

CALL YOUR DOCTOR IF

- You have symptoms of Lyme disease.
- New, unexplained symptoms develop. The drugs used in treatment may produce side effects.

ILLNESSES & DISORDERS

LYMPHOGRANULOMA VENEREUM
(LGV; Lymphogranuloma Inguinale)

BASIC INFORMATION FOR OLDER ADULTS

DESCRIPTION—Lymphogranuloma venereum is a contagious, sexually transmitted disease found mostly in tropical and subtropical areas. It is rare in North America. Body parts involved: The genitals; the lymph glands.

SPECIAL CONSIDERATIONS FOR AGING
- The immune system becomes less effective, opening the way for viral, bacterial and other infections; malignancies; immune disorders; and allergies.
- Decreased nutrition, common among chronically ill older people, increases the risk of any disease or disorder.
- Stress from any emotional cause—fear, worry, anxiety, sadness, loneliness or anger—affects all aspects of any illness or disorder.

SIGNS & SYMPTOMS—The following begin 1 to 4 weeks after exposure and progress in order:
- A painless blister on the genitals which ulcerates and heals quickly.
- Enlarged lymph glands in the groin that form large, red, tender masses.
- Multiple areas of deep infection that discharge thick pus and blood-stained material.

Other symptoms include:
- Fever.
- Muscle aches and pain, including backache.
- Headaches.
- Joint pain.
- Appetite loss.
- Vomiting.

CAUSES & RISK FACTORS—Caused by the germ chlamydia, which is transmitted by sexual activity. Risk factors include:
- Travel and sexual activity with new partners in a country with a tropical or subtropical climate.
- Crowded or unsanitary living conditions.

DOCTOR'S TREATMENT & DIAGNOSTIC TESTS
- Medical history and physical exam.
- Laboratory studies such as a blood study to rule out syphilis, a culture of the discharge from the lesions and a Frei test (see Glossary).
- Surgery to drain the affected lymph glands or remove abscesses and fistulas.

HOME TREATMENT BY SELF OR CARE-GIVER

GENERAL INSTRUCTIONS—No specific instructions except those listed under other headings.

MEDICATION (ADJUSTED FOR AGING)
- For minor discomfort, you may use non-prescription drugs such as acetaminophen.
- Your doctor may prescribe:
  Antibiotics or sulfa drugs to fight infection.
  Pain relievers.
- *Note:* Adverse reactions and side effects may be more frequent and severe in older persons. Remind your doctor of any medicines you already take.

ACTIVITY FOR OLDER PATIENTS
- After treatment, resume your normal activities as soon as your symptoms improve. Don't resume sexual relations until you are completely healed.
- See Appendix 20 regarding physical fitness for the active older adult.

FOOD & BEVERAGE
- No special diet is required.
- See Appendix 1 regarding good nutrition for people over 50.

FUTURE CONSIDERATIONS FOR THE AGING ADULT

POSSIBLE COMPLICATIONS
- Chronic infection.
- Interference with bowel and bladder function.
- Impotence (sometimes).

PROBABLE OUTCOME—Usually curable in 6 months if treatment is successful. If not, the disorder is incurable, although it does not reduce life expectancy.

PREVENTING RECURRENCE
- Use condoms during sexual intercourse with new partners.
- Don't engage in sexual activity with an infected person.

CALL YOUR DOCTOR IF

- You have symptoms of lymphogranuloma venereum.
- Any of the following occurs during treatment:
  Your fever spikes to 101F (38.3C) or higher.
  Your pain cannot be relieved with simple pain medicine.
  You develop symptoms of malabsorption (see Malabsorption in the Illnesses section).
- New, unexplained symptoms develop. The drugs used in treatment may produce side effects.

LYMPHOMA, NON-HODGKIN'S
(Lymphosarcoma; Reticulum-Cell Sarcoma)

BASIC INFORMATION FOR OLDER ADULTS

DESCRIPTION—Non-Hodgkin's lymphoma is a malignant tumor of the lymph glands. This is more common than Hodgkin's disease. Body parts involved: The lymphocytes (white blood cells), lymph glands (glands which fight infection and produce immune substances), and spleen (a large lymph gland).

SPECIAL CONSIDERATIONS FOR AGING
- The immune system becomes less effective, opening the way for viral, bacterial and other infections; malignancies; immune disorders; and allergies.
- Malignant diseases are less likely to spread rapidly.
- Unusual and unexpected reactions to drugs and medications are more likely.
- Stress from any emotional cause—fear, worry, anxiety, sadness, loneliness or anger—affects all aspects of any illness or disorder.

SIGNS & SYMPTOMS
- Swollen, rubbery, non-tender, distinct lymph glands anywhere in the body—but most commonly in the armpit, neck or groin.
- Weight loss; a general ill feeling.
- Anemia.
- Bleeding from the gastrointestinal tract.
- Jaundice (yellow skin and eyes).

CAUSES & RISK FACTORS—The cause is unknown, but research suggests that a virus infection may be a factor. The risk increases in adults over 40.

DOCTOR'S TREATMENT & DIAGNOSTIC TESTS
- Medical history and physical exam.
- Laboratory studies of blood and bone marrow.
- Lymphangiogram (see Glossary).
- Biopsy (see Glossary) of lymph nodes.
- X-rays of various body parts that may be involved.
- CT scan (see Glossary).
- Hospitalization for short periods for treatment.
- Surgery to discover the extent of disease. Advancing age alone is not a deterrent.
- Radiation therapy.
- Self-care instructions focused on the older patient.

HOME TREATMENT BY SELF OR CARE-GIVER

GENERAL INSTRUCTIONS
- Medical treatment will depend on the extent of the cancer and your age.
- Maintain as positive an attitude as possible during treatment.
- Treatment may cause side effects, but they are usually temporary.

- The pain can be controlled. Don't hesitate to ask your doctor for pain medication.
- Fear may be your worst enemy.
- Call on family members and friends for whatever support and help you need.

MEDICATION (ADJUSTED FOR AGING)
- Your doctor may prescribe anticancer drugs (chemotherapy). Medication may cause side effects or adverse reactions in some people. New symptoms may be caused by the medicine, the original disorder or a new illness. Side effects caused by medicine usually disappear when your body adjusts to the drug or when the drug is discontinued.
- *Note:* Adverse reactions and side effects may be more frequent and severe than in younger persons. Remind your doctor of any medicines you already take.

ACTIVITY FOR OLDER PATIENTS
- Remain as active as your strength allows.
- See Appendix 20 regarding physical fitness for the active older adult.

FOOD & BEVERAGE
- No special diet is required.
- See Appendix 1 regarding good nutrition for people over 50.

FUTURE CONSIDERATIONS FOR THE AGING ADULT

POSSIBLE COMPLICATIONS—Spread of lymphoma to other parts of the body.

PROBABLE OUTCOME—Usually treatable with radiation therapy and anticancer drugs. If you are cured, your life expectancy is normal. The potential for cure varies according to the cell type discovered from biopsy of the lymph nodes and the extent and spread of the disease when it is diagnosed. Consult your doctor.

PREVENTING RECURRENCE—There are no specific preventive measures.

CALL YOUR DOCTOR IF

- You have symptoms of lymphoma.
- Any of the following occurs during treatment:
  Fever.
  Signs of infection (redness, swelling, pain or tenderness) anywhere in the body.
  Swelling of the feet and ankles.
  Discomfort when urinating or decreased daily urine output.
- You think your medicine is causing symptoms.
- New, unexplained symptoms develop. The drugs used in treatment may produce side effects.

MALABSORPTION
(Malabsorptive Syndrome)

BASIC INFORMATION FOR OLDER ADULTS

DESCRIPTION—Malabsorption is the poor absorption of nutrients, vitamins or minerals from the intestinal tract into the bloodstream. Body parts involved: The intestinal tract; liver; pancreas.

SPECIAL CONSIDERATIONS FOR AGING
- The stomach produces less acid.
- The total digestive system becomes more sluggish.
- Characteristic signs and symptoms of many disorders are frequently changed or absent.

SIGNS & SYMPTOMS
- Diarrhea.
- Weakness.
- Weight loss.
- Gas and vague abdominal discomfort.
- Bad-smelling, copious stools.
- Mild anemia (sometimes).

CAUSES & RISK FACTORS
Causes include:
- Deficiency of intestinal enzymes.
- Inadequate digestion caused by disease of the pancreas (such as cystic fibrosis), gallbladder or liver.
- Change in the bacteria that normally live in the intestinal tract.
- Disease of the intestinal walls, including worms or parasites, tropical sprue and celiac disease.
- Surgery that reduces the intestinal tract, decreasing the area for absorption.

Risk factors include:
- A family history of malabsorption or cystic fibrosis.
- Excessive alcohol consumption.
- The use of drugs such as mineral oil and other laxatives.
- Travel to foreign countries.
- Intestinal surgery.

DOCTOR'S TREATMENT & DIAGNOSTIC TESTS
- Medical history and physical exam.
- Laboratory studies of the stool, chromosomes and blood.
- X-rays of the intestinal tract.
- Self-care instructions focused on the older patient.

HOME TREATMENT BY SELF OR CARE-GIVER

GENERAL INSTRUCTIONS—You may need injections of vitamin B-12 and iron because neither is absorbed well with any malabsorptive disorder.

MEDICATION (ADJUSTED FOR AGING)
- Your doctor may prescribe:
  Enzymes to replace missing intestinal enzymes.

Antispasmodics to reduce discomfort. Supplements to replace lost nutrients, vitamins or minerals.
- *Note:* Adverse reactions and side effects may be more frequent and severe in older persons. Remind your doctor of any medicines you already take.

ACTIVITY FOR OLDER PATIENTS
- No restrictions are necessary. Resume your normal activities as soon as your symptoms improve.
- See Appendix 20 regarding physical fitness for the active older adult.

FOOD & BEVERAGE
- Don't drink alcohol.
- You will need a special diet, depending on the cause of your illness. Your doctor or nutritionist will provide specific information. For a gluten-free diet for sprue and celiac disease, see Appendix 5. For a milk-free diet for lactase deficiency, see Appendix 4.

FUTURE CONSIDERATIONS FOR THE AGING ADULT

POSSIBLE COMPLICATIONS
- Prolonged illness.
- Additional illness caused by nutritional, vitamin or mineral deficiency.

PROBABLE OUTCOME—The degree to which the symptoms can be controlled depends on the cause of the disorder, but many things are common to all malabsorptive disorders. The onset is usually slow and difficult to diagnose. These disorders may be present for months or years before being recognized. Treatment is long and complicated and may need to be changed often. Patience and a positive attitude are important in curing these disorders.

PREVENTING RECURRENCE
- Avoid prolonged dependence on mineral oil and other laxatives.
- Avoid excessive alcohol consumption.

CALL YOUR DOCTOR IF

- You have symptoms of malabsorption.
- You have black, tarry bowel movements.
- You have a fever of 101F (38.3C) or higher.
- You have severe abdominal pain.
- You have muscle cramps.
- New, unexplained symptoms develop. The drugs used in treatment may produce side effects.

MALARIA

BASIC INFORMATION FOR OLDER ADULTS

DESCRIPTION—Malaria is an infection caused by a single-cell parasite that is transmitted by the bite of an anopheles mosquito. Body parts involved: The blood cells; blood vessels; liver; central nervous system.

SPECIAL CONSIDERATIONS FOR AGING
- The immune system becomes less effective, opening the way for viral, bacterial and other infections; malignancies; immune disorders; and allergies.
- Characteristic signs and symptoms of many disorders are frequently changed or absent.
- The percentage of muscle tissue decreases.

SIGNS & SYMPTOMS—The first episode of the following symptoms usually occurs about 8 to 30 days after the mosquito bite:
- Headache.
- Fatigue.
- Nausea and vomiting.
- Hard, shaking chills with fever for 12 to 24 hours.
- Rapid breathing.
- Heavy sweating, accompanied by a drop in temperature.

Episodes may recur every 2 or 3 days until the disease is treated. Without treatment, the disease can continue for years.

CAUSES & RISK FACTORS—There are 4 types of malarial parasites. They are transferred from person to person by a mosquito bite. The mosquito becomes infected with malaria after biting a person with the disease. The organisms multiply in the mosquito, then enter the bloodstream of the next person the mosquito bites. Once in a person's bloodstream, the parasites travel to the liver, where they thrive and multiply rapidly. After several days, thousands re-enter the bloodstream and destroy red blood cells. Some parasites remain in the liver, continue to multiply and are released again at intervals into the bloodstream. Risk factors include:
- Crowded or unsanitary living conditions.
- Hot, humid climates.
- Geographic locations such as Latin America, Asia and Africa. Malaria is uncommon in the U.S., but it often affects travelers or military personnel stationed in foreign countries.

DOCTOR'S TREATMENT & DIAGNOSTIC TESTS
- Medical history and physical exam. Tell your doctor of recent travel.
- Laboratory studies such as studies of blood smears to identify the parasite.
- After diagnosis, self-care instructions focused on the older patient.
- Hospitalization (in severe cases).

HOME TREATMENT BY SELF OR CARE-GIVER

GENERAL INSTRUCTIONS
- Protect yourself from secondary bacterial infection while you are ill with malaria. Wash your hands and bathe often.
- Make your environment mosquito-free so your infection cannot be transmitted to others. See Preventing Recurrence.

MEDICATION (ADJUSTED FOR AGING)
- Your doctor may prescribe antimalarial drugs to kill the parasite.
- *Note:* Adverse reactions and side effects may be more frequent and severe in older persons. Remind your doctor of any medicines you already take.

ACTIVITY FOR OLDER PATIENTS
- Rest in bed until the fever and chills subside. Resume your normal activities gradually as the symptoms improve.
- See Appendix 20 regarding physical fitness for the active older adult.

FOOD & BEVERAGE
- No special diet is required. Take vitamin and mineral supplements until you recover.
- See Appendix 1 regarding good nutrition for people over 50.

FUTURE CONSIDERATIONS FOR THE AGING ADULT

POSSIBLE COMPLICATIONS
- Anemia caused by blood cell destruction.
- Clumping of blood cells, which may cause brain or kidney damage.

PROBABLE OUTCOME—Usually curable in 2 weeks with treatment. Malaria can be fatal without treatment in persons who don't receive adequate nourishment or have low resistance to disease.

PREVENTING RECURRENCE
- Take antimalarial drugs before visiting an area where malaria is prevalent. Continue to take the drugs after you return. The public health department or your doctor can give you instructions.
- If you are in a mosquito-infested area, destroy mosquito breeding areas, install window screens and mosquito nets over beds and use insect repellants.

CALL YOUR DOCTOR IF

- You have symptoms of malaria.
- You are weak for a prolonged time after an attack. This may indicate anemia.
- The symptoms of malaria recur after treatment.
- New, unexplained symptoms develop. The drugs used in treatment may produce side effects.

MARCH FRACTURE
(Stress Fracture)

BASIC INFORMATION FOR OLDER ADULTS

DESCRIPTION—A march fracture is a fracture of a bone in the foot that develops after repeated stress, such as from prolonged standing, walking or running. Body parts involved: The bones in the feet (the metatarsal bones).

SPECIAL CONSIDERATIONS FOR AGING
- Years of weight bearing cause wear and tear on the bones, joints and ligaments.
- Coordination and balance become impaired.
- Bone strength lessens.

SIGNS & SYMPTOMS
- Severe, unexplained foot pain when standing or walking. The pain disappears when the load is taken off the feet.
- Swelling and increased warmth and tenderness over the painful area.

CAUSES & RISK FACTORS—Caused by fatigue of the foot bone(s) due to repeated overload, as with playing tennis, dancing, walking, running or jogging. The risk increases with fatigue or overwork, especially standing or walking on a hard surface (such as concrete) for prolonged periods.

DOCTOR'S TREATMENT & DIAGNOSTIC TESTS
- Medical history and physical exam.
- X-rays of both feet. X-rays are often normal for 10 to 24 days after the symptoms begin. Then they show a fracture line across one or more metatarsal bones.
- A bone scan if the symptoms are typical but the x-rays are negative.
- Self-care instructions focused on the older patient.

HOME TREATMENT BY SELF OR CARE-GIVER

GENERAL INSTRUCTIONS—Your doctor will probably apply a short, weight-bearing leg cast. For care of casts, see Appendix 17.

MEDICATION (ADJUSTED FOR AGING)
- You may use non-prescriptions drugs such as aspirin or other non-steroidal anti-inflammatory drugs to relieve minor pain.
- Your doctor may prescribe stronger pain relievers if necessary.
- *Note:* Adverse reactions and side effects may be more frequent and severe in older persons. Remind your doctor of any medicines you already take.

ACTIVITY FOR OLDER PATIENTS
- Don't bear weight on the injured foot. Learn to walk with crutches and prop your foot up whenever possible. Resume your normal activities when the cast is removed.
- See Appendix 20 regarding physical fitness for the active older adult.

FOOD & BEVERAGE
- No special diet is required.
- See Appendix 1 regarding good nutrition for people over 50.

FUTURE CONSIDERATIONS FOR THE AGING ADULT

POSSIBLE COMPLICATIONS—Complete fracture from continued foot abuse after symptoms begin.

PROBABLE OUTCOME—Complete healing in 6 to 8 weeks with treatment.

PREVENTING RECURRENCE—Heed early warnings of impending fracture, such as foot pain after extended standing or walking. Adjust your activities *before* a fracture occurs.

CALL YOUR DOCTOR IF

- You have symptoms of a march fracture.
- Your toes become dark, blue, cold or numb while the cast is on.
- New, unexplained symptoms develop. The drugs used in treatment may produce side effects.

MELANOMA, MALIGNANT

BASIC INFORMATION FOR OLDER ADULTS

DESCRIPTION—Malignant melanoma is a type of skin cancer that spreads to other areas of the body, primarily the lymph nodes, liver, lungs and central nervous system. Most melanomas begin in a mole or another pre-existing skin lesion. Body parts involved: Usually the skin of the head, neck, legs or back. Melanoma rarely appears in the eyes, mouth, vagina or anus.

SPECIAL CONSIDERATIONS FOR AGING
- Malignant diseases are less likely to spread rapidly.
- The skin becomes thinner.
- The responsiveness of the skin's immune system decreases.
- Stress from any emotional cause—fear, worry, anxiety, sadness, loneliness or anger—affects all aspects of any illness or disorder.

SIGNS & SYMPTOMS
- A flat or slightly raised skin lesion that can be black, brown, blue, red, white or a mixture of all colors. Its borders are often irregular and may bleed.
- Itching and bleeding may occur with advanced lesions.

CAUSES & RISK FACTORS—Caused by the uncontrolled growth of the cells that give the skin its brownish color (melanocytes). When the cells grow down into deep skin layers, they invade blood vessels and lymph vessels and are spread to other body areas. Risk factors include:
- Moles on the skin.
- Occupations or activities involving excessive sun exposure, such as farming, construction work, athletics or sunbathing.
- Genetic factors. Malignant melanoma is most common in light-complexioned blonde people. It is rare in black people.
- Radiation treatment or excessive exposure to ultraviolet light, as with sun lamps.

DOCTOR'S TREATMENT & DIAGNOSTIC TESTS
- Medical history and physical exam.
- Biopsy (see Glossary) of suspicious lesions. The melanoma's depth must be established to determine appropriate treatment.
- Surgery to remove suspicious skin lesions or to remove nearby lymph glands if the tumor has spread.
- Hospitalization for radiation treatment if the tumor has spread. Advancing age alone is not a deterrent.
- Self-care instructions focused on the older patient.

HOME TREATMENT BY SELF OR CARE-GIVER

GENERAL INSTRUCTIONS—No specific instructions except those listed under other headings.

MEDICATION (ADJUSTED FOR AGING)
- Your doctor may prescribe anticancer (chemotherapy) drugs.
- *Note:* Adverse reactions and side effects may be more frequent and severe in older persons. Remind your doctor of any medicines you already take.

ACTIVITY FOR OLDER PATIENTS
- No restrictions are necessary.
- See Appendix 20 regarding physical fitness for the active older adult.

FOOD & BEVERAGE
- No special diet is required.
- See Appendix 1 regarding good nutrition for people over 50.

FUTURE CONSIDERATIONS FOR THE AGING ADULT

POSSIBLE COMPLICATIONS—Fatal spread of the malignancy to the lungs, liver, brain or other internal organs.

PROBABLE OUTCOME—Varies greatly. Early melanomas that have not grown downward are curable with surgical removal. Once the tumor has spread to distant organs, this condition is currently considered incurable and is fatal in a short time. However, the symptoms can be relieved or controlled. Scientific research into causes and treatment continues, so there is hope for increasingly effective treatment and a cure.

PREVENTING RECURRENCE
- Protect yourself from excessive sun exposure. Wear broad-rimmed hats and protective clothing. Use maximum-protection sun-block preparations daily on exposed skin. Make a habit of applying it every morning.
- Examine your skin, including the soles of your feet, regularly for changes in pigmented areas. Ask a family member to examine your back. See your doctor about any skin area (especially brown or black) that becomes multicolored, develops irregular edges or surfaces, bleeds or changes in any way.

CALL YOUR DOCTOR IF

- You have symptoms of malignant melanoma.
- During treatment, changes occur in another skin area.
- New, unexplained symptoms develop. The drugs used in treatment may produce side effects.

ILLNESSES & DISORDERS

MENIERE'S DISEASE

BASIC INFORMATION FOR OLDER ADULTS

DESCRIPTION—Meniere's disease is characterized by increased fluid in the semicircular canals of the inner ear, which help maintain balance. Excess fluid produces pressure in the inner ear, disturbing balance and sometimes reducing hearing. Body parts involved: The semicircular canals of the inner ear, usually on one side only.

SPECIAL CONSIDERATIONS FOR AGING
- Nerve cell loss begins at age 20 to 40 and continues throughout life. Cells in the brain and other parts of the central nervous system cannot reproduce or replace themselves.
- Some degree of hearing loss occurs.
- Degenerative changes in the nerves and other body parts concerned with balance occurs in 90% of older people.
- Stress from any emotional cause—fear, worry, anxiety, sadness, loneliness or anger—affects all aspects of any illness or disorder.

SIGNS & SYMPTOMS
The following occur with every acute attack:
- Severe dizziness.
- Noises in the affected ear, such as ringing or buzzing.
- Hearing loss that increases with each attack.
Possible accompanying symptoms include:
- Vomiting.
- Sweating.
- Jerky eye movements.
- Loss of balance.
- A feeling of pain or pressure in the ear.

CAUSES & RISK FACTORS—The cause is
unknown. Theories include:
- Spasms of the blood vessels to the inner ear.
- Fluid retention in the inner ear.
- Allergic reactions.

DOCTOR'S TREATMENT & DIAGNOSTIC TESTS
- Medical history and physical exam.
- Laboratory studies such as audiometry and ice-water ("caloric") tests (see Glossary for both).
- X-rays of the head.
- Self-care instructions focused on the older patient.
- Surgical destruction of the affected inner ear (rare). Advancing age alone is not a deterrent.

HOME TREATMENT BY SELF OR CARE-GIVER

GENERAL INSTRUCTIONS
- Avoid glaring light and don't read during attacks.
- Equip risk areas of your home (e.g., bathrooms) with handrails and good lighting.

MEDICATION (ADJUSTED FOR AGING)
- Your doctor may prescribe:
  Antinausea drugs.
  Tranquilizers to reduce dizziness.
  Antihistamines, which lessen the symptoms in some persons.
  Diuretics to decrease fluid in the inner ear.
- *Note:* Adverse reactions and side effects may be more frequent and severe in older persons. Remind your doctor of any medicines you already take.

ACTIVITY FOR OLDER PATIENTS
- Rest quietly in bed.
- Until dizziness and nausea disappear:
  Don't walk without assistance.
  Avoid sudden changes in position.
  Don't drive, climb ladders or work around dangerous machinery.
- Resume your normal activities as soon as the symptoms disappear.
- See Appendix 20 regarding physical fitness for the active older adult.

FOOD & BEVERAGE
- No special diet is required, but you should decrease your salt and fluid intake.
- See Appendix 1 regarding good nutrition for people over 50.

FUTURE CONSIDERATIONS FOR THE AGING ADULT

POSSIBLE COMPLICATIONS
- Permanent hearing loss.
- Chronic noises in the ear.
- Falls due to dizziness.

PROBABLE OUTCOME—Attacks of Meniere's disease usually recur over many years. Some symptoms can be controlled. The condition is frustrating but not life-threatening.

PREVENTING RECURRENCE—There are no specific preventive measures.

CALL YOUR DOCTOR IF

- You have symptoms of Meniere's disease.
- Any of the following occurs during treatment:
  Decreased hearing in either ear.
  Persistent vomiting.
  Convulsions.
  Fainting.
  A fever of 101F (38.3C) or higher.
- New, unexplained symptoms develop. The drugs used in treatment may produce side effects.

MENINGITIS, ASEPTIC
(Viral Meningitis; Non-Bacterial Meningitis)

BASIC INFORMATION FOR OLDER ADULTS

DESCRIPTION—Aseptic meningitis is an inflammation of the meninges (the thin membranes that cover the brain and spinal cord). This is contagious. Body parts involved: The brain and spinal cord.

SPECIAL CONSIDERATIONS FOR AGING
- The immune system becomes less effective, opening the way for viral, bacterial and other infections; malignancies; immune disorders; and allergies.
- Decreased nutrition increases the risk of infections.
- Characteristic signs and symptoms of many disorders are frequently changed or absent.

SIGNS & SYMPTOMS
- Fever.
- Headache.
- Irritability.
- Eyes that are sensitive to light.
- Stiff neck.
- Vomiting.
- Confusion, lethargy and drowsiness.

CAUSES & RISK FACTORS
Causes include:
- Viruses of several types, including the polio virus.
- Fungi, including yeasts.
- A reaction—probably an autoimmune response—following various viral illnesses, such as measles.

Risk factors include:
- Recent measles, German measles or various types of flu.
- Immunosuppressive treatment, such as for cancer or following an organ transplant.
- Poor nutrition.
- Recent illness that has lowered resistance.
- Meningitis epidemics. The disease becomes more virulent as it spreads from person to person.

DOCTOR'S TREATMENT & DIAGNOSTIC TESTS
- Medical history and physical exam.
- Laboratory studies such as blood cell counts and lumbar puncture (see Glossary) to examine the cerebrospinal fluid.
- Hospitalization in severe cases.
- Self-care instructions focused on the older patient.

HOME TREATMENT BY SELF OR CARE-GIVER

GENERAL INSTRUCTIONS—No special instructions except those listed under other headings.

MEDICATION (ADJUSTED FOR AGING)
- If aseptic meningitis is caused by a virus, there is no medication for it. The body's defenses will usually cure it, although a polio virus may leave permanent damage.
- If meningitis is caused by a fungus, your doctor may prescribe antifungal drugs, such as amphotericin B.
- Avoid aspirin for pain, as it may cause bleeding.
- *Note:* Adverse reactions and side effects may be more frequent and severe in older persons. Remind your doctor of any medicines you already take.

ACTIVITY FOR OLDER PATIENTS
- Rest in bed in a darkened room.
- Resume your normal activities as soon as your symptoms improve.
- See Appendix 20 regarding physical fitness for the active older adult.

FOOD & BEVERAGE
- No special diet is required. Drink 6 to 8 glasses of fluid daily, even if you don't feel like it.
- See Appendix 1 regarding good nutrition for people over 50.

FUTURE CONSIDERATIONS FOR THE AGING ADULT

POSSIBLE COMPLICATIONS
- Permanent brain damage (rare).
- Muscle impairment or paralysis (if caused by poliomyelitis).

PROBABLE OUTCOME—Most patients recover fully from aseptic meningitis without specific therapy. This is not the case with bacterial meningitis, in which antibiotics may be life-saving.

PREVENTING RECURRENCE—Talk to your doctor about keeping immunizations up to date against all viruses for which vaccines are available. See Appendix 16 for an immunization schedule.

CALL YOUR DOCTOR IF

- You have symptoms of aseptic meningitis.
- New, unexplained symptoms develop. The drugs used in treatment may produce side effects.

MENINGITIS, BACTERIAL
(Spinal Meningitis)

BASIC INFORMATION FOR OLDER ADULTS

DESCRIPTION—Bacterial meningitis is a bacterial infection or inflammation of the meninges (the thin membranes that cover the brain and spinal cord). Body part involved: The central nervous system. (THIS IS AN EMERGENCY; SEEK MEDICAL CARE IMMEDIATELY!)

SPECIAL CONSIDERATIONS FOR AGING
- The immune system becomes less effective, opening the way for viral, bacterial and other infections; malignancies; immune disorders; and allergies.
- Decreased nutrition increases the risk of infections.
- Characteristic signs and symptoms of many disorders are frequently changed or absent.

SIGNS & SYMPTOMS—A sore throat or other signs of respiratory illness may precede the other symptoms, which are as follows:
- Fever, chills and sweating (may be absent in critically ill persons).
- Headache.
- Irritability.
- Sensitivity of the eyes to light.
- Pupils of different sizes (possibly).
- Stiff neck.
- Vomiting.
- Red or purple skin rash.
- Confusion, lethargy, drowsiness or unconsciousness.

CAUSES & RISK FACTORS
Caused by bacteria from the following sources:
- An infection in another body part, such as the lung, ear, nose, throat or sinus, that spreads to the meninges.
- A head injury, such as a fractured skull, that allows infection to enter.
Risk factors include:
- Illness that has lowered resistance.
- Poor nutrition.
- The use of drugs that decrease the body's immune responses, such as anticancer drugs.

DOCTOR'S TREATMENT & DIAGNOSTIC TESTS
- Medical history and physical exam.
- Laboratory studies such as blood sugar tests and cultures of the blood and the secretions of the throat, nose or other infection sites.
- Lumbar puncture (see Glossary) to examine the cerebrospinal fluid.
- Hospitalization.
- After hospitalization, self-treatment instructions focused on the older patient.

HOME TREATMENT BY SELF OR CARE-GIVER

GENERAL INSTRUCTIONS—Restrict visitors until the doctor determines that the disease is no longer contagious.

MEDICATION (ADJUSTED FOR AGING)
- Your doctor may prescribe antibiotics, depending on what type of bacteria is causing the meningitis.
- *Note:* Adverse reactions and side effects may be more frequent and severe in older persons. Remind your doctor of any medicines you already take.

ACTIVITY FOR OLDER PATIENTS—While in the hospital, you will need bed rest in a darkened room. After a 2- to 3-week recovery, you should be as active as your strength allows.

FOOD & BEVERAGE—You may be given intravenous nutrients in the hospital. At home, eat a normal, well-balanced diet. Vitamin and mineral supplements should not be necessary unless you have a deficiency or cannot eat normally.

FUTURE CONSIDERATIONS FOR THE AGING ADULT

POSSIBLE COMPLICATIONS—Death or permanent brain damage—including paralysis, hearing loss, speech difficulty and intellectual impairment—if not treated quickly.

PROBABLE OUTCOME—Full recovery is likely in 2 to 3 weeks with treatment if no complications arise.

PREVENTING RECURRENCE
- Consult your doctor for treatment of any infection in your body to prevent its spread.
- Avoid contact with anyone who has meningitis (depending on the type of bacteria). Those who have had close contact with a person with meningitis may need preventive antibiotic treatment even if they have no symptoms.
- Talk to your doctor about possible vaccination for meningitis.

CALL YOUR DOCTOR IF

- You have symptoms of bacterial meningitis. *This is an emergency!*
- Your temperature rises to 101F (38.3C) or higher during treatment.
- New, unexplained symptoms develop. The drugs used in treatment may produce side effects.
- You have had contact with someone who has meningitis.

MENOPAUSE & POST-MENOPAUSE

BASIC INFORMATION FOR OLDER ADULTS

DESCRIPTION—Menopause is the permanent cessation of menstruation. This occurs as early as age 35 or as late as age 55 and usually spans 1 to 2 years. It is usually diagnosed in females after 1 year of absent periods. Menopause is only one event in the "climacteric," a biological change in all body tissues and body systems that occurs in both sexes between the mid-40s and the mid-60s. Body parts involved: The female reproductive system, with secondary effects in other body parts.

SPECIAL CONSIDERATIONS FOR AGING—Many body changes occur as a result of estrogen deficiency beginning at menopause. These include vaginal dryness, shortening and narrowing of the vagina, greater susceptibility to vaginal infections, frequent bladder infections, reductions in the size of the clitoris and increased facial hair. Changes in other systems of the body may lead to a greater tendency to osteoporosis, hardening of the arteries and other disorders.

SIGNS & SYMPTOMS—Physical changes (directly associated with decreased blood levels of female hormones):
- Menstrual irregularity.
- Hot flashes or flushes—sensations of heat spreading from the waist or chest toward the neck, face and upper arms.
- Headaches; dizziness; night sweats.
- Rapid or irregular heartbeat.
- Vaginal dryness, itching, burning or discomfort during intercourse, beginning a few years after menopause.
- Bloating in the upper abdomen.
- Bladder irritability; breast tenderness.

Emotional changes (associated with lower hormone levels *and* conflicting feelings about aging and loss of fertility):
- Mood changes; sleeping difficulty.
- Pronounced tension and anxiety.
- Depression or melancholy and fatigue.
- Loss of sexual desire.
- Lack of concentration and memory difficulty.

CAUSES & RISK FACTORS
- Caused by a normal decline in the function of the ovaries that results in decreased levels of the female hormones, estrogen and progesterone.
- Surgical removal of both ovaries.

DOCTOR'S TREATMENT & DIAGNOSTIC TESTS
- Medical history and physical exam.
- Laboratory blood studies of hormone levels.
- Diagnosis to rule out other causes of the symptoms.
- Self-care instructions focused on the older patient.
- Psychotherapy or counseling if emotional changes interfere with personal relationships or work.

HOME TREATMENT BY SELF OR CARE-GIVER

GENERAL INSTRUCTIONS
- Reduce stress as much as possible. See Appendix 13.
- If you take estrogen replacement therapy (ERT), have a Pap smear every 6 months.

MEDICATION (ADJUSTED FOR AGING)
- Most women require no medication. If the symptoms are severe, your doctor may prescribe estrogen replacement therapy (female hormones). Because this type of hormone treatment has risks as well as benefits, learn all you can about ERT before deciding on treatment.
- Don't take hormones if you have diabetes mellitus, breast cancer or high blood pressure and are obese. Hormones may aggravate the underlying condition and complicate treatment.
- Beta blocker drugs may be prescribed if you are unable to take ERT.

ACTIVITY FOR OLDER PATIENTS
- No restrictions are necessary.
- To prevent osteoporosis, an active exercise program is important (see Appendix 20) along with adequate calcium intake.

FOOD & BEVERAGE
- No special diet is required.
- See Appendix 1 regarding good nutrition for people over 50.

FUTURE CONSIDERATIONS FOR THE AGING ADULT

POSSIBLE COMPLICATIONS
- Increased irritability and susceptibility to infection in the urinary tract.
- Diminished breast size.
- Decreased skin elasticity.
- Increased risk of hardening of the arteries, heart disease, stroke and osteoporosis after menopause.

PROBABLE OUTCOME—Menopause is a normal process—not an illness. Most women make an easy transition without crisis.

PREVENTING RECURRENCE—Take estrogen replacement therapy, beginning before menopause and extending throughout life, to prevent symptoms.

CALL YOUR DOCTOR IF

- You have symptoms of menopause. Other causes should be ruled out.
- Bleeding appears 6 months or more after your last period.
- New, unexplained symptoms develop. Estrogen replacement therapy used in treatment may produce side effects.
- The symptoms of menopause return while taking estrogen replacement therapy.

ILLNESSES & DISORDERS

BASIC INFORMATION FOR OLDER ADULTS

DESCRIPTION—Mitral valve prolapse is a disorder characterized by a bulging of the leaflets of the mitral valve of the heart into the atrium. This bulging causes a crisp click and murmur which can be heard with a stethoscope. Body parts involved: The heart.

SPECIAL CONSIDERATIONS FOR AGING
- The coronary arteries nourishing the heart are less healthy. They become thicker and lose their elasticity.
- The total heart functions less efficiently—especially among smokers.

SIGNS & SYMPTOMS—Usually none, but the following may occur:
- Fatigue.
- Chest pains.
- Shortness of breath.
- Palpitations (caused by rhythm problems).

CAUSES & RISK FACTORS
- Diseases of the mitral heart valves.
- Marfan syndrome (see Glossary).
- Defects in the walls of the heart chambers.

DOCTOR'S TREATMENT & DIAGNOSTIC TESTS
- Medical history and physical exam.
- Laboratory blood studies and urinalysis.
- ECG (see Glossary).
- Radioactive studies of heart muscle efficiency.
- Angiography; heart catheterization.
- Self-care instructions focused on the older patient.

HOME TREATMENT BY SELF OR CARE-GIVER

GENERAL INSTRUCTIONS—None.

MEDICATION (ADJUSTED FOR AGING)
- Your doctor may prescribe:
  Beta-adrenergic-blocking agents.
  Anticoagulants.
  Digitalis.
- *Note:* Adverse reactions and side effects may be more frequent and severe in older persons. Remind your doctor of any medicines you already take.

ACTIVITY FOR OLDER PATIENTS
- No restrictions are necessary.
- Arise from sitting or lying positions slowly.
- See Appendix 20 regarding physical fitness for the active older adult.

FOOD & BEVERAGE
- No special diet is required.
- See Appendix 1 regarding good nutrition for people over 50.

FUTURE CONSIDERATIONS FOR THE AGING ADULT

POSSIBLE COMPLICATIONS
- Heartbeat irregularities (arrhythmias).
- Rupture of the chordae tendineae (the cords inside the heart).
- Blood clots to the brain (extremely rare).

PROBABLE OUTCOME—The symptoms can usually be controlled.

PREVENTING RECURRENCE—Your doctor may suggest prophylactic antibiotics before dental or surgical procedures.

CALL YOUR DOCTOR IF

- You have symptoms of mitral valve prolapse.
- Your diagnosis has been confirmed and you are going in for elective dentistry or surgery.

MOTION SICKNESS
(Car, Sea or Air Sickness)

BASIC INFORMATION FOR OLDER ADULTS

DESCRIPTION—Motion sickness is an unpleasant, temporary disturbance that occurs while traveling that is characterized by dizziness and stomach upset. Body parts involved: The semicircular canals of the inner ear. These fluid-filled canals maintain balance.

SPECIAL CONSIDERATIONS FOR AGING
- Nerve cell loss begins at age 20 to 40 and continues throughout life. Cells in the brain and other parts of the central nervous system cannot reproduce or replace themselves.
- Degenerative changes in the nerves and other body parts concerned with balance occur in 90% of older people.
- Medications for treatment are much more likely to cause significant side effects. Beware.

SIGNS & SYMPTOMS
- Loss of appetite.
- Nausea and vomiting.
- A spinning sensation.
- Weakness and unsteadiness.
- Paleness; sweating.

CAUSES & RISK FACTORS—Caused by travel by any means, especially airplane, boat or car. Irregular motion causes fluid changes in the semicircular canals of the inner ear, which transmit signals to the brain's vomiting center. Risk factors include:
- Stress.
- Ear disorders.
- A smoky environment or poor ventilation.
- Excessive alcohol consumption.
- A full stomach.

DOCTOR'S TREATMENT & DIAGNOSTIC TESTS
- Medical history and physical exam if motion sickness is recurrent and interferes with your life.
- Self-care instructions focused on the older patient.
- Doctor's treatment if you have a chronic illness that may be worsened by vomiting.
- Psychotherapy or counseling if your occupation or lifestyle requires travel and you usually develop motion sickness.

OTHER—Some airlines have developed behavior modification techniques for those who are afraid to fly or have motion sickness. Contact the airline or your travel agent for information.

HOME TREATMENT BY SELF OR CARE-GIVER

GENERAL INSTRUCTIONS
- Psychological factors contribute to motion sickness. Try to resolve concerns about travel before leaving home. Maintain a positive attitude.

- Accupressure bands worn on the wrists are becoming popular as a preventive. They are available at marine supply stores and sporting goods stores or through travel agents.

MEDICATION (ADJUSTED FOR AGING)
- For minor discomfort, you may use non-prescription drugs such as dimenhydrate before and during travel.
- Your doctor may prescribe scopolamine patches to control the symptoms. Remove them promptly. Long-term use may cause mental illness. The usefulness of scopolamine has proven to be disappointing for many people. Longer-acting antihistamines (promethazine, phenergan or medizine) may also be prescribed.
- *Note:* Adverse reactions and side effects may be more frequent and severe in older persons. Remind your doctor of any medicines you already take.

ACTIVITY FOR OLDER PATIENTS—To minimize symptoms during travel, rest in a reclining position and fix your gaze on a distant object.

FOOD & BEVERAGE
- Eat lightly or not at all before and during brief trips. For longer trips, don't take large drinks, but sip frequently on beverages to maintain your fluid intake.
- See Appendix 1 regarding good nutrition for people over 50.

FUTURE CONSIDERATIONS FOR THE AGING ADULT

POSSIBLE COMPLICATIONS
- Dehydration from vomiting.
- Falls and injuries from unsteadiness.

PROBABLE OUTCOME—Spontaneous recovery when the trip is over.

PREVENTING RECURRENCE
- Don't eat large meals or drink alcohol before or during travel.
- Sit in areas of an airplane (usually over the wings) or boat with the least motion.
- Recline in your seat if possible.
- Breathe slowly and deeply.
- Avoid areas where others are smoking if possible.
- On an airplane or bus, turn on the overhead air vent to improve air circulation.
- Take medication to prevent motion sickness before you travel.

CALL YOUR DOCTOR IF

You plan to travel and have had disabling motion sickness in the past.

MOUTH OR TONGUE TUMOR, BENIGN

BASIC INFORMATION FOR OLDER ADULTS

DESCRIPTION—A benign mouth or tongue tumor is an abnormal new growth in the mouth or tongue that is unlikely to spread to other body parts. Such tumors usually occur singly and grow very slowly over 2 to 6 years. Body parts involved: The lips; gums; palate; tongue; membrane covering the lips and cheeks; floor of the mouth.

SPECIAL CONSIDERATIONS FOR AGING
- Malignant diseases are less likely to spread rapidly.
- Characteristic signs and symptoms of many disorders are frequently changed or absent.
- Decreased nutrition increases the risk of infections.

SIGNS & SYMPTOMS—A lump in any part of the mouth or tongue with the following characteristics:
- It may ulcerate and bleed.
- It may interfere with the way dentures fit.
- It may interfere with speech or swallowing.

CAUSES & RISK FACTORS—The cause is unknown, although it is most common in people who smoke cigarettes, cigars or pipes or who use chewing tobacco or snuff. The risk increases with:
- The use of tobacco.
- Poorly fitting dentures.

DOCTOR'S TREATMENT & DIAGNOSTIC TESTS
- Medical history and physical exam.
- Biopsy (see Glossary) of the tumor.
- Treatment by a dentist or doctor.
- Self-care instructions focused on the older patient.
- Surgery to remove the tumor. Advancing age alone is not a deterrent.

HOME TREATMENT BY SELF OR CARE-GIVER

GENERAL INSTRUCTIONS—After surgery, cleanse the mouth 3 to 4 times a day with a soothing salt-water solution (1 teaspoon salt in 8 oz. warm water).

MEDICATION (ADJUSTED FOR AGING)
- For minor discomfort, you may use non-prescription drugs such as acetaminophen.
- Your doctor may prescribe antibiotics if infection exists.
- *Note:* Adverse reactions and side effects may be more frequent and severe in older persons. Remind your doctor of any medicines you already take.

ACTIVITY FOR OLDER PATIENTS
- No restrictions are necessary.
- See Appendix 20 regarding physical fitness for the active older adult.

FOOD & BEVERAGE
- No special diet is required after recovery. A liquid diet may be necessary for several days after surgery.
- See Appendix 1 regarding good nutrition for people over 50.

FUTURE CONSIDERATIONS FOR THE AGING ADULT

POSSIBLE COMPLICATIONS
- A cancerous change in the tumor (rare).
- Bleeding from the tumor.
- Infection in the tumor.

PROBABLE OUTCOME—Curable with surgical removal. Normal facial appearance can usually be restored by plastic surgery.

PREVENTING RECURRENCE
- Don't smoke or use tobacco.
- See your dentist for annual dental exams and for problems with the fit of dentures.

CALL YOUR DOCTOR IF

- You have symptoms of a mouth or tongue tumor.
- Any of the following occurs after surgery:
  Fever.
  Bleeding at the surgical site.
  Unbearable pain.
- New, unexplained symptoms develop. The drugs used in treatment may produce side effects.

MULTIPLE MYELOMA
(Primary Bone Marrow Cancer)

BASIC INFORMATION FOR OLDER ADULTS

DESCRIPTION—Multiple myeloma is a malignancy that begins in the plasma cells of the bone marrow. It occurs much more often in persons over 50. The plasma cells normally produce antibodies to help destroy germs and protect against infection. With myeloma, this function becomes impaired and the body cannot deal effectively with infection. Body parts involved: The bone marrow of all bones, but most commonly those of the thigh, back, pelvis or upper arms.

SPECIAL CONSIDERATIONS FOR AGING
- Malignant diseases are less likely to spread rapidly.
- The immune system becomes less effective, opening the way for viral, bacterial and other infections and malignancies.
- Stress from any emotional cause affects all aspects of any illness or disorder.

SIGNS & SYMPTOMS
- Pain in the affected bone. The pain is severe, boring and deep. If the bone collapses, the pain spreads to other parts of the body.
- Weight loss.
- Symptoms of anemia, such as weakness, paleness, tiredness and breathlessness.
- Frequent infections; sensitivity to cold.
- Mental confusion; carpal tunnel syndrome.

CAUSES & RISK FACTORS—The bone pain is caused by the cancerous plasma cells. The anemia is caused by damaged red blood cells and decreased platelets. The causes of the disorder itself may include:
- Exposure to radiation.
- Chronic disease, such as cholecystitis, osteomyelitis or rheumatoid arthritis.
- Exposure to asbestos or a viral illness.

DOCTOR'S TREATMENT & DIAGNOSTIC TESTS
- Medical history and physical exam.
- Laboratory blood studies.
- Biopsy (see Glossary) of bone marrow.
- X-rays of painful bones.
- Plasmapheresis (see Glossary).
- Self-care instructions focused on the older patient.
- Radiation therapy to relieve the bone pain. Advancing age alone is not a deterrent.
- Hospitalization for blood transfusion to lessen the anemia and in the late stages of the disease.

HOME TREATMENT BY SELF OR CARE-GIVER

GENERAL INSTRUCTIONS—No specific instructions except those listed under other headings.

MEDICATION (ADJUSTED FOR AGING)
- Your doctor may prescribe:
  Anticancer and cortisone drugs (chemotherapy).
  Pain relievers.
  Antibiotics to fight infections.
- *Note:* Adverse reactions and side effects may be more frequent and severe in older persons. Remind your doctor of any medicines you already take.

ACTIVITY FOR OLDER PATIENTS
- Stay as active as the pain or bone complications allow. Activity may help prevent further bone loss.
- Special corsets or braces may be worn to relieve back pain.
- See Appendix 20 regarding physical fitness for the active older adult.

FOOD & BEVERAGE
- No special diet is required.
- Drink plenty of fluids daily to maintain an increased urine output.
- See Appendix 1 regarding good nutrition for people over 50.

FUTURE CONSIDERATIONS FOR THE AGING ADULT

POSSIBLE COMPLICATIONS
- Recurrent infections.
- Kidney failure.
- Spontaneous bleeding.

PROBABLE OUTCOME—This condition is currently considered incurable. However, the pain can be relieved or controlled. Some persons live up to 5 years after the symptoms appear, and medical literature cites a few instances of unexplained recovery. Scientific research into causes and treatment continues, so there is hope for increasingly effective treatment and a cure.

PREVENTING RECURRENCE—There are no specific preventive measures.

CALL YOUR DOCTOR IF

- You have symptoms of multiple myeloma.
- Any of the following occurs during treatment:
  Fever.
  Any sign of infection (pain, swelling, redness, tenderness or warmth) anywhere in the body.
  Swelling of the feet and ankles.
  Urination discomfort or decreased urine output in 1 day.
  Unexplained bleeding from any part of the body.
- New, unexplained symptoms develop. The drugs used in treatment may produce side effects.

MUSCLE, PULLED OR TORN

BASIC INFORMATION FOR OLDER ADULTS

DESCRIPTION—A pulled or torn muscle is a muscle whose fibers are stretched or torn. Body parts involved: The muscles attached to bones anywhere in the body.

SPECIAL CONSIDERATIONS FOR AGING
- Muscle bulk and power decrease.
- Characteristic signs and symptoms of many disorders in older people are frequently changed or absent.
- Muscle tone decreases.

SIGNS & SYMPTOMS
- Pain or tenderness in the injury area.
- Gradual stiffening or contraction of the injured muscle.
- Swelling, redness or bruising at the injury site.

CAUSES & RISK FACTORS—Caused by injury due to the overuse or stress of a muscle group. Risk factors include:
- Poor nutrition, especially an electrolyte imbalance or vitamin deficiencies.
- Poor physical condition.
- Strenuous activity following excessive alcohol consumption.
- Obesity.
- Fatigue or overwork.
- The improper lifting of heavy weights.

DOCTOR'S TREATMENT & DIAGNOSTIC TESTS
- Medical history and physical exam.
- X-rays of the painful area (seldom necessary).
- Self-care instructions focused on the older patient.
- Doctor's treatment for severe injuries or if self-care is not successful.
- Rehabilitation and treatment by a physical therapist or athletic trainer.

HOME TREATMENT BY SELF OR CARE-GIVER

GENERAL INSTRUCTIONS
- Apply ice to the injured area during the first 24 hours. Place ice in a plastic bag and separate it from the skin with a thin towel. Hold it against the muscle with your hand or an elastic bandage. Keep the ice pack on the area as long as you can tolerate the cold.
- Wrap the area with a support bandage. Don't wrap it too tightly. If there is swelling *below* the bandage, loosen it. Elevate the injured part whenever possible.
- After 24 hours, apply heat in any form or continue ice packs, whichever feels better. Ice is usually more beneficial. For heat, use a heating pad, heat lamp, whirlpool, ultrasound, hot baths or hot compresses.

MEDICATION (ADJUSTED FOR AGING)
- You may take non-prescription pain relievers. If your pain is severe or the affected area becomes badly swollen, your doctor may prescribe stronger pain relievers or muscle relaxants.
- *Note:* Adverse reactions and side effects may be more frequent and severe in older persons. Remind your doctor of any medicines you already take.

ACTIVITY FOR OLDER PATIENTS
- Don't use the pulled muscle as long as it is painful. However, keep uninjured parts of the body active. Severe leg injuries may require crutches and severe arm injuries may require slings.
- Physical therapy, with a graduated exercise program, may be necessary to restore normal use and strength.
- See Appendix 20 regarding physical fitness for the active older adult.

FOOD & BEVERAGE
- Eat a normal, well-balanced diet.
- See Appendix 1 regarding good nutrition for people over 50.

FUTURE CONSIDERATIONS FOR THE AGING ADULT

POSSIBLE COMPLICATIONS—Permanent weakness in the affected muscle.

PROBABLE OUTCOME—The healing time for a pulled muscle depends on your age, general physical condition, previous injuries and the severity of the injury. Most partial tears or pulls heal with treatment within 1 month. Muscle function will be poor until the torn fibers heal. If the muscle is ruptured (torn in two), surgery may be necessary.

PREVENTING RECURRENCE—Avoid vigorous exercise if you are not accustomed to it. If you are out of condition, begin an exercise program to strengthen your muscles gradually and prevent future injury. See Appendix 20.

CALL YOUR DOCTOR IF

You have symptoms of a pulled or torn muscle, especially if any of the following occur:
- You become unable to use the affected muscle.
- The pain becomes intolerable.
- The swelling or bruising increase after 24 hours.
- You think a medicine is causing symptoms.

MYASTHENIA GRAVIS

BASIC INFORMATION FOR OLDER ADULTS

DESCRIPTION—Myasthenia gravis is a disorder of the muscles, especially those of the face and head, with increasing fatigue and weakness as the muscles are used. Body parts involved: The muscles, especially those around the eyes, mouth and throat and those of the extremities.

SPECIAL CONSIDERATIONS FOR AGING
- Characteristic signs and symptoms of many disorders are frequently changed or absent.
- Neurological diseases become more likely.

SIGNS & SYMPTOMS
- Drooping eyelids.
- Double vision.
- Loss of normal facial expression.
- Swallowing difficulty.
- Weakness of the arms and legs.
- Difficulty speaking clearly.
- Breathing difficulty.

Most flare-ups appear after a brief period of normal muscle function and worsen as the muscle is used.

CAUSES & RISK FACTORS
Causes include:
- An autoimmune disorder (probably).
- A tumor of the thymus.

Risk factors include:
- A medical history of other autoimmune diseases.
- Some cancers, especially cancers of the thymus and lung.

DOCTOR'S TREATMENT & DIAGNOSTIC TESTS
- Medical history and physical exam.
- Laboratory studies of antibodies in the blood and electrical muscle tests.
- X-rays of the chest; CT scan or MRI imaging (see Glossary for both).
- Therapeutic trial of anticholinesterase drugs.
- Pulmonary function tests and nerve conduction studies.
- Surgery to remove a thymus tumor if present.
- Plasmapheresis during crisis (see Glossary).
- Self-care instructions focused on the older patient.

HOME TREATMENT BY SELF OR CARE-GIVER

GENERAL INSTRUCTIONS
- Maintain as normal a life as possible. See Appendix 13.
- Join a support group.
- Frequent monitoring by a medical professional is necessary to detect signs of complications.

- Myasthenia gravis is a complicated, serious disorder. This page can cover only the main points of diagnosis and treatment. Your doctor, nurse or librarian can provide sources of supplemental information.

MEDICATION (ADJUSTED FOR AGING)
- Your doctor may prescribe: Anticholinesterase drugs to restore normal muscle function. Excessive doses may cause weakness.
  Cortisone drugs at times when the symptoms worsen. Dosage levels start low and are increased gradually to optimal levels.
- *Note:* Adverse reactions and side effects may be more frequent and severe in older persons. Remind your doctor of any medicines you already take.

ACTIVITY FOR OLDER PATIENTS
- No restrictions are necessary. Remain as active as possible.
- See Appendix 20 regarding physical fitness for the active older adult.

FOOD & BEVERAGE
- No special diet is required.
- See Appendix 1 regarding good nutrition for people over 50.

FUTURE CONSIDERATIONS FOR THE AGING ADULT

POSSIBLE COMPLICATIONS
- Choking due to swallowing difficulty.
- Respiratory paralysis.
- Osteoporosis; cataracts; diabetes; infections; high blood pressure; excessive weight gain.

PROBABLE OUTCOME—This condition is currently considered incurable. However, the symptoms can be relieved or controlled. Worsening may be followed by improvement. Life expectancy is reduced, but patients usually live many years with the disease. Scientific research into causes and treatment continues, so there is hope for increasingly effective treatment and a cure.

PREVENTING RECURRENCE—Cannot be prevented at present.

CALL YOUR DOCTOR IF

- You have symptoms of myasthenia gravis.
- You develop swallowing or breathing difficulty. (You should have emergency medications—anticholinesterase drugs—available at all times to use if these symptoms develop.)

MYOCARDITIS

BASIC INFORMATION FOR OLDER ADULTS

DESCRIPTION—Myocarditis is an inflammation of the heart muscle (myocardium) that usually occurs as a complication of underlying illness, such as hypersensitive immune reactions, injury, radiation therapy, infection or toxic reactions to drugs. Body part involved: The heart muscle.

SPECIAL CONSIDERATIONS FOR AGING
- The immune system becomes less effective, opening the way for viral, bacterial and other infections; immune disorders; and allergies.
- Decreased nutrition increases the risk of any disease or disorder.
- Characteristic signs and symptoms of many disorders are frequently changed or absent.

SIGNS & SYMPTOMS
Typical symptoms include:
- Fatigue; shortness of breath.
- Irregular heartbeat.
- Fever; other symptoms caused by the underlying disorder.

If myocarditis causes congestive heart failure, the following symptoms may also occur:
- Swollen feet and ankles.
- Distended neck veins.
- Rapid heartbeat, even when at rest.
- Breathing difficulty while resting or lying down.

CAUSES & RISK FACTORS
Causes include:
- Viral infections, such as measles, influenza or adenovirus; parasite infections.
- Bacterial infections, such as tetanus, gonorrhea, typhoid fever, tuberculosis or diphtheria.
- Heart surgery; rheumatic fever.
- Radiation therapy for cancers in the chest, such as lung or breast cancer.

Risk factors include:
- Excessive alcohol consumption.
- Geographic location. Parasite infections are more common in underdeveloped countries.

DOCTOR'S TREATMENT & DIAGNOSTIC TESTS
- Medical history and physical exam.
- Laboratory blood studies.
- ECG (see Glossary); other studies appropriate for the underlying disorder.
- Self-care instructions focused on the older patient.
- Hospitalization for the underlying disorder (frequently).
- Heart transplantation may be the only effective treatment for some types of myocarditis.

HOME TREATMENT BY SELF OR CARE-GIVER

GENERAL INSTRUCTIONS—During the acute stages, complete rest is required. Obtain complete nursing care, including help with bathing and eating.

MEDICATION (ADJUSTED FOR AGING)
- Your doctor may prescribe:
  Antibiotics to fight infection if the myocarditis is caused by a bacterial infection.
  Cortisone drugs to reduce inflammation.
  Appropriate medications if myocarditis develops into congestive heart failure. These include diuretics to reduce fluid retention, digitalis to stimulate a stronger heartbeat, anticoagulants to prevent clot formation and medications to reduce the heart's workload.
- *Note:* Adverse reactions and side effects may be more frequent and severe in older persons. Remind your doctor of any medicines you already take.

ACTIVITY FOR OLDER PATIENTS
- Rest in bed until the symptoms disappear. Recovery time varies, depending on the underlying cause. You may read or watch TV.
- Use a bedside commode for bowel movements while at complete bed rest. This causes less stress than using a bedpan.
- After recovery, resume your normal activities gradually.
- See Appendix 20 regarding physical fitness for the active older adult.

FOOD & BEVERAGE—Eat a low-salt diet (see Appendix 9).

FUTURE CONSIDERATIONS FOR THE AGING ADULT

POSSIBLE COMPLICATIONS—Even with excellent treatment of the underlying disorder, a few patients develop congestive heart failure; permanent damage to the heart muscle or valves; a blood clot inside the heart muscle that can break away and lodge elsewhere in the body (this may be life-threatening).

PROBABLE OUTCOME—Often curable with detection and treatment of the underlying cause.

PREVENTING RECURRENCE
- Don't drink more than 1 or 2 alcoholic drinks—if any—a day.
- Keep immunizations current against diphtheria, tetanus, measles, German measles and polio. See Appendix 16.

CALL YOUR DOCTOR IF

- You have symptoms of myocarditis.
- Any of the following occurs during treatment:
  Recurrence of fever or chills.
  Increased shortness of breath.
- New, unexplained symptoms develop. The drugs used in treatment may produce side effects.

NAILBED INFECTION
(Paronychia)

BASIC INFORMATION FOR OLDER ADULTS

DESCRIPTION—Paronychia is an inflammation of tissue folds that surround the fingernail or toenail. The inflammation can be bacterial or fungal and is not contagious. Body parts involved: The fingernails or toenails.

SPECIAL CONSIDERATIONS FOR AGING
- The immune system becomes less effective, opening the way for viral, bacterial and other infections; malignancies; immune disorders; and allergies.
- Decreased nutrition, common among chronically ill older people, increases the risk of any disease or disorder.
- The skin's reactions to injury or infection increase in intensity and duration.

SIGNS & SYMPTOMS
Bacterial paronychia:
- Pain or tenderness, redness, warmth and swelling of the tissue adjacent to the nail or nail.
- Central whitish area produced by pus.

Fungal paronychia:
- Redness and swelling around the nail.
- No pain, warmth, itching or pus.

CAUSES & RISK FACTORS—Bacterial
paronychia is preceded by injury, such as a torn hangnail. The infecting germ is usually staphylococcus. Fungal paronychia is caused by a fungus or yeast infection. Risk factors include:
- Injury around the nail.
- Occupational exposure to constant wetness, such as that experienced by dishwashers, bartenders and housewives.
- Poor circulation.
- Diabetes mellitus, psoriasis or eczema.

DOCTOR'S TREATMENT & DIAGNOSTIC TESTS
- Medical history and physical exam.
- Laboratory studies, such as a culture of the discharge, to identify the germ.
- Self-care instructions focused on the older patient.

HOME TREATMENT BY SELF OR CARE-GIVER

GENERAL INSTRUCTIONS
- Wear heavy-duty rubber or vinyl gloves to prevent contact with irritating substances such as water, soap, detergent, metal scrubbing pads, scouring pads, scouring powder and other chemicals.
- Dry the insides of gloves after use. Discard the gloves if they develop holes. A glove with a hole harms the hand more than not wearing a glove.
- Wear gloves when you peel or squeeze lemons, oranges, grapefruit, tomatoes or potatoes.

- Wear leather or heavy-duty fabric gloves for housework or gardening.
- Use a dishwashing machine or ask someone else to wash dishes.
- Avoid contact with irritating chemicals such as paint, paint thinner, turpentine and polish for cars, floors, shoes, furniture or metal.
- Wear rubber sandals in public showers, and wear shoes outdoors.
- Use lukewarm water and very little mild soap to shower or bathe. All soaps are irritating. Expensive soaps offer no more protection against irritation than less expensive ones.
- For bacterial paronychia, apply warm soaks. Dry your hands or feet thoroughly when you are finished.

MEDICATION (ADJUSTED FOR AGING)
- For minor pain, you may use non-prescription drugs such as aspirin or acetaminophen.
- Your doctor may prescribe antibiotics or antifungal medicines (depending on the type of infection).
- *Note:* Adverse reactions and side effects may be more frequent and severe in older persons. Remind your doctor of any medicines you already take.

ACTIVITY FOR OLDER PATIENTS—No
restrictions are necessary.

FOOD & BEVERAGE
- No special diet is required.
- See Appendix 1 regarding good nutrition for people over 50.

FUTURE CONSIDERATIONS FOR THE AGING ADULT

POSSIBLE COMPLICATIONS—If untreated, the disorder may permanently damage the nail and the nail bed and the infection may enter the bones or the bloodstream.

PROBABLE OUTCOME
- Bacterial paronychia is curable with treatment in 2 weeks.
- Fungal paronychia is chronic and may require 6 months to heal.
- Recurrence is common with both forms.

PREVENTING RECURRENCE
- Protect your hands and feet from wetness.
- Leave hangnails alone.
- Avoid injury to the fingertips and toetips.

CALL YOUR DOCTOR IF

- You have symptoms of paronychia.
- A fever develops.
- The pain is not relieved by treatment.

NAIL SPLITTING

BASIC INFORMATION FOR OLDER ADULTS

DESCRIPTION—This disorder is characterized by the splitting of the fingernails and toenails. Body parts involved: The fingernails and toenails.

SPECIAL CONSIDERATIONS FOR AGING—Nails grow more slowly and are thinner, softer and more brittle.

SIGNS & SYMPTOMS—Painless splitting of the nails. Cracks may be parallel to the length of the fingers or toes, or flakes may chip off the ends of the nails.

CAUSES & RISK FACTORS
- Unknown (usually).
- Scar formation from injury to the nail bed (sometimes).
- A family history of nail splitting.
- Iron-deficiency anemia (rare).

DOCTOR'S TREATMENT & DIAGNOSTIC TESTS
- Medical history and physical exam.
- Self-care instructions focused on the older patient.
- Treatment of the diagnosed disorder if the splitting becomes severe.

HOME TREATMENT BY SELF OR CARE-GIVER

GENERAL INSTRUCTIONS
- Apply multiple layers of clear fingernail polish so that cracks, fissures and flakes will be cemented together. This can provide a splint or shield to protect the nails. Nail polishes that contain nylon fibers will thicken and strengthen the nails.
- Don't remove nail polish too often. Polish remover has a drying effect and may increase splitting. Instead, patch chips in the nail polish as they occur.
- Wear rubber gloves with cotton linings for housework that involves water.
- Use a hand cream often. Massage it into the skin around the nails.
- Several options are available to improve the cosmetic appearance of the nails. Check beauty shops, drugstores or cosmetic counters in department stores.

MEDICATION (ADJUSTED FOR AGING)—Medicine is usually not necessary for this disorder.

ACTIVITY FOR OLDER PATIENTS
- No restrictions are necessary.
- See Appendix 20 regarding physical fitness for the active older adult.

FOOD & BEVERAGE
- No special diet is required. Many people say the condition improves if they drink large quantities of liquid containing plain gelatin each day. Evidence does not support this theory.
- See Appendix 1 regarding good nutrition for people over 50.

FUTURE CONSIDERATIONS FOR THE AGING ADULT

POSSIBLE COMPLICATIONS—None are expected.

PROBABLE OUTCOME—Splitting may never disappear completely, but it may improve from time to time.

PREVENTING RECURRENCE—Protect your nails from trauma, especially excessive irritation from soap and water.

CALL YOUR DOCTOR IF

- You have severe nail splitting that has become a problem.
- Self-care produces no improvement in 6 months.

NAILS, RINGWORM INFECTION OF
(Onychomycosis; Tinea Unguium)

BASIC INFORMATION FOR OLDER ADULTS

DESCRIPTION—A ringworm infection of the nails is a fungus infection of the toenails or fingernails in which the nails become pliable, opaque, white and thickened. This is contagious. Body parts involved: The toenails (usually) or fingernails.

SPECIAL CONSIDERATIONS FOR AGING
- The immune system becomes less effective, opening the way for viral, bacterial and other infections; malignancies; immune disorders; and allergies.
- Decreased nutrition, common among chronically ill older people, increases the risk of any disease or disorder.
- Decreased nutrition increases the risk of infections.

SIGNS & SYMPTOMS
- This disorder begins with a small separation between the end of the nail and the nail bed.
- Soft yellow material gradually builds up in the separation.
- The nail becomes thickened and yellow.
- The disorder usually doesn't itch, and it is painless unless the area is extensive and becomes infected.
- Eventually the entire nail is separated, resulting in a partially destroyed, misshapen, yellow nail.

CAUSES & RISK FACTORS—Caused by infection with the trichophyton fungus. Fingernail infections occur only if the nail has been injured or the nail is affected by another skin disease on the hand. Toenail infections can occur with or without injury. Risk factors include:
- Exposure to occupational heat, wetness and humidity, such as that experienced by cooks, dishwashers and housewives.
- Hot, humid weather.
- Poor circulation.
- Diabetes mellitus.

DOCTOR'S TREATMENT & DIAGNOSTIC TESTS
- Medical history and physical exam.
- Laboratory fungal cultures of the material under the nails.
- Self-care instructions focused on the older patient.
- Surgical removal of the nail.

HOME TREATMENT BY SELF OR CARE-GIVER

GENERAL INSTRUCTIONS
- Dry your feet and hands with extra care after bathing—even after the infection clears.
- Wear light footwear, such as sandals, to allow free air circulation. Don't wear socks or shoes made of synthetic materials. During acute phases, go barefoot as much as possible. Keep your feet and hands cool, dry and exposed to sunlight.
- Wear cotton-lined latex or rubber gloves for dishwashing or other cleaning jobs that require the immersion of the hands in water or chemicals.

MEDICATION (ADJUSTED FOR AGING)
- Non-prescription antifungal ointments, creams and powders are available, but they are ineffective in curing these infections. Your doctor may prescribe oral antifungal drugs to cure the infection, but therapy may be long and expensive.
- *Note:* Adverse reactions and side effects may be more frequent and severe in older persons. Remind your doctor of any medicines you already take.

ACTIVITY FOR OLDER PATIENTS
- No restrictions are necessary, but avoid heat and excessive sweating.
- See Appendix 20 regarding physical fitness for the active older adult.

FOOD & BEVERAGE
- No special diet is required.
- See Appendix 1 regarding good nutrition for people over 50.

FUTURE CONSIDERATIONS FOR THE AGING ADULT

POSSIBLE COMPLICATIONS—Permanent nail loss or deformity.

PROBABLE OUTCOME—Most fingernail infections are curable with 6 months of continuous treatment. Toenails require 12 to 24 months of treatment because of their slower growth rate. Most fingernail infections respond well to treatment, but toenail infections are more resistant to treatment. Recurrence is likely.

PREVENTING RECURRENCE
- Keep your feet cool, dry and exposed to sunlight as much as possible.
- Wear cotton or wool socks. Avoid footwear made from synthetic fibers.
- Wear roomy shoes.

CALL YOUR DOCTOR IF

- You have a minor nail infection that becomes a problem.
- The symptoms fail to improve after 2 weeks of medication.
- The skin adjacent to the nail becomes red of inflamed or drains pus.
- New, unexplained symptoms develop. The drugs used in treatment may produce side effects.

NARCOLEPSY

 ## BASIC INFORMATION FOR OLDER ADULTS

DESCRIPTION—Narcolepsy is a rare sleep disorder characterized by uncontrollable episodes of falling asleep at any place or time. After a 10- or 15-minute sleep attack, the person feels rested only briefly, then returns to an uncomfortable feeling of sleepiness. Attacks may occur while driving, talking or working. Body part involved: The central nervous system.

SPECIAL CONSIDERATIONS FOR AGING
- Neurological diseases become more likely.
- Nerve cells in aging people are especially susceptible to the action of drugs—particularly mind-altering drugs such as narcotics, alcohol, sleep inducers, pain killers, antihistamines, muscle relaxants, antinausea medications and others.

SIGNS & SYMPTOMS—Any of the following (10% of people with narcolepsy have all signs):
- Sleep attacks that may occur up to 10 times a day. These can occur during conversations or other activities. An attack leaves the person feeling refreshed, but another may occur again quickly.
- Vivid dreams, sounds or hallucinations at the beginning of a sleep attack or upon awakening.
- Temporary paralysis (sudden loss of muscle strength) when one is falling asleep or just before complete awakening.
- Momentary paralysis that is not related to sleep when one is feeling sudden emotion, such as anger, fear or joy.
- Irresistible drowsiness during the day.

CAUSES & RISK FACTORS—The cause is unknown. Occasionally it follows a brain infection or a head injury. Risk factors include a a family history of narcolepsy. Either of the following may trigger an attack:
- Monotonous activity.
- Prolonged laughter.

DOCTOR'S TREATMENT & DIAGNOSTIC TESTS
- Medical history and physical exam.
- EEG (see Glossary).
- Studies performed in a sleep laboratory.
- Self-care instructions focused on the older patient.

 ## HOME TREATMENT BY SELF OR CARE-GIVER

GENERAL INSTRUCTIONS—Wear a Medic Alert bracelet or pendant (see Glossary).

MEDICATION (ADJUSTED FOR AGING)
- Your doctor may prescribe stimulants or antidepressants (but not both).
- *Note:* Adverse reactions and side effects may be more frequent and severe in older persons. Remind your doctor of any medicines you already take.

ACTIVITY FOR OLDER PATIENTS
- Don't engage in any activity that carries the risk of injury from a sudden sleep attack. These include activities such as driving long distances, climbing ladders or working around dangerous machinery.
- Regularly scheduled naps may be helpful.
- See Appendix 20 regarding physical fitness for the active older adult.

FOOD & BEVERAGE
- No special diet is required.
- See Appendix 1 regarding good nutrition for people over 50.

 ## FUTURE CONSIDERATIONS FOR THE AGING ADULT

POSSIBLE COMPLICATIONS—Accidental injury during a sudden sleep attack.

PROBABLE OUTCOME—This disorder lasts throughout life, but it has no effect on life expectancy. Medication can decrease the frequency of sleep attacks.

PREVENTING RECURRENCE—You can reduce the frequency of attacks by avoiding the risk factors listed above if possible.

 ## CALL YOUR DOCTOR IF

- You have symptoms of narcolepsy.
- New, unexplained symptoms develop. The drugs used in treatment may produce side effects.

NASAL ALLERGY
(Hay Fever; Allergic Rhinitis)

BASIC INFORMATION FOR OLDER ADULTS

DESCRIPTION—Hay fever is an allergic response to airborne allergens that affects the eyes and upper respiratory tract. Body parts involved: The nose; eyes; sinuses; throat; mouth; lungs.

SPECIAL CONSIDERATIONS FOR AGING
- The immune system becomes less effective, opening the way for viral, bacterial and other infections; immune disorders; and allergies.
- Characteristic signs and symptoms of many disorders are frequently changed or absent.
- Stress from any emotional cause affects all aspects of any illness or disorder.

SIGNS & SYMPTOMS
- Itching, watery eyes.
- Frequent sneezing in sudden attacks; stuffy nose with a clear, watery discharge.
- Itching in the roof of the mouth.
- Wheezing (sometimes).
- Sore throat (sometimes).
- Headaches (worse at night).

CAUSES & RISK FACTORS—Caused by an allergic sensitivity to airborne allergens such as:
- Pollen from weeds, flowers, grasses and trees (seasonal).
- Mold; dust; mites; dog or cat hair.
- Tobacco smoke and other air pollutants.
Risk factors include:
- A medical history of allergic reactions, such as eczema or asthma; smoking.
- Spring and autumn. Most plants produce pollen during these seasons.

DOCTOR'S TREATMENT & DIAGNOSTIC TESTS
- Medical history and physical exam.
- Laboratory tests such as a blood count and allergy skin tests (see Glossary).
- Self-care instructions focused on the older patient.

HOME TREATMENT BY SELF OR CARE-GIVER

GENERAL INSTRUCTIONS—Eliminate as many allergens from your environment as possible. Prepare your bedroom and other rooms as follows:
- Empty the room of furniture, rugs or carpet and drapes or curtains.
- Clean the walls, woodwork and floors with a damp mop. Wax the floor.
- Take the mattress and box springs outside and vacuum or clean them.
- Cover the box springs, mattress and pillows with plastic covers.
- Use only rugs that can be washed once a week.
- Use bedclothes that can be washed often,

such as cotton sheets, washable mattress pads and synthetic fiber blankets. Don't use chenille bedspreads, quilts or comforters.
- Use wood or plastic chairs. Don't use stuffed chairs.
- Use plastic curtains or blinds if possible. Dust them daily.
- Use a vacuum cleaner, damp rags and a damp or oiled mop to clean the bedroom thoroughly once a week.
- Keep windows and doors closed as much as possible.
- Don't handle objects that are very dusty, such as books or stored clothing.
- Don't keep stuffed animals or toys in the house.
- Remove *all pets* (except fish) from the house.

MEDICATION (ADJUSTED FOR AGING)—To reduce the body's allergic response, your doctor may prescribe:
- Antihistamines; decongestants; cortisone eye drops or nasal spray; cortisone tablets (severe cases only); cromolyn nasal spray; cromolyn nose and eye drops. These medications relieve the symptoms, but they don't cure hay fever. Some of them cause drowsiness; be sure you know the side effects.
- Desensitization injections for known allergens for severe or year-round cases.

ACTIVITY FOR OLDER PATIENTS—No restrictions are necessary.

FOOD & BEVERAGE—Avoid foods that cause allergic reactions.

FUTURE CONSIDERATIONS FOR THE AGING ADULT

POSSIBLE COMPLICATIONS—Sleeping difficulty and chronic fatigue; sinus infection.

PROBABLE OUTCOME—The symptoms can be controlled with treatment.

PREVENTING RECURRENCE
- Change furnace or air conditioner filters often.
- Wear a filter face mask during exposure to allergens.
- Install an air purification unit in your home's heating and air conditioning system.

CALL YOUR DOCTOR IF

- You have severe symptoms of nasal allergy that are interfering with your normal activities.
- Signs of infection appear, such as fever, headache, muscle aches or thick, discolored nasal discharge. A sinus infection may be complicating the allergy.
- New, unexplained symptoms develop. Drugs used in treatment may produce side effects.

BASIC INFORMATION FOR OLDER ADULTS

DESCRIPTION—Nasal polyps are non-malignant growths in the nasal cavities, usually in both sides of the nose. Body parts involved: The nasal mucous membranes.

SPECIAL CONSIDERATIONS FOR AGING
- The immune system becomes less effective, opening the way for viral, bacterial and other infections; malignancies; immune disorders; and allergies.
- Decreased nutrition, common among chronically ill older people, increases the risk of any disease or disorder.
- Characteristic signs and symptoms of many disorders are frequently changed or absent.

SIGNS & SYMPTOMS
- A chronic "stuffy nose" feeling due to the obstruction of the air's passage through the nose.
- An impaired sense of smell.
- Feelings of fullness in the face.
- Nasal discharge (sometimes).
- Facial pain (sometimes).
- Headaches (sometimes).

CAUSES & RISK FACTORS—Caused by
chronic infection or allergy in the nose (allergic rhinitis) that makes the nasal mucous membranes swell and produce excess fluid in the nasal cells. The risk increases with sinusitis or chronic nasal infection.

DOCTOR'S TREATMENT & DIAGNOSTIC TESTS
- Medical history and physical exam.
- Laboratory skin tests to identify allergies.
- Self-care instructions focused on the older patient.
- Surgery to remove polyps under local anesthesia—a minor surgical procedure. Advancing age alone is not a deterrent.

HOME TREATMENT BY SELF OR CARE-GIVER

GENERAL INSTRUCTIONS—If nosebleeds occur, see the treatment described under Nosebleed in the Illnesses section.

MEDICATION (ADJUSTED FOR AGING)
- For minor pain, you may use acetaminophen. Avoid aspirin, which may increase the tendency to bleed and may cause an allergic reaction.
- Your doctor may prescribe cortisone drugs or cromolyn in nasal spray or oral form for a short while before surgery to shrink the polyps.
- *Caution:* Don't use over-the-counter nasal sprays.
- *Note:* Adverse reactions and side effects may be more frequent and severe in older persons. Remind your doctor of any medicines you already take.

ACTIVITY FOR OLDER PATIENTS
- Resume your normal activities gradually after surgery.
- See Appendix 20 regarding physical fitness for the active older adult.

FOOD & BEVERAGE
- No special diet is required.
- See Appendix 1 regarding good nutrition for people over 50.

FUTURE CONSIDERATIONS FOR THE AGING ADULT

POSSIBLE COMPLICATIONS
- Repeated infections.
- Nosebleeds.

PROBABLE OUTCOME—The symptoms can be controlled with treatment (usually surgery). Recurrence was once common, even with surgical treatment, but improved techniques are making this less likely.

PREVENTING RECURRENCE—Obtain medical treatment for the underlying allergy. Consult your doctor about allergy testing and desensitizing procedures.

CALL YOUR DOCTOR IF

- You have symptoms of nasal polyps.
- Any of the following occurs during treatment:
  Nosebleeds that cannot be stopped.
  Fever.
  Pain that persists despite the use of acetaminophen.

NOSE FRACTURE

BASIC INFORMATION FOR OLDER ADULTS

DESCRIPTION—A nose fracture is a fracture or damage to the bones and cartilage of the nose. This often happens when other facial bones are also fractured. Body part involved: The nose.

SPECIAL CONSIDERATIONS FOR AGING
- Bone strength lessens.
- The nasal mucous membrane becomes thinner and less elastic.

SIGNS & SYMPTOMS
- Pain in the nose.
- Nosebleed.
- A swollen, discolored nose.
- Inability to breathe through the nose.
- A crooked or misshapen nose (sometimes).

CAUSES & RISK FACTORS—Caused by an injury to the nose. The risk increases with a previous nose injury.

DOCTOR'S TREATMENT & DIAGNOSTIC TESTS
- Medical history and physical exam.
- Laboratory blood tests if bleeding is heavy.
- X-ray of the nose.
- After diagnosis of minor injuries, self-care instructions focused on the older patient.
- Emergency-room treatment for heavy bleeding.
- Surgery if the nose is crooked or breathing is impaired.

HOME TREATMENT BY SELF OR CARE-GIVER

GENERAL INSTRUCTIONS
- Apply ice packs to the nose immediately after injury to minimize swelling.
- If the nosebleed is heavy or cannot be stopped, obtain emergency medical treatment.

MEDICATION (ADJUSTED FOR AGING)
- For minor discomfort, you may use non-prescription drugs such as acetaminophen.
- Your doctor may prescribe:
  Stronger pain relievers if needed.
  Antibiotics if infection develops.
- *Note:* Adverse reactions and side effects may be more frequent and severe in older persons. Remind your doctor of any medicines you already take.

ACTIVITY FOR OLDER PATIENTS
- Rest until any bleeding stops.
- See Appendix 20 regarding physical fitness for the active older adult.

FOOD & BEVERAGE
- No special diet is required.
- See Appendix 1 regarding good nutrition for people over 50.

FUTURE CONSIDERATIONS FOR THE AGING ADULT

POSSIBLE COMPLICATIONS
- Infection of the nose and sinuses.
- Shock from loss of blood (rare).
- Permanent breathing difficulty.
- Permanent change in appearance.
- Deviated nasal septum.

PROBABLE OUTCOME—Minor fractures with no deformity usually heal in 4 weeks. Major fractures can be repaired with surgery. If surgery is necessary, it should be done within 2 weeks or not until 6 months after injury.

PREVENTING RECURRENCE—Protect your nose from injury whenever possible. Wear protective headgear when riding a bicycle or motorcycle. Wear auto seat belts.

CALL YOUR DOCTOR IF

- You have symptoms of a fractured nose, especially bleeding that is heavy or cannot be stopped.
- You have had a fractured nose and think surgery is needed.

NOSEBLEED
(Epistaxis)

BASIC INFORMATION FOR OLDER ADULTS

DESCRIPTION—Epistaxis is bleeding from the nose. Body parts involved: The blood vessels (arteries and veins) in the nose. Nosebleeds occur close to the nasal opening or deeper in the nose.

SPECIAL CONSIDERATIONS FOR AGING
- The nasal mucous membrane becomes thinner and less elastic.
- The immune system becomes less effective, opening the way for infections and allergies.
- The walls of the veins become thinner.

SIGNS & SYMPTOMS
- Blood oozing from a nostril. If the nosebleed is close to the nostril, the blood is bright red. If the nosebleed is deeper in the nose, the blood may be bright or dark.
- Lightheadedness from the loss of a large amount of blood.
- Rapid heartbeat, shortness of breath and pallor (with significant blood loss only).
- Black stool from swallowed blood.

CAUSES & RISK FACTORS
Causes include:
- An injury to the nose or nasal polyps—even simple injury caused by picking the nose.
- A nasal or sinus infection.
- A foreign body in the nose.
- Scarlet fever, malaria or typhoid fever.
- Dry mucous membranes in the nose from any cause, such as low humidity.
- Atherosclerosis; high blood pressure.
- Bleeding tendencies associated with aplastic anemia, leukemia, thrombocytopenia or liver disease.

Risk factors include:
- Any disorder listed as a cause.
- Hodgkin's disease; scurvy; rheumatic fever.
- Blood disorders, including leukemia and hemophilia.
- The use of certain drugs, such as anticoagulants or aspirin, or the prolonged use of nose drops.
- Exposure to irritating chemicals.
- High altitude or dry climate.

DOCTOR'S TREATMENT & DIAGNOSTIC TESTS
- Medical history and physical exam.
- Laboratory blood studies.
- Self-care instructions focused on the older patient.
- Doctor's treatment or emergency room treatment if self-care is unsuccessful. Gauze packing may be inserted to absorb blood, stop dripping and exert pressure on the ruptured blood vessels. Continued or recurrent bleeding may require cauterization (see Glossary).
- Surgery (for severe bleeding only) to tie off the artery feeding the bleeding area.

HOME TREATMENT BY SELF OR CARE-GIVER

GENERAL INSTRUCTIONS
- Sit up with your head bent forward.
- Pinch your nose closed with your fingers for 5 uninterrupted minutes. During this time, breathe through your mouth.
- If the bleeding stops and then recurs, pinch your nose firmly on both sides for 8 to 10 minutes. Holding your nose tightly closed allows the blood to clot and seal the damaged blood vessels. You may apply cold compresses at the same time.
- Don't blow your nose for 12 hours after the bleeding stops to avoid dislodging the blood clot.
- Don't swallow the blood. It may upset your stomach or make you "gag," causing you to inhale blood.
- Don't talk (also to avoid gagging).

MEDICATION (ADJUSTED FOR AGING)—Your doctor may prescribe drugs to treat any underlying serious disorder.

ACTIVITY FOR OLDER PATIENTS—Resume your normal activities as soon as your symptoms improve.

FOOD & BEVERAGE—No special diet.

FUTURE CONSIDERATIONS FOR THE AGING ADULT

POSSIBLE COMPLICATIONS—Bleeding severe enough to require transfusion.

PROBABLE OUTCOME—The symptoms can be controlled with treatment. Severe bleeding requires hospitalization. It is usually caused by an underlying disorder, such as liver disease, blood disease or hypertension, which should also be treated.

PREVENTING RECURRENCE
- Avoid injury if possible.
- Obtain medical treatment for the underlying cause.
- Humidify the air if you live in a dry climate or at high altitude.
- Avoid picking or blowing your nose.
- Avoid aspirin if you have frequent nosebleeds.

CALL YOUR DOCTOR IF

- You have a nosebleed that won't stop with the self-care instructions described above.
- After the nosebleed, you become nauseous or vomit.
- After the nose has been packed, your temperature rises to 101F (38.3C) or higher.

OBESITY

BASIC INFORMATION FOR OLDER ADULTS

DESCRIPTION—Obesity is the storage of excess fat in the body. A person is considered obese if his or her body weight is 20% or more above a desirable weight. Body parts involved: The total body.

SPECIAL CONSIDERATIONS FOR AGING
- Physical activity tends to decrease.
- Stress from any emotional cause affects all aspects of any illness or disorder.

SIGNS & SYMPTOMS—Over 25% body fat composition in women, over 20% in men. Most obese persons have no symptoms except associated emotional problems and poor exercise tolerance. Excess weight increases the heart's work.

CAUSES & RISK FACTORS
Causes include:
- Eating more food than the body can use (the most common cause). Any excess is converted to fat and is stored. One pound of fat represents about 3,500 excess calories, depending on individual metabolism.
- Diseases of the central nervous system, such as a brain tumor or stroke (rare).
- Disorders of the endocrine glands (rare).
Risk factors include:
- Excessive alcohol consumption.
- Genetic factors. Some people remain thin despite a large food intake.
- A decrease in exercise with no corresponding decrease in food intake.
- Stress, depression, nervous tension, boredom, frustration or dissatisfaction.
- Poor eating habits learned in childhood.

DOCTOR'S TREATMENT & DIAGNOSTIC TESTS
- Medical history and physical exam.
- Laboratory blood studies of endocrine function.
- Self-care instructions focused on the older patient.
- Psychotherapy or counseling.
- Surgical procedures to reduce weight, such as bypassing part of the intestine or stomach, cutting away fat, fat suctioning or wiring the jaw shut, are desperate measures. They are used only in extreme circumstances.

HOME TREATMENT BY SELF OR CARE-GIVER

GENERAL INSTRUCTIONS
- See Food & Beverage.
- Join a support group for overweight persons. Many people find it easier to follow a reduction diet and exercise program if they join a group of people with similar problems.

MEDICATION (ADJUSTED FOR AGING)—Most doctors don't recommend medication to aid weight loss. Medications often cause harmful side effects or adverse reactions. At best, they control appetite only for short time periods and don't help you change your eating habits.

ACTIVITY FOR OLDER PATIENTS—Increase your level of activity. Daily exercise (bicycle riding, walking, swimming and others) helps you lose weight, feel better and control your appetite. See Appendix 20.

FOOD & BEVERAGE
- See Appendix 10 for a reducing diet. This diet is varied and balanced. Choose foods you like so you can establish eating patterns you can maintain indefinitely.
- Some nutritionists suggest eating 4 or 5 small meals a day rather than 3. Skipping meals does not help you lose weight in the long run.
- Diets that are not nutritionally balanced can cause more problems than the obesity. Crash diets and fad diets don't produce long-term results. Schemes which promise easy weight loss are usually unsuccessful.
- During your diet and exercise program, there may be periods when you don't lose weight. This is normal; don't stop the program. Weight loss will begin again in a week or two.
- A realistic weight loss is 1 to 2-1/2 pounds a week. This may seem slow, but 1 pound of fat lost per week totals 52 pounds in 1 year!

FUTURE CONSIDERATIONS FOR THE AGING ADULT

POSSIBLE COMPLICATIONS
- Obesity may contribute to the development of diabetes, high blood pressure, heart disease and gallbladder disease. It complicates the treatment and decreases the chances of survival of patients with stroke, kidney disease and other disorders.
- Extra weight also places strain on the knees and the back.
- Obese women are more prone to cancer of the breast, cervix and uterus.
- Obese men run an increased risk of cancer of the colon, rectum and prostate.

PROBABLE OUTCOME—Obesity can be controlled if your motivation stays high for life.

PREVENTING RECURRENCE
- Avoid a sedentary lifestyle. Exercise daily or at least 3 times a week.
- Eat less food that is high in fat and sugar. Concentrate on not gaining weight rather than on gaining and then reducing.
- Limit your alcohol consumption to 1 or 2 drinks a day—if any.

CALL YOUR DOCTOR IF

Your weight increases despite self-help.

OBSTRUCTIVE PULMONARY DISEASE, CHRONIC
(COPD; Cor Pulmonale; Pulmonary Hypertension)

BASIC INFORMATION FOR OLDER ADULTS

DESCRIPTION—Chronic obstructive pulmonary disease (COPD) is congestive heart failure resulting from raised blood pressure in the lungs. This is a complication of disorders that slow or block the blood flow in the lungs. Body parts involved: The lungs, heart and blood vessels.

SPECIAL CONSIDERATIONS FOR AGING
- Characteristic signs and symptoms of many disorders are frequently changed or absent.
- Obstruction of the airways becomes more common, especially among people who have smoked tobacco for many years.
- The chest muscles used for breathing become weaker.

SIGNS & SYMPTOMS
Early stages:
- No symptoms (usually).

Later stages:
- Weakness and fatigue.
- Shortness of breath with exertion.
- Frequent fainting.
- Swelling of the ankles and feet caused by fluid retention.
- Distended neck veins.
- Bluish skin.
- Chest pain.
- Enlarged liver and swollen abdomen.

CAUSES & RISK FACTORS
Causes include:
- Severe chronic obstructive lung disease, such as emphysema, recurrent pneumonia, bronchiectasis, silicosis, lung cancer, tuberculosis or collagen diseases.
- Small blood clots that travel to the lung from another body site—usually a deep vein in the calf of the leg—and obstruct the blood vessels in the lung.
- Primary diseases of the heart, including rheumatic heart disease and congenital heart disease.

Risk factors include:
- Prolonged bed rest for any illness. This increases the chance of blood clot formation.
- Smoking.

DOCTOR'S TREATMENT & DIAGNOSTIC TESTS
- Medical history and physical exam.
- Laboratory studies of blood and lung function.
- X-rays of the lungs.
- Surgery to correct problems caused by congenital or acquired disorders, such as replacing damaged heart valves (sometimes). Advancing age alone is not a deterrent.
- Self-care instructions focused on the older patient.

HOME TREATMENT BY SELF OR CARE-GIVER

GENERAL INSTRUCTIONS
- You may need oxygen. Your doctor or an oxygen therapist can arrange for the type of oxygen that allows you to be up and about.
- Weigh daily and keep a record. Any sudden increase may indicate increased fluid retention.

MEDICATION (ADJUSTED FOR AGING)—
Your doctor may prescribe:
- Diuretics to prevent fluid accumulation.
- Digitalis to strengthen the force of the heart muscle's contractions.
- Antibiotics for recurrent infections.

ACTIVITY FOR OLDER PATIENTS—No restrictions are necessary. Be as active as your condition allows, but don't overexert. Rest between activities.

FOOD & BEVERAGE—Eat a diet that is low in salt (see Appendix 9).

FUTURE CONSIDERATIONS FOR THE AGING ADULT

POSSIBLE COMPLICATIONS—Irreversible congestive heart failure and death.

PROBABLE OUTCOME—This condition is currently considered incurable by time or medical means. Many persons live 10 or 15 years after diagnosis, but disability will slowly increase. However, the symptoms can be relieved or controlled. Lung transplants may be curative. Scientific research into causes and treatment continues, so there is hope for increasingly effective treatment and a cure.

PREVENTING RECURRENCE
- Don't smoke.
- Obtain regular medical treatment for any underlying disorder that can be corrected with surgery or medical treatment.

CALL YOUR DOCTOR IF

- You have symptoms of chronic obstructive pulmonary disease.
- Any of the following occurs during treatment:
  A temperature of 101F (38.3C) or higher.
  A weight gain of 3 to 4 pounds in 1 or 2 days.
  Increased shortness of breath.
  Increased swelling of the ankles.
  A cough with sputum that is discolored or tinged with blood.

ORAL CANCER

BASIC INFORMATION FOR OLDER ADULTS

DESCRIPTION—Oral cancer is a growth of malignant cells in the mouth or tongue. These are rare but dangerous. Any sore, ulcer or lump in the mouth which doesn't heal in 2 weeks should be examined by a doctor. Body parts involved: The lips; gums; palate; tongue; membranes inside the lip or cheek; floor of the mouth; tonsillar area.

SPECIAL CONSIDERATIONS FOR AGING
- Malignant diseases are less likely to spread rapidly.
- The oral mucous membrane becomes thinner and less elastic.
- Stress from any emotional cause—fear, worry, anxiety, sadness, loneliness or anger—affects all aspects of any illness or disorder.

SIGNS & SYMPTOMS—A pale lump—usually painless—with a hard rim that appears in any part of the mouth or tongue. It has the following characteristics:
- It enlarges, ulcerates and bleeds easily.
- It may prevent dentures from fitting properly.
- It may make the tongue stiff and difficult to control, causing speaking and swallowing difficulty.

CAUSES & RISK FACTORS—The cause is unknown. The risk increases with:
- The use of tobacco in any form.
- A family history of oral cancer.
- A past history of oral cancer.
- Heavy alcohol consumption.
- Poor oral hygiene.
- Ill-fitting dentures or jagged teeth.

DOCTOR'S TREATMENT & DIAGNOSTIC TESTS
- Medical history and physical exam.
- Laboratory blood studies.
- Biopsy (see Glossary) of the lump.
- X-rays of the head.
- Self-care instructions focused on the older patient.
- Surgery to remove the cancerous area. Advancing age alone is not a deterrent.
- Reconstructive surgery may be necessary if facial disfigurement results.
- Radiation therapy.
- Speech therapy if surgery impairs speech.

HOME TREATMENT BY SELF OR CARE-GIVER

GENERAL INSTRUCTIONS
- After surgery, cleanse the mouth 3 to 4 times a day with a soothing salt-water solution (1 teaspoon salt to 8 oz. warm water).

- Oral cancer is a complicated, serious disorder. This page can cover only the main points of diagnosis and treatment. Your doctor, nurse or librarian can provide sources of supplemental information.

MEDICATION (ADJUSTED FOR AGING)
- Your doctor may prescribe:
  Anticancer drugs.
  Pain relievers after surgery.
  Antibiotics if infection coexists.
- *Note:* Adverse reactions and side effects may be more frequent and severe in older persons. Remind your doctor of any medicines you already take.

ACTIVITY FOR OLDER PATIENTS
- Resume your normal activities gradually after surgery.
- See Appendix 20 regarding physical fitness for the active older adult.

FOOD & BEVERAGE
- No special diet is required after recovery. A liquid diet may be necessary for several days after surgery.
- See Appendix 1 regarding good nutrition for people over 50.

FUTURE CONSIDERATIONS FOR THE AGING ADULT

POSSIBLE COMPLICATIONS
- Slow healing after surgery.
- Spread to lymph nodes in the neck, requiring radical head and neck surgery.
- Permanent disfigurement.
- Permanent speech impairment.

PROBABLE OUTCOME—Usually curable with early detection and treatment. Normal facial appearance can often be restored by plastic surgery.

PREVENTING RECURRENCE—Don't use tobacco.

CALL YOUR DOCTOR IF

- You have signs of a mouth or tongue tumor.
- Any of the following occurs after surgery:
  Increasing pain.
  Fever.
  New lumps.
  Excessive bleeding.

OSTEOARTHRITIS
(Degenerative Joint Disease; Hypertrophic Arthritis)

BASIC INFORMATION FOR OLDER ADULTS

DESCRIPTION—Osteoarthritis is characterized by the degeneration of cartilage at a joint and the growth of bone "spurs" that inflame the surrounding tissue. Body parts involved: All joints, but most commonly those of the fingers, feet, knees, hips and spine.

SPECIAL CONSIDERATIONS FOR AGING
- Years of weight bearing and work cause wear and tear on bones, ligaments and joints.
- The total weight and density of bone decrease.

SIGNS & SYMPTOMS
- Joint stiffness and pain, including backache. Weather changes—especially cold, damp weather—may increase aching.
- Limited movement and loss of dexterity in the affected joints; no redness, heat or fever in the affected joints (usually).
- Swelling of the affected joints (sometimes), especially the finger joints; cracking or grating sounds with joint movement (sometimes).

CAUSES & RISK FACTORS
Causes include:
- Stress on the joints caused by activity and aging (almost all people over age 50 have some osteoarthritis); injury to the joint linings.
Risk factors include:
- Poor posture; obesity.
- Occupations that stress the joints, such as dancing; football playing; needlework.
- Diseases such as diabetes mellitus and other joint disorders.

DOCTOR'S TREATMENT & DIAGNOSTIC TESTS
- Medical history and physical exam.
- Laboratory blood studies to rule out inflammatory forms of arthritis.
- X-rays of painful joints.
- Self-care instructions focused on the older patient.
- Physical therapy for muscle and joint rehabilitation; acupuncture (sometimes).
- Arthroscopic surgery (sometimes).
- Joint replacement arthroplasty. Replacement surgery is available for joints in the hip, knee, shoulder, elbow, wrist, finger, toe and ankle.
- Arthrodesis surgery to immobilize the joint.

HOME TREATMENT BY SELF OR CARE-GIVER

GENERAL INSTRUCTIONS
- To relieve the pain, apply heat to painful and stiff joints for 20 minutes 2 or 3 times a day. Use hot towels, hot tubs, infrared heat lamps, electric heating pads or deep-heating ointments or lotions. Swim often in a heated pool or move around in a whirlpool spa.
- If osteoarthritis of the neck causes pain in the arms, wear a soft, immobilizing collar (a Thomas collar). If this isn't helpful, buy or rent a neck traction device for home use.
- For pain in the back, a special corset can be worn. Ask your doctor about this possibility.
- Massage the muscles around painful joints. Massaging the joint itself is not helpful.
- If osteoarthritis affects the spine, sleep on your back on a very firm mattress or place 3/4-inch plywood between your box springs and mattress. Waterbeds help some people.
- Avoid chilling. Wear thermal underwear or avoid outdoor activity in cold weather.
- Consider moving to a warm, dry climate, such as southwest desert areas of the U.S.
- Keep a positive outlook on life. Don't think of yourself as an invalid. Remain active to prevent wasting of the muscles.

MEDICATION (ADJUSTED FOR AGING)
- Your doctor may prescribe:
  Aspirin or other non-steroidal anti-inflammatory drugs.
  Cortisone injections into painful, stiff joints. These may provide temporary relief.
- Don't take oral cortisone drugs. They are not effective for long-term relief and have many harmful side effects.

ACTIVITY FOR OLDER PATIENTS
- Rest is important only during acute phases of the disease when joints are very painful. Resume your normal activity as soon as your symptoms improve.
- Follow physical therapy guidelines recommended by your doctor or physical therapist.

FOOD & BEVERAGE—If you are overweight, lose weight. A reducing diet appears in Appendix 10.

FUTURE CONSIDERATIONS FOR THE AGING ADULT

POSSIBLE COMPLICATIONS—Crippling (sometimes); the muscles around the affected joints may become smaller and weaker because of decreased use due to pain.

PROBABLE OUTCOME—The symptoms can usually be relieved, but the joint changes are permanent. The pain may begin as a minor irritant, but it can become severe enough to interfere with daily activities and sleep. As degeneration occurs, the pain may decrease.

PREVENTING RECURRENCE—Maintain a normal weight; be physically active, but avoid activities that lead to joint injury (try regular stretching or yoga exercises).

CALL YOUR DOCTOR IF

- You have joint pain or stiffness.
- New, unexplained symptoms develop. The drugs used in treatment may produce side effects.

OSTEOMYELITIS

BASIC INFORMATION FOR OLDER ADULTS

DESCRIPTION—Osteomyelitis is an infection of the bone and bone marrow. It may be acute or chronic. Body parts involved: Any bone in the body. Among older adults, the pelvis or spine is usually affected.

SPECIAL CONSIDERATIONS FOR AGING
- Decreased nutrition, common among chronically ill older people, increases the risk of any disease or disorder.
- The immune system becomes less effective, opening the way for viral, bacterial and other infections; malignancies; immune disorders; and allergies.

SIGNS & SYMPTOMS
- Fever. Sometimes this is the only symptom.
- Pain, swelling, redness, warmth and tenderness in the area over the infected bone, especially when moving a nearby joint. Nearby joints—especially the knee—may also be red, warm and swollen.
- Pus drainage through a skin abscess, without fever or severe pain (in chronic osteomyelitis only).
- A general ill feeling.

CAUSES & RISK FACTORS—Usually caused by a staphylococcal infection, but many other bacteria may be responsible. The bacteria may spread to the bone through the bloodstream in the following ways:
- A compound fracture or other injury.
- A boil, carbuncle or any break in the skin.
- A middle ear infection.
- Pneumonia.
- Infection following an operation.

Risk factors include:
- Illness that has lowered resistance.
- Radiotherapy.
- Diabetes mellitus; atherosclerosis; heart disease; tuberculosis.

DOCTOR'S TREATMENT & DIAGNOSTIC TESTS
- Medical history and physical exam.
- Laboratory blood studies and blood cultures to identify the bacteria.
- X-rays of the bone. X-rays often don't show changes until 2 to 3 weeks after the infection begins.
- CT scan (see Glossary).
- Hospitalization for surgery to drain abscesses or to remove pockets of infected bone and to administer high doses of antibiotics—sometimes intravenously.
- Chronic osteomyelitis may require surgery to remove the affected bone, followed by a bone graft to replace it.
- Self-care instructions focused on the older patient.

HOME TREATMENT BY SELF OR CARE-GIVER

GENERAL INSTRUCTIONS
- Wear sterile gloves to change dressings.
- Keep the involved limb level or slightly elevated and immobilized with pillows. Don't let it dangle.
- Keep unaffected parts of the body as active as possible to prevent pressure sores during required prolonged bed rest.

MEDICATION (ADJUSTED FOR AGING)—Your doctor may prescribe:
- Large doses of antibiotics. With powerful new antibiotics, intravenous administration, once a necessity, may no longer be needed. Antibiotics may be necessary—either orally or by injection—for 8 to 10 weeks.
- Pain relievers.
- Laxatives if constipation develops during prolonged bed rest.

ACTIVITY FOR OLDER PATIENTS—Rest in bed until 2 to 3 weeks after the symptoms disappear. Resume your normal activities gradually.

FOOD & BEVERAGE
- No special diet is required. Eat heartily. Take vitamin and mineral supplements.
- See Appendix 1 regarding good nutrition for people over 50.

FUTURE CONSIDERATIONS FOR THE AGING ADULT

POSSIBLE COMPLICATIONS
- An abscess that breaks through the skin and won't heal until the underlying bone heals.
- Permanent stiffness in a nearby joint (rare).
- Blood poisoning that makes amputation necessary (rare).

PROBABLE OUTCOME—Usually curable with prompt and aggressive treatment.

PREVENTING RECURRENCE—Obtain prompt medical treatment of any bacterial infection to prevent its spread to the bones or other body parts.

CALL YOUR DOCTOR IF

- You have symptoms of osteomyelitis.
- Any of the following occurs during treatment: An abscess forms over the infected bone or drainage from an existing abscess increases. A fever develops.
  The pain becomes intolerable.
- New, unexplained symptoms develop. The drugs used in treatment may produce side effects.

OSTEOPOROSIS

BASIC INFORMATION FOR OLDER ADULTS

DESCRIPTION—Osteoporosis is a loss of normal bone density, mass and strength, leading to increased porousness and vulnerability to fracture. Osteoporosis is more common in women. Body parts involved: The bones.

SPECIAL CONSIDERATIONS FOR AGING
- Many body changes occur as a result of estrogen deficiency beginning at menopause. Changes in other systems of the body may lead to a greater tendency to osteoporosis, hardening of the arteries and other disorders.
- Characteristic signs and symptoms of many disorders are frequently changed or absent.
- Bone density declines.

SIGNS & SYMPTOMS
Early symptoms:
- Backache.
- No symptoms (often).

Late symptoms:
- Fractures that occur with minor injury, especially of the hip or arm (often the first sign).
- Sudden back pain with a cracking sound indicating fracture; loss of height.
- A deformed spinal column with humps.

CAUSES & RISK FACTORS—Caused by the loss of bone structure and strength. Risk factors include prolonged lack of adequate calcium and protein in the diet; low estrogen levels after menopause; decreased activity with increased age; smoking; the use of cortisone drugs; prolonged disease, including alcoholism; vitamin deficiency (especially of vitamin C); hyperthyroidism; cancer; the use of steroid-type medications; surgery to remove the ovaries; radiation treatment for ovarian cancer; chronic or recurrent urinary tract or other pelvic infections; chronic lung disorders such as bronchitis and emphysema; a family history of osteoporosis; and body type (thin women with small frames are more susceptible).

DOCTOR'S TREATMENT & DIAGNOSTIC TESTS
- Medical history and physical exam.
- X-rays of the bones; blood test or bone biopsy (to exclude other problems).
- Thyroid function tests; bone density measurement.
- Self-care instructions focused on the older patient.

HOME TREATMENT BY SELF OR CARE-GIVER

GENERAL INSTRUCTIONS
- Avoid all circumstances which may lead to injury. Stay off icy streets and wet or waxed floors. Hold banisters when using stairs, and make sure the banisters are sturdy.
- Make your home as accident-proof as possible.
- Use canes or walkers if movement is difficult.

- If estrogen is prescribed, visit your doctor for regular pelvic exams and Pap smears. Examine your breasts for lumps once a month. Report any vaginal bleeding or discharge.
- Use heat or ice in any form to ease the pain.
- Sleep on a firm mattress.
- Use a back brace if prescribed by your doctor.
- Use correct posture when lifting.
- Avoid mind-altering medications, such as sedatives or tranquilizers, which may cause falls and fractures.

MEDICATION (ADJUSTED FOR AGING)
- For minor pain, you may use non-prescription drugs such as acetaminophen.
- Your doctor may prescribe calcium, vitamin D supplements, estrogen or fluoride.

ACTIVITY FOR OLDER PATIENTS
- Stay active, but avoid the risk of falls.
- Exercise—especially weight-bearing exercise such as walking—helps maintain bone strength.
- If walking isn't feasible for you, ask your doctor about an exercise program.

FOOD & BEVERAGE—Eat a normal, well-balanced diet that is high in protein, calcium and vitamin D. See Appendix 1.

FUTURE CONSIDERATIONS FOR THE AGING ADULT

POSSIBLE COMPLICATIONS—Bone fracture, especially of the hip or spine, after a fall. Sometimes a bone will break or collapse without injury or a fall.

PROBABLE OUTCOME—Bone deterioration can be halted—even reversed—by a proper diet, calcium and fluoride supplements, vitamin D, exercise and estrogen. Fractures will heal with standard treatment.

PREVENTING RECURRENCE
- Ensure an adequate calcium intake—up to 1500mg a day—by consuming milk and milk products. Talk to your doctor about calcium supplements.
- Get regular exercise, such as brisk walking, which is better for preventing osteoporosis than swimming.
- Protect yourself against falls, especially in the home.
- Consult your doctor about taking estrogen, calcium and fluoride after menopause begins or the ovaries have been removed.
- Drink little or no alcohol.

CALL YOUR DOCTOR IF

- You have symptoms of osteoporosis.
- Pain develops, especially after injury.
- New, unexplained symptoms develop, such as vaginal bleeding. The drugs used in treatment may produce side effects.

OTOSCLEROSIS

BASIC INFORMATION FOR OLDER ADULTS

DESCRIPTION—Otosclerosis is the slow formation of abnormal spongy bone growth in the middle ear. The growth prevents one of the small bones in the middle ear from vibrating sound waves, leading to hearing loss. Body parts involved: The bones in the middle ear and the nerves in the ear that allow us to hear. Otosclerosis usually affects both ears.

SPECIAL CONSIDERATIONS FOR AGING
- Some degree of hearing loss occurs.
- Hearing decreases in 50% of people 65 or older.
- Stress from any emotional cause—fear, worry, anxiety, sadness, loneliness or anger—affects all aspects of any illness or disorder.

SIGNS & SYMPTOMS
- Slow, progressive hearing loss.
- Ringing in the ears.
- Hearing that is better in noisy environments than quiet ones.
- Dizziness.

CAUSES & RISK FACTORS—Oteosclerosis is inherited. It is a dominant genetic trait. Risk factors include:
- A family history of hearing loss.
- Caucasian heritage. Otosclerosis affects about 10% of all white people to some degree.

DOCTOR'S TREATMENT & DIAGNOSTIC TESTS
- Medical history and physical exam.
- Laboratory studies such as an audiogram and Rinne test (see Glossary).
- Surgery to remove the stapes (a bone in the middle ear) or other surgical procedures may help. Advancing age alone is not a deterrent.
- Self-care instructions focused on the older patient.

HOME TREATMENT BY SELF OR CARE-GIVER

GENERAL INSTRUCTIONS
- A hearing aid may be useful if surgery is not recommended or desired.
- To prevent complications after surgery:
  Don't blow your nose for 1 week.
  Avoid unnecessary contact with persons who have respiratory infections, such as colds, flu or bronchitis.
  Protect your ears against cold.
  Avoid activities that might cause dizziness, such as bending, lifting or straining.
  Avoid loud noises and sudden pressure changes (flying or scuba diving) for 6 months or until healing is complete.

- Otosclerosis is a complicated, serious disorder. This page can cover only the main points of diagnosis and treatment. Your doctor, nurse or librarian can provide sources of supplemental information.

MEDICATION (ADJUSTED FOR AGING)
- Your doctor may prescribe antibiotics after surgery.
- *Note:* Adverse reactions and side effects may be more frequent and severe in older persons. Remind your doctor of any medicines you already take.

ACTIVITY FOR OLDER PATIENTS
- After surgery, resume your normal activities gradually.
- See Appendix 20 regarding physical fitness for the active older adult.

FOOD & BEVERAGE
- No special diet is required.
- See Appendix 1 regarding good nutrition for people over 50.

FUTURE CONSIDERATIONS FOR THE AGING ADULT

POSSIBLE COMPLICATIONS—Total deafness in 10 to 15 years without treatment. The younger the patient, the more rapid the hearing loss.

PROBABLE OUTCOME—In most cases, hearing is at least partially restored with surgery.

PREVENTING RECURRENCE—Cannot be prevented at present. Obtain genetic counseling before starting a family if you or your spouse has otosclerosis.

CALL YOUR DOCTOR IF

- You have symptoms of otosclerosis.
- Signs of infection, such as fever, pain or excessive dizziness, develop after treatment.

OVARIAN CANCER

BASIC INFORMATION FOR OLDER ADULTS

DESCRIPTION—Ovarian cancer is a malignant growth in the ovary that is likely to spread to other body parts and threaten life. Body parts involved: One or both ovaries. It may spread to the lungs and bone.

SPECIAL CONSIDERATIONS FOR AGING
- Malignant diseases are less likely to spread rapidly.
- The immune system becomes less effective, opening the way for viral, bacterial and other infections; malignancies; immune disorders; and allergies.
- Characteristic signs and symptoms of many disorders are frequently changed or absent.
- Stress from any emotional cause—fear, worry, anxiety, sadness, loneliness or anger—affects all aspects of any illness or disorder.

SIGNS & SYMPTOMS—Frequently no symptoms occur until the tumor becomes large. The earliest symptoms include:
- Vague discomfort or swelling in the lower abdomen.
- Gastrointestinal upsets.

Later symptoms include:
- A deep voice.
- Excessive hair growth.
- Unexplained weight loss.
- An enlarged, hard and sometimes tender mass in the lower abdomen.
- Pain with intercourse.
- Anemia.

CAUSES & RISK FACTORS—Unknown.

DOCTOR'S TREATMENT & DIAGNOSTIC TESTS
- Medical history and physical exam.
- Laboratory blood studies.
- Sonogram (see Glossary) of the abdomen.
- X-rays of the abdomen.
- Surgical diagnostic procedures such as culdoscopy and laparoscopy (see Glossary).
- Surgery to remove the cancerous ovary and other affected areas, including the Fallopian tubes, the uterus, the other ovary (sometimes) and the nearby lymph glands. Advancing age alone is not a deterrent.
- Radiation treatment and/or chemotherapy.
- Psychotherapy or counseling to help you learn to accept and cope with cancer.
- Self-care instructions focused on the older patient.

HOME TREATMENT BY SELF OR CARE-GIVER

GENERAL INSTRUCTIONS
- Ovarian cancer is a complicated, serious disorder. This page can cover only the main points of diagnosis and treatment. Your doctor, nurse or librarian can provide sources of supplemental information.
- For an explanation of surgery and post-operative care, see Hysterectomy in the Surgeries section.

MEDICATION (ADJUSTED FOR AGING)
- Your doctor may prescribe:
  Anticancer (chemotherapy) drugs.
  Pain relievers.
  Female hormones if menopause has not yet begun.
- *Note:* Adverse reactions and side effects may be more frequent and severe in older persons. Remind your doctor of any medicines you already take.

ACTIVITY FOR OLDER PATIENTS
- No restrictions are necessary after recovery from surgery.
- See Appendix 20 regarding physical fitness for the active older adult.

FOOD & BEVERAGE
- Eat a normal, well-balanced diet that is high in protein to promote the repair of body tissues.
- See Appendix 1 regarding good nutrition for people over 50.

FUTURE CONSIDERATIONS FOR THE AGING ADULT

POSSIBLE COMPLICATIONS—Death from the spread of cancer to other body parts.

PROBABLE OUTCOME—25% to 50% of women with ovarian cancer survive at least 5 years after treatment.

PREVENTING RECURRENCE—Have yearly pelvic examinations, which offer the best chance of early detection and cure.

CALL YOUR DOCTOR IF

- You have symptoms of an ovarian tumor.
- Any of the following occurs after surgery:
  Increased pain, swelling, redness or drainage from the surgical wound.
  Pain or swelling in the legs.
  Signs of infection, such as fever, chills, headache or muscle aches.

OVARIAN CYST

BASIC INFORMATION FOR OLDER ADULTS

DESCRIPTION—An ovarian cyst is a closed cavity or sac containing liquid or semisolid material which develops in the ovary. Ovarian cysts are rarely cancerous. Body parts involved: The ovaries; Fallopian tubes; peritoneum; colon.

SPECIAL CONSIDERATIONS FOR AGING—Many body changes occur as a result of estrogen deficiency beginning at menopause. These include vaginal dryness, shortening and narrowing of the vagina, greater susceptibility to vaginal infections, frequent bladder infections, reductions in the size of the clitoris and increased facial hair. Changes in other systems of the body may lead to a greater tendency to osteoporosis, hardening of the arteries and other disorders.

SIGNS & SYMPTOMS—Some cysts produce no symptoms. Others produce any of the following:
- Swelling without pain in the lower abdomen.
- Painful sexual intercourse.
- Stinging or burning on urination (if the cyst presses on the bladder).
- Difficulty emptying the bladder completely.
- Brownish vaginal discharge.
- Increased hairiness (if the cyst produces excess hormones).

The following may occur if the cyst twists, bleeds or breaks:
- Severe abdominal pain.
- Fever.
- Vomiting.

CAUSES & RISK FACTORS—Hormone disturbance. The risk increases with taking hormones for any purpose.

DOCTOR'S TREATMENT & DIAGNOSTIC TESTS
- Medical history and physical exam—including a complete pelvic examination—by a doctor.
- X-ray of the abdomen.
- Pelvic ultrasonography (see Glossary).
- Laparoscopy, a surgical diagnostic procedure (see Glossary).
- Surgery to drain the cyst (sometimes) or to remove the ovary. Advancing age alone is not a deterrent.
- Self-care instructions focused on the older patient.

HOME TREATMENT BY SELF OR CARE-GIVER

GENERAL INSTRUCTIONS—Ask your doctor for an explanation of the surgery and postoperative care.

MEDICATION (ADJUSTED FOR AGING)—Medicine is usually not necessary for this disorder. For minor discomfort, you may use non-prescription drugs such as acetaminophen.

ACTIVITY FOR OLDER PATIENTS
- No restrictions are necessary. If surgery is necessary, resume your normal activities gradually.
- See Appendix 20 regarding physical fitness for the active older adult.

FOOD & BEVERAGE
- No special diet is required.
- See Appendix 1 regarding good nutrition for people over 50.

FUTURE CONSIDERATIONS FOR THE AGING ADULT

POSSIBLE COMPLICATIONS
- Rupture of the cyst or twisting of the cyst's stalk. This requires emergency surgery.
- Urinary obstruction.
- Increased risk of ovarian cancer.

PROBABLE OUTCOME—Ovarian cysts are curable with surgery, but they may recur.

PREVENTING RECURRENCE—Cannot be prevented at present.

CALL YOUR DOCTOR IF

- You have symptoms of an ovarian cyst.
- Any of the following occurs after diagnosis:
  You lose weight for no apparent reason.
  You feel generally ill.
  You have pain in the lower abdomen.
  You have severe abdominal pain, nausea and fever that come on suddenly. This may indicate the rupture of a cyst.

ILLNESSES & DISORDERS

OVARIAN TUMOR, BENIGN

BASIC INFORMATION FOR OLDER ADULTS

DESCRIPTION—A benign ovarian tumor is a cystic (saclike) growth on the ovary that contains fluid or semisolid material. Such tumors are usually small, but in some cases they may grow large enough to make a woman appear to be pregnant. Ovarian tumors are usually benign, but a few undergo malignant change. Body parts involved: One or both ovaries.

SPECIAL CONSIDERATIONS FOR AGING
- Many body changes occur as a result of estrogen deficiency beginning at menopause. These include vaginal dryness, shortening and narrowing of the vagina, greater susceptibility to vaginal infections, frequent bladder infections, reductions in the size of the clitoris and increased facial hair. Changes in other systems of the body may lead to a greater tendency to osteoporosis, hardening of the arteries and other disorders.
- Characteristic signs and symptoms of many disorders are frequently changed or absent.

SIGNS & SYMPTOMS—May not cause
symptoms. If symptoms occur, they may include:
- Mild pelvic pain.
- Pain in the lower back.
- Discomfort with sexual intercourse.
- Excessive hair growth, a deep voice and weight gain (sometimes).

If a large ovarian tumor twists or ruptures, the following will occur in the lower abdomen:
- Severe pain.
- Rigid muscles.
- Swelling.

CAUSES & RISK FACTORS—The cause is
unknown, but it is probably related to abnormalities in the production and secretion of female hormone.

DOCTOR'S TREATMENT & DIAGNOSTIC TESTS
- Medical history and physical exam.
- Laboratory blood studies.
- Ultrasound or MRI (see Glossary for both).
- Laparoscopy, a surgical diagnostic procedure. A small tube is inserted through a small incision into the abdomen under local anesthesia. The tube allows the doctor to see the organs and biopsy or drain the tumor if necessary.
- Surgery (laparotomy) to remove the tumor or diseased ovary (sometimes). Advancing age alone is not a deterrent.
- Self-care instructions focused on the older patient.

HOME TREATMENT BY SELF OR CARE-GIVER

GENERAL INSTRUCTIONS
- A benign ovarian tumor is a complicated, serious disorder. This page can cover only the main points of diagnosis and treatment. Your doctor, nurse or librarian can provide sources of supplemental information.
- Have yearly medical checkups and pelvic exams to detect tumors early. Treatment may not be necessary, except to have regular pelvic examinations so the tumor's growth can be monitored.

MEDICATION (ADJUSTED FOR AGING)
- Your doctor may prescribe female hormones. These help shrink or destroy some tumors.
- *Note:* Adverse reactions and side effects may be more frequent and severe in older persons. Remind your doctor of any medicines you already take.

ACTIVITY FOR OLDER PATIENTS
- No restrictions are necessary if surgery is not necessary.
- See Appendix 20 regarding physical fitness for the active older adult.

FOOD & BEVERAGE
- No special diet is required.
- See Appendix 1 regarding good nutrition for people over 50.

FUTURE CONSIDERATIONS FOR THE AGING ADULT

POSSIBLE COMPLICATIONS—Twisting, rupture or bleeding of a tumor, which will require emergency abdominal surgery.

PROBABLE OUTCOME
- Most ovarian tumors require no treatment and disappear spontaneously within 2 months.
- Some tumors require surgery to diagnose them accurately, ruling out malignancy, or to treat them.

PREVENTING RECURRENCE—There are no specific preventive measures.

CALL YOUR DOCTOR IF

- You have symptoms of an ovarian tumor, especially severe pain, rigidity and abdominal distention.
- New, unexplained symptoms develop. The drugs used in treatment may produce side effects.

PAGET'S DISEASE
(Osteitis Deformans)

BASIC INFORMATION FOR OLDER ADULTS

DESCRIPTION—Paget's disease is a gradual, progressive bone disease characterized by the bones breaking down and regenerating excessively. The new bone is fragile and weak. It is not cancerous. Body parts involved: The bones of the skull, spine, legs, collarbone and pelvis.

SPECIAL CONSIDERATIONS FOR AGING
- The immune system becomes less effective, opening the way for viral, bacterial and other infections; malignancies; immune disorders; and allergies.
- Characteristic signs and symptoms of many disorders are frequently changed or absent.
- Stress from any emotional cause—fear, worry, anxiety, sadness, loneliness or anger—affects all aspects of any illness or disorder.

SIGNS & SYMPTOMS
Early stages:
- Mild bone pain or none.

Later stages:
- The affected bones are chronically painful—especially at night—and are enlarged, misshapen, tender and warm.
- Movement is impaired.
- Spinal curvature compresses the sensory nerves.
- Fractures occur from minor trauma and heal slowly with deformity.
- Headache, vertigo and deafness if the skull bones are involved.

CAUSES & RISK FACTORS—The cause is unknown, although a virus may be involved. The risk increases with a family history of Paget's disease. Geographic location may also have a bearing. For instance, New York City has 4 times the number of cases that Atlanta has.

DOCTOR'S TREATMENT & DIAGNOSTIC TESTS
- Medical history and physical exam.
- X-rays of affected bones.
- Laboratory blood and urine studies to determine levels of serum alkaline phosphatase and urinary calcium.
- Self-care instructions focused on the older patient.
- Bone surgery (sometimes). Advancing age alone is not a deterrent.

HOME TREATMENT BY SELF OR CARE-GIVER

GENERAL INSTRUCTIONS
- Use heat to relieve the pain, including hot compresses, hot soaks (see Appendix 18) or heat lamps.
- Try aspirin or non-steroidal anti-inflammatory drugs for pain.

- If you don't have a firm bed, place 3/4-inch plywood under your mattress.
- Accident-proof your home as much as possible. Avoid throw rugs and slippery floors. Install hand rails next to the tub.

MEDICATION (ADJUSTED FOR AGING)—Your doctor may prescribe etidronate disodium, pain relievers or calcitonin injections. All relieve the pain, but none cure the disease.

ACTIVITY FOR OLDER PATIENTS
- Rest in bed during active phases. Move or turn often to prevent pressure sores. Resume your normal activities during remissions.
- See Appendix 20 regarding physical fitness for the active older adult.

FOOD & BEVERAGE
- No special diet is required.
- See Appendix 1 regarding good nutrition for people over 50.

FUTURE CONSIDERATIONS FOR THE AGING ADULT

POSSIBLE COMPLICATIONS
- Blindness or hearing loss caused by the skull pressing on the brain.
- High blood pressure.
- Kidney stones; gout; bone cancer.
- Congestive heart failure. The heart is strained by the greatly increased blood flow through diseased bones.
- Misdiagnosis of Paget's disease as an overactive parathyroid gland or as the spread of cancer from the prostate gland, breast or bone marrow.

PROBABLE OUTCOME—Paget's disease is currently considered incurable. However, the symptoms can be relieved or controlled. The disease has a pattern of remissions and flare-ups that become progressively worse. Sometimes adjacent joints become involved. Life expectancy is reduced, but most persons live with the disease for at least 10 to 15 years. Scientific research into causes and treatment continues, so there is hope for increasingly effective treatment and a cure.

PREVENTING RECURRENCE—There are no specific preventive measures.

CALL YOUR DOCTOR IF

- You have symptoms of Paget's disease.
- Any of the following occurs during treatment: A fever of 101F (38.3C) or higher. Unbearable pain. Weight loss. Worsening symptoms.
- New, unexplained symptoms develop. The drugs used in treatment may produce side effects.

BASIC INFORMATION FOR OLDER ADULTS

DESCRIPTION—Cancer of the pancreas is an uncontrolled growth of malignant cells in the pancreas. This is the 4th leading cause of cancer deaths in the U.S. Older adults account for 80% of the cases. Body part involved: The pancreas, an organ in the back of the upper abdomen. The pancreas produces intestinal enzymes to help digest food and insulin to control blood sugar.

SPECIAL CONSIDERATIONS FOR AGING
- Malignant diseases are less likely to spread rapidly.
- The immune system becomes less effective, opening the way for viral, bacterial and other infections; malignancies; immune disorders; and allergies.
- Stress from any emotional cause—fear, worry, anxiety, sadness, loneliness or anger—affects all aspects of any illness or disorder.

SIGNS & SYMPTOMS
- Depression.
- Rapid, unexplained weight loss.
- Pain in the back or upper abdomen that is often relieved by bending forward.
- Blood clots in veins anywhere, especially the arms and legs. This is often an early sign.
- Jaundice (yellow skin and eyes) from blockage of the nearby bile duct. The jaundice is usually accompanied by intense itching.
- Nausea and vomiting.

CAUSES & RISK FACTORS—The cause is
unknown. Risk factors include:
- Chronic pancreatitis; diabetes mellitus.
- Genetic factors. This disorder is more common in blacks than in Caucasians.
- Smoking; excessive alcohol consumption.
- Geographic location. The incidence is higher in Israel, the U.S., Sweden and Canada than in other parts of the world.
- Poor nutrition, especially a diet that is high in fat, protein and processed foods containing many food additives.
- Exposure to industrial chemicals, such as urea, naphthalene or benzidine.

DOCTOR'S TREATMENT & DIAGNOSTIC TESTS
- Medical history and physical exam.
- Laboratory blood chemistry studies of the pancreas, liver and gallbladder and blood sugar tests.
- Needle biopsy (see Glossary) of the liver.
- Exploratory abdominal surgery (laparotomy).
- X-rays of the abdomen, liver, gallbladder and blood vessels (angiography).
- Ultrasonography (see Glossary) of the pancreas.
- CT scan (see Glossary) of the pancreas.
- Psychotherapy or counseling to help you adjust to incurable illness.
- Chemotherapy and/or radiation therapy.

- Surgery to remove the tumor if it is small, to relieve any bile duct blockage or to relieve or prevent bowel obstruction. Advancing age alone is not a deterrent.
- Self-care instructions focused on the older patient.

HOME TREATMENT BY SELF OR CARE-GIVER

GENERAL INSTRUCTIONS—No specific instructions except those listed under other headings.

MEDICATION (ADJUSTED FOR AGING)—
Your doctor may prescribe:
- Antibiotics for coexisting infections.
- Pain relievers; sedatives for sleep.
- Anticancer (chemotherapy) drugs.
- Pancreatic enzymes to replace those the pancreas cannot manufacture.

ACTIVITY FOR OLDER PATIENTS—Remain as active as your strength allows.

FOOD & BEVERAGE—No special diet.

FUTURE CONSIDERATIONS FOR THE AGING ADULT

POSSIBLE COMPLICATIONS—Hemorrhage into the intestinal tract; pancreas infections; spread of the cancer to the liver, other abdominal organs and the lungs.

PROBABLE OUTCOME—This condition is currently considered incurable. The chances of survival for more than 1 or 2 years are unlikely. However, the symptoms can be relieved or controlled. Scientific research into causes and treatment continues, so there is hope for increasingly effective treatment and a cure.

PREVENTING RECURRENCE—Cannot be prevented. To reduce the risk:
- Don't smoke.
- Don't drink more than 1 or 2 alcoholic drinks—if any—a day.
- Eat more poultry, fish, fresh fruits and vegetables, and eat less red meat, processed foods and fat in any form.
- Avoid exposure to harmful chemicals.

CALL YOUR DOCTOR IF

- You have symptoms of pancreatic cancer.
- Any of the following occurs during treatment:
  Fever and headache.
  Muscle aches and fatigue.
  Nausea and vomiting.
  Severe abdominal pain and swelling.
  Black, tarry stools.
- New, unexplained symptoms develop. The drugs used in treatment may produce side effects.

PANCREATITIS

BASIC INFORMATION FOR OLDER ADULTS

DESCRIPTION—Pancreatitis is an inflammation of the pancreas. Chronic pancreatitis usually follows recurrent attacks of acute pancreatitis, because the pancreas does not recover completely between attacks. It gradually becomes unable to supply the digestive juices and hormones necessary for good health. Body part involved: The pancreas, an organ in the back of the upper abdomen.

SPECIAL CONSIDERATIONS FOR AGING
- The immune system becomes less effective, opening the way for viral, bacterial and other infections; malignancies; immune disorders; and allergies.
- Decreased nutrition, common among chronically ill older people, increases the risk of any disease or disorder.

SIGNS & SYMPTOMS
Severe acute pancreatitis:
- Sudden, extreme abdominal pain that may spread to the back.
- Vomiting and weakness.
- Abdominal swelling and gas.
- Fever; muscle aches.
- A drop in blood pressure.

Chronic pancreatitis:
- Persistent, mild or severe pain, often after meals, in the upper abdomen, sometimes radiating to the back or generalized. The pain is aching, burning, gnawing or stabbing. Episodes of pain may last days or weeks, but rarely less than 1 day.
- Mild jaundice (yellow skin and eyes) sometimes.
- Rapid weight loss.

CAUSES & RISK FACTORS
Causes include:
- Alcoholism.
- Disease of the gallbladder or bile ducts.
- Obstruction of the pancreatic duct by stones, scarring or slow-growing cancer (rare).
- Abdominal injury.
- Viral infection.
- Hyperlipidemia.

Risk factors include:
- Poor nutrition.
- Obesity.
- Excessive alcohol consumption.
- The use of drugs such as sulfa drugs, azathioprine, chlorothiazide, tetracycline or cortisone drugs.

DOCTOR'S TREATMENT & DIAGNOSTIC TESTS
- Medical history and physical exam. This may be difficult to diagnose.
- Laboratory studies such as blood and urine tests and radioisotope scans (see Glossary).
- X-rays of the pancreas.
- CT scan (see Glossary) of the pancreas.
- Hospitalization, in severe cases, to replace lost fluids.
- Surgery if a perforated peptic ulcer or common duct stone is suspected. Advancing age alone is not a deterrent.
- Self-care instructions focused on the older patient.

HOME TREATMENT BY SELF OR CARE-GIVER

GENERAL INSTRUCTIONS—Use heat from a heat lamp or hot compresses to relieve the pain.

MEDICATION (ADJUSTED FOR AGING)
- Your doctor may prescribe:
  Pain relievers.
  Digestive enzymes that the damaged pancreas cannot manufacture.
  Antibiotics if bacterial infection develops.
  Stomach acid (H_2) blockers.
- *Note:* Adverse reactions and side effects may be more frequent and severe in older persons. Remind your doctor of any medicines you already take.

ACTIVITY FOR OLDER PATIENTS
- No restrictions are necessary after recovery from an attack.
- See Appendix 20 regarding physical fitness for the active older adult.

FOOD & BEVERAGE
- Totally abstain from drinking alcohol.
- Eat a low-fat diet. See Appendix 8.

FUTURE CONSIDERATIONS FOR THE AGING ADULT

POSSIBLE COMPLICATIONS—Diabetes mellitus; chronic calcium deficiency; secondary bacterial infection in the pancreas; massive hemorrhage and destruction of the pancreas; cyst or abscess of the pancreas.

PROBABLE OUTCOME
- Acute pancreatitis is often curable with intensive care. Treatment includes resting the gastro-intestinal tract completely and providing intravenous fluids and nourishment. About 5% of cases don't respond to treatment and are fatal.
- Chronic pancreatitis may cause recurrent attacks for many years.

PREVENTING RECURRENCE—Don't drink alcoholic drinks.

CALL YOUR DOCTOR IF

- You have symptoms of acute pancreatitis.
- Any of the following occurs during or after treatment:
  Jaundice.
  Fever of 101F (38.3C) or higher.
  Continued weight loss.
  Signs of calcium deficiency, such as muscle cramps or seizures.

PARAPLEGIA OR QUADRIPLEGIA

BASIC INFORMATION FOR OLDER ADULTS

DESCRIPTION—Paraplegia is the partial or complete paralysis of both legs. Quadriplegia is the partial or complete paralysis of both arms *and* legs. Early treatment (within hours of injury) is essential to minimize damage. Body parts involved: The spinal cord and all body parts below the damage to the spinal cord.

SPECIAL CONSIDERATIONS FOR AGING—Decreased hearing and vision open the way for more frequent and serious accidents.

SIGNS & SYMPTOMS—The following vary, depending on the site and the extent of damage to the spinal cord:
- Loss of movement and sensation in the affected arms or legs.
- Loss of urinary and bowel control.
- Impaired sexual function.
- Loss of normal blood pressure.
- Loss of body temperature control.
- Constipation.

CAUSES & RISK FACTORS—Paraplegia is caused by damage to the spinal cord in the back. Quadriplegia is caused by damage to the spinal cord in the neck. Spinal cord damage results from accidents or spinal cord tumors. Risk factors include:
- Occupations, sports or other activities with a high risk of injury.
- Excessive alcohol consumption or drug use. These increase the risk of accidents—especially vehicle accidents.

DOCTOR'S TREATMENT & DIAGNOSTIC TESTS
- Medical history and physical exam.
- Laboratory studies of the blood and urine.
- X-rays of the injured area.
- Surgery to limit further damage to the spinal cord or to remove bones or a tumor.
- Time in an extended-care facility or nursing home (sometimes).
- Occupational and physical rehabilitation.
- Self-care instructions focused on the older patient.
- Psychotherapy or counseling for depression or for sexual problems.
- Recent studies show that the injection of methylprednisolone shortly after the spinal injury seems to lessen the degree of paralysis.

HOME TREATMENT BY SELF OR CARE-GIVER

GENERAL INSTRUCTIONS
- If someone is in an accident and has neck pain or a possible spinal cord injury, *don't move the person unless absolutely necessary.* Splint the neck to avoid movement and additional damage.

- If you have a spinal cord injury, you will need emotional support from family members and friends. Don't be afraid to ask for help.
- Wear thigh-high elastic stockings during convalescence—and knee-high stockings later—to reduce the chance of deep-vein blood clots.
- Sleep on a waterbed or egg-crate foam mattress to reduce the chance of pressure sores.
- You may need to wear a corset or orthopedic collar for support and to relieve the pain.

MEDICATION (ADJUSTED FOR AGING)—No medication can heal a damaged spinal cord. Your doctor may prescribe:
- Antibiotics to fight infection. Urinary tract infections are most common.
- Stool softeners and laxatives to prevent constipation.

ACTIVITY FOR OLDER PATIENTS
- Stay as active as your strength and condition allow. The body can be retrained to compensate for or restore some lost functions, including sexual abilities.
- Follow the recommendations of your physical therapist to achieve the highest possible level of fitness.

FOOD & BEVERAGE
- Eat a high-fiber diet to prevent constipation.
- If you have a urinary catheter, drink up to 16 glasses of water a day to prevent bladder stones and urinary tract infections.

FUTURE CONSIDERATIONS FOR THE AGING ADULT

POSSIBLE COMPLICATIONS—Kidney infections, especially if a urinary catheter is needed; lung infections; fecal impaction; pressure sores; deep-vein blood clots; depression.

PROBABLE OUTCOME—Depends on the extent of the injury. A damaged spinal cord is limited in its ability to recover from injury. With rehabilitation, uninjured areas can take over some lost functions.

PREVENTING RECURRENCE
- Observe safety precautions and don't take risks.
- Don't dive into shallow swimming pools or into water of unknown depth.
- Don't drive after drinking alcohol or using mind-altering drugs.
- Use seat belts in cars.
- Wear protective headgear during contact sports or while riding a bicycle or motorcycle.

CALL YOUR DOCTOR IF

- You observe signs of a neck or spine injury in someone.
- Signs of infection occur during treatment. These include fever, chills, cloudy urine, muscle aches and headache.

PARATHYROID, OVERACTIVE
(Hyperparathyroidism)

BASIC INFORMATION FOR OLDER ADULTS

DESCRIPTION—Hyperparathyroidism is characterized by the increased production of hormones by the parathyroid glands, causing a high level of calcium in the blood. Body parts involved: The parathyroid glands in the neck; the teeth; the blood, which affects all body tissues, especially the heart, blood vessels, bones, kidneys, gastrointestinal tract, central nervous system and skin.

SPECIAL CONSIDERATIONS FOR AGING
- The immune system becomes less effective, opening the way for viral, bacterial and other infections; malignancies; immune disorders; and allergies.
- Decreased nutrition, common among chronically ill older people, increases the risk of any disease or disorder.

SIGNS & SYMPTOMS
- Often none. May be discovered as part of a routine blood screening.
- Severe flank pain caused by kidney stones.
- Chronic low back pain caused by softening of the bones.
- Easy bone fractures caused by decreased calcium in the bones.
- Upper abdominal pain caused by a peptic ulcer or pancreatitis.
- Depression.

CAUSES & RISK FACTORS
Causes include:
- Benign tumors of the parathyroid glands, which are located next to the thyroid gland in the neck.
- Recent illness, especially an endocrine disorder.
Risk factors include:
- A medical history of rickets or vitamin D deficiency.
- Kidney failure.
- The use of laxatives.
- The use of digitalis.

DOCTOR'S TREATMENT & DIAGNOSTIC TESTS
- Medical history and physical exam.
- Laboratory blood and urine studies.
- X-rays of the bones.
- Surgery to remove parathyroid tumors if they are present.
- After treatment or surgery, self-care instructions focused on the older patient.

HOME TREATMENT BY SELF OR CARE-GIVER

GENERAL INSTRUCTIONS—To prevent fractures:
- Use a walker or cane until the blood studies return to normal. This may take up to 6 months.
- Install safety rails near the tub, shower and toilet.
- Tape rugs down around the edges.
- Keep the house—especially stairs—brightly lit to avoid stumbling.

MEDICATION (ADJUSTED FOR AGING)
- Your doctor may prescribe:
  Diuretics to force the excretion of sodium and calcium.
  Vitamin D.
- Don't take antacids that contain calcium.
- *Note:* Adverse reactions and side effects may be more frequent and severe in older persons. Remind your doctor of any medicines you already take.

ACTIVITY FOR OLDER PATIENTS
- No restrictions are necessary.
- See Appendix 20 regarding physical fitness for the active older adult.

FOOD & BEVERAGE
- Drink extra water to prevent kidney stones.
- Limit your intake of calcium-containing foods, such as milk and cheese.
- Avoid highly seasoned or spicy food, especially if you have an ulcer.
- See Appendix 1 regarding good nutrition for people over 50.

FUTURE CONSIDERATIONS FOR THE AGING ADULT

POSSIBLE COMPLICATIONS
- Cataracts.
- Kidney damage.
- Peptic ulcer.
- Pancreatitis.
- Psychosis.
- Underactive parathyroid caused by the removal of too much parathyroid tissue during surgery.
- Underactive thyroid if the thyroid gland is injured inadvertently during surgery on the parathyroid glands.

PROBABLE OUTCOME—Curable with surgery.

PREVENTING RECURRENCE—There are no specific preventive measures except those listed under other headings.

CALL YOUR DOCTOR IF

- You have symptoms of an overactive parathyroid.
- Any of the following occurs:
  Muscle cramps, numbness or weakness.
  Breathing difficulty.
  Persistent heartburn or pain in the upper abdomen.
  Drastic mood or behavior changes.

ILLNESSES & DISORDERS

PARATHYROID, UNDERACTIVE
(Hypoparathyroidism)

BASIC INFORMATION FOR OLDER ADULTS

DESCRIPTION—Hypoparathyroidism is characterized by the decreased production of hormones by the parathyroid glands, causing a low level of calcium in the blood. Body parts involved: The parathyroid glands in the neck; the teeth; the blood, which affects all body tissues, especially the heart, blood vessels, bones, kidneys, gastrointestinal tract, central nervous system and skin.

SPECIAL CONSIDERATIONS FOR AGING—
Usual signs and symptoms may be absent and be replaced by symptoms of confusion, dizziness, failure to thrive, falling, incontinence, increasing dementia, refusal to eat or drink, weight loss, depression, paranoia, hypochondriasis, psychosis or threats of suicide.

SIGNS & SYMPTOMS
Acute phase:
- Tingling fingertips.
- Muscle tension and spasms in the hands and feet.
- Spasms of the larynx and throat muscles, causing breathing difficulty.

Chronic phase:
- Scaling skin.
- Splitting nails.
- Poor tooth development.
- Seizures.
- Mental retardation in children.
- Psychosis in adults.

CAUSES & RISK FACTORS
Causes include:
- A complication of surgery on the parathyroid glands, the thyroid glands or other neck tissues.
- A genetic autoimmune disorder (possibly).
- Radiation of the thyroid gland.
- Hemochromatosis (see Glossary).
- Tuberculosis.
- Neck injury.

Risk increases with:
- Recent infection of any kind.
- The use of diuretic drugs.

DOCTOR'S TREATMENT & DIAGNOSTIC TESTS
- Medical history and physical exam.
- Laboratory blood and urine studies.
- ECG (see Glossary).
- X-rays of bones.
- Treatment during the acute stage.
- After diagnosis during the chronic stage, self-care instructions focused on the older patient.
- Hospitalization for severe muscle spasms.

HOME TREATMENT BY SELF OR CARE-GIVER

GENERAL INSTRUCTIONS
- If muscle cramps start, place a paper bag over your mouth. Blow into it and rebreathe the air. This will raise the carbon dioxide level in your blood and decrease the muscle spasms.
- Apply lubricating creams or ointments to dry, scaling skin.
- Keep your nails trimmed to prevent splitting.

MEDICATION (ADJUSTED FOR AGING)
- Your doctor may prescribe:
  Vitamin D and calcium supplements in high doses. Intravenous calcium supplements during hospitalization for severe muscle spasms. Sedatives and anticonvulsants for frequent muscle spasms.
- *Note:* Adverse reactions and side effects may be more frequent and severe in older persons. Remind your doctor of any medicines you already take.

ACTIVITY FOR OLDER PATIENTS
- No restrictions are necessary.
- See Appendix 20 regarding physical fitness for the active older adult.

FOOD & BEVERAGE—Eat a high-calcium, low-phosphorous diet. Your doctor or dietitian will provide specific instructions.

FUTURE CONSIDERATIONS FOR THE AGING ADULT

POSSIBLE COMPLICATIONS
- Cataracts.
- Brain damage.
- Heartbeat abnormalities and congestive heart failure.
- Treatment needs to be monitored carefully to avoid development of toxic levels of calcium.

PROBABLE OUTCOME—This condition is currently considered incurable. It requires lifelong replacement therapy to control the symptoms. Without treatment, it is fatal. Scientific research into causes and treatment continues, so there is hope for increasingly effective treatment and a cure.

PREVENTING RECURRENCE—There are no specific preventive measures.

CALL YOUR DOCTOR IF

- You have unexplained muscle spasms of the hands, feet or throat or have numbness or tingling in the hands or feet.
- The muscle spasms don't decrease in 1 week despite treatment.

PARKINSON'S DISEASE

BASIC INFORMATION FOR OLDER ADULTS

DESCRIPTION—Parkinson's disease is a disease of the central nervous system characterized by gradual, progressive muscle rigidity, tremors and clumsiness. Body parts involved: The area of the brain that regulates movement; the muscles.

SPECIAL CONSIDERATIONS FOR AGING
- Neurological diseases become more likely.
- This is one of the diseases that is common only in older adults.

SIGNS & SYMPTOMS
- Tremors, especially when not moving.
- General muscle stiffness and slowness.
- An awkward or shuffling walk.
- Stooped posture.
- Loss of facial expression.
- Voice changes. The voice becomes weak and high-pitched.
- Swallowing difficulty.
- Slow deterioration of intellectual ability, but only in the advanced stages.
- Shaking of the head.
- Depression and anxiety.
- Seborrhea of the scalp and face.

CAUSES & RISK FACTORS—The causes and risk factors are usually unknown. Some cases may be caused by medications such as phenothiazine tranquilizers; brain injury; tumors; post-influenza encephalitis; slow virus infection; carbon monoxide poisoning (possibly).

DOCTOR'S TREATMENT & DIAGNOSTIC TESTS
- Medical history and physical exam.
- Laboratory blood studies.
- EEG (see Glossary).
- Psychotherapy or counseling to help relieve depression.
- Physical therapy if muscle rigidity is severe.
- Speech therapy.
- Surgery using heat, cold or radiation to destroy the areas of the brain that cause Parkinson's disease (rare). Advancing age alone is not a deterrent.
- Self-care instructions focused on the older patient.

HOME TREATMENT BY SELF OR CARE-GIVER

GENERAL INSTRUCTIONS
- Take frequent warm baths and have massages to forestall muscle rigidity.
- Shave with an electric razor.
- Use special tableware with large handles.
- Use devices to amplify the voice if it becomes weak.
- Wear shoes without laces, such as loafers or those with zipper or Velcro fasteners.

- Accident-proof your home to prevent falls and injuries.
- The gradual restrictions of the disease may frustrate you. Seek professional help and ask your family for support in finding ways to remain active and useful.
- Consider joining a Parkinson's support group.

MEDICATION (ADJUSTED FOR AGING)
- Your doctor may prescribe antidepressants; anticholinergics; antihistamines; antiviral drugs, such as amantadine; or antiparkinson medications, including bromocriptine, levodopa and carbidopa. All these decrease the tremors and reduce muscle rigidity, but they often have significant side effects.
- A new medication, selegiline, appears to be very effective in providing relief of some symptoms.

ACTIVITY FOR OLDER PATIENTS—Remain as active as possible, and rest often. Physical abilities vary greatly between persons with this disease. The only restrictions are those imposed by muscle rigidity. Physical therapy helps reduce this.

FOOD & BEVERAGE
- No special diet is required, but soft foods may be necessary if swallowing becomes difficult. Add bulk or fiber to the diet and increase fluid intake to prevent constipation.
- See Appendix 1 regarding good nutrition for people over 50.

FUTURE CONSIDERATIONS FOR THE AGING ADULT

POSSIBLE COMPLICATIONS
- Depression, sometimes severe.
- Pneumonia.
- Severe constipation.
- Urine retention caused by medication.
- Falls and fractures.

PROBABLE OUTCOME—This condition is currently considered incurable. However, the symptoms can be relieved or controlled, and life expectancy is not significantly reduced. Scientific research into causes and treatment continues, so there is hope for increasingly effective treatment and a cure.

PREVENTING RECURRENCE—There are no specific preventive measures.

CALL YOUR DOCTOR IF

- You have symptoms of Parkinson's disease or the symptoms worsen during treatment.
- New, unexplained symptoms develop, especially urination difficulty, confusion or blurred vision. The drugs used in treatment may produce side effects.

PARROT FEVER
(Psittacosis; Ornithosis)

BASIC INFORMATION FOR OLDER ADULTS

DESCRIPTION—Parrot fever is an infectious form of pneumonia transmitted by birds. Body parts involved: The lungs.

SPECIAL CONSIDERATIONS FOR AGING
- The immune system becomes less effective, opening the way for viral, bacterial and other infections; malignancies; immune disorders; and allergies.
- Decreased nutrition, common among chronically ill older people, increases the risk of any disease or disorder.

SIGNS & SYMPTOMS
- Fever, chills and muscle pain.
- A general ill feeling.
- Appetite loss.
- A cough without sputum that progresses to a cough with occasional discolored sputum.
- Shortness of breath.
- Severe headache.

CAUSES & RISK FACTORS—Caused by infection from the germ chlamydia. Microscopic chlamydia organisms are not bacteria, viruses or fungi. However, they can be destroyed with antibiotics. Psittacosis is found in psittacine birds (parrots, parakeets and lovebirds), poultry, pigeons, canaries and some sea birds. The germs enter the human body when you inhale air that contains the germ or receive a bite from an infected bird. The incubation time is 1 to 3 weeks after exposure. The risk increases with exposure to birds, especially in zoos or pet shops or on farms.

DOCTOR'S TREATMENT & DIAGNOSTIC TESTS
- Medical history and physical exam.
- Laboratory blood studies and sputum culture.
- X-rays of the lungs.
- Self-care instructions focused on the older patient.

HOME TREATMENT BY SELF OR CARE-GIVER

GENERAL INSTRUCTIONS
- Remain isolated to avoid transmitting the disease through cough droplets and sputum.
- Use a cool-mist humidifier to increase the air moisture and loosen lung secretions. Use pure water; don't put medication in the humidifier.
- Use warm compresses on the chest to relieve the pain.
- Don't smoke.

MEDICATION (ADJUSTED FOR AGING)
- Your doctor may prescribe tetracycline (an antibiotic) for at least 10 days to control the fever and other symptoms.

- Don't suppress the cough if it produces sputum. It is performing a useful function in ridding the lungs of mucus. If the cough is non-productive and painful, you may suppress it with prescribed medication.
- For minor pain, take non-prescription drugs such as aspirin or acetaminophen.
- *Note:* Adverse reactions and side effects may be more frequent and severe in older persons. Remind your doctor of any medicines you already take.

ACTIVITY FOR OLDER PATIENTS
- Bed rest is necessary until the fever, pain and shortness of breath have been gone at least 48 hours. Then you may resume your normal activities gradually. Fatigue and weakness may persist for a long time, so don't expect a quick return to normal strength.
- See Appendix 20 regarding physical fitness for the active older adult.

FOOD & BEVERAGE
- No special diet is required. Increase your fluid intake to at least 1 glass of fluid every hour. This helps to thin lung secretions so they can be coughed up more easily.
- See Appendix 1 regarding good nutrition for people over 50.

FUTURE CONSIDERATIONS FOR THE AGING ADULT

POSSIBLE COMPLICATIONS
- Severe or fatal pneumonia.
- Myocarditis.

PROBABLE OUTCOME—Usually curable in 7 to 14 days with early diagnosis and treatment. The fever may remain for 2 or 3 weeks before falling slowly unless antibiotics are used.

PREVENTING RECURRENCE
- Avoid dust from bird feathers and cage contents.
- Don't handle any sick bird. Imported psittacine birds must be treated for 45 days with feed that contains chlortetracycline. This eliminates the organisms from the birds' blood and feces.

CALL YOUR DOCTOR IF

- You have symptoms of psittacosis.
- Any of the following occurs during treatment:
  A fever develops.
  The pain is not relieved by heat or prescribed medication.
  The shortness of breath increases.
  Your fingernails become dark or bluish.
  Blood appears in the sputum.
  You experience nausea, vomiting or diarrhea.

PELVIC INFLAMMATORY DISEASE
(PID)

BASIC INFORMATION FOR OLDER ADULTS

DESCRIPTION—Pelvic inflammatory disease is an infection of the female internal reproductive organs. This is contagious if it is caused by a sexually transmitted organism. Body parts involved: The Fallopian tubes; cervix; uterus; ovaries; urinary bladder.

SPECIAL CONSIDERATIONS FOR AGING
- The immune system becomes less effective, opening the way for viral, bacterial and other infections; malignancies; immune disorders; and allergies.
- Decreased nutrition, common among chronically ill older people, increases the risk of any disease or disorder.
- Characteristic signs and symptoms of many disorders are frequently changed or absent.

SIGNS & SYMPTOMS
Early symptoms (up to 1 week):
- Pain in the lower pelvis on one or both sides.
- Pain with intercourse.
- Bad-smelling vaginal discharge.
- A general ill feeling.
- Low fever.
- Frequent, painful urination.

Later symptoms (1 to 3 weeks later):
- Severe pain and tenderness in the lower abdomen.
- High fever.
- Increased amount of bad-smelling vaginal discharge.

CAUSES & RISK FACTORS
Causes include:
- Infection with a bacterium (chlamydia, gonorrhea or mycoplasma) or a virus; this may be transmitted by an infected sexual partner.
- Pelvic surgery.

Risk factors include:
- Many sexual partners.
- Previous episode of PID.

DOCTOR'S TREATMENT & DIAGNOSTIC TESTS
- Medical history and physical exam.
- Laboratory blood studies and culture of the vaginal discharge.
- Surgical diagnostic procedures such as laparoscopy or culdocentesis (see Glossary).
- Ultrasonography (see Glossary).
- Self-care instructions focused on the older patient.
- Hospitalization if your fever is high or pelvic abscess is suspected.
- Surgery to drain a pelvic abscess (sometimes).

OTHER—Your sexual partner may also need examination and treatment.

HOME TREATMENT BY SELF OR CARE-GIVER

GENERAL INSTRUCTIONS
- Use heat to relieve the pain:
  Place a heating pad or hot water bottle on your abdomen or back.
  Take frequent warm baths. This may reduce the bad odor of the vaginal discharge as well as relax the muscles and relieve your discomfort. Sit in a tub of warm water for 10 to 15 minutes as often as needed.
- Use sanitary pads to absorb the discharge.
- Don't douche during treatment.

MEDICATION (ADJUSTED FOR AGING)—
Your doctor may prescribe:
- Oral antibiotics to treat early or mild PID.
- Intravenous antibiotics to fight infection if hospitalization is required. Oral antibiotics may be necessary for about 1 month following hospitalization.
- Pain relievers.

ACTIVITY FOR OLDER PATIENTS—Avoid sexual intercourse until you are well. Rest in bed until the fever subsides. Sit and lie in different positions until you find one that is comfortable for you. Recovery may take 2 to 3 months.

FOOD & BEVERAGE
- No special diet is required. Be sure to drink plenty of fluids.
- See Appendix 1 regarding good nutrition for people over 50.

FUTURE CONSIDERATIONS FOR THE AGING ADULT

POSSIBLE COMPLICATIONS—Pelvic abscess and rupture, which can be life-threatening; adhesions (bands of scar tissue) inside the pelvis; infertility; blood poisoning; thrombophlebitis (blood clots that break off and travel to the lungs).

PROBABLE OUTCOME—Usually curable with early treatment. Complications may be fatal. The illness lasts from 1 to 6 weeks, depending on its severity.

PREVENTING RECURRENCE—Use rubber condoms with a spermicide to reduce the risk of infection.

CALL YOUR DOCTOR IF

- You have symptoms of pelvic inflammatory disease.
- Your symptoms recur after treatment.
- New, unexplained symptoms develop. The drugs used in treatment may produce side effects.

BASIC INFORMATION FOR OLDER ADULTS

DESCRIPTION—Cancer of the penis is a malignant tumor of the penis. Body parts involved: The penis, including the glans (tip), corona (rounded border of the glans) or prepuce (foreskin covering the glans).

SPECIAL CONSIDERATIONS FOR AGING
- The immune system becomes less effective, opening the way for viral, bacterial and other infections; malignancies; immune disorders; and allergies.
- Malignant diseases are less likely to spread rapidly.
- Stress from any emotional cause—fear, worry, anxiety, sadness, loneliness or anger—affects all aspects of any illness or disorder.

SIGNS & SYMPTOMS
Early stages:
- A small circular lesion (resembling a pimple) or persistent, painless sore on the penis. The lesion is easily visible in a circumcised male, but it may go unnoticed in an uncircumcised male.

Later stages:
- Pain, bleeding or discharge from the tumor.
- Discomfort with urination.
- Enlarged lymph nodes in the groin.

CAUSES & RISK FACTORS—The cause is unknown, but penile cancer is rare in men who are circumcised at birth or shortly thereafter. This may explain why it is rare among Jews, Muslims, and men in other cultures where early circumcision is customary. Risk factors include:
- Previous leukoplakia of the penis, balanitis or epithelial horn on the penis.
- Personal uncleanliness, especially of the genitals in uncircumcised males.
- Viral infection.
- The smoking of tobacco.

DOCTOR'S TREATMENT & DIAGNOSTIC TESTS
- Medical history and physical exam.
- Laboratory studies such as culture of the tumor discharge, urinalysis and blood tests.
- Biopsy (see Glossary).
- Self-care instructions focused on the older patient.
- Hospitalization and surgery to remove the tumor. Advancing age alone is not a deterrent. Local tumors of the foreskin may require circumcision only. Invasive tumors require total removal of the penis and the regional lymph nodes.
- Radiation or chemotherapy treatment after surgery.
- Psychotherapy or counseling after surgery to help you learn to cope with an altered self-image.

HOME TREATMENT BY SELF OR CARE-GIVER

GENERAL INSTRUCTIONS—A bladder catheter will be necessary for a prolonged period—sometimes permanently—after surgery and radiation treatment.

MEDICATION (ADJUSTED FOR AGING)
- Your doctor may prescribe:
  Pain relievers if necessary.
  Anticancer (chemotherapy) drugs for wide-spread cancer. However, the effectiveness of presently available drugs is only temporary.
- *Note:* Adverse reactions and side effects may be more frequent and severe in older persons. Remind your doctor of any medicines you already take.

ACTIVITY FOR OLDER PATIENTS
- Resume your normal activities as soon as possible after treatment. Sexual relations are possible if enough penile tissue remains following surgery.
- See Appendix 20 regarding physical fitness for the active older adult.

FOOD & BEVERAGE
- No special diet is required.
- See Appendix 1 regarding good nutrition for people over 50.

FUTURE CONSIDERATIONS FOR THE AGING ADULT

POSSIBLE COMPLICATIONS—This form of cancer spreads quickly to nearby lymph nodes, but slowly to distant sites or organs. Many men delay treatment due to denial or fear of disfigurement and loss of sexual function. This increases the likelihood that the cancer will spread and cause death.

PROBABLE OUTCOME—Often curable with early diagnosis, surgery and radiation treatment. Without treatment, this condition is incurable, and the 5-year survival rate is less than 40%.

PREVENTING RECURRENCE—Examine the penis and testicles monthly to detect possible cancers early, when treatment is most successful. Seek medical treatment for any sign of infection or sore on the penis.

CALL YOUR DOCTOR IF

- You have any lump or sore on the penis.
- Excessive bleeding occurs at the surgical site.
- New, unexplained symptoms develop. The drugs used in treatment may produce side effects.

PENIS INFECTION
(Balanitis)

BASIC INFORMATION FOR OLDER ADULTS

DESCRIPTION—Balanitis occurs when the foreskin and head of the penis become infected and inflamed, usually in an uncircumcised male. Body parts involved: The penis and foreskin.

SPECIAL CONSIDERATIONS FOR AGING
- The immune system becomes less effective, opening the way for viral, bacterial and other infections; malignancies; immune disorders; and allergies.
- Decreased nutrition increases the risk of infections.

SIGNS & SYMPTOMS
- Pain, redness, moistness and swelling of the head of the penis.
- Inflammation of the foreskin.
- Ulceration of the penis.
- Enlarged lymph glands in the groin.
- Chills and fever (rare).
- Discharge from the penis (rare).
- Burning on urination (rare).

CAUSES & RISK FACTORS—Caused by infection with bacteria under the foreskin of the penis that invade the head of the penis. The risk increases with:
- Inadequate cleansing under the foreskin.
- Trauma or minor injury to the foreskin and penis, as from excessive masturbation or vigorous intercourse.
- Irritation from chemicals in clothing.

DOCTOR'S TREATMENT & DIAGNOSTIC TESTS
- Medical history and physical exam.
- Laboratory culture of the discharge from the infected area.
- Surgery to circumcise the penis if penis infections recur frequently. Advancing age alone is not a deterrent.
- Self-care instructions focused on the older patient.

HOME TREATMENT BY SELF OR CARE-GIVER

GENERAL INSTRUCTIONS—Use warm-water soaks (see Appendix 18) to relieve the pain.

MEDICATION (ADJUSTED FOR AGING)
- Your doctor may prescribe:
  Steroid creams to control swelling.
  Topical or oral antibiotics to fight infection.
  Aspirin or acetaminophen to relieve minor pain and fever.

- *Note:* Adverse reactions and side effects may be more frequent and severe in older persons. Remind your doctor of any medicines you already take.

ACTIVITY FOR OLDER PATIENTS
- Rest in bed if you have a fever. You may read or watch TV. Avoid sexual intercourse during treatment.
- Resume your normal activities when the infection is cured.
- See Appendix 20 regarding physical fitness for the active older adult.

FOOD & BEVERAGE
- No special diet is required.
- See Appendix 1 regarding good nutrition for people over 50.

FUTURE CONSIDERATIONS FOR THE AGING ADULT

POSSIBLE COMPLICATIONS
- Ulceration of the penis.
- Spread of the infection to deeper skin layers of the penis shaft.
- Blood poisoning.

PROBABLE OUTCOME—Usually curable in 1 to 2 weeks with medical treatment.

PREVENTING RECURRENCE
- Wash daily with soap and water, especially after sexual intercourse. Cleanse under the foreskin.
- Stretch a tight foreskin with daily gentle retraction.
- Use a condom during intercourse.

CALL YOUR DOCTOR IF

- You have symptoms of a penis infection.
- Your symptoms don't improve in 3 days despite treatment.
- The penis infection recurs. Consider circumcision.

PERICARDITIS, ACUTE

BASIC INFORMATION FOR OLDER ADULTS

DESCRIPTION—Acute pericarditis is an inflammation of the pericardium (the thin membrane around the heart). This is not contagious or cancerous unless it is caused by the spread of cancer elsewhere. Body part involved: The pericardium.

SPECIAL CONSIDERATIONS FOR AGING
- The immune system becomes less effective, opening the way for viral, bacterial and other infections; malignancies; immune disorders; and allergies.
- Decreased nutrition increases the risk of infections.

SIGNS & SYMPTOMS
- Dull or sharp pain in the front of the chest, radiating to the neck and shoulder. The pain worsens with movement and eases when sitting up or leaning forward.
- Rapid breathing.
- A cough.
- Fever and chills.
- Weakness.
- Anxiety.
- The most important signs are apparent only with medical examination: a friction rub heard through a stethoscope; elevated white blood cell count; rapid sedimentation rate (see Glossary); abnormal ECG (see Glossary).

CAUSES & RISK FACTORS—The cause is sometimes unknown. The most common known causes are:
- Viral, bacterial or fungal infections.
- Rheumatic fever and other diseases of the connective tissue, such as lupus erythematosus.
- Chronic kidney failure.
- A complication of a heart attack.
- A complication following heart surgery.
- A complication of a chest injury, including the use of a cardiac catheter.
- The spread of cancer to the pericardium.
- Drug toxicity.

Risk factors include:
- Recent illness, such as a heart attack, viral illness, autoimmune disease, uremia or rheumatic fever.
- A medical history of tuberculosis.
- Radiation treatment.

DOCTOR'S TREATMENT & DIAGNOSTIC TESTS
- Medical history and physical exam.
- ECG (see Glossary).
- Echocardiograph (see Glossary).
- Chest x-ray.
- Pericardiocentesis (the removal of fluid from the pericardial sac). This procedure may be diagnostic or therapeutic.
- Surgery to remove fluid through a needle if fluid collects in the pericardium (sometimes).
- Surgery to remove thickened pericardium (rare).
- Self-care instructions focused on the older patient.

HOME TREATMENT BY SELF OR CARE-GIVER

GENERAL INSTRUCTIONS—Apply warm compresses to the chest to relieve the pain.

MEDICATION (ADJUSTED FOR AGING)
- Your doctor may prescribe steroid drugs if the pericarditis is a complication of heart attack, connective tissue disease or a metabolic disorder. No medication is needed if the pericarditis is caused by a virus.
- You may use non-prescriptions drugs such as acetaminophen for minor pain.
- *Note:* Adverse reactions and side effects may be more frequent and severe in older persons. Remind your doctor of any medicines you already take.

ACTIVITY FOR OLDER PATIENTS
- Rest in bed until the fever and pain subside. You may read or watch TV.
- Resume your normal activities gradually.
- Resume sexual relations when the fever and pain disappear.
- See Appendix 20 regarding physical fitness for the active older adult.

FOOD & BEVERAGE
- No special diet is required.
- See Appendix 1 regarding good nutrition for people over 50.

FUTURE CONSIDERATIONS FOR THE AGING ADULT

POSSIBLE COMPLICATIONS—Fluid in the pericardium may cause pressure on the heart. This can be fatal unless the fluid is removed quickly.

PROBABLE OUTCOME—Usually curable in 6 months unless the pericarditis is caused by cancer. After it is cured, there should be no functional disability.

PREVENTING RECURRENCE—There are no specific preventive measures except medical treatment of the disorders that cause pericarditis.

CALL YOUR DOCTOR IF

- You have symptoms of pericarditis.
- Any of the following occurs during treatment:
  Fever.
  Shortness of breath and rapid heartbeat.
  Cough with blood.
  Unexplained weight loss.
  Pain that is not controlled by acetaminophen.
- New, unexplained symptoms develop. Steroids used in treatment may produce side effects, especially restlessness.

PERIODONTITIS
(Gum Inflammation)

BASIC INFORMATION FOR OLDER ADULTS

DESCRIPTION—Periodontitis is an inflammation and infection of the gums causing loss of supporting bone. Periodontitis is responsible for more tooth loss than tooth decay. It is not contagious. Body parts involved: The gums and jawbones.

SPECIAL CONSIDERATIONS FOR AGING
- The immune system becomes less effective, opening the way for viral, bacterial and other infections; malignancies; immune disorders; and allergies.
- The oral mucous membrane becomes thinner and more fragile.

SIGNS & SYMPTOMS
- An unpleasant taste in the mouth.
- Bad breath.
- Loosening of the teeth in the sockets.
- Aching teeth and gums when eating hot, cold or sweet food.
- Bleeding gums.
- If an abscess develops, tenderness, swelling, pain and fever will also occur.

CAUSES & RISK FACTORS—Poor oral hygiene leads to gingivitis, which causes pockets between the gums and the teeth. Plaque (a sticky deposit of food, bacteria and mucus) forms in these pockets and destroys the bone that surrounds and supports the teeth. The risk increases with any illness that has lowered resistance.

DOCTOR'S TREATMENT & DIAGNOSTIC TESTS
- Medical history and physical exam by a dentist.
- X-rays of the mouth.
- A dentist's care.
- Surgery to remove unhealthy gum tissue and reshape the underlying bone to eliminate pockets. Advancing age alone is not a deterrent.
- Self-care instructions focused on the older patient.

HOME TREATMENT BY SELF OR CARE-GIVER

GENERAL INSTRUCTIONS
- Brush your teeth daily. Scrub the clear, sticky plaque off your teeth with a soft toothbrush. A soft brush is less likely to damage the teeth and gums than a hard brush. Place the brush at the gum line and gently rotate it, pointing the bristles toward the gum. Brush one section of teeth at a time.
- Floss your teeth daily. Wind waxed or unwaxed dental floss around one finger on each hand. Force the dental floss between the teeth. Gently clean the tooth surfaces with a back-and-forth sawing motion at the gum line. Floss between all lower teeth, using your fingers as guides. Next loosen the floss and place it on the tops of your thumbs. Floss between all upper teeth, using your thumbs as guides.
- Use mouthwash. Your dentist can recommend an effective one.

MEDICATION (ADJUSTED FOR AGING)
- For minor pain, you may use non-prescription drugs such as acetaminophen.
- *Note:* Adverse reactions and side effects may be more frequent and severe in older persons. Remind your doctor of any medicines you already take.

ACTIVITY FOR OLDER PATIENTS
- No restrictions are necessary.
- See Appendix 20 regarding physical fitness for the active older adult.

FOOD & BEVERAGE
- No special diet is required, except to avoid sweets.
- See Appendix 1 regarding good nutrition for people over 50.

FUTURE CONSIDERATIONS FOR THE AGING ADULT

POSSIBLE COMPLICATIONS—Without treatment, the teeth loosen so much in their bony sockets that they must be extracted.

PROBABLE OUTCOME—Usually curable with a combination of dental treatment and strict adherence to a good oral hygiene program (see General Instructions).

PREVENTING RECURRENCE
- Practice good oral hygiene (see General Instructions).
- Avoid sweet snacks, which contribute to the formation of plaque.
- Visit your dentist regularly to have your teeth cleaned. Ask your dentist about the level of fluoride in the local drinking water. Fluoride supplements may provide added protection.

CALL YOUR DOCTOR IF

You have symptoms of periodontitis.

PERIPHERAL NEUROPATHY
(Peripheral Neuritis)

BASIC INFORMATION FOR OLDER ADULTS

DESCRIPTION—Peripheral neuropathy is characterized by a group of symptoms that are caused by abnormalities in the sensory or motor nerves. Body parts involved: Many of the nerves that end in muscles, blood vessels and skin. This usually affects the fingers, toes, hands, feet, lower arms and legs, and it may affect bladder or bowel control.

SPECIAL CONSIDERATIONS FOR AGING
- Neurological diseases become more likely
- Decreased nutrition increases the risk of infections.
- The number of autoantibodies (see Glossary) increases.
- Stress from any emotional cause—fear, worry, anxiety, sadness, loneliness or anger—affects all aspects of any illness or disorder.

SIGNS & SYMPTOMS—These symptoms
usually appear gradually over many months:
- Tingling and numbness that begins in the hands and feet and spreads gradually.
- Gradual muscle weakness throughout the body—often in same place on both sides of the body.
- Shooting pains that are often worse at night. The pains are aggravated by touch or temperature changes.
- Painless ulcers on the toes or fingers.
- Pale, dry skin that becomes sensitive to the touch.
- Weight loss.
- Severe back pain or loss of bladder or bowel control if the disorder is caused by intervertebral disk disease.

CAUSES & RISK FACTORS
Causes include:
- Reactions to drugs or chemicals, including emetine, hexobarbital, chlorbutanol, sulfonamides, phenytoin, nitrofurantoin, heavy metals, carbon monoxide, solvents or industrial poisons.
- Interactions of drugs required by people with cardiovascular disease.
- A complication of an underlying disorder, such as diabetes mellitus, alcoholism, vitamin deficiency, vitamin B-12 deficiency anemia or thyroid disorder.
- Poor nutrition; malabsorption disorders; autoimmune reaction; trauma or pressure on a nerve; excessive vomiting; decreased thyroid function; acute porphyria; a complication of dialysis treatment; cancer; a ruptured intervertebral disc.

Risk factors include:
- The use of drugs listed under Causes, especially multiple medications.
- Exposure to chemicals listed under Causes.
- Poor nutrition, such as in alcoholism.
- Poor control of diabetes.

DOCTOR'S TREATMENT & DIAGNOSTIC TESTS
- Medical history and physical exam.
- Laboratory studies of blood, urine, vitamin B-12 levels, thyroid function and spinal fluid.
- Electromyography (see Glossary).
- Hospitalization (sometimes).
- Surgery to relieve pressure if the nerves are compressed. Advancing age alone is not a deterrent.
- Self-care instructions focused on the older patient.

HOME TREATMENT BY SELF OR CARE-GIVER

GENERAL INSTRUCTIONS
- If peripheral neuropathy is caused by an incurable disorder, obtain biofeedback training to help you learn relaxation techniques that relieve pain.
- If peripheral neuropathy is interfering with normal activities, consult a physical therapist.
- If you have difficulty maintaining balance, walk with a cane or other support.
- Install rails next to the bathtub.
- Inspect your hands and feet daily for unnoticed wounds.
- Keep your feet clean and your toenails trimmed properly; wear shoes that fit well.

MEDICATION (ADJUSTED FOR AGING)—For minor pain, you may use non-prescription drugs such as aspirin or acetaminophen.

ACTIVITY FOR OLDER PATIENTS—Stay as active as possible.

FOOD & BEVERAGE
- No special diet is required. Vitamin and mineral supplements will probably be necessary. Pyridoxine (vitamin B-6) may help.
- See Appendix 1 regarding good nutrition for people over 50.

FUTURE CONSIDERATIONS FOR THE AGING ADULT

POSSIBLE COMPLICATIONS—Chronic pain and disability.

PROBABLE OUTCOME—Mild cases can be cured if the underlying cause is diagnosed and treated. Serious cases may be incurable, but the symptoms can improve.

PREVENTING RECURRENCE—Avoid as many causes and risks as possible.

CALL YOUR DOCTOR IF

- You have symptoms of peripheral neuropathy.
- The symptoms (especially muscle weakness) persist or worsen despite treatment.
- You develop a severe bruise or open sore.

PERITONITIS

BASIC INFORMATION FOR OLDER ADULTS

DESCRIPTION—Peritonitis is a serious infection or inflammation of part or all of the peritoneum, the covering of the intestinal tract. Body parts involved: The abdomen, including the intestines and the peritoneum. (THIS IS AN EMERGENCY; SEEK MEDICAL CARE IMMEDIATELY!)

SPECIAL CONSIDERATIONS FOR AGING
- The immune system becomes less effective, opening the way for viral, bacterial and other infections; malignancies; immune disorders; and allergies.
- Decreased nutrition, common among chronically ill older people, increases the risk of any disease or disorder.
- Characteristic signs and symptoms of many disorders are frequently changed or absent.
- Usual signs and symptoms may be absent and be replaced by symptoms of confusion, dizziness, failure to thrive, falling, incontinence, increasing dementia, refusal to eat or drink, weight loss, depression, paranoia, hypochondriasis, psychosis or threats of suicide.

SIGNS & SYMPTOMS
- Pain in one area or throughout the abdomen. The pain usually starts suddenly and becomes increasingly severe. It may be crampy at first, and then steady. The patient often prefers to lie quietly on the back because movement or pressure on the abdomen increases the pain.
- Shoulder pain (sometimes).
- Chills and fever (often high).
- Dizziness and weakness.
- Rapid heartbeat.
- Low blood pressure.
- Vomiting and dehydration.

CAUSES & RISK FACTORS—Peritonitis occurs when foreign materials enter the abdominal cavity. These foreign materials include bacteria or gastrointestinal contents, such as digestive juices, blood, partly digested food or feces. These materials enter the abdomen following:
- The rupture or perforation of any organ in the abdomen, such as an inflamed appendix, peptic ulcer or infected diverticulum or gallbladder.
- Injury to the abdominal wall, such as from a knife or bullet wound.
- Pelvic inflammatory disease.
Risk factors include:
- A delay in the treatment of the causes listed above.
- Recent abdominal surgery.

DOCTOR'S TREATMENT & DIAGNOSTIC TESTS
- Medical history and physical exam.
- Laboratory white blood cell count to detect inflammation, red blood cell count to detect bleeding and measurement of fluid and electrolyte levels.
- Surgical diagnostic procedures, such as passing a small needle into the abdomen to obtain fluid, blood or other material.
- X-rays of the abdomen.
- Exploratory surgery (laparotomy) if the cause is unknown. Advancing age alone is not a deterrent.
- Hospitalization.
- Intravenous fluids for dehydration.
- Surgery to repair the organ damage or the injury that allowed the foreign materials to get into the abdomen.
- Self-care instructions focused on the older patient.

HOME TREATMENT BY SELF OR CARE-GIVER

GENERAL INSTRUCTIONS—Early diagnosis and treatment of the underlying disorder, such as appendicitis or ulcer, are essential. If abdominal pain develops, don't waste valuable time with home treatments—especially laxative use, which may cause inflamed abdominal organs to rupture.

MEDICATION (ADJUSTED FOR AGING)—Your doctor may prescribe:
- Antibiotics to fight infection.
- Pain relievers (sometimes) after diagnosis or surgery.

ACTIVITY FOR OLDER PATIENTS—Rest in bed after treatment until the symptoms disappear. You may read or watch TV. If surgery is necessary, resume your activities gradually after surgery.

FOOD & BEVERAGE—Don't eat or drink anything so the intestinal tract can rest until the acute infection subsides. You may be given intravenous nourishment and fluids.

FUTURE CONSIDERATIONS FOR THE AGING ADULT

POSSIBLE COMPLICATIONS—Shock; blood poisoning (septicemia); intestinal obstruction caused by later adhesions (bands of scar tissue).

PROBABLE OUTCOME—Usually curable with early diagnosis and treatment. Treatment delay and complications can be fatal.

PREVENTING RECURRENCE—Obtain prompt medical treatment for underlying disorders.

CALL YOUR DOCTOR IF

- You have symptoms of peritonitis. *This is an emergency!*
- Any of the following occurs during treatment: Constipation.
  Signs of new infection, including fever, chills, muscle aches, dizziness, headache and increasing abdominal pain.
- New, unexplained symptoms develop. The drugs used in treatment may produce side effects.

PHARYNGITIS

BASIC INFORMATION FOR OLDER ADULTS

DESCRIPTION—Pharyngitis is a throat inflammation and infection from any of a variety of germs. Body parts involved: The throat area, including the tonsils.

SPECIAL CONSIDERATIONS FOR AGING
- The immune system becomes less effective, opening the way for viral, bacterial and other infections; malignancies; immune disorders; and allergies.
- Decreased nutrition, common among chronically ill older people, increases the risk of any disease or disorder.

SIGNS & SYMPTOMS
- Sore throat; swallowing difficulty.
- A tickle or "lump" in the throat.
- Swollen glands in the neck (sometimes).
- A throat that is red or covered with a grayish membrane (sometimes).
- Fever; generalized aching; earache.

CAUSES & RISK FACTORS—Caused by an infection from bacteria, viruses or fungi. Following are the most common germs:
- Bacteria—streptococci, diphtheria, gonococci, hemophilus, pneumococci or staphylococci.
- Viruses—Epstein-Barr and many types of respiratory viruses.
- Fungi—monilial.

Risk factors include:
- Illness that has lowered resistance.
- Fatigue or overwork.
- Diabetes mellitus; immune deficiencies.
- Smoking; excessive alcohol consumption.
- Oral sex.
- Epidemics, during which all persons are at increased risk.
- Swallowing a substance that can scald, corrode or scratch the throat.

DOCTOR'S TREATMENT & DIAGNOSTIC TESTS
- Medical history and physical exam.
- Laboratory throat culture and blood count.
- Self-care instructions focused on the older patient.
- Hospitalization for pharyngitis caused by diphtheria or hemophilus bacteria.

HOME TREATMENT BY SELF OR CARE-GIVER

GENERAL INSTRUCTIONS
- Use gargles to relieve throat pain. Prepare double-strength tea, hot or cold, or a salt-water solution (1 teaspoon salt in 8 oz. warm water), and use it to gargle as often as you wish.
- Use a cool-mist humidifier to increase the air moisture. This will relieve the dry, tight feeling in your throat.
- If the glands are large and tender, apply moist, warm soaks (see Appendix 18) at least

4 times a day for 30 to 60 minutes. The compresses will be more effective if they are kept warm. Be careful not to burn the skin.

MEDICATION (ADJUSTED FOR AGING)
- For minor discomfort, you may use non-prescription drugs such as acetaminophen.
- Your doctor may prescribe antibiotics or antifungal agents to fight bacterial or fungal infections.
- Be sure to finish the entire course of prescribed antibiotics to avoid complications to heart or kidneys.

ACTIVITY FOR OLDER PATIENTS
- Activities should be adjusted to suit your feeling of well-being. Bed rest may be necessary for treating an underlying disease.
- See Appendix 20 regarding physical fitness for the active older adult.

FOOD & BEVERAGE
- Extra fluids are necessary—at least 8 glasses of water daily, more for high fevers. If swallowing solid food is painful, a liquid diet may be necessary. See Appendix 7.
- See Appendix 1 regarding good nutrition for people over 50.

FUTURE CONSIDERATIONS FOR THE AGING ADULT

POSSIBLE COMPLICATIONS
- Epiglottitis, leading to complete breathing obstruction; pneumonia.
- Rheumatic fever, scarlet fever or glomerulonephritis if the pharyngitis is caused by strep bacteria and does not receive adequate antibiotic treatment.

PROBABLE OUTCOME—Spontaneous recovery for most cases of viral pharyngitis. Other cases are curable with antibiotic or antifungal drugs.

PREVENTING RECURRENCE
- Avoid close contact with anyone with a sore throat.
- Keep your immunizations, including those for diphtheria, up to date. An immunization schedule appears in Appendix 16.

CALL YOUR DOCTOR IF

- You have symptoms of pharyngitis.
- Any of the following occurs during treatment:
  Breathing or swallowing difficulty.
  Fever; severe headache.
  Thick mucus drainage from the nose.
  A cough that produces green, yellow, brown or bloody sputum.
  A skin rash.
  Dark urine.
  Chest pain.

PILONIDAL CYST

BASIC INFORMATION FOR OLDER ADULTS

DESCRIPTION—A pilonidal cyst is a small, hair-containing sac of skin at the base of the spine. The cyst looks like a small opening—sometimes no more than a dimple—with a few hairs protruding (sometimes). It is prone to infection. Pilonidal cysts are uncommon in black people. Body part involved: The skin.

SPECIAL CONSIDERATIONS FOR AGING
- The immune system becomes less effective, opening the way for viral, bacterial and other infections; malignancies; immune disorders; and allergies.
- Decreased nutrition, common among chronically ill older people, increases the risk of any disease or disorder.

SIGNS & SYMPTOMS—There are no symptoms when the cyst is not infected. When infected, it causes:
- Pain, redness, tenderness and swelling in the area.
- Fever and chills.
- A discharge of pus.

CAUSES & RISK FACTORS
The cyst is a minor abnormality that occurs during fetal development. Infection is usually caused by staphylococcal bacteria. Risk factors include:
- Heavy perspiration. Obesity increases perspiration.
- Tight clothing.

DOCTOR'S TREATMENT & DIAGNOSTIC TESTS
- Medical history and physical exam.
- Laboratory culture of the discharge.
- Self-care instructions focused on the older patient.
- Surgery to remove the cyst if it repeatedly becomes infected.

HOME TREATMENT BY SELF OR CARE-GIVER

GENERAL INSTRUCTIONS
- If the cyst is infected, take warm baths to relieve the pain. Sit in a tub of warm water for 10 to 15 minutes as often as it feels good.
- If surgery is necessary, see Pilonidal Cyst Removal in the Surgeries section for an explanation of the surgery and postoperative care.

MEDICATION (ADJUSTED FOR AGING)
- Your doctor may prescribe antibiotics to fight infection.
- *Note:* Adverse reactions and side effects may be more frequent and severe in older persons. Remind your doctor of any medicines you already take.

ACTIVITY FOR OLDER PATIENTS—No restrictions are necessary, unless the cyst becomes infected. Then, limit activities until the infection is cured.

FOOD & BEVERAGE
- Lose weight if you are overweight. A reducing diet appears in Appendix 10.
- See Appendix 1 regarding good nutrition for people over 50.

FUTURE CONSIDERATIONS FOR THE AGING ADULT

POSSIBLE COMPLICATIONS—Spread of the infection (rare).

PROBABLE OUTCOME—Curable with antibiotic treatment.

PREVENTING RECURRENCE
- Bathe or shower daily to keep the area clean. Warm tub baths seem more effective in preventing the infection of the cyst.
- Wear light, loose-fitting clothing.
- Avoid being overweight.

CALL YOUR DOCTOR IF

- You have symptoms of a pilonidal cyst. It should be diagnosed.
- After diagnosis, a cyst shows signs of infection.

PINKEYE
(Conjunctivitis)

BASIC INFORMATION FOR OLDER ADULTS

DESCRIPTION—Pinkeye is an inflammation of the eyelid's underside and the white part of the eye. Body parts involved: The eye and the underside of the eyelid.

SPECIAL CONSIDERATIONS FOR AGING
- The immune system becomes less effective, opening the way for viral, bacterial and other infections; malignancies; immune disorders; and allergies.
- Decreased nutrition increases the risk of infections.
- Injured tissues repair more slowly.

SIGNS & SYMPTOMS—The following symptoms may affect one or both eyes:
- Clear, green or yellow discharge from the eye.
- After sleeping, crusts on the lashes that cause the eyelids to stick together.
- Eye pain.
- Swollen eyelids.
- Sensitivity to bright light.
- Redness and a gritty feeling in the eye.
- Intense itching (with allergic conjunctivitis only).

CAUSES & RISK FACTORS
Caused by:
- Viral infections. Pinkeye may accompany colds.
- Bacterial infections.
- Chemical irritation or wind, dust, smoke and other types of air pollution.
- Allergies caused by cosmetics, pollen or other allergens.
- A partially closed tear duct.
- Intense light, such as from sunlamps, snow reflection or electric arcs used in welding.
Risk factors include:
- Crowded or unsanitary living conditions.
- Exposure to others in public places.

DOCTOR'S TREATMENT & DIAGNOSTIC TESTS
- Medical history and physical exam.
- Laboratory culture of the discharge from the eye.
- Self-care instructions focused on the older patient.

HOME TREATMENT BY SELF OR CARE-GIVER

GENERAL INSTRUCTIONS
- Wash your hands often with antiseptic soap, and use paper towels to dry. Don't touch your eyes. Gently wipe the discharge from the eye using disposable tissues. Infections are frequently spread by contaminated fingers, towels, handkerchiefs or washcloths that have touched the infected eye.
- Use warm-water soaks (see Appendix 18) to reduce the discomfort.
- Don't use eye makeup.

MEDICATION (ADJUSTED FOR AGING)
- Your doctor may prescribe antibiotic eye drops, sulfa eye drops, steroid eye drops or an antibiotic ointment to fight the infection. Use 3 times daily.
- If the infection does not improve in 2 or 3 days, it may be caused by an insensitive bacteria, virus or allergy. At this point, an ophthalmologist may need to culture the conjunctivae or make special studies to determine the cause. Most ophthalmologists believe steroid eye drops should not be used until a diagnosis is definite. If the infection is caused by the herpes simplex virus, steroids may spread it from the conjunctiva to the cornea, damaging the eye.
- *Note:* Adverse reactions and side effects may be more frequent and severe in older persons. Remind your doctor of any medicines you already take.

ACTIVITY FOR OLDER PATIENTS
- Resume your normal activities as soon as your symptoms improve.
- See Appendix 20 regarding physical fitness for the active older adult.

FOOD & BEVERAGE
- No special diet is required.
- See Appendix 1 regarding good nutrition for people over 50.

FUTURE CONSIDERATIONS FOR THE AGING ADULT

POSSIBLE COMPLICATIONS—If untreated, pinkeye may spread and damage the cornea permanently, impairing vision.

PROBABLE OUTCOME
- Allergic pinkeye can be cured if the allergen is removed. It is likely to recur.
- Other forms are curable in 1 to 2 weeks with treatment.

PREVENTING RECURRENCE
- Wash your hands frequently with soap and warm water.
- Avoid exposure to eye irritants.

CALL YOUR DOCTOR IF

- You have symptoms of pinkeye.
- The infection does not improve in 48 hours despite treatment.
- A fever develops.
- Your pain increases.
- Your vision is affected.

PINWORMS
(Enterobiasis; Seatworm; Threadworm; Oxyuriasis)

BASIC INFORMATION FOR OLDER ADULTS

DESCRIPTION—Pinworms are intestinal parasites. Pinworm infestations are more a nuisance than a major health problem. Body parts involved: The cecum (the pouchlike beginning of the large intestine on the right side, to which the appendix is attached); large intestine; anus; skin around the anus.

SPECIAL CONSIDERATIONS FOR AGING
- The immune system becomes less effective, opening the way for viral, bacterial and other infections; malignancies; immune disorders; and allergies.
- Decreased nutrition, common among chronically ill older people, increases the risk of any disease or disorder.

SIGNS & SYMPTOMS
- Skin irritation and painful itching around the anus, especially during sleep.
- Restless sleep.
- Vaginal discharge, itching and discomfort if the pinworms migrate into the vaginal opening.
- Poor appetite and stomach pain (rare).
- Paleness (sometimes).

CAUSES & RISK FACTORS—Caused by the infestation of the cecum by a very small worm (oxyuria) that measures only 10mm in its adult form. Pinworms travel from the cecum to the rectum to lay their eggs around the anus and buttocks. The tiny eggs are picked up on the fingers by scratching. The eggs are transferred to others on toilet seats or by hand-to-hand or hand-to-mouth contact. They also drift in the air, where they are inhaled or swallowed. The eggs hatch in the small intestine. The larvae travel to the cecum, where they mature, mate and repeat the cycle. Risk factors include:
- Poor personal hygiene.
- Dishwater that is not hot enough to kill the eggs.

DOCTOR'S TREATMENT & DIAGNOSTIC TESTS
- Medical history and physical exam.
- Microscopic study of the worms or eggs.
- Home care after diagnosis.
- Self-care instructions focused on the older patient.

HOME TREATMENT BY SELF OR CARE-GIVER

GENERAL INSTRUCTIONS—The following should be done on the day the family is treated with medicine:
- Clean the house with extra care. Wash the sheets and clothing with extra bleach or ammonia or boil them.
- If there are children in the home, scrub washable toys. Sterilize metal toys and similar objects in a hot oven.
- Cut and clean your fingernails.
- Change towels.
- Scrub toilet bowls.
- Take extra-long showers.

About 2 weeks after treatment, your doctor will probably check to be sure that all parasites have been destroyed.

MEDICATION (ADJUSTED FOR AGING)
- Your doctor may prescribe antiworm medicine. Follow the directions carefully. Take the medicine on an empty stomach. The medicine may cause nausea, vomiting and diarrhea. It is not absorbed by the stomach or intestines, so the bowel movement following treatment will probably be the color of the medicine.
- *Note:* Adverse reactions and side effects may be more frequent and severe in older persons. Remind your doctor of any medicines you already take.

ACTIVITY FOR OLDER PATIENTS
- No restrictions are necessary.
- See Appendix 20 regarding physical fitness for the active older adult.

FOOD & BEVERAGE
- No special diet is required.
- See Appendix 1 regarding good nutrition for people over 50.

FUTURE CONSIDERATIONS FOR THE AGING ADULT

POSSIBLE COMPLICATIONS—No serious complications are expected.

PROBABLE OUTCOME—Usually curable in one treatment—two treatments at the most. Treatment should include all family members at once. Recurrence is common. If more worms reappear soon after treatment, they usually represent a new infection—not treatment failure.

PREVENTING RECURRENCE
- Wash your hands carefully after using the toilet and before meals.
- Keep your nails short and clean.
- Wash the anus and genitals at least once a day. Rinse well, preferably under a shower.
- Don't scratch the anus or put your fingers near your nose or mouth.
- Use very hot water to wash dishes.

CALL YOUR DOCTOR IF

- Anyone in your family has symptoms of pinworms.
- Pinworms reappear after treatment.
- You think the medicine used in treatment is causing side effects that don't disappear quickly.

PITUITARY GLAND, UNDERACTIVE
(Hypopituitarism)

BASIC INFORMATION FOR OLDER ADULTS

DESCRIPTION—Hypopituitarism is the underactivity of the pituitary gland, which results in inadequate amounts of hormones produced by the pituitary. The anterior lobe of the pituitary produces the following hormones:
- Growth hormone.
- Prolactin, which stimulates the breasts to produce milk.
- Thyroid-stimulating hormone:
- Adrenal-stimulating hormone.
- Ovarian- or testicular-stimulating hormones.

The posterior lobe of the pituitary gland produces two hormones:
- Antidiuretic hormone, which affects the kidneys in regulating the concentration and quantity of urine.
- Oxytocin, which stimulates contractions of the uterus during childbirth and releases milk during breast feeding.

Body parts involved: The pituitary gland (located at the base of the brain) and the body parts mentioned above.

SPECIAL CONSIDERATIONS FOR AGING—Neurological diseases become more likely.

SIGNS & SYMPTOMS
- Unusual vaginal bleeding.
- Impotence; infertility.
- Low blood sugar and weakness; low blood pressure.
- Cold intolerance.
- Mental changes, including psychosis.
- Extreme lethargy.
- Persistent headaches.

CAUSES & RISK FACTORS—The causes are unknown (sometimes). Known causes include the following:
- Serious head injury with pressure (usually from bleeding) on the pituitary gland.
- A tumor of the pituitary gland.
- An infection in the brain.
- An aneurysm of the blood vessels in the base of the brain.

The risk increases with a family history of pituitary disorders.

DOCTOR'S TREATMENT & DIAGNOSTIC TESTS
- Medical history and physical exam.
- Laboratory blood studies of hormone levels and function.
- CT scan, MRI (see Glossary for both) or x-ray of the head.
- Angiogram (see Glossary).
- Visual field testing (see Glossary).
- Close supervision of continuing treatment.

- Surgery to remove underlying tumors or blood clots if necessary.
- Radiation therapy (sometimes).
- Self-care instructions focused on the older patient.

HOME TREATMENT BY SELF OR CARE-GIVER

GENERAL INSTRUCTIONS—No specific instructions except those listed under other headings.

MEDICATION (ADJUSTED FOR AGING)
- Your doctor may prescribe:
  Hormones to replace those the pituitary gland is not producing.
  Pain relievers after surgery.
  Antibiotics or antiviral medications if an infection is causing the disorder.
- *Note:* Adverse reactions and side effects may be more frequent and severe in older persons. Remind your doctor of any medicines you already take.

ACTIVITY FOR OLDER PATIENTS
- Stay as active as your condition allows.
- See Appendix 20 regarding physical fitness for the active older adult.

FOOD & BEVERAGE—See Appendix 1 regarding good nutrition for people over 50.

FUTURE CONSIDERATIONS FOR THE AGING ADULT

POSSIBLE COMPLICATIONS—Hormonal failure and death without treatment.

PROBABLE OUTCOME—Usually treatable with surgery or replacement therapy of pituitary, thyroid, adrenal and sex hormones.

PREVENTING RECURRENCE—Obtain medical treatment for the underlying injury, infection or tumor if possible.

CALL YOUR DOCTOR IF

- You have symptoms of an underactive pituitary gland.
- After surgery, you develop signs of infection, such as fever, lethargy and muscle aches.
- New, unexplained symptoms develop. The drugs used in treatment may produce side effects.

PITUITARY TUMOR

BASIC INFORMATION FOR OLDER ADULTS

DESCRIPTION—A pituitary tumor is an abnormal growth in the pituitary gland that leads to the overactivity of other endocrine glands. Pituitary tumors may be benign or malignant—but even malignant pituitary tumors rarely spread to other body parts. Body parts involved: The pituitary gland, which is located at the base of the brain.

SPECIAL CONSIDERATIONS FOR AGING
- The immune system becomes less effective, opening the way for viral, bacterial and other infections; malignancies; immune disorders; and allergies.
- Malignant diseases are less likely to spread rapidly.
- Characteristic signs and symptoms of many disorders are frequently changed or absent.
- Stress from any emotional cause—fear, worry, anxiety, sadness, loneliness or anger—affects all aspects of any illness or disorder.

SIGNS & SYMPTOMS
- Blurred vision, double vision, dizziness or a drooping eyelid caused by the pressure of the tumor on the nerves to the eye.
- A headache in the forehead.
- Nausea and vomiting.
- Seizures.
- A runny nose.
- Excessive thirst.
- Unexplained weight gain.
- Low blood sugar.
- Low blood pressure.
- Loss of peripheral vision.
- Symptoms of abnormalities in other endocrine glands. See Thyroid, Overactive; Parathyroid, Overactive; Cushing's Syndrome; and Ovarian Tumor in the Illnesses section.

CAUSES & RISK FACTORS—The cause is unknown, but it may be caused by a dominant genetic trait.

DOCTOR'S TREATMENT & DIAGNOSTIC TESTS
- Medical history and physical exam.
- Laboratory studies of cerebrospinal fluid and blood.
- X-rays of the skull.
- CT scan or MRI (see Glossary for both).
- Angiogram (see Glossary).
- Visual field testing (see Glossary).
- Surgery to remove the tumor (see Craniotomy). Advancing age alone is not a deterrent.
- Postoperative radiation therapy.
- Self-care instructions focused on the older patient.

HOME TREATMENT BY SELF OR CARE-GIVER

GENERAL INSTRUCTIONS
- No specific instructions except those listed under other headings.
- A pituitary tumor is a complicated, serious disorder. This page can cover only the main points of diagnosis and treatment. Your doctor, nurse or librarian can provide sources of supplemental information.

MEDICATION (ADJUSTED FOR AGING)
- Your doctor may prescribe:
  Pain relievers.
  Hormone replacement medication for life. This may require frequent dosage adjustments.
  Anticancer (chemotherapy) drugs.
- *Note:* Adverse reactions and side effects may be more frequent and severe in older persons. Remind your doctor of any medicines you already take.

ACTIVITY FOR OLDER PATIENTS
- Resume your normal activities gradually after surgery.
- See Appendix 20 regarding physical fitness for the active older adult.

FOOD & BEVERAGE
- No special diet is required.
- See Appendix 1 regarding good nutrition for people over 50.

FUTURE CONSIDERATIONS FOR THE AGING ADULT

POSSIBLE COMPLICATIONS—The following complications may diminish or be reversed after surgery:
- Blindness.
- Loss of the sense of smell.
- Extreme hormone imbalance.

PROBABLE OUTCOME—Curable with surgery if the tumor has not spread from the pituitary gland. If it has, fatal complications usually develop.

PREVENTING RECURRENCE—There are no specific preventive measures.

CALL YOUR DOCTOR IF

- You have symptoms of a pituitary tumor.
- Any of the following occurs after surgery:
  Bleeding at the surgical site.
  Signs of general infection, such as fever, chills, muscle aches and headache.
  A clear discharge from the nose.

ILLNESSES & DISORDERS

PITYRIASIS ROSEA

BASIC INFORMATION FOR OLDER ADULTS

DESCRIPTION—Pityriasis rosea is a non-contagious inflammatory skin disorder with a faint rash that lasts 3 to 4 weeks. Body parts involved: The skin, especially that of the chest and abdomen (the area a T-shirt would cover).

SPECIAL CONSIDERATIONS FOR AGING
- The skin's reactions to injury or infection increase in intensity and duration.
- The skin becomes more permeable to bacteria, oil and water.

SIGNS & SYMPTOMS
- A faint rash—often found in skin creases—of oval or round, pale pink or brown areas. One larger patch (the "herald patch") may appear first.
- Mild fatigue.
- Itching, usually mild.
- Occasional slight fever and headache.

CAUSES & RISK FACTORS—The cause is unknown, but it may be caused by a virus or an autoimmune disorder. The risk increases with the fall and spring seasons. Simultaneous breakouts in the same household have been reported.

DOCTOR'S TREATMENT & DIAGNOSTIC TESTS
- Medical history and physical exam to rule out other disorders.
- Self-care instructions focused on the older patient.
- Doctor's treatment if severe itching occurs.

HOME TREATMENT BY SELF OR CARE-GIVER

GENERAL INSTRUCTIONS
- Bathe as usual with a mild soap. Avoid hot baths or showers. You don't need to sterilize the tub or shower after bathing.
- Expose the skin to moderate amounts of sunlight. This may decrease the rash.

MEDICATION (ADJUSTED FOR AGING)
- For minor discomfort, you may use non-prescriptions drugs such as:
  Calamine lotion to decrease the itching.
  Acetaminophen to reduce the fever.
- Your doctor may prescribe antihistamine drugs for more severe itching or topical steroids (cortisone or hydrocortisone) for acute skin irritations.
- *Note:* Adverse reactions and side effects may be more frequent and severe in older persons. Remind your doctor of any medicines you already take.

ACTIVITY FOR OLDER PATIENTS
- Usually no restrictions. Be as active as your strength allows.
- See Appendix 20 regarding physical fitness for the active older adult.

FOOD & BEVERAGE
- No special diet is required.
- See Appendix 1 regarding good nutrition for people over 50.

FUTURE CONSIDERATIONS FOR THE AGING ADULT

POSSIBLE COMPLICATIONS—Secondary bacterial infection of the rash area.

PROBABLE OUTCOME—Pityriasis rosea usually runs its natural course in 5 weeks to 4 months. No medication or treatment is available to shorten its course, but the itching and discomfort can be relieved. The skin eruptions won't leave scars unless complicated by a secondary infection. New rash areas continue to break out for several weeks.

PREVENTING RECURRENCE—Cannot be prevented at present.

CALL YOUR DOCTOR IF

- You have symptoms of pityriasis rosea.
- Any of the following occurs during treatment:
  Fever over 101F (38.3C).
  Signs of infection (warmth, redness, tenderness, pain and swelling) in the rash area.

PLEURISY

BASIC INFORMATION FOR OLDER ADULTS

DESCRIPTION—Pleurisy is the inflammation and irritation of the pleura, a thin, two-layered membrane that encloses the lung and lines the inside of the chest. Pleurisy is not a disease, but it may be a manifestation of many different diseases. Body part involved: The pleura.

SPECIAL CONSIDERATIONS FOR AGING
- The immune system becomes less effective, opening the way for viral, bacterial and other infections; malignancies; immune disorders; and allergies.
- Decreased nutrition, common among chronically ill older people, increases the risk of any disease or disorder.
- Characteristic signs and symptoms of many disorders are frequently changed or absent.

SIGNS & SYMPTOMS
- Sudden chest pain that worsens with breathing and coughing. The pain varies from a vague discomfort that occurs only with deep breathing or coughing to an intense, stabbing pain. The pain is usually over the area of pleura inflammation, but it may also occur in the shoulder, lower chest or abdomen.
- Fever (sometimes).
- Discomfort on moving the affected side.
- Rapid, shallow breathing.

If fluid develops at the site of inflammation between the two membrane layers, the liquid is called pleural effusion. When this happens, the pleurisy pain usually subsides, but breathlessness worsens.

CAUSES & RISK FACTORS
Pleurisy is a complication of:
- Lung or chest infections, such as pneumonia or tuberculosis.
- Bronchiectasis.
- Collapse of part of the lung.
- A blood clot in the lung.
- Injury to the chest or a rib fracture.
- Cancer in other parts of the body.
- Collagen vascular disease, such as systemic lupus erythematosus or rheumatoid arthritis.
- Congestive heart failure.
- Kidney and liver disorders.

Risk factors include:
- Obesity.
- Smoking.
- The use of immunosuppressive drugs.

DOCTOR'S TREATMENT & DIAGNOSTIC TESTS
- Medical history and physical exam.
- Laboratory blood studies to detect infection or autoimmune disease.
- X-rays of the chest.
- Biopsy (sometimes).
- Examination of the pleural fluid (if any).
- Self-care instructions focused on the older patient.

HOME TREATMENT BY SELF OR CARE-GIVER

GENERAL INSTRUCTIONS
- For chest pain, wrap the entire chest loosely with 2 or 3 non-adhesive elastic bandages 6 inches wide.
- For coughing, use a cool-mist humidifier to help loosen bronchial secretions so they can be coughed up easily.

MEDICATION (ADJUSTED FOR AGING)
- Your doctor may prescribe antibiotics or pain relievers after diagnosis of the underlying disorder. You may take simple pain relievers, such as acetaminophen or aspirin, to relieve the pain if no complicating disorders exist.
- *Note:* Adverse reactions and side effects may be more frequent and severe in older persons. Remind your doctor of any medicines you already take.

ACTIVITY FOR OLDER PATIENTS
- Reduce your activity level until the pain and fever disappear. Then resume your normal activities gradually.
- See Appendix 20 regarding physical fitness for the active older adult.

FOOD & BEVERAGE
- No special diet is required.
- See Appendix 1 regarding good nutrition for people over 50.

FUTURE CONSIDERATIONS FOR THE AGING ADULT

POSSIBLE COMPLICATIONS
- Pneumonia.
- Lung compression or collapse and impaired breathing from the leakage of pleural effusion.
- Scarring and adhesions at the site of inflammation that restrict lung expansion.

PROBABLE OUTCOME—The successful treatment of pleurisy depends on the successful treatment of the disorder causing it. Often, symptoms without complications clear completely and spontaneously in 2 weeks.

PREVENTING RECURRENCE—Obtain medical treatment for the underlying disorder.

CALL YOUR DOCTOR IF

- You have symptoms of pleurisy.
- Any of the following occurs during treatment:
  Fever.
  Increased pain.
  Increased breathlessness.
  A cough that is dry and non-productive.
  Blue or dark fingernails, toenails or lips.
  Blood in the sputum.

PNEUMOCONIOSIS

BASIC INFORMATION FOR OLDER ADULTS

DESCRIPTION—Pneumoconiosis is an inflammation of the lung caused by breathing industrial dusts. This is not contagious. It may lead to lung cancer. Body parts involved: The lungs.

SPECIAL CONSIDERATIONS FOR AGING
- The immune system becomes less effective, opening the way for viral, bacterial and other infections; malignancies; immune disorders; and allergies.
- Decreased nutrition, common among chronically ill older people, increases the risk of any disease or disorder.
- Characteristic signs and symptoms of many disorders are frequently changed or absent.

SIGNS & SYMPTOMS
Early symptoms:
- Shortness of breath.
- A cough that produces little or no sputum.
- A general ill feeling.

Late symptoms:
- Fitful sleep.
- Appetite and weight loss.
- Chest pain; hoarseness; coughing blood.
- Symptoms of congestive heart failure.
- Bluish nails.
- Shadows on the lungs (visible with chest x-rays).

CAUSES & RISK FACTORS—At least 20 years of exposure to small particles of industrial dusts causes the following forms of pneumoconiosis:
- Coal dust causes black lung disease (coal miner's pneumoconiosis or anthracosis).
- Beryllium and its compounds—once used in manufacturing fluorescent lamp bulbs, ceramics and chemicals—cause berylliosis.
- Talc, iron, cotton, synthetic fiber and aluminum dusts cause a rare form of pneumoconiosis.
- Asbestos and silica cause asbestosis and silicosis. These are described separately in the Illnesses section.

Risk factors include:
- Poor nutrition; smoking.
- Excessive alcohol consumption.

DOCTOR'S TREATMENT & DIAGNOSTIC TESTS
- Medical history and physical exam.
- X-rays of the chest.
- Pulmonary function tests.
- Self-care instructions focused on the older patient.

HOME TREATMENT BY SELF OR CARE-GIVER

GENERAL INSTRUCTIONS—The following measures may relieve the symptoms and protect against recurrent lung infections:
- Obtain medical treatment for any respiratory infection, including the common cold.
- Consider moving to a warm, dry climate if your disease is advanced.
- Practice bronchial drainage. Your doctor will provide instructions.
- Use a cool-mist humidifier to loosen bronchial secretions so they may be coughed up easily.

MEDICATION (ADJUSTED FOR AGING)
- Your doctor may prescribe:
  Antibiotics for infections.
  Bronchodilators (inhaled or oral) with inhalation therapy (supervised at first by an inhalation therapist) to open bronchial tubes to the maximum.
- For minor discomfort, you may use non-prescription drugs such as acetaminophen or aspirin.

ACTIVITY FOR OLDER PATIENTS
- Rest in bed with infections. You may read or watch TV.
- After treatment, resume normal activity as soon as your symptoms improve.
- See Appendix 20 regarding physical fitness for the active older adult.

FOOD & BEVERAGE
- No special diet is required.
- See Appendix 1 regarding good nutrition for people over 50.

FUTURE CONSIDERATIONS FOR THE AGING ADULT

POSSIBLE COMPLICATIONS—Congestive heart failure; lung collapse; pleurisy; tuberculosis in the late stages; cancer.

PROBABLE OUTCOME—This condition is currently considered incurable. However, the symptoms can be relieved or controlled. Pneumoconiosis reduces life expectancy, but many patients live into their 60s and 70s. Scientific research into causes and treatment continues, so there is hope for increasingly effective treatment and a cure.

PREVENTING RECURRENCE
- During exposure to industrial dusts, wear a protective mask or a hood supplied with external air.
- Don't smoke.
- Participate in a regular physical exercise program to maintain good cardiopulmonary fitness.
- Avoid lung irritants such as cigarette smoke or dust.

CALL YOUR DOCTOR IF

- You have symptoms of pneumoconiosis.
- Any of the following occurs during treatment:
  A temperature spike of 101F (38.3C) or more.
  Increased chest pain or breathlessness.
  Blood in the sputum.
  Continuing weight loss.
- New, unexplained symptoms develop. The drugs used in treatment may produce side effects.

BASIC INFORMATION FOR OLDER ADULTS

DESCRIPTION—Bacterial pneumonia is an infection and inflammation of the lungs with bacterial germs. Pneumonias are one of the most frequent and severe health problems for older adults. Body parts involved: The lungs and bronchial tubes.

SPECIAL CONSIDERATIONS FOR AGING
- The immune system becomes less effective, opening the way for viral, bacterial and other infections.
- Decreased nutrition, common among chronically ill older people, increases the risk of any disease or disorder.
- Characteristic signs and symptoms of many disorders are frequently changed or absent.
- The vital capacity of the lungs decreases.
- The chest muscles used for breathing become weaker.

SIGNS & SYMPTOMS
- A high fever (over 102F or 38.9C) and chills.
- Shortness of breath; rapid breathing.
- A cough with sputum that may contain blood or blood streaks.
- Chest pain that worsens with inhalations.
- Abdominal pain; fatigue.
- Bluish lips and nails (rare).

CAUSES & RISK FACTORS—Caused by infection with bacteria such as pneumococci, hemophili, streptococci or staphylococci. Risk factors include:
- The use of anticancer drugs; smoking.
- Illness that has lowered resistance, such as heart disease, recent surgery, cancer, tuberculosis, congestive heart failure, diabetes, alcoholism or chronic lung disease.
- Poor general health from any cause.
- Crowded or unsanitary living conditions.
- Institutional living (e.g., in a nursing home) or hospitalization.
- Immunosuppressant drugs.

DOCTOR'S TREATMENT & DIAGNOSTIC TESTS
- Medical history and physical exam.
- Laboratory studies such as a sputum culture, blood culture and blood count.
- X-rays of the lungs.
- Self-care instructions focused on the older patient.
- Hospitalization (in severe cases only).
- Respiratory or chest physical therapy (sometimes).

HOME TREATMENT BY SELF OR CARE-GIVER

GENERAL INSTRUCTIONS
- Use a cool-mist humidifier to increase the air moisture. Putting medicine in the humidifier probably will not help.
- Don't suppress the cough with medicine if the cough produces sputum or mucus. It is useful in ridding the body of lung secretions.
- Suppress the cough with medicine if it is dry, non-productive and painful. Consult your doctor about a cough suppressant.
- Use warm compresses to help relieve the chest pain.

MEDICATION (ADJUSTED FOR AGING)
- Your doctor may prescribe antibiotics to fight infection.
- You may use non-prescriptions drugs such as acetaminophen, to relieve minor discomfort.

ACTIVITY FOR OLDER PATIENTS—Rest in bed until the fever declines and the pain and shortness of breath disappear. You may read or watch TV. After treatment, resume normal activity as soon as possible.

FOOD & BEVERAGE
- No special diet is required. Increase your fluid intake; drink at least 1 glass of water or other beverage every hour. Extra fluid helps thin lung secretions so they are easier to cough up.
- See Appendix 1 regarding good nutrition for people over 50.

FUTURE CONSIDERATIONS FOR THE AGING ADULT

POSSIBLE COMPLICATIONS
- Pleurisy; pleural effusion (fluid between the membranes that cover the lung).
- Spread of the infection to the brain or meninges (meningitis).
- Failure to respond to treatment, which can lead to respiratory failure and death.

PROBABLE OUTCOME—Usually curable in 1 to 2 weeks with treatment, but it may take longer for the elderly.

PREVENTING RECURRENCE
- Obtain prompt medical treatment for respiratory infections.
- Arrange for pneumococcal and influenza immunizations. Vaccines appear to be more effective if they are given at age 55 up to age 65 before someone becomes debilitated by a chronic disease.

CALL YOUR DOCTOR IF
- You have symptoms of pneumonia.
- Any of the following occurs during treatment:
  Fever.
  Pain that is not relieved by heat or prescribed medication.
  Increased shortness of breath.
  Dark or bluish fingernails, skin or toenails.
  Blood in the sputum.
  Nausea, vomiting or diarrhea.
- New, unexplained symptoms develop. The drugs used in treatment may produce side effects.

PNEUMONIA, MYCOPLASMA
(Primary Atypical Pneumonia; "Walking Pneumonia"; Eaton-Agent Pneumonia)

BASIC INFORMATION FOR OLDER ADULTS

DESCRIPTION—Mycoplasma pneumonia is a contagious lung inflammation caused by mycoplasma bacteria. This germ can cause infection in other body parts. Body parts involved: The upper respiratory system.

SPECIAL CONSIDERATIONS FOR AGING
- The immune system becomes less effective, opening the way for viral, bacterial and other infections.
- Decreased nutrition, common among chronically ill older people, increases the risk of any disease or disorder.
- Characteristic signs and symptoms of many disorders are frequently changed or absent.
- The vital capacity of the lungs decreases.
- The chest muscles used for breathing become weaker.

SIGNS & SYMPTOMS
- A cough (with or without sputum).
- A fever.
- Labored breathing.
- Chest pain.
- Abdominal pain.
- Bluish skin (severe cases).

CAUSES & RISK FACTORS—Caused by a preceding mycoplasma infection in the nose, throat or bronchial tubes. Risk factors include:
- Stress.
- Illness that has lowered resistance.
- Exposure to cold, harsh weather.
- Crowded or unsanitary living conditions.

DOCTOR'S TREATMENT & DIAGNOSTIC TESTS
- Medical history and physical exam.
- Laboratory culture of sputum and blood studies.
- Chest x-rays.
- Self-care instructions focused on the older patient.

HOME TREATMENT BY SELF OR CARE-GIVER

GENERAL INSTRUCTIONS
- Use a cool-mist humidifier to increase air moisture. Putting medicine in the humidifier probably will not help.
- Don't suppress the cough with medicine if it produces sputum or mucus. Coughing is useful in ridding the body of lung secretions.
- Suppress the cough with medicine if it is dry, non-productive and painful. Consult your doctor about a cough suppressant.
- Use warm compresses to help relieve the chest pain.
- Catch sneezes and coughs with disposable tissue.

MEDICATION (ADJUSTED FOR AGING)
- Your doctor may prescribe:
  Antibiotics, such as erythromycin, to fight the infection.
  Cough medicine to make the cough more tolerable.
  Nose drops, sprays or oral decongestants to reduce congestion in the upper respiratory system.
- *Note:* Adverse reactions and side effects may be more frequent and severe in older persons. Remind your doctor of any medicines you already take.

ACTIVITY FOR OLDER PATIENTS
- Bed rest is necessary until the fever subsides. Resume your normal activities gradually.
- See Appendix 20 regarding physical fitness for the active older adult.

FOOD & BEVERAGE
- No special diet is required. Increase your intake of fluids to at least 1 glass of water or other beverage every hour. Extra fluid helps thin the lung secretions so they can be coughed up more easily.
- See Appendix 1 regarding good nutrition for people over 50.

FUTURE CONSIDERATIONS FOR THE AGING ADULT

POSSIBLE COMPLICATIONS—Prolonged illness.

PROBABLE OUTCOME—This form of pneumonia is characteristically slow to heal. It is usually curable in 4 to 6 weeks with treatment. The lungs should not have residual scars.

PREVENTING RECURRENCE
- Avoid exposure to persons who are ill with respiratory infections.
- Don't get chilled or wet in cold weather.

CALL YOUR DOCTOR IF

- You have symptoms of mycoplasma pneumonia.
- Any of the following occurs during treatment:
  Fever.
  Pain that is not relieved by heat or prescribed medication.
  Increased shortness of breath.
  Dark or bluish fingernails, skin or toenails.
  Blood in the sputum.
  Nausea, vomiting or diarrhea.
- New, unexplained symptoms develop. The drugs used in treatmentpmay produce side effects.

PNEUMONIA, VIRAL

BASIC INFORMATION FOR OLDER ADULTS

DESCRIPTION—Viral pneumonia is a lung infection caused by a virus. It is unlikely that others will develop pneumonia from exposure to a person with viral pneumonia. Pneumonias are one of the most frequent and severe health problems for older adults. Body parts involved: The lower respiratory tract (bronchial tubes, bronchioles and lungs) and the upper respiratory tract (nose, throat, tonsils, sinuses, trachea and larynx).

SPECIAL CONSIDERATIONS FOR AGING
- The immune system becomes less effective, opening the way for viral, bacterial and other infections; malignancies; immune disorders; and allergies.
- Decreased nutrition, common among chronically ill older people, increases the risk of any disease or disorder.
- Characteristic signs and symptoms of many disorders are frequently changed or absent.
- The vital capacity of the lungs decreases.
- The chest muscles used for breathing become weaker.

SIGNS & SYMPTOMS
- Fever and chills.
- Muscle aches and fatigue.
- A cough, with or without sputum or "croup."
- Rapid, labored (sometimes) breathing.
- Chest pain.
- Sore throat.
- Loss of appetite.
- Enlarged lymph glands in the neck.

CAUSES & RISK FACTORS
—Caused by virus infections including influenza, chickenpox, respiratory viruses, measles and cytomegalovirus. Risk factors include:
- Asthma.
- Cystic fibrosis.
- Inhalation of a foreign body into the lung.
- Smoking or alcoholism.
- Crowded or unsanitary living conditions.
- Institutional living (e.g., in a nursing home) or hospitalization.
- Immunosuppressant drugs.

DOCTOR'S TREATMENT & DIAGNOSTIC TESTS
- Medical history and physical exam.
- Laboratory studies such as a sputum culture, blood culture and blood count.
- X-rays of the chest.
- Self-care instructions focused on the older patient.
- Hospitalization (in severe cases only).

HOME TREATMENT BY SELF OR CARE-GIVER

GENERAL INSTRUCTIONS
- Use a cool-mist humidifier to increase the air moisture. Putting medicine in the vaporizer probably will not help.
- Use a warm compress on the chest to relieve the chest pain.

MEDICATION (ADJUSTED FOR AGING)
- If the cough produces sputum, it is ridding the lungs of secretions and should not be suppressed with medicine. If the cough is dry, non-productive and painful, you may suppress it with non-prescription cough medicine that contains dextromethorphan.
- For minor pain and fever, you may use non-prescription drugs such as acetaminophen or decongestant nose drops, nasal sprays or tablets.
- Your doctor may prescribe:
  Antibiotics to fight secondary bacterial infections (they do not help viral pneumonia).
  Antiviral drugs.
- *Note:* Adverse reactions and side effects may be more frequent and severe in older persons. Remind your doctor of any medicines you already take.

ACTIVITY FOR OLDER PATIENTS
- Bed rest is necessary until the fever, pain and shortness of breath have been gone at least 48 hours. Then normal activity may be resumed slowly. Many people are fatigued and weak for up to 6 weeks after recovery, so don't expect a quick return to normal strength.
- See Appendix 20 regarding physical fitness for the active older adult.

FOOD & BEVERAGE
- No special diet is required, but do everything possible to maintain a normal intake of nutritious foods and drinks. Drink at least 1 full glass of fluid each hour. This helps thin lung secretions so they are easier to cough up.
- See Appendix 1 regarding good nutrition for people over 50.

FUTURE CONSIDERATIONS FOR THE AGING ADULT

POSSIBLE COMPLICATIONS
- Secondary bacterial infections of the lungs.
- Post-infectious depression.

PROBABLE OUTCOME—Usually curable in 4 weeks.

PREVENTING RECURRENCE—There are no specific preventive measures.

CALL YOUR DOCTOR IF

- You have symptoms of pneumonia.
- Any of the following occurs during treatment:
  Temperature spikes over 102F (38.9C).
  Intolerable pain despite medication and heat treatment.
  Increasing shortness of breath.
  Increasing blueness of nails and skin.
  Blood in the sputum.
  Nausea, vomiting or diarrhea.

BASIC INFORMATION
FOR OLDER ADULTS

DESCRIPTION—Pneumothorax is the collapse of part or all of a lung caused by pressure from free air in the chest between the two layers of the pleura (the thin membrane that covers the lungs). The pain is sometimes confused with that of a heart attack. Body parts involved: The lungs and the pleura. (THIS IS AN EMERGENCY; SEEK MEDICAL CARE IMMEDIATELY!)

SPECIAL CONSIDERATIONS FOR AGING
- Decreased nutrition, common among chronically ill older people, increases the risk of any disease or disorder.
- Characteristic signs and symptoms of many disorders in older people are frequently changed or absent.

SIGNS & SYMPTOMS—The following
symptoms vary according to the degree of lung collapse and the extent of the underlying lung disease. The symptoms may be less acute if pneumothorax develops slowly:
- Sharp chest pain. The pain may extend to a shoulder or across the chest or abdomen.
- Shortness of breath.
- A dry, hacking cough (occasionally).

CAUSES & RISK FACTORS
- Spontaneous pneumothorax is caused by the rupture of a small air sac in the lung resulting from asthma; lung abscess or empyema; or physical exertion, such as diving, high-altitude flying or stretching. Causes related to activity occur most often in healthy persons.
- Pneumothorax due to trauma is caused by: Penetrating wounds to the chest, which permit outside air to rush into the pleural space and cause the lung to collapse. A complication of removing fluid from the lung (thoracentesis). A complication of inserting a catheter into the neck for artificial feeding or diagnostic procedures.
- Risk factors include: Chest injury. Chronic lung disease. Smoking.

DOCTOR'S TREATMENT
& DIAGNOSTIC TESTS
- Medical history and physical exam.
- X-rays of the chest to confirm the diagnosis.
- Self-care instructions focused on the older patient.
- Hospitalization if the extent of lung collapse is disabling.
- Placement of a tube in the chest to remove air from the pleural cavity.

HOME TREATMENT BY
SELF OR CARE-GIVER

GENERAL INSTRUCTIONS
- Don't smoke.

- Try not to cough.
- Avoid loud talking, laughing or singing.
- You may be more comfortable if you rest in a sitting position.

MEDICATION (ADJUSTED FOR AGING)
- Medication is usually not necessary. However, you may use non-prescription drugs such as acetaminophen for minor pain. For severe pain, your doctor may prescribe stronger pain relievers.
- *Note:* Adverse reactions and side effects may be more frequent and severe in older persons. Remind your doctor of any medicines you already take.

ACTIVITY FOR OLDER PATIENTS
- Stay as active as your strength allows. Rest often. Resume your normal activities as soon as possible. Allow about 2 weeks for recovery.
- See Appendix 20 regarding physical fitness for the active older adult.

FOOD & BEVERAGE
- No special diet is required.
- See Appendix 1 regarding good nutrition for people over 50.

FUTURE CONSIDERATIONS
FOR THE AGING ADULT

POSSIBLE COMPLICATIONS
- Respiratory failure.
- Lung infection.

PROBABLE OUTCOME
- A small pneumothorax is inconsequential and heals itself. However, if the collapse is extensive and it occurs in someone whose lungs are damaged by asthma, chronic bronchitis or emphysema, it can lead to respiratory failure and critical illness.
- Treatment depends on the size of the pneumothorax and the condition of the lungs. The disorder may heal itself, but hospitalization and treatment may be necessary to remove the air.

PREVENTING RECURRENCE
- Obtain medical treatment for lung disorders, such as asthma or emphysema.
- Don't smoke.
- People with spontaneous pneumothorax may have a recurrence.

CALL YOUR DOCTOR IF

- You have symptoms of pneumothorax. *This is an emergency!*
- Any of the following occurs during treatment: Your temperature rises to 101F (38.3C). Your chest pain or shortness of breath increases. Painful, debilitating coughing or sputum production begins.

POLYARTERITIS
(Polyarteritis Nodosa; Periarteritis Nodosa; Necrotizing Angiitis)

BASIC INFORMATION FOR OLDER ADULTS

DESCRIPTION—Polyarteritis is a rare disorder of the connective tissue that is one of several related diseases of collagen tissue. Collagen is a protein molecule that forms the major part of all connective tissue. Polyarteritis causes an inflammation of the small and medium arteries, decreasing the blood supply to organs supplied by the affected blood vessels. It is not contagious. Body parts involved: All body parts.

SPECIAL CONSIDERATIONS FOR AGING
- The immune system becomes less effective, opening the way for viral, bacterial and other infections.
- Decreased nutrition increases the risk of any disease or disorder.
- Characteristic signs and symptoms of many disorders are frequently changed or absent.
- Stress from any emotional cause affects all aspects of any illness or disorder.

SIGNS & SYMPTOMS—Depend on which organ is affected by the decreased blood supply. The most common include:
- Chest pain (heart involvement).
- Shortness of breath (lung involvement).
- Abdominal pain, nausea and vomiting (intestinal and liver involvement).
- Blood in the urine (kidney involvement).
- Numbness and tingling of the hands and feet (nerve involvement).

The course may be acute, with fever, weight loss and rapid deterioration. If the course is chronic, body tissues will waste away over several years.

CAUSES & RISK FACTORS—Polyarteritis is considered a disease of autoimmunity or hypersensitivity, although the cause is uncertain. In many persons, no predisposing factors can be found. Following are the most common predisposing factors.
- Bacterial infections; viral infections.
- The use of certain drugs, including sulfa drugs, penicillin, antithyroid drugs, gold and thiazide diuretics; vaccines.

Risk factors include:
- A family history of collagen or hypersensitivity disease.
- Smoking; a hepatitis B infection.

DOCTOR'S TREATMENT & DIAGNOSTIC TESTS
- Medical history and physical exam.
- Laboratory studies of the kidneys and blood, including sedimentation rate (see Glossary).
- Biopsy of tissue from affected organs.
- Angiogram (see Glossary).

- Self-care instructions focused on the older patient.
- Surgery to remove part of the intestines if they are involved. Advancing age alone is not a deterrent.
- Hospitalization (in severe cases).

HOME TREATMENT BY SELF OR CARE-GIVER

GENERAL INSTRUCTIONS—No specific instructions except those listed under other headings.

MEDICATION (ADJUSTED FOR AGING)—Your doctor may prescribe:
- Cortisone drugs in high doses until the acute symptoms diminish. Then symptoms may be controlled by 1 dose of cortisone every other day. Take cortisone only as long as necessary. Its long-term use produces serious adverse effects.
- Drugs to treat disorders of the organs involved with this serious disease, such as heart medications for heart involvement or antihypertensives for high blood pressure.
- Immunosuppressive drugs—either alone or with steroids—if other drugs fail. These drugs pose additional risks, including severe generalized septic bacterial infections.

ACTIVITY FOR OLDER PATIENTS
- Resume your normal activities gradually as the symptoms improve.
- See Appendix 20 regarding physical fitness for the active older adult.

FOOD & BEVERAGE—Eat a low-salt diet (see Appendix 9).

FUTURE CONSIDERATIONS FOR THE AGING ADULT

POSSIBLE COMPLICATIONS—Kidney failure and death despite treatment.

PROBABLE OUTCOME—This condition is currently considered incurable. However, the symptoms can be relieved or controlled. Many patients live several years with the disease, and medical literature cites a few instances of unexplained recovery. Scientific research into causes and treatment continues, so there is hope for increasingly effective treatment and a cure.

PREVENTING RECURRENCE—There are no specific preventive measures.

CALL YOUR DOCTOR IF

- You have symptoms of polyarteritis.
- New, unexplained symptoms develop. The drugs used in treatment may produce side effects.

POLYCYTHEMIA

BASIC INFORMATION FOR OLDER ADULTS

DESCRIPTION—Polycythemia is an increase in the red blood cells in the body. The disease has 3 forms:
- Polycythemia vera, which involves the overproduction of red blood cells, white blood cells and platelets.
- Secondary polycythemia (pseudo-polycythemia), which is a complication of diseases or factors other than blood cell disorders.
- Stress polycythemia (pseudo-polycythemia), which involves decreased blood plasma.

Body parts involved: The blood-forming organs—the bone marrow, spleen, lymph glands and lymph channels.

SPECIAL CONSIDERATIONS FOR AGING
- Malignant diseases are less likely to spread rapidly.
- The immune system becomes less effective, opening the way for viral, bacterial and other infections; malignancies; immune disorders; and allergies.
- There is less efficient response to physical stress (fright and flight) due to the decreased responsiveness of the adrenal glands.
- Stress from any emotional cause—fear, worry, anxiety, sadness, loneliness or anger—affects all aspects of any illness or disorder.

SIGNS & SYMPTOMS—Some patients have no symptoms. Others have any of the following:
- Fatigue; headache; drowsiness; dizziness.
- Itching or flushed skin.
- An enlarged spleen.
- Unexplained bleeding.
- Visual disturbances.

CAUSES & RISK FACTORS
Causes include:
- Polycythemia vera—Unknown.
- Secondary polycythemia—Congenital heart disease; chronic lung disease; cigarette or cigar smoking; living at high altitude.
- Stress polycythemia—The use of diuretic drugs; smoking; dehydration.

Risk factors include:
- Smoking; stress.
- Heart or lung disease.
- A family history of polycythemia.

DOCTOR'S TREATMENT & DIAGNOSTIC TESTS
- Medical history and physical exam.
- Laboratory studies of bone marrow and blood (red blood cell count, measurement of hematocrit).
- X-rays of the kidneys.
- Radioactive chromium studies. Your doctor may use 1 of 3 forms of treatment available to keep the hematocrit range (see Glossary) near normal and prevent clotting or hemorrhage: phlebotomy (the withdrawal of blood); radioisotope therapy (see Glossary); or drug therapy. The treat-ment chosen will depend upon your symptoms and their response to treatment. More than one form of treatment may be needed.
- Self-care instructions focused on the older patient.

HOME TREATMENT BY SELF OR CARE-GIVER

GENERAL INSTRUCTIONS—No specific instructions except those under other headings.

MEDICATION (ADJUSTED FOR AGING)—
Your doctor may prescribe:
- Aspirin to decrease clotting and reduce the chance of stroke or heart attack.
- Radioactive phosphorus or cytotoxic drugs.
- Allopurinol for elevated uric acid.
- Anti-itching medications.

ACTIVITY FOR OLDER PATIENTS
- After treatment, resume normal activity as soon as possible.
- See Appendix 20 regarding physical fitness for the active older adult.

FOOD & BEVERAGE
- No special diet is required. Drink 6 to 8 oz. of fluid every 2 hours to maintain adequate body fluid.
- See Appendix 1 regarding good nutrition for people over 50.

FUTURE CONSIDERATIONS FOR THE AGING ADULT

POSSIBLE COMPLICATIONS—Clots in veins or arteries; gout; stroke; heart attack; peptic ulcer; kidney stones; chronic leukemia.

PROBABLE OUTCOME
- Polycythemia vera is incurable, but the symptoms can be controlled. Survival with the disease is about 10 to 15 years. Death is more likely to result from complications such as stroke.
- The other forms of polycythemia can be cured if the causes can be eliminated. For example, descending from a high-altitude environment to sea level can return the blood to normal.

PREVENTING RECURRENCE
- Polycythemia vera cannot be prevented at present.
- To prevent secondary polycythemia or stress polycythemia, don't smoke, avoid dehydration and obtain medical treatment for heart or lung disease.

CALL YOUR DOCTOR IF

- You have symptoms of polycythemia.
- You have symptoms of complications (refer to the specific disorder in the Illnesses section).
- New, unexplained symptoms develop. The drugs used in treatment may produce side effects.

POLYMYALGIA RHEUMATICA OR TEMPORAL ARTERITIS
(Giant-Cell Arteritis; Cranial Arteritis)

BASIC INFORMATION FOR OLDER ADULTS

DESCRIPTION—Polymyalgia rheumatica or temporal arteritis is an inflammatory disease of the large arteries, especially those in the head and neck. The symptoms of polymyalgia rheumatica and temporal arteritis are the same, so the two diseases may be identical. Body parts involved: The muscles; temporal arteries; eyes; connective tissue. (THIS IS AN EMERGENCY; SEEK MEDICAL CARE IMMEDIATELY!)

SPECIAL CONSIDERATIONS FOR AGING
- Neurological diseases become more likely.
- The blood vessels nourishing the brain become thicker and lose their elasticity.
- The number of autoantibodies (see Glossary) increases.
- The immune system becomes less effective.

SIGNS & SYMPTOMS—The following symptoms may resemble those of an infection such as influenza:
- A low-grade fever (under 101F).
- Muscle stiffness, aches and pains—especially in the morning. The muscles involved are usually those of the trunk, upper arms and legs.
- A severe, throbbing headache (usually in one temple); redness, swelling, tenderness and pulsating nodules along the temporal artery on one side of the head.
- Appetite loss.

CAUSES & RISK FACTORS—This is an auto-immune disorder in which the body's immune system attacks and destroys its own tissues (especially connective tissues). The underlying cause is unknown. It is rare before age 50 and affects twice as many women as men.

DOCTOR'S TREATMENT & DIAGNOSTIC TESTS
- Medical history and physical exam.
- Laboratory studies such as a test of sedimentation rate (see Glossary), a white blood cell count and blood tests for anemia.
- Biopsy (see Glossary) of the temporal artery and muscle.
- Self-care instructions focused on the older patient.
- Treatment for problems associated with this disorder. These may include heart disease, high blood pressure or decreased blood supply to the bowel.
- Surgery if the bowel develops intestinal gangrene. Advancing age alone is not a deterrent.

HOME TREATMENT BY SELF OR CARE-GIVER

GENERAL INSTRUCTIONS
- Apply heat to the painful side of the head. You may use warm compresses or a heat lamp.
- Gently massage the back of the neck and sore muscles.

MEDICATION (ADJUSTED FOR AGING)—
Your doctor may prescribe:
- Cortisone drugs in high doses until the acute phase ends. These dramatically relieve the symptoms by altering the inflammation causing them. For continuing treatment with cortisone, the lowest possible single dose taken every other day may keep the symptoms under control.
- Immunosuppressive drugs—either alone or with cortisone—if other treatment is not successful. These drugs impose additional risks, including severe those of generalized bacterial infections.
- Heart medications (if the heart is involved).
- Antihypertensive drugs (if high blood pressure is part of the problem).

ACTIVITY FOR OLDER PATIENTS—No restrictions are necessary.

FOOD & BEVERAGE—No special diet.

FUTURE CONSIDERATIONS FOR THE AGING ADULT

POSSIBLE COMPLICATIONS
- Without treatment—Loss of vision if the blood vessels to the eyes are involved (*this is an emergency!*); coronary artery disease; stroke; poor blood circulation to the arms and legs.
- With treatment—Cortisone drugs may be necessary for many months. The complications of long-term cortisone use are significant, including osteoporosis and peptic ulcer disease.

PROBABLE OUTCOME—Usually curable, but relapse is possible. The course of the disease runs 1 to 2 years, but it may stay active for several years in some people.

PREVENTING RECURRENCE—There are no specific preventive measures.

CALL YOUR DOCTOR IF

- You have symptoms of polymyalgia rheumatica or temporal arteritis. *This is an emergency!*
- Any of the following occurs during treatment: A temperature of 101F (38.3C). Blood in the urine. Shortness of breath. Chest pain. Bloody bowel movements. Severe abdominal pain. Any illness with fever.
- New, unexplained symptoms develop. The drugs used in treatment may produce side effects.

POLYMYOSITIS & DERMATOMYOSITIS

BASIC INFORMATION FOR OLDER ADULTS

DESCRIPTION—Polymyositis and dermatomyositis are inflammations of the connective tissue with degenerative changes in the muscles (polymyositis) and skin (dermatomyositis). This causes weakness and muscle wasting, especially in the arms and legs. This disease has many similarities to rheumatoid arthritis and lupus erythematosus. Body parts involved: The muscles, including the large muscles of the skeleton and the tiny muscles that control the small arteries; the skin; connective tissue.

SPECIAL CONSIDERATIONS FOR AGING
- The number of autoantibodies (see Glossary) increases.
- The immune system becomes less effective, opening the way for viral, bacterial and other infections; malignancies; immune disorders; and allergies.
- Characteristic signs and symptoms of many disorders are frequently changed or absent.

SIGNS & SYMPTOMS—Sudden or slow onset of the following:
- Weakness in the pelvic girdle and shoulder girdle muscles.
- A skin rash that may itch on the face, shoulders, arms and over joints.
- Cold hands and feet.
- Frequent falls and difficulty in getting up.
- Speaking or swallowing difficulty.
- Infection with fever, muscle weakness, weight loss and joint pain (sometimes) preceding other symptoms.
- Swollen upper eyelids.

CAUSES & RISK FACTORS—This is probably a disorder of hypersensitivity or autoimmunity, although the cause is uncertain. This disorder has been associated with preceding bacterial infections and viral infections and with the use of certain drugs and vaccines. Women comprise 2/3 of the patients. Risk factors include:
- Allergies.
- The use of sulfa drugs, penicillin, antithyroid drugs, gold and thiazide diuretics.
- A family history of hypersensitivity diseases from drugs or illness, such as lupus.
- Cancer of the lung, colon or breast.

DOCTOR'S TREATMENT & DIAGNOSTIC TESTS
- Medical history and physical exam.
- Laboratory blood studies to measure antinuclear antibodies (ANA) and muscle enzymes.
- Surgical diagnostic procedures, such as a biopsy of affected muscle tissue and an electromyography (see Glossary for both).
- Self-care instructions focused on the older patient.
- Hospitalization during the early, active phases.
- Surgery if intestinal obstruction occurs.
- Time in an extended-care facility for physical therapy and rehabilitation.

HOME TREATMENT BY SELF OR CARE-GIVER

GENERAL INSTRUCTIONS
- The patient may need a wheelchair and attendants to help with his or her daily routine.
- If confined to bed, the patient should be moved frequently to prevent pressure sores.
- Passive exercise (see Glossary) should be provided to prevent contractures (muscle shortening).
- Cool-water compresses may relieve itching.

MEDICATION (ADJUSTED FOR AGING)—
Your doctor may prescribe:
- Cortisone drugs in high doses until the acute symptoms diminish, then in lower doses.
- Immunosuppressive drugs if other treatment is not effective. These drugs impose additional risks, including life-threatening septic bacterial infections.

ACTIVITY FOR OLDER PATIENTS—No restrictions are necessary, except those imposed by muscle weakness.

FOOD & BEVERAGE—No special diet.

FUTURE CONSIDERATIONS FOR THE AGING ADULT

POSSIBLE COMPLICATIONS—Muscle and body wasting; congestive heart failure; high blood pressure; intestinal obstruction; kidney damage.

PROBABLE OUTCOME—The disease may begin suddenly or gradually. About 50% of patients recover in a few years. Some patients become wheelchair-bound or bedridden because of muscle weakness. Some symptoms can be controlled briefly with treatment, but the disease can eventually affect the lungs and other organs and lead to death. However, remissions or spontaneous recovery can occur. Scientific research into causes and treatment continues, so there is hope for increasingly effective treatment and a cure.

PREVENTING RECURRENCE—There are no specific preventive measures.

CALL YOUR DOCTOR IF

- You have symptoms or polymyositis and dermatomyositis.
- Any of the following occurs during treatment:
  Blood in the urine.
  Shortness of breath.
  Chest pain.
  Bloody bowel movements.
  Severe abdominal pain.
  Fever.

POMPHOLYX
(Dyshidrosis; Dyshydrotic Eczema)

BASIC INFORMATION FOR OLDER ADULTS

DESCRIPTION—Pompholyx is a skin condition characterized by small blisters on the hands or feet that are apparently related to stress. Body parts involved: The tips and sides of the fingers and toes; the palms and soles.

SPECIAL CONSIDERATIONS FOR AGING
- The skin's reactions to injury or infection increase in intensity and duration.
- The skin becomes thinner.

SIGNS & SYMPTOMS—Small blisters with the following characteristics:
- The blisters are very small (1mm or less in diameter). They appear on the tips and sides of fingers, toes, palms and soles.
- The blisters are opaque and deep-seated; they are either flush with the skin or slightly elevated. They don't break easily. Eventually, small blisters come together and form large blisters.
- The blisters may itch, cause pain or produce no symptoms. They worsen after contact with soap, water or irritating substances.

CAUSES & RISK FACTORS—The causes are unknown, but they are probably related to periods of anxiety, stress and frustration in ambitious people who internalize their emotions. Persons with pompholyx have difficulty relaxing—even during non-stressful periods. This problem is not caused by sweat retention, as was once believed. Risk factors include:
- Stress and internalized frustration or irritation.
- An obsessive-compulsive personality.

DOCTOR'S TREATMENT & DIAGNOSTIC TESTS
- Medical history and physical exam.
- After diagnosis, self-care instructions.
- Psychotherapy or counseling to help you learn to cope with stress more effectively.

HOME TREATMENT BY SELF OR CARE-GIVER

GENERAL INSTRUCTIONS
- Keep heat and moisture away from the affected areas whenever possible.
- Wear cotton socks and leather-soled shoes. Don't wear tennis shoes or other footwear made of man-made materials.
- Remove your shoes and socks frequently to allow sweat to evaporate.
- Wear heavy-duty, cotton-lined vinyl gloves to prevent contact of the hands with irritating substances such as water, soap, detergent, metal scrubbing pads, scouring powder, and other chemicals.
- Dry the insides of gloves after use. Discard gloves if they develop holes.

- Wear gloves when you peel or squeeze acid fruits and vegetables.
- Wear leather or heavy-duty fabric gloves for housework or gardening.
- Use a dishwashing machine to wash dishes if possible. If not, ask someone else to wash them.
- Avoid contact with irritating chemicals such as paint, paint thinner and polish for cars, floors, shoes, furniture and metal.
- Remove rings before doing housework or washing your hands hands.
- Use lukewarm water and very little mild soap to shower or bathe.

MEDICATION (ADJUSTED FOR AGING)
- You may use non-prescription topical steroid preparations to reduce the inflammation and decrease the itching. Apply it once or twice a day after bathing unless directed otherwise. If this is not effective, your doctor may prescribe stronger steroid preparations.
- *Note:* Adverse reactions and side effects may be more frequent and severe in older persons. Remind your doctor of any medicines you already take.

ACTIVITY FOR OLDER PATIENTS—No restrictions are necessary.

FOOD & BEVERAGE
- No special diet is required.
- See Appendix 1 regarding good nutrition for people over 50.

FUTURE CONSIDERATIONS FOR THE AGING ADULT

POSSIBLE COMPLICATIONS—Secondary bacterial infection (sometimes).

PROBABLE OUTCOME—The symptoms can be controlled with treatment, but recurrence is common. Persons with mild problems have occasional attacks, and the skin returns to normal between episodes. Persons with severe problems have more severe symptoms—sometimes with persistent peeling and fissuring of the involved skin.

PREVENTING RECURRENCE—Follow the instructions under General Instructions. These are helpful in preventing recurrences, as well as in treating active episodes.

CALL YOUR DOCTOR IF

- You have symptoms of pompholyx.
- Signs of infection (swelling, redness, tenderness or warmth) appear around the blisters.
- Your symptoms don't improve after 1 week despite treatment.
- Improvement begins, and then the symptoms recur.

POTASSIUM IMBALANCE
(Hyperkalemia; Hypokalemia)

BASIC INFORMATION FOR OLDER ADULTS

DESCRIPTION—Potassium imbalance is characterized by above-normal or below-normal levels of potassium in the blood, body fluids and body cells. Body parts involved: The blood, which affects all body cells and body fluids.

SPECIAL CONSIDERATIONS FOR AGING
- Many diseases become more common with age, and all may present themselves in unusual ways.
- There is less efficient response to physical stress (fright and flight) due to the decreased responsiveness of the adrenal glands.

SIGNS & SYMPTOMS
For above-normal levels (hyperkalemia):
- Weakness and paralysis.
- Dangerously rapid, irregular heartbeat or slow heartbeat (sometimes); nausea and diarrhea.

For below-normal levels (hypokalemia):
- Weakness and paralysis.
- Confusion and disorientation.
- Low blood pressure.
- Drowsiness, dizziness and fatigue.
- Life-threatening rapid, irregular heartbeat. This is more severe than with hyperkalemia.

CAUSES & RISK FACTORS
Causes of hyperkalemia include:
- Chronic kidney disease with kidney failure. Failing kidneys eliminate potassium too slowly, causing an excess in the body.
- The use of oral potassium supplements.
- Burns or crushing injuries. These may release potassium from body tissues into body fluids.
- Addison's disease.

Causes of hypokalemia include:
- The use of diuretic drugs for hypertension or heart failure.
- The prolonged loss of body fluids from vomiting or diarrhea.
- Chronic kidney disease with kidney failure. At certain stages, this may cause the body to lose potassium.
- Chronic laxative use.

Risk factors for both hyperkalemia and hypokalemia include:
- Diabetes mellitus; adrenal disease.
- The use of drugs such as diuretics, potassium supplements and digitalis. Low potassium levels—especially in persons who take digitalis—often lead to serious heartbeat disturbances.

DOCTOR'S TREATMENT & DIAGNOSTIC TESTS
- Your own observation of the symptoms, especially muscle weakness and heart rhythm changes.
- Medical history and physical exam.
- Laboratory blood and urine studies of potassium and other electrolytes.

- ECG (see Glossary).
- Self-care instructions focused on the older patient.
- Hospitalization (in severe cases).

OTHER—A normal to high blood level of potassium may help protect against coronary artery disease.

HOME TREATMENT BY SELF OR CARE-GIVER

GENERAL INSTRUCTIONS—If you take diuretics *and* digitalis, your friends and family members should learn cardiopulmonary resuscitation (CPR). Learn to count your own pulse at the wrist or neck.

MEDICATION (ADJUSTED FOR AGING)—Your doctor may prescribe:
- Oral potassium supplements to raise low levels.
- Diuretics to increase urination and decrease high potassium levels.
- Intravenous fluids to correct a serious imbalance.
- Medications appropriate for the underlying disease.

ACTIVITY FOR OLDER PATIENTS—Resume your normal activities as soon as your symptoms improve.

FOOD & BEVERAGE—Depends on the condition. Mild hypokalemia can be corrected by increasing the consumption of potassium-containing foods, such as orange juice and bananas.

FUTURE CONSIDERATIONS FOR THE AGING ADULT

POSSIBLE COMPLICATIONS—Cardiac arrest and death.

PROBABLE OUTCOME—Usually can be corrected with intravenous fluids and treatment of the underlying disorder.

PREVENTING RECURRENCE
- If you have a disorder or take drugs that affect potassium levels (see Causes & Risk Factors), learn as much as you can about your condition, your drugs and how you can prevent a potassium imbalance.
- If you take digitalis *and* diuretics, have frequent blood studies to monitor potassium levels.
- Obtain medical care for prolonged vomiting or diarrhea.

CALL YOUR DOCTOR IF

You have symptoms of a potassium imbalance or are having problems with a disorder that affects potassium levels.

PRIAPISM

BASIC INFORMATION FOR OLDER ADULTS

DESCRIPTION—Priapism is a problem involving the penis that is characterized by a painful, persistent, abnormal penile erection. There is no accompanying sexual excitement or desire. The corpora cavernosa (the columns of tissue on the back and side of the penis) become choked with dark venous blood of the consistency of motor oil. Body part involved: The penis.

SPECIAL CONSIDERATIONS FOR AGING—Decreased nutrition, common among chronically ill older people, increases the risk of any disease or disorder.

SIGNS & SYMPTOMS
- Abnormally painful penile erection.
- Persistent penile erection.

CAUSES & RISK FACTORS
- Blood clots in the pelvic blood vessels.
- May be secondary to prolonged sex, leukemia, sickle-cell trait or pelvic tumor.
- Prostatitis.
- Urethritis.
- Cystitis.
- Bladder stones.
- Adverse effects of drugs such as trazodone, chlorpromazine, methaqualone, prazosin, tolbutamide, some antihypertensives, anticoagulants or corticosteroids.

DOCTOR'S TREATMENT & DIAGNOSTIC TESTS
- Medical history and physical exam.
- Laboratory blood studies and urinalysis.
- X-rays of the pelvis.
- Hospitalization (in severe cases).
- Surgery (sometimes). Advancing age alone is not a deterrent.

HOME TREATMENT BY SELF OR CARE-GIVER

GENERAL INSTRUCTIONS
- There is no effective self-care.
- If hospitalized, follow your doctor's discharge instructions.

MEDICATION (ADJUSTED FOR AGING)—No medication is helpful.

ACTIVITY FOR OLDER PATIENTS—Bed rest until the priapism is relieved.

FOOD & BEVERAGE
- No special diet is required.
- See Appendix 1 regarding good nutrition for people over 50.

FUTURE CONSIDERATIONS FOR THE AGING ADULT

POSSIBLE COMPLICATIONS—Destruction of sexual function for life.

PROBABLE OUTCOME—Curable if treated quickly and effectively.

PREVENTING RECURRENCE—Avoid the drugs listed under Causes & Risk Factors.

CALL YOUR DOCTOR IF

- You have symptoms of priapism.
- There is any early sign of recurrence.

PROSTATE CANCER

BASIC INFORMATION FOR OLDER ADULTS

DESCRIPTION—Prostate cancer is a growth of malignant cells in the prostate gland, the gland at the base of the urinary bladder in men that helps form semen. Many prostate cancers grow very slowly and never cause symptoms or spread. Body part involved: The prostate.

SPECIAL CONSIDERATIONS FOR AGING
- Characteristic signs and symptoms of many disorders are frequently changed or absent.
- The immune system becomes less effective, opening the way for viral, bacterial and other infections; malignancies; immune disorders; and allergies.
- Stress from any emotional cause—fear, worry, anxiety, sadness, loneliness or anger—affects all aspects of any illness or disorder.

SIGNS & SYMPTOMS
Early stages:
- No symptoms (usually). Most prostate cancers are discovered during a routine rectal examination.

Later stages:
- Difficulty in starting urination.
- A decreased amount of urine.
- Frequent urination.
- Pain in the low back or pelvis from the spread of cancer.

CAUSES & RISK FACTORS—The cause is unknown. Prostate cancer does *not* seem to be related to an enlarged prostate, a common condition in older men.

DOCTOR'S TREATMENT & DIAGNOSTIC TESTS
- Your own observation of the symptoms, especially urinary problems.
- Medical history and physical exam, including a rectal examination.
- Laboratory blood tests for enzymes (acid phosphatase), which appear in higher quantities in the blood if the cancer has spread to bone.
- Needle biopsy (see Glossary) of the prostate.
- X-rays of bone.
- Ultrasound scan (see Glossary).
- Psychotherapy or counseling if sexual difficulties occur after treatment.
- Surgery to remove the prostate gland and testes (sometimes) if the cancer has not spread. Advancing age alone is not a deterrent.
- Radiation or hormone treatment if the cancer has spread. May be administered on an outpatient basis or in a hospital.

HOME TREATMENT BY SELF OR CARE-GIVER

GENERAL INSTRUCTIONS—No appropriate self-care. Surgery or radiation is the usual treatment unless pre-existing medical conditions such as chronic heart, lung, kidney or liver disease prohibit it. A yearly rectal examination after age 40 is the best way to detect early prostate cancer.

MEDICATION (ADJUSTED FOR AGING)
- Your doctor may prescribe:
  Hormones (usually estrogens) to slow malignant growth in the bones.
  Analgesics to control the pain.
- *Note:* Adverse reactions and side effects may be more frequent and severe in older persons. Remind your doctor of any medicines you already take.

ACTIVITY FOR OLDER PATIENTS
- Resume your normal activities gradually after surgery. Resume sexual relations when you are able.
- See Appendix 20 regarding physical fitness for the active older adult.

FOOD & BEVERAGE
- No special diet is required.
- See Appendix 1 regarding good nutrition for people over 50.

FUTURE CONSIDERATIONS FOR THE AGING ADULT

POSSIBLE COMPLICATIONS
- Fatal spread to bone and the bladder and other organs.
- Urinary incontinence.
- Sexual impotence after surgery (sometimes).

PROBABLE OUTCOME—Often curable with surgery or radiation if it is treated before the cancer spreads. Even after it spreads, therapy can relieve the symptoms and prolong your life.

PREVENTING RECURRENCE
- There are no specific preventive measures.
- All men over 40 should have an annual exam to screen for prostate cancer.

CALL YOUR DOCTOR IF

- You have symptoms of prostate cancer.
- During treatment, any sign of urinary tract infection occurs, such as frequent, difficult or painful urination; fever and chills; aching around the genitals or rectum; or backache.
- New, unexplained symptoms develop. The drugs used in treatment may produce side effects.

PROSTATE, ENLARGED
(Prostate Hypertrophy;
Benign Prostatic Hypertrophy, BPH)

BASIC INFORMATION FOR OLDER ADULTS

DESCRIPTION—Prostate hypertrophy is an enlargement of the prostate (a golf ball-sized gland surrounding the neck of the bladder and urethra in the male). The enlargement may obstruct the flow of urine from the bladder, but it is not cancerous. Body parts involved: The prostate gland; bladder; urethra.

SPECIAL CONSIDERATIONS FOR AGING
- All men who live long enough will have enlarged prostates.
- Older people are more likely to have multiple disorders.
- As men age, the prostate increases in size and begins to compress on the urethra.

SIGNS & SYMPTOMS
- Increased urinary urgency and frequency, especially at night; a weak urinary stream.
- Straining and dribbling on urination.
- Feeling that the bladder cannot be emptied completely; burning on urination.
- Urine of abnormal color; impotence (sometimes).
- Abdominal pain (rare).

CAUSES & RISK FACTORS
Causes include:
- Overgrowth of the prostate due to hormonal changes that accompany aging.
- Diminishing sex life with few or no ejaculations (believed by some experts).
The risk of obstruction increases with:
- Stress; smoking.
- Excessive alcohol consumption.
- Cold, moist weather.
- The use of many drugs, including atropine, antihistamines, muscle relaxers, beta-adrenergic blockers and calcium channel blockers.

DOCTOR'S TREATMENT & DIAGNOSTIC TESTS
- Medical history and physical exam, including a rectal examination.
- Laboratory studies such as urinalysis and blood enzyme studies.
- Ultrasound scan or pyelography (see Glossary for both) to provide information about the obstruction. If the symptoms are mild, your doctor may delay any action to see if they clear up without treatment.
- Hospitalization for surgery to remove the prostate. Surgery is recommended for these conditions: Inability to empty the bladder completely, leading to chronic infection of the urinary tract. One or more episodes of urinary retention (complete inability to empty the bladder). Kidney failure caused by the obstruction, swelling or destruction of the kidney as revealed by x-ray.

Persistent bleeding from the prostate. Recurrent prostate infection.

HOME TREATMENT BY SELF OR CARE-GIVER

GENERAL INSTRUCTIONS
- Urinate as soon as you feel the urge. Don't let the bladder become too full before emptying it. Relax during urination.
- Sit on hard chairs rather than soft ones whenever possible.
- Avoid exposure to dampness or cold temperatures.

MEDICATION (ADJUSTED FOR AGING)
- Your doctor may prescribe antibiotics if you develop a urinary tract infection.
- Your doctor may reduce or discontinue medications that may be causing the symptoms.

ACTIVITY FOR OLDER PATIENTS
- Engage in frequent sexual intercourse. Avoid sexual stimulation and arousal without ejaculation.
- Avoid long bus, train or plane rides unless restrooms are available so you can urinate at any time.

FOOD & BEVERAGE—No special diet is required. Avoid spicy foods and pepper, which irritate the urethra. Avoid drinking fluids at bedtime.

FUTURE CONSIDERATIONS FOR THE AGING ADULT

POSSIBLE COMPLICATIONS—Any of the conditions listed above requiring surgery.

PROBABLE OUTCOME—Treatable with surgery. Repeat surgery may be necessary within 5 years for a small percentage of patients.

PREVENTING RECURRENCE
- Maintain physical fitness (see Appendix 20).
- Continue an active sex life or masturbation during your older years.
- Drink alcohol in moderation—1 to 2 drinks a day—if at all.
- Take only medication that is essential for your health.

CALL YOUR DOCTOR IF

- You cannot urinate.
- You develop a fever.
- You have an enlarged prostate and the symptoms are worsening.

PROSTATITIS

BASIC INFORMATION FOR OLDER ADULTS

DESCRIPTION—Prostatitis is an inflammation or infection of the prostate (the gland surrounding the neck of the bladder and urethra). Prostatitis is not contagious. It may rarely accompany cancer of the prostate. Body part involved: The prostate gland.

SPECIAL CONSIDERATIONS FOR AGING
- The immune system becomes less effective, opening the way for viral, bacterial and other infections; malignancies; immune disorders; and allergies.
- Decreased nutrition, common among chronically ill older people, increases the risk of any disease or disorder.

SIGNS & SYMPTOMS
- Urgency to urinate.
- Burning with urination.
- Frequent urination; waking to urinate at night.
- Difficulty starting urination and emptying the bladder completely.
- Fever; chills.
- Discharge from the penis.
- Pain between the scrotum and anus.
- Joint and muscle aches.
- Blood in the urine (sometimes) or semen.
- Low back pain.
- Pain with a doctor's rectal examination.

CAUSES & RISK FACTORS
Causes include:
- A bacterial infection, usually from gram-negative germs such as those found in feces. These may reach the prostate through the bloodstream, the lymphatic system or directly from the urethra.
- An infection caused by prostate cancer (rare).
Risk factors include:
- A recent urinary tract infection.
- Smoking.
- Excessive alcohol consumption.

DOCTOR'S TREATMENT & DIAGNOSTIC TESTS
- Medical history and physical exam, including a rectal examination.
- Laboratory studies such as urinalysis and culture of secretions obtained at the time of the doctor's prostate exam.
- Self-care instructions focused on the older patient.
- Treatment may include prostate massage for chronic forms after the acute symptoms subside.
- Hospitalization for 3 to 4 days in serious cases if blood poisoning is suspected.
- Surgery to drain an abscess of the prostate (rare).

HOME TREATMENT BY SELF OR CARE-GIVER

GENERAL INSTRUCTIONS—Sit in a tub with 6 or 8 inches of warm water (106F or 41.1C) for 15 minutes at least 3 times a day. Use a whirlpool bath if possible.

MEDICATION (ADJUSTED FOR AGING)
- Your doctor may prescribe:
  Antibiotics to fight infection (usually for at least 30 days).
  Pain relievers.
  Stool softeners.
- *Note:* Adverse reactions and side effects may be more frequent and severe in older persons. Remind your doctor of any medicines you already take.

ACTIVITY FOR OLDER PATIENTS
- Rest in bed until the fever and pain subside. Then resume your normal activities gradually.
- The ability to be sexually active during acute prostatitis depends on the degree of disability. The symptoms are usually relieved in 1 to 10 days, so during convalescence let your sense of well-being be your guide.
- See Appendix 20 regarding physical fitness for the active older adult.

FOOD & BEVERAGE
- No special diet is required, but don't drink alcoholic or caffeinated drinks or eat spicy foods. These irritate the urethra. Drink 8 to 10 glasses of water a day to ensure an adequate urine flow.
- See Appendix 1 regarding good nutrition for people over 50.

FUTURE CONSIDERATIONS FOR THE AGING ADULT

POSSIBLE COMPLICATIONS—If untreated, prostatitis may lead to:
- Blood poisoning.
- Chronic bacterial or non-bacterial prostate infections. These have similar symptoms, but they are more likely to recur and respond less readily to treatment.

PROBABLE OUTCOME—Usually curable with treatment, but recurrence is common.

PREVENTING RECURRENCE—Some experts believe men who have never had prostatitis are less likely to develop it if they are sexually active. Men who have prostatitis at least once may decrease the likelihood of recurrence by maintaining an active sex life with frequent ejaculations.

CALL YOUR DOCTOR IF

- You have symptoms of prostatitis.
- Your symptoms worsen or you have a fever during treatment.
- Your symptoms don't improve after 3 days of treatment.
- Your symptoms recur after treatment.

PSEUDOMEMBRANOUS ENTEROCOLITIS

BASIC INFORMATION FOR OLDER ADULTS

DESCRIPTION—Pseudomembranous enterocolitis is a rare, severe illness in the small and large intestines. It usually follows 5 to 7 days after extensive gastrointestinal surgery and antibiotic treatment in a person who was debilitated before surgery. It is characterized by the inflammation and tissue death of the membrane lining the intentines and deeper layers of the intestines. Body parts involved: The large and small intestines.

SPECIAL CONSIDERATIONS FOR AGING
- The immune system becomes less effective, opening the way for viral, bacterial and other infections; malignancies; immune disorders; and allergies.
- Injured tissues repair more slowly.

SIGNS & SYMPTOMS
- Watery diarrhea (sometimes bloody) with abdominal cramps.
- Fever.
- A drop in blood pressure, sometimes to shock levels, with weak pulse and rapid heartbeat.
- Nausea and vomiting.
- Disorientation.

CAUSES & RISK FACTORS—Caused by an infection from bacteria, usually the germ *clostridium difficile*, which manufactures a toxin that causes the symptoms, or by the staphylococcus germ. These germs normally inhabit the intestinal tract. They cause enterocolitis when other normal bacteria of the intestinal tract have been killed by the heavy use of broad-spectrum antibiotics. This upsets the bacterial balance of the intestinal tract. The illness usually occurs as a complication of surgery. Risk factors include:
- Recent surgery with a drop in blood pressure during surgery.
- Kidney failure; obesity; poor nutrition.
- The use of antibiotics, especially lincomycin, clindamycin, ampicillin, chloramphenicol, cephalosporins, penicillin or sulfa drugs.

DOCTOR'S TREATMENT & DIAGNOSTIC TESTS
- Medical history and physical exam.
- Biopsy (see Glossary) of the membrane lining of the large intestine through a colonoscope (see Glossary).
- Hospitalization for intravenous nutrition and intensive care.
- During convalescence after hospitalization, self-care instructions focused on the older patient.
- Surgery (a colectomy or ileostomy) rarely. Advancing age alone is not a deterrent.

HOME TREATMENT BY SELF OR CARE-GIVER

GENERAL INSTRUCTIONS
- The most important treatment is to discontinue the use of the antibiotic causing the illness.

- Pseudomembranous enterocolitis is a complicated, serious disorder. This page can cover only the main points of diagnosis and treatment. Your doctor, nurse or librarian can provide sources of supplemental information.

MEDICATION (ADJUSTED FOR AGING)
- Your doctor may prescribe: Vancomycin or metronidazole to prevent secondary, non-bacterial infections that occur when the balance of intestinal organisms is upset. High doses of cortisone for a short time to decrease inflammation.
- Don't take antidiarrheal drugs unless they are prescribed by your doctor. They may contribute to intestinal perforation.
- *Note:* Adverse reactions and side effects may be more frequent and severe in older persons. Remind your doctor of any medicines you already take.

ACTIVITY FOR OLDER PATIENTS
- Rest in bed until all symptoms of the illness disappear. Flex your legs often while in bed to decrease the likelihood of deep-vein blood clots. Resume your normal activities gradually.
- See Appendix 20 regarding physical fitness for the active older adult.

FOOD & BEVERAGE
- Intravenous nourishment will be necessary at first, progressing to a liquid diet, a soft diet and finally to a normal diet.
- See Appendix 1 regarding good nutrition for people over 50.

FUTURE CONSIDERATIONS FOR THE AGING ADULT

POSSIBLE COMPLICATIONS—The following occur only if the problem is not recognized and treated: shock and severe dehydration; peritonitis caused by perforation of the intestine; death.

PROBABLE OUTCOME—The symptoms will usually disappear in 1 to 2 weeks after the offending antibiotic is discontinued. A substitute antibiotic is usually not prescribed; the body's defense mechanisms must take over for the withdrawn antibiotic. The worst cases are fatal.

PREVENTING RECURRENCE—There are no specific preventive measures.

CALL YOUR DOCTOR IF

- You have symptoms of pseudomembranous enterocolitis following intestinal surgery.
- The symptoms return after treatment.
- New, unexplained symptoms develop. The drugs used in treatment may produce side effects.

PSORIASIS

BASIC INFORMATION FOR OLDER ADULTS

DESCRIPTION—Psoriasis is a chronic, scaly skin disorder characterized by frequent remissions and recurrences. Approximately 3% of patients acquire it after age 60. Body parts involved: The skin, especially that of the scalp, elbows, knees, chest, back, arms, legs, toenails, fingernails and the fold between the buttocks.

SPECIAL CONSIDERATIONS FOR AGING
- The skin becomes dryer and rougher.
- The responsiveness of the skin's immune system decreases.
- Stress from any emotional cause—fear, worry, anxiety, sadness, loneliness or anger—affects all aspects of any illness or disorder.

SIGNS & SYMPTOMS
- Skin areas that are slightly raised, have red borders and are covered with large white or silver-white scales. The areas crack and become painful.
- Itching (sometimes).
- Joint pain.

CAUSES & RISK FACTORS—The cause is unknown, but psoriasis is probably caused by an autoimmune disorder. Risk factors include:
- Rheumatoid arthritis.
- Local injury.
- Infections (viral and bacterial) elsewhere in the body.
- A family history of psoriasis.
- Stress.
- Cold climates.
- Genetic factors. Persons with psoriasis have HLA antigens, and the incidence is highest among Caucasians.

DOCTOR'S TREATMENT & DIAGNOSTIC TESTS
- Medical history and physical exam.
- Laboratory blood tests.
- Self-care instructions focused on the older patient.
- Psychotherapy or counseling (sometimes) to help you adapt to the disorder.

HOME TREATMENT BY SELF OR CARE-GIVER

GENERAL INSTRUCTIONS
- Move to a warm climate if possible. The severity of psoriasis increases during cold weather.
- Maintain good skin hygiene with daily baths or showers.
- Avoid skin injury, including harsh scrubbing, which can trigger new outbreaks.
- Avoid skin dryness to decrease the frequency of recurrences. To reduce scaling, use non-prescription waterless cleansers and hair preparations containing coal tar or cortisone.
- Expose your skin to moderate amounts of sunlight as often as possible.
- Oatmeal baths may loosen the scales. Use 1 cup of oatmeal to a tub of warm water.
- If your motion is limited (as from arthritis), you may need help in getting ointments or creams to affected parts of the body.
- Psoriasis is a complicated, serious disorder. This page can cover only the main points of diagnosis and treatment. Your doctor, nurse or librarian can provide sources of supplemental information.

MEDICATION (ADJUSTED FOR AGING)
- Your doctor may prescribe the following to decrease the inflammation and scaling:
  Ointments containing coal tar.
  Topical cortisone drugs to use under plastic dressings.
  High-intensity ultraviolet light.
  Immunosuppressive drugs (in the severest cases).
  Methotrexate which, taken orally, may help if other treatments fail.
- *Note:* Adverse reactions and side effects may be more frequent and severe in older persons. Remind your doctor of any medicines you already take.

ACTIVITY FOR OLDER PATIENTS
- No restrictions are necessary.
- See Appendix 20 regarding physical fitness for the active older adult.

FOOD & BEVERAGE
- No special diet is required.
- See Appendix 1 regarding good nutrition for people over 50.

FUTURE CONSIDERATIONS FOR THE AGING ADULT

POSSIBLE COMPLICATIONS
- Secondary bacterial infection in the affected area.
- Generalized secondary bacterial infection—sometimes fatal—characterized by the eruption of many pustules, fever and joint pain.

PROBABLE OUTCOME—The symptoms can be controlled but not cured. The disease may have long periods of inactivity.

PREVENTING RECURRENCE—Cannot be prevented at present.

CALL YOUR DOCTOR IF

- You have symptoms of psoriasis or the symptoms recur after treatment.
- During an outbreak, pustules erupt on the skin accompanied by fever, muscle aches and fatigue.
- New, unexplained symptoms develop. The drugs used in treatment may produce side effects.

PSORIATIC ARTHRITIS

BASIC INFORMATION FOR OLDER ADULTS

DESCRIPTION—Psoriatic arthritis is a type of joint inflammation that accompanies psoriasis lesions in nearby nails and skin. Body parts involved: The joints in any part of the body, but especially the finger joints and the joints in the lower back and neck; skin or nails that have psoriasis lesions and are close to the affected joint. Sometimes additional skin sites include the scalp, navel, underarms and groin.

SPECIAL CONSIDERATIONS FOR AGING
- The immune system becomes less effective, opening the way for viral, bacterial and other infections; malignancies; immune disorders; and allergies.
- Decreased nutrition, common among chronically ill older people, increases the risk of any disease or disorder.

SIGNS & SYMPTOMS
- Pain, swelling, restricted movement, tenderness and warmth in the affected joint.
- Scaling skin.
- Pitted, ridged, yellow nails.
- In 80% of cases, psoriasis precedes psoriatic arthritis.

CAUSES & RISK FACTORS
Causes include:
- Physical or emotional trauma (rare).
- An immunological response to a streptococcal infection.
- Unknown (usually).
Risk factors include:
- Strep infections (rare).
- A family history of rheumatoid arthritis or psoriasis.

DOCTOR'S TREATMENT & DIAGNOSTIC TESTS
- Medical history and physical exam.
- Laboratory blood studies to detect a rheumatic factor and measure antinuclear antibodies (ANAs).
- X-rays to distinguish psoriatic arthritis from other forms of arthritis.
- Self-care instructions focused on the older patient.

HOME TREATMENT BY SELF OR CARE-GIVER

GENERAL INSTRUCTIONS
- Immobilize inflamed joints with splints.
- Use heat to relieve the joint pain. Hot soaks (see Glossary), whirlpool treatments, heat lamps, ultrasound or diathermy (see Glossary) are all effective.
- Schedule periods for regular, moderate exposure to sunlight.
- For proper treatment of the skin and nails, see Psoriasis in the Illnesses section.
- Use high-intensity ultraviolet light.

MEDICATION (ADJUSTED FOR AGING)
- For minor discomfort, you may use non-prescription drugs such as aspirin.
- To reduce joint inflammation, your doctor may prescribe:
  Non-steroidal anti-inflammatory drugs.
  Cortisone injections into inflamed joints (occasionally).
  Immunosuppressive drugs (sometimes) such as methotrexate.
  Gold therapy.
- *Note:* Adverse reactions and side effects may be more frequent and severe in older persons. Remind your doctor of any medicines you already take.

ACTIVITY FOR OLDER PATIENTS
- Rest inflamed joints during flare-ups, then resume your normal activities gradually. Try to increase your outdoor activity in the sunshine.
- See Appendix 20 regarding physical fitness for the active older adult.

FOOD & BEVERAGE—See Appendix 1 regarding good nutrition for people over 50.

FUTURE CONSIDERATIONS FOR THE AGING ADULT

POSSIBLE COMPLICATIONS—Permanent joint deformity and crippling—although this is less likely than with rheumatoid arthritis.

PROBABLE OUTCOME—This condition is currently considered incurable. It is characterized by acute flare-ups and remissions. However, the symptoms can be relieved or controlled, and medical literature cites a few instances of unexplained recovery. Scientific research into causes and treatment continues, so there is hope for increasingly effective treatment and a cure.

PREVENTING RECURRENCE—Obtain prompt antibiotic treatment for strep infections.

CALL YOUR DOCTOR IF

- You have symptoms of psoriatic arthritis.
- New, unexplained symptoms develop. The drugs used in treatment may produce side effects.

PULMONARY EDEMA

BASIC INFORMATION FOR OLDER ADULTS

DESCRIPTION—Pulmonary edema is characterized by a set of dramatic, life-threatening symptoms caused by congestive heart failure. Body parts involved: The lungs and heart. (THIS IS AN EMERGENCY; SEEK MEDICAL CARE IMMEDIATELY!)

SPECIAL CONSIDERATIONS FOR AGING
- Older people are more likely to have multiple disorders.
- Characteristic signs and symptoms of many disorders are frequently changed or absent.
- The lungs lose their ability to defend themselves against infection.
- Stress from any emotional cause—fear, worry, anxiety, sadness, loneliness or anger—affects all aspects of any illness or disorder.

SIGNS & SYMPTOMS—The following
symptoms often begin suddenly in the middle of the night and worsen rapidly:
- Extreme shortness of breath, sometimes with wheezing.
- Rapid breathing.
- Restlessness and anxiety.
- Paleness; sweating.
- Bluish nails and lips.
- Low blood pressure.
- A cough. This may be unproductive at first, but later it can produce a frothy, blood-stained sputum.

CAUSES & RISK FACTORS—Caused by the
failure of the heart's left ventricle to pump well enough to supply all body cells with oxygen. The underlying cause of heart failure includes many forms of heart disease, especially heart rhythm disturbances or hypertension with atherosclerosis or narrowing of the aortic valve. Risk factors include:
- Stress; obesity; smoking.
- A recent heart attack.
- High blood pressure or any form of heart disease.
- Fatigue or overwork.

DOCTOR'S TREATMENT & DIAGNOSTIC TESTS
- Medical history and physical exam.
- Laboratory blood studies and ECG (see Glossary).
- X-rays of the chest.
- Echocardiography or angiography (see Glossary for both) to determine the cause.
- Hospitalization for oxygen and medication.

HOME TREATMENT BY SELF OR CARE-GIVER

GENERAL INSTRUCTIONS
- Self-care is not appropriate for pulmonary edema. This is a medical emergency requiring intensive medical care. Delay can lead to death.

- Pulmonary edema is a complicated, serious disorder. This page can cover only the main points of diagnosis and treatment. Your doctor, nurse or librarian can provide sources of supplemental information.

MEDICATION (ADJUSTED FOR AGING)
- Your doctor may prescribe:
  Narcotics to relieve anxiety, decrease the blood flow to the lungs and reduce the oxygen demand of the body.
  Diuretics to decrease excess fluid circulating in the bloodstream and lessen fluid accumulated in the lungs.
  Digitalis to stimulate a stronger heartbeat.
  Antibiotics (if the pulmonary edema has been triggered by infection).
  Medications such as beta blockers, ACE inhibitors, nitrates and calcium channel blockers to reduce the workload of the heart.
- *Note:* Adverse reactions and side effects may be more frequent and severe in older persons. Remind your doctor of any medicines you already take.

ACTIVITY FOR OLDER PATIENTS
- Rest in bed until your condition stabilizes. You may read or watch TV. After treatment, resume your normal activities gradually. Resume sexual relations when the symptoms disappear and your strength returns.
- See Appendix 20 regarding physical fitness for the active older adult.

FOOD & BEVERAGE—Consume a low-salt, low-fat diet (see Appendices 8 and 9).

FUTURE CONSIDERATIONS FOR THE AGING ADULT

POSSIBLE COMPLICATIONS
- Death (if treatment is delayed or unsuccessful).
- Misdiagnosis as asthma, resulting in inappropriate treatment.

PROBABLE OUTCOME—In most cases, the symptoms can be controlled with treatment. The treatment for pulmonary edema usually brings dramatic and effective relief. However, the underlying heart disease causing pulmonary edema will require lifelong treatment.

PREVENTING RECURRENCE—If you have any form of heart disease, obtain prompt treatment for less dramatic signs of congestive heart failure. The treatment will include a low-salt diet, cessation of smoking, maintenance of an ideal weight, adequate rest and prescription drugs.

CALL YOUR DOCTOR IF

You have symptoms of pulmonary edema. *This is an emergency!*

PULMONARY EMBOLISM

BASIC INFORMATION FOR OLDER ADULTS

DESCRIPTION—A pulmonary embolism is a blood clot or an accumulation of fat cells (rarely) in one of the arteries carrying blood to the lungs. The blood clot begins in a deep vein of the leg or pelvis. A fat embolus often begins at a fracture site. The embolus moves through the bloodstream, passing through the heart and lodging in the branch of an artery that nourishes the lungs. This blockage decreases breathing ability and sometimes destroys lung tissue. Body parts involved: The veins, especially those in the legs; the pulmonary artery and smaller artery branches that nourish the lungs; broken bone. (THIS IS AN EMERGENCY; SEEK MEDICAL CARE IMMEDIATELY!)

SPECIAL CONSIDERATIONS FOR AGING
- Characteristic signs and symptoms of many disorders are frequently changed or absent.
- Older people are more likely to have multiple disorders.

SIGNS & SYMPTOMS
- Sudden shortness of breath.
- Faintness or fainting.
- Pain in the chest; low fever.
- A cough (sometimes with bloody sputum).
- Rapid heartbeat.

These symptoms are often preceded by swelling and pain in the leg.

CAUSES & RISK FACTORS—Caused by deep-vein thrombosis, which can occur any time that blood pools in a vein. Risk factors include:
- Any injury or illness that requires prolonged bed rest.
- Sitting in one position for prolonged periods, as on airplane flights.
- Recent surgery; bone fractures.
- Congestive heart failure.
- Heart rhythm disturbances.
- Polycythemia; hemolytic anemia.
- Obesity; smoking.

DOCTOR'S TREATMENT & DIAGNOSTIC TESTS
- Medical history and physical exam.
- Laboratory blood studies to measure coagulation factors, prothrombin time and arterial blood gases.
- X-rays of the chest; radioactive lung scan.
- ECG to show heart activity changes.
- Venous thrombosis study to help determine the course of the embolus.
- Hospitalization for anticoagulation and oxygen.
- Surgery to tie off the big vein leading to the heart and lungs (the vena cava) or to insert a filter to trap recurrent clots (rare).
- Self-care instructions focused on the older patient.

HOME TREATMENT BY SELF OR CARE-GIVER

GENERAL INSTRUCTIONS
- Wear elastic stockings or leg wraps with elastic bandages.
- Don't sit with your legs or ankles crossed.
- Elevate your feet higher than your hips when sitting for long periods.
- Elevate the foot of your bed.

MEDICATION (ADJUSTED FOR AGING)
- Your doctor may prescribe anticoagulant drugs to dissolve and prevent clots. The anticoagulant level must be monitored to keep it in a safe range.
- Thrombolytic drugs (blood clot-dissolving drugs) may be used to speed the process of dissolving clots.

ACTIVITY FOR OLDER PATIENTS—Rest in bed until all symptoms and signs of clot inflammation disappear. While in bed, passive (see Glossary) or active leg exercises help prevent thrombosis.

FOOD & BEVERAGE—See Appendix 1 regarding good nutrition for people over 50.

FUTURE CONSIDERATIONS FOR THE AGING ADULT

POSSIBLE COMPLICATIONS
- Rapid death from a large clot that obstructs more than 50% of the blood to the lungs.
- Massive bleeding in the lungs caused by smaller clots.

PROBABLE OUTCOME—Usually curable in 10 to 14 days with intensive care.

PREVENTING RECURRENCE
- Avoid prolonged bed rest during illnesses. Wear elastic stockings during recuperation—in or out of bed.
- Start moving your lower limbs and walking as soon as possible after surgery.
- Don't smoke.
- Avoid needless surgery. Get a second opinion.
- When traveling, stand and walk every 1 to 2 hours.
- Taking one aspirin a day may prevent recurrence. Ask your doctor.

CALL YOUR DOCTOR IF

- You have symptoms of pulmonary embolism. *This is an emergency!*
- Any of the following occurs during treatment: Chest pain; coughing up blood. Shortness of breath. Increased swelling and pain in the leg despite treatment.
- You take anticoagulants and develop any signs of bleeding.

RABIES
(Hydrophobia)

BASIC INFORMATION FOR OLDER ADULTS

DESCRIPTION—Rabies is a serious virus infection of the central nervous system that is transmitted by the bite of an infected animal or by a lick over a break in the skin. Body parts involved: The brain and central nervous system; body parts bitten by the rabid animal.

SPECIAL CONSIDERATIONS FOR AGING
- The immune system becomes less effective, opening the way for viral, bacterial and other infections; malignancies; immune disorders; and allergies.
- Older people are less able to flee from animals.

SIGNS & SYMPTOMS—The symptoms may appear 3 to 7 weeks after the bite or lick over a break in the skin or as long as 1 year later.
Early symptoms:
- Restlessness and irritability; fatigue.
- Slight fever; cough; sore throat.
- Increased saliva and tears.
2 to 10 days later:
- Violent spasms of the throat muscles that make swallowing impossible.
- Hyperactivity and violent behavior.
- Confusion; high fever; intense thirst.
- Irregular heartbeat; irregular breathing.

CAUSES & RISK FACTORS—Caused by a virus in the saliva of infected animals that passes to humans through broken skin or a mucous membrane. The virus travels slowly from the bite area to the brain. Animals that are commonly infected include dogs (especially wild dogs), bats, skunks, foxes, coyotes and raccoons. Other animals can also be infected, so consult your local health department after *any* animal bite. Risk factors include:
- Multiple bites or bites on the face, head, neck or upper body.
- Outdoor activities that involve exposure to wild animals, especially cave exploration and hunting (in which animals are handled).
- Travel to countries where rabies is prevalent.

DOCTOR'S TREATMENT & DIAGNOSTIC TESTS
- Your own observation of the animal's behavior. Determine if the animal was provoked. Animals that attack without provocation are more likely to be infected.
- Medical history and physical exam.
- Laboratory blood tests and fluid and electrolyte measurements.
- Pathological exam of the animal's tissue.
- Surgery to clean and repair the bite wound (sometimes). The wound should not be stitched.
- Hospitalization if symptoms develop.
- Self-care instructions focused on the older patient.

HOME TREATMENT BY SELF OR CARE-GIVER

GENERAL INSTRUCTIONS
- Wash the bite area for 10 minutes with soap and water to remove all saliva.
- Cover the wound with a clean bandage.
- Call your doctor or local emergency room for advice.
- Call your local animal control center to catch the animal if possible.
- If the animal is killed, remove the head and refrigerate or freeze it until it can be examined by pathologists.
- Don't panic. The incubation period allows time for diagnosis and treatment.

MEDICATION (ADJUSTED FOR AGING)
- Your doctor may prescribe one of the following: An injection of rabies-immune globulin. Injections of human diploid-cell strain vaccine if the animal is proven rabid. The course of injections lasts several weeks. A tetanus booster.
- Painful injections in the abdomen are no longer necessary.
- *Note:* Adverse reactions and side effects may be more frequent and severe in older persons. Remind your doctor of any medicines you already take.

ACTIVITY FOR OLDER PATIENTS—No restrictions are necessary unless symptoms begin. If they do, bed rest in a hospital is necessary.

FOOD & BEVERAGE—No special diet is required during outpatient treatment before symptoms begin. Intravenous fluids and nutrients are necessary during hospitalization.

FUTURE CONSIDERATIONS FOR THE AGING ADULT

POSSIBLE COMPLICATIONS—Dehydration and shock; coma; paralysis and death.

PROBABLE OUTCOME—Rabies can be prevented with early treatment following animal bites. Once symptoms begin, survival is unlikely.

PREVENTING RECURRENCE
- Vaccinate your dog or cat against rabies.
- Report stray animals in the neighborhood.
- Have a rabies immunization if your work involves animals.
- Keep tetanus immunizations up-to-date. See Appendix 16 for an immunization schedule.

CALL YOUR DOCTOR IF

Anyone is bitten by an animal.

RADIATION SICKNESS

BASIC INFORMATION FOR OLDER ADULTS

DESCRIPTION—Radiation sickness is a set of side effects that accompany radiation treatment for cancer or the after-effects of accidental exposure to radiation. Body parts involved: Depend on the location of treatment or exposure. See Signs & Symptoms below.

SPECIAL CONSIDERATIONS FOR AGING
- Characteristic signs and symptoms of many disorders are frequently changed or absent.
- Decreased nutrition, common among chronically ill older people, increases the risk of any disease or disorder.

SIGNS & SYMPTOMS—The following vary widely and are often temporary, depending on the radiation dosage and the area radiated:
- Nausea, vomiting and diarrhea.
- Headache; rapid heartbeat.
- Fatigue and shortness of breath.
- Anxiety and disorientation.
- Yeast infection in the mouth.
- Dry mouth and loss of taste.
- Swallowing difficulty.
- Worsening of tooth or gum disease.
- Hair loss; dry cough; anemia.
- Heart inflammation with chest pain.
- Burning, inflammation or scarring of the skin.
- Permanent skin darkening; sexual impotence.
- Bleeding spots anywhere under the skin.

CAUSES & RISK FACTORS—Caused by radiation damage to the immune system and to healthy tissues. The risk of after-effects from radiation treatment increases with:
- Poor nutrition.
- Illness that has lowered resistance.
- Large dosages given to large areas over the abdomen.

DOCTOR'S TREATMENT & DIAGNOSTIC TESTS
- Laboratory blood studies of hemoglobin, platelet counts and white blood cell counts.
- X-rays of the treated areas.
- Psychotherapy or counseling to reduce the stress of radiation treatment.
- Hospitalization for radiation treatment or complications.
- Bone marrow transplant. Advancing age alone is not a deterrent.

HOME TREATMENT BY SELF OR CARE-GIVER

GENERAL INSTRUCTIONS
- Join a support group of people with similar experiences.
- During radiation treatment, keep your doctor informed of how you are feeling. Treatments can sometimes be interrupted until you feel better.
- If you lose your hair, wear a wig until hair growth resumes.

MEDICATION (ADJUSTED FOR AGING)
- Your doctor may prescribe:
  Antinausea drugs. Unfortunately, no really effective drug is available for this type of nausea.
  Pain relievers.
  Blood transfusions for anemia.
  Antibiotics to fight infections.
- *Note:* Adverse reactions and side effects may be more frequent and severe in older persons. Remind your doctor of any medicines you already take.

ACTIVITY FOR OLDER PATIENTS—Be as active as your strength allows. Rest often.

FOOD & BEVERAGE—Eat a balanced diet. You may temporarily need a liquid diet (see Appendix 7) or want to prepare food in a blender if you have trouble swallowing. Intravenous feeding or the use of a small stomach tube is also possible until you resume normal eating. A dietitian can help.

FUTURE CONSIDERATIONS FOR THE AGING ADULT

POSSIBLE COMPLICATIONS
- Susceptibility to infections due to decreased resistance.
- Increased susceptibility to cancer—especially bone marrow cancer or leukemia.
- With radiation treatment, other complications depend on the area involved. Your doctor will explain possible complications. Modern radiation equipment makes serious complications unlikely.

PROBABLE OUTCOME
- Most side effects or complications of radiation treatment disappear gradually afterward.
- The after-effects of radiation accidents may not appear for years.

PREVENTING RECURRENCE
- Have a thorough dental checkup to detect tooth or gum disease before head or neck radiation.
- Eat well before radiation treatment to be in optimal nutritional condition.
- If you work around radiation, learn and observe safety regulations.

CALL YOUR DOCTOR IF

- You are accidentally exposed to radiation.
- You feel very ill during radiation treatment, especially if you have unexpected symptoms.
- After exposure or treatment you develop signs of infection, such as fever and chills, muscle aches, headache and dizziness.
- New, unexplained symptoms develop. Drugs used in treatment may produce side effects.

RAPE-CRISIS SYNDROME

BASIC INFORMATION FOR OLDER ADULTS

DESCRIPTION
Rape-crisis syndrome is characterized by the physical and emotional after-effects of rape (forced sexual entry into the body). Fewer than 1% of rapes occur in women over 50. Body parts involved: The genitals; rectum; mouth; brain.

SPECIAL CONSIDERATIONS FOR AGING
- Older women are less able to protect themselves against assailants.
- Characteristic signs and symptoms of many disorders are frequently changed or absent.
- Denial is common.
- Stress from any emotional cause—fear, worry, anxiety, sadness, loneliness or anger—affects all aspects of any illness or disorder.

SIGNS & SYMPTOMS
- Cuts, bruises or other injuries, including vaginal and rectal tears.
- Effects of exposure to the elements if the attack occurred outdoors or in a remote place.
- Fear, anger, crying or unusual behavior such as laughter for no reason.
- Unwarranted self-blame and guilt.
- Depression and withdrawal, even from family members and friends.
- Fear of revenge.
- Sleep disorders.
- No outward signs (sometimes).

CAUSES & RISK FACTORS—Rape is not a sexual act for pleasure. It is a show of power and an attempt to degrade or humiliate the victim. Some rapists have previously been victims of sexual abuse. Many know their victims—at least casually—and their attacks may be planned, not impulsive. Risk factors include:
- Economically depressed areas.
- Excessive alcohol consumption or drug abuse by the potential rapist.

DOCTOR'S TREATMENT & DIAGNOSTIC TESTS
- Medical history and physical exam.
- Laboratory studies such as cultures and blood tests for gonorrhea or other venereal disease.
- Detailed examination of the body for evidence from the rapist, such as hair, sperm or bits of clothing.
- X-rays if fractures are suspected.
- Doctor's treatment *always*—regardless of whether there are physical injuries.
- Surgery to repair any wounds.
- Hospitalization (rare).
- Psychotherapy or counseling to help you learn to cope with fear, sexual trauma and unrealistic feelings of guilt or worthlessness.

HOME TREATMENT BY SELF OR CARE-GIVER

GENERAL INSTRUCTIONS—If you are raped:
- Report the rape to police or a rape-crisis center. If you don't, the rapist will probably attack others.
- Call your doctor or go to the nearest emergency room. Many cities have rape-crisis teams to help you through the stress of the medical examination.
- Don't bathe, douche or change clothes.
- Talk over your feelings with trusted friends and family members. Suppressing your feelings will increase your distress.

MEDICATION (ADJUSTED FOR AGING)—
Your doctor may prescribe:
- Antibiotics if a sexually transmitted disease is suspected or diagnosed.
- Sedatives or tranquilizers for a short time to reduce your anxiety.
- A tetanus booster if lacerations were inflicted.

ACTIVITY FOR OLDER PATIENTS—Resume your normal life as quickly as possible.

FOOD & BEVERAGE—No special diet.

FUTURE CONSIDERATIONS FOR THE AGING ADULT

POSSIBLE COMPLICATIONS—Prolonged psychological trauma; sexually transmitted disease.

PROBABLE OUTCOME—Complete physical and psychological recovery is often possible with professional treatment.

PREVENTING RECURRENCE
At home:
- Keep doors and windows locked.
- Install security devices.
Away from home:
- Avoid dark, quiet or isolated places. Stay within sight of others.
- Never hitchhike; always lock your car.
- Check the back seat of your car before getting in.
- Take a self-defense course.
- If you are threatened with rape, remain calm. Panic may worsen the situation. Sometimes a rapist can be stopped by unexpected behavior, such as asking for help with a task.
- Carry a rape siren or whistle. Most authorities don't recommend that you carry a weapon.

CALL YOUR DOCTOR IF

You or someone you know has been raped.

RAYNAUD'S DISEASE

BASIC INFORMATION FOR OLDER ADULTS

DESCRIPTION—Raynaud's disease is a primary disorder of the circulatory system that affects blood circulation to the fingers and occasionally to the toes. This is different from Raynaud's phenomenon, which is a disorder of the circulatory system that occurs as a complication of other diseases. Body parts involved: The small arteries to the hands and feet.

SPECIAL CONSIDERATIONS FOR AGING—50% of people over 60 have x-ray evidence of narrowing of the coronary arteries, yet only 50% of those people have symptoms.

SIGNS & SYMPTOMS
Early symptoms:
- Fingers that turn pale when exposed to cold or stress. The paleness is followed by a bluish tinge, then redness. Pain, numbness and tingling accompany the color changes. Warmth relieves these symptoms.

Late symptoms:
- Chronic infections around the fingernails and toenails.
- Ulcers on the fingertips caused by inadequate blood circulation in the fingers.

The symptoms of Raynaud's disease develop gradually over a period of years. With Raynaud's phenomenon, the symptoms may begin suddenly.

CAUSES & RISK FACTORS—Caused by spasms of the arteries that supply blood to the fingers and toes due to extreme sensitivity to cold. The sensitivity may be due to poor function of the autoimmune system. Risk factors include:
- Stress; cold, wet weather.
- Smoking, which impairs circulation to the extremities.

DOCTOR'S TREATMENT & DIAGNOSTIC TESTS
- Medical history and physical exam.
- Laboratory blood studies.
- X-rays of the hands and feet.
- Self-care instructions focused on the older patient.
- Biofeedback training (see Glossary).
- Surgery to sever the sympathetic nerves to the involved extremities. Surgery usually relieves the symptoms for 1 to 2 years before they recur. Advancing age alone is not a deterrent.

OTHER—There are many similarities between Raynaud's disease and Raynaud's phenomenon. Diagnosis of one or the other may require years of observation.

HOME TREATMENT BY SELF OR CARE-GIVER

GENERAL INSTRUCTIONS
- Stop smoking. Your symptoms will improve if you do.
- Avoid exposure to cold in any form. Wear mittens and gloves outdoors and when handling ice or frozen foods.
- Wear comfortable, roomy shoes and wool socks.
- Avoid stressful situations. See Appendix 13.
- Move to a warm climate if possible.
- Raynaud's disease is a complicated, serious disorder. This page can cover only the main points of diagnosis and treatment. Your doctor, nurse or librarian can provide sources of supplemental information.

MEDICATION (ADJUSTED FOR AGING)
- Your doctor may prescribe: Vasodilator drugs to dilate the small arteries and improve the circulation. Sedatives to reduce stress.
- *Note:* Adverse reactions and side effects may be more frequent and severe in older persons. Remind your doctor of any medicines you already take.

ACTIVITY FOR OLDER PATIENTS
- No restrictions are necessary, except to keep warm. Avoid becoming chilled while participating in active sports.
- See Appendix 20 regarding physical fitness for the active older adult.

FOOD & BEVERAGE
- No special diet is required.
- Because alcohol dilates the blood vessels and may temporarily improve circulation slightly, you may have an occasional alcoholic drink.
- See Appendix 1 regarding good nutrition for people over 50.

FUTURE CONSIDERATIONS FOR THE AGING ADULT

POSSIBLE COMPLICATIONS—Permanent weakness and numbness in the toes and fingers; gangrene and amputation (in the worst cases only).

PROBABLE OUTCOME—This condition is currently considered incurable. The disease worsens gradually over many years. However, the symptoms can be relieved or controlled. Most persons cope well with Raynaud's disease and live a normal life span if complications don't arise. Scientific research into causes and treatment continues, so there is hope for increasingly effective treatment and a cure.

PREVENTING RECURRENCE—Don't smoke. Tobacco triggers the problem. This disease is rare among non-smokers.

CALL YOUR DOCTOR IF

- You have symptoms of Raynaud's disease.
- Your discomfort worsens despite treatment.
- Ulcers appear on the fingers or toes and do not heal.

RAYNAUD'S PHENOMENON

BASIC INFORMATION FOR OLDER ADULTS

DESCRIPTION—Raynaud's phenomenon is a disorder of the circulatory system affecting the fingers and toes that is a complication of an underlying disease or emotional disturbance. This is different from Raynaud's disease, which is a primary disease. Symptoms arise suddenly with Raynaud's phenomenon. With Raynaud's disease, they appear slowly over several years. Body parts involved: The small arteries to the hands and feet.

SPECIAL CONSIDERATIONS FOR AGING—50% of people over 60 have x-ray evidence of narrowing of the coronary arteries, yet only 50% of those people have symptoms.

SIGNS & SYMPTOMS
Early symptoms:
- Fingers that turn pale when exposed to cold or stress. Paleness is followed by a bluish tinge and then redness. Numbness and tingling accompany the color changes. The symptoms are relieved by warmth.

Late symptoms:
- Ulcers on the fingertips caused by a lack of normal blood flow to the fingers.
- Chronic infections under and around the fingernails and toenails.

CAUSES & RISK FACTORS—Caused by spasms of the arteries that supply blood to the fingers and toes. The spasms may be due to scleroderma, lupus erythematosus or other connective tissue disorders; Buerger's disease; cor pulmonale; certain medications, including ergot preparations, antihypertensives, alpha- and beta-adrenergic blockers and calcium channel blockers. Risk factors include:
- Stress; smoking; cold, wet weather.
- Occupations or hobbies that involve work with heavy equipment that vibrates forcefully, such as a chain saw or pneumatic drill. This disorder is occasionally seen in typists, pianists and others whose fingers are subject to continued trauma.

DOCTOR'S TREATMENT & DIAGNOSTIC TESTS
- Medical history and physical exam.
- Laboratory blood studies.
- X-rays of the hands and feet.
- Self-care instructions focused on the older patient.
- Surgery to sever the sympathetic nerves to the affected extremities. Surgery sometimes relieves the symptoms for 1 or 2 years before they recur. Advancing age alone is not a deterrent.

OTHER—Because of the similarities between Raynaud's disease and Raynaud's phenomenon, an accurate diagnosis of one or the other may require years of observation.

HOME TREATMENT BY SELF OR CARE-GIVER

GENERAL INSTRUCTIONS
- Don't smoke.
- Avoid exposure to cold in any form. Wear mittens and gloves outdoors and when handling ice or frozen food.
- Wear comfortable, roomy shoes and wool socks. Don't go barefoot outdoors.
- Avoid stress. See Appendix 13.
- Move to a warm climate if possible.
- Raynaud's phenomenon is a complicated, serious disorder. This page can cover only the main points of diagnosis and treatment. Your doctor, nurse or librarian can provide sources of supplemental information.

MEDICATION (ADJUSTED FOR AGING)
- Your doctor may prescribe: Vasodilator drugs to dilate the small arteries and improve the circulation. Sedatives to relieve tension and anxiety.
- *Note:* Adverse reactions and side effects may be more frequent and severe in older persons. Remind your doctor of any medicines you already take.

ACTIVITY FOR OLDER PATIENTS—No restrictions are necessary, except to keep warm. Avoid becoming chilled, which may happen following any active recreational sport.

FOOD & BEVERAGE—No special diet is required. Alcohol dilates the blood vessels and may temporarily improve the circulation slightly, so an occasional alcoholic beverage may be helpful.

FUTURE CONSIDERATIONS FOR THE AGING ADULT

POSSIBLE COMPLICATIONS—Permanent weakness and numbness in the toes and fingers caused by blockage of the blood supply; gangrene that necessitates amputation due to a loss of blood supply (in the worst cases only).

PROBABLE OUTCOME—Curable if the underlying cause can be cured.

PREVENTING RECURRENCE
- Don't smoke; avoid exposure to cigarette smoke from other people.
- Avoid exposure to the cold.
- Obtain medical treatment for the diseases listed as causes.

CALL YOUR DOCTOR IF

- You have symptoms of Raynaud's phenomenon.
- Your discomfort worsens despite treatment.
- Ulcers appear on the fingers or toes and do not heal.

RECTAL PROLAPSE

BASIC INFORMATION FOR OLDER ADULTS

DESCRIPTION—Rectal prolapse is a protrusion of rectal tissues outside the anus. This disorder is somewhat common in older adults. Mucosal prolapse involves only the mucosa, while complete prolapse involves all layers of the rectum. Body parts involved: The anus and rectum.

SPECIAL CONSIDERATIONS FOR AGING
- Muscle bulk and power decrease.
- Constipation is more common among older people.

SIGNS & SYMPTOMS
- A vague sense of fullness in the lower abdomen or rectal area.
- A mucus discharge from the rectum—sometimes tinged with blood.
- A firm mass of tissue that can be felt at the anus after a bowel movement.

CAUSES & RISK FACTORS
Causes include:
- Weak pelvic muscles.
- Abdominal pressure caused by:
  Chronic cough.
  Prolonged constipation and straining to have bowel movements.
  Standing or walking for long periods.
Risk factors include:
- Previous surgery on the rectum or vagina.
- Age. The older you are, the more likely you are to develop rectal prolapse.

DOCTOR'S TREATMENT & DIAGNOSTIC TESTS
- Medical history and physical exam.
- Examination of the rectal area by anoscope or sigmoidoscope (see Glossary for both).
- Self-care instructions focused on the older patient.
- For complete prolapse, surgery to provide support or strengthen the tissues that support the rectum. Advancing age alone is not a deterrent.
- Mucosal prolapse may be treated surgically by excising the protruding tissue. This is similar to hemorrhoid surgery.

HOME TREATMENT BY SELF OR CARE-GIVER

GENERAL INSTRUCTIONS
- Occasional minor prolapse can often be reversed by gently pushing the protruding tissue back into the rectum.
- Temporary help using conservative therapy may delay surgery, but it will eventually be necessary.
- Use sanitary napkins or absorbent pads to absorb the mucus discharge.
- Women can learn to recognize, control and develop the muscles of the pelvic floor. These are the ones you use to interrupt urination in mid-stream. The following exercises

(Kegel exercises) strengthen these muscles so you can control or relax them completely: To identify which muscles are involved, alternately start and stop urinating when using the toilet.
Practice tightening and releasing these muscles while sitting, standing, walking, driving, watching TV or listening to music. Tighten the muscles a small amount at a time—"like an elevator going up to the 10th floor." Then release very slowly—"one floor at a time."
Tighten the muscles from front to back, including the anus, as in the previous exercise.
Practice these exercises every morning, afternoon and evening. Start with 5 each time, and gradually work up to 20 or 30 each time.

MEDICATION (ADJUSTED FOR AGING)
- Your doctor may prescribe stool softeners to prevent constipation.
- *Note:* Adverse reactions and side effects may be more frequent and severe in older persons. Remind your doctor of any medicines you already take.

ACTIVITY FOR OLDER PATIENTS
- Avoid standing or walking for long periods; this increases abdominal pressure.
- Practice pelvis-strengthening exercises to prevent a recurrence. See General Instructions.
- See Appendix 20 regarding physical fitness for the active older adult.

FOOD & BEVERAGE
- No special diet is required. Drink at least 8 glasses of water a day and eat a diet that is high in fiber to prevent constipation.
- See Appendix 1 regarding good nutrition for people over 50.

FUTURE CONSIDERATIONS FOR THE AGING ADULT

POSSIBLE COMPLICATIONS
- Ulceration and bleeding of tissue that protrudes permanently.
- Bowel incontinence.

PROBABLE OUTCOME—Surgery can cure both complete prolapse and mucosal prolapse.

PREVENTING RECURRENCE
- Women can practice pelvis-strengthening exercises to prevent recurrences. See General Instructions.
- Do not strain when having bowel movements.

CALL YOUR DOCTOR IF

- Rectal tissue remains outside the anus.
- Rectal pain or bleeding occur.
- Fever or chills develop, indicating infection.

RETINAL DETACHMENT

BASIC INFORMATION FOR OLDER ADULTS

DESCRIPTION—Retinal detachment is a separation or tear of the retina (the light-sensitive tissue at the back of the eye) from the remainder of the eye. Body parts involved: The eye(s). (THIS IS AN EMERGENCY; SEEK MEDICAL CARE IMMEDIATELY!)

SPECIAL CONSIDERATIONS FOR AGING—The skin becomes thinner.

SIGNS & SYMPTOMS—The following usually affect one eye, but sometimes both are affected:
- Light flashes in the field of vision.
- Floating spots in the field of vision.
- Blurred vision.
- Wavy visual images (sometimes).
- Gradual loss of vision. This may not be noticed because it is so gradual.
- No pain.

CAUSES & RISK FACTORS
Causes include:
- Extreme nearsightedness (myopia).
- Complications of eye surgery.
- Eye injury.
- An inherited tendency (possibly).
Risk factors include:
- Age.
- Diabetes mellitus.
- Vascular disease.
- Previous retinal detachment.
- A family history of retinal detachment.

DOCTOR'S TREATMENT & DIAGNOSTIC TESTS
- Medical history and physical exam.
- Ophthalmologist's treatment.
- Surgery to reattach the retina using special lasers or cryotherapy (see Glossary) or to change the shape of the eye (sometimes).
- Self-care instructions focused on the older patient.

HOME TREATMENT BY SELF OR CARE-GIVER

GENERAL INSTRUCTIONS—The following instructions apply after surgery:
- Both eyes will be patched for a time. Your family and friends can help overcome the stress this will cause by providing companionship and assistance.
- Use dark glasses after the patches are removed.
- Don't rub your eyes.
- Don't bend over.
- Avoid straining, such as from constipation, heavy lifting or hard coughing. This may increase the pressure in the eyes.

MEDICATION (ADJUSTED FOR AGING)
- Your doctor may prescribe: Mydriatic eye drops to dilate the pupil. Dilation reduces eye activity during healing. If you cannot instill the drops, ask someone to be available to help at the appropriate times. Sedatives or tranquilizers to reduce your anxiety during convalescence.
- *Note:* Adverse reactions and side effects may be more frequent and severe in older persons. Remind your doctor of any medicines you already take.

ACTIVITY FOR OLDER PATIENTS
- After surgery, lie on your back in bed with your head elevated. Move your legs frequently to prevent blood clots from forming in the deep veins. Resume your normal activities when your ophthalmologist considers it safe.
- See Appendix 20 regarding physical fitness for the active older adult.

FOOD & BEVERAGE
- No special diet is required.
- See Appendix 1 regarding good nutrition for people over 50.

FUTURE CONSIDERATIONS FOR THE AGING ADULT

POSSIBLE COMPLICATIONS
- Without treatment—Partial or complete blindness in the affected eye.
- With delayed treatment—Detachment which extends to the macula (the area of most detailed vision). This causes permanent loss of detailed (central) vision.

PROBABLE OUTCOME—Often treatable with early surgical treatment using laser surgery.

PREVENTING RECURRENCE
- Wear protective eye shields when participating in sports.
- If you have diabetes mellitus or vascular disease, obtain medical treatment to control the disorder. See an ophthalmologist at least once a year.

CALL YOUR DOCTOR IF

- You have flashes or floating spots in your field of vision. *This is an emergency!*
- Any sign of infection (bleeding, redness, pain, swelling or fever) occurs after surgery.
- Your vision worsens after full recovery from surgery.

RINGWORM

BASIC INFORMATION FOR OLDER ADULTS

DESCRIPTION—Ringworm is an infection of the skin by a fungus (tinea) and is fairly common in this age group. Ringworm is transmitted by person-to-person contact, exposure to an infected animal or contact with infected surfaces, such as towels, shoes or shower stalls. Body parts involved: The scalp (tinea capitis); skin (tinea corporis); groin skin (tinea cruris); nails (tinea unguium); feet (tinea pedis); skin under the beard (tinea barbae).

SPECIAL CONSIDERATIONS FOR AGING
- The immune system becomes less effective, opening the way for viral, bacterial and other infections; malignancies; immune disorders; and allergies.
- Decreased nutrition, common among chronically ill older people, increases the risk of any disease or disorder.

SIGNS & SYMPTOMS—Lesions that itch (sometimes) and have the following characteristics:
- On the scalp, the lesions cause patchy hair loss and scaling scalp.
- On body skin, the lesions are red, circular, flat and scaling and have well-defined borders.
- On the bearded area of the face, lesions cause an itchy, scaling rash under the beard.
- On the feet—See Athlete's Foot in the Illnesses section.
- Of the nails—See Nailbed Infection (paronychia) in the Illnesses section.

CAUSES & RISK FACTORS—Caused by a fungus infection with one or more of 5 different fungi. Risk factors include:
- Diabetes mellitus.
- Exposure to darkness, moisture and warmth.
- Crowded or unsanitary living conditions.
- Exposure to infected animals (especially cats).

DOCTOR'S TREATMENT & DIAGNOSTIC TESTS
- Medical history and physical exam.
- Microscopic exam of skin scrapings in potassium hydroxide solution.
- Laboratory culture of skin scrapings.
- Examination with ultraviolet light (Wood's lamp) for ringworm on the scalp.
- Self-care instructions focused on the older patient.

HOME TREATMENT BY SELF OR CARE-GIVER

GENERAL INSTRUCTIONS
For ringworm on the body:
- Boil or chemically sterilize all clothing, towels or bed linens that have touched the lesions.
- Keep the skin dry. Moist areas favor fungus growth.
- Wear cotton underwear. Change more than once a day. Avoid tight clothes.

- If the area is red, swollen and weeping, use compresses made of 1 teaspoon salt to 1 pint water. Apply 4 times a day for 2 to 3 days before starting the local antifungal medication.

For ringworm of the scalp:
- Shampoo the hair every day.
- Have the hair cut short, but don't shave the scalp. Place large sheets of paper under and around the hair and chair to catch all the clippings. Place a cloth drape around your shoulders, chest and back. Don't wear street clothes for a haircut. Wear something that can be sterilized, such as pajamas, a housecoat or a smock. Repeat this procedure every 2 weeks or whenever the hair grows back.

MEDICATION (ADJUSTED FOR AGING)
- Your doctor may prescribe oral or topical antifungal drugs.
- *Note:* Adverse reactions and side effects may be more frequent and severe in older persons. Remind your doctor of any medicines you already take.

ACTIVITY FOR OLDER PATIENTS
- No restrictions are necessary.
- See Appendix 20 regarding physical fitness for the active older adult.

FOOD & BEVERAGE
- No special diet is required.
- See Appendix 1 regarding good nutrition for people over 50.

FUTURE CONSIDERATIONS FOR THE AGING ADULT

POSSIBLE COMPLICATIONS—Secondary bacterial infection of the ringworm lesions.

PROBABLE OUTCOME—Usually curable in 6 weeks with treatment, but recurrence is common. Ringworm becomes chronic in 20% of cases.

PREVENTING RECURRENCE—The fungi are so prevalent that total prevention is impossible. To minimize risk:
- Avoid continuous exposure to overheated humid environments.
- Avoid contact with pets that have skin problems. Have infected pets treated.
- Carefully dry your feet after bathing in a tub or shower or after swimming.

CALL YOUR DOCTOR IF

- You have symptoms of ringworm.
- The ringworm lesions become redder and painful and ooze pus.
- Your symptoms don't improve in 3 or 4 weeks despite treatment.
- New, unexplained symptoms develop. The drugs used in treatment may produce side effects.

ROCKY MOUNTAIN SPOTTED FEVER
(Tick Fever; Tick Typhus; Spotted Fever)

BASIC INFORMATION FOR OLDER ADULTS

DESCRIPTION—Rocky Mounted spotted fever is an acute illness with fever caused by a germ transmitted by infected ticks. This is not contagious from person to person. Body parts involved: The skin; central nervous system; gastrointestinal tract; muscles.

SPECIAL CONSIDERATIONS FOR AGING
- The immune system becomes less effective, opening the way for viral, bacterial and other infections; malignancies; immune disorders; and allergies.
- Repair from injury or disease is complete and effective, but recovery takes longer in older people.
- Characteristic signs and symptoms of many disorders are frequently changed or absent.

SIGNS & SYMPTOMS—The following occur 2 to 5 days after a tick bite:
- Fever, often high, with chills.
- A red skin rash that begins on the hands and feet and spreads to the ankles, wrists, legs, trunk and abdomen.
- Headache.
- Muscle aches and weakness; stiff back.
- Nausea and vomiting.
- Mental confusion; coma.

CAUSES & RISK FACTORS—Caused by rickettsia germs that live inside ticks. People are infected through tick bites, usually in the spring or summer. Rickettsia also infect rodents, squirrels and chipmunks. Rocky Mountain spotted fever has characteristics similar to those of Lyme disease. The disease occurs in all states of the U.S., especially on the Eastern seaboard from Georgia to Maryland, and in heavy brushy areas. The risk increases with outdoor activities in tick-infested areas.

DOCTOR'S TREATMENT & DIAGNOSTIC TESTS
- Medical history and physical exam.
- Laboratory studies such as blood counts and serological tests (see Glossary).
- Doctor's treatment. This may be a medical emergency.
- Self-care instructions focused on the older patient.

HOME TREATMENT BY SELF OR CARE-GIVER

GENERAL INSTRUCTIONS—No specific instructions except those listed under other headings.

MEDICATION (ADJUSTED FOR AGING)
- Your doctor may prescribe antibiotics, such as tetracycline or chloramphenicol.
- *Note:* Adverse reactions and side effects may be more frequent and severe in older persons. Remind your doctor of any medicines you already take.

ACTIVITY FOR OLDER PATIENTS
- Rest in bed until the fever and other symptoms disappear. You may read or watch TV. Resume your normal activities gradually.
- See Appendix 20 regarding physical fitness for the active older adult.

FOOD & BEVERAGE
- No special diet is required.
- See Appendix 1 regarding good nutrition for people over 50.

FUTURE CONSIDERATIONS FOR THE AGING ADULT

POSSIBLE COMPLICATIONS—Rocky Mountain spotted fever is often fatal if untreated.

PROBABLE OUTCOME—Curable if antibiotic treatment is begun in the early stages.

PREVENTING RECURRENCE
- Wear protective clothing in tick-infested areas, and use insect repellant.
- During outdoor activity, carefully inspect the body frequently to remove ticks. Don't crush them during removal; the whole tick must be removed. Hold a lighted cigarette near the tick or apply gasoline, kerosene or oil to the tick's body. Pull it off with tweezers.

CALL YOUR DOCTOR IF
- You have symptoms of Rocky Mountain spotted fever.
- New, unexplained symptoms develop. The drugs used in treatment may produce side effects.

ROUNDWORMS
(Ascariasis)

BASIC INFORMATION FOR OLDER ADULTS

DESCRIPTION—Roundworms are intestinal parasites shaped like earthworms that can be seen easily without a microscope. Roundworms thrive in the gastrointestinal tract and are contagious. Body parts involved: The gastrointestinal tract; the lungs (sometimes).

SPECIAL CONSIDERATIONS FOR AGING
- The immune system becomes less effective, opening the way for viral, bacterial and other infections; malignancies; immune disorders; and allergies.
- Characteristic signs and symptoms of many disorders are frequently changed or absent.
- Decreased nutrition, common among chronically ill older people, increases the risk of any disease or disorder.

SIGNS & SYMPTOMS
- Irritability.
- Restlessness at night.
- Erratic or poor appetite.
- Frequent fatigue.
- Weight loss or lack of weight gain.
- Colicky abdominal discomfort.
- Diarrhea (sometimes).
- A cough and wheezing (rare).

CAUSES & RISK FACTORS—Caused by a parasite called ascaris whose eggs enter the human body through contaminated water, food or soil-contaminated hands.
The risk increases with crowded or unsanitary living conditions.

DOCTOR'S TREATMENT & DIAGNOSTIC TESTS
- Medical history and physical exam.
- Laboratory studies to identify the worm.
- X-rays of the chest to check if the worms have migrated.
- Self-care instructions focused on the older patient.

OTHER—Worms may sometimes be seen in bowel movements. One may be vomited or coughed up rarely.

HOME TREATMENT BY SELF OR CARE-GIVER

GENERAL INSTRUCTIONS
- Wash your hands carefully after using the toilet or before meals. Keep your fingers away from your mouth. Keep your nails short and clean.
- Wash the anus and genitals with warm soap and water at least twice a day. Rinse well, preferably under a shower. Don't take tub baths.
- If possible, boil all soiled linen, nightclothes, underwear, towels and washcloths that have been used by anyone with roundworms. Fabrics that cannot be boiled can be soaked in an ammonia solution (1 cup of household ammonia to 5 gallons of cold water).
- After treatment, scrub all toilet seats, bathroom floors and fixtures. Vacuum rugs, table tops, curtains, sofas and chairs carefully. If there are children in the household, sterilize metal toys or similar objects in a hot oven.

MEDICATION (ADJUSTED FOR AGING)
- Your doctor may prescribe drugs to kill roundworms, such as pyrantel pamoate, piperazine or mebendazole.
- *Note:* Adverse reactions and side effects may be more frequent and severe in older persons. Remind your doctor of any medicines you already take.

ACTIVITY FOR OLDER PATIENTS
- Resume your normal activities as soon as your symptoms improve.
- See Appendix 20 regarding physical fitness for the active older adult.

FOOD & BEVERAGE
- No special diet is required.
- See Appendix 1 regarding good nutrition for people over 50.

FUTURE CONSIDERATIONS FOR THE AGING ADULT

POSSIBLE COMPLICATIONS—If untreated:
- Anemia or malnutrition.
- Intestinal obstruction (rare).

PROBABLE OUTCOME—Usually curable in 1 week with treatment.

PREVENTING RECURRENCE
- Wash your hands frequently—*always* before eating.
- Keep your fingers away from your mouth.
- Have pets treated for worms. Avoid strange animals.

CALL YOUR DOCTOR IF

- You have symptoms of roundworms.
- Roundworms reappear after treatment.
- New, unexplained symptoms develop. The drugs used in treatment may produce side effects.

SALIVARY DUCT STONE

BASIC INFORMATION FOR OLDER ADULTS

DESCRIPTION—A salivary duct stone is a tiny hard particle that forms in a salivary gland duct (usually a salivary gland under the tongue). Chemicals in the saliva cause crusting in the duct. The disorder is not contagious or cancerous, but the symptoms of stones and tumors may be identical. Body parts involved: The salivary ducts or glands under the tongue or in the cheeks.

SPECIAL CONSIDERATIONS FOR AGING
- Some studies show decreased saliva production in older people.
- The mucous membranes of the mouth are more permeable.

SIGNS & SYMPTOMS
- Pain and swelling in the salivary gland (between the ear and jaw), especially during meals.
- Redness and tenderness in the floor of the mouth and under the jaw.
- Swollen, tender lymph glands in the neck or under the jaw.
- Fever (if infection is present).

CAUSES & RISK FACTORS—Caused by a chemical in the secretions of the salivary glands for unknown reasons. Infections and injuries sometimes precede stone formation. Risk factors include:
- Smoking.
- A recent infection in the salivary gland.

DOCTOR'S TREATMENT & DIAGNOSTIC TESTS
- Medical history and physical exam.
- X-rays of the salivary duct (sialography).
- Surgery to remove the stone—generally under local anesthesia.
- Self-care instructions focused on the older patient.

HOME TREATMENT BY SELF OR CARE-GIVER

GENERAL INSTRUCTIONS—Use warm-water or cool-water soaks (see Appendix 18)—whichever feels better—to relieve the pain and hasten healing.

MEDICATION (ADJUSTED FOR AGING)
- Your doctor may prescribe antibiotics if infection is present with the stone.
- For minor pain, you may use non-prescription drugs such as acetaminophen.
- *Note:* Adverse reactions and side effects may be more frequent and severe in older persons. Remind your doctor of any medicines you already take.

ACTIVITY FOR OLDER PATIENTS
- After surgery, resume normal activities as soon as possible.
- See Appendix 20 regarding physical fitness for the active older adult.

FOOD & BEVERAGE
- No special diet is required.
- See Appendix 1 regarding good nutrition for people over 50.

FUTURE CONSIDERATIONS FOR THE AGING ADULT

POSSIBLE COMPLICATIONS—Recurrence of the stone. If it recurs, a surgeon can permanently open the duct so the saliva drains from the gland directly into the mouth.

PROBABLE OUTCOME—Many stones pass spontaneously. Others are usually curable with surgery.

PREVENTING RECURRENCE
- Brush and floss your teeth regularly to prevent infection in the mouth.
- Visit your dentist regularly for checkups.

CALL YOUR DOCTOR IF

- You have symptoms of a salivary duct stone.
- The symptoms worsen or don't improve in 4 days despite treatment.
- You develop a fever.

SALIVARY GLAND INFECTION

BASIC INFORMATION FOR OLDER ADULTS

DESCRIPTION—This disorder is the infection of a salivary gland caused by an infectious organism other than the virus that causes mumps. Body parts involved: The salivary glands and ducts.

SPECIAL CONSIDERATIONS FOR AGING
- Some studies show decreased saliva production in older persons.
- The immune system becomes less effective, opening the way for viral, bacterial and other infections; malignancies; immune disorders; and allergies.
- Decreased nutrition, common among chronically ill older people, increases the risk of any disease or disorder.

SIGNS & SYMPTOMS
- Pain and swelling of the parotid (behind the ear) or the sublingual (under the tongue) salivary glands.
- Pain and swelling of the lymph glands in the neck (below the jaw).
- Bitter pus in the mouth from the infected gland.
- Fever.
- Dry mouth.

CAUSES & RISK FACTORS—Caused by staphylococci or another of many strains of bacteria. Risk factors include:
- Smoking.
- Dehydration.
- Poor nutrition, especially vitamin deficiency.
- Recent or chronic illness that has lowered resistance, especially mouth infection.
- The use of drugs that affect salivation, such as analgesics, antidepressants, antihistamines, antihypertensives, diuretics, narcotics and cytotoxics.
- Thyroid disorders.

DOCTOR'S TREATMENT & DIAGNOSTIC TESTS
- Medical history and physical exam.
- Laboratory studies such as culture of pus from the infected gland.
- X-rays of the salivary gland (sialography).
- Self-care instructions focused on the older patient.

HOME TREATMENT BY SELF OR CARE-GIVER

GENERAL INSTRUCTIONS—Apply warm-water soaks (see Appendix 18) or a heating pad on the low setting to ease the pain and hasten healing.

MEDICATION (ADJUSTED FOR AGING)
- Your doctor may prescribe antibiotics to fight bacterial infection.
- For minor pain, you may use non-prescription drugs such as acetaminophen.
- If your problem is drug-related, your doctor may reduce the dosage or use an alternate medication.
- *Note:* Adverse reactions and side effects may be more frequent and severe in older persons. Remind your doctor of any medicines you already take.

ACTIVITY FOR OLDER PATIENTS
- No restrictions are necessary. Resume your normal activities when the fever disappears.
- See Appendix 20 regarding physical fitness for the active older adult.

FOOD & BEVERAGE
- No special diet is required. Drink at least 6 to 8 glasses of fluid a day.
- See Appendix 1 regarding good nutrition for people over 50.

FUTURE CONSIDERATIONS FOR THE AGING ADULT

POSSIBLE COMPLICATIONS—Complete, permanent blockage of the salivary gland duct, which requires surgery.

PROBABLE OUTCOME—Usually curable in 2 weeks with treatment. If the gland becomes blocked with a stone or scar tissue, surgery is necessary before the infection can clear.

PREVENTING RECURRENCE
- Brush and floss your teeth often and use antiseptic mouthwash, especially when you are ill.
- Visit your dentist regularly for checkups.

CALL YOUR DOCTOR IF

- You have symptoms of a salivary gland infection.
- The infection does not improve in 4 days or the symptoms worsen despite treatment.
- The fever persists despite treatment or recurs after treatment.

SALIVARY GLAND TUMOR

BASIC INFORMATION FOR OLDER ADULTS

DESCRIPTION—A salivary gland tumor is an abnormal growth in the salivary gland. Most salivary gland tumors are benign and require several years to develop. Even malignant tumors rarely spread to distant body parts. Body parts involved: The parotid glands (the salivary glands in the jaw); the submaxillary and sublingual glands (the salivary glands in the floor of the mouth).

SPECIAL CONSIDERATIONS FOR AGING
- Some studies show decreased saliva production in older adults.
- Decreased nutrition, common among chronically ill older people, increases the risk of any disease or disorder.
- Stress from any emotional cause—fear, worry, anxiety, sadness, loneliness or anger—affects all aspects of any illness or disorder.

SIGNS & SYMPTOMS—A soft, painful swelling or firm mass above the angle of either jaw or in the floor of the mouth.

CAUSES & RISK FACTORS—The cause is unknown. Risk factors include:
- Dehydration.
- Poor oral hygiene.
- Smoking.
- A salivary duct stone.
- Dentures.

DOCTOR'S TREATMENT & DIAGNOSTIC TESTS
- Medical history and physical exam.
- X-rays of the salivary glands.
- MRI or CT scan (see Glossary for both).
- Biopsy of tissue.
- Surgery to remove the tumor and the lymph glands in the neck if malignant cells have spread. Advancing age alone is not a deterrent.
- Self-care instructions focused on the older patient.

HOME TREATMENT BY SELF OR CARE-GIVER

GENERAL INSTRUCTIONS
- After surgery, keep your mouth clean with salt-water mouthwashes. At least 3 or 4 times a day, rinse the mouth with a solution of 1 teaspoon salt in 8 oz. of warm water.
- A salivary gland tumor is a complicated, serious disorder. This page can cover only the main points of diagnosis and treatment. Your doctor, nurse or librarian can provide sources of supplemental information.

MEDICATION (ADJUSTED FOR AGING)
- Your doctor may prescribe:
  Pain relievers.
  Antibiotics if infection is present.
  Anticancer (chemotherapy) drugs if surgery and radiation treatment don't destroy a malignant tumor.
- *Note:* Adverse reactions and side effects may be more frequent and severe in older persons. Remind your doctor of any medicines you already take.

ACTIVITY FOR OLDER PATIENTS
- Resume your normal activities as soon as possible after surgery.
- See Appendix 20 regarding physical fitness for the active older adult.

FOOD & BEVERAGE
- After surgery, a liquid diet (see Appendix 7) will be necessary until your mouth heals so you can eat normally.
- See Appendix 1 regarding good nutrition for people over 50.

FUTURE CONSIDERATIONS FOR THE AGING ADULT

POSSIBLE COMPLICATIONS
- Infection at the surgical site.
- Disfigurement after surgery.
- Fatal spread to other organs.

PROBABLE OUTCOME
- Malignant salivary tumors are usually curable with surgery, radiation treatment and anticancer drugs.
- Benign tumors are usually curable with surgery alone.

PREVENTING RECURRENCE—Some salivary gland tumors can't be prevented, but the risk can be minimized by:
- Not smoking.
- Brushing and flossing your teeth at least twice a day to keep your mouth healthy.

CALL YOUR DOCTOR IF

- You have symptoms of a salivary gland tumor.
- After surgery, signs of infection develop in your mouth, including increased warmth, redness, pain or tenderness and swelling.
- New, unexplained symptoms develop. The drugs used in treatment may produce side effects.

SALMONELLA INFECTION

BASIC INFORMATION FOR OLDER ADULTS

DESCRIPTION—A salmonella infection is a general infection caused by germs in the salmonella family. Body parts involved: The gastrointestinal tract; lymphatic system.

SPECIAL CONSIDERATIONS FOR AGING
- The immune system becomes less effective, opening the way for viral, bacterial and other infections; malignancies; immune disorders; and allergies.
- Characteristic signs and symptoms of many disorders are frequently changed or absent.
- Decreased nutrition, common among chronically ill older people, increases the risk of any disease or disorder.

SIGNS & SYMPTOMS
- Diarrhea, often accompanied by abdominal cramps. In mild cases, the diarrhea may be only 2 or 3 loose bowel movements a day. In severe cases, it may be watery diarrhea as often as every 10 or 15 minutes.
- Vomiting (occasionally); fever.
- Blood in the stool (sometimes).

A relatively mild salmonella infection may be mistaken for simple gastroenteritis.

CAUSES & RISK FACTORS—Caused by an infection with salmonella bacteria after eating meat that contains the bacteria. Salmonella bacteria survive freezing, but thorough cooking kills them. Pet turtles can also carry salmonella bacteria. Salmonella epidemics often occur when many people eat the same contaminated food at a picnic, social gathering or restaurant. The infection can be transmitted from person to person. Risk factors include:
- Recent gastrointestinal illness.
- Crowded or unsanitary living conditions.

DOCTOR'S TREATMENT & DIAGNOSTIC TESTS
- Medical history and physical exam.
- Laboratory stool studies.
- Self-care instructions focused on the older patient.
- Doctor's treatment if the symptoms continue longer than 48 hours or for complications.
- Hospitalization (rare).

HOME TREATMENT BY SELF OR CARE-GIVER

GENERAL INSTRUCTIONS
- Isolate the ill person if possible.
- Use warm compresses or a hot water bottle to relieve abdominal cramps.
- If the diarrhea is severe, use a bedside commode.

MEDICATION (ADJUSTED FOR AGING)
- Medicine is usually not necessary for mild cases. Antidiarrhea medications may retard recovery. For severe cases or if your have an underlying chronic illness, your doctor may prescribe anti-diarrhea medication, antibiotics to fight infection and intravenous fluids for severe dehydration.
- *Note:* Adverse reactions and side effects may be more frequent and severe in older persons. Remind your doctor of any medicines you already take.

ACTIVITY FOR OLDER PATIENTS
- Stay in bed, except for trips to the bathroom, until at least 3 days after the diarrhea, fever and other symptoms disappear. Then resume your normal activities gradually. Flex your legs regularly in bed to prevent the formation of blood clots.
- See Appendix 20 regarding physical fitness for the active older adult.

FOOD & BEVERAGE
- Drink diluted electrolyte solutions until the diarrhea stops. Then eat a high-calorie, well-balanced diet. Vitamin and mineral supplements may be helpful after prolonged illness.
- See Appendix 1 regarding good nutrition for people over 50.

FUTURE CONSIDERATIONS FOR THE AGING ADULT

POSSIBLE COMPLICATIONS
- Dehydration from excessive diarrhea and vomiting. Severe dehydration can be fatal.
- Infection of other organs, such as the kidneys, gallbladder, spleen and lungs, from salmonella bacteria in the bloodstream (rare).

PROBABLE OUTCOME—Most salmonella infections are mild and curable with treatment in 24 to 48 hours. Patients with severe infections require hospitalization and isolation. The infection may last 2 to 3 weeks.

PREVENTING RECURRENCE
- Follow these recommendations in any area with a substandard water supply: Drink purified water, boil water for drinking or add 2 to 4 drops of 4% to 6% chlorine bleach to each quart of water 30 minutes before use. If you are in a hotel, draw hot water from the faucet, let it cool and use it as drinking water. Don't use ice. Don't eat raw fruits and vegetables unless you can peel them.
- Drink only pasteurized milk.
- Wash your hands after bowel movements and before handling food.
- Isolate anyone in the family who has the infection.
- Ask your doctor about preventive antibiotics before traveling in countries with unsanitary water and food supplies.

CALL YOUR DOCTOR IF

- You have symptoms of a salmonella infection that persist longer than 48 hours.
- Any of the following occurs during the illness: a fever of 102F (38.9C) or higher; jaundice; a cough with blood; worsening diarrhea.

SCABIES

BASIC INFORMATION FOR OLDER ADULTS

DESCRIPTION—Scabies is a disease of the skin caused by a mite (the "itch" mite) with a characteristic pattern of distribution. Scabies is contagious from person to person (by shared clothing or bed linen) and from one site to another in the same person. Body parts involved: The skin of the finger webs and underarms and the folds of the arms, breasts, elbows, genitals and buttocks.

SPECIAL CONSIDERATIONS FOR AGING
- Characteristic signs and symptoms of many disorders are frequently changed or absent.
- The immune system becomes less effective, opening the way for viral, bacterial and other infections; malignancies; immune disorders; and allergies.
- The responsiveness of the skin's immune system decreases.

SIGNS & SYMPTOMS
- Small, itchy blisters (usually in a thin line) in several parts of the body. The blisters break easily when scratched.
- Broken blisters leave scratch marks and thickened skin, crisscrossed by grooves and scaling.

CAUSES & RISK FACTORS—Caused by a mite that burrows into the deep skin layers, where the female mite deposits eggs. The eggs mature into adult mites in 3 weeks. Mites are 0.1mm in diameter and can be seen under a microscope. Scratching collects mites and eggs under the fingernails, so they spread to other parts of the body. The risk increases with crowded, institutional or unsanitary living conditions.

DOCTOR'S TREATMENT & DIAGNOSTIC TESTS
- Medical history and physical exam. The diagnosis is confirmed by discovering the mite, lifting it from its burrow and identifying it under a microscope.
- Self-care instructions focused on the older patient.

HOME TREATMENT BY SELF OR CARE-GIVER

GENERAL INSTRUCTIONS
- All household members and close personal contacts must be treated.
- Apply the medicinal lotion or cream prescribed by your doctor as follows:
  Bathe thoroughly before applying.
  Apply from the neck down, and cover the entire body. You will need assistance in applying the lotion or cream, since all parts of the body must be covered.

Wait 15 minutes before dressing.
Leave the medicine on the skin for 24 hours before bathing.
Repeat in 1 week.
- Carefully wash all clothes and bedding used prior to or during treatment. You don't need to clean furniture or floors with special care.

MEDICATION (ADJUSTED FOR AGING)
- Your doctor will prescribe a topical medicinal lotion or cream (pediculicide) and may prescribe topical corticosteroids for itching. In severe cases, oral corticosteroids may be prescribed.
- *Note:* Adverse reactions and side effects may be more frequent and severe in older persons. Remind your doctor of any medicines you already take.

ACTIVITY FOR OLDER PATIENTS
- No restrictions are necessary.
- See Appendix 20 regarding physical fitness for the active older adult.

FOOD & BEVERAGE
- No special diet is required.
- See Appendix 1 regarding good nutrition for people over 50.

FUTURE CONSIDERATIONS FOR THE AGING ADULT

POSSIBLE COMPLICATIONS—Secondary bacterial infections of the mite-infested areas.

PROBABLE OUTCOME—The itching usually disappears quickly, and evidence of the disease is gone in 1 to 2 weeks with treatment. In 20% of cases, re-treatment is necessary in 20 days. If the skin irritation persists longer than this, oral antihistamines or topical steroids may be necessary to break the itch-scratch cycle. Scabies may occur in a community in a 7-year cycle—the "seven-year itch."

PREVENTING RECURRENCE
- Avoid contact with persons or linen and clothing that you suspect may be infected with scabies.
- Maintain personal cleanliness:
  Bathe daily or at least 2 to 3 times a week.
  Wash your hands before eating.
  Launder your clothes often.

CALL YOUR DOCTOR IF
- You have symptoms of scabies.
- After treatment, the lesions show signs of infection (redness, pus, swelling or pain).
- New, unexplained symptoms develop. The drugs used in treatment may produce side effects.

SCLERODERMA
(Progressive Systemic Sclerosis)

BASIC INFORMATION FOR OLDER ADULTS

DESCRIPTION—Scleroderma is a widespread connective tissue disease in which the skin and other body parts gradually degenerate, thicken and become stiff. It is most likely to appear between ages 40 and 60. Body parts involved: The skin; joints; digestive system, especially the esophagus; heart; kidneys; lungs; blood vessels; fingers; toes.

SPECIAL CONSIDERATIONS FOR AGING
- The number of autoantibodies (see Glossary) increases.
- The immune system becomes less effective, opening the way for viral, bacterial and other infections; malignancies; immune disorders; and allergies.

SIGNS & SYMPTOMS
- Fingers—Hardening and thickening of the skin, stiffness, poor circulation, numbness and fingertip ulceration.
- Digestive system—Swallowing difficulty, poor food absorption, bloating after eating, weight loss, heartburn and a feeling that food sticks in the chest.
- Skin—Hardening and thickening, especially in the face, which becomes tight and loses its elasticity.
- Muscle aches; fever; anemia.
- Weakness and fatigue.
- Joint pain, stiffness and swelling.
- Symptoms vary widely from person to person.

CAUSES & RISK FACTORS—The causes and risk factors are unknown, but scleroderma may be an autoimmune disorder. The connective tissue (the framework for all body tissues and blood vessels) thickens, becoming stiff and inflexible.

DOCTOR'S TREATMENT & DIAGNOSTIC TESTS
- Medical history and physical exam.
- Laboratory blood tests to detect anemia and measure antibodies.
- Urinalysis to detect red cells in the urine.
- ECG (see Glossary).
- X-rays of the hands, esophagus and chest.
- Biopsy of skin tissue to confirm diagnosis.
- Self-care instructions focused on the older patient.
- Psychotherapy or counseling to help you adjust to living with an incurable disease.
- Hospitalization for heart, lung or kidney complications.
- Physical therapy to relieve joint pain.
- Dialysis may be necessary if your kidneys are severely damaged as part of the disease.

HOME TREATMENT BY SELF OR CARE-GIVER

GENERAL INSTRUCTIONS
- Because of poor circulation, wear warm clothing—especially socks and gloves.
- Avoid exposure to extreme cold.
- Protect yourself from burns and cuts.
- Sleep on 2 or 3 pillows or raise the head of your bed 5 to 8 inches to prevent stomach acid from going back into the esophagus.
- Learn biofeedback techniques to increase circulation to the extremities.

MEDICATION (ADJUSTED FOR AGING)
- You may take non-prescription antacids to relieve heartburn or indigestion and aspirin or ibuprofen to relieve muscle aches and joint pain.
- Use skin lotions, lubricants and bath oil to soften your skin.
- Your doctor may prescribe cortisone drugs to relieve inflammatory symptoms, antibiotics to fight infections, vasodilators to help breathing and antihypertensives to treat high blood pressure.
- *Note:* Adverse reactions and side effects may be more frequent and severe in older persons. Remind your doctor of any medicines you already take.

ACTIVITY FOR OLDER PATIENTS—Be as active as your strength permits. Poor circulation in the legs may restrict exercise.

FOOD & BEVERAGE—Eat frequent, small meals to minimize bloating, heartburn and gastrointestinal discomfort. Use additional fluids to help with swallowing. A dietitian can help you plan a nutritious diet. Consult your doctor about taking vitamin and mineral supplements.

FUTURE CONSIDERATIONS FOR THE AGING ADULT

POSSIBLE COMPLICATIONS—Poor wound healing and gangrene; bleeding tendencies; heart rhythm disturbances; congestive heart failure; kidney failure; high blood pressure; lung destruction.

PROBABLE OUTCOME—This condition is currently considered incurable, but the symptoms can be controlled for a while with treatment. With treatment, most patients live at least 5 years.

PREVENTING RECURRENCE—Cannot be prevented at present.

CALL YOUR DOCTOR IF

- You have symptoms of scleroderma.
- Any of the following occurs during treatment: Unexplained bruising or bleeding under the skin. Slow healing of a wound.

SEBACEOUS CYST
(Epidermoid Cyst; Wen)

BASIC INFORMATION FOR OLDER ADULTS

DESCRIPTION—A sebaceous cyst is a dome-shaped cyst filled with semisolid material (keratin, the same material that forms the skin, hair and nails). The name *sebaceous cyst* is in error, because a real sebaceous cyst would be filled with material called sebum that is manufactured in the hair follicles. Body parts involved: The skin of the trunk, face, neck and scalp.

SPECIAL CONSIDERATIONS FOR AGING—The skin becomes thinner.

SIGNS & SYMPTOMS—A cyst with the following characteristics:
- The cyst has sloped "shoulders" or a dome-shaped, nodular appearance and a smooth surface.
- The cyst is whitish or skin-colored.
- The cyst is from 1cm to 4cm in diameter.
If the cyst becomes injured or infected, it may become bright red and painful.

CAUSES & RISK FACTORS—Sebaceous cysts are caused by plugged ducts in malformed hair follicles. They may enlarge due to hormonal stimulation or injury. Risk factors include skin injury.

DOCTOR'S TREATMENT & DIAGNOSTIC TESTS
- Medical history and physical exam.
- Self-care instructions focused on the older patient.
- Surgery to remove the cyst (sometimes). Small cysts can be removed through a simple incision, but rupture of the cyst—and corresponding incomplete removal—frequently results in recurrence. Large cysts do better if incised and drained in an initial procedure, with total removal of the cyst at another time.

HOME TREATMENT BY SELF OR CARE-GIVER

GENERAL INSTRUCTIONS—Before surgery, apply warm compresses to the cyst to reduce its inflammation and size.

MEDICATION (ADJUSTED FOR AGING)
- Medicine usually is not necessary for this disorder. If a cyst becomes infected, your doctor may prescribe antibiotics.
- *Note:* Adverse reactions and side effects may be more frequent and severe in older persons. Remind your doctor of any medicines you already take.

ACTIVITY FOR OLDER PATIENTS
- Resume your normal activities as soon as your symptoms improve.
- See Appendix 20 regarding physical fitness for the active older adult.

FOOD & BEVERAGE
- No special diet is required.
- See Appendix 1 regarding good nutrition for people over 50.

FUTURE CONSIDERATIONS FOR THE AGING ADULT

POSSIBLE COMPLICATIONS
- Infection of a cyst.
- Injury to a cyst, causing rupture or inflammation.

PROBABLE OUTCOME—Cysts which cause no symptoms require no medical treatment. Those that are unsightly or are repeatedly injured can be removed. Infected cysts may require incision, drainage and packing with gauze.

PREVENTING RECURRENCE—Cannot be prevented at present.

CALL YOUR DOCTOR IF

- After removal, signs of infection (pain, redness, warmth and increased tenderness) occur at the surgical site.
- A fever of 101F (38.3C) or higher develops.
- The treated area does not appear to be healing well within 1 week.
- You are taking antibiotics and new, unexplained symptoms develop. Antibiotics may produce side effects.

SEIZURES
(Seizure Disorders; Convulsions; Epilepsy)

BASIC INFORMATION FOR OLDER ADULTS

DESCRIPTION—Seizure disorders are disorders of the brain's functioning characterized by sudden seizures, brief attacks of inappropriate behavior, changes in one's state of consciousness or bizarre movements. Seizures—also called fits or convulsions—are a symptom, not a disease. Seizure disorders are not contagious. Some forms occur only during childhood, while others may occur throughout life. Body part involved: The brain.

SPECIAL CONSIDERATIONS FOR AGING
- The brain shrinks in volume. The older the person, the more the shrinkage.
- Neurological diseases become more likely.
- The blood vessels nourishing the brain become thicker and lose their elasticity.
- Nerve cells in aging people are especially susceptible to the action of drugs.

SIGNS & SYMPTOMS—There are several forms of seizures, each with its own characteristics:
- Petit mal seizure, which mostly affects children. The person stops activity and stares around for a minute or so, unaware of what is happening.
- Grand mal seizure, which affects all ages. The person loses consciousness, stiffens, then twitches and jerks uncontrollably. He or she may lose bladder control. The seizure lasts several minutes and is often followed by deep sleep or mental confusion. Prior to the seizure, the person may have warning signals—a tense feeling, visual disturbances, smelling a bad odor or hearing strange noises.
- Focal seizure, in which a small part of the body begins twitching uncontrollably. The twitching spreads until it may involve the whole body. The person does not lose consciousness.
- Temporal lobe seizure, in which the person suddenly behaves out of character or inappropriately, becoming suddenly violent or angry, laughing for no reason, or making agitated or bizarre body movements, including odd chewing movements.

CAUSES & RISK FACTORS—Seizures are characteristic of more than 50 brain disorders, but the organic cause can be determined in only 25% of cases. Common causes include brain damage at or before birth; drug or alcohol abuse; alcohol or drug withdrawal; adverse reactions to some drugs, particularly overdose; chemical poisoning; severe head injury; brain infection; a brain tumor or an expanding lesion that compresses the brain (occasionally). The risk increases with:
- A family history of seizure disorders.
- Excessive alcohol consumption.
- The use of mind-altering drugs.
- Exposure to toxic fumes; low blood sugar.

DOCTOR'S TREATMENT & DIAGNOSTIC TESTS
- Medical history and physical exam.
- Laboratory blood studies; x-rays of the head.
- CT scan; EEG (see Glossary for both).
- Surgery to remove any tumor, scar or abscess if one is causing seizures.
- Psychotherapy or counseling to help you understand and live with the disorder.
- Self-care instructions focused on the older patient.

HOME TREATMENT BY SELF OR CARE-GIVER

GENERAL INSTRUCTIONS
- Request and carry a Medic Alert bracelet or pendant that shows you have epilepsy in case you have a seizure.
- Avoid any circumstance that has triggered a seizure previously.
- If you are with a person who is having a seizure, loosen the clothing, lay the person flat and protect him or her from injury. Although frightening, seizures are rarely harmful in themselves.

MEDICATION (ADJUSTED FOR AGING)
- Your doctor will prescribe anticonvulsant drugs. Your response to treatment will be monitored. Medication changes or adjustments are often necessary.
- Learn as much as you can about your medication. The drugs used cause significant side effects, in addition to suppressing seizures.

ACTIVITY FOR OLDER PATIENTS—No restrictions are necessary. Most states allow persons to drive a vehicle after being seizure-free for 1 year.

FOOD & BEVERAGE—No special diet. Don't drink alcohol. It may decrease the effectiveness of your medication and provoke seizures.

FUTURE CONSIDERATIONS FOR THE AGING ADULT

POSSIBLE COMPLICATIONS—Continuing seizures (despite treatment); mental deterioration (rare).

PROBABLE OUTCOME—Seizure disorders are frequently incurable, except in relatively rare cases when they are caused by treatable brain damage, tumors or infections. However, anticonvulsant drugs can prevent most seizures and allow you to lead a nearly normal life.

PREVENTING RECURRENCE—Avoid alcohol or drug abuse; vigorously treat any infection anywhere in the body.

CALL YOUR DOCTOR IF

- You have a seizure, no matter what the expected cause.
- New, unexplained symptoms develop during treatment. The drugs used in treatment may produce side effects.

ILLNESSES & DISORDERS

479

BASIC INFORMATION FOR OLDER ADULTS

DESCRIPTION—Female sexual dysfunction is characterized by a woman's difficulty in becoming sexually aroused or achieving orgasm. Body parts involved: The brain and central nervous system; the autonomic nervous system.

SPECIAL CONSIDERATIONS FOR AGING

- Many body changes occur as a result of estrogen deficiency beginning at menopause. These include vaginal dryness, shortening and narrowing of the vagina, greater susceptibility to vaginal infections, frequent bladder infections, reductions in the size of the clitoris and increased facial hair. Changes in other systems of the body may lead to a greater tendency to osteoporosis, hardening of the arteries and other disorders.
- Stress from any emotional cause—fear, worry, anxiety, sadness, loneliness or anger—affects all aspects of any illness or disorder.

SIGNS & SYMPTOMS

- Lack of sexual desire; inability to enjoy sex.
- Failure to achieve orgasm, even when sexually aroused.

CAUSES & RISK FACTORS

Causes include:
- Inadequate foreplay; exhaustion.
- Anxiety, preoccupation and worry about other important issues.
- Worry about the health of your partner.
- Worry about the loss of a youthful appearance.
- Psychological problems, including depression and poor self-esteem.
- Feelings of shame or guilt about sex.
- The proximity of other people in a household.
- Acute illness, including vaginal infections.
- Chronic illness, especially of the central nervous system or the endocrine system, as with multiple sclerosis or hypothyroidism.
- Inadequate information about sexuality on the part of either partner.
- Repressed anger toward your sexual partner, which may result from feelings of being used as a sexual object, physical or emotional abuse, jealousy or fears of disloyalty, or lack of true intimacy.

Risk factors include:
- Previous sexual abuse or sexual trauma.
- Alcoholism.
- The use of some drugs, such as female hormones, including oral contraceptives (although these heighten sexual pleasure in some women); antihypertensives; antihistamines; beta-adrenergic blockers; and calcium channel blockers.
- Withdrawal from the long-term use of mind-altering drugs, including narcotics, psychedelics, hallucinogens, marijuana, sedatives, hypnotics or cocaine.

DOCTOR'S TREATMENT & DIAGNOSTIC TESTS

- Medical history (including a sexual history) and physical exam.

- Self-care instructions focused on the older patient.
- Counseling with a professional trained in sex therapy. Your doctor can assist you in finding help.

HOME TREATMENT BY SELF OR CARE-GIVER

GENERAL INSTRUCTIONS

- Admit the problem and try to establish open communication with your partner. Pretending that you are aroused or have orgasms leaves the problem unsolved.
- Wear cotton underwear and avoid tight clothing to help prevent infection in the vaginal area.
- Use a lubricant such as baby oil or a lubricating jelly to help prevent painful intercourse.
- See Appendix 13 for recommendations to reduce stress in your life.

MEDICATION (ADJUSTED FOR AGING)

- Your doctor may prescribe estrogen replacement therapy to relieve the symptoms of menopause.
- Medication is not necessary unless the sexual problem is due to some underlying medical condition. There is no known aphrodisiac that is effective and safe.
- *Note:* Adverse reactions and side effects may be more frequent and severe in older persons. Remind your doctor of any medicines you already take.

ACTIVITY FOR OLDER PATIENTS—No

restrictions are necessary. Exercise regularly (see Appendix 20) to reduce stress and improve your self-image. A healthy body and mind make enjoyable sex more likely.

FOOD & BEVERAGE

- Eat a well-balanced diet. Vitamin and mineral supplements may be helpful. Consult your doctor.
- See Appendix 1 regarding good nutrition for people over 50.

FUTURE CONSIDERATIONS FOR THE AGING ADULT

POSSIBLE COMPLICATIONS

- Permanent inability to enjoy sex.
- Damage to interpersonal relationships.

PROBABLE OUTCOME—With open communication between partners and professional counseling when necessary, most sexual problems can be resolved.

PREVENTING RECURRENCE

- Talk with your partner about your sexual needs and feelings.
- Seek counseling to resolve your feelings about past sexual trauma or abuse.

☎ CALL YOUR DOCTOR IF

You have sexual problems and you want help in resolving them.

BASIC INFORMATION FOR OLDER ADULTS

DESCRIPTION—Uncomfortable sexual intercourse means difficult or painful sexual intercourse, usually in females. Body parts involved: The vaginal muscles; uterus (sometimes); penis (rare); brain.

SPECIAL CONSIDERATIONS FOR AGING
- The female vagina changes shape, its flexibility decreases and vaginal lubrication decreases or stops.
- Many body changes occur as a result of estrogen deficiency beginning at menopause. These include vaginal dryness, shortening and narrowing of the vagina, greater susceptibility to vaginal infections, frequent bladder infections, reductions in the size of the clitoris and increased facial hair.
- Stress from any emotional cause affects all aspects of any illness or disorder.

SIGNS & SYMPTOMS—Pain in the genital area during sexual activity, including foreplay, intercourse or attempted intercourse. The pain may be mild or severe, and it may vary with different intercourse positions.

CAUSES & RISK FACTORS
Physical causes include:
- Infection of the genitals, including herpes and others involving the vagina, cervix, Fallopian tubes or ovaries in women and the penis in men.
- Pressure against the vaginal wall caused by scarring from operations or radiation treatment.
- A fibroid or other uterine tumor.
- Endometriosis.
- A bruised opening to the urethra.
- Inadequate vaginal or condom lubrication.
- Allergic reactions to diaphragms, condoms or contraceptive foams and jellies.
- Dryness and thinness of the vaginal wall after menopause.
- Pelvic inflammatory disease.
- In men, pain may be caused by anatomical abnormalities.

Psychological and emotional causes include:
- Lack of sexual arousal and vaginal lubrication caused by inadequate or insufficient sexual foreplay, aversion to a sexual partner, fatigue or anxiety.
- Past sexual injury or psychological trauma.
- Temporary lack of desire for a particular sexual partner.

Risk factors include:
- Stress; fatigue or overwork; recent illness.

DOCTOR'S TREATMENT & DIAGNOSTIC TESTS
- Medical history and physical exam.
- Laboratory studies such as a Pap smear (see Glossary) and culture of any vaginal discharge.

- Psychotherapy or counseling (sometimes) if the cause is psychological.
- Self-care instructions focused on the older patient.

HOME TREATMENT BY SELF OR CARE-GIVER

GENERAL INSTRUCTIONS
- Sitz baths frequently relieve tenderness. Sit in a tub of hot water for 10 to 15 minutes. Repeat baths as often as 3 or 4 times a day.
- Use a non-prescription lubricant such as baby oil or a lubricating jelly during sexual intercourse.
- Your doctor may provide instructions for exercises or techniques to dilate the vagina.
- Try different positions for sexual intercourse to discover new ones that might reduce penile penetration and be pain-free.

MEDICATION (ADJUSTED FOR AGING)—Your doctor may prescribe antibiotic, antiviral or antifungal medications for underlying infections.

ACTIVITY FOR OLDER PATIENTS
- No restrictions are necessary. Resume sexual relations as soon as possible.
- See Appendix 20 regarding physical fitness for the active older adult.

FOOD & BEVERAGE—No special diet.

FUTURE CONSIDERATIONS FOR THE AGING ADULT

POSSIBLE COMPLICATIONS—Damage to personal relationships; permanent inability to enjoy sexual experiences; loss of self-esteem.

PROBABLE OUTCOME—Depends on the cause. Medical disorders are usually curable with treatment. Psychological problems can often be cured with therapy, and interpersonal problems can improve with communication and patience.

PREVENTING RECURRENCE
- Obtain prompt medical treatment if you have symptoms of infection of the reproductive organs.
- Obtain professional counseling to resolve feelings about past sexual trauma.
- Discuss your lack of sexual arousal with your partner, including ways to improve foreplay. Enlist your partner's support and patience to overcome the problem. Use a lubricant if necessary.

CALL YOUR DOCTOR IF

- You have symptoms of uncomfortable sexual intercourse.
- The pain worsens despite treatment.
- The symptoms don't disappear after 3 months of treatment.

ILLNESSES & DISORDERS

SHINGLES
(Herpes Zoster)

BASIC INFORMATION FOR OLDER ADULTS

DESCRIPTION—Shingles is an uncomfortable and sometimes very painful eruption of the skin caused by a viral infection of the central nervous system. Shingles is contagious to persons who have not had chickenpox and frequently to patients who require immunosuppressant drugs for any illness. The peak incidence of shingles occurs between ages 50 and 70 in both men and women. Body parts involved: The sensory nerves of the skin on one side of the body only.

SPECIAL CONSIDERATIONS FOR AGING—This disease causes much more pain and disability in the older age group because:
- The skin is thinner and more sensitive.
- The circulation is less efficient.
- The capillaries are more fragile.
- Healing is slower.
- The immune system becomes less effective, opening the way for viral, bacterial and other infections; malignancies; immune disorders; and allergies.
- Stress from any emotional cause—fear, worry, anxiety, sadness, loneliness or anger—affects all aspects of any illness or disorder.

SIGNS & SYMPTOMS
- Painful red blisters that appear along the course of a sensory nerve on one side of the body on the face, chest or abdomen. These blisters generally appear in crops beginning 4 to 5 days after the pain begins. The blisters appear on a broad streak of reddened skin.
- Mild chills and low-grade fever.
- A general ill feeling (malaise).
- Mild nausea, abdominal cramps or diarrhea.
- Chest pain, face pain or burning pain in the skin of the abdomen, depending on the affected area.

CAUSES & RISK FACTORS—Shingles is caused by the *varicella zoster* virus, the same virus that causes chickenpox. It may lie dormant in the spinal cord until triggered by risk factors, including:
- Aging; the stress of everyday living.
- Illness that has lowered resistance.
- Hodgkin's disease; the use of immuno-suppressive or anticancer drugs.

DOCTOR'S TREATMENT & DIAGNOSTIC TESTS
- Medical history and physical exam.
- Biopsy or laboratory test of blister tissue.
- Self-care instructions focused on the older patient.

HOME TREATMENT BY SELF OR CARE-GIVER

GENERAL INSTRUCTIONS
- Avoid chilling drafts.
- When bathing, wash the blisters gently.
- Don't bandage the sores.
- Apply heat or moist compresses if this decreases the pain.

MEDICATION (ADJUSTED FOR AGING)
- For minor discomfort, you may use non-prescription drugs such as acetaminophen or aspirin.
- Your doctor may prescribe:
  Pain relievers.
  Tranquilizers for a short time.
  Cortisone drugs to relieve the pain in severe cases.
  Antiviral drugs such as acyclovir.
- *Note:* Adverse reactions and side effects may be more frequent and severe in older persons. Remind your doctor of any medicines you already take.

ACTIVITY FOR OLDER PATIENTS
- No restrictions are necessary. Stay as active mentally and physically as possible.
- Bed rest doesn't help and may be harmful.
- See Appendix 20 regarding physical fitness for the active older adult.

FOOD & BEVERAGE
- No special diet is required.
- See Appendix 1 regarding good nutrition for people over 50.

FUTURE CONSIDERATIONS FOR THE AGING ADULT

POSSIBLE COMPLICATIONS
- Delayed recovery. The older you are, the greater the likelihood of a prolonged healing time.
- Secondary infection in the shingles blisters.
- Chronic pain that persists for months or years in the sensory nerves where the blisters have been. The older you are, the greater the likelihood of prolonged pain.

PROBABLE OUTCOME—Most patients recover spontaneously without lasting complications, except for mild scarring. One attack usually provides immunity against shingles, but a few older persons have had more than one attack.

PREVENTING RECURRENCE—Cannot be prevented at present. Having had chickenpox may confer immunity.

CALL YOUR DOCTOR IF

- You have symptoms of shingles.
- The pain is intolerable despite treatment.
- New, unexplained symptoms develop. The drugs used in treatment may produce side effects.

SHOCK

BASIC INFORMATION FOR OLDER ADULTS

DESCRIPTION—Shock is low blood pressure that is too low for the body to maintain vital functions. Shock does not include a person's reaction to emotional trauma, which is a totally different disorder. Body parts involved: The heart; blood vessels; blood. (THIS IS AN EMERGENCY; SEEK MEDICAL CARE IMMEDIATELY!)

SPECIAL CONSIDERATIONS FOR AGING
- There is less efficient response to physical stress (fright and flight) due to the decreased responsiveness of the adrenal glands.
- Side effects of medication and adverse reactions are more frequent and worse.

SIGNS & SYMPTOMS
- Cold hands and feet.
- Fast, weak pulse.
- Disorientation or confusion.
- Anxiety with feelings of impending doom.
- Skin that is pale, moist and sweaty.
- Shortness of breath and rapid breathing.
- Lack of urination.
- Low blood pressure. This may be so low that it cannot be measured by usual means.

CAUSES & RISK FACTORS—Causes include the sudden loss of blood from an injury or disorders such as a bleeding peptic ulcer, ruptured aneurysm or ruptured ectopic pregnancy (hypovolemic shock); fluid loss, such as that which occurs with severe burns, fluid and electrolyte imbalance or peritonitis; impaired heart-pumping function from heart attack, heart rhythm irregularities, pericarditis or pulmonary embolism (cardiogenic shock); blood poisoning, which causes the blood vessels to greatly expand, as occurs with toxic shock syndrome or major infections (septic shock); some endocrine diseases, such as Addison's disease or diabetes mellitus. Risk factors include:
- Recent serious injury or surgery.
- Anemia; infection; cancer.
- The use of drugs that cause anaphylactic (allergic) shock as an adverse reaction, such as penicillin, local anesthetics and many others.
- Overdose of mind-altering drugs.
- Excessive alcohol consumption.

DOCTOR'S TREATMENT & DIAGNOSTIC TESTS
- Medical history and physical exam.
- Laboratory blood studies to measure the amount of blood in circulation and to measure fluids and electrolytes.
- Surgery to stop hemorrhaging.
- Hospitalization for intravenous fluids and medications to raise blood pressure and treat the underlying cause.

HOME TREATMENT BY SELF OR CARE-GIVER

GENERAL INSTRUCTIONS—If you observe signs of shock in someone, do the following until medical help arrives:
- Stop external bleeding by applying pressure.
- Keep the victim lying down with legs elevated. Cover the victim for warmth.
- Make sure the victim's airway is open to allow breathing. If breathing stops, give mouth-to-mouth resuscitation. If breathing *and* pulse stop, give cardiopulmonary resuscitation.

MEDICATION (ADJUSTED FOR AGING)—Depends on the underlying disorder:
- If the shock is from blood or fluid loss, treatment includes blood transfusion or intravenous fluids.
- If the blood pressure low enough to be life-threatening, hypertensive drugs may be given to raise blood pressure.
- If infection is present, antibiotics will be used.
- *Note:* Adverse reactions and side effects may be more frequent and severe in older persons. Remind your doctor of any medicines you already take.

ACTIVITY FOR OLDER PATIENTS
- Rest in bed until you have completely recovered. Move your legs actively while in bed to decrease the likelihood of deep-vein blood clots.
- See Appendix 20 regarding physical fitness for the active older adult.

FOOD & BEVERAGE
- No special diet is required.
- See Appendix 1 regarding good nutrition for people over 50.

FUTURE CONSIDERATIONS FOR THE AGING ADULT

POSSIBLE COMPLICATIONS—Cardiac arrest; respiratory arrest; permanent brain damage.

PROBABLE OUTCOME—Usually curable with early diagnosis and treatment. Without treatment, shock can be fatal.

PREVENTING RECURRENCE—Avoid the causes and risk factors listed above when possible.

CALL YOUR DOCTOR IF

- You have symptoms of shock or observe them in someone else. Call immediately. *This is an emergency!*
- New, unexplained symptoms develop. The drugs used in treatment may produce side effects.

ILLNESSES & DISORDERS

SHOULDER, FROZEN
(Adhesive Capsulitis)

BASIC INFORMATION FOR OLDER ADULTS

DESCRIPTION—Frozen shoulder is characterized by pain and stiffness in the shoulder joint that progresses to inability to use the shoulder. In this case, "frozen" does not relate to freezing temperatures. Body parts involved: The shoulder tendons, bursa, joint capsule, muscles, blood vessels and nerves.

SPECIAL CONSIDERATIONS FOR AGING
- Muscle bulk and power decrease.
- Characteristic signs and symptoms of many disorders in older people are frequently changed or absent.

SIGNS & SYMPTOMS
Early stages:
- Pain in the shoulder, often slight, that progresses to severe pain that interferes with sleep and normal activities. The pain worsens with shoulder movement.
- Stiffness in the shoulder that prevents normal movement. Reduced movement increases the stiffness.

Later stages:
- Pain in the arm or neck.
- Inability to move the shoulder.
- Intolerable shoulder pain.

CAUSES & RISK FACTORS—Caused by minor shoulder injury or inflammation, such as bursitis or tendinitis, that worsens from lack of use of the shoulder. Adhesions (constricting bands of tissue) form with disuse in 7 to 10 days and result in increased disuse. After 3 weeks of disuse, the adhesions become so severe that the joint cannot move. Risk factors include:
- Neglect of minor injuries, including bursitis or tendinitis.
- Poor nutrition, especially lack of adequate protein.
- Poor physical conditioning and occasional athletic activity.
- Chronic illness such as rheumatoid arthritis or osteoarthritis.

DOCTOR'S TREATMENT & DIAGNOSTIC TESTS
- Medical history and physical exam.
- X-rays of the shoulder.
- Self-care instructions focused on the older patient.
- Doctor's treatment, including manipulation of the shoulder to break up adhesions. This is done in a hospital or outpatient surgical facility under general anesthesia.
- Physical therapy and exercises.

HOME TREATMENT BY SELF OR CARE-GIVER

GENERAL INSTRUCTIONS
- After treatment and rehabilitation begin, your doctor will prescribe ice treatment and exercises.
- Frozen shoulder is a complicated, serious disorder. This page can cover only the main points of diagnosis and treatment. Your doctor, nurse or librarian can provide sources of supplemental information.

MEDICATION (ADJUSTED FOR AGING)
- Your doctor may prescribe:
  Pain relievers.
  Non-steroidal anti-inflammatory drugs.
  Injections of cortisone and local anesthesia into the shoulder to reduce the pain and inflammation.
- For minor pain, you may use non-prescription drugs such as aspirin.
- *Note:* Adverse reactions and side effects may be more frequent and severe in older persons. Remind your doctor of any medicines you already take.

ACTIVITY FOR OLDER PATIENTS
- Resume your normal activities as soon as your symptoms improve.
- See Appendix 20 regarding physical fitness for the active older adult.

FOOD & BEVERAGE
- No special diet is required. Vitamin and mineral supplements don't help unless you can't eat a normal, well-balanced diet.
- See Appendix 1 regarding good nutrition for people over 50.

FUTURE CONSIDERATIONS FOR THE AGING ADULT

POSSIBLE COMPLICATIONS—Permanent shoulder disability and pain without treatment or with delayed treatment.

PROBABLE OUTCOME—Usually curable with treatment and rehabilitation.

PREVENTING RECURRENCE—Obtain medical treatment for bursitis and tendinitis, including exercises to prevent the formation of adhesions.

CALL YOUR DOCTOR IF

- You have symptoms of a frozen shoulder.
- You have persistent shoulder pain that indicates possible bursitis or tendinitis.
- New, unexplained symptoms develop. The drugs used in treatment may produce side effects.

SILICOSIS

BASIC INFORMATION FOR OLDER ADULTS

DESCRIPTION—Silicosis is an inflammation of the lungs due to breathing silica (quartz) dust. It primarily affects workers over age 50. Silicosis may lead to lung cancer. Body parts involved: The lungs.

SPECIAL CONSIDERATIONS FOR AGING
- The immune system becomes less effective, opening the way for viral, bacterial and other infections; malignancies; immune disorders; and allergies.
- Decreased nutrition, common among chronically ill older people, increases the risk of any disease or disorder.

SIGNS & SYMPTOMS
Early symptoms:
- Shortness of breath.
- A cough that produces little or no sputum.
- A general ill feeling.

Late symptoms:
- Fitful sleep; appetite loss.
- Chest pain; hoarseness.
- Coughing up blood.
- Symptoms of heart failure.
- Bluish nails.

CAUSES & RISK FACTORS—Caused by 20 to 30 years of exposure to small particles of silica in work such as mining, granite cutting, pottery manufacturing, metal grinding and sand blasting. Risk factors include:
- Poor nutrition; smoking.
- Excessive alcohol consumption.

DOCTOR'S TREATMENT & DIAGNOSTIC TESTS
- Medical history and physical exam.
- X-rays of the chest.
- Pulmonary function test.

HOME TREATMENT BY SELF OR CARE-GIVER

GENERAL INSTRUCTIONS—The following measures may relieve the symptoms and protect against recurrent lung infections:
- Obtain medical treatment for any respiratory infection, including the common cold.
- Consider moving to a warm, dry climate if you have advanced disease.
- Practice bronchial drainage. Your physician will provide instructions.
- Use a cool-mist humidifier to loosen the bronchial secretions so they may be coughed up easily.
- Avoid further exposure to the dust.

MEDICATION (ADJUSTED FOR AGING)
- Your doctor may prescribe:
  Antibiotics for infections.
  Bronchodilators (inhaled or oral) with inhalation therapy (supervised at first by an inhalation therapist) to open the bronchial tubes to the maximum.
- For minor discomfort, you may use non-prescription drugs such as acetaminophen or aspirin.
- *Note:* Adverse reactions and side effects may be more frequent and severe in older persons. Remind your doctor of any medicines you already take.

ACTIVITY FOR OLDER PATIENTS
- Rest in bed with infections. You may read or watch TV.
- After treatment, resume normal activity as soon as your symptoms improve.
- See Appendix 20 regarding physical fitness for the active older adult.

FOOD & BEVERAGE
- No special diet is required.
- See Appendix 1 regarding good nutrition for people over 50.

FUTURE CONSIDERATIONS FOR THE AGING ADULT

POSSIBLE COMPLICATIONS—Tuberculosis (in the late stages of silicosis); heart failure due to lung disease; lung collapse; pleurisy; lung cancer.

PROBABLE OUTCOME—This condition is currently considered incurable. Life expectancy is reduced, and it causes increasing respiratory disability. However, the symptoms can be relieved or controlled. Scientific research into causes and treatment continues, so there is hope for increasingly effective treatment and a cure.

PREVENTING RECURRENCE
- During exposure to silica, wear a protective mask or a hood supplied with external air.
- Don't smoke.
- Participate in a regular physical exercise program to maintain good cardiopulmonary fitness.
- The overall incidence of this disease is falling because of increased preventive measures.

CALL YOUR DOCTOR IF

- You have symptoms of silicosis.
- Any of the following occurs during treatment:
  Fever.
  Increased chest pain or breathlessness.
  Blood in the sputum.
  Continuing weight loss.
  Confusion or lethargy.
- New, unexplained symptoms develop. The drugs used in treatment may produce side effects.

SINUS INFECTION
(Sinusitis)

BASIC INFORMATION FOR OLDER ADULTS

DESCRIPTION—Sinusitis is an inflammation of the sinuses adjacent to the nose. The germs that cause sinusitis are contagious. Body parts involved: The sinuses.

SPECIAL CONSIDERATIONS FOR AGING
- The immune system becomes less effective, opening the way for viral, bacterial and other infections and allergies.
- Decreased nutrition increases the risk of any disease or disorder.

SIGNS & SYMPTOMS
Early stages:
- Nasal congestion with greenish-yellow (sometimes blood-tinged) discharge.
- A feeling of pressure inside the head.
- Eye pain; post-nasal drip.
- A headache that is worse in the morning or when bending forward.
- Cheek pain that may resemble a toothache.
- A cough (sometimes) that is usually non-productive; disturbed sleep (sometimes).
- Fever (sometimes); diminished sense of smell.

Late stages:
- Complete blockage of the sinus openings, blocking the discharge and increasing pain.

CAUSES & RISK FACTORS
Causes include:
- An infection, usually initiated by a common cold, influenza or other upper respiratory infection. The infection may be complicated by a bacterial invasion of organisms that normally inhabit the nose and throat.
- Irritation of the nasal passages due to allergies, smoking, hard sneezing with the mouth closed, fatigue, getting chilled, and swimming, especially jumping into the water without holding your nose.
- Abscess in an upper tooth.

Risk factors include:
- Illness that has lowered resistance; smoking.
- Exposure to cold, damp weather outdoors and dry heat indoors.
- Exposure to others in public places.
- Excessive nose blowing during an upper respiratory infection.

DOCTOR'S TREATMENT & DIAGNOSTIC TESTS
- Medical history and physical exam.
- X-rays of the sinuses.
- Laboratory study of nasal discharge to identify the type of bacteria (sometimes).
- Self-care instructions focused on the older patient.
- Surgery to drain blocked sinuses (rare).
- Hospitalization (if outpatient treatment fails) for intravenous antibiotics and possible surgical drainage.

HOME TREATMENT BY SELF OR CARE-GIVER

GENERAL INSTRUCTIONS
- Use a cool-mist humidifier to help thin secretions so they will drain more easily.
- Apply heat to relieve the pain in your sinuses and nose. Use an electric heating pad or warm compresses.
- Don't allow other persons to use your nose drops. They will be contaminated by the infection. Discard the drops after treatment.
- Avoid non-prescription nose drops or sprays. Use prescribed drops only for the recommended time. They can interfere with normal nasal and sinus function and become addictive, causing a rebound phenomenon (see Glossary).

MEDICATION (ADJUSTED FOR AGING)
- Your doctor may prescribe:
  Nasal sprays, nose drops or decongestant medicines to reduce the congestion.
  Antibiotics to fight the infection.
- For minor pain, you may use non-prescription drugs such as acetaminophen.

ACTIVITY FOR OLDER PATIENTS
- Resume your normal activities gradually.
- See Appendix 20 regarding physical fitness for the active older adult.

FOOD & BEVERAGE
- No special diet is required, but drink extra fluids to help thin secretions.
- See Appendix 1 regarding good nutrition for people over 50.

FUTURE CONSIDERATIONS FOR THE AGING ADULT

POSSIBLE COMPLICATIONS—Meningitis or brain abscess (rare); small benign tumors of the mucous glands; infection of the skull.

PROBABLE OUTCOME—Usually curable with intense treatment. Recurrence is common.

PREVENTING RECURRENCE
- Keep the humidity level at 45% to 50% in heated buildings during the winter.
- Don't stifle sneezes.

CALL YOUR DOCTOR IF

- You have symptoms of sinusitis.
- Any of the following occurs during treatment:
  Fever; bleeding from the nose.
  Swelling of the face (the forehead, eyes, side of the nose or cheek).
  Severe headache; blurred vision.

SKIN, BACTERIAL INFECTION OF
(Impetigo; Pyoderma)

BASIC INFORMATION FOR OLDER ADULTS

DESCRIPTION—Impetigo is a common contagious infection that affects the superficial layers of the skin. Body parts involved: The skin of the face, arms and legs.

SPECIAL CONSIDERATIONS FOR AGING
- The immune system becomes less effective, opening the way for viral, bacterial and other infections; malignancies; immune disorders; and allergies.
- Decreased nutrition increases the risk of infections.
- The total state of well-being in many older people makes them increasingly susceptible to infections and impairs their ability to prevent infections from spreading.

SIGNS & SYMPTOMS
- A red rash with many small blisters. Some blisters contain pus, and yellow-brown crusts form when they break. The blisters don't hurt, but they may itch.
- A slight fever (sometimes).
- Tiredness.
- Enlarged, hard lymph glands (sometimes).

CAUSES & RISK FACTORS—Caused by staphylococci or streptococci bacteria growing in the upper skin layers. Risk factors include:
- Skin that is sensitive to sun and irritants such as soap and makeup.
- Poor nutrition.
- Illness that has lowered resistance.
- Warm, moist weather.
- Crowded or unsanitary living conditions.
- Poor hygiene.
- A cut in the skin or a cold sore.

DOCTOR'S TREATMENT & DIAGNOSTIC TESTS
- Medical history and physical exam.
- Laboratory skin culture to identify the germ causing the infection.
- Self-care instructions focused on the older patient.

HOME TREATMENT BY SELF OR CARE-GIVER

GENERAL INSTRUCTIONS
- Follow the suggestions listed under Preventing Recurrence.
- Gently wash the lesions with gauze and antiseptic soap. Break any pustules. Remove all crusts, and expose and cleanse all lesions. If the crusts are difficult to remove, soak them in warm soapy water and scrub them gently.
- Cover the sores with gauze and tape to keep your hands away from them.
- Treat new lesions the same way, even if you are not sure they are impetigo.

- If possible, separate and boil bed linen and towels, clothes and other items that have touched the sores.
- Men should shave around sores on the face, not over them. Use an aerosol shaving cream and change razor blades each day. Don't use a shaving brush, as it may harbor germs.

MEDICATION (ADJUSTED FOR AGING)
- Your doctor may prescribe:
  Oral antibiotics. To avoid complications, take the antibiotics for 10 days even if the symptoms disappear.
  Antibiotic ointments for very small areas of infection. Rub the ointment into the lesions for 60 seconds at least 4 times a day. If your doctor has not prescribed an ointment, you may use a non-prescription ointment containing neomycin and bacitracin.
- Avoid cortisone ointments.
- *Note:* Adverse reactions and side effects may be more frequent and severe in older persons. Remind your doctor of any medicines you already take.

ACTIVITY FOR OLDER PATIENTS
- No restrictions are necessary.
- See Appendix 20 regarding physical fitness for the active older adult.

FOOD & BEVERAGE
- No special diet is required.
- See Appendix 1 regarding good nutrition for people over 50.

FUTURE CONSIDERATIONS FOR THE AGING ADULT

POSSIBLE COMPLICATIONS
- Penetration of the infection to deeper skin layers (ecthyma or cellulitis). This may cause scarring. The treatment is the same.
- Acute glomerulonephritis.

PROBABLE OUTCOME—Curable in 10 days with treatment.

PREVENTING RECURRENCE
- Bathe daily with soap and water.
- Keep your fingernails short. Don't scratch the blisters.
- If there is an outbreak in the family, urge all members to use antibacterial soap.
- Use separate towels for each family member or substitute paper towels temporarily.
- Don't share razors with other people.

CALL YOUR DOCTOR IF

- You have symptoms of bacterial skin infection.
- You develop a fever.
- The sores continue to spread or don't begin to heal in 3 days despite treatment.

SKIN CANCER, BASAL-CELL

BASIC INFORMATION FOR OLDER ADULTS

DESCRIPTION—This is a type of skin cancer that affects the skin's basal layer (the 5th layer). Basal-cell skin cancer invades areas under the skin, but it does not spread to distant areas. Body parts involved: The skin of the face, ears, backs of the hands, shoulders and arms.

SPECIAL CONSIDERATIONS FOR AGING
- The immune system becomes less effective, opening the way for viral, bacterial and other infections; malignancies; immune disorders; and allergies.
- Malignant diseases are less likely to spread rapidly.
- Usual signs and symptoms may be absent and be replaced by symptoms of confusion, dizziness, failure to thrive, falling, incontinence, increasing dementia, refusal to eat or drink, weight loss, depression, paranoia, hypochondriasis, psychosis or threats of suicide.
- Stress from any emotional cause—fear, worry, anxiety, sadness, loneliness or anger—affects all aspects of any illness or disorder.

SIGNS & SYMPTOMS—A small skin lesion that does not heal in 3 weeks with the following characteristics:
- The lesion appears flat and "pearly." Its edges are translucent and rounded or rolled. The edges may have small, curvy, new blood vessels. The ulcer in the center is dimpled.
- The lesion's size varies from 4mm to 6mm, but it may grow larger if untreated.
- The lesion occurs on skin that is exposed to the sun and shows evidence of sun damage.
- The lesion grows slowly. It does not hurt or itch.

CAUSES & RISK FACTORS—Caused by skin damage from the sun that has occurred many years prior to the cancer's appearance. Risk factors include:
- Excessive exposure to sunlight.
- Fair skin complexion.

DOCTOR'S TREATMENT & DIAGNOSTIC TESTS
- Medical history and physical exam.
- Pathological exam of tissue after removal to confirm diagnosis.
- Removal of the cancer by one of the following methods. The treatment method is chosen in a doctor-patient conference: Surgery in the doctor's office or an outpatient surgical unit of the hospital. Advancing age alone is not a deterrent. Electrosurgery (see Glossary). Cryosurgery (see Glossary). Radiation treatment.
- Self-care instructions focused on the older patient.

HOME TREATMENT BY SELF OR CARE-GIVER

GENERAL INSTRUCTIONS—After surgery:
- Apply rubbing alcohol to the scab twice a day.
- Apply an adhesive bandage to the scab during the day. Leave it uncovered at night.
- Wash the wound as usual. Dry it gently and completely after bathing or swimming.

MEDICATION (ADJUSTED FOR AGING)
- For minor pain, you may use non-prescription drugs such as acetaminophen or aspirin.
- If the scab cracks or oozes, apply a non-prescription antibiotic ointment several times a day.
- Your doctor may prescribe an antibiotic ointment to prevent infection of the wound.
- *Note:* Adverse reactions and side effects may be more frequent and severe in older persons. Remind your doctor of any medicines you already take.

ACTIVITY FOR OLDER PATIENTS
- No restrictions are necessary.
- See Appendix 20 regarding physical fitness for the active older adult.

FOOD & BEVERAGE
- No special diet is required.
- See Appendix 1 regarding good nutrition for people over 50.

FUTURE CONSIDERATIONS FOR THE AGING ADULT

POSSIBLE COMPLICATIONS—Without treatment, these cancers may enlarge, ulcerate and disfigure. Fewer than 1% spread to other sites, but they should be removed to prevent local damage.

PROBABLE OUTCOME—Curable in 2 weeks if the cancer is removed. This disorder does not become life-threatening unless it is ignored completely.

PREVENTING RECURRENCE—Limit your exposure to the sun. Protect your skin from exposure to the sun with a hat, clothing and sunscreen with a protective factor of 15 or more.

CALL YOUR DOCTOR IF

- You have symptoms of basal-cell skin cancer.
- The wound bleeds after surgery and the bleeding cannot be stopped by applying pressure for 10 minutes.
- The wound shows signs of infection, such as pain, redness, swelling or increased tenderness.

SKIN CANCER, SQUAMOUS-CELL

BASIC INFORMATION FOR OLDER ADULTS

DESCRIPTION—Squamous-cell skin cancer is a malignant growth of the epithelial layer (external surface) of the skin. Body parts involved: The skin in areas that are exposed to the sun, such as the face, ears, hands or arms.

SPECIAL CONSIDERATIONS FOR AGING
- The immune system becomes less effective, opening the way for viral, bacterial and other infections; malignancies; immune disorders; and allergies.
- Malignant diseases are less likely to spread rapidly.
- Usual signs and symptoms may be absent and be replaced by symptoms of confusion, dizziness, failure to thrive, falling, incontinence, increasing dementia, refusal to eat or drink, weight loss, depression, paranoia, hypochondriasis, psychosis or threats of suicide.
- Stress from any emotional cause—fear, worry, anxiety, sadness, loneliness or anger—affects all aspects of any illness or disorder.

SIGNS & SYMPTOMS—A small, disfiguring, scaling, raised bump on the skin with a crusting ulcer in the center. The bump doesn't hurt or itch.

CAUSES & RISK FACTORS
Causes include:
- Excessive exposure to sunlight.
- Overexposure to x-rays.
Risk factors include:
- Light complexion.
- Recent illness with chronic skin ulcers from any cause.
- An outdoor occupation.
- An occupation or treatment requiring exposure to x-rays.
- The use of immunosuppressant drugs.

DOCTOR'S TREATMENT & DIAGNOSTIC TESTS
- Medical history and physical exam.
- Biopsy (see Glossary).
- Treatment with any of the following methods:
  Surgical removal.
  Scraping and electrocautery (see Glossary).
  Radiation therapy. This may be used on some growths or in cases in which surgery is not suitable.
- Self-care instructions focused on the older patient.

HOME TREATMENT BY SELF OR CARE-GIVER

GENERAL INSTRUCTIONS—After removal of the tumor, keep the area clean, dry and protected from clothing until it heals. Your doctor will provide additional instructions, depending on the treatment used.

MEDICATION (ADJUSTED FOR AGING)
- For minor discomfort, you may use non-prescription drugs such as acetaminophen.
- Your doctor may prescribe topical antibiotic ointment or cream to prevent infection after surgery.
- *Note:* Adverse reactions and side effects may be more frequent and severe in older persons. Remind your doctor of any medicines you already take.

ACTIVITY FOR OLDER PATIENTS
- After treatment, resume normal activity as soon as possible.
- See Appendix 20 regarding physical fitness for the active older adult.

FOOD & BEVERAGE
- No special diet is required.
- See Appendix 1 regarding good nutrition for people over 50.

FUTURE CONSIDERATIONS FOR THE AGING ADULT

POSSIBLE COMPLICATIONS
- The cancer must be treated again in 10% of cases.
- The cancer will spread to other tissue if untreated.

PROBABLE OUTCOME—This type of skin cancer responds well to treatment. It is usually curable in 2 weeks with treatment.

PREVENTING RECURRENCE—Wear sunscreen with a protective factor of 15 or more or a hat and protective clothing to protect your skin from sun damage.

CALL YOUR DOCTOR IF

- You have symptoms of squamous-cell skin cancer.
- Any of the following occurs after treatment:
  Redness, swelling, bleeding or tenderness at the treatment site.
  Pain that is not controlled by non-prescription pain relievers.
- The sore has not healed 3 weeks after treatment.

BASIC INFORMATION FOR OLDER ADULTS

DESCRIPTION—Benign skin lesions are noncancerous growths or areas of pigment or color change on the skin. Body part involved: The skin.

SPECIAL CONSIDERATIONS FOR AGING
- The immune system becomes less effective, opening the way for viral, bacterial and other infections; malignancies; immune disorders; and allergies.
- The skin becomes dryer and rougher.
- The responsiveness of the skin's immune system decreases.

SIGNS & SYMPTOMS—Benign skin lesions fall into the following categories:
- Tags—Soft, flesh-colored buds, often on stalks, found on the neck, armpits or groin.
- Moles—Flat or raised lesions with clearly defined borders. Moles may be black, blue, red, yellow or brown.
- Cherry spots—Pinhead-sized, bright red lesions on the chest or back.
- Strawberry marks—Bright red raised areas in infants that grow until they are removed.
- Keloids—Thick, pale, irregular growths that begin at the site of a scar and gradually increase in size.
- Dermatofibromas—Rounded nodules, usually brownish and usually on the legs.
- Freckles—Flat, brownish spots of pinhead size or larger.

CAUSES & RISK FACTORS—The cause is unknown, but most people have a few benign skin lesions. The risk increases with a family history of benign skin lesions.

DOCTOR'S TREATMENT & DIAGNOSTIC TESTS
- Medical history and physical exam.
- Skin biopsy (see Glossary).
- Self-care instructions focused on the older patient.
- Surgery to remove lesions that enlarge, bleed, change color, are slow to heal or are unsightly.
- Radiation treatment following removal of keloids to prevent their recurrence.

HOME TREATMENT BY SELF OR CARE-GIVER

GENERAL INSTRUCTIONS
- Examine skin lesions—especially those that are constantly rubbed or irritated by clothing—regularly for signs of growth, color change, pain, infection or bleeding.
- If a lesion is removed, cover the area with a clean dressing and protect it against injury. Ointments are rarely needed.

MEDICATION (ADJUSTED FOR AGING)—
Medicine is usually not necessary for this disorder. Makeup may be helpful in covering unsightly blemishes.

ACTIVITY FOR OLDER PATIENTS
- No restrictions are necessary.
- See Appendix 20 regarding physical fitness for the active older adult.

FOOD & BEVERAGE
- No special diet is required.
- See Appendix 1 regarding good nutrition for people over 50.

FUTURE CONSIDERATIONS FOR THE AGING ADULT

POSSIBLE COMPLICATIONS
- Malignant change in moles.
- Bleeding in strawberry marks.

PROBABLE OUTCOME—Treatment is usually unnecessary because most skin lesions are harmless. Suspicious or unsightly lesions can be removed surgically. If the affected area is large or in a prominent place, plastic surgery may be necessary after removal.

PREVENTING RECURRENCE—To decrease the number of freckles, avoid excessive exposure to the sun. Other forms cannot be prevented.

CALL YOUR DOCTOR IF

You have a skin lesion that enlarges, bleeds, changes color, is painful or doesn't heal.

SLEEP APNEA IN ADULTS

BASIC INFORMATION FOR OLDER ADULTS

DESCRIPTION—Sleep apnea in adults is a temporary cessation of breathing (lasting 10 seconds or longer) while in deep sleep. Typically it affects men who are middle-aged and older. Women are much less likely to have sleep apnea. Body parts involved: The central nervous system.

SPECIAL CONSIDERATIONS FOR AGING
- Obstruction of the airways becomes more common, especially among people who have smoked tobacco for many years.
- The chest muscles used for breathing become weaker.

SIGNS & SYMPTOMS
- Long periods (usually 20 to 30 seconds, but possibly up to 1 or 2 minutes) of not breathing while asleep. Sleep apnea must be observed by others; it is most reliably recorded in a sleep laboratory.
- Choking while asleep due to obstruction in the back of the throat by the uvula and other loose tissues. This causes cycles of sleep, choking, startled awakening, drowsiness and sleep. The cycles often continue throughout the day because poor sleep causes chronic sleepiness.

CAUSES & RISK FACTORS—The cause is often unknown. Known causes include:
- Airway obstruction, especially in obese patients.
- Chronic disease of the respiratory system.
- A disorder of the central nervous system, such as a brain tumor, viral brain infection or stroke.

Risk factors include:
- Stress, including anxiety and depression.
- A recent stroke; senility.
- Obesity; smoking; allergies.
- Excessive alcohol consumption.
- The use of mind-altering drugs.
- Nasal polyps or a previous nose fracture.
- Sleeping on the back.

DOCTOR'S TREATMENT & DIAGNOSTIC TESTS
- Observation of the symptoms by someone close to you.
- Medical history and physical exam.
- Laboratory studies to measure the amount of oxygen in the blood, chest wall movement and air flow through the nose.
- EEG (see Glossary).
- Studies in a sleep laboratory.
- Self-care instructions focused on the older patient.
- Surgery (a tracheostomy) to advance the chin, remove the uvula and implant a pacemaker to stimulate the diaphragm.
- Other options, which may be suggested after a complete workup in a sleep laboratory, include continuous positive airway pressure (CPAP; see General Instructions), low-flow oxygen, tongue-retaining devices or weight loss. A tracheostomy is the only measure that guarantees total success.

HOME TREATMENT BY SELF OR CARE-GIVER

GENERAL INSTRUCTIONS
- Try to always sleep on your side.
- If sleep apnea occurs only when you sleep on your back, sew a ping-pong ball or tennis ball to the back of your pajamas. This forces you to sleep on your side.
- For a description of surgery and postoperative care, see Tracheostomy in the Surgeries section.
- A new treatment—continuous positive airway pressure or CPAP—involves wearing a mask over the nose and mouth during sleep. A compressor forces air into the airway to keep it open. Ask your doctor about it.

MEDICATION (ADJUSTED FOR AGING)—Various medicines have been used for this disorder, but all have had mixed results. Consult your doctor about withdrawing medications that may be causing sleep apnea.

ACTIVITY FOR OLDER PATIENTS—No restrictions are necessary. Engage in regular physical exercise to become physically fit, but don't exercise vigorously before bedtime.

FOOD & BEVERAGE—Lose weight if you are obese. A reducing diet appears in Appendix 10.

FUTURE CONSIDERATIONS FOR THE AGING ADULT

POSSIBLE COMPLICATIONS
- Impaired productivity and depression caused by sleep deprivation.
- Permanent brain damage caused by recurrent episodes of inadequate oxygen to the brain.
- Heartbeat irregularities and congestive heart failure.

PROBABLE OUTCOME—If sleep laboratory studies reveal significant sleep disturbance, surgery (a tracheostomy) is sometimes necessary to cure the sleep apnea—no matter what the underlying cause.

REDUCING RISK OF RECURRENCE
- If you have an underlying disease listed as a cause of sleep apnea, avoid as many risk factors as possible to decrease the chance of triggering the disorder.
- Lose weight.

CALL YOUR DOCTOR IF

- You suspect you have sleep apnea.
- You observe signs of sleep apnea in another family member.

BASIC INFORMATION FOR OLDER ADULTS

DESCRIPTION—This page describes the effects of a bite from a poisonous snake. Bites on the extremities are most common, but bites on the head and trunk are most dangerous. Not all bites involve the actual injection of venom. Body parts involved: The affected skin; the blood and lymphatic system. **(THIS IS AN EMERGENCY; SEEK MEDICAL CARE IMMEDIATELY!)**

SPECIAL CONSIDERATIONS FOR AGING—Older people are less able to see snakes or flee from them.

SIGNS & SYMPTOMS
Early symptoms:
- Severe pain and swelling around the bite.

Late symptoms:
- Fever and nausea.
- Skin discoloration that resembles bruising around the bite.
- Bleeding spots under the skin all over the body.
- Numbness and tingling around the mouth and in the hands and feet.
- Excessive sweating and thirst.
- Low blood pressure and shock.
- Breathing difficulty.
- Blurred vision and dizziness.
- Headache; seizures; coma.

Signs:
- Multiple fang marks and small cuts if the bite is from a coral snake. Symptoms may not appear for 3 to 4 hours.
- Deep single or double fang marks if the bite is from another snake. Symptoms begin quickly.

CAUSES & RISK FACTORS—Caused by a bite from a poisonous snake, such as a rattlesnake, copperhead, water moccasin or coral snake. The risk increases with outdoor activities during warm months in areas where poisonous snakes are abundant.

DOCTOR'S TREATMENT & DIAGNOSTIC TESTS
- Identification of the snake. Kill and preserve it if possible.
- Immediate self-care.
- Doctor's treatment as soon as possible.
- Surgery (sometimes) to remove injured or gangrenous tissue 2 to 3 days after the bite.
- In severe cases, dialysis to treat renal failure and breathing support may be necessary.

HOME TREATMENT BY SELF OR CARE-GIVER

GENERAL INSTRUCTIONS
- Don't panic! The venom will spread more quickly through the body if you run or become excited.
- Remain still if possible with the bitten part in a horizontal position.
- Don't drink alcohol or take stimulants.
- Don't pack the affected part in ice.
- Before giving first aid, try to identify the snake.
- Apply a pad or sterile dressing to the wound.
- Incision and suction by an unskilled person may cause more harm. Don't perform this procedure unless you have had training.
- Go to the nearest emergency facility.

MEDICATION (ADJUSTED FOR AGING)
- Your doctor may prescribe:
  Antivenin to neutralize the snake poison.
  A tetanus booster injection.
  Antibiotics to prevent infection.
  Pain relievers. (Narcotics cannot be used for bites by coral snakes. They may cause shock.)
- *Note:* Adverse reactions and side effects may be more frequent and severe in older persons. Remind your doctor of any medicines you already take.

ACTIVITY FOR OLDER PATIENTS
- Resume your normal activities as soon as your symptoms improve.
- See Appendix 20 regarding physical fitness for the active older adult.

FOOD & BEVERAGE
- No special diet is required.
- See Appendix 1 regarding good nutrition for people over 50.

FUTURE CONSIDERATIONS FOR THE AGING ADULT

POSSIBLE COMPLICATIONS—Gangrene, requiring amputation of the affected part (rare); DIC (disseminated intravascular coagulation); a severe immunological response if you have had a previous venomous snakebite.

PROBABLE OUTCOME—Usually curable with rapid medical care. Severe bites involving a large amount of poisonous venom may be fatal—even with treatment. After one snakebite, succeeding snakebites may produce more severe reaction.

PREVENTING RECURRENCE—Wear protective shoes, boots and clothing for hiking, camping, fishing and hunting. Prevent complications by carrying a snakebite kit and instructions.

CALL YOUR DOCTOR IF

- You or someone you are with receives a snakebite. *This is an emergency!*
- New, unexplained symptoms develop. The drugs used in treatment may produce side effects.

SODIUM, TOO LITTLE IN BLOOD
(Hyponatremia)

BASIC INFORMATION FOR OLDER ADULTS

DESCRIPTION—Hyponatremia is a below-normal level of sodium in the blood. Sodium is necessary to regulate the body's water balance and maintain a normal heart rhythm, and it is responsible for nerve impulse conduction and muscle contraction. Body parts involved: All body cells.

SPECIAL CONSIDERATIONS FOR AGING
- Electrolyte imbalances are more likely.
- Older people are more likely to have multiple disorders.
- TBW (total body water) decreases.

SIGNS & SYMPTOMS
- Confusion.
- Restlessness and anxiety.
- Weakness.
- Muscle cramps (usually in the legs).
- Changes in pulse rate and blood pressure.
- Tissue swelling (edema).
- Stupor or coma (if the imbalance is severe).

Sodium imbalance may be part of a disease with other symptoms that predominate, such as fever, vomiting, diarrhea or excessive sweating.

CAUSES & RISK FACTORS
- Prolonged loss of body fluids from vomiting or diarrhea.
- Addison's disease.
- Congestive heart failure.
- The use of diuretics.
- Prolonged, excessive drinking of water. (This is usually a psychiatric condition.)
- Some cancers of the adrenal glands.
- Infections with high fever.
- Formula diets.

DOCTOR'S TREATMENT & DIAGNOSTIC TESTS
- Medical history and physical exam.
- Laboratory blood and urine studies of sodium and other electrolytes.
- Oral water-loading test to measure urine volume.
- Self-care instructions focused on the older patient.
- Hospitalization (sometimes).

HOME TREATMENT BY SELF OR CARE-GIVER

GENERAL INSTRUCTIONS—If you have a disorder or take drugs that affect sodium balance, learn as much as possible about your drugs, your condition and how to prevent a sodium imbalance.

MEDICATION (ADJUSTED FOR AGING)
- Your doctor may prescribe:
  Intravenous sodium.
  Medications to correct underlying disorders.
  Increased salt intake.
- *Note:* Adverse reactions and side effects may be more frequent and severe in older persons. Remind your doctor of any medicines you already take.

ACTIVITY FOR OLDER PATIENTS
- Resume your normal activities after recovery.
- See Appendix 20 regarding physical fitness for the active older adult.

FOOD & BEVERAGE—No special diet is required. Your fluid intake may be restricted to maintain the sodium concentration in the total body water.

FUTURE CONSIDERATIONS FOR THE AGING ADULT

POSSIBLE COMPLICATIONS—Shock and death.

PROBABLE OUTCOME—Usually can be corrected with intravenous fluids and treatment of the underlying disorder.

PREVENTING RECURRENCE—Because sodium imbalance may be a result of underlying disease, obtain early medical treatment to prevent a sodium imbalance.

CALL YOUR DOCTOR IF

- You have symptoms of a sodium imbalance.
- You are having problems with a disorder that affects sodium levels.

SODIUM, TOO MUCH IN BLOOD
(Hypernatremia)

BASIC INFORMATION FOR OLDER ADULTS

DESCRIPTION—Hypernatremia is an above-normal level of sodium in the blood. Sodium is necessary to regulate the body's water balance and maintain a normal heart rhythm, and it is responsible for nerve impulse conduction and muscle contraction. Body parts involved: All body cells.

SPECIAL CONSIDERATIONS FOR AGING
- Electrolyte imbalances are more likely.
- Older people are more likely to have multiple disorders.
- TBW (total body water) decreases.

SIGNS & SYMPTOMS
- Confusion.
- Restlessness and anxiety.
- Weakness.
- Muscle cramps (usually in the legs).
- Changes in pulse rate and blood pressure.
- Tissue swelling (edema).
- Stupor or coma (if the imbalance is severe).
Sodium imbalance may be part of a disease with other symptoms that predominate, such as fever, vomiting, diarrhea or excessive sweating.

CAUSES & RISK FACTORS
Causes include:
- An inability to drink water, as with a stroke or gastrointestinal diseases.
- The use of cortisone drugs.
- Excessive intake of salty food or liquid, as with near drowning in salt water.
Risk factors include:
- Diabetes mellitus.
- Congestive heart failure.
- The use of diuretics.
- Kidney diseases. Healthy kidneys can usually control sodium levels.
- Increased water loss due to diarrhea or sweating.

DOCTOR'S TREATMENT & DIAGNOSTIC TESTS
- Medical history and physical exam.
- Laboratory blood and urine studies of sodium and other electrolytes.
- Self-care instructions focused on the older patient.
- Hospitalization (sometimes).

HOME TREATMENT BY SELF OR CARE-GIVER

GENERAL INSTRUCTIONS—If you have a disorder or take drugs that affect sodium balance, learn as much as possible about your drugs, your condition and how to prevent a sodium imbalance.

MEDICATION (ADJUSTED FOR AGING)
- Your doctor may prescribe:
  Diuretics to decrease high sodium levels.
  Medications to correct underlying disorders.
  Decreased oral sodium intake.
- *Note:* Adverse reactions and side effects may be more frequent and severe in older persons. Remind your doctor of any medicines you already take.

ACTIVITY FOR OLDER PATIENTS
- Resume your normal activities after recovery.
- See Appendix 20 regarding physical fitness for the active older adult.

FOOD & BEVERAGE—Most persons with high sodium levels benefit from a low-salt diet (see Appendix 9). Low-salt diets contain enough sodium to prevent hyponatremia (too little sodium). However, sodium levels are not influenced by diet alone.

FUTURE CONSIDERATIONS FOR THE AGING ADULT

POSSIBLE COMPLICATIONS
- Shock and death.
- Increased risk of heart disease, stroke and kidney damage.
- Fluid retention that could cause swelling of the legs and dizziness.

PROBABLE OUTCOME—Usually can be corrected with intravenous fluids and treatment of the underlying disorder.

PREVENTING RECURRENCE—Because sodium disturbance may be a result of underlying disease, obtain early medical treatment to prevent a sodium imbalance.

CALL YOUR DOCTOR IF

- You have symptoms of a sodium imbalance.
- You are having problems with a disorder that affects sodium levels.

SORES, PRESSURE
(Bed Sores; Decubitus Ulcers)

BASIC INFORMATION FOR OLDER ADULTS

DESCRIPTION—Pressure sores are skin ulcerations, usually in an area of pressure over a bony prominence. Pressure sores are not contagious or cancerous. Approximately 70% to 90% of all pressure sores occur in people over 65. Body parts involved: The skin over pressure points in the lower back, buttocks, elbows, knees, shoulders, heels, ankles and other areas with bony prominences.

SPECIAL CONSIDERATIONS FOR AGING
- The fatty layer of tissue under the skin becomes thinner.
- The skin becomes thinner.

SIGNS & SYMPTOMS—Spots of skin that are red and shiny. The spots progress to blisters, then ulcers, leading to a breakdown of the tissue under the ulcer. The ulcers are usually painless.

CAUSES & RISK FACTORS—Caused by constant pressure on the skin, especially over bony areas. Pressure reduces the blood supply, causing death of the tissue layers. Pressure sores usually develop in persons who cannot move because of chronic illness or disability that confines them to bed. Risk factors include:
- Poor circulation.
- Decreased or absent sensation.
- Malnutrition; incontinence.
- Obesity; low body weight.
- An illness or accident requiring prolonged bed confinement, especially with unsanitary living conditions and wrinkled or wet bed linen.
- Sitting or lying for long periods of time.

DOCTOR'S TREATMENT & DIAGNOSTIC TESTS
- Medical history and physical exam.
- Self-care instructions focused on the older patient.
- Surgery to remove dead tissue (sometimes).

HOME TREATMENT BY SELF OR CARE-GIVER

GENERAL INSTRUCTIONS
- Provide good nursing care for the patient (see Preventing Recurrence).
- Provide warm whirlpool treatments if a pressure sore is on an arm, hand, foot or leg.
- Apply lotions or ointment if prescribed by your doctor. Apply a thin layer of the cream, ointment or lotion 3 or 4 times daily. A heavy layer wastes medicine and is no more beneficial than a thin layer. Rub it in gently for several minutes until it disappears.

MEDICATION (ADJUSTED FOR AGING)
- Your doctor may prescribe: Antibiotics to fight infection.

Ointments, dressings and drying agents, such as zinc oxide, povidone-iodine packs or 3% hydrogen peroxide.
- Avoid harsh soaps, tincture of benzoin or hexachlorophene.

ACTIVITY FOR OLDER PATIENTS—Return to whatever level of activity is attainable once the symptoms improve.

FOOD & BEVERAGE
- Eat a normal, well-balanced diet that includes extra protein. Vitamin and mineral supplements may be necessary.
- Proper nutrition is vital, and special supplements may be necessary. Ask your doctor for nutritional information and instructions.

FUTURE CONSIDERATIONS FOR THE AGING ADULT

POSSIBLE COMPLICATIONS—Local or general infection; infection of the bones (osteomyelitis) adjacent to the ulcer.

PROBABLE OUTCOME—Usually curable with treatment. The sores may heal very slowly. The healing time varies with the site and size of the ulcer and the patient's general health.

PREVENTING RECURRENCE—Provide good nursing care for the disabled, including:
- Frequent changes of position in bed. Teach the patient to change position or make small body shifts.
- Protective, soft padding, such as gel flotation pads or sheepskin, over bony areas.
- A water mattress, egg-crate rubber mattress or alternating-pressure mattress.
- Clean, dry, smooth bed linen.
- Frequent inspection of the skin areas at risk. Keep the skin clean and dry.
- Limiting the time the patient sits up in a chair.
- Range-of-motion exercises to maintain the patient's mobility and muscle mass to prevent contractures (muscle shortening) and improve circulation.
- Heel and elbow protectors made of sheepskin or synthetic material.

CALL YOUR DOCTOR IF

- You have symptoms of pressure sores or observe them in someone else.
- Any of the following occurs during treatment: Skin inflammation or breakdown. Fever; signs of infection, such as pain, redness, tenderness, swelling or increased warmth of the affected area.

SPASTIC COLON
(Irritable Bowel Syndrome; Colitis; Mucous Colitis)

BASIC INFORMATION FOR OLDER ADULTS

DESCRIPTION—Spastic colon is an irritative and inflammatory disorder of the intestine. It is not contagious, inherited or cancerous. Body parts involved: The small and large intestines.

SPECIAL CONSIDERATIONS FOR AGING
- Stress from any emotional cause—fear, worry, anxiety, sadness, loneliness or anger—affects all aspects of any illness or disorder.
- Decreased nutrition, common among chronically ill older people, increases the risk of any disease or disorder.

SIGNS & SYMPTOMS—The following symptoms usually begin in early adult life. Episodes may last for days, weeks or months.
- Cramp-like pain in the middle or to one side of the lower abdomen. The pain is usually relieved with bowel movements.
- Nausea.
- Bloating and gas.
- Headache.
- Rectal pain.
- Backache.
- Occasional appetite loss that may lead to weight loss.
- Diarrhea or constipation, usually alternating.
- Fatigue.
- Depression.
- Anxiety.
- Difficulty concentrating.

CAUSES & RISK FACTORS—Caused by stress and emotional conflict resulting in anxiety or depression. Situations that often precede an attack include obsessive worry about everyday problems, marital tension, fear of loss of a beloved person or object or the death of a loved one. Symptoms may also be triggered by eating, though no specific food has been identified as responsible. The risk increases with:
- Stress; improper diet; smoking.
- Excessive alcohol consumption.
- The use of drugs.
- Fatigue or overwork.
- Poor physical fitness.

DOCTOR'S TREATMENT & DIAGNOSTIC TESTS
- Medical history and physical exam.
- Laboratory studies, including stool studies, to rule out other disorders such as lactose intolerance, ulcers, parasites, enzyme deficiency and ulcerative colitis.
- X-rays of the colon (barium enema).
- Colonoscopy.

HOME TREATMENT BY SELF OR CARE-GIVER

GENERAL INSTRUCTIONS—Medication, exercise, diet changes and adequate rest can help, but the cure is more dependent on defining, confronting and solving conflicts in day-to-day living. See Appendix 13.

MEDICATION (ADJUSTED FOR AGING)
- Medication may help, but it will not cure this disorder. Your doctor may prescribe: Antispasmodics to relieve severe abdominal cramps.
  Short-term tranquilizers to reduce anxiety.
- *Note:* Adverse reactions and side effects may be more frequent and severe in older persons. Remind your doctor of any medicines you already take.

ACTIVITY FOR OLDER PATIENTS—No restrictions are necessary. Good physical fitness improves bowel function.

FOOD & BEVERAGE
- Increase the amount of fiber in your diet to promote good bowel function. See Appendix 1.
- Don't eat foods that aggravate the symptoms.
- Avoid gas-producing foods.

FUTURE CONSIDERATIONS FOR THE AGING ADULT

POSSIBLE COMPLICATIONS—Psychological fixation on bowel function, leading to psychological disability.

PROBABLE OUTCOME—Curable if the underlying causes can be eliminated or modified. If not, the symptoms can be controlled with treatment.

PREVENTING RECURRENCE—Reduce stress or try to modify your response to it. See Appendix 13.

CALL YOUR DOCTOR IF

- A fever develops.
- Your stools are black or tarry looking.
- You begin vomiting.
- You experience an unexplained weight loss of 5 pounds or more.
- Your symptoms don't improve despite treatment.

SPINAL CORD TUMOR

BASIC INFORMATION FOR OLDER ADULTS

DESCRIPTION—A spinal cord tumor is an abnormal growth that compresses the spinal cord or its nerve roots. The growth may be benign or malignant, but a non-malignant tumor may be as disabling as a malignant tumor unless it is treated appropriately. Body parts involved: The spinal cord and the nerves below the level of the spinal cord tumor.

SPECIAL CONSIDERATIONS FOR AGING
- Malignant diseases are less likely to spread rapidly.
- Neurological diseases become more likely.
- 50% of people over 60 have x-ray evidence of narrowing of the coronary arteries, yet only 50% of those people have symptoms.
- Stress from any emotional cause—fear, worry, anxiety, sadness, loneliness or anger—affects all aspects of any illness or disorder.

SIGNS & SYMPTOMS
- Progressive weakness, numbness and wasting of the muscles whose nerve supply comes from the affected area of the spinal cord.
- Difficult urination or bowel movements; incontinence.
- Chronic back pain.

CAUSES & RISK FACTORS—Tumors originating in the spinal cord (primary tumors) are rare, and their cause is unknown. A spinal cord tumor usually results from cancer that has spread from another part of the body, such as the lung, breast, intestinal tract, prostate, kidney, thyroid or lymphatic system. The risk increases with cancer in any of the body parts listed above.

DOCTOR'S TREATMENT & DIAGNOSTIC TESTS
- Medical history and physical exam.
- Laboratory studies of the blood and spinal fluid.
- X-rays of the spine.
- MRI or CT scan (see Glossary for both).
- Self-care instructions focused on the older patient.
- Surgery to remove tumors and surrounding bone that compress the spinal cord. Advancing age alone is not a deterrent.
- Radiation therapy following surgery.
- Physical therapy.

HOME TREATMENT BY SELF OR CARE-GIVER

GENERAL INSTRUCTIONS
- No specific instructions except those listed under other headings.
- A spinal cord tumor is a complicated, serious disorder. This page can cover only the main points of diagnosis and treatment. Your doctor, nurse or librarian can provide sources of supplemental information.

MEDICATION (ADJUSTED FOR AGING)
- Your doctor may prescribe:
  Pain relievers.
  Cortisone drugs to decrease the swelling around the tumor and reduce the pressure on the spinal cord.
  Anticancer (chemotherapy) drugs if the tumor is malignant.
- *Note:* Adverse reactions and side effects may be more frequent and severe in older persons. Remind your doctor of any medicines you already take.

ACTIVITY FOR OLDER PATIENTS
- Stay as active as your strength allows. Work and exercise moderately. Rest when you tire.
- See Appendix 20 regarding physical fitness for the active older adult.

FOOD & BEVERAGE
- Eat a normal, well-balanced diet. Vitamin and mineral supplements should not be necessary unless you show evidence of deficiency or cannot eat normally.
- See Appendix 1 regarding good nutrition for people over 50.

FUTURE CONSIDERATIONS FOR THE AGING ADULT

POSSIBLE COMPLICATIONS—Total paralysis caused by a blockage of the blood vessels that nourish the cells of the spinal cord.

PROBABLE OUTCOME—The success of treatment depends on the type, size and location of the growth.
- Surgery to remove bone surrounding the cord can relieve pressure on the spinal nerves and the nerve pathways. This operation generally relieves the pain and other symptoms immediately, but it may impair motor function. Physical therapy and rehabilitation may restore lost function.
- If the tumor originated on the exterior of the spinal cord and has not spread, surgery restores a normal life expectancy.

PREVENTING RECURRENCE
- Because spinal cord tumors frequently result from the spread of cancer, be alert to early symptoms of cancer in other organs.
- Don't smoke.
- Eat a high-fiber diet to reduce the likelihood of intestinal cancer.
- Be alert to enlargement of the thyroid gland.
- For men, request a prostate exam with your annual physical.
- For women, practice breast self-examination (see Appendix 14).

CALL YOUR DOCTOR IF

You have any symptoms of a spinal cord tumor.

SPOROTRICHOSIS

BASIC INFORMATION FOR OLDER ADULTS

DESCRIPTION—Sporotrichosis is an infectious fungal disease that causes ulcers and abscesses of the skin, lymph nodes and lymph channels. Farm laborers, florists and gardeners are most often infected. Sporotrichosis is not contagious from person to person. Body parts involved: The skin; lymph system; lungs; joints; bones (rare).

SPECIAL CONSIDERATIONS FOR AGING
- The immune system becomes less effective, opening the way for viral, bacterial and other infections; malignancies; immune disorders; and allergies.
- Decreased nutrition, common among chronically ill older people, increases the risk of any disease or disorder.

SIGNS & SYMPTOMS
Early stages:
- A small, movable, non-tender nodule appears under the skin of the fingers. The nodule enlarges slowly, becomes pink and ulcerates.

In a few days or weeks:
- Dark nodules appear along the lymphatic channel that drains the area.
- A cough with sputum begins if the organism reaches the lungs (rare).
- Usually sporotrichosis produces no other symptoms, unlike other fungal diseases, which cause fever, chills, a general ill feeling and appetite loss.

CAUSES & RISK FACTORS—Caused by infection from a fungus, *sporothrix schenckii,* that lives in soil, sphagnum moss, weeds and decaying organic vegetation. Infection is most often contracted through a skin wound. Risk factors include:
- A medical history of sarcoidosis or tuberculosis.
- Occupations that involve work with plants and soil, such as farming, nursery work and horticulture.

DOCTOR'S TREATMENT & DIAGNOSTIC TESTS
- Medical history and physical exam.
- Laboratory culture of pus from the lesions.
- Self-care instructions focused on the older patient.
- Hospitalization if complications occur.

HOME TREATMENT BY SELF OR CARE-GIVER

GENERAL INSTRUCTIONS
- Because sporotrichosis is not contagious, the patient does not need to be isolated.
- Cover the lesions with loose-fitting bandages to prevent secondary infection with bacteria.
- Weigh daily and keep a record.

MEDICATION (ADJUSTED FOR AGING)
- Your doctor may prescribe:
  A saturated solution of potassium iodide. Dilute this in water, fruit juice or other beverages and take it 3 times a day after meals. Drink this with a straw to prevent the discoloration of the teeth.
  Antifungal medicine, such as amphotericin B. This medication is potent and may cause severe adverse reactions. It is reserved for serious cases. Hospitalization is necessary so the drug can be administered intravenously.
- *Note:* Adverse reactions and side effects may be more frequent and severe in older persons. Remind your doctor of any medicines you already take.

ACTIVITY FOR OLDER PATIENTS
- No restrictions are necessary unless you develop signs of widespread infection.
- See Appendix 20 regarding physical fitness for the active older adult.

FOOD & BEVERAGE
- No special diet is required.
- See Appendix 1 regarding good nutrition for people over 50.

FUTURE CONSIDERATIONS FOR THE AGING ADULT

POSSIBLE COMPLICATIONS—Spread of the fungi throughout the body, causing widespread, life-threatening infection (rare).

PROBABLE OUTCOME—With treatment, usually curable within 1 to 2 months after the lesions heal, but recovery may require 6 or 7 months. The fatality rate is high if the infection spreads throughout the body.

PREVENTING RECURRENCE
- Wear gloves when working with soil.
- Don't go barefoot.

CALL YOUR DOCTOR IF

- You have symptoms of sporotrichosis.
- Any of the following occurs during treatment: An unexplained weight loss.
  A fever of 101F (38.3C) measured orally.
- New, unexplained symptoms develop. The antifungal drugs used in treatment may produce side effects, including skin rash, tongue and mouth irritation and cough.

SPRAINS & STRAINS

BASIC INFORMATION FOR OLDER ADULTS

DESCRIPTION—Sprains and strains are injuries to the ligaments that hold the joints together and in position. A sprain is a stretched ligament. A strain is a stretched and torn muscle. Sprains occur most often in the ankles, knees or fingers, although any joint can be sprained. Sprained joints can function—but only with pain. Body parts involved: Any ligament (tendon) attached to any joint.

SPECIAL CONSIDERATIONS FOR AGING
- Muscle tone decreases.
- Years of weight bearing cause wear and tear on the bones, joints and ligaments.

SIGNS & SYMPTOMS
- Pain or tenderness in the area of injury; the severity varies with the extent of injury.
- Swelling of the affected joint.
- Redness or bruising in the area of injury, either immediately or several hours after injury.
- Loss of normal mobility in the injured joint.

CAUSES & RISK FACTORS—Caused by the overuse or stress of a ligament or membrane around a joint. A sprain usually occurs when the body weight is abnormally placed on ligaments, causing them to stretch and tear. The ankle is injured most often because of its anatomical weakness, its exposed position and the stress it sustains in athletic and recreational activities. The risk increases with obesity.

DOCTOR'S TREATMENT & DIAGNOSTIC TESTS
- Medical history and physical exam.
- X-rays of the injured area.
- If the injury is not severe, self-care instructions focused on the older patient.
- Doctor's treatment if the joint cannot move or bear weight normally.
- A cast for a severely sprained joint.
- Surgery to repair badly torn ligaments.
- Physical therapy to help you regain strength and the normal use of the joint.

HOME TREATMENT BY SELF OR CARE-GIVER

GENERAL INSTRUCTIONS—The same treatment applies to a sprain or strain:
- Apply ice to the injured joint during the first 24 hours. Place the ice in a plastic bag and separate it from the skin with a thin towel. Hold it against the joint with your hand or an elastic bandage. Keep the ice pack on the joint for up to 2 hours at a time—either constantly or intermittently—depending on your ability to tolerate the cold. Continue the ice treatment at 2-hour intervals for 24 hours.
- After 24 hours, some doctors recommend continued ice treatment. Others recommend heat.

- To use heat, soak the joint in hot water or apply heat for 15 minutes every 2 hours or whenever possible. Don't apply heat during the first 24 hours. It may increase the bleeding and swelling and prolong healing time.
- Whenever possible, elevate the joint so fluid can drain and diminish swelling.
- A cast may be necessary for severe sprains or following surgery. See Appendix 17. Following cast removal, you will wear support bandages for a while.
- Learn how to use crutches if needed.

MEDICATION (ADJUSTED FOR AGING)
- You may use non-prescription pain relievers such as acetaminophen or ibuprofen. If the sprain is severe, your doctor may prescribe a stronger pain reliever.
- *Note:* Adverse reactions and side effects may be more frequent and severe in older persons. Remind your doctor of any medicines you already take.

ACTIVITY FOR OLDER PATIENTS
- Allow the joint to rest for 1 or 2 days. Then begin exercising it gently, without putting weight on it.
- See Appendix 20 regarding physical fitness for the active older adult.

FOOD & BEVERAGE
- No special diet is required.
- See Appendix 1 regarding good nutrition for people over 50.

FUTURE CONSIDERATIONS FOR THE AGING ADULT

POSSIBLE COMPLICATIONS—Permanent weakness if the sprain is severe or if a joint is sprained repeatedly.

PROBABLE OUTCOME—Strains usually heal in 1 to 2 weeks. Sprains generally heal in 2 weeks without complications.

PREVENTING RECURRENCE—To avoid injury:
- Wrap weak joints with support bandages before strenuous activity.
- Stretch your muscles before and after exercise.
- Strengthen weak muscles with rehabilitative exercises to prevent a recurrence. Consult your doctor or a physical therapist for exercises.
- Accident-proof your home.

CALL YOUR DOCTOR IF

- You have a sprained joint that won't bear weight or move normally.
- The pain becomes intolerable.
- The swelling or bruising increases despite treatment.

STOMACH CANCER
(Gastric Carcinoma)

BASIC INFORMATION FOR OLDER ADULTS

DESCRIPTION—Stomach cancer is an uncontrolled growth of malignant cells in the stomach. It is a common cancer that occurs most often in men over 40. Body part involved: The stomach.

SPECIAL CONSIDERATIONS FOR AGING
- Malignant diseases are less likely to spread rapidly.
- Characteristic signs and symptoms of many disorders are frequently changed or absent.
- The immune system becomes less effective, opening the way for viral, bacterial and other infections; malignancies; immune disorders; and allergies.
- Stress from any emotional cause—fear, worry, anxiety, sadness, loneliness or anger—affects all aspects of any illness or disorder.

SIGNS & SYMPTOMS
Early stages:
- Vague symptoms of indigestion, such as fullness, burping, nausea and poor appetite.
Later stages:
- Unexplained weight loss.
- Vomiting blood; black stools.
- Fullness after eating small amounts.
- Anemia; pain in the upper abdomen.
- A mass in the upper abdomen that can be felt (sometimes).

CAUSES & RISK FACTORS—The cause is unknown. Risk factors include:
- A family history of stomach cancer.
- Blood type. This is most common in people with type A blood.
- Pernicious anemia.
- Excessive alcohol consumption.
- The absence of normal stomach acid, previous stomach surgery or partial stomach removal.
- A diet that includes many smoked, pickled and salted meats.

DOCTOR'S TREATMENT & DIAGNOSTIC TESTS
- Medical history and physical exam.
- Laboratory blood studies for anemia, stomach tests for acid and stool tests for bleeding.
- Surgical diagnostic procedures such as biopsy through a gastroscope (see Glossary).
- X-rays of the stomach, esophagus and small intestine.
- Surgery to remove part or all of the stomach. Advancing age alone is not a deterrent.
- Radiation treatment.
- Self-care instructions focused on the older patient.

HOME TREATMENT BY SELF OR CARE-GIVER

GENERAL INSTRUCTIONS
- No specific instructions except those listed under other headings.
- Stomach cancer is a complicated, serious disorder. This page can cover only the main points of diagnosis and treatment. Your doctor, nurse or librarian can provide sources of supplemental information.

MEDICATION (ADJUSTED FOR AGING)—
Your doctor may prescribe:
- Anticancer (chemotherapy) drugs (sometimes).
- Pain relievers.

ACTIVITY FOR OLDER PATIENTS
- Resume your normal activities as soon as your symptoms improve after surgery or chemotherapy.
- See Appendix 20 regarding physical fitness for the active older adult.

FOOD & BEVERAGE—Eat frequent, small meals of soft foods. Try to maintain a high calorie intake. Consult a dietician for menu planning.

FUTURE CONSIDERATIONS FOR THE AGING ADULT

POSSIBLE COMPLICATIONS—Internal bleeding; misdiagnosis as a stomach ulcer; fatal spread to the liver, bones and lungs.

PROBABLE OUTCOME—In about 10% of the cases, stomach cancer is curable with surgery. With early diagnosis and treatment, the 5-year survival rate is 65%. Scientific research into causes and treatment continues, so there is hope for increasingly effective treatment and a cure.

PREVENTING RECURRENCE
- Don't ignore symptoms of indigestion that last more than a few days.
- Avoid eating processed or smoked meats, such as bacon, prepared ham and lunch meats.
- Decrease your alcohol consumption if you drink more than 1 or 2 drinks a day.
- Examine your stools yearly or more often with home tests for blood in the stool.

CALL YOUR DOCTOR IF

- You have symptoms of stomach cancer.
- Indigestion occurs after surgery and does not respond to medication in a few days.
- New, unexplained symptoms develop. The drugs used in treatment may produce side effects.

STOMACH EROSION
(Gastric Erosion)

BASIC INFORMATION FOR OLDER ADULTS

DESCRIPTION—Stomach erosion is a slight break in the innermost lining of the stomach. If the break goes deeper, it becomes a duodenal ulcer. This is not contagious or cancerous. Body part involved: The stomach.

SPECIAL CONSIDERATIONS FOR AGING
- Older people frequently drink an inadequate amount of water.
- The stomach produces less acid.
- Stress from any emotional cause—fear, worry, anxiety, sadness, loneliness or anger—affects all aspects of any illness or disorder.

SIGNS & SYMPTOMS
- Vomiting blood. The blood may be bright red or it may resemble black coffee grounds.
- Blood in the stool. The blood will appear black or "tarry."

CAUSES & RISK FACTORS—Probably caused by drugs that irritate the stomach lining. The most likely drugs are alcohol; caffeine; tobacco; aspirin; non-steroidal anti-inflammatory drugs used to treat arthritis and gout; and cortisone drugs used to treat asthma, Addison's disease or other conditions. Risk factors include:
- Stress.
- The use of *any* oral medication.

DOCTOR'S TREATMENT & DIAGNOSTIC TESTS
- Medical history and physical exam.
- Laboratory studies of the stool and blood tests for anemia.
- X-rays of the upper digestive tract.
- Self-care instructions focused on the older patient.

HOME TREATMENT BY SELF OR CARE-GIVER

GENERAL INSTRUCTIONS
- Check your stool every day for signs of bleeding. If the stool is black, remove a stool portion from the toilet bowl and take it to your doctor's office for examination.
- Avoid stressful situations (see Appendix 13).
- Don't smoke or drink alcoholic beverages.

MEDICATION (ADJUSTED FOR AGING)
- Your doctor may prescribe H_2 blockers to reduce the production of stomach acid.
- For minor pain, you may use non-prescription antacids.

- *Note:* Adverse reactions and side effects may be more frequent and severe in older persons. Remind your doctor of any medicines you already take.

ACTIVITY FOR OLDER PATIENTS
- Resume your normal activities as soon as your symptoms improve.
- See Appendix 20 regarding physical fitness for the active older adult.

FOOD & BEVERAGE
- Avoid hot and spicy foods. Eat small, frequent meals for 2 weeks. Don't drink alcohol.
- See Appendix 1 regarding good nutrition for people over 50.

FUTURE CONSIDERATIONS FOR THE AGING ADULT

POSSIBLE COMPLICATIONS
- Bleeding is an uncommon but dangerous complication, especially in the elderly. Another major complication is perforation, in which the erosion penetrates the stomach wall. Surgery is necessary to correct either complication. It involves little risk except for those over 70 years of age.
- The loss of blood may be slight, but it can cause anemia.

PROBABLE OUTCOME—Curable in 2 weeks with treatment if the cause is eliminated. Recurrence is common.

PREVENTING RECURRENCE
- Don't take medicines without enteric (protective) coatings.
- Don't drink alcohol if you have had stomach erosion. It may trigger bleeding.

CALL YOUR DOCTOR IF

- You have the signs of bleeding described under Signs & Symptoms.
- You develop diarrhea. This may represent an adverse reaction to drugs used in treatment. The prescription may need adjustment.
- You have severe pain that is not relieved by treatment.
- You are unusually weak, pale or lightheaded.
- The symptoms of gastric erosion recur after treatment.

ILLNESSES & DISORDERS

STOMACH INFLAMMATION
(Gastritis)

BASIC INFORMATION FOR OLDER ADULTS

DESCRIPTION—Gastritis is a mild irritation, erosion or infection of the stomach lining. It may be confused with a peptic ulcer. Body part involved: The stomach.

SPECIAL CONSIDERATIONS FOR AGING
- Older people frequently drink an inadequate amount of water.
- The stomach produces less acid.
- Stress from any emotional cause—fear, worry, anxiety, sadness, loneliness or anger—affects all aspects of any illness or disorder.

SIGNS & SYMPTOMS
- Abdominal pain and cramps.
- Vomiting (occasionally).
- Appetite loss; weakness; fever.
- A swollen abdomen.
- A sharp, dull or annoying pain in the chest.
- An acid taste in the mouth.
- Mild nausea and diarrhea (rare).
- Belching or gas.

CAUSES & RISK FACTORS
Causes include:
- Excess stomach acid caused by heavy drinking, smoking or overeating (especially of foods you don't digest easily).
- Virus infection. This form may be contagious.
- Adverse reaction to alcohol, caffeine or drugs.
- Unknown (sometimes).

Risk factors include:
- Stress; fatigue or overwork.
- Improper diet; smoking.
- Illness that has lowered resistance.
- The use of drugs such as aspirin, non-steroidal anti-inflammatories, cortisone, caffeine and many more.
- Excessive alcohol consumption.

DOCTOR'S TREATMENT & DIAGNOSTIC TESTS
- Medical history and physical exam.
- Laboratory studies to measure stomach acid.
- Biopsy of stomach tissue.
- Self-care instructions focused on the older patient.

HOME TREATMENT BY SELF OR CARE-GIVER

GENERAL INSTRUCTIONS—Consider lifestyle changes (see Appendix 12).

MEDICATION (ADJUSTED FOR AGING)
- For minor discomfort, you may use non-prescription antacids and acetaminophen. Don't take aspirin.

- Your doctor may prescribe additional medication depending on the cause of your gastritis.
- *Note:* Adverse reactions and side effects may be more frequent and severe in older persons. Remind your doctor of any medicines you already take.

ACTIVITY FOR OLDER PATIENTS
- Resume your normal activities as soon as your symptoms improve.
- See Appendix 20 regarding physical fitness for the active older adult.

FOOD & BEVERAGE
- Don't eat solid food on the first day of the attack. Drink liquids frequently, preferably milk or water. Resume a normal diet slowly, but avoid hot and spicy foods until your symptoms disappear.
- See Appendix 1 regarding good nutrition for people over 50.

FUTURE CONSIDERATIONS FOR THE AGING ADULT

POSSIBLE COMPLICATIONS
- Bleeding is an uncommon but dangerous complication, especially in the elderly. Another major complication is ulceration or perforation, in which stomach acid erodes into or through the stomach wall. Surgery is necessary to correct either complication. Stomach inflammation involves little risk except for those over 70 years of age.
- Chronic stomach inflammation if you continue to smoke or drink alcohol.

PROBABLE OUTCOME—Usually curable in several days if the cause is eliminated.

PREVENTING RECURRENCE
- Eat and drink moderately. Several (4 to 5) small meals a day may be better than 3 regular-size meals.
- Don't skip meals or eat irregularly.
- Avoid foods you find hard to digest.
- Don't smoke anything or drink alcohol.
- Discuss with your doctor all medicines you take. Avoid medicines that irritate your stomach if possible.

CALL YOUR DOCTOR IF

- You vomit blood.
- Your bowel movements become black or tarry.
- The pain becomes severe.
- You develop signs of dehydration, such as a dry mouth, wrinkled skin, excessive thirst or decreased urination.

STOMACH & INTESTINAL INFLAMMATION
(Gastroenteritis)

BASIC INFORMATION FOR OLDER ADULTS

DESCRIPTION—Gastroenteritis is an irritation and infection of the digestive tract for any reason, including dysentery, typhoid fever, cholera, food poisoning and traveler's diarrhea. This condition may be confused with spastic colitis. Body parts involved: The stomach; small intestine; colon.

SPECIAL CONSIDERATIONS FOR AGING
- Older people frequently drink an inadequate amount of water.
- The immune system becomes less effective, opening the way for infections.
- The number of autoantibodies (see Glossary) increases.
- Stress from any emotional cause affects all aspects of any illness or disorder.

SIGNS & SYMPTOMS
- Nausea that sometimes causes vomiting.
- Diarrhea that ranges from 2 or 3 loose stools to many watery stools.
- Abdominal cramps, pain or tenderness.
- Appetite loss; fever; weakness.

CAUSES & RISK FACTORS
Causes include:
- Infection (viral, bacterial or parasitic).
- Food poisoning; food allergy; emotional upset.
- Excessive alcohol consumption.
- The use of harsh laxatives.
- A change in the bacteria that normally live in the intestinal tract.

Risk factors include:
- Improper diet; excessive alcohol consumption.
- The use of drugs such as aspirin, non-steroidal anti-inflammatories, antibiotics, laxatives, cortisone or caffeine.
- Travel to foreign countries.

DOCTOR'S TREATMENT & DIAGNOSTIC TESTS
- Medical history and physical exam.
- Laboratory studies such as blood counts and stool studies.
- Self-care instructions focused on the older patient.
- Hospitalization if dehydration is severe.

HOME TREATMENT BY SELF OR CARE-GIVER

GENERAL INSTRUCTIONS—It is not necessary to isolate persons with stomach and intestinal inflammation.

MEDICATION (ADJUSTED FOR AGING)—Medicine is usually not necessary. If the stomach and intestinal inflammation is severe or prolonged, your doctor may prescribe antinausea and antidiarrhea medication. Some antidiarrhea medicines may prolong diarrhea and irritation.

ACTIVITY FOR OLDER PATIENTS—Rest in bed until the nausea, vomiting, diarrhea and fever are gone. Gradually increase your activity.

FOOD & BEVERAGE
- Suck ice chips or drink an electrolyte replenisher or rehydration liquid (mix 4 teaspoons sugar and 1/4 teaspoon salt in 1 pint of cold water).
- After the diarrhea and vomiting stop, drink small amounts of clear liquids such as tea, "flat" ginger ale or lemon-lime soda, broth and gelatin.
- If you tolerate liquids for 12 hours, eat small amounts of soft foods such as cooked cereal, rice, eggs, custard, baked potato and yogurt.
- If you tolerate soft food for 2 or 3 days, gradually return to a normal diet. Avoid alcohol, spicy food (such as pizza, spaghetti and onions), gravy, raw vegetables, raw fruit, salad dressing, cream soup, coffee and milk for several more days.

FUTURE CONSIDERATIONS FOR THE AGING ADULT

POSSIBLE COMPLICATIONS
- Serious dehydration that requires intravenous fluids.
- Serious illness that may be overlooked because the symptoms of stomach and intestinal inflammation mimic those of other disorders.

PROBABLE OUTCOME—The vomiting and diarrhea usually disappear in 2 to 5 days, but adults may feel weak, fatigued and depressed for about 1 week.

PREVENTING RECURRENCE
- Wash your hands frequently if you or someone around you has stomach and intestinal inflammation.
- Avoid as many of the causes and risk factors mentioned above as possible.

CALL YOUR DOCTOR IF

- The symptoms of stomach and intestinal inflammation persist longer than 2 days.
- Any of the following occurs during treatment: Mucus or blood in the stool. A fever of 101F (38.3C) or higher. Abdominal swelling. Severe pain in the abdomen or rectum, especially pain that begins in the center and moves to the lower right side.
- The vomiting and diarrhea recur after treatment.
- You develop signs of dehydration, such as a dry mouth, wrinkled skin, excessive thirst or decreased urination.

STREP THROAT
(Streptococcal Sore Throat)

BASIC INFORMATION FOR OLDER ADULTS

DESCRIPTION—Strep throat is the infection and inflammation of the pharynx by streptococcal bacteria. Strep throat is contagious. One out of 4 family members usually catches it within 2 to 7 days after exposure. Body parts involved: The throat; the tonsils.

SPECIAL CONSIDERATIONS FOR AGING
- The immune system becomes less effective, opening the way for viral, bacterial and other infections; malignancies; immune disorders; and allergies.
- The total state of well-being in many older people makes them increasingly susceptible to infections and impairs their ability to prevent infections from spreading.
- Decreased nutrition increases the risk of infections.

SIGNS & SYMPTOMS
- Fever; rapid onset of throat pain.
- Throat pain that is worse when swallowing.
- Appetite loss; headache.
- A general ill feeling.
- Ear pain when swallowing (sometimes).
- Swollen glands in the neck.
- Bright red tonsils that may have specks of pus.

CAUSES & RISK FACTORS—Caused by
streptococcal bacteria. Risk factors include:
- A recent strep infection in the household.
- Smoking; fatigue.
- Cold, wet weather.
- Crowded living conditions.

DOCTOR'S TREATMENT & DIAGNOSTIC TESTS
- Medical history and physical exam.
- Laboratory studies such as a throat culture and blood count. A throat culture is the only way to diagnose a strep throat infection. It is an inexpensive, quick, painless procedure in a doctor's office.
- Self-care instructions focused on the older patient.

HOME TREATMENT BY SELF OR CARE-GIVER

GENERAL INSTRUCTIONS
- Prepare a soothing gargle with warm salt-water or tea. Double the usual strength of tea, and gargle it warm or cold as often as it feels good.
- Use a cool-mist humidifier to provide moisture. This relieves the dry, tight feeling in the throat.
- Use warm-water soaks (see Appendix 18) to relieve the pain in swollen glands.

MEDICATION (ADJUSTED FOR AGING)
- Your doctor may prescribe penicillin or another antibiotic to take orally or by injection.
- When the infection appears to be streptococcal, treatment is often started prior to the completion of a culture.
- *Note:* Adverse reactions and side effects may be more frequent and severe in older persons. Remind your doctor of any medicines you already take.

ACTIVITY FOR OLDER PATIENTS
- Rest in bed until the fever subsides. You may read or watch TV.
- After treatment, resume your normal activities as your symptoms improve.

FOOD & BEVERAGE
- A liquid diet may be necessary while the throat is sore. Drink as many fluids as possible, including milk shakes, soups, tea, carbonated drinks and iced coffee. Any type and amount of solid food is acceptable as long as it can be swallowed without too much pain.
- See Appendix 1 regarding good nutrition for people over 50.

FUTURE CONSIDERATIONS FOR THE AGING ADULT

POSSIBLE COMPLICATIONS
- Dehydration (if the throat is too sore to swallow liquid).
- The following complications can be prevented with at least 10 days of treatment with penicillin or other effective antibiotics: abscess next to the tonsil; rheumatic fever; glomerulonephritis; sinusitis, otitis media or mastoiditis.

PROBABLE OUTCOME—Usually curable in 10 to 12 days with antibiotic treatment.

PREVENTING RECURRENCE—Avoid contact with infected people.

CALL YOUR DOCTOR IF

- You have symptoms of a strep throat.
- Any of the following occurs during treatment:
  Your temperature is normal for 1 or 2 days and then a fever develops.
  New symptoms appear, such as nausea, vomiting, earache, cough, swollen glands, skin rash, severe headache, nasal drainage or shortness of breath.
  Your joints become red or painful.
  You experience dark urine, a rash, chest pain or fatigue. These may occur as much as 3 to 4 weeks later.

STROKE
(Cerebrovascular Accident, CVA)

 BASIC INFORMATION FOR OLDER ADULTS

DESCRIPTION—Stoke is a sudden decrease in the blood supply to part of the brain that damages the area so it cannot function normally. Body parts involved: The central nervous system; the musculoskeletal system. (THIS IS AN EMERGENCY; SEEK MEDICAL CARE IMMEDIATELY!)

SPECIAL CONSIDERATIONS FOR AGING
- The blood vessels nourishing the brain become thicker and lose their elasticity.
- 50% of people over 60 have x-ray evidence of narrowing of the coronary arteries, yet only 50% of those people have symptoms.

SIGNS & SYMPTOMS—The following symptoms may vary according to the site of brain damage:
- Inability to speak or move part of the body.
- Loss of consciousness.
- Sudden heaviness in an arm or leg or numbness and an inability to control some muscles.
- Headache; vision disturbances.
- Confusion; dizziness.
- Loss of bowel and bladder control.

CAUSES & RISK FACTORS—Usually caused by hardening of the arteries (atherosclerosis) or high blood pressure. These may result in the following:
- Thrombosis, in which blood flow is blocked by a narrow or closed artery.
- Embolism, in which a small part of an artery wall or a small blood clot from a diseased artery or the heart travels to the brain.
- Cerebral hemorrhage, in which a blood vessel to the brain ruptures and bleeds into surrounding brain tissue.
- Rupture of an aneurysm of a small artery to the brain.

Risk factors include:
- Smoking; obesity; high blood pressure.
- A diet that is high in fat or salt.
- Diabetes mellitus; coronary artery disease.
- Previous transient ischemic attacks.
- A family history of stroke.
- Excessive alcohol consumption.

DOCTOR'S TREATMENT & DIAGNOSTIC TESTS
- Medical history and physical exam.
- Laboratory studies of the spinal fluid and blood.
- MRI or CT scan (see Glossary for both).
- X-rays of the head; lumbar puncture (see Glossary) to rule out meningitis.
- ECG and angiogram (see Glossary for both).
- Self-care instructions focused on the older patient.
- Hospitalization.
- Surgery (sometimes) to remove a clot in an artery (carotid) to the brain.
- Nursing home care (sometimes).
- Physical therapy and speech therapy.

 HOME TREATMENT BY SELF OR CARE-GIVER

GENERAL INSTRUCTIONS
- Following a stroke, consider installing ramps at entries to your house and handbars next to tubs and toilets.
- The loss of function due to stroke varies considerably. Impaired speech or movement can be improved with therapy. A positive attitude is important. Conferences with your doctor and therapists will help you determine the most suitable rehabilitation therapy.

MEDICATION (ADJUSTED FOR AGING)—Your doctor may prescribe:
- Anticoagulant drugs to reduce the chance of clot formation.
- Antihypertensive drugs if you have high blood pressure.

ACTIVITY FOR OLDER PATIENTS—If you have lost muscle control, therapy will help you learn to use the affected limbs to regain basic skills such as eating, dressing and toilet functions.

FOOD & BEVERAGE—Eat a diet that is low in salt and fat (see Appendices 8 and 9).

 FUTURE CONSIDERATIONS FOR THE AGING ADULT

POSSIBLE COMPLICATIONS—Pneumonia; depression; pressure sores from prolonged bed rest; permanent paralysis or disability.

PROBABLE OUTCOME—Stroke causes death, permanent damage or disability in 2/3 of all cases. In the rest, complete recovery without long-term disability is possible. A mild stroke may be the forerunner of more severe attacks. For stroke survivors, partial paralysis may last for months.

PREVENTING RECURRENCE
- Exercise regularly. See Appendix 20.
- Eat a diet that is low in salt and fat.
- Don't smoke.
- Have your blood pressure checked regularly. If it is high, consult your doctor.
- Ask your doctor about taking 1 aspirin daily. Recent studies indicate this may decrease the chance of cerebral thrombosis or embolism.

 CALL YOUR DOCTOR IF

- You have symptoms of a stroke or observe them in someone else. *This is an emergency!*
- Any of the following occurs during treatment: fever; pressure sores; worsening symptoms.

ILLNESSES & DISORDERS

STY
(Hordeolum)

BASIC INFORMATION FOR OLDER ADULTS

DESCRIPTION—A sty is a small abscess of a hair follicle gland in the eyelid. Body parts involved: The eyelid; eyelashes; conjunctiva (white of the eye).

SPECIAL CONSIDERATIONS FOR AGING
- The immune system becomes less effective, opening the way for viral, bacterial and other infections; malignancies; immune disorders; and allergies.
- The total state of well-being in many older people makes them increasingly susceptible to infections and impairs their ability to prevent infections from spreading.
- Decreased nutrition, common among chronically ill older people, increases the risk of any disease or disorder.

SIGNS & SYMPTOMS
- Redness, swelling, warmth, tenderness or pain on the edge of the top or bottom eyelid. The head of the sty is usually on the outside, but it may be on the underside of the lid.
- Increased tear production.
- Sensitivity to bright light.
- A gritty feeling in the eye.

CAUSES & RISK FACTORS
CAUSES & RISK FACTORS—Caused by a bacterial infection (usually staphylococcal). The infection may be limited to the eyelid or may have spread from somewhere else in the body. A sty may result from general poor health or may occasionally indicate a need for glasses. Risk factors include:
- Stress.
- Illness that has lowered resistance.
- Eye irritation from smoking.
- Exposure to chemical or environmental irritants.
- Crowded or unsanitary living conditions.
- Poor nutrition.

DOCTOR'S TREATMENT & DIAGNOSTIC TESTS
- Medical history and physical exam.
- Laboratory culture of the discharge from the sty.
- Self-care instructions focused on the older patient.
- Surgery to drain the abscess (sometimes).

HOME TREATMENT BY SELF OR CARE-GIVER

GENERAL INSTRUCTIONS—Use warm-water soaks (see Appendix 18) to relieve the pain and inflammation and hasten healing. Apply the soaks for 20 minutes, then rest at least 1 hour. Repeat as often as needed.

MEDICATION (ADJUSTED FOR AGING)
- Your doctor may prescribe: Antibiotic eye drops to prevent the spread of infection to other parts of the eye. Oral antibiotics or antibiotic injections are usually not needed.
  Topical antibiotic ointments or creams, such as erythromycin or bacitracin. Apply a thin layer of medication to the eyelid edge 3 or 4 times daily. A heavy layer wastes medicine and is no more beneficial than a thin layer.
- Both eyes may be treated to avoid the spread of infection.
- *Note:* Adverse reactions and side effects may be more frequent and severe in older persons. Remind your doctor of any medicines you already take.

ACTIVITY FOR OLDER PATIENTS
- No restrictions are necessary.
- See Appendix 20 regarding physical fitness for the active older adult.

FOOD & BEVERAGE
- No special diet is required.
- See Appendix 1 regarding good nutrition for people over 50.

FUTURE CONSIDERATIONS FOR THE AGING ADULT

POSSIBLE COMPLICATIONS—Spread of the infection to other glands in the eyelid.

PROBABLE OUTCOME—Usually curable within 1 week after the sty discharges its pus. Sties frequently recur, even with treatment.

PREVENTING RECURRENCE
- Wash your hands frequently, and dry them with clean towels.
- Avoid environments with excessive dust or other irritating substances.
- Eat a normal, well-balanced diet.

CALL YOUR DOCTOR IF

- A ripened sty does not drain spontaneously or after the gentle removal of the affected eyelash.
- Pain occurs in the *eye*.
- Your vision changes.

SUBARACHNOID HEMORRHAGE

BASIC INFORMATION FOR OLDER ADULTS

DESCRIPTION—A subarachnoid hemorrhage is a sudden bleeding into the subarachnoid space (the area between 2 of the membranes that cover the brain). The space is normally filled with cerebrospinal fluid. Body parts involved: The brain; meninges (membranes that cover the brain); blood vessels to the brain. (THIS IS AN EMERGENCY; SEEK MEDICAL CARE IMMEDIATELY!)

SPECIAL CONSIDERATIONS FOR AGING
- The blood vessels nourishing the brain are less healthy. They become thicker and lose their elasticity.
- 50% of people over 60 have x-ray evidence of narrowing of the coronary arteries, yet only 50% of those people have symptoms.

SIGNS & SYMPTOMS
- Acute, severe headache, often followed by unconsciousness.
- Drowsiness, dizziness, convulsions or coma.
- Eye pain with extreme sensitivity to light.
- Vomiting; fever.
- Rapid heartbeat and breathing.
- A stiff neck with pain on movement.
- Numbness, weakness or inability to move an arm or leg.

CAUSES & RISK FACTORS
Causes include:
- Head injury (the most common cause).
- Hardening of the arteries.
- Infection in any part of the central nervous system.
- Rupture of an aneurysm (weakened part of an artery) that has been present since birth. A rupture is often preceded by high blood pressure or hardening of the arteries.
- A bleeding disorder such as sickle-cell anemia, leukemia or any that is a side effect of prescription drugs.
Risk factors include:
- Atherosclerosis (hardening of the arteries) or high blood pressure.
- A family history of bleeding disorders.
- A family history of subarachnoid hemorrhage. Cerebral aneurysms run in families.
- Unaccustomed physical exercise.

DOCTOR'S TREATMENT & DIAGNOSTIC TESTS
- Medical history and physical exam.
- Laboratory studies of the blood and cerebrospinal fluid.
- X-rays of the skull.
- CT scan (see Glossary).
- Angiography (see Glossary).
- Surgery to stop the bleeding and remove collected blood.
- Long-term rehabilitation in a nursing home or other facility.
- Self-care instructions focused on the older patient.

HOME TREATMENT BY SELF OR CARE-GIVER

GENERAL INSTRUCTIONS—Ongoing care and medical treatment will be tailored to the individual circumstances. Your doctor will need to provide detailed, written instructions and follow-up assistance. Home visits by specially trained nurses can help you find ways to modify your living arrangements, furniture placement, bathroom facilities and other areas to accommodate you.

MEDICATION (ADJUSTED FOR AGING)—Your doctor may prescribe:
- Cortisone drugs to reduce the brain's swelling and pressure.
- Pain relievers for headaches.
- Laxatives or stool softeners to prevent straining.

ACTIVITY FOR OLDER PATIENTS
- If you have lost some motor functions, occupational and physical therapists will help you use the affected limbs to regain basic skills such as eating, dressing and toilet functions.
- After recovery, resume as many of your former activities as your strength and sense of well-being allow. Allow 6 to 12 months for recovery.

FOOD & BEVERAGE—No special diet is required. Vitamin and mineral supplements should not be necessary unless you cannot eat normally.

FUTURE CONSIDERATIONS FOR THE AGING ADULT

POSSIBLE COMPLICATIONS—Death or permanent disability if treatment does not begin soon enough.

PROBABLE OUTCOME—If surgery is possible, the chances of recovery are good. Partial paralysis, weakness or numbness and speech and visual difficulties may remain in some cases. The damaged area of the brain cannot be restored. However, undamaged areas of the brain often can be taught the lost functions. This usually requires rehabilitation, including physical therapy or speech therapy. Determination and a positive attitude greatly affect the success of the rehabilitation process.

PREVENTING RECURRENCE
- Avoid head injury. Use seat belts in cars and protective head gear while biking.
- Have your blood pressure checked regularly. If it is high, consult your doctor for treatment to reduce it.

CALL YOUR DOCTOR IF

- You have any symptoms of a subarachnoid hemorrhage. *This is an emergency!*
- Your symptoms recur after surgery.

SUBCONJUNCTIVAL HEMORRHAGE

BASIC INFORMATION FOR OLDER ADULTS

DESCRIPTION—A subconjunctival hemorrhage is characterized by the sudden appearance of blood in the white area of the eye. Although the bleeding may be frightening, it is not painful or serious. Body parts involved: The conjunctiva (white of the eye).

SPECIAL CONSIDERATIONS FOR AGING
- 50% of people over 60 have x-ray evidence of narrowing of the coronary arteries, yet only 50% of those people have symptoms.
- Decreased nutrition, common among chronically ill older people, increases the risk of any disease or disorder.
- Stress from any emotional cause—fear, worry, anxiety, sadness, loneliness or anger—affects all aspects of any illness or disorder.

SIGNS & SYMPTOMS—A small, painless collection of bright red blood over the white of the eye. Swelling may occur in the affected area of the conjunctiva. The blood changes color gradually to brown or green before disappearing. The condition doesn't interfere with vision.

CAUSES & RISK FACTORS—Usually caused by spontaneous bleeding with no known cause. It may follow coughing, sneezing, vomiting or direct injury to the eye. Risk factors include:
- The use of mind-altering drugs.
- The use of anticoagulant drugs.

DOCTOR'S TREATMENT & DIAGNOSTIC TESTS
- Medical history and physical exam (sometimes).
- Self-care instructions focused on the older patient.
- Treatment if there has been injury or a change in vision.

HOME TREATMENT BY SELF OR CARE-GIVER

GENERAL INSTRUCTIONS
- Use cold compresses for several days to prevent additional bleeding. Fold a clean cloth in several layers, dip it in ice water and wring it out a little. Apply it to the eye for 10 minutes every hour.
- Use warm compresses when the signs of bleeding have been stopped for 2 days. This will hasten blood absorption. Dip the compress in warm water instead of cold water. Apply it to the eye for 10 minutes 3 times a day.

MEDICATION (ADJUSTED FOR AGING)—Medicine is usually not necessary for this disorder.

ACTIVITY FOR OLDER PATIENTS
- No restrictions are necessary.
- See Appendix 20 regarding physical fitness for the active older adult.

FOOD & BEVERAGE
- No special diet is required.
- See Appendix 1 regarding good nutrition for people over 50.

FUTURE CONSIDERATIONS FOR THE AGING ADULT

POSSIBLE COMPLICATIONS—None are expected.

PROBABLE OUTCOME—The blood should be absorbed in 2 or 3 weeks. It is very unlikely that any scarring will occur.

PREVENTING RECURRENCE—There are no specific preventive measures.

CALL YOUR DOCTOR IF

You have symptoms of subconjunctival hemorrhage, especially if you have eye pain or your vision changes.

SUBDURAL HEMORRHAGE & HEMATOMA

BASIC INFORMATION FOR OLDER ADULTS

DESCRIPTION—Subdural hemorrhage and hematoma is bleeding (hemorrhage) that causes blood to collect and form a clot (hematoma) beneath the outermost of 3 membranes that cover the brain (meninges). There are 2 types of subdural hematomas. An acute subdural hematoma occurs soon after a severe head injury. A chronic subdural hematoma is a complication that may develop weeks after a head injury. The injury may have been so minor that the patient does not remember it. Both types occur most often in people who have fallen. Body parts involved: The brain; meninges; blood vessels to the brain. **(THIS IS AN EMERGENCY; SEEK MEDICAL CARE IMMEDIATELY!)**

SPECIAL CONSIDERATIONS FOR AGING
- The blood vessels nourishing the brain are less healthy. They become thicker and lose their elasticity.
- 50% of people over 60 have x-ray evidence of narrowing of the coronary arteries, yet only 50% of those people have symptoms.
- Neurological diseases become more likely.
- There is a bit more space between the membranes in which blood can pool.

SIGNS & SYMPTOMS
- Recurrent headaches that worsen each day.
- Fluctuating drowsiness, dizziness, mental changes or confusion.
- Weakness or numbness on one side of the body.
- Vision disturbances.
- Vomiting without nausea.
- Pupils of different sizes (sometimes).

CAUSES & RISK FACTORS—Caused by head injury. Risk factors include:
- The use of anticoagulant drugs.
- Excessive alcohol consumption.
- The use of mind-altering drugs.

DOCTOR'S TREATMENT & DIAGNOSTIC TESTS
- Medical history and physical exam.
- Laboratory studies of the blood and cerebrospinal fluid.
- Hospital diagnostic tests such as x-ray, angiography, MRI scan, PET scan and CT scan (see Glossary for all).
- Surgical exploration and removal of the clot.

HOME TREATMENT BY SELF OR CARE-GIVER

GENERAL INSTRUCTIONS—There is no self-treatment. The suggestions under Activity for Older Patients and Food & Beverage apply to care at home following surgery.

MEDICATION (ADJUSTED FOR AGING)
- Your doctor may prescribe cortisone drugs to reduce the swelling inside the skull.
- *Note:* Adverse reactions and side effects may be more frequent and severe in older persons. Remind your doctor of any medicines you already take.

ACTIVITY FOR OLDER PATIENTS—Stay as active as your strength allows. Work and exercise moderately. Rest when you tire. If your speech or muscle control has been damaged, you may need physical therapy or speech therapy.

FOOD & BEVERAGE
- Eat a normal, well-balanced diet. Vitamin and mineral supplements should not be necessary unless you cannot eat normally.
- See Appendix 1 regarding good nutrition for people over 50.

FUTURE CONSIDERATIONS FOR THE AGING ADULT

POSSIBLE COMPLICATIONS—Death or permanent brain damage, including partial or complete paralysis, behavioral and personality changes and speech problems.

PROBABLE OUTCOME—The degree of recovery depends upon your general health and age, the severity of the injury, the rapidity of the treatment and the extensiveness of the bleeding or clot. After the clot is removed, the brain tissue that has been compressed usually expands slowly to fill its original space. The outlook is good under the best circumstances.

PREVENTING RECURRENCE—Avoid head injury in the following ways:
- Use seat belts in cars.
- Wear protective head gear while riding a bicycle or motorcycle.
- Don't drink alcohol or use mind-altering drugs and drive.

CALL YOUR DOCTOR IF

- You have had a head injury—even if it seems minor—and you develop any symptoms of subdural hemorrhage. *This is an emergency!*
- Any of the following occurs during or after treatment:
  You develop a fever.
  The surgical wound becomes red, swollen or tender.
  Your headache worsens.

SUN POISONING
(Photosensitivity)

BASIC INFORMATION FOR OLDER ADULTS

DESCRIPTION—Sun poisoning is an abnormal reaction to the sun. Body parts involved: The skin in the areas most exposed to sunlight.

SPECIAL CONSIDERATIONS FOR AGING
- The skin becomes thinner.
- The skin becomes less elastic.
- Injured tissues repair more slowly.

SIGNS & SYMPTOMS
- A red skin rash, sometimes with small blisters, in areas exposed to sunlight.
- Fever.
- Fatigue or dizziness.

CAUSES & RISK FACTORS—Sun poisoning is most likely to occur during hot seasons when ultraviolet light is strongest. It is triggered by exposure to the sun, usually in conjunction with sunburn. It is especially likely in persons who take medications that cause photosensitivity (increased sensitivity to ultraviolet light). The most common drugs include tetracycline antibiotics, thiazide diuretics, sulfa drugs and oral contraceptives. Some cosmetics, including lipstick, perfume and soaps, can also cause a photosensitive reaction. Risk factors include:
- Underlying infection.
- Previous episodes of sun poisoning.
- Metabolic disorders such as diabetes mellitus, lupus erythematosus or thyroid disease.
- The use of immunosuppressive drugs or any drugs listed under Causes.

DOCTOR'S TREATMENT & DIAGNOSTIC TESTS
- Medical history and physical exam.
- Self-care instructions focused on the older patient.

HOME TREATMENT BY SELF OR CARE-GIVER

GENERAL INSTRUCTIONS
- Stay out of the sun during the hours of strongest ultraviolet light (10 a.m. to 4 p.m.).
- If you must go out in the sun, wear protective clothing and the most protective sun-screen preparation available.

MEDICATION (ADJUSTED FOR AGING)
- Your doctor may prescribe:
  Beta-carotene to reduce your discomfort.
  Chloroquine prior to sun exposure to prevent a recurrence of symptoms.
- *Note:* Adverse reactions and side effects may be more frequent and severe in older persons. Remind your doctor of anymedicines you already take.

ACTIVITY FOR OLDER PATIENTS
- No restrictions are necessary, except to avoid prolonged sun exposure.
- See Appendix 20 regarding physical fitness for the active older adult.

FOOD & BEVERAGE
- No special diet is required. Drink extra fluids to prevent dehydration.
- See Appendix 1 regarding good nutrition for people over 50.

FUTURE CONSIDERATIONS FOR THE AGING ADULT

POSSIBLE COMPLICATIONS—Recurrence of the rash and other symptoms when you are exposed to the sun—even for short periods—especially in the spring and summer.

PROBABLE OUTCOME—The symptoms can be controlled with treatment if you stay out of the sun. Allow up to 1 week for recovery.

PREVENTING RECURRENCE
- Stay out of the sun when possible if you have a history of sun poisoning.
- When exposed to the sun, use sunscreen lotions with a skin protective factor (SPF) of 15 or more.

CALL YOUR DOCTOR IF

- You have symptoms of sun poisoning.
- New, unexplained symptoms develop. The drugs used in treatment may produce side effects.

SUNBURN

BASIC INFORMATION FOR OLDER ADULTS

DESCRIPTION—Sunburn is an inflammation of the skin that follows overexposure to the sun, sun lamps or occupational light sources. Body part involved: Exposed skin.

SPECIAL CONSIDERATIONS FOR AGING
- The skin becomes thinner.
- The skin becomes less elastic.

SIGNS & SYMPTOMS
- Red, swollen, painful and sometimes blistered skin.
- Fever (occasionally).
- Nausea and vomiting (with severe burns).
- Delirium (with severe, extensive burns).
- Tanning or peeling of the skin after recovery, depending on the severity of the burn.

CAUSES & RISK FACTORS—Caused by excessive exposure to ultraviolet (UV) light. This is not screened out by thin clouds on overcast days, but it is partially screened by smoke and smog. A great deal of ultraviolet light reflects from snow, water, sand and sidewalks. Risk factors include:
- Genetic factors, especially fair skin, blue eyes and red or blonde hair.
- Exposure to industrial light sources, such as welding arcs.
- The use of drugs, including sulfa, tetracyclines, amoxicillin or oral contraceptives.

DOCTOR'S TREATMENT & DIAGNOSTIC TESTS
- Medical history and physical exam.
- For minor sunburn, self-care instructions focused on the older patient.
- Doctor's treatment for severe sunburn.

HOME TREATMENT BY SELF OR CARE-GIVER

GENERAL INSTRUCTIONS
- To reduce the heat and pain, dip gauze or towels in cool water and lay these on the burned areas.
- After the skin's swelling subsides, apply cold cream or baby lotion.
- For badly blistered skin, apply a light coating of petroleum jelly. This prevents anything from sticking to the blisters.

MEDICATION (ADJUSTED FOR AGING)
- Use non-prescription drugs such as aspirin or acetaminophen to relieve the pain and reduce the fever. Non-prescription burn remedies that contain local anesthetics, such as benzocaine or lidocaine, may be useful, but they produce allergic reactions in some.
- Your doctor may prescribe pain relievers or cortisone drugs to use briefly.

ACTIVITY FOR OLDER PATIENTS—Rest in any comfortable position until your fever and discomfort diminish. Cover yourself with an upside-down "cradle" or tent of cardboard or other material to keep bed linens off the burned skin.

FOOD & BEVERAGE
- No special diet is required. Increase your fluid intake.
- See Appendix 1 regarding good nutrition for people over 50.

FUTURE CONSIDERATIONS FOR THE AGING ADULT

POSSIBLE COMPLICATIONS—Skin changes leading to skin cancer, including life-threatening malignant melanoma; keratoses, premalignant skin lesions; premature wrinkling and loss of the skin's elasticity; temporary delirium in the worst cases.

PROBABLE OUTCOME—Spontaneous recovery in 3 days to 3 weeks, depending on the severity of the sunburn.

PREVENTING RECURRENCE
- Avoid the sun from 10 a.m. to 4 p.m.
- Use a sun-block preparation for outdoor activity. Products with a skin protective value of 15 or more protect almost totally. Those with lower values offer partial protection and allow minimal tanning. Some of these resist water and perspiration, but reapply them after swimming or prolonged exposure to the sun. Baby oil, mineral oil or cocoa butter offer no protection from the sun.
- For maximum protection, use a physical barrier agent such as zinc oxide ointment. Reapply it after swimming and at frequent intervals during exposure. Barrier agents are especially helpful on skin areas that are most susceptible to burns, such as the nose, ears, backs of the legs and back of the neck.
- If you rarely burn, use a sunscreen product that permits tanning and provides minimal protection.
- Wear muted colors such as tan. Avoid brilliant colors and whites, which reflect the sun into your face.
- If you insist on tanning, limit your sun exposure on the 1st day to 5 to 10 minutes on each side. Add 5 minutes per side each day.

CALL YOUR DOCTOR IF

Any of the following occurs after sunburn:
- A temperature spike to 101F (38.3C).
- Vomiting or diarrhea.
- Delirium.
- Pain and fever that persist longer than 48 hours.

SURGICAL WOUND, INFECTION OF

BASIC INFORMATION FOR OLDER ADULTS

DESCRIPTION—This disorder involves an infection from bacterial contamination during or after a surgical procedure. Infections occur following surgery in 1.5% to 30% of cases, depending on the type of procedure. Body parts involved: Any body part with a surgical incision.

SPECIAL CONSIDERATIONS FOR AGING
- The immune system becomes less effective, opening the way for viral, bacterial and other infections; malignancies; immune disorders; and allergies.
- Decreased nutrition increases the risk of infections.
- Repair from injury or disease is complete and effective, but recovery takes longer in older people.

SIGNS & SYMPTOMS—The following usually begin within 5 to 10 days after surgery, but in some cases they begin months later:
- Pain and redness around the surgical wound.
- Pus and other collections of fluid around the incision, making the sutures tighter.
- Fever (sometimes).

CAUSES & RISK FACTORS
Causes include:
- Infection with bacteria, including streptococci, staphylococci or other germs. These sometimes cause infection, in spite of elaborate precautions against them and scrupulous surgical technique.
- Infection from any material left in the surgical area, including instruments or gauze.

Risk factors include:
- Poor nutrition.
- Any chronic illness, especially diabetes mellitus.
- Gastrointestinal surgery.
- The use of immunosuppressive drugs.
- Obesity.

DOCTOR'S TREATMENT & DIAGNOSTIC TESTS
- Medical history and physical exam.
- Laboratory culture of pus from the infection site.
- Surgery to incise and drain a wound abscess.
- Self-care instructions focused on the older patient.

HOME TREATMENT BY SELF OR CARE-GIVER

GENERAL INSTRUCTIONS
- Use heat to relieve the pain. Use a warm compress 3 or 4 times a day for 30 to 40 minutes.
- Change dressings frequently if the wound oozes.

MEDICATION (ADJUSTED FOR AGING)
- Your doctor may prescribe:
  Antibiotics to fight the infection.
  Vitamin and mineral supplements to hasten healing.
  Pain relievers. You may use non-prescription drugs such as acetaminophen to relieve minor pain.
- *Note:* Adverse reactions and side effects may be more frequent and severe in older persons. Remind your doctor of any medicines you already take.

ACTIVITY FOR OLDER PATIENTS—Rest in bed until all signs of infection disappear. You may read or watch TV.

FOOD & BEVERAGE—Your surgeon will prescribe a diet.

FUTURE CONSIDERATIONS FOR THE AGING ADULT

POSSIBLE COMPLICATIONS
- Peritonitis.
- Blood poisoning.
- Interference with normal healing of the incision after surgery, sometimes necessitating further surgery and repairs.

PROBABLE OUTCOME—Usually curable in most patients with drainage of pus and antibiotic treatment. Allow about 2 weeks for the infection to heal.

PREVENTING RECURRENCE—Skillful surgeons use techniques and presurgical procedures that include the following:
- The use of certain antibiotics, such as neomycin, before gastrointestinal surgery to sterilize the intestinal tract.
- Meticulous cleansing of the skin before surgery.
- The use of as few sutures as possible.

CALL YOUR DOCTOR IF

- You have symptoms of an infection of a surgical wound.
- You develop a high fever and a general ill feeling or the infection seems to worsen after treatment.
- New, unexplained symptoms develop. The drugs used in treatment may produce side effects.

SWEATING, EXCESSIVE
(Hyperhidrosis)

BASIC INFORMATION FOR OLDER ADULTS

DESCRIPTION—Sweating is a normal body function that helps maintain an even body temperature. Excessive sweating serves no purpose and often creates social embarrassment because of odor or stained clothes. In extreme cases, excessive sweating can ruin clothes and shoes. Body parts involved: The skin, especially that of the underarms, palms and soles.

SPECIAL CONSIDERATIONS FOR AGING
- The fatty layer of tissue under the skin becomes thinner.
- The responsiveness of the skin's immune system decreases.

SIGNS & SYMPTOMS
- Heavy perspiration from the underarms, soles and palms—and, to a lesser degree, from other body parts.
- Unpleasant odor, which is caused by the bacteria in sweat.

CAUSES & RISK FACTORS
Causes include:
- Stress or chronic anxiety.
- Fever and infection.
- Malignancy, such as lymphoma.
- Hyperthyroidism.
- Heart attack.
- Menopause.
- Some drugs and medicines, such as narcotics.
- Withdrawal from addicting drugs.
- Unknown in some cases.
The risk increases with:
- Stress.
- Strenuous activity.
- Hot weather.

DOCTOR'S TREATMENT & DIAGNOSTIC TESTS
- Medical history and physical exam.
- Self-care instructions focused on the older patient.
- Treatment for underlying conditions or if self-care is unsuccessful.
- Psychotherapy or counseling if stress is a major factor.
- Surgery to remove sweat glands or sever the nerves to major sweat-producing areas (rare).

HOME TREATMENT BY SELF OR CARE-GIVER

GENERAL INSTRUCTIONS
- Bathe frequently.
- Change clothes frequently.

- Wear loose-fitting clothes made of natural fibers such as cotton rather than man-made materials.
- Use underarm sweat shields.
- Use antiperspirants and deodorants.
- Use drying powders.
- Wear cotton socks.
- Wear shoes or sandals made of leather rather than man-made materials.
- Use topical foot powders daily.
- Electrical devices temporarily reduce sweating of the palms, underarms or feet. Ask your doctor.
- Shave underarm hair.

MEDICATION (ADJUSTED FOR AGING)
- Your doctor may prescribe:
  Tranquilizers or anticholinergics to reduce the activity of the central nervous system. Don't use these if you have glaucoma or prostate disease.
  Special solutions to reduce sweating, such as topical applications of aluminum chloride.
  Beta-adrenergic blockers may occasionally help.
  Note: Adverse reactions and side effects may be more frequent and severe in older persons. Remind your doctor of any medicines you already take.

ACTIVITY FOR OLDER PATIENTS
- No restrictions are necessary.
- See Appendix 20 regarding physical fitness for the active older adult.

FOOD & BEVERAGE
- No special diet is required. Drink at least 8 glasses of water a day—more in hot weather.
- See Appendix 1 regarding good nutrition for people over 50.

FUTURE CONSIDERATIONS FOR THE AGING ADULT

POSSIBLE COMPLICATIONS
- Psychological distress caused by social embarrassment.
- Rashes from deodorants or antiperspirants.
- Dehydration if your fluid intake is insufficient to replace the water lost in sweat.

PROBABLE OUTCOME—The symptoms can be controlled with treatment.

PREVENTING RECURRENCE—Resolve tension-causing conditions. See Appendix 13.

CALL YOUR DOCTOR IF

Excessive sweating is causing you problems at work or in social situations.

SYPHILIS

BASIC INFORMATION FOR OLDER ADULTS

DESCRIPTION—Syphilis is a contagious sexually transmitted disease that causes widespread tissue destruction. Syphilis is known as the "great mimic," because its symptoms resemble those of many other diseases. Body parts involved: The genitals; skin; central nervous system.

SPECIAL CONSIDERATIONS FOR AGING
- The immune system becomes less effective, opening the way for viral, bacterial and other infections; malignancies; immune disorders; and allergies.
- Decreased nutrition, common among chronically ill older people, increases the risk of any disease or disorder.
- Stress from any emotional cause—fear, worry, anxiety, sadness, loneliness or anger—affects all aspects of any illness or disorder.

SIGNS & SYMPTOMS
First stage (contagious; appears 3 to 6 days after contact):
- A painless, red sore (chancre) on the genitals, mouth or rectum. The sore usually affects the penis in males and the vagina or cervix in females.

Second stage (contagious; begins 6 or more weeks after the chancre appears):
- Enlarged lymph glands in the neck, armpit or groin.
- Headache.
- A rash on skin and mucous membranes of the penis, vagina or mouth. The rash has small, red, scaly bumps.
- Fever (sometimes).

Third stage (non-contagious; may appear years after the first and second stages):
- Mental deterioration.
- Sexual impotence.
- Loss of balance.
- Loss of feeling or shooting pains in the legs.
- Heart disease.

CAUSES & RISK FACTORS—The infecting germ is *treponema pallidum*. It is spread by intimate sexual contact with someone who has syphilis in the first or second stages. The risk increases with many sexual partners.

DOCTOR'S TREATMENT & DIAGNOSTIC TESTS
- Medical history and physical exam.
- Laboratory studies such as a blood serum test for syphilis, a microscopic exam of discharge from the chancre and a study of the spinal fluid. These tests are repeated after treatment.
- Self-care instructions focused on the older patient.

HOME TREATMENT BY SELF OR CARE-GIVER

GENERAL INSTRUCTIONS
- Make sure that all your sexual partners obtain treatment. The public health department will work with you to notify them confidentially and help them obtain treatment.
- After treatment, have blood studies done each month for 6 months to check for recurrence. Have these studies repeated every 3 months for 2 years.

MEDICATION (ADJUSTED FOR AGING)—Your doctor will probably prescribe penicillin by injection unless you are allergic to it. If penicillin cannot be used, other antibiotics can be equally as effective.

ACTIVITY FOR OLDER PATIENTS—Avoid sexual intercourse for at least 2 months after treatment begins. Then use rubber condoms during sexual intercourse.

FOOD & BEVERAGE—No special diet.

FUTURE CONSIDERATIONS FOR THE AGING ADULT

POSSIBLE COMPLICATIONS—Widespread tissue destruction and death without treatment.

PROBABLE OUTCOME—Usually curable in 3 months with treatment. In spite of treatment, syphilis returns within 1 year in 10% of patients. If this happens, re-treatment is necessary.

PREVENTING RECURRENCE
- Use rubber condoms during intercourse.
- Avoid any sexual contact if you suspect a partner is infectious.

CALL YOUR DOCTOR IF

- You have symptoms of syphilis.
- Any of the following occurs during or after treatment:
  A fever.
  A skin rash, sore throat or swelling in any joint, such as the ankle or knee.
- New, unexplained symptoms develop. The drugs used in treatment may produce side effects.
- You once had syphilis and have not had a medical checkup in the past year.
- You have had sexual contact with someone who has syphilis.

TAPEWORM

BASIC INFORMATION FOR OLDER ADULTS

DESCRIPTION—This disorder is an infestation of the intestinal tract by the tapeworm, a parasite. This is not contagious from person to person. Body part involved: The intestinal tract.

SPECIAL CONSIDERATIONS FOR AGING
- Signs and symptoms may differ significantly from those listed below.
- Decreased nutrition increases the risk of infections.
- Stress from social isolation increases the risk of infection.

SIGNS & SYMPTOMS—Most people with this problem have no symptoms. However, some experience the following:
- Pain in the upper abdomen.
- Diarrhea.
- Unexplained weight loss.
- Symptoms of anemia (weakness, fatigue and shortness of breath).
- Bowel movements containing worm eggs and worm body parts.

CAUSES & RISK FACTORS—Caused by an intestinal parasite called *taenia saginata*. People become infected by eating improperly cooked or raw beef muscle, pork or fish that is infected with the parasite. Risk factors include travel to Africa, the Middle East, Eastern Europe, Mexico and South America. Tapeworm is uncommon in the U.S., except in California and New England.

DOCTOR'S TREATMENT & DIAGNOSTIC TESTS
- Medical history and physical exam.
- Laboratory stool studies to identify the worm.
- Self-care instructions focused on the older patient.

HOME TREATMENT BY SELF OR CARE-GIVER

GENERAL INSTRUCTIONS
- Wash your hands before eating.
- Have all family members examined by a doctor for possible infection.

MEDICATION (ADJUSTED FOR AGING)
- Your doctor may prescribe an anthelminthic drug to kill the parasite. The drug cures with a single dose. A disintegrating worm should be passed within 48 hours.
- *Note:* Adverse reactions and side effects may be more frequent and severe in older persons. Remind your doctor of any medicines you already take.

ACTIVITY FOR OLDER PATIENTS
- No restrictions are necessary.
- See Appendix 20 regarding physical fitness for the active older adult.

FOOD & BEVERAGE
- No special diet is required.
- See Appendix 1 regarding good nutrition for people over 50.

FUTURE CONSIDERATIONS FOR THE AGING ADULT

POSSIBLE COMPLICATIONS—Anemia.

PROBABLE OUTCOME—Usually curable in 1 day with treatment.

PREVENTING RECURRENCE
- Cook beef, pork and fish according to recipe directions.
- Buy only meat that has been inspected.

CALL YOUR DOCTOR IF

- You have symptoms of a tapeworm.
- New, unexplained symptoms develop. The drugs used in treatment may produce side effects.

TELOGEN EFFLUVIUM

BASIC INFORMATION FOR OLDER ADULTS

DESCRIPTION—Telogen effluvium is a type of generalized hair loss in which numerous scattered hair follicles simultaneously change from the growing phase to the resting stage of the hair-growth cycle.
Persons with this disorder rarely progress to significant baldness, and it is not contagious.
Body parts involved: The hair and scalp.

SPECIAL CONSIDERATIONS FOR AGING
- The responsiveness of the skin's immune system decreases.
- The skin loses hair bulbs and the hair shafts become thinner.
- Characteristic signs and symptoms of many disorders in older people are frequently changed or absent.

SIGNS & SYMPTOMS
- Hair loss at 4 to 5 times the normal rate. Normal hair loss is approximately 400 hairs a day, mostly during washing or brushing.
- No itching or pain.

CAUSES & RISK FACTORS
Causes include:
- Hormonal changes.
- Severe psychological stress—including that of serious illness, such as high fever, heart attack or stroke.

Risk factors include:
- Stress.
- Iron deficiency.
- Menopause.
- "Crash dieting" or malnutrition.

DOCTOR'S TREATMENT & DIAGNOSTIC TESTS
- Medical history and physical exam (for severe, prolonged cases only).
- Self-care instructions focused on the older patient.

HOME TREATMENT BY SELF OR CARE-GIVER

GENERAL INSTRUCTIONS
- Continue to wash and brush your hair as usual.
- Confront and define areas of conflict in your family life and in your occupational and leisure-time activities. If you cannot resolve conflicts, ask for help from family members, friends or competent counselors.
- Aim for a balance of work, recreation, reflection and rest.
- Concentrate on feeling positive. A good attitude toward yourself and others is a powerful asset.

MEDICATION (ADJUSTED FOR AGING)—Medicine is usually not necessary for this disorder.

ACTIVITY FOR OLDER PATIENTS
- No restrictions are necessary. Engage in a regular exercise program at least 3 times a week to reduce stress and maintain good overall fitness.
- See Appendix 20 regarding physical fitness for the active older adult.

FOOD & BEVERAGE
- No special diet or supplements are required. Eat a normal, well-balanced diet to provide the nutrients necessary for healthy hair growth.
- See Appendix 1 regarding good nutrition for people over 50.

FUTURE CONSIDERATIONS FOR THE AGING ADULT

POSSIBLE COMPLICATIONS—None are expected.

PROBABLE OUTCOME—Spontaneous recovery in 6 to 12 months.

PREVENTING RECURRENCE—There are no specific preventive measures.

CALL YOUR DOCTOR IF

- Hair loss doesn't improve in 4 months.
- Signs of infection (pain, redness, tenderness or swelling) begin at the site of hair loss.

TEMPERATURE, TOO LOW
(Hypothermia)

BASIC INFORMATION FOR OLDER ADULTS

DESCRIPTION—Hypothermia is a dangerous cooling of the body from exposure to cold air or water. Body parts involved: All major organ systems, as there is decreased blood flow through the kidneys and brain. (THIS IS AN EMERGENCY; SEEK MEDICAL CARE IMMEDIATELY!)

SPECIAL CONSIDERATIONS FOR AGING
- The temperature regulation mechanism (thalamus) becomes less efficient.
- Signs and symptoms may differ significantly from those listed below.
- The metabolism decreases.
- The amount of body fat decreases.
- Poor nutrition is more common.
- One's perception of cold diminishes.

SIGNS & SYMPTOMS
Early symptoms:
- Poor muscle coordination; mental confusion.
- Shivering and low body temperature (95F to 98F or 35C to 36.7C) measured rectally.
- Slow pulse; sleepiness.
Late symptoms:
- Rigid muscles; loss of consciousness.
- Temperature drop to 77F to 84F (25C to 28.9C).
- Purple fingers, toes and nail beds.

CAUSES & RISK FACTORS—Caused by prolonged exposure to cold temperatures, especially outdoors with a high wind-chill factor. Risk factors include:
- Thin or wet clothing.
- Slender body. Slender persons lose heat more rapidly than obese persons.
- Smoking, which decreases circulation to the extremities; excessive alcohol consumption.
- Mental impairment.
- Diseases that diminish activity, such as arthritis or Parkinson's disease; increase heat loss, such as inflammatory dermatitis or Paget's disease; or impair one's perception of cold, such as stroke or diabetes.

DOCTOR'S TREATMENT & DIAGNOSTIC TESTS
- Medical history and physical exam.
- Laboratory studies such as kidney function studies; temperature reading with a low-reading thermometer.
- Hospitalization. Arrange transportation to the nearest emergency center immediately.

HOME TREATMENT BY SELF OR CARE-GIVER

GENERAL INSTRUCTIONS
- *Note:* The victim may be confused and resist helpful measures.

- Call for emergency help at once.
- If you have access to shelter:
  Place the victim in bed and cover him or her with a blanket or an electric blanket set at normal body temperature.
  A warm (not hot) bath may be helpful; call the nearest emergency center for advice.
- If you are outdoors:
  Cover the victim with blankets or shield him or her from the wind.
- If possible, warm the victim with direct body heat.
- Do not warm the victim too quickly. This can cause abnormal heart rhythms which could be fatal.

MEDICATION (ADJUSTED FOR AGING)—The doctor may prescribe medicine to support the blood pressure if the victim's condition is critical.

ACTIVITY FOR OLDER PATIENTS—After treatment, normal activity should be resumed gradually.

FOOD & BEVERAGE—Don't give alcohol to a person with hypothermia. It is of no help and may be harmful.

FUTURE CONSIDERATIONS FOR THE AGING ADULT

POSSIBLE COMPLICATIONS—Shock; pneumonia; death.

PROBABLE OUTCOME—Sometimes fatal, depending on the length and amount of temperature loss. The chances of survival are excellent if the patient is conscious on arrival at the emergency center.

PREVENTING RECURRENCE
- Obtain warm housing and adequate clothing before winter.
- In cold weather, wear windproof clothing in many layers, including a scarf, hat and mittens.
- In rain, change to dry clothing as soon as possible.
- Keep moving to generate body heat.
- Don't leave your home during a severe winter storm.
- Don't skate or fish on ice unless you have determined that the ice is safe.
- Persons who are unable to care for themselves fully, such as the mentally impaired or alcoholic, should be visited or cared for during cold weather.

CALL YOUR DOCTOR IF

You observe symptoms of hypothermia in someone. *This is an emergency!*

TEMPOROMANDIBULAR JOINT SYNDROME
(TMJ; Myofascial Pain Dysfunction Syndrome, MPD)

BASIC INFORMATION FOR OLDER ADULTS

DESCRIPTION—TMJ is pain and inflammation in the temporomandibular joint (the joint on either side of the jaw that opens and closes the mouth) and the adjoining muscles. Body parts involved: The temporomandibular joint; facial muscles; sensory nerves.

SPECIAL CONSIDERATIONS FOR AGING
- The total weight and density of bone decrease.
- For many reasons, older people are less likely to maintain a good level of physical conditioning.
- Years of weight bearing cause wear and tear on the bones, joints and ligaments.
- Characteristic signs and symptoms of many disorders in older people are frequently changed or absent.
- Stress from any emotional cause—fear, worry, anxiety, sadness, loneliness or anger—affects all aspects of any illness or disorder.

SIGNS & SYMPTOMS
- Dull, aching pain on one side of the jaw (below the ear) that radiates to the temples, the back of the head and the jaw line.
- Tenderness of the muscles used to chew.
- "Clicking" or "popping" sounds when opening the mouth.
- Inability to open the jaw completely.
- Headache.

CAUSES & RISK FACTORS—Caused by grinding the teeth and contracting the jaw muscles in an unconscious attempt to:
- Relieve muscle tension caused by stress.
- Correct a faulty alignment ("bite") between the upper and lower jaws.

Risk factors include:
- Stress.
- Osteoarthritis.
- Jaw dislocation due to injury of the jaw, head or neck.

DOCTOR'S TREATMENT & DIAGNOSTIC TESTS
- Medical history and physical exam by a doctor or dentist.
- X-rays of the temporomandibular joint.
- Self-care instructions focused on the older patient.
- Your dentist may manufacture, fit and install a night-guard prosthesis to prevent tooth grinding while you are asleep. A night-guard prosthesis consists of removable splints that fit over the tops of the teeth to eliminate incorrect biting pressure.
- Psychotherapy or counseling, including biofeedback training, to help you learn new ways to cope with stress.

- Surgery to reconstruct the joint (in severe cases that do not respond to simpler measures).

HOME TREATMENT BY SELF OR CARE-GIVER

GENERAL INSTRUCTIONS
- Ice and/or moist heat may be of slight benefit in relieving the discomfort, but it will not cure the disorder.
- Massage the muscles.

MEDICATION (ADJUSTED FOR AGING)
- Your doctor may prescribe:
  Tranquilizers or muscle relaxants for a short time.
  Non-steroidal anti-inflammatory drugs.
- For minor pain, you may use non-prescription drugs such as aspirin or acetaminophen.
- *Note:* Adverse reactions and side effects may be more frequent and severe in older persons. Remind your doctor of any medicines you already take.

ACTIVITY FOR OLDER PATIENTS
- No restrictions are necessary.
- See Appendix 20 regarding physical fitness for the active older adult.

FOOD & BEVERAGE
- Eat a soft diet (see Appendix 11) until your symptoms subside.
- See Appendix 1 regarding good nutrition for people over 50.

FUTURE CONSIDERATIONS FOR THE AGING ADULT

POSSIBLE COMPLICATIONS—Without treatment, bone in the temporomandibular joint may erode and deteriorate.

PROBABLE OUTCOME—With treatment, the symptoms can be controlled and the behavior that produces the symptoms can be modified. A jaw misalignment can also be corrected.

PREVENTING RECURRENCE—Don't grind your teeth. Learn techniques for relaxing your muscles and relieving tension, such as biofeedback, meditation and exercise.

CALL YOUR DOCTOR IF

- You have symptoms of temporomandibular joint syndrome.
- New, unexplained symptoms develop. The drugs used in treatment may produce side effects.

TENDINITIS

BASIC INFORMATION FOR OLDER ADULTS

DESCRIPTION—Tendinitis is the painful inflammation of a tendon (ligament). Tendon fibers merge into muscle fibers. A typical skeletal muscle has a tendon on each end that attaches to bone. The force of a muscle contraction is transmitted through the tendon to produce movement. Body parts involved: The tendons; bones; joints.

SPECIAL CONSIDERATIONS FOR AGING
- Years of weight bearing cause wear and tear on the bones, joints and ligaments.
- Bone strength lessens.
- Muscle tone decreases.

SIGNS & SYMPTOMS
- Restricted movement, tenderness and swelling around the inflamed tendon. Common sites are the shoulder, elbow, Achilles' tendon and hamstring.
- Weakness in the tendon caused by calcium deposits that often accompany tendinitis.

CAUSES & RISK FACTORS
Causes include:
- Injury, usually from strenuous athletic activity.
- Musculoskeletal disorders, including congenital defects and rheumatism.
- Poor posture.

Risk factors include:
- Overuse of certain tendons and joints from participation in active competitive sports.
- Incorrect movement and strain during activity. For example, repeatedly holding and swinging a tennis racket incorrectly may cause tendinitis at the elbow (see Tennis Elbow in the Illnesses section).

DOCTOR'S TREATMENT & DIAGNOSTIC TESTS
- Medical history and physical exam.
- X-rays of the involved area.
- Ultrasound therapy (see Glossary).
- For mild cases, self-care instructions focused on the older patient.

HOME TREATMENT BY SELF OR CARE-GIVER

GENERAL INSTRUCTIONS—Treatment varies with the cause, severity and duration of the condition:
- If you have severe pain, stiffness and tenderness, relax completely with the injured area resting in a splint or on a pillow until the pain becomes more bearable.
- Apply ice packs to the affected area during the acute stage or after receiving injections (see Medication).
- When the pain diminishes, wear a sling or use crutches until the pain becomes bearable.

- After the acute phase, apply heat. Take hot showers, apply hot compresses, use a heat lamp or heating pad or rub in deep-heating ointment.
- If you have a shoulder injury, perform shoulder exercises that your doctor or physical therapist will give you. If done conscientiously, these exercises will help prevent stiffness and increase strength.
- Elastic bandages may help. Consult your doctor.

MEDICATION (ADJUSTED FOR AGING)
- Your doctor may prescribe: Anti-inflammatory drugs. Pain relievers. Injections of local anesthetics. Injections of cortisone into painful and calcified tendons. This reduces the pain and inflammation and allows movement, preventing a frozen joint.
- *Note:* Adverse reactions and side effects may be more frequent and severe in older persons. Remind your doctor of any medicines you already take.

ACTIVITY FOR OLDER PATIENTS
- Resume your normal activities as soon as your symptoms improve.
- See Appendix 20 regarding physical fitness for the active older adult.

FOOD & BEVERAGE
- No special diet is required.
- See Appendix 1 regarding good nutrition for people over 50.

FUTURE CONSIDERATIONS FOR THE AGING ADULT

POSSIBLE COMPLICATIONS—Large deposits of calcium in the inflamed tendon, leading to permanent impairment ("frozen joint").

PROBABLE OUTCOME—Usually curable with treatment and rest of the tendon. Allow 6 weeks for healing.

PREVENTING RECURRENCE
- Precondition your body and build up strength gradually for a sport before beginning it on a regular, competitive basis.
- Warm up before each workout.
- Learn the proper techniques for any sport you intend to play regularly.

CALL YOUR DOCTOR IF

- You have symptoms of tendinitis.
- The pain and swelling increase despite treatment.
- New, unexplained symptoms develop. The drugs used in treatment may produce side effects.

TENNIS ELBOW
(Epicondylitis)

BASIC INFORMATION FOR OLDER ADULTS

DESCRIPTION—Tennis elbow is an inflammation of bony areas of the elbow. Body parts involved: The elbow muscles, tendons and epicondyle (a bony prominence on the outside of the elbow where the muscles of the forearm attach to the bone of the upper arm).

SPECIAL CONSIDERATIONS FOR AGING
- Years of weight bearing cause wear and tear on the bones, joints and ligaments.
- Bone strength lessens.
- Muscle tone decreases.

SIGNS & SYMPTOMS
- Pain and tenderness over the epicondyle.
- A weak grip.
- Pain when twisting the hand and arm, as in using a screwdriver, lifting a heavy object or playing tennis.

CAUSES & RISK FACTORS—Caused by a partial tear of the tendon and the attached covering of the bone due to:
- Chronic stress on the tissues that attach the muscles of the forearm to the elbow.
- Sudden strain on the forearm.

Risk factors include:
- Occupations or hobbies that require strenuous forearm movement, such as mechanics, gardening or carpentry.
- Participation in sports that require strenuous forearm movement, such as tennis.
- Poor physical conditioning.

DOCTOR'S TREATMENT & DIAGNOSTIC TESTS
- Medical history and physical exam.
- X-rays of the elbow.
- Self-care instructions focused on the older patient.
- Physical therapy.
- Surgery (rare). Advancing age alone is not a deterrent.

HOME TREATMENT BY SELF OR CARE-GIVER

GENERAL INSTRUCTIONS
- Use heat to relieve the pain. Use warm soaks (see Appendix 18) or a heat lamp or soak in a whirlpool.
- You may receive diathermy (see Glossary), ultrasound (see Glossary) or massage treatments in your doctor's office or a physical therapy facility. These may bring quicker symptom relief and healing.
- You may need to wear a forearm splint to immobilize the elbow.

- Do the following exercise 3 or 4 times a day while wearing the splint: Stretch your arm, flex your wrist, then press the back of your hand against a wall. Hold for 1 minute.

MEDICATION (ADJUSTED FOR AGING)
- Your doctor may prescribe: Non-steroidal anti-inflammatory drugs to reduce inflammation. Injections of anesthetics or cortisone drugs. Cortisone reduces inflammation, and anesthetics temporarily relieve pain. Caution: Repeated injections may weaken the muscle ligament.
- *Note:* Adverse reactions and side effects may be more frequent and severe in older persons. Remind your doctor of any medicines you already take.

ACTIVITY FOR OLDER PATIENTS
- Don't repeat the activity that caused tennis elbow until the symptoms disappear. Then resume your normal activities gradually after proper conditioning.
- See Appendix 20 regarding physical fitness for the active older adult.

FOOD & BEVERAGE
- No special diet is required.
- See Appendix 1 regarding good nutrition for people over 50.

FUTURE CONSIDERATIONS FOR THE AGING ADULT

POSSIBLE COMPLICATIONS—Complete ligament tear, requiring surgery to repair.

PROBABLE OUTCOME—Usually curable, but treatment may require 3 to 6 months.

PREVENTING RECURRENCE
- Don't play sports such as tennis for long periods until you are in excellent condition. Take frequent rest periods.
- Do forearm conditioning exercises to build your strength gradually.
- Warm up slowly and completely before participating in sports—especially before competition.
- Use a tennis elbow strap when you resume normal activity after treatment.
- Consult a tennis instructor about your playing technique and the size of the grip on your racket.

CALL YOUR DOCTOR IF

- You have symptoms of tennis elbow.
- Your symptoms don't improve in 2 weeks despite treatment.
- New, unexplained symptoms develop. The drugs used in treatment may produce side effects.

TETANUS
(Lockjaw)

BASIC INFORMATION FOR OLDER ADULTS

DESCRIPTION—Tetanus is an infection in a wound or injury that causes severe muscle spasms. Tetanus is not contagious from person to person. Few cases occur in the U.S., but the majority of these cases occur in non-immunized people over age 50. Body parts involved: The injured tissue; the muscles throughout the body, especially the jaw, neck, back and abdomen.

SPECIAL CONSIDERATIONS FOR AGING
- The immune system becomes less effective, opening the way for viral, bacterial and other infections; malignancies; immune disorders; and allergies.
- The total state of well-being in many older people makes them increasingly susceptible to infections and impairs their ability to prevent infections from spreading.

SIGNS & SYMPTOMS
- Muscle pain, irritability and frequent, severe spasms.
- Severe swallowing difficulty.
- Fever.
- Difficulty using the chest muscles to breathe.
- Stiffness in the abdominal and back muscles.

CAUSES & RISK FACTORS—
Caused by a bacterium (*clostridium tetani*) that is present almost everywhere—especially in soil, manure or dust. The bacteria may enter through any break in the skin, including burns or puncture wounds. Toxins produced by the bacteria travel to nerves the that control muscle contraction, producing muscle spasms and seizures. The risk increases with:
- Diabetes mellitus.
- The lack of up-to-date tetanus immunizations.
- Warm, humid weather.
- Crowded or unsanitary living conditions.
- The use of street drugs administered with unclean needles and syringes.

DOCTOR'S TREATMENT & DIAGNOSTIC TESTS
- Medical history and physical exam.
- Surgery to remove the infected tissue.
- Hospitalization in a quiet, dark room. Treatment may include the use of breathing tubes, a respirator and 24-hour nursing care.
- Self-care instructions focused on the older patient.

HOME TREATMENT BY SELF OR CARE-GIVER

GENERAL INSTRUCTIONS—Provide the patient with reassurance and psychological support. Despite the seriousness of tetanus, patients are usually conscious.

MEDICATION (ADJUSTED FOR AGING)
- Your doctor may prescribe: Antitoxins to neutralize the nerve toxin. Muscle relaxants to control spasms. Sedatives to relieve anxiety.
- *Note:* Adverse reactions and side effects may be more frequent and severe in older persons. Remind your doctor of any medicines you already take.

ACTIVITY FOR OLDER PATIENTS
- During hospitalization, bed rest is necessary with as little disturbance as possible. During recovery, resume your normal activities gradually.
- See Appendix 20 regarding physical fitness for the active older adult.

FOOD & BEVERAGE
- During hospitalization, intravenous fluids will be necessary because of swallowing difficulty.
- See Appendix 1 regarding good nutrition for people over 50.

FUTURE CONSIDERATIONS FOR THE AGING ADULT

POSSIBLE COMPLICATIONS
- Pneumonia.
- Pressure sores.
- Irregular heartbeat.
- Respiratory paralysis and death.

PROBABLE OUTCOME—The death rate from tetanus is 40%. With early diagnosis and treatment, however, full recovery is likely. Allow 4 weeks for recovery.

PREVENTING RECURRENCE
- Obtain a tetanus immunization with boosters every 10 years afterwards. An additional booster shot may be necessary at the time of injury. Private doctors or local health departments may provide immunizations at little or no cost.
- Clean any wound carefully and use an antiseptic on it.

CALL YOUR DOCTOR IF

- You have symptoms of tetanus or observe them in someone else. Call immediately. *This is an emergency!*
- You or someone in your family needs basic or booster tetanus immunizations.
- You have a puncture wound or injury that breaks the skin and you have not had an immunization or booster in 5 years.
- New, unexplained symptoms develop. The drugs used in treatment may produce side effects.

THALASSEMIA
(Mediterranean Anemia; Hereditary Leptocytosis)

BASIC INFORMATION FOR OLDER ADULTS

DESCRIPTION—Thalassemia an inherited form of anemia in which the red blood cells contain less hemoglobin than normal. Body part involved: The blood.

SPECIAL CONSIDERATIONS FOR AGING—Older people have decreased reserve power for heart function, making symptoms more pronounced.

SIGNS & SYMPTOMS—The minor form may produce no symptoms, but when symptoms occur, they may include:
- Fatigue.
- Paleness.
- Breathlessness.
- Irregular heartbeat, especially with exertion.
- Bloody or dark urine.
- Jaundice (yellow skin and eyes).
- Leg ulcers.
- An enlarged spleen.

CAUSES & RISK FACTORS
Causes include:
- Destruction of abnormal blood cells in the spleen and other sites.
- Inadequate manufacture of normal amounts of hemoglobin-A.

Risk factors include:
- Poor nutrition, especially a diet likely to produce other anemias.
- Obesity.
- A family history of thalassemia.
- Genetic factors, including absence of the gene necessary to manufacture hemoglobin-A. The disorder first appeared in persons of Mediterranean heritage; it also affects people from the Middle East and Far East.

DOCTOR'S TREATMENT & DIAGNOSTIC TESTS
- Medical history and physical exam.
- Laboratory blood tests and bone marrow examinations.
- Self-care instructions focused on the older patient.
- Hospitalization for repeated transfusions as needed.

HOME TREATMENT BY SELF OR CARE-GIVER

GENERAL INSTRUCTIONS—The only treatment for thalassemia is periodic hospitalization for blood transfusions when the symptoms become disabling.

MEDICATION (ADJUSTED FOR AGING)
- Medicine is usually not necessary for this disorder. For minor pain, you may use nonprescription drugs such as acetaminophen.
- *Note:* Adverse reactions and side effects may be more frequent and severe in older persons. Remind your doctor of any medicines you already take.

ACTIVITY FOR OLDER PATIENTS
- After treatment, resume your normal activities as soon as possible.
- See Appendix 20 regarding physical fitness for the active older adult.

FOOD & BEVERAGE
- No special diet is required. Don't take iron supplements; they make the symptoms worse.
- See Appendix 1 regarding good nutrition for people over 50.

FUTURE CONSIDERATIONS FOR THE AGING ADULT

POSSIBLE COMPLICATIONS
- Many years of thalassemia produce gallstones.
- Transmission of blood-borne diseases.
- Repeated transfusions increase the risk of transfusion reaction or kidney damage due to thalassemia.

PROBABLE OUTCOME—Varies. This condition is currently considered incurable. However, the symptoms can be relieved or controlled. It usually causes death by early adulthood or middle age, depending on the severity of the symptoms. Some forms are consistent with a normal or nearly normal lifespan. Scientific research into causes and treatment continues, so there is hope for increasingly effective treatment and a cure.

PREVENTING RECURRENCE—Cannot be prevented at present, especially if the mother *and* the father have thalassemia or the thalassemia genetic trait.

CALL YOUR DOCTOR IF

- You have symptoms of anemia (fatigue, paleness, irregular heartbeat and breathlessness).
- New, unexplained symptoms develop. The drugs used in treatment may produce side effects.

THORACIC OUTLET OBSTRUCTION SYNDROME
(Cervical Rib Syndrome)

BASIC INFORMATION FOR OLDER ADULTS

DESCRIPTION—Thoracic outlet obstruction syndrome is characterized by pain and weakness from the compression of the nerves in the neck that affect the shoulders, arms and hands. Body parts involved: The nerves and blood vessels that supply the neck, shoulders, arms and hands.

SPECIAL CONSIDERATIONS FOR AGING
- Repair from injury or disease is complete and effective, but recovery takes longer in older people.
- 50% of people over 60 have x-ray evidence of narrowing of the coronary arteries, yet only 50% of those people have symptoms.
- Characteristic signs and symptoms of many disorders in older people are frequently changed or absent.

SIGNS & SYMPTOMS
- Pain, numbness and tingling in the neck, shoulders, arms and hands.
- Weakness in the arms and hands.
- Poor blood circulation characterized by coldness, swelling and blueness in the hands and fingers (rare).
- Absent pulse in the wrist when raising the arm and turning the head toward the opposite shoulder.

CAUSES & RISK FACTORS—The nerves and blood vessels that supply the shoulder, arms and hands start in the neck and pass as a bundle near the cervical ribs and the collarbone. Pressure on this nerve and bundle of blood vessels creates the symptoms. The pressure may be caused by:
- An extra rib in the lower neck or overdeveloped neck muscles.
- Muscle weakness and drooping in the shoulder.
- Holding the neck or arm in an abnormal position for a long time, as during surgery with general anesthesia.
- Injury from overextending the arm or shoulder.
- A tumor that has spread to the head and neck area from another part of the body.

Risk factors include:
- Recent unconsciousness from illness, injury or alcohol or drug use.
- Recent surgery with general anesthesia.
- Lifting and carrying heavy loads.

DOCTOR'S TREATMENT & DIAGNOSTIC TESTS
- Medical history and physical exam.
- X-rays of the neck and shoulder area to look for an extra cervical rib or a tumor.
- Surgery to relieve the pressure on the nerves and blood vessels (rare). Advancing age alone is not a deterrent.
- Exercise and physical therapy.
- Self-care instructions focused on the older patient.

HOME TREATMENT BY SELF OR CARE-GIVER

GENERAL INSTRUCTIONS
- Use hot showers or warm compresses to relieve the pain.
- Your doctor or physical therapist may recommend bracing the shoulder to improve your posture.
- Large-breasted women need to wear strong, supportive bras.

MEDICATION (ADJUSTED FOR AGING)—You may use non-prescription drugs such as acetaminophen or aspirin to relieve the pain. Medication cannot correct the underlying condition.

ACTIVITY FOR OLDER PATIENTS—Your doctor will prescribe physical therapy and exercises. Avoid physical activities that aggravate the condition.

FOOD & BEVERAGE—No special diet.

FUTURE CONSIDERATIONS FOR THE AGING ADULT

POSSIBLE COMPLICATIONS—If the disorder is caused by a tumor or an extra cervical rib, treatment may be unsuccessful. These can cause permanent numbness, loss of full arm or hand strength or gangrene in the fingers (rare).

PROBABLE OUTCOME—Usually curable in most patients with physical therapy or surgery.

PREVENTING RECURRENCE
- Avoid shoulder and neck injury whenever possible. Wear seat belts and use padded headrests in cars.
- Don't use mind-altering drugs or drink excessive amounts of alcohol.

CALL YOUR DOCTOR IF

- You have symptoms of thoracic outlet obstruction syndrome.
- Your symptoms don't improve in 2 weeks despite treatment.
- New, unexplained symptoms develop. The drugs used in treatment may produce side effects.

BASIC INFORMATION FOR OLDER ADULTS

DESCRIPTION—Thrombocytopenia is a reduction of the platelets in the blood, which reduces blood clotting and increases the risk of bleeding. Body part involved: The blood, which affects all body parts.

SPECIAL CONSIDERATIONS FOR AGING
- Unusual and unexpected reactions to drugs and medications are more likely.
- The immune system becomes less effective, opening the way for viral, bacterial and other infections; malignancies; immune disorders; and allergies.
- Decreased nutrition, common among chronically ill older people, increases the risk of any disease or disorder.
- Characteristic signs and symptoms of many disorders in older people are frequently changed or absent.

SIGNS & SYMPTOMS
- Abnormal bleeding in the mouth.
- A rash of pinpoint-sized dots that doesn't fade when the skin is pressed.
- Unexplained bruising.
- Spontaneous nosebleeds.
- Blood in the urine.
- Unexplained vaginal bleeding.
- Black, tarry stools.
- Signs of anemia (weakness, fatigue and paleness) if the bleeding is prolonged.

CAUSES & RISK FACTORS—The cause is frequently unknown. The following often precede the disorder:
- Allergies; virus infections.
- The use of medications such as non-steroidal anti-inflammatory drugs, tricyclic antidepressants, antihistamines and phenothiazines.
- Collagen disorders such as lupus erythematosus.
- Blood transfusions and surgery.
- Blood poisoning; liver disease.
- Radiation treatment or x-rays.
- An enlarged spleen from any cause.
- Uremia; scurvy; leukemia.
- Pernicious anemia; alcoholism.

Risk factors include:
- A family history of bleeding disorders.
- The use of any drug; poor nutrition.

DOCTOR'S TREATMENT & DIAGNOSTIC TESTS
- Medical history and physical exam.
- Laboratory blood studies.
- Hospitalization to transfuse platelets (sometimes).
- Self-care instructions focused on the older patient.

HOME TREATMENT BY SELF OR CARE-GIVER

GENERAL INSTRUCTIONS
- To stop bleeding at any accessible site, apply cold compresses or ice packs and pressure until the bleeding stops.
- Inform any doctor or dentist who treats you that you have thrombocytopenia.
- Avoid surgery, including dental surgery, unless it is essential.
- Avoid injections. If a shot is necessary, apply pressure continuously to the injection site for 5 minutes.
- Avoid injury whenever possible.

MEDICATION (ADJUSTED FOR AGING)
- Talk with your doctor about discontinuing all drugs, including non-prescription drugs (especially aspirin) and vitamins.
- Your doctor may prescribe cortisone drugs to reduce the body's autoimmune response.
- *Note:* Adverse reactions and side effects may be more frequent and severe in older persons. Remind your doctor of any medicines you already take.

ACTIVITY FOR OLDER PATIENTS
- Don't engage in contact sports.
- Avoid overexertion or dehydration.
- If your occupation involves a risk of injury, don't go to work until you are cured.
- See Appendix 20 regarding physical fitness for the active older adult.

FOOD & BEVERAGE
- No special diet is required.
- See Appendix 1 regarding good nutrition for people over 50.

FUTURE CONSIDERATIONS FOR THE AGING ADULT

POSSIBLE COMPLICATIONS—The spleen may enlarge and require surgical removal.

PROBABLE OUTCOME—Usually curable in 2 to 3 weeks if the cause can be treated.

PREVENTING RECURRENCE
- Avoid any medication which has lowered your platelet count in the past.
- Take only medications that are necessary.
- Eat a well-balanced diet.

CALL YOUR DOCTOR IF

- You have symptoms of thrombocytopenia.
- Any of the following occurs during treatment:
  Bleeding that can't be stopped.
  Enlargement of the abdomen.
  Black, tarry stools or vomit that looks like coffee grounds.
  A rash (described under Signs & Symptoms)—especially if fever is present.
- New, unexplained symptoms develop. The drugs used in treatment may produce side effects.

THROMBOPHLEBITIS, SUPERFICIAL
(Phlebitis; Phlebothrombosis)

BASIC INFORMATION FOR OLDER ADULTS

DESCRIPTION—Superficial thrombophlebitis is characterized by inflammation and small blood clots in a superficial vein and is usually caused by infection or injury. This type of inflammation seldom causes clots to break loose and flow in the bloodstream, as does deep-vein thrombosis. Body parts involved: The superficial veins, usually in the legs.

SPECIAL CONSIDERATIONS FOR AGING
- 50% of people over 60 have x-ray evidence of narrowing of the coronary arteries, yet only 50% of those people have symptoms.
- The immune system becomes less effective, opening the way for viral, bacterial and other infections; malignancies; immune disorders; and allergies.
- Characteristic signs and symptoms of many disorders in older people are frequently changed or absent.

SIGNS & SYMPTOMS
- A hard superficial vein (it feels like a cord).
- Redness, tenderness, swelling and pain in the affected area.
- Fever (sometimes).

CAUSES & RISK FACTORS—Caused by increased fibrin and clotting of the red blood cells in a vein due to:
- Injury to the vein's membrane lining from injections, which allows bacteria to enter.
- The spread of malignant blood cancer.
- The pooling of blood following surgery or prolonged bed rest.

Risk factors include:
- Illness with prolonged bed confinement.
- Smoking.

DOCTOR'S TREATMENT & DIAGNOSTIC TESTS
- Medical history and physical exam.
- Laboratory blood studies if the cause is not immediately apparent.
- Self-care instructions focused on the older patient.
- Minor surgery to close off the vein (sometimes).

OTHER—Repeated episodes may indicate pancreatic, lung or ovarian cancer.

HOME TREATMENT BY SELF OR CARE-GIVER

GENERAL INSTRUCTIONS
- Stop smoking.
- Wear elastic stockings or wrapped elastic bandages to hasten the blood flow through the veins, relieving the discomfort and helping prevent further clot formation. Don't

wear garters or knee-high hosiery.
- To relieve the pain, use wrapped soaks (see Appendix 18).

MEDICATION (ADJUSTED FOR AGING)
- Your doctor may prescribe: Non-steroidal anti-inflammatory drugs, including aspirin, to decrease the inflammation and pain. Antibiotics if bacterial infection is suspected (rare).
- *Note:* Adverse reactions and side effects may be more frequent and severe in older persons. Remind your doctor of any medicines you already take.

ACTIVITY FOR OLDER PATIENTS
- Bed rest with the affected limb elevated may be helpful for 1 or 2 days. Move your feet, ankles and legs often. When the inflammation begins to subside, resume your normal activities slowly. Rest often. Don't sit or stand for prolonged periods, and don't cross your legs.
- See Appendix 20 regarding physical fitness for the active older adult.

FOOD & BEVERAGE
- No special diet is required.
- See Appendix 1 regarding good nutrition for people over 50.

FUTURE CONSIDERATIONS FOR THE AGING ADULT

POSSIBLE COMPLICATIONS—Embolism, in which part of a clot breaks off and travels through the bloodstream, lodging in the lung or elsewhere (extremely rare).

PROBABLE OUTCOME—Usually curable in 2 weeks.

PREVENTING RECURRENCE
- Don't smoke.
- If you are confined to bed for any reason, move your legs as much as possible to prevent the pooling of blood in the veins.
- Don't use any drug intravenously if you can avoid it.

CALL YOUR DOCTOR IF

- You have symptoms of superficial thrombophlebitis.
- Any of the following occurs during treatment: A fever of 102F (38.9C) or higher. Intolerable pain. Coughing up blood. Shortness of breath. Chest pain.
- New, unexplained symptoms develop. The drugs used in treatment may produce side effects.

ILLNESSES & DISORDERS

THROMBOSIS, DEEP-VEIN

BASIC INFORMATION FOR OLDER ADULTS

DESCRIPTION—Deep-vein thrombosis is the formation of a blood clot inside a deep vein. It may partially or completely block the the blood flow or break off and travel to the lung (embolus). This is different from a clot in a superficial vein, where clots rarely break off. Body parts involved: Usually the lower legs (calves) or the lower abdomen, but occasionally other veins in the body.

SPECIAL CONSIDERATIONS FOR AGING
- The skin becomes thinner.
- Characteristic signs and symptoms of many disorders in older people are frequently changed or absent.

SIGNS & SYMPTOMS
- Swelling and pain in the area drained by the vein, usually the ankle, calf or thigh. The swelling in the leg includes everything below the clot, extending to the toes.
- Tenderness and redness of the affected parts.
- Soreness or pain when walking. The soreness does not disappear with rest.
- Pain when raising the leg and flexing the foot (sometimes).
- Fever (sometimes); increased heartbeat (sometimes).

CAUSES & RISK FACTORS—Caused by the pooling of blood in the vein, which triggers blood-clotting mechanisms. The pooling may occur after prolonged bed rest following surgery or following illness, such as a heart attack, stroke or bone fracture. The risk increases with:
- Obesity; smoking.
- The use of estrogen for any reason, such as replacement therapy after menopause. This is especially hazardous if estrogen use is combined with smoking.

DOCTOR'S TREATMENT & DIAGNOSTIC TESTS
- Medical history and physical exam.
- Laboratory studies such as ultrasound, radioactive fibrinogen and prothrombin time (see Glossary for all); x-rays of the veins after dye is injected into a foot vein.
- Hospitalization for anticoagulant injections.
- Self-care instructions focused on the older patient.

HOME TREATMENT BY SELF OR CARE-GIVER

GENERAL INSTRUCTIONS—The following suggestions apply after hospitalization or if the condition can be treated safely at home:
- Wear fitted elastic stockings or wrapped elastic bandages, but don't wear garters or knee-high hosiery.
- Don't cross your legs or ankles while sitting, lying in bed or traveling.
- Elevate your feet higher than your hips when sitting for long periods.
- Elevate the foot of your bed.

MEDICATION (ADJUSTED FOR AGING)
- After hospitalization, your doctor may prescribe oral anticoagulant drugs such as coumadin. To minimize the danger of pulmonary embolism, blood tests to monitor the anticoagulant level are mandatory. Oral anticoagulants may be necessary for up to 6 months.
- *Note:* Adverse reactions and side effects may be more frequent and severe in older persons. Remind your doctor of any medicines you already take.

ACTIVITY FOR OLDER PATIENTS
- Rest in bed until all signs of inflammation have disappeared. While resting, make it a habit to move your legs, bend your ankles and wiggle your toes.
- See Appendix 20 regarding physical fitness for the active older adult.

FOOD & BEVERAGE
- No special diet is required.
- If you are overweight, lose weight. See Appendix 10 for a reducing diet.

FUTURE CONSIDERATIONS FOR THE AGING ADULT

POSSIBLE COMPLICATIONS—Pulmonary embolism, in which the clot breaks away and travels to the lung. The lung's blood supply is blocked, causing the affected lung tissue to die.

PROBABLE OUTCOME—Usually curable with anticoagulant treatment if pulmonary embolism can be avoided.

PREVENTING RECURRENCE
- Avoid prolonged bed rest during illnesses. Start moving the lower limbs as soon as possible after any surgical procedure or during any illness requiring bed confinement.
- On long auto or airplane trips, exercise your legs at least every 1 or 2 hours.
- Stop smoking, especially if you take estrogen for any purpose.

CALL YOUR DOCTOR IF

- You have symptoms of deep-vein thrombosis.
- Any of the following occurs during treatment:
  Unexpected bleeding anywhere.
  Chest pain.
  Coughing up blood.
  Shortness of breath.
  Continued or increased swelling and pain despite treatment.
- New, unexplained symptoms develop. The drugs used in treatment may produce side effects.

THROMBOSIS & EMBOLUS, ARTERIAL

BASIC INFORMATION FOR OLDER ADULTS

DESCRIPTION—Arterial thrombosis is the formation of a blood clot in an artery (thrombosis) that may travel to distant organs (embolus). Body parts involved: The large or medium arteries anywhere in the body, especially the arteries in the neck or those to the brain, intestines, legs, arms or kidneys. (THIS IS AN EMERGENCY; SEEK MEDICAL CARE IMMEDIATELY!)

SPECIAL CONSIDERATIONS FOR AGING
- 50% of people over 60 have x-ray evidence of narrowing of the coronary arteries, yet only 50% of those people have symptoms.
- Characteristic signs and symptoms of many disorders are frequently changed or absent.

SIGNS & SYMPTOMS—The following depend on where the embolus lodges:
- Brain—Temporary blindness, speaking difficulty, partial paralysis, hearing loss, headache and dizziness.
- Extremities—Pain in the arm or calf after exercise (subsides with rest); weakness, numbness, burning and tingling sensations; weak or absent pulse beyond the blocked blood flow. These symptoms subside with rest.
- Intestines—Abdominal pain, nausea, vomiting and shock.

CAUSES & RISK FACTORS—Clots may form with any condition that damages the smooth lining of the heart or that of a blood vessel. As the clot grows, small or large portions break away and are carried by the bloodstream to the brain, abdomen, extremities or other areas. Conditions that damage the blood vessel lining include atherosclerosis (hardening of the arteries), injury to a blood vessel from accident or surgery, heart valve disease, heat attack and atrial fibrillation. Risk factors include:
- Smoking; high blood pressure; diabetes mellitus.
- Previous transient ischemic attacks.

DOCTOR'S TREATMENT & DIAGNOSTIC TESTS
- Medical history and physical exam.
- Laboratory studies of blood clotting and blood flow; x-rays of the arteries (angiography) and ECG (see Glossary for both).
- Self-care instructions focused on the older patient.
- Surgery to repair or replace damaged blood vessels or to remove an embolus by suction or bypass. Advancing age alone is not a deterrent.

HOME TREATMENT BY SELF OR CARE-GIVER

GENERAL INSTRUCTIONS—Follow the suggestions under Activity for Older Patients and Food & Beverage to maintain a healthy lifestyle.

MEDICATION (ADJUSTED FOR AGING)
- Your doctor may prescribe:
  Anticoagulants to thin the blood and reduce the chance of embolus.
  Aspirin (1 tablet a day). This has been shown to reduce the chance of small clots to the brain in men over 45.
  Vasodilators to widen the blood vessels.
- *Note:* Adverse reactions and side effects may be more frequent and severe in older persons. Remind your doctor of any medicines you already take.

ACTIVITY FOR OLDER PATIENTS
- Complete rest is necessary until the circulation is re-established by surgery or other treatment.
- See Appendix 20 regarding physical fitness for the active older adult.

FOOD & BEVERAGE
- No special diet is required during recovery. However, atherosclerosis and diabetes require dietary control.
- See Appendix 1 regarding good nutrition for people over 50.

FUTURE CONSIDERATIONS FOR THE AGING ADULT

POSSIBLE COMPLICATIONS—Tissue death or gangrene in the cells deprived of oxygen by a clot.

PROBABLE OUTCOME—Depends on the organs affected, the size of the affected blood vessel and the size of the embolus. Clots in the extremities can be removed with surgery, relieving the symptoms. Clots to the brain, kidney and intestines may cause death or permanent disability before they can be removed.

PREVENTING RECURRENCE
- Follow the suggestions for preventing atherosclerosis under that heading in the Illnesses section.
- If you have high blood pressure or diabetes mellitus, adhere to your treatment program to control the disease.
- Take anticoagulant drugs for a short time after injury or surgery to prevent blood clots.
- Exercise regularly (see Appendix 20) to keep the blood vessels healthy.

CALL YOUR DOCTOR IF

- You have symptoms of arterial thrombosis or embolus. *This is an emergency!*
- The symptoms return after surgery.
- New, unexplained symptoms develop. The drugs used in treatment may produce side effects.

THRUSH
(Oral Thrush)

BASIC INFORMATION FOR OLDER ADULTS

DESCRIPTION—Thrush is a common fungus infection of the mouth that frequently infects denture wearers. Body parts involved: The mouth; gums; tongue; soft palate; cheeks; lips.

SPECIAL CONSIDERATIONS FOR AGING
- The immune system becomes less effective, opening the way for viral, bacterial and other infections; malignancies; immune disorders; and allergies.
- Decreased nutrition increases the risk of infections.
- Characteristic signs and symptoms of many disorders in older people are frequently changed or absent.

SIGNS & SYMPTOMS—Patches appear in the mouth with the following characteristics:
- The patches are white to creamy yellow and slightly raised. They are similar to milk curds, but they don't wipe off.
- The patches are not painful unless they are rubbed off. Then they leave small, painful ulcers.
- The mouth is dry.

CAUSES & RISK FACTORS—Caused by a fungus called *candida albicans,* which may develop from treatment with antibiotics. This may upset the natural balance of organisms in the mouth and allow thrush to develop. Risk factors include:
- Poor nutrition.
- Illness that has lowered resistance.
- AIDS.
- Diabetes.
- Irritation from dentures.
- The use of immunosuppressive drugs.

DOCTOR'S TREATMENT & DIAGNOSTIC TESTS
- Medical history and physical exam.
- Culture of material from the white patches to confirm the diagnosis.
- Self-care instructions focused on the older patient.

HOME TREATMENT BY SELF OR CARE-GIVER

GENERAL INSTRUCTIONS
- To avoid transmitting thrush to others, boil your eating utensils or use disposable items. Boil anything that touches your mouth or saliva.
- Rinse your mouth with a salt solution (1/2 teaspoon salt to 8 ounces water) 3 times a day or more after eating.
- Clean your dentures carefully because they can be contaminated with the fungus.

MEDICATION (ADJUSTED FOR AGING)
- Gently swab patches of thrush in the mouth with antiseptic mouthwash or non-prescription 1% gentian violet solution.
- If these simple medicines don't cure the infection, your doctor may prescribe an antifungal drug to apply to the patches.
- *Note:* Adverse reactions and side effects may be more frequent and severe in older persons. Remind your doctor of any medicines you already take.

ACTIVITY FOR OLDER PATIENTS
- No restrictions are necessary.
- See Appendix 20 regarding physical fitness for the active older adult.

FOOD & BEVERAGE
- Maintain an adequate fluid intake with milk, liquid gelatin, ice cream, custard, water, tea or other beverages and foods that are easy to swallow. Use a straw for drinking if the patches are painful. Once your symptoms disappear, return to a regular diet.
- See Appendix 1 regarding good nutrition for people over 50.

FUTURE CONSIDERATIONS FOR THE AGING ADULT

POSSIBLE COMPLICATIONS—Can spread to the vagina, skin, larynx, gastrointestinal tract or respiratory system.

PROBABLE OUTCOME—Treatment usually clears this infection in 3 days. It is not dangerous or serious, but it has a tendency to recur.

PREVENTING RECURRENCE
- If you have had thrush and must take antibiotics, drink buttermilk or eat yogurt during treatment to replenish helpful bacteria in the digestive tract.
- See your dentist about poor-fitting or problem dentures.

CALL YOUR DOCTOR IF

- You experience unexplained weight loss.
- A fever develops.
- Lesions appear on the skin or vagina.
- You develop signs of a secondary bacterial infection (pain, redness, tenderness, swelling and sometimes fever) in your mouth.
- New, unexplained symptoms develop. The drugs used in treatment may produce side effects.

THYROID, OVERACTIVE
(Hyperthyroidism; Thyrotoxicosis; Toxic Goiter)

BASIC INFORMATION FOR OLDER ADULTS

DESCRIPTION—Hyperthyroidism is the over-activity of the thyroid, an endocrine gland that regulates all body functions. Body parts involved: The thyroid gland, a hormone-producing organ at the base of the neck next to the trachea (windpipe), and most other body organs, especially the endocrine system, which includes the pituitary gland, parathyroid glands, pancreas, adrenal glands and ovaries or testicles.

SPECIAL CONSIDERATIONS FOR AGING—Usual signs and symptoms may be absent and be replaced by symptoms of confusion, dizziness, failure to thrive, falling, incontinence, increasing dementia, refusal to eat or drink, weight loss, depression, paranoia, hypochondriasis, psychosis or threats of suicide.

SIGNS & SYMPTOMS
- Hyperactivity.
- Feeling warm or hot all the time.
- Tremors.
- Sweating.
- Itching skin.
- Pounding, rapid, irregular heartbeat.
- Weight loss despite overeating.
- Marked anxiety and restlessness.
- Sleeplessness.
- Fatigue and weakness.
- Protruding eyes (exophthalmos) and double vision (sometimes).
- Diarrhea (sometimes).
- Hair loss (sometimes).
- Goiter (sometimes).

CAUSES & RISK FACTORS
Causes include:
- Grave's disease.
- Thyroid nodules or tumors.
- Thyroid infection or inflammation (goiter).
- Pituitary disorders.
- Ovarian disorders.
Risk factors include:
- A family history of hyperthyroidism.
- Stress.

DOCTOR'S TREATMENT & DIAGNOSTIC TESTS
- Medical history and physical exam.
- Laboratory blood studies, including radioimmunoassays (see Glossary).
- ECG (see Glossary).
- Self-care instructions focused on the older patient.
- Surgery to remove part of the thyroid if medication does not control the disorder. Advancing age alone is not a deterrent.

HOME TREATMENT BY SELF OR CARE-GIVER

GENERAL INSTRUCTIONS—Since this condition develops gradually, the symptoms may be difficult to recognize. If your family members and friends mention changes in your behavior or appearance, consult your doctor.

MEDICATION (ADJUSTED FOR AGING)
- Your doctor may prescribe:
  Antithyroid drugs to depress thyroid activity.
  Beta-adrenergic blockers to decrease a rapid heartbeat.
  Radioactive iodine, which selectively destroys thyroid cells.
- *Note:* Adverse reactions and side effects may be more frequent and severe in older persons. Remind your doctor of any medicines you already take.

ACTIVITY FOR OLDER PATIENTS
- Rest in bed as much as possible until the disorder is cured.
- Ask your doctor to recommend activity levels as you adjust to the medication and improve.

FOOD & BEVERAGE
- Eat a diet that is high in protein to replace tissue lost from thyroid overactivity.
- See Appendix 1 regarding good nutrition for people over 50.

FUTURE CONSIDERATIONS FOR THE AGING ADULT

POSSIBLE COMPLICATIONS
- Congestive heart failure.
- "Thyroid storm," a sudden worsening of all symptoms. *This is a life-threatening emergency!*
- Misdiagnosis as a psychiatric anxiety reaction.

PROBABLE OUTCOME—Usually curable with medication or surgery. Allow 6 months of treatment for the condition to stabilize. Some forms may return to normal without treatment.

PREVENTING RECURRENCE—There are no specific preventive measures.

CALL YOUR DOCTOR IF

- You have symptoms of overactive thyroid.
- The symptoms worsen suddenly, especially after surgery.
- New, unexplained symptoms develop. The drugs used in treatment may produce side effects.

THYROID TUMOR

BASIC INFORMATION FOR OLDER ADULTS

DESCRIPTION—A thyroid tumor is a benign or malignant thyroid nodule. Benign tumors are unlikely to spread to other body parts. These growths may be cystic or solid (thyroid adenoma). Malignant thyroid nodules can spread and threaten life. Body part involved: The thyroid gland, a hormone-producing organ at the base of the neck next to the trachea (windpipe).

SPECIAL CONSIDERATIONS FOR AGING
- The immune system becomes less effective, opening the way for viral, bacterial and other infections; malignancies; immune disorders; and allergies.
- Malignant diseases (especially in the colon, lung and breast) represent difficult-to-diagnose problems.
- Cancerous growth tends to be somewhat faster.
- Stress from any emotional cause—fear, worry, anxiety, sadness, loneliness or anger—affects all aspects of any illness or disorder.

SIGNS & SYMPTOMS
- A swelling or lump in the thyroid gland.
- Pain and tenderness in the thyroid gland.
- Swallowing difficulty; hoarseness.
- Breathing difficulty (rare).
- Symptoms of underactive thyroid or overactive thyroid (both described in the Illnesses section).
The early symptoms of both benign and malignant thyroid tumors are the same.

CAUSES & RISK FACTORS—The cause is
unknown. The risk increases with:
- Radiation treatment during childhood—even in small doses—to the head, neck and upper chest.
- A family history of thyroid tumors.

DOCTOR'S TREATMENT & DIAGNOSTIC TESTS
- Medical history and physical exam.
- Laboratory tests such as radioactive iodine uptake studies, a CAT scan (see Glossary for both) and blood studies of thyroid function.
- Biopsy (see Glossary).
- Home care instructions after diagnosis.
- Surgery to aspirate a cystic tumor or to remove a solid tumor and the affected lobe of the thyroid. Advancing age alone is not a deterrent.
- Radioactive iodine treatment (see Glossary).
- Speech therapy if the voice is affected after surgery.
- Self-care instructions focused on the older patient.

HOME TREATMENT BY SELF OR CARE-GIVER

GENERAL INSTRUCTIONS
- For an explanation of surgery and postoperative care, see Thyroid Gland Removal in the Surgeries section.

- If you lose your voice, special equipment is available from the telephone company and other agencies to assist you with speech.
- After thyroid surgery, when rising from a lying to a sitting position, put a pillow under your head and support it with your hands to prevent neck muscle strain.

MEDICATION (ADJUSTED FOR AGING)
- Your doctor may prescribe:
  Antithyroid medications *or* replacement thyroid hormone.
  Radioactive iodine to treat the cancer.
  Pain relievers.
- *Note:* Adverse reactions and side effects may be more frequent and severe in older persons. Remind your doctor of any medicines you already take.

ACTIVITY FOR OLDER PATIENTS
- Resume your normal activities as soon as your symptoms improve after surgery.
- See Appendix 20 regarding physical fitness for the active older adult.

FOOD & BEVERAGE
- No special diet is required.
- See Appendix 1 regarding good nutrition for people over 50.

FUTURE CONSIDERATIONS FOR THE AGING ADULT

POSSIBLE COMPLICATIONS
- Spread of a malignant tumor to adjacent parts requiring radical surgery to remove the lymph nodes and muscles of one side of the neck.
- Hypothyroidism or hypoparathyroidism caused by inadvertent injury to the thyroid or parathyroid glands during surgery.
- Permanent hoarseness and loss of voice following surgery for some thyroid cancers.

PROBABLE OUTCOME—Usually curable with surgery or a combination of surgery and radioactive iodine treatment.

PREVENTING RECURRENCE—Avoid radiation treatments to the neck for acne, tonsillitis, an enlarged thymus gland or other minor conditions.

CALL YOUR DOCTOR IF

- You have symptoms of thyroid nodules or thyroid enlargement.
- Any of the following occurs after surgery:
  Symptoms of hypothyroidism (fatigue, puffy face, rapid weight gain, coarse hair and decreased sex drive).
  Bleeding, pain or swelling at the surgical site.
  Fever; twitching muscles.
  Breathing difficulty.
- New, unexplained symptoms develop. The drugs used in treatment may produce side effects.

THYROID, UNDERACTIVE
(Hypothyroidism)

BASIC INFORMATION FOR OLDER ADULTS

DESCRIPTION—Hypothyroidism is thyroid hormone deficiency due to an underactive thyroid gland. Body parts involved: The thyroid gland, a hormone-producing organ at the base of the neck next to the trachea (windpipe); endocrine system; pituitary gland.

SPECIAL CONSIDERATIONS FOR AGING—Usual signs and symptoms may be absent and be replaced by symptoms of confusion, dizziness, failure to thrive, falling, incontinence, increasing dementia, refusal to eat or drink, weight loss, depression, paranoia, hypochondriasis, psychosis or threats of suicide.

SIGNS & SYMPTOMS—It is unlikely that one person will have all the following symptoms, but most will have several:
- Decreased tolerance for cold.
- Decreased sweating.
- Decreased appetite.
- Constipation; chest pain.
- Coarse or slow-growing hair.
- Slow, rapid or irregular heartbeat.
- Weight gain or extreme thinness.
- Placidity or nervousness.
- Sleepiness or insomnia.
- Mental impairment, including depression, psychosis or poor memory.
- Fluid retention, especially around the eyes.
- Dull facial expression and droopy eyelids.
- Coarse skin; anemia.
- Decreased tolerance for medication.
- Decreased sex drive and infertility.
- Numbness and tingling in the hands and feet.
- Deepened or hoarse voice.

CAUSES & RISK FACTORS—The cause is sometimes unknown. Following are the most common known causes:
- Autoimmune disease, in which the body's immune system functions abnormally and attacks the thyroid gland.
- Radioactive iodine treatment.
- Surgery for overactive thyroid (hyperthyroidism).
- Iodine deficiency in the diet.
- Decreased activity of the pituitary gland, which secretes a thyroid-stimulating hormone.
- The use of drugs, such as lithium, that may depress thyroid function.
- Natural substances found in some foods, such as rutabagas, cabbage and cranberries.
Risk factors include:
- Obesity; x-ray treatments.
- Surgery for an overactive thyroid (hyperthyroidism).

DOCTOR'S TREATMENT & DIAGNOSTIC TESTS
- Medical history and physical exam.
- Laboratory blood studies of the thyroid hormones.

Lab studies can confirm the diagnosis of hypothyroidism, but they cannot indicate how much replacement therapy is needed.
- Self-care instructions focused on the older patient.

HOME TREATMENT BY SELF OR CARE-GIVER

GENERAL INSTRUCTIONS—No special instructions except those listed under other headings.

MEDICATION (ADJUSTED FOR AGING)
- Your doctor will prescribe thyroid replacement hormones. The dosages will be increased gradually until full replacement levels are reached. This may take 1 to 2 months.
- *Note:* Adverse reactions and side effects may be more frequent and severe in older persons. Remind your doctor of any medicines you already take.

ACTIVITY FOR OLDER PATIENTS
- No restrictions are necessary.
- See Appendix 20 regarding physical fitness for the active older adult.

FOOD & BEVERAGE
- No special diet is required.
- See Appendix 1 regarding good nutrition for people over 50.

FUTURE CONSIDERATIONS FOR THE AGING ADULT

POSSIBLE COMPLICATIONS—Without treatment, the symptoms will continue.

PROBABLE OUTCOME—Usually curable with careful thyroid replacement therapy. The goal of treatment is to provide the body with enough thyroid substance for efficient body function. Medical evaluation may be necessary for several months to establish the correct dose of thyroid replacement. The usual result is a return to robust good health.

PREVENTING RECURRENCE
- Use iodized salt.
- Take replacement thyroid for life after thyroid surgery or destruction of the thyroid gland by radiation treatment.

CALL YOUR DOCTOR IF

- You have symptoms of an underactive thyroid.
- The symptoms don't improve within 3 weeks after treatment begins.
- New, unexplained symptoms develop. The drugs used in treatment may produce side effects.

THYROIDITIS

BASIC INFORMATION FOR OLDER ADULTS

DESCRIPTION—Thyroiditis is an inflammation of the thyroid gland. Body part involved: The thyroid gland, a hormone-producing organ at the base of the neck next to the trachea (windpipe).

SPECIAL CONSIDERATIONS FOR AGING
- The immune system becomes less effective, opening the way for viral, bacterial and other infections; malignancies; immune disorders; and allergies.
- Usual signs and symptoms may be absent and be replaced by symptoms of confusion, dizziness, failure to thrive, falling, incontinence, increasing dementia, refusal to eat or drink, weight loss, depression, paranoia, hypochondriasis, psychosis or threats of suicide.
- Decreased nutrition, common among chronically ill older people, increases the risk of any disease or disorder.
- Stress from any emotional cause—fear, worry, anxiety, sadness, loneliness or anger—affects all aspects of any illness or disorder.

SIGNS & SYMPTOMS
- An enlarged, painful, tender thyroid gland.
- Fever.
- Pain in the jaw or ears (sometimes).
- Hyperthyroidism (rapid heartbeat, nervousness, tremor and rapid weight loss).

CAUSES & RISK FACTORS—Caused by a disorder of the autoimmune system, accompanied by one of the following:
- Various viruses, such as mumps or influenza.
- Rheumatoid arthritis.
- Bacterial infection of the thyroid gland (rare).
Risk factors include:
- Recent illness, such as tuberculosis or any infection.
- A family history of thyroiditis.
- Previous thyroid disorders.

DOCTOR'S TREATMENT & DIAGNOSTIC TESTS
- Medical history and physical exam.
- Laboratory blood counts and tests of thyroid function.
- Self-care instructions focused on the older patient.
- Consultation with an endocrinologist may be valuable.
- Hospitalization (rare).
- Surgery to relieve pressure on the adjacent areas of the neck or to drain an abscess (rare). Advancing age alone is not a deterrent.

HOME TREATMENT BY SELF OR CARE-GIVER

GENERAL INSTRUCTIONS—No specific instructions except those listed under other headings.

MEDICATION (ADJUSTED FOR AGING)
- Your doctor may prescribe:
  Antithyroid medication or thyroid replacement hormones, depending on the activity of your thyroid hormones.
  Beta-adrenergic blockers to suppress the symptoms of an overactive thyroid.
  Antibiotics to fight infection if necessary.
  Cortisone drugs to decrease the inflammation (rare).
  Aspirin in high doses to help the inflammation subside.
- *Note:* Adverse reactions and side effects may be more frequent and severe in older persons. Remind your doctor of any medicines you already take.

ACTIVITY FOR OLDER PATIENTS
- Resume your normal activities as soon as your symptoms improve.
- See Appendix 20 regarding physical fitness for the active older adult.

FOOD & BEVERAGE
- No special diet is required.
- See Appendix 1 regarding good nutrition for people over 50.

FUTURE CONSIDERATIONS FOR THE AGING ADULT

POSSIBLE COMPLICATIONS—Permanent loss of thyroid function requiring lifelong thyroid hormone replacement.

PROBABLE OUTCOME—Usually curable with treatment. Some persons recover spontaneously. Regular medical follow-up is recommended after the condition is apparently cured.

PREVENTING RECURRENCE—There are no specific preventive measures.

CALL YOUR DOCTOR IF

- You have symptoms of thyroiditis.
- Any of the following occurs during treatment: Fever and redness of the thyroid gland. Lethargy.
- New, unexplained symptoms develop. The drugs used in treatment may produce side effects.

TIC DOULOUREUX
(Trigeminal Neuralgia)

BASIC INFORMATION FOR OLDER ADULTS

DESCRIPTION—Tic douloureux is a nerve condition that causes brief, but often severe, face pain. Tic douloureux is more common in middle and later life. Body parts involved: The nerve branches from the trigeminal or 5th cranial nerve (the nerve from the brain that supplies sensation to the face, scalp, teeth, mouth and nose).

SPECIAL CONSIDERATIONS FOR AGING
- The immune system becomes less effective, opening the way for viral, bacterial and other infections; malignancies; immune disorders; and allergies.
- Decreased nutrition, common among chronically ill older people, increases the risk of any disease or disorder.
- Neurological diseases become more likely.
- The blood vessels nourishing the brain are less healthy. They become thicker and lose their elasticity.

SIGNS & SYMPTOMS—Severe face pain, often described as "jabbing" or "searing." The pain is often triggered by touching or stroking the face, brushing the teeth, shaving, chewing or exposure to wind. Bouts of pain usually last 1 to 15 minutes. Attacks may occur several times a day or may disappear for weeks or months. Between bouts, there is little or no discomfort.

CAUSES & RISK FACTORS
Causes include:
- Pressure on the nerve from adjacent blood vessels (sometimes).
- Unknown (often).
The risk increases with multiple sclerosis.

DOCTOR'S TREATMENT & DIAGNOSTIC TESTS
- Medical history and physical exam.
- X-rays or CT scan (see Glossary) of the head to rule out other conditions, such as brain tumor.
- Self-care instructions focused on the older patient.
- Surgery to relieve pressure on the nerve if medication is unsuccessful.
- Nerve destruction by electrocoagulation or ultrasound treatments (high-frequency sound waves).

HOME TREATMENT BY SELF OR CARE-GIVER

GENERAL INSTRUCTIONS
- Following are suggestions for ways to prevent sudden pain:
  Avoid blasts of hot or cold air.
  Chew on the unaffected side of the mouth.
  Grow a beard.
- Maintain good oral health with dental checkups at least twice a year.

MEDICATION (ADJUSTED FOR AGING)
- Your doctor may prescribe anticonvulsant medication to prevent painful attacks.
- *Note:* Adverse reactions and side effects may be more frequent and severe in older persons. Remind your doctor of any medicines you already take.

ACTIVITY FOR OLDER PATIENTS
- No restrictions are necessary.
- See Appendix 20 regarding physical fitness for the active older adult.

FOOD & BEVERAGE
- No special diet is required.
- See Appendix 1 regarding good nutrition for people over 50.

FUTURE CONSIDERATIONS FOR THE AGING ADULT

POSSIBLE COMPLICATIONS
- Interference with normal activities due to frequent severe episodes of pain.
- Addiction to analgesics.

PROBABLE OUTCOME—Most patients obtain pain relief with anticonvulsant medication. Destruction of the nerve by electrocoagulation will relieve the pain but cause annoying numbness. Surgery will relieve the pain, but it often returns within 5 to 10 years when the nerves regenerate.

PREVENTING RECURRENCE—There are no specific preventive measures.

CALL YOUR DOCTOR IF

- You have symptoms of tic douloureux.
- New, unexplained symptoms develop. The drugs used in treatment may produce side effects.

TOENAIL, INGROWN

BASIC INFORMATION FOR OLDER ADULTS

DESCRIPTION—Ingrown toenail is a disorder in which the sharp edge of a toenail grows into the flesh of the toe, usually the great (big) toe. Body parts involved: The toes.

SPECIAL CONSIDERATIONS FOR AGING
- The immune system becomes less effective, opening the way for viral, bacterial and other infections; malignancies; immune disorders; and allergies.
- Decreased nutrition, common among chronically ill older people, increases the risk of any disease or disorder.

SIGNS & SYMPTOMS—Pain, tenderness, redness, swelling and heat in the toe where the sharp nail edge pierces the surrounding fold of tissue. Once the tissue surrounding the nail becomes inflamed, infection usually develops in the injured area.

CAUSES & RISK FACTORS—An ingrown toenail is likely to accompany one of the following conditions:
- The nail is more curved than normal.
- The toenail is clipped back too far, allowing tissue to grow up over it.
- The shoes fit poorly, forcing the toe of the shoe against the nail and the surrounding tissue.
- The person participates in activities that require sudden stops ("toe jamming").

DOCTOR'S TREATMENT & DIAGNOSTIC TESTS
- Medical history and physical exam.
- Self-care instructions focused on the older patient.
- Surgery to remove the nail.

HOME TREATMENT BY SELF OR CARE-GIVER

GENERAL INSTRUCTIONS—The following home treatment is appropriate either before or after surgery:
- Use immersion soaks (see Appendix 18).
- Lift the nail corners free of surrounding inflamed tissue by wedging a small piece of cotton under the nail around the edges. Protect the inflamed tissue from further injury.
- If you have trouble cutting your toenails, get someone to do it for you.

MEDICATION (ADJUSTED FOR AGING)
- Your doctor may prescribe antibiotics to fight the infection.
- *Note:* Adverse reactions and side effects may be more frequent and severe in older persons. Remind your doctor of any medicines you already take.

ACTIVITY FOR OLDER PATIENTS
- Resume your normal activities as soon as your symptoms improve. You may need to wear a shoe with the toe cut out until the toe heals.
- See Appendix 20 regarding physical fitness for the active older adult.

FOOD & BEVERAGE
- No special diet is required.
- See Appendix 1 regarding good nutrition for people over 50.

FUTURE CONSIDERATIONS FOR THE AGING ADULT

POSSIBLE COMPLICATIONS—Chronic infection that cannot be cured without surgery.

PROBABLE OUTCOME—Curable with treatment. Oral antibiotics usually relieve the symptoms of infection within 1 week. Then part or all of the toenail is removed surgically and the nail bed is scraped so the problem will not recur. The nail should grow back, but it probably won't look the same.

PREVENTING RECURRENCE
- Wear roomy, low-heeled, well-fitting shoes made of a flexible material.
- Cut toenails carefully. Persons with diabetes mellitus or peripheral vascular disease should be especially careful in trimming toenails. Foot injury is dangerous with these disorders because of impaired blood circulation to the feet.

CALL YOUR DOCTOR IF

- You have symptoms of an ingrown toenail.
- Any of the following occurs during treatment or after surgery:
  Fever.
  Increased pain.
  Signs of infection (pain, redness, tenderness, swelling or heat) in the toe.
- New, unexplained symptoms develop. The drugs used in treatment may produce side effects.

TONGUE INFLAMMATION
(Glossitis)

 BASIC INFORMATION FOR OLDER ADULTS

DESCRIPTION—Glossitis is an acute or chronic inflammation of the tongue from a variety of causes. This is sometimes contagious, but not cancerous. Body parts involved: The tongue and adjacent parts of the mouth.

SPECIAL CONSIDERATIONS FOR AGING
- The immune system becomes less effective, opening the way for viral, bacterial and other infections; malignancies; immune disorders; and allergies.
- Decreased nutrition, common among chronically ill older people, increases the risk of any disease or disorder.
- Characteristic signs and symptoms of many disorders in older people are frequently changed or absent.

SIGNS & SYMPTOMS—Any of the following:
- A bright red, swollen tongue.
- Ulcers on the tongue.
- A hairy-looking tongue.
- A tongue with a red tip and edges.

CAUSES & RISK FACTORS
Causes include:
- Infections, including herpes.
- Burns; injuries from jagged teeth, ill-fitting dentures, breathing through the mouth or repeated biting of the tongue during convulsive seizures.
- Excessive consumption of alcohol, tobacco, hot food or spices.
- Poor dental health.
- An allergy to toothpaste, mouthwash (especially mouthwash containing peroxide), candy, dye or materials used in dental work.
- A lack of B vitamins resulting in pellagra, B-12-deficiency anemia or iron-deficiency anemia.
- Adverse reaction to antibiotic drugs.
Risk factors include:
- Poor nutrition, especially vitamin deficiencies.
- Smoking; chemical or environmental exposure to irritating or corrosive chemicals.

DOCTOR'S TREATMENT & DIAGNOSTIC TESTS
- Medical history and physical exam.
- Self-care instructions focused on the older patient.

 HOME TREATMENT BY SELF OR CARE-GIVER

GENERAL INSTRUCTIONS
- Observe if there is an association between eating specific foods and tongue inflammation. Irritating foods may include chocolate, citrus, acidic foods (such as vinegar and pickles), salted nuts or potato chips.
- Rinse your mouth 3 or more times a day with a salt solution (1/2 teaspoon salt to 8 oz. water).

- If the tongue inflammation is caused by a rough tooth or denture, consult your dentist. The inflammation won't heal until the cause is eliminated.

MEDICATION (ADJUSTED FOR AGING)
- For minor pain, you may use non-prescription drugs such as anesthetic mouthwashes or acetaminophen.
- For infection and pain, your doctor may prescribe antibiotics or topical anesthetics.
- *Note:* Adverse reactions and side effects may be more frequent and severe in older persons. Remind your doctor of any medicines you already take.

ACTIVITY FOR OLDER PATIENTS—No restrictions are necessary.

FOOD & BEVERAGE
- No special diet is required, except to avoid foods that aggravate inflammation. Drink as many fluids and eat as well-balanced a diet as possible while healing. To minimize the pain, sip liquids through straws. Foods that cause the least pain are milk, liquid gelatin, yogurt, ice cream and custard.
- See Appendix 1 regarding good nutrition for people over 50.

 FUTURE CONSIDERATIONS FOR THE AGING ADULT

POSSIBLE COMPLICATIONS—Tongue inflammation can become chronic if it is not adequately treated.

PROBABLE OUTCOME—Usually curable in 2 weeks with treatment.

PREVENTING RECURRENCE
- Practice good oral hygiene. Brush your teeth and tongue at least twice a day, and floss your teeth daily. Get regular dental checkups.
- Don't smoke.
- Prevent tongue injury by wearing protective headgear for cycling.

 CALL YOUR DOCTOR IF

- A fever develops.
- Your symptoms don't improve in 3 days despite treatment.
- The pain is unbearable and isn't relieved by treatment.
- A skin rash appears.
- Weight loss occurs.
- The tongue swells and interferes with swallowing.
- New, unexplained symptoms develop. The drugs used in treatment may produce side effects.

TOOTH ABSCESS
(Periapical Abscess; Periodontal Abscess)

BASIC INFORMATION FOR OLDER ADULTS

DESCRIPTION—This disorder is an abscess around a tooth root which is imbedded in bone of the upper or lower jaw. Body parts involved: The gums; the jawbone.

SPECIAL CONSIDERATIONS FOR AGING
- The immune system becomes less effective, opening the way for viral, bacterial and other infections; malignancies; immune disorders; and allergies.
- Decreased nutrition, common among chronically ill older people, increases the risk of any disease or disorder.
- Characteristic signs and symptoms of many disorders in older people are frequently changed or absent.

SIGNS & SYMPTOMS
- Persistent toothache or throbbing, extreme pain upon biting or chewing.
- Swelling and tenderness in the neck glands and on the side of the face.
- Earache; fever; a general ill feeling.
- A foul taste in the mouth and bad breath (if the abscess opens spontaneously).

CAUSES & RISK FACTORS
Causes include:
- Tartar beneath the gum.
- Deep decay which has entered the tooth nerve. The infection spreads down the nerve and into surrounding bone and gum tissue, but does not affect the adjacent teeth.
Risk factors include:
- Poor nutrition; improper diet.
- Inadequate fluoride in the drinking water.
- Injury to a tooth.

DOCTOR'S TREATMENT & DIAGNOSTIC TESTS
- Medical history and physical exam by a dentist or doctor.
- X-rays of the mouth.
- Self-care instructions focused on the older patient.
- Draining the abscess in one of 3 ways:
  If the tooth has poor bone and gum support, the tooth can be extracted, allowing the abscess to drain through the socket and heal.
  A hole can be drilled through the top of the tooth and a tiny metal or plastic wick can be inserted into the narrow nerve canal through the center of the tooth. This allows the abscess to drain.
  An incision can be made in the gum at the site of infection, which dramatically relieves the pain and pressure. Your dentist may place a small rubber wick in the incision for a few days. When the infection improves, your dentist can perform root canal therapy.

HOME TREATMENT BY SELF OR CARE-GIVER

GENERAL INSTRUCTIONS
- Rinse your mouth with warm water to reduce the infection from the abscess. Repeat each hour or as often as it feels good.
- Don't chew on the affected side of your mouth for at least 2 days.
- If a tube has been used to drain the abscess, keep the hole free of infection and food.
- If a drain has been placed in the gum, return to your dentist to have it removed.

MEDICATION (ADJUSTED FOR AGING)
- For minor pain, you may use non-prescription drugs such as acetaminophen.
- Your doctor or dentist may prescribe: Antibiotics to control the infection. Pain relievers.

ACTIVITY FOR OLDER PATIENTS—Resume your normal activities as soon as possible.

FOOD & BEVERAGE
- A liquid diet may be necessary for 1 or 2 days until the pain subsides.
- See Appendix 1 regarding good nutrition for people over 50.

FUTURE CONSIDERATIONS FOR THE AGING ADULT

POSSIBLE COMPLICATIONS—Rupture into the sinus of an abscess in the upper jaw; loss of the tooth; spread of the infection to other body parts.

PROBABLE OUTCOME—Usually curable with oral surgery.

PREVENTING RECURRENCE
- Prevent decay with good brushing and flossing: Use a soft-bristle toothbrush to remove plaque from the front and back surfaces of the teeth, especially at the gum line. Learn to use dental floss correctly. Ask your dentist or hygienist to demonstrate the technique.
- Use fluoride mouthwash, toothpaste, tablets or liquid supplements if your dentist recommends them.
- Reduce your sugar consumption. Tooth decay increases as sugar consumption increases.
- Have a dental checkup at least once a year.

CALL YOUR DOCTOR IF

- You have symptoms of a tooth abscess.
- Any of the following occurs during treatment: Your fever spikes to 101F (38.3C) or higher. The pain becomes unbearable.
- New, unexplained symptoms develop. The drugs used in treatment may produce side effects.

TOOTH DECAY
(Caries; Dental Decay; Cavities)

BASIC INFORMATION FOR OLDER ADULTS

DESCRIPTION—Tooth decay is a disintegration of the tooth enamel that allows injury to the dentin (the layer of the tooth below the enamel) and eventual involvement of the pulp (the layer below the dentin), which contains nerves and blood vessels. Tooth decay and the common cold are the most common human disorders. Body parts involved: The teeth.

SPECIAL CONSIDERATIONS FOR AGING
- Characteristic signs and symptoms of many disorders in older people are frequently changed or absent.
- Decreased nutrition, common among chronically ill older people, increases the risk of any disease or disorder.

SIGNS & SYMPTOMS
- Tooth sensitivity to heat and cold.
- Tooth discomfort after eating sugar.
- Darkening on or between the teeth (cavity) when the decay has progressed enough to be seen. The most common tooth cavity sites are the gum line, the biting surfaces and the surfaces between adjacent teeth.
- An unpleasant taste in the mouth and bad breath from stagnant food and bacteria trapped in the cavity.
- Persistent tooth pain (in the final stages of decay when the pulp becomes inflamed).

CAUSES & RISK FACTORS—Cavities are caused by acid destruction of tooth material. Acid is produced by the bacteria in the mouth. The bacteria feed on food debris—usually sugar—and produce the acid that dissolves tooth material. The combination of sugars from food debris, bacteria and chemicals in the saliva form a substance called plaque. Plaque becomes a localized site of acid production that forms continuously at the neck of each tooth. This plaque must be thoroughly cleaned away at the gum line daily or it fosters tooth decay. The risk increases with:
- Poor nutrition and improper diet.
- Poor dental hygiene.

DOCTOR'S TREATMENT & DIAGNOSTIC TESTS
- Examination by a dentist. The decayed area feels soft when the dentist probes it with a sharp instrument.
- X-rays of the teeth and mouth.
- Dentist's treatment to remove all decay in the tooth and replace it with a restorative material (filling). The filling prevents further decay.
- Self-care instructions focused on the older patient.

HOME TREATMENT BY SELF OR CARE-GIVER

GENERAL INSTRUCTIONS—No specific instructions except those listed under other headings.

MEDICATION (ADJUSTED FOR AGING)
- For minor pain, you may use non-prescription drugs such as acetaminophen.
- Your dentist may prescribe stronger pain relievers or fluoride supplements.
- *Note:* Adverse reactions and side effects may be more frequent and severe in older persons. Remind your doctor of any medicines you already take.

ACTIVITY FOR OLDER PATIENTS—No restrictions are necessary.

FOOD & BEVERAGE
- For 48 hours after your dentist fills the decayed tooth, don't put pressure on the tooth, such as by eating apples, hard candy, raw vegetables or chewing on ice. Avoid very hot or cold foods. The tooth remains sensitive for 48 hours to 10 days after a cavity has been filled.
- See Appendix 1 regarding good nutrition for people over 50.

FUTURE CONSIDERATIONS FOR THE AGING ADULT

POSSIBLE COMPLICATIONS
- Abscess around a decayed tooth.
- Death of the tooth, caused by destruction of the tooth pulp that contains the tooth's nerve and blood supply.

PROBABLE OUTCOME—Usually curable with dental treatment.

PREVENTING RECURRENCE
- Brush and floss your teeth regularly.
- Consult your dentist about using fluoride mouthwash, liquid or tablets or having fluoride treatments once or twice a year.
- Sealants may help prevent enamel erosion.
- Have a dental checkup at least once a year.

CALL YOUR DOCTOR IF

- You have symptoms of tooth decay.
- Any of the following occurs after treatment: Fever; increased pain that is not relieved by non-prescription medication.
  Discomfort with hot or cold food that persists longer than 2 weeks after the filling procedure.
  Brown spots on the tops of any other teeth.
- New, unexplained symptoms develop. The drugs used in treatment may produce side effects.

TOOTH GRINDING
(Bruxism)

BASIC INFORMATION FOR OLDER ADULTS

DESCRIPTION—Bruxism is the habit of grinding the teeth. Tooth grinding is often done while one is asleep, but grinding or tapping the teeth during the day is also common. Continual tooth grinding may erode the gums and supporting bones in the mouth. Body parts involved: The teeth; gums; temporomandibular joints.

SPECIAL CONSIDERATIONS FOR AGING—Years of wear and tear make the teeth and supporting structures more susceptible to damage and destruction.

SIGNS & SYMPTOMS
- Frequent contraction of the muscles on the side of the face.
- Annoying tooth-grinding noises at night. These may be loud enough to awaken others.
- Damaged teeth, supporting gums and bone (apparent in a dental exam).
- Headaches.

CAUSES & RISK FACTORS
Causes include:
- Anxiety.
- Unconscious attempts to correct a faulty "bite" (the contact between the upper and lower teeth when the jaws are closed).

The risk increases with stress, anxiety or alcoholism.

DOCTOR'S TREATMENT & DIAGNOSTIC TESTS
- Medical history and physical exam by a dentist.
- X-rays of the mouth.
- Self-care instructions focused on the older patient.
- Your dentist may manufacture, fit and install a night-guard prosthesis to prevent you from grinding your teeth while you are asleep. A night-guard prosthesis consists of removable splints which fit over the tops of the teeth to eliminate incorrect biting pressure.
- Biofeedback training (relaxation exercises) or counseling to help you learn ways to cope more effectively with stress.

HOME TREATMENT BY SELF OR CARE-GIVER

GENERAL INSTRUCTIONS—No specific instructions except those listed under other headings.

MEDICATION (ADJUSTED FOR AGING)
- Medicine usually is not necessary for this disorder. A tranquilizer for short-term treatment may help.
- *Note:* Adverse reactions and side effects may be more frequent and severe in older persons. Remind your doctor of any medicines you already take.

ACTIVITY FOR OLDER PATIENTS
- No restrictions are necessary.
- See Appendix 20 regarding physical fitness for the active older adult.

FOOD & BEVERAGE
- No special diet is required.
- See Appendix 1 regarding good nutrition for people over 50.

FUTURE CONSIDERATIONS FOR THE AGING ADULT

POSSIBLE COMPLICATIONS—Without treatment, the teeth, bones and gums may erode from the pressure of grinding.

PROBABLE OUTCOME—Usually curable in 6 months with treatment.

PREVENTING RECURRENCE—Avoid stressful situations if possible. See Appendix 13.

CALL YOUR DOCTOR IF
- You grind your teeth at night.
- You develop pain around your ears, dizziness or ringing in the ears.
- You develop pain or clicking in your jaw.
- You lose or break your night-guard prosthesis.

TORTICOLLIS
(Wryneck)

BASIC INFORMATION FOR OLDER ADULTS

DESCRIPTION—Torticollis is a shortening of the neck muscles or a chronic neck muscle spasm that causes the head to turn and bend. Body parts involved: The brain and central nervous system; the muscular system.

SPECIAL CONSIDERATIONS FOR AGING—Characteristic signs and symptoms of many disorders in older people are frequently changed or absent.

SIGNS & SYMPTOMS—The following may be permanent or intermittent:
- A head that turns sideways and bends down.
- Neck muscle spasms that are sometimes painful.

CAUSES & RISK FACTORS
The causes of constant torticollis include:
- A minor neck injury or a burn that has caused the skin to shrink.
- An inflammation of the neck muscle.
The causes of intermittent torticollis include:
- Stress and psychological conflict.
Risk factors include:
- Sleeping in an awkward position.
- Emotional disturbances, such as neurosis or hypochondriasis.

DOCTOR'S TREATMENT & DIAGNOSTIC TESTS
- Medical history and physical exam.
- Laboratory blood tests for infection and inflammation.
- X-rays of the spinal column in the neck.
- Self-care instructions focused on the older patient.
- Psychotherapy, biofeedback or counseling if the cause is stress-related.
- Surgery to lengthen the neck muscles if the cause is congenital.
- Physical therapy (sometimes), including gentle massage.
- Ultrasound therapy (see Glossary).

HOME TREATMENT BY SELF OR CARE-GIVER

GENERAL INSTRUCTIONS—For non-congenital forms of torticollis:
- Your doctor may recommend that you wear a neck brace.
- Relieve the pain of neck spasms with heat or massage. Take hot showers or use hot compresses, deep-heating ointments or heat lamps.

MEDICATION (ADJUSTED FOR AGING)
- If the condition is caused by injury or inflammation, your doctor may prescribe muscle relaxants and pain relievers.
- *Note:* Adverse reactions and side effects may be more frequent and severe in older persons. Remind your doctor of any medicines you already take.

ACTIVITY FOR OLDER PATIENTS
- You may resume your normal activities as soon as your symptoms improve.
- See Appendix 20 regarding physical fitness for the active older adult.

FOOD & BEVERAGE
- No special diet is required.
- See Appendix 1 regarding good nutrition for people over 50.

FUTURE CONSIDERATIONS FOR THE AGING ADULT

POSSIBLE COMPLICATIONS—Without treatment, the congenital form becomes permanent, causing an unattractive, abnormal appearance of the head and neck.

PROBABLE OUTCOME
- Congenital torticollis can usually be corrected with muscle-stretching exercises or surgery.
- Other forms will improve or heal with treatment. Healing time varies. Some cases require treatment for several years.

PREVENTING RECURRENCE—Stress-related forms can be prevented with stress-reduction techniques, including biofeedback.

CALL YOUR DOCTOR IF

- You have neck pain or spasms that persist longer than 1 week.
- New, unexplained symptoms develop. The drugs used in treatment may produce side effects.

TRANSIENT ISCHEMIC ATTACK
(TIA)

 BASIC INFORMATION FOR OLDER ADULTS

DESCRIPTION—A TIA is a temporary decrease in the blood supply to part of the brain. The affected part of the brain is temporarily (for a few minutes to 24 hours) unable to function normally. Body parts involved: The blood vessels to the brain and the part of the brain supplied by the affected blood vessels.

SPECIAL CONSIDERATIONS FOR AGING
- Characteristic signs and symptoms of many disorders in older people are frequently changed or absent.
- 50% of people over 60 have x-ray evidence of narrowing of the coronary arteries, yet only 50% of those people have symptoms.
- The total heart functions less efficiently—especially among smokers.

SIGNS & SYMPTOMS—The following symptoms are brief, lasting from several minutes to a few hours.
- Loss of muscle function on one side of the body.
- Headache; dizziness; confusion; vision disturbance or temporary blindness in one eye.
- Tingling in the arms and legs; numbness.
- Faintness without loss of consciousness.
- Slurred speech or inability to speak.

CAUSES & RISK FACTORS—TIAs are caused by a partial blockage in a small artery in the brain or a larger artery (usually the carotid artery in the neck) that supplies blood to the arteries of the brain. The blockage is often caused by a small clot from a piece of heart or blood vessel that breaks away and is carried into the brain. This temporarily decreases the blood flow to an area of the brain and causes strokelike symptoms. Risk factors include:
- Smoking; diabetes; heart attack.
- A personal or family medical history of high blood pressure and atherosclerosis.

DOCTOR'S TREATMENT & DIAGNOSTIC TESTS
- Medical history and physical exam.
- Laboratory blood studies to analyze cholesterol and other fats.
- X-rays (angiography), CT scan or sonograms (see Glossary for all) of the blood vessels in the neck or brain.
- Self-care instructions focused on the older patient.
- Surgery to remove plaques (fatty deposits) from the carotid arteries in the neck (sometimes).
- Treatment of the underlying condition.

 HOME TREATMENT BY SELF OR CARE-GIVER

GENERAL INSTRUCTIONS—No specific instructions except those listed under other headings.

MEDICATION (ADJUSTED FOR AGING)
- Your doctor may prescribe:
  Anticoagulants, such as warfarin, to decrease the formation of blood clots. These drugs must be monitored with laboratory studies of prothrombin time (see Glossary).
  1 or 2 aspirin tablets a day. Recent medical experiments indicate that aspirin can decrease blood clotting enough to reduce the likelihood of TIAs developing into a stroke. The aspirin seems more effective in men than in women.
- *Note:* Adverse reactions and side effects may be more frequent and severe in older persons. Remind your doctor of any medicines you already take.

ACTIVITY FOR OLDER PATIENTS
- If you have frequent TIAs, don't drive, work in high places or operate machinery.
- See Appendix 20 regarding physical fitness for the active older adult.

FOOD & BEVERAGE—Eat a normal, well-balanced diet that is low in salt and fat, especially saturated fat (see Appendices 8 and 9).

 FUTURE CONSIDERATIONS FOR THE AGING ADULT

POSSIBLE COMPLICATIONS—Stroke. Without treatment, about 50% of persons who have TIAs have strokes within 5 years.

PROBABLE OUTCOME—Transient ischemic attacks are often signals of an impending stroke. They should be treated to attempt to prevent a stroke, which may cause serious brain damage. TIAs are likely to recur. A person may have several attacks daily or only 2 or 3 over several years. The symptoms of each attack may be similar or quite different from others. In some patients symptoms appear repeatedly without leaving permanent damage.

PREVENTING RECURRENCE
- Exercise at least 3 times a week to maintain good cardiovascular fitness.
- Follow the recommendations under Food & Beverage; don't smoke.
- Have your blood pressure checked regularly. If it is high, consult your doctor for treatment to reduce it.
- Daily aspirin may help. Ask your doctor.

 CALL YOUR DOCTOR IF

- You have your first symptoms of a TIA.
- The symptoms of a TIA recur after diagnosis and persist longer than 2 hours.
- New, unexplained symptoms develop. The drugs used in treatment may produce side effects.

TRENCH MOUTH

(Necrotizing Ulcerative Gingivitis; Vincent's Disease; Fusospirochetosis)

BASIC INFORMATION FOR OLDER ADULTS

DESCRIPTION—Trench mouth is an infection of the tissues between the teeth. This is not contagious or cancerous. Body parts involved: The gums. If untreated, trench mouth can spread to the lymph glands in the neck and to the tonsils, vocal cords, bronchial tubes, rectum or vagina.

SPECIAL CONSIDERATIONS FOR AGING
- The immune system becomes less effective, opening the way for viral, bacterial and other infections; malignancies; immune disorders; and allergies.
- Decreased nutrition, common among chronically ill older people, increases the risk of any disease or disorder.
- Characteristic signs and symptoms of many disorders in older people are frequently changed or absent.

SIGNS & SYMPTOMS
- Painful gums; bad breath.
- Gums that bleed when pressed.
- Excessive salivation.
- Ulcers on the gums covered with gray membrane.
- Difficulty swallowing or speaking.

CAUSES & RISK FACTORS
Causes include:
- Spirochetes; fusiform bacteria.
- Tartar, plaque or food debris between the teeth.
Risk factors include:
- Poor nutrition; smoking; stress.
- Illness that has lowered resistance.
- Inadequate sleep; alcoholism.
- Viral or bacterial infections.

DOCTOR'S TREATMENT & DIAGNOSTIC TESTS
- Medical history and physical exam.
- Laboratory culture to identify the infecting germs.
- Self-care instructions focused on the older patient.
- Scaling of the teeth by a dentist to remove plaque.
- Frequent dental checkups—up to once a month—after treatment.

HOME TREATMENT BY SELF OR CARE-GIVER

GENERAL INSTRUCTIONS
- Rinse your mouth every 2 hours, alternating the following rinses:
  A mixture of 1 teaspoon salt in a large glass of very warm water.
  A mixture of equal parts 2% hydrogen peroxide and warm water.
- Don't smoke.
- Avoid any gum irritation until the gums heal completely.

MEDICATION (ADJUSTED FOR AGING)
- Your doctor may prescribe penicillin or another antibiotic to fight infection.
- You may use non-prescription drugs such as acetaminophen for minor pain.

ACTIVITY FOR OLDER PATIENTS
- Rest at home for the first 2 days of treatment, then resume normal activities.
- See Appendix 20 regarding physical fitness for the active older adult.

FOOD & BEVERAGE
- A liquid diet (see Appendix 7) may be necessary for 2 or 3 days because of gum tenderness. When the pain subsides, eat many fresh fruits and vegetables. Don't eat spicy or hot (temperature) food.
- Drink juices and 4 to 6 glasses of water each day. Don't drink carbonated beverages or alcohol.
- See Appendix 1 regarding good nutrition for people over 50.

FUTURE CONSIDERATIONS FOR THE AGING ADULT

POSSIBLE COMPLICATIONS—Surgery may be necessary to trim rough, infected gums.

PROBABLE OUTCOME—Usually curable in 2 weeks with treatment.

PREVENTING RECURRENCE
- Maintain good oral hygiene.
  Brush clear, sticky plaque off your teeth daily with a soft toothbrush. Place the brush at the gum line and gently rotate, pointing the bristles toward the gum. Brush one section of teeth at a time. Then brush your tongue. A soft brush is less likely to damage the teeth and gums than a hard brush.
  Floss your teeth using waxed or unwaxed dental floss according to the instructions on the package label or your dentist's instructions.
- Eat a well-balanced diet.
- Don't smoke.

CALL YOUR DOCTOR IF

- You have symptoms of trench mouth.
- Any of the following occurs during treatment:
  Fever.
  Swelling of the neck or face.
  Swallowing difficulty.
  Inability to eat.
- New, unexplained symptoms develop. The drugs used in treatment may produce side effects.

ILLNESSES & DISORDERS

TRICHINOSIS

BASIC INFORMATION FOR OLDER ADULTS

DESCRIPTION—Trichinosis is an infection caused by the larvae of parasites that live in the intestines of pigs and bears and are transmitted to humans who eat undercooked meat of the infected animals. Body parts involved: The gastrointestinal tract (where the larvae enter); the lymphatic system and bloodstream (through which they are transported); and the large muscles of the body, especially the diaphragm (the large muscle used in breathing that separates the chest from the abdomen).

SPECIAL CONSIDERATIONS FOR AGING
- The immune system becomes less effective, opening the way for viral, bacterial and other infections; malignancies; immune disorders; and allergies.
- Characteristic signs and symptoms of many disorders in older people are frequently changed or absent.
- Decreased nutrition, common among chronically ill older people, increases the risk of any disease or disorder.

SIGNS & SYMPTOMS
Early stages (usually beginning in 7 to 10 days):
- Appetite loss, nausea, vomiting, diarrhea and abdominal cramps.
Later stages:
- Puffy eyelids and face.
- Muscle pain; sweating.
- Itching, burning skin.
- High fever (102F to 104F or 38.9C to 40C).
Late stages:
- The symptoms subside, but some muscle tissues remain permanently infected with microscopic cysts. In rare cases, these cause disorders of the heart and central nervous system.

CAUSES & RISK FACTORS—Caused by infection with a parasite, *trichina spiralis*, which is transmitted to people when they eat the meat of infected animals. Thorough cooking kills the parasite and makes infected meat safe to eat. The parasites pass from animal to animal in contaminated food, usually in raw garbage. The risk increases with:
- Eating improperly cooked or raw pork or bear meat.
- The use of immunosuppressive drugs.

DOCTOR'S TREATMENT & DIAGNOSTIC TESTS
- Medical history and physical exam.
- Laboratory blood studies.
- Muscle biopsy to detect larvae.
- Self-care instructions focused on the older patient.
- Hospitalization (worst cases).

HOME TREATMENT BY SELF OR CARE-GIVER

GENERAL INSTRUCTIONS—Reduce a high fever.

MEDICATION (ADJUSTED FOR AGING)
- Your doctor may prescribe anthelminthic drugs (usually thiabendazole) to kill the parasites.
- You may take non-prescription drugs such as acetaminophen to reduce your fever and discomfort.
- *Note:* Adverse reactions and side effects may be more frequent and severe in older persons. Remind your doctor of any medicines you already take.

ACTIVITY FOR OLDER PATIENTS
- Rest in bed until your symptoms subside. While confined to bed, move your legs frequently to reduce the likelihood of deep-vein blood clots. Resume your normal activities gradually.
- See Appendix 20 regarding physical fitness for the active older adult.

FOOD & BEVERAGE
- Consume a special high-protein diet to help rebuild damaged muscle tissue. The diet will be prescribed by your doctor and explained by a dietitian. Usually you may progress to an unrestricted, well-balanced diet within 6 months.
- See Appendix 1 regarding good nutrition for people over 50.

FUTURE CONSIDERATIONS FOR THE AGING ADULT

POSSIBLE COMPLICATIONS—Overwhelming infection, which can lead to congestive heart failure; respiratory failure; permanent damage of the central nervous system.

PROBABLE OUTCOME—Usually curable in most persons without treatment or with antiparasite drugs. In severe cases, expert medical care will need to be continued. Some deaths have been reported. Allow up to 6 months for recovery.

PREVENTING RECURRENCE—Don't eat raw or undercooked pork (including sausage) or bear meat. Cook all meats thoroughly.

CALL YOUR DOCTOR IF

- You have symptoms of trichinosis.
- Any of the following occurs during treatment:
  A fever spike to over 104F (40C).
  Irregular heartbeat.
  Shortness of breath.
  Puffy ankles.
  Clumsy finger or thumb movement.
- New, unexplained symptoms develop. The drugs used in treatment may produce side effects, especially nausea, vomiting, skin rash or fever.

TUBERCULOSIS
(TB)

BASIC INFORMATION FOR OLDER ADULTS

DESCRIPTION—TB is an acute or chronic contagious bacterial infection. Persons over 65 now account for 25% to 30% of new cases. In the U.S., AIDS cases have caused an increase in the total number of people who are ill with tuberculosis. Body parts involved: Primarily the lungs, but the infection may spread to other organs.

SPECIAL CONSIDERATIONS FOR AGING
- Characteristic signs and symptoms of many disorders in older people are frequently changed or absent.
- Decreased nutrition increases the risk of any disease or disorder.
- The immune system becomes less effective, opening the way for viral, bacterial and other infections.
- Signs and symptoms may differ significantly from those listed below.
- Stress from any emotional cause affects all aspects of any illness or disorder.

SIGNS & SYMPTOMS
Early stages:
- No symptoms (often).
- Symptoms that resemble those of influenza.

Next stages:
- Low fever; weight loss; chronic fatigue.
- Heavy sweating, especially at night.

Later stages:
- A cough with sputum that becomes progressively bloody, yellow, thick or gray.
- Chest pain; shortness of breath.
- Reddish or cloudy urine (sometimes).

CAUSES & RISK FACTORS—Caused by infection from the germ *mycobacterium tuberculosis*. The germ is transmitted in the air from one person to another. Cattle are also susceptible and can transmit TB through non-pasteurized milk. The risk increases with:
- Chronic illness that has lowered resistance.
- The use of cortisone or immunosuppressive drugs (these may reactivate inactive TB).
- Crowded, institutional or unsanitary living conditions.
- HIV (human immunodeficiency virus) infection with or without AIDS.

DOCTOR'S TREATMENT & DIAGNOSTIC TESTS
- Medical history and physical exam.
- Tuberculin skin test; x-rays of the chest.
- Laboratory cultures of the sputum and urine.
- Self-care instructions focused on the older patient.
- Bronchoscopy (see Glossary) or biopsy of lymph tissue (rare).

OTHER—Health authorities recommend vaccination and preventive treatment for the following groups:
- Persons who have positive reactions to TB tests, but show no symptoms of disease.
- Persons traveling to countries where TB is prevalent.
- Persons who must take immunosuppressive or cortisone drugs for a long time.
- Post-gastrectomy patients whose x-rays show evidence of inactive TB.
- Persons with silicosis.

HOME TREATMENT BY SELF OR CARE-GIVER

GENERAL INSTRUCTIONS
- It may not be necessary to isolate or hospitalize a person with TB. The disease is usually spread before diagnosis. Patients are probably not infectious after 10 days to 2 weeks of treatment.
- Occasionally you will need to collect a 24-hour sputum specimen for laboratory analysis to see if the TB is still active.
- Get regular follow-up x-rays.

MEDICATION (ADJUSTED FOR AGING)—Your doctor may prescribe antitubercular drugs.

ACTIVITY FOR OLDER PATIENTS—Rest in bed until your symptoms disappear and tests show that the TB germs are gone. You may need to restrict your activities for 6 months.

FOOD & BEVERAGE—No special diet is required. See Appendix 1 regarding good nutrition for people over 50.

FUTURE CONSIDERATIONS FOR THE AGING ADULT

POSSIBLE COMPLICATIONS—Lung abscess; bronchiectasis; COPD (see Glossary); spread of the infection to other organs (the brain, bone, spine and kidneys); respiratory failure.

PROBABLE OUTCOME
- Usually curable with treatment. Relapse rates are less than 5%. Without treatment, TB can be fatal.
- The most common reason for treatment failure is lack of patient adherence to prescribed regimens.

PREVENTING RECURRENCE
- Vaccination with BCG, a strain of tuberculosis bacteria. This may prevent infection or shorten and diminish the severity of the infection.
- Preventive treatment for several months with isonicotinic acid if a tuberculin skin test is positive.

CALL YOUR DOCTOR IF

- You have symptoms of TB.
- The symptoms persist or worsen despite treatment.
- New, unexplained symptoms develop. The drugs used in treatment may produce side effects.

TYPHOID FEVER

BASIC INFORMATION FOR OLDER ADULTS

DESCRIPTION—Typhoid fever is a bacterial infection of the gastrointestinal tract. Body parts involved: The gastrointestinal tract; skin; central nervous system.

SPECIAL CONSIDERATIONS FOR AGING
- The immune system becomes less effective, opening the way for viral, bacterial and other infections.
- Characteristic signs and symptoms of many disorders are frequently changed or absent.
- Signs and symptoms may differ significantly from those listed below.

SIGNS & SYMPTOMS
- Diarrhea. In mild cases, this may be only 2 or 3 loose bowel movements a day. In severe cases, it may be watery diarrhea as often as every 10 or 15 minutes.
- Vomiting; fever; headache; muscle aches.
- A rose-colored skin rash on the abdomen.
- Abdominal cramps (sometimes).
- Blood in the stool (sometimes).

A relatively mild attack may be mistaken for simple gastroenteritis.

CAUSES & RISK FACTORS—Infection with one type of salmonella, a bacterium found in infected animals and transmitted to persons in contaminated food or water. Thorough cooking kills the germ. The infection can also be transmitted by ill persons or by carriers who aren't ill who handle food without careful hand washing after bowel movements. The risk increases with:
- Illness that has lowered resistance.
- Crowded or unsanitary living conditions.
- Travel to countries where the disease is endemic.

DOCTOR'S TREATMENT & DIAGNOSTIC TESTS
- Medical history and physical exam.
- Laboratory studies such as stool studies and a blood culture; sigmoidoscopy (see Glossary).
- X-rays of the gastrointestinal tract.
- During the convalescent stage, self-care instructions focused on the older patient.
- Hospitalization for severe cases.

HOME TREATMENT BY SELF OR CARE-GIVER

GENERAL INSTRUCTIONS
- Isolate ill persons and have them use bedside commodes or a separate bathroom.
- Use a heating pad or hot water bottle to relieve abdominal cramps.
- Wash your hands carefully and often.
- Turn patients frequently in bed.
- Apply lukewarm wet towels to the groin and underarms to reduce the fever. *Don't* use aspirin or acetaminophen; both irritate the gastrointestinal tract.

MEDICATION (ADJUSTED FOR AGING)—Your doctor may prescribe antibiotics.

ACTIVITY FOR OLDER PATIENTS—Bed rest is necessary until all your symptoms have been gone at least 3 days. Flex your legs often in bed to prevent the formation of deep-vein blood clots.

FOOD & BEVERAGE—A diet of clear liquids is necessary during the diarrhea phase. Later a high-calorie, well-balanced diet is necessary (see Appendix 20). Vitamin and mineral supplements may be helpful.

FUTURE CONSIDERATIONS FOR THE AGING ADULT

POSSIBLE COMPLICATIONS—Dehydration; perforation of the intestines; gastrointestinal hemorrhage or abscess; deep-vein blood clots; pneumonia; bone infection; congestive heart failure.

PROBABLE OUTCOME—Usually curable in 2 to 3 weeks with treatment. Without treatment, it can be fatal.

PREVENTING RECURRENCE
- Follow these recommendations in any area with a substandard water supply:
  Drink purified water, boil the water for 15 to 20 minutes or add 2 to 4 drops of 4% to 6% chlorine bleach to each quart of water 30 minutes before use.
  If your are in a hotel, draw hot water from the faucet, let it cool and then use it as drinking water; don't use ice.
  Don't eat raw fruits and vegetables unless you can peel them.
- Drink only pasteurized milk.
- Wash your hands after bowel movements and before handling food.
- Obtain a vaccination if you are exposed to typhoid or may travel to a country where the risk of typhoid is high.

CALL YOUR DOCTOR IF

- You have symptoms of typhoid fever.
- Any of the following occurs during treatment:
  Fever; sore throat.
  Severe cough or coughing up blood.
  Shortness of breath.
  Severe abdominal pain or swelling.
  Rectal bleeding.
  Pain in the calf or leg.
  Headache, earache or swollen joints.
- New, unexplained symptoms develop. The drugs used in treatment may produce side effects.

ULCER, DUODENAL
(Peptic Ulcer, Duodenal)

BASIC INFORMATION FOR OLDER ADULTS

DESCRIPTION—A duodenal ulcer is an ulcer (or "sore") in the duodenum which causes symptoms similar to those of a stomach ulcer. An ulcer is not contagious or cancerous. Body parts involved: The duodenum (the first 12 inches of the small intestine beyond the stomach).

SPECIAL CONSIDERATIONS FOR AGING
- Characteristic signs and symptoms of many disorders are frequently changed or absent.
- Signs and symptoms may differ significantly from those listed below.
- Decreased nutrition increases the risk of any disease or disorder.
- Stress from any emotional cause affects all aspects of any illness or disorder.
- This type of ulcer occurs more often in younger individuals, but is more serious in older adults.

SIGNS & SYMPTOMS
- Pain that has the following characteristics: The pain is a burning, boring or gnawing feeling that lasts 30 minutes to 3 hours. It is often interpreted as heartburn, indigestion or hunger. The pain is usually in the upper abdomen, but occasionally it is below the breastbone. The pain occurs in some persons immediately after eating; in others, it may not occur until hours later. It frequently awakens one at night. The pain comes and goes. Weeks of intermittent pain may alternate with short pain-free periods. The pain may be relieved by drinking milk, eating, resting or taking antacids.
- Appetite and weight loss.
- Recurrent vomiting.
- Blood in the stool; anemia.
- Belching and bloating.

CAUSES & RISK FACTORS—The cause is unknown. An ulcer can develop wherever stomach acid comes in contact with the gastrointestinal lining—especially at the lower end of the esophagus and in the stomach and the duodenum. Recent experimental work implicates the possibility of a bacterial infection smoldering in the stomach lining. An ulcer is most likely to develop in an anxious, tense or worried person. A person with an ulcer usually has an overactive stomach that manufactures too much hydrochloric acid. In addition, persons with ulcers often have irregular living habits. Risk factors include:
- A family history of ulcers; stress; improper diet.
- Irregular mealtimes and skipped meals.
- Smoking; fatigue or overwork.
- Excessive alcohol consumption.
- The use of medications containing aspirin, caffeine or alcohol, which irritate the stomach.

DOCTOR'S TREATMENT & DIAGNOSTIC TESTS
- Medical history and physical exam.
- Gastroscopy (see Glossary) to determine the ulcer's size and location; barium x-ray.
- Self-care instructions focused on the older patient.
- Hospitalization (for complications).
- Surgery for obstruction, pain or bleeding (rare).

HOME TREATMENT BY SELF OR CARE-GIVER

GENERAL INSTRUCTIONS
- Don't smoke; avoid aspirin and non-steroidal anti-inflammatory drugs.
- Check your stool daily for bleeding. If the stool is black, remove it from the toilet and take it to your doctor's office for analysis.

MEDICATION (ADJUSTED FOR AGING)—Your doctor may prescribe:
- Antacids to help neutralize excess stomach acid.
- H_2 blockers to reduce the amount of stomach acid.
- Medications to coat the ulcer area.
- Combined antibiotics (experimental treatment).

ACTIVITY FOR OLDER PATIENTS—Resume your normal activities as soon as your symptoms improve.

FOOD & BEVERAGE
- A full liquid diet may help during the acute phase.
- Eat small, frequent meals on a regular schedule recommended by your doctor.
- Don't drink alcohol; avoid coffee, tea, cola drinks and decaffeinated beverages.
- Eliminate any foods that cause irritation.
- See Appendix 1 regarding good nutrition for people over 50.

FUTURE CONSIDERATIONS FOR THE AGING ADULT

POSSIBLE COMPLICATIONS—Perforation (erosion of the ulcer through the intestinal wall) or dangerous bleeding; unrelenting pain, failure to heal and scarring; extensive peptic ulcer disease; increased likelihood of stomach cancer.

PROBABLE OUTCOME—Usually curable with lifestyle changes and medical treatment. However, recurrence is not uncommon.

PREVENTING RECURRENCE—Avoid as many risk factors as possible.

CALL YOUR DOCTOR IF

- You have symptoms of an ulcer.
- Vomiting begins that is bloody or looks like coffee grounds.
- Your stools are bloody, black or tarry looking.
- Diarrhea begins which may be caused by antacids.
- The pain is severe despite treatment.
- You are unusually weak or pale.
- New, unexplained symptoms develop. The drugs used in treatment may produce side effects.

ULCER, STOMACH
(Peptic Ulcer; Gastric Ulcer)

BASIC INFORMATION FOR OLDER ADULTS

DESCRIPTION—A stomach ulcer is a raw spot that develops in the stomach lining. Body part involved: The stomach, including the stomach lining.

SPECIAL CONSIDERATIONS FOR AGING
- Characteristic signs and symptoms of many disorders are frequently changed or absent.
- Signs and symptoms may differ significantly from those listed below.
- Decreased nutrition increases the risk of any disease or disorder.
- Stress from any emotional cause affects all aspects of any illness or disorder.

SIGNS & SYMPTOMS
- Pain with the following characteristics:
  The pain is a burning, gnawing pain in the upper abdomen or the lower chest below the breastbone. It is often interpreted as indigestion, heartburn or hunger and may be relieved temporarily with milk, antacids or bland food. The pain lasts 30 minutes to 3 hours. It may occur immediately after eating or hours later. The pain comes and goes. Weeks of intermittent pain may alternate with short pain-free periods.
- Loss of appetite; weight loss.
- Anemia; occasional vomiting.

Sometimes the symptoms are not typical, and diagnostic procedures are necessary.

CAUSES & RISK FACTORS—The cause is unknown. Persons with ulcers often have irregular living habits. Many doctors believe emotional tension causes ulcers. An infectious bacterial component may contribute to ulcer formation. Risk factors include.
- Stress; smoking.
- Improper diet or irregular meals.
- Excessive consumption of alcohol or caffeine-containing drinks.
- The use of drugs such as cortisone, aspirin or other non-steroidal anti-inflammatory drugs.
- A family history of ulcers; type "O" blood.

DOCTOR'S TREATMENT & DIAGNOSTIC TESTS
- Medical history and physical exam.
- Laboratory studies to measure stomach acid.
- X-rays of the stomach.
- Gastroscopy (see Glossary).
- Self-care instructions focused on the older patient.
- Hospitalization (sometimes) during the initial treatment.
- Psychotherapy or counseling.
- Surgery to remove part of the stomach or cut the nerves that stimulate acid production if conservative treatment fails. Advancing age alone is not a deterrent.

HOME TREATMENT BY SELF OR CARE-GIVER

GENERAL INSTRUCTIONS
- Don't smoke during convalescence.
- Examine your stool daily for signs of bleeding. If the stool is black, take a specimen to your doctor's office.

MEDICATION (ADJUSTED FOR AGING)
- Don't take aspirin or other non-steroidal anti-inflammatory drugs.
- Your doctor may prescribe:
  Antacids to reduce stomach acid.
  H_2 blockers to decrease the stomach's production of hydrochloric acid.
  Medications that coat the ulcer.
  Combined antibiotics (experimental).
- Don't medicate yourself with antacids unless your doctor prescribes them and you are under medical supervision.

ACTIVITY FOR OLDER PATIENTS—Rest as needed to rebuild your energy.

FOOD & BEVERAGE
- Eat small, frequent meals for 2 weeks.
- Don't drink alcohol. After recovery, don't drink more than 1 or 2 alcoholic drinks a day.

FUTURE CONSIDERATIONS FOR THE AGING ADULT

POSSIBLE COMPLICATIONS—Bleeding; perforation, in which the ulcer erodes through the stomach wall; scarring and obstruction in the stomach caused by recurrent ulcers; malignant change in an ulcer; anemia.

PROBABLE OUTCOME--Usually curable with 6 to 8 weeks of treatment. If an ulcer doesn't heal in that time or if recovery is only temporary, surgery may be necessary. For perforation or hemorrhaging, surgery is mandatory. It usually results in a complete cure.

PREVENTING RECURRENCE—See Appendices 12 and 13 for suggestions for a healthy lifestyle.

CALL YOUR DOCTOR IF

- You have symptoms of a stomach ulcer or your symptoms recur after treatment.
- You have signs of bleeding, such as passing a black stool or are vomiting blood or material that looks like coffee grounds.
- Diarrhea begins; the pain becomes intolerable.
- You become unusually weak or pale.
- New, unexplained symptoms develop. The drugs used in treatment may produce side effects.

URETHRITIS

BASIC INFORMATION FOR OLDER ADULTS

DESCRIPTION—Urethritis is an inflammation or infection of the urethra (the tube through which urine travels from the bladder to the outside of the body), frequently accompanied by bladder infection or inflammation (cystitis). The female urethra is much shorter than the male and more susceptible to injury and infection. Body parts involved: The urethra; the bladder (sometimes).

SPECIAL CONSIDERATIONS FOR AGING
- The immune system becomes less effective, opening the way for viral, bacterial and other infections.
- The total state of well-being in many older people impairs their ability to prevent infections from spreading.
- Signs and symptoms may differ significantly from those listed below.
- Stress from any emotional cause affects all aspects of any illness or disorder.

SIGNS & SYMPTOMS
- Painful or burning urination with a cloudy yellow-green discharge of mucus from the urethra.
- A frequent urge to urinate, even when there is not much urine in the bladder.
- Painful sexual intercourse or temporary impotence in males; dribbling of urine in men.

CAUSES & RISK FACTORS—Caused by a bacterial infection. In women the infection is associated with bacteria that enter the urethra from the skin around the genitals and anal area and bruising during sexual intercourse. In men the infection is associated with non-specific urethritis, which may be caused by sexual contact or irritation of the urethra, and infections that reach the urethra through the bloodstream from the prostate gland or through the penis. In both sexes the infection may be associated with gonorrhea, which is spread by contact with an infected sexual partner. Risk factors include:
- The use of a urinary catheter.
- The use of drugs to which the bacteria causing infection have become resistant.
- Multiple sexual partners.
- Previous kidney stones, prostatitis, epididymitis or genital injury.
- The use of antiseptics or other chemical irritants.

DOCTOR'S TREATMENT & DIAGNOSTIC TESTS
- Medical history and physical exam.
- Urinalysis and urine culture.
- Self-care instructions focused on the older patient.

HOME TREATMENT BY SELF OR CARE-GIVER

GENERAL INSTRUCTIONS
- To relieve the pain, take sitz baths by sitting in a tub of hot water for 15 minutes at least twice a day.

- Women—Pouring a glass of warm water over the genital area during urination may lessen the burning sensation.
- Men—Don't irritate the urethra by pulling the skin of the penis down to open it and see if the discharge is still present. The penis may be inspected, but don't squeeze it.
- Keep the area around the genitals clean. Use plain unscented soap.

MEDICATION (ADJUSTED FOR AGING)—Your doctor may prescribe antibiotics to fight the infection. Be sure to finish the prescribed dose, even if your symptoms subside sooner.

ACTIVITY FOR OLDER PATIENTS—No restrictions are necessary. Avoid sexual excitement and intercourse until you have been free of symptoms for 2 weeks.

FOOD & BEVERAGE
- Drink 8 glasses of water every day.
- Avoid caffeine and alcohol during treatment.
- Drink cranberry juice to acidify the urine. Some drugs are more effective with acid urine.

FUTURE CONSIDERATIONS FOR THE AGING ADULT

POSSIBLE COMPLICATIONS—Chronic urethritis and cystitis if treatment is inadequate; spread of the infection to the ureters and kidneys.

PROBABLE OUTCOME—Urethritis is usually "low grade," seldom producing serious, long-term illness. Recurrence is common.

PREVENTING RECURRENCE
- For causes related to sexual activity:
  Drink a glass of water before sexual intercourse, and urinate within 15 minutes afterward.
  Use a rubber condom.
  Use a water-soluble lubricant.
  Use varying sexual positions to decrease the chance of trauma to the female urethra.
- For causes related only to women:
  After bowel movements, wipe from the front to the back and wash with soap and water.
  Take showers rather than tub baths.
- For both sexes:
  Drink 8 glasses of water every day.

CALL YOUR DOCTOR IF

- You have symptoms of urethritis.
- Any of the following occurs during treatment:
  An oral temperature of 101F (38.3C) or higher.
  Bleeding from the urethra or blood in urine.
  No improvement in 1 week despite treatment.
- New, unexplained symptoms develop. The drugs used in treatment may produce side effects.

ILLNESSES & DISORDERS

UTERINE CANCER

BASIC INFORMATION FOR OLDER ADULTS

DESCRIPTION—Uterine cancer is an abnormal growth in the the uterus. Approximately 40,000 to 50,000 new cases are reported each year, and they occur most often in women ages 50 to 70. Body parts involved: The uterus and, if the cancer spreads, the adjacent organs.

SPECIAL CONSIDERATIONS FOR AGING
- The immune system becomes less effective, opening the way for viral, bacterial and other infections; malignancies; immune disorders; and allergies.
- Decreased nutrition, common among chronically ill older people, increases the risk of any disease or disorder.
- Stress from any emotional cause—fear, worry, anxiety, sadness, loneliness or anger—affects all aspects of any illness or disorder.

SIGNS & SYMPTOMS
Early stages:
- Bleeding or spotting, especially after sexual intercourse. This often occurs after menstrual activity has ceased for 12 months or more. A watery or blood-streaked vaginal discharge may precede bleeding or spotting.
- An enlarged uterus. It is sometimes large enough to be felt externally.

Later stages:
- Spread of the cancer to other organs, causing abdominal pain, chest pain and weight loss.

CAUSES & RISK FACTORS—The cause is unknown. Risk factors include:
- Diabetes mellitus; obesity.
- High blood pressure.
- The use of estrogen without also using progesterone.
- A family history of breast or ovarian cancer.
- A history of menstrual cycles without ovulation, uterine polyps or other signs of hormone imbalance.

DOCTOR'S TREATMENT & DIAGNOSTIC TESTS
- Your own observation of your symptoms, especially abnormal bleeding.
- Medical history and physical exam.
- Laboratory blood studies and a Pap smear (although this is only 40% accurate in detecting this condition).
- MRI scan (see Glossary), x-ray and cystoscopy to determine the extent of the disease.
- Surgical diagnostic procedures such as uterine biopsy or dilatation and curettage (see Glossary for both).
- Psychotherapy or counseling for depression.
- Surgery to remove the uterus and usually the ovaries and Fallopian tubes. Advancing age alone is not a deterrent.
- Hospitalization; radiation therapy.
- Self-care instructions focused on the older patient.

HOME TREATMENT BY SELF OR CARE-GIVER

GENERAL INSTRUCTIONS—During treatment, maintain an optimistic outlook. Counseling may help.

MEDICATION (ADJUSTED FOR AGING)
- Your doctor may prescribe: Anticancer (chemotherapy) drugs, including cortisone drugs. Hormone replacement therapy.
- *Note:* Adverse reactions and side effects may be more frequent and severe in older persons. Remind your doctor of any medicines you already take.

ACTIVITY FOR OLDER PATIENTS
- Resume your normal activities as soon as your symptoms improve after treatment. Discuss concerns regarding sexual activity with your partner and your doctor. In most cases, you can resume full sexual activity as soon as possible after therapy.
- See Appendix 20 regarding physical fitness for the active older adult.

FOOD & BEVERAGE
- No special diet is required, but eat a well-balanced diet—even if you lose your appetite from radiation or drug therapy. Vitamin and mineral supplements are helpful. Work with a dietitian to plan nutritious and appetizing meals.
- See Appendix 1 regarding good nutrition for people over 50.

FUTURE CONSIDERATIONS FOR THE AGING ADULT

POSSIBLE COMPLICATIONS—Fatal spread of cancer to the bladder, rectum and distant organs.

PROBABLE OUTCOME—With early diagnosis and treatment, 90% of patients survive at least 5 years.

PREVENTING RECURRENCE
- See your doctor for pelvic examinations every 6 to 12 months.
- Obtain medical care for any uterine bleeding or spotting after menopause.

CALL YOUR DOCTOR IF

- You have symptoms of uterine cancer.
- Any of the following occurs after surgery: Excessive bleeding (soaking a pad or tampon at least once an hour). Signs of infection, such as fever, muscle aches and headache.
- New, unexplained symptoms develop. The drugs used in treatment may produce side effects.

UTERINE PROLAPSE

BASIC INFORMATION FOR OLDER ADULTS

DESCRIPTION—Uterine prolapse is characterized by a uterus that has fallen or sunk from its normal location, causing it to bulge into the vagina. In its most pronounced form, it projects outside the vagina. Body parts involved: The uterus; ligaments that suspend the uterus; vagina.

SPECIAL CONSIDERATIONS FOR AGING
- The percentage of muscle tissue decreases.
- For many reasons, older people are less likely to maintain a good level of physical conditioning.
- Characteristic signs and symptoms of many disorders in older people are frequently changed or absent.

SIGNS & SYMPTOMS
- A lump in front or back of the vagina or projecting outside it.
- Vague discomfort in the pelvic region.
- Backache that worsens with lifting.
- Discomfort with urinating.
- Occasional stress incontinence (urine leakage when laughing, sneezing or coughing).
- Difficulty in moving the bowels.
- Pain with sexual intercourse.
- Inability to walk comfortably because of the protrusion.

CAUSES & RISK FACTORS—Prolapse occurs when the muscles and ligaments at the base of the abdomen become extremely stretched, usually as a result of childbirth or aging. Risk factors include:
- Poor nutrition; obesity.
- Poor physical fitness.
- Repeated childbirth, although one pregnancy and vaginal delivery can weaken the area enough to lead to prolapse eventually.
- Straining to have bowel movements.

DOCTOR'S TREATMENT & DIAGNOSTIC TESTS
- Medical history and physical examination.
- Self-care instructions focused on the older patient (Kegel exercises; see General Instructions).
- Treatment to fit a pessary (see Glossary).
- Surgery to remove the uterus (sometimes). Advancing age alone is not a deterrent.

HOME TREATMENT BY SELF OR CARE-GIVER

GENERAL INSTRUCTIONS—Learn to recognize, control and develop the pelvic muscles. These are the ones you use to interrupt urination in mid-stream. The following exercises (Kegel exercises) strengthen these muscles so you can control or relax them completely:
- To identify which muscles are involved, alternately start and stop urinating when using the toilet.
- Practice tightening and releasing these muscles while sitting, standing, walking, driving, watching TV or listening to music.
- Tighten the muscles a small amount at a time, "like an elevator going up to the 10th floor." Then release very slowly, "one floor at a time."
- Tighten the muscles from front to back, including the anus.
- Practice these exercises every morning, afternoon and evening. Start with 5 each times, and gradually work up to 20 or 30 each time.

MEDICATION (ADJUSTED FOR AGING)—Medicine is not necessary. Your doctor may prescribe a pessary made of rubber or other material to fit inside the vagina to support the uterus.

ACTIVITY FOR OLDER PATIENTS
- No restrictions are necessary. If surgery is necessary, resume your normal activities gradually.
- See Appendix 20 regarding physical fitness for the active older adult.

FOOD & BEVERAGE
- Lose weight if you are obese. A reducing diet appears in Appendix 10.
- Eat a diet that is high in fiber to prevent constipation.
- See Appendix 1 regarding good nutrition for people over 50.

FUTURE CONSIDERATIONS FOR THE AGING ADULT

POSSIBLE COMPLICATIONS
- Total prolapse, requiring surgery.
- Ulceration of the cervix.
- Increased risk of infection or injury to the pelvic organs.

PROBABLE OUTCOME—Aggressive treatment is not always necessary because prolapse is not a health risk. Exercise can often improve muscle function. If the prolapse is severe, it can be cured with surgery.

PREVENTING RECURRENCE
- Maintain an appropriate weight.
- Practice Kegel exercises (see General Instructions).
- Eat a normal, well-balanced diet.
- Engage in a regular exercise program to maintain good muscle strength.

CALL YOUR DOCTOR IF

- You have symptoms of uterine prolapse.
- The symptoms don't improve in 3 months despite treatment or exercise or the symptoms become intolerable and you wish to consider surgery.
- Any of the following occurs if a pessary is fitted: unusual vaginal bleeding, discomfort or urination difficulty.

BASIC INFORMATION FOR OLDER ADULTS

DESCRIPTION—Cancer of the vagina or vulva is an uncontrolled growth of malignant cells in the vagina or on the vulva (the lips of the vagina). This form of cancer is rare. Body parts involved: The vagina; the vulva.

SPECIAL CONSIDERATIONS FOR AGING
- The immune system becomes less effective, opening the way for viral, bacterial and other infections; malignancies; immune disorders; and allergies.
- Malignant diseases (especially in the colon, lung and breast) represent difficult-to-diagnose problems.
- Stress from any emotional cause—fear, worry, anxiety, sadness, loneliness or anger—affects all aspects of any illness or disorder.

SIGNS & SYMPTOMS
- Itching.
- Abnormal vaginal bleeding.
- Discomfort or bleeding with intercourse.
- A firm, ulcerated, painless lesion (either small or large) of the vulva. Cancers on the vulva have thick, raised edges and bleed easily.
- Uncomfortable urination if the cancer spreads to the bladder.
- Rectal bleeding if it spreads to the rectum.

CAUSES & RISK FACTORS—The cause is unknown. Risk factors include:
- A family history of cancer of the reproductive organs.
- Being the daughter of a mother who took estrogen during pregnancy.
- A long history of untreated genital warts.

DOCTOR'S TREATMENT & DIAGNOSTIC TESTS
- Medical history and physical exam.
- Laboratory studies such as a Pap smear and colposcopy (see Glossary for both).
- Surgical diagnostic procedures such as dilatation and curettage (D&C; see Glossary).
- Surgery (usually) to remove the cancerous area. The clitoris and uninvolved areas may be spared if the cancer is not invasive. Advancing age alone is not a deterrent.
- Radiation treatment (sometimes). External radiation shrinks the primary tumor. Internal radiation (implants) affects any cancer that has spread to adjoining tissues. Implants of radium or cesium are used for 48 to 72 hours.
- Self-care instructions focused on the older patient.

HOME TREATMENT BY SELF OR CARE-GIVER

GENERAL INSTRUCTIONS—No specific instructions except those listed under other headings.

MEDICATION (ADJUSTED FOR AGING)—Your doctor may prescribe:
- Pain relievers.
- Antibiotics if a urinary tract infection results from the use of a bladder catheter during radiation treatment.
- Stool softeners beginning a week after treatment.

ACTIVITY FOR OLDER PATIENTS
- A catheter will remain in the bladder for about 2 weeks following surgery or during radiation treatment.
- If you have radiation implants, lie on your back while the radiation source is in place. Move your arms and legs often to prevent the formation of deep-vein blood clots.
- After radiation treatment—internal or external—resume your normal activities in about 5 days.
- After surgery, resume your normal activities gradually, allowing 6 weeks for full recovery.
- Resume sexual relations when healing is complete, in 8 to 10 weeks.

FOOD & BEVERAGE—No special diet is required after treatment.

FUTURE CONSIDERATIONS FOR THE AGING ADULT

POSSIBLE COMPLICATIONS—Fatal spread of the cancer to other body parts. Common sites of spread are the lymph nodes in the groin, the wall of the pelvis, the bladder, rectum, bone, lungs or liver.

PROBABLE OUTCOME—This condition is currently considered incurable, but early detection and treatment offer a good chance for normal life expectancy. The symptoms can be relieved or controlled during treatment. Scientific research into causes and treatment continues, so there is hope for increasingly effective treatment and a cure.

PREVENTING RECURRENCE
- There are no specific preventive measures. Have a yearly pelvic exam to detect the disease during the early stages when treatment is most effective.
- Become familiar with the appearance of your genitals. (Use a mirror and examine them once a month.)

CALL YOUR DOCTOR IF

- You have symptoms of cancer of the vagina or vulva.
- Any of the following occurs at the treatment site after surgery or radiation treatment: Signs of infection, such as increasing pain, fever and swelling. Excessive bleeding.
- New, unexplained symptoms develop. The drugs used in treatment may produce side effects.

VAGINAL BLEEDING, POST-MENOPAUSAL

BASIC INFORMATION FOR OLDER ADULTS

DESCRIPTION—Post-menopausal vaginal bleeding is unexpected, menstrual-like bleeding that begins 6 months or more after menopause. Body parts involved: The vulva (vaginal lips); vagina; cervix (lower third of the uterus); endometrium (inner uterine lining).

SPECIAL CONSIDERATIONS FOR AGING
- The vagina develops fragile blood vessels and the lining becomes thinner.
- Characteristic signs and symptoms of many disorders in older people are frequently changed or absent.
- The immune system becomes less effective, opening the way for viral, bacterial and other infections; malignancies; immune disorders; and allergies.
- Stress from any emotional cause—fear, worry, anxiety, sadness, loneliness or anger—affects all aspects of any illness or disorder.

SIGNS & SYMPTOMS
- Bleeding from the uterus through the vagina, either a light brownish discharge or heavy red blood with or without clots. Mucus may accompany the bleeding. The bleeding episodes vary in length; there is no expected range.
- Pelvic pain.

CAUSES & RISK FACTORS—Causes include cancer of the reproductive system; irritation, infection or thinning of the membranes lining the vulva; injury or trauma to the vagina associated with reduced estrogen levels; polyps or benign tumors of the cervix; polyps on the inner uterine lining (myomas; see Glossary) or fibroid tumors of the uterus; hormone therapy that stimulates the endometrium (the uterine lining), causing sloughing similar to that of normal menstruation (estrogens—female hormones—taken irregularly are a common cause of this); disorders of the blood cells, lymphatic system or bone marrow; high blood pressure; congestive heart failure; liver disorders; anticoagulant or aspirin-containing drugs; and recent vaginal infection.

DOCTOR'S TREATMENT & DIAGNOSTIC TESTS
- Medical history and physical exam.
- Laboratory studies such as a Pap smear (see Glossary) and blood studies.
- Surgical diagnostic procedures such as dilatation and curettage (D&C) and colposcopy (see Glossary for both). Advancing age alone is not a deterrent.
- Biopsy (see Glossary) of suspicious areas.
- Surgery (a hysterectomy) to remove the uterus (sometimes).
- Psychotherapy or counseling to reduce your anxiety about the bleeding.

HOME TREATMENT BY SELF OR CARE-GIVER

GENERAL INSTRUCTIONS
- Use heat to relieve the pain. Place a heating pad or hot water bottle on your abdomen or back.
- Take frequent hot baths to relax your muscles and relieve any discomfort. Sit in a tub of hot water for 10 to 15 minutes as often as necessary.
- Use sanitary pads instead of tampons.

MEDICATION (ADJUSTED FOR AGING)
- Your doctor may prescribe: Hormones. Be sure to follow the dosage regimen. Medication to treat the underlying disorder, such as antihypertensives for high blood pressure.
- *Note:* Adverse reactions and side effects may be more frequent and severe in older persons. Remind your doctor of any medicines you already take.

ACTIVITY FOR OLDER PATIENTS
- Resume your normal activities as soon as your symptoms improve.
- Resume sexual relations as soon as possible after diagnosis and treatment.
- See Appendix 20 regarding physical fitness for the active older adult.

FOOD & BEVERAGE
- No special diet is required.
- See Appendix 1 regarding good nutrition for people over 50.

FUTURE CONSIDERATIONS FOR THE AGING ADULT

POSSIBLE COMPLICATIONS
- Anemia.
- If cancer is the cause, it may spread to other body parts and cause death.

PROBABLE OUTCOME—Depends on the underlying cause and the treatment chosen. A hysterectomy cures the bleeding immediately. Hormone treatment may require up to 6 months.

PREVENTING RECURRENCE—There are no specific preventive measures.

CALL YOUR DOCTOR IF

- You have post-menopausal vaginal bleeding.
- The bleeding persists for 1 week despite treatment.
- Your bleeding becomes excessive, saturating a pad more frequently than once each hour.
- You develop signs of infection, such as fever, a general feeling of ill health, headache, dizziness and muscle aches.
- New, unexplained symptoms develop. The drugs used in treatment may produce side effects.

ILLNESSES & DISORDERS

VAGINISMUS

BASIC INFORMATION FOR OLDER ADULTS

DESCRIPTION—Vaginismus is a spasm of the muscles around the opening of the vagina. Body parts involved: The muscles surrounding the vagina and the muscles of the lower vagina.

SPECIAL CONSIDERATIONS FOR AGING
- Characteristic signs and symptoms of many disorders in older people are frequently changed or absent.
- Many body changes occur as a result of estrogen deficiency beginning at menopause. These include vaginal dryness, shortening and narrowing of the vagina, greater susceptibility to vaginal infections, frequent bladder infections, reductions in the size of the clitoris and increased facial hair. Changes in other systems of the body may lead to a greater tendency to osteoporosis, hardening of the arteries and other disorders.
- Stress from any emotional cause—fear, worry, anxiety, sadness, loneliness or anger—affects all aspects of any illness or disorder.

SIGNS & SYMPTOMS—Involuntary contraction of the muscles around the vagina and rectum. The vagina closes so tightly that your partner's penis cannot penetrate for sexual intercourse.

CAUSES & RISK FACTORS
Causes include:
- An unconscious desire to prevent penile penetration because of emotional or psychological factors. These may include fear, anxiety, hostility, anger or a distaste for sex.
- An insensitive sexual partner, insufficient or unskillful foreplay or inadequate vaginal lubrication prior to attempted penetration.
- Physical disorders (rare) such as infections or allergic reactions.
Risk factors include:
- Previous sexual trauma; stress.
- Chronic vaginitis.

DOCTOR'S TREATMENT & DIAGNOSTIC TESTS
- Medical history and physical exam.
- Self-care instructions focused on the older patient.
- Your doctor or nurse will probably teach you how to dilate the vaginal opening gently and gradually with rubber or glass dilators. Office treatments will probably be necessary 3 times a week, and you should practice at home at least twice a day.
- Psychotherapy or counseling if medical treatment is unsuccessful.

HOME TREATMENT BY SELF OR CARE-GIVER

GENERAL INSTRUCTIONS
- Learn dilation techniques and practice them twice daily at home.
- Prior to dilation exercises or attempted intercourse, sit in a tub of hot water for 10 to 15 minutes. Baths often relax your muscles and relieve any discomfort. Repeat the baths as often as is helpful.
- Before attempting intercourse, you and your partner should use a lubricant such as a lubricating jelly or baby oil.

MEDICATION (ADJUSTED FOR AGING)
- Medicine is usually not necessary for vaginismus, but your doctor may prescribe mild sedatives or tranquilizers for short periods of time.
- *Note:* Adverse reactions and side effects may be more frequent and severe in older persons. Remind your doctor of any medicines you already take.

ACTIVITY FOR OLDER PATIENTS
- No restrictions are necessary.
- See Appendix 20 regarding physical fitness for the active older adult.

FOOD & BEVERAGE
- No special diet is required.
- See Appendix 1 regarding good nutrition for people over 50.

FUTURE CONSIDERATIONS FOR THE AGING ADULT

POSSIBLE COMPLICATIONS
- Psychological trauma caused by guilt, anxiety or loss of self-esteem and feelings of inadequacy; interpersonal problems resulting from the disorder.
- Painful intercourse for your sexual partner.

PROBABLE OUTCOME—Usually curable if the underlying cause can be cured or a coping method can be developed through medical treatment and psychological counseling.

PREVENTING RECURRENCE—Pelvic examination by a doctor and counseling prior to beginning sexual activity.

CALL YOUR DOCTOR IF

- You have symptoms of vaginismus.
- The symptoms don't improve after 3 weeks despite treatment,
- The symptoms recur after treatment.

VAGINITIS, BACTERIAL OR NON-SPECIFIC

BASIC INFORMATION FOR OLDER ADULTS

DESCRIPTION—Vaginitis is an infection or inflammation of the vagina. Non-specific vaginitis implies that any of several germs has caused the infection, including gardnerella, *escherichia coli*, mycoplasma, streptococci, staphylococci and viruses. These infections are contagious. Body parts involved: Vagina; urethra; bladder; skin around the genitals.

SPECIAL CONSIDERATIONS FOR AGING
- The immune system becomes less effective, opening the way for viral, bacterial and other infections; malignancies; immune disorders; and allergies.
- Decreased nutrition increases the risk of infections.
- Signs and symptoms may differ significantly from those listed below.
- Stress from any emotional cause—fear, worry, anxiety, sadness, loneliness or anger—affects all aspects of any illness or disorder.

SIGNS & SYMPTOMS—The severity of the following symptoms varies between women and from time to time in the same woman:
- Vaginal discharge that has an unpleasant odor.
- Genital itching; vaginal discomfort.
- A change in the color of the vagina from pale pink to red.
- Discomfort during sexual intercourse.

CAUSES & RISK FACTORS—The germs normally present in the vagina can multiply and cause infection when the pH and hormone balance of the vagina and surrounding tissue are disturbed. *Escherichia coli* bacteria normally inhabit the rectum and can cause infection if they spread to the vagina. The following conditions increase the likelihood of non-specific and gardnerella infections:
- General poor health.
- Hot weather; non-ventilating clothing, especially underwear; or any other condition that increases genital moisture, warmth and darkness. These foster the growth of germs.

Risk factors include:
- Diabetes mellitus; menopause.
- Illness that has lowered resistance.

DOCTOR'S TREATMENT & DIAGNOSTIC TESTS
- Medical history and physical exam (including a pelvic exam).
- Laboratory studies such as a Pap smear (see Glossary) and culture of the vaginal discharge.
- Self-care instructions focused on the older patient.

HOME TREATMENT BY SELF OR CARE-GIVER

GENERAL INSTRUCTIONS
- Follow the first 4 instructions under Preventing Recurrence.
- Don't douche unless your doctor recommends it.
- If urinating causes burning:

Urinate through a tubular device such as a toilet paper roll or a plastic cup with the end cut out.
Urinate while bathing.
Pour a glass of warm water over the vaginal area while urinating.

MEDICATION (ADJUSTED FOR AGING)—Your doctor may prescribe:
- Antibiotics or antiparasitic drugs for both partners.
- Soothing vaginal creams or lotions for non-specific forms of vaginitis. Use a thin sanitary pad to protect your clothing from creams or suppositories. Keep creams or lotions in the refrigerator. After treatment, you may want to keep a refill of the medication so you can begin treatment quickly if the infection recurs. Follow the prescription directions carefully.

ACTIVITY FOR OLDER PATIENTS—Avoid overexertion, heat and excessive sweating. Delay sexual relations until after treatment.

FOOD & BEVERAGE
- No special diet is required.
- See Appendix 1 regarding good nutrition for people over 50.

FUTURE CONSIDERATIONS FOR THE AGING ADULT

POSSIBLE COMPLICATIONS—Secondary bacterial infection of the vagina.

PROBABLE OUTCOME—Usually curable in 2 weeks with treatment. Your sexual partner will also need treatment.

PREVENTING RECURRENCE
- Keep the genital area clean. Use plain unscented soap.
- Take showers rather than tub baths.
- Wear cotton panties or pantyhose with a cotton crotch. Avoid panties made from non-ventilating materials such as nylon.
- Don't sit around in wet clothing—especially a wet bathing suit.
- After urination or bowel movements, cleanse by wiping or washing from front to back (vagina to anus).
- Lose weight if you are obese.
- Avoid frequent douches.
- If you have diabetes, adhere strictly to your treatment program.

CALL YOUR DOCTOR IF

- You have symptoms of vaginitis.
- The symptoms persist longer than 1 week or worsen despite treatment.
- You experience unusual vaginal bleeding or swelling.
- New, unexplained symptoms develop. The drugs used in treatment may produce side effects.

ILLNESSES & DISORDERS

VAGINITIS, MONILIAL
(Vaginal Yeast Infection; Vaginal Candidiasis)

BASIC INFORMATION FOR OLDER ADULTS

DESCRIPTION—Monilial vaginitis is an infection or inflammation of the vagina caused by a yeastlike fungus (monilia or *candida albicans*). It causes at least 50% of the infections in the vagina. Body parts involved: The vagina and adjacent skin.

SPECIAL CONSIDERATIONS FOR AGING
- The immune system becomes less effective, opening the way for viral, bacterial and other infections.
- Decreased nutrition increases the risk of infections.
- Signs and symptoms may differ significantly from those listed below.
- Stress from any emotional cause affects all aspects of any illness or disorder.

SIGNS & SYMPTOMS—The severity of the following symptoms varies between women and from time to time in the same woman:
- A white, "curdy" vaginal discharge that resembles lumps of cottage cheese. The odor may be unpleasant, but not foul.
- Swollen, red, tender, itching vaginal lips (labia) and surrounding skin.
- Burning on urination; a change in the color of the vagina from pale pink to red.

CAUSES & RISK FACTORS—Monilia (or candida) live in small numbers in a healthy vagina. When the vagina's hormone and pH balance is disturbed, the organisms multiply and cause infections. Factors that may disturb the vagina's balance include diabetes mellitus; antibiotic treatment; high carbohydrate intake; hot weather or non-ventilating clothing, which increase moisture, warmth and darkness and foster fungal growth; and immunosuppression from drugs or disease.

DOCTOR'S TREATMENT & DIAGNOSTIC TESTS
- Medical history and physical exam (including a pelvic exam).
- Laboratory studies such as a Pap smear (see Glossary) and a culture and microscopic exam of the vaginal discharge.
- Self-care instructions focused on the older patient.

HOME TREATMENT BY SELF OR CARE-GIVER

GENERAL INSTRUCTIONS
- Follow the first 4 instructions under Preventing Recurrence.
- Don't douche unless your doctor recommends it.
- If urination causes burning:
  Urinate through a tubular device such as a toilet paper roll or a plastic cup with the end cut out.
  Urinate while bathing.
  Pour a glass of warm water over the vaginal area while urinating.

- Your sexual partner may also need to be treated. Ask your doctor.

MEDICATION (ADJUSTED FOR AGING)—Your doctor may prescribe antifungal drugs, either in oral form or in the form of vaginal creams or suppositories (usually). Keep these creams or suppositories in the refrigerator. After treatment, you may keep a refill of the medication so you can begin treatment quickly if the infection recurs. Follow the prescription carefully.

ACTIVITY FOR OLDER PATIENTS—Avoid overexertion, heat and excessive sweating. Delay sexual relations until your symptoms cease.

FOOD & BEVERAGE
- Increase your consumption of yogurt, buttermilk or sour cream.
- See Appendix 1 regarding good nutrition for people over 50.

FUTURE CONSIDERATIONS FOR THE AGING ADULT

POSSIBLE COMPLICATIONS—Secondary bacterial infections of the vagina and other pelvic organs.

PROBABLE OUTCOME—Usually curable with 2 weeks of treatment. Recurrence is common.

PREVENTING RECURRENCE
- Keep the genital area clean. Use plain unscented soap.
- Take showers rather than tub baths.
- Wear cotton panties or pantyhose with a cotton crotch. Avoid panties made from non-ventilating materials.
- Don't sit around in wet clothing—especially a wet bathing suit.
- Avoid frequent douches.
- Limit your intake of sweets and alcohol.
- Ask your doctor about eating yogurt, sour cream or buttermilk or taking acidophilus tablets when you take antibiotics.
- After urination or bowel movements, cleanse by wiping or washing from front to back.
- Lose weight if you are obese.
- If you have diabetes, adhere strictly to your treatment program.
- Avoid broad-spectrum antibiotics unless they are absolutely necessary.

CALL YOUR DOCTOR IF

- You have symptoms of monilial vaginitis.
- The symptoms worsen or persist longer than 1 week despite treatment.
- You experience unusual vaginal bleeding or swelling.
- The symptoms recur after treatment.
- New, unexplained symptoms develop. The drugs used in treatment may produce side effects.

VAGINITIS, POST-MENOPAUSAL
(Atrophic Vaginitis)

BASIC INFORMATION FOR OLDER ADULTS

DESCRIPTION—Post-menopausal vaginitis is an infection or inflammation of the vagina caused by lowered estrogen levels that upset the vagina's normal hormone and pH balance. Post-menopausal vaginitis is not contagious. Body part involved: The vagina.

SPECIAL CONSIDERATIONS FOR AGING
- The immune system becomes less effective, opening the way for viral, bacterial and other infections.
- Decreased nutrition increases the risk of infections.
- Signs and symptoms may differ significantly from those listed below.
- Stress from any emotional cause affects all aspects of any illness or disorder.

SIGNS & SYMPTOMS—The severity of the following symptoms varies greatly between women and from time to time in the same woman:
- Bad-smelling vaginal discharge. The discharge is usually thin, whitish and sometimes tinged with blood.
- Genital pain and itching; a change in the color of the vagina from pale pink to red.
- Discomfort during sexual intercourse.

CAUSES & RISK FACTORS—Germs that inhabit a healthy vagina cause infection when the normal physiology of the vagina is disturbed. After menopause, the estrogen level that helped maintain a normal vaginal environment decreases, leaving the vagina more vulnerable to infection. The following conditions increase the likelihood of post-menopausal vaginitis:
- General poor health.
- Hot weather; non-ventilating clothing, especially underwear; or any other condition that increases genital moisture, warmth and darkness and foster the growth of germs.
Risk factors include:
- Diabetes; illness that has lowered resistance.
- More frequent sexual intercourse.

DOCTOR'S TREATMENT & DIAGNOSTIC TESTS
- Medical history and physical exam (including pelvic exam) by a doctor.
- Laboratory studies such as a Pap smear (see Glossary) and a microscopic exam and culture of the vaginal discharge.
- Self-care instructions focused on the older patient.

HOME TREATMENT BY SELF OR CARE-GIVER

GENERAL INSTRUCTIONS
- Follow the first 4 instructions under Preventing Recurrence.
- Don't douche unless your doctor recommends it.

- If urinating causes burning:
  Urinate through a tubular device such as a toilet paper roll or a plastic cup with the end cut out.
  Urinate while bathing.
  Pour a glass of warm water over vaginal area while urinating.

MEDICATION (ADJUSTED FOR AGING)—Your doctor may prescribe:
- Topical or oral estrogen. If you use a cream or suppository, use a small sanitary pad to protect your clothing. Keep creams or suppositories in the refrigerator. After treatment, you may want to keep a refill of the medication so you can begin treatment quickly if the infection recurs. Follow the prescription directions carefully.
- Other creams, ointments or suppositories to suppress the organisms causing the infection.

ACTIVITY FOR OLDER PATIENTS—Avoid overexertion, heat and excessive sweating. Delay sexual relations until you are well.

FOOD & BEVERAGE
- No special diet is required.
- See Appendix 1 regarding good nutrition for people over 50.

FUTURE CONSIDERATIONS FOR THE AGING ADULT

POSSIBLE COMPLICATIONS—Secondary bacterial infection in any pelvic organ.

PROBABLE OUTCOME—Usually curable in 10 days with treatment.

PREVENTING RECURRENCE
- Keep the genital area clean. Use plain unscented soap.
- Take showers rather than tub baths.
- Wear cotton panties or pantyhose with a cotton crotch. Avoid panties made from non-ventilating materials such as nylon.
- Don't sit around in wet clothing—especially a wet bathing suit.
- After urination or bowel movements, cleanse by wiping or washing from front to back (vagina to anus).
- Avoid frequent douches.
- Lose weight if you are obese; if you have diabetes, adhere strictly to your treatment program.
- Ask your doctor about replacement estrogen.

CALL YOUR DOCTOR IF

- You have symptoms of vaginitis.
- The symptoms persist longer than 1 week or worsen despite treatment.
- Unusual vaginal bleeding or swelling develops.
- Symptoms recur after treatment.
- New, unexplained symptoms develop. The drugs used in treatment may produce side effects.

VAGINITIS, TRICHOMONAL
(Trichomoniasis)

BASIC INFORMATION FOR OLDER ADULTS

DESCRIPTION—Trichomonal vaginitis is an infection or inflammation of the vagina caused by a parasite that lives in the lower genitourinary tract of males and females. This is very contagious between sexual partners. Body parts involved: The vagina, urethra and bladder.

SPECIAL CONSIDERATIONS FOR AGING
- The immune system becomes less effective, opening the way for viral, bacterial and other infections; malignancies; immune disorders; and allergies.
- Decreased nutrition increases the risk of infections.
- Signs and symptoms may differ significantly from those listed below.
- Stress from any emotional cause—fear, worry, anxiety, sadness, loneliness or anger—affects all aspects of any illness or disorder.

SIGNS & SYMPTOMS
- Foul-smelling, frothy vaginal discharge.
- Vaginal itching and pain.
- Redness of the vaginal lips (labia) and vagina.
- Painful urination if urine touches inflamed tissue. The severity of discomfort varies greatly from woman to woman and from time to time in the same woman.

CAUSES & RISK FACTORS—Caused by infection from a tiny parasite, *trichomonas vaginalis*. The parasite passes from person to person during sexual intercourse. It may live in its host for years without producing symptoms. Then, perhaps due to altered resistance, it will suddenly multiply rapidly and cause distressing symptoms. Since it thrives in both men and women, both sexual partners must receive treatment. The risk increases with number of sexual partners.

DOCTOR'S TREATMENT & DIAGNOSTIC TESTS
- Medical history and physical exam (including a pelvic exam).
- Microscopic exam of the vaginal discharge.
- Self-care instructions focused on the older patient.
- Both sexual partners require simultaneous treatment.

HOME TREATMENT BY SELF OR CARE-GIVER

GENERAL INSTRUCTIONS
- Follow the first 4 instructions under Preventing Recurrence.
- Don't douche unless it is recommended by your doctor.
- If urinating causes burning:
  Urinate through a tubular device such as a toilet paper roll or a plastic cup with the end cut out. Urinate while bathing.

MEDICATION (ADJUSTED FOR AGING)—Your doctor may prescribe metronidazole for you and your sexual partner or partners. Follow the directions carefully. *Don't drink alcohol or use vinegar when you take metronidazole.* Alcohol or vinegar and metronidazole interact to cause a violent reaction causing nausea, vomiting, sweating, weakness and other symptoms.

ACTIVITY FOR OLDER PATIENTS—Avoid overexertion, heat and excessive sweating. Delay sexual relations until you are well. Allow about 10 days for recovery.

FOOD & BEVERAGE
- No special diet is required.
- See Appendix 1 regarding good nutrition for people over 50.

FUTURE CONSIDERATIONS FOR THE AGING ADULT

POSSIBLE COMPLICATIONS—Secondary bacterial infections.

PROBABLE OUTCOME—Usually curable with treatment.

PREVENTING RECURRENCE
- Keep the genital area clean. Use plain unscented soap.
- Take showers rather than tub baths.
- Wear cotton panties or pantyhose with a cotton crotch. Avoid panties made from non-ventilating materials such as nylon.
- Don't sit around in wet clothing—especially a wet bathing suit.
- After urination or bowel movements, cleanse by wiping or washing from front to back (vagina to anus).
- Lose weight if you are obese.
- Avoid frequent douches.
- If you have diabetes, adhere strictly to your treatment program.
- Ask your doctor about replacement estrogen.
- Use condoms during sexual intercourse.

CALL YOUR DOCTOR IF

- You have symptoms of trichomonal vaginitis.
- The symptoms persist longer than 1 week or worsen despite treatment.
- You experience unusual vaginal bleeding or swelling.
- The symptoms recur after treatment.
- New, unexplained symptoms develop. The drugs used in treatment may produce side effects.

VALLEY FEVER
(San Joaquin Valley Fever; Coccidioidomycosis; "Cocci")

BASIC INFORMATION FOR OLDER ADULTS

DESCRIPTION—Valley fever is an infection caused by a fungus whose spores are found in soil. It is not contagious from person to person. Body parts involved: The upper respiratory tract; the lymph glands.

SPECIAL CONSIDERATIONS FOR AGING
- The immune system becomes less effective, opening the way for viral, bacterial and other infections; malignancies; immune disorders; and allergies.
- Decreased nutrition increases the risk of infections.

SIGNS & SYMPTOMS—The infection is usually so mild that it produces no symptoms. In a few cases the symptoms may be quite severe. They include:
- Cough; sore throat.
- Chills and fever.
- Chest pain; headache.
- Muscle and joint aches.
- Shortness of breath.
- Skin rash; depression.
- A general ill feeling.
- Sweating at night.
- Weight loss.
- Stiff neck (sometimes).

CAUSES & RISK FACTORS—Caused by an infection from the fungus *coccidioides immitis*, which thrives in soil—especially soil that lines rodent burrows. Susceptible persons become infected when they breathe the dust from such soil, and the fungi lodge in the lungs. Incubation time is 1 to 4 weeks after exposure. Risk factors include:
- Geographic location. The disease is most common in California's San Joaquin Valley, scattered regions in southern and central Arizona and southwest Texas.
- Occupational or environmental exposure to dust, such as from construction or archeological sites.
- Illness that has lowered resistance, especially uremia, diabetes mellitus, chronic lung disease, tuberculosis, Hodgkin's disease, leukemia or severe burns.
- The use of immunosuppressive drugs, cortisone drugs or antimetabolites.
- Genetic factors. Blacks, Filipinos and Mexicans are most likely to have severe complications from valley fever.

DOCTOR'S TREATMENT & DIAGNOSTIC TESTS
- Medical history and physical exam.
- Laboratory skin tests and blood studies.
- X-rays of the chest.
- Self-care instructions focused on the older patient.
- Hospitalization and possible surgery (in severe cases only).

HOME TREATMENT BY SELF OR CARE-GIVER

GENERAL INSTRUCTIONS
- Use a cool-mist humidifier, without medicine added, to increase the moisture in the air and help relieve a cough and sore throat.
- Keep a daily weight chart.

MEDICATION (ADJUSTED FOR AGING)
- Medicine is usually not necessary. For severe infection, hospitalization may be necessary for treatment with intravenous antifungal drugs. These drugs are potent and have potential severe adverse reactions.
- *Note:* Adverse reactions and side effects may be more frequent and severe in older persons. Remind your doctor of any medicines you already take.

ACTIVITY FOR OLDER PATIENTS
- Stay as active as your strength allows. Rest often.
- See Appendix 20 regarding physical fitness for the active older adult.

FOOD & BEVERAGE
- No special diet is required.
- See Appendix 1 regarding good nutrition for people over 50.

FUTURE CONSIDERATIONS FOR THE AGING ADULT

POSSIBLE COMPLICATIONS—Spread of the infection throughout the body and severe illness, especially in the brain or the membranes that cover the brain.

PROBABLE OUTCOME—Spontaneous recovery in 3 to 6 weeks. Most persons continue to feel ill for 3 to 6 weeks after the signs of infection disappear. Antifungal drugs are reserved for persons with severe, widespread infection, in which case they are life-saving.

PREVENTING RECURRENCE—Cannot be prevented at present.

CALL YOUR DOCTOR IF

- You have symptoms of valley fever.
- Any of the following occurs during treatment:
  Continued weight loss.
  Fever.
  Diarrhea that cannot be controlled.
  Stiff neck with severe headache.

VARICOSE VEINS

BASIC INFORMATION FOR OLDER ADULTS

DESCRIPTION—Varicose veins are veins, usually in the legs, that become permanently dilated and twisted. Body parts involved: The veins in the legs, including the superficial veins, deep veins and veins that connect the superficial and deep veins. Veins in the esophagus, scrotum and those around the anus (hemorrhoids) may also become varicose.

SPECIAL CONSIDERATIONS FOR AGING
- 50% of people over 60 have x-ray evidence of narrowing of the coronary arteries, yet only 50% of those people have symptoms.
- Characteristic signs and symptoms of many disorders in older people are frequently changed or absent.

SIGNS & SYMPTOMS
- Enlarged, disfiguring, snakelike bluish veins that are visible under the skin upon standing. They appear most often in the back of the calf or on the inside of the leg from the ankle to groin.
- Vague discomfort and aching in the legs, especially after standing.
- Fatigue.
- Swelling of feet and legs.
- Persistent itching of the skin.

CAUSES & RISK FACTORS—The veins of the legs contain one-way valves every few inches to help the blood return against gravity to the heart. If the valves leak, the blood pressure in the veins prevents blood from draining properly. The valves may fail because of:
- Previous vein disease, such as thrombophlebitis.
- Prolonged standing.
- Pressure on the veins in the pelvis from tumors or fluid in the abdomen.

Risk factors include:
- A family history of varicose veins.
- Occupations that require prolonged standing.
- Hormonal changes at menopause.

DOCTOR'S TREATMENT & DIAGNOSTIC TESTS
- Medical history and physical exam.
- X-rays of the veins (venogram).
- Self-care instructions focused on the older patient.
- Sclerotherapy (injection into the vein of a solution that causes it to close. Other veins take over the work).
- Surgery to remove enlarged veins. Advancing age alone is not a deterrent.
- Hospitalization for complications.

HOME TREATMENT BY SELF OR CARE-GIVER

GENERAL INSTRUCTIONS
- Exercise to keep the circulation and leg muscles in good condition. Walking is ideal.
- Wear elastic support stockings.

- Rest often with your legs slightly elevated to promote good circulation.
- Don't sit with your legs crossed.
- Don't wear girdles, garters or pantyhose with tight elastic tops that obstruct the blood flow.
- If the skin over a varicose vein breaks and the vein bleeds, lie down and press on it with your hand in a cloth until the bleeding stops.
- Don't stretch the skin over varicose veins.
- Elevate the foot of your bed with 2-inch blocks to help the circulation in your legs at night.

MEDICATION (ADJUSTED FOR AGING)
- Medicine usually is not necessary for this disorder. However, your doctor may inject a chemical into small varicose veins to make them clot and scar (sometimes). Other veins will take over the circulation in the area. Some doctors recommend 1 aspirin daily to reduce the risk of clot formation.
- *Note:* Adverse reactions and side effects may be more frequent and severe in older persons. Remind your doctor of any medicines you already take.

ACTIVITY FOR OLDER PATIENTS
- No restrictions are necessary.
- See Appendix 20 regarding physical fitness for the active older adult.

FOOD & BEVERAGE
- No special diet is required.
- See Appendix 1 regarding good nutrition for people over 50.

FUTURE CONSIDERATIONS FOR THE AGING ADULT

POSSIBLE COMPLICATIONS
- An ulcer near the ankle (stasis dermatitis) caused by poor circulation to the skin. This may be slow to heal.
- A deep-vein blood clot.
- Bleeding under the skin or externally.
- Skin problems adjacent to the varicose veins that resemble eczema.

PROBABLE OUTCOME—The symptoms can be controlled with treatment or cured with surgery.

PREVENTING RECURRENCE—Exercise regularly, especially by walking, swimming or bicycling, to keep the circulation healthy. Additional varicose veins may develop even after surgery or scleropathy.

CALL YOUR DOCTOR IF

- You have varicose veins.
- After diagnosis the varicose veins begin causing circulation problems in your feet, especially stasis dermatitis.

VITAMIN A DEFICIENCY

BASIC INFORMATION FOR OLDER ADULTS

DESCRIPTION—Vitamin A deficiency is rare in the United States. Vitamin A is necessary for healthy skin, for normal vision and cell structure and to protect the linings of the respiratory, digestive and urinary tracts against infection.

SPECIAL CONSIDERATIONS FOR AGING
- Characteristic signs and symptoms of many disorders are frequently changed or absent.
- Decreased nutrition, common among chronically ill older people, increases the risk of any disease or disorder.

SIGNS & SYMPTOMS
- Poor night vision.
- Dry, inflamed eyes.
- Dry, rough skin.
- Loss of appetite.
- Diarrhea.
- Lowered resistance to infection.
- Weak bones and teeth (with a severe deficiency).

CAUSES & RISK FACTORS—The intestines don't absorb enough of the vitamin, which may be caused by:
- Cystic fibrosis.
- Bile duct obstruction.
- Long-term treatment with lipid-lowering drugs.
- A diet that is extremely poor in nutritional value.

DOCTOR'S TREATMENT & DIAGNOSTIC TESTS
- Medical history and physical exam.
- Laboratory studies to measure the blood level of vitamin A.
- Self-care instructions focused on the older patient.

HOME TREATMENT BY SELF OR CARE-GIVER

GENERAL INSTRUCTIONS—No specific instructions except those listed under other headings.

MEDICATION (ADJUSTED FOR AGING)
- Your doctor may prescribe vitamin A supplements and medication for any underlying cause.
- *Note:* Adverse reactions and side effects may be more frequent and severe in older persons. Remind your doctor of any medicines you already take.

ACTIVITY FOR OLDER PATIENTS
- No restrictions are necessary.
- See Appendix 20 regarding physical fitness for the active older adult.

FOOD & BEVERAGE
- Eat a well-balanced diet and avoid fad reducing diets. Good sources of vitamin A include liver, egg yolk, milk and dairy products, carrots and celery.
- See Appendix 1 regarding good nutrition for people over 50.

FUTURE CONSIDERATIONS FOR THE AGING ADULT

POSSIBLE COMPLICATIONS—Severe eye disorders (rare).

PROBABLE OUTCOME—Curable with proper diet.

PREVENTING RECURRENCE
- Eat a well-balanced diet.
- Take vitamin supplements if your diet is inadequate.

CALL YOUR DOCTOR IF

You have symptoms of vitamin A deficiency.

VITAMIN B DEFICIENCY

BASIC INFORMATION FOR OLDER ADULTS

DESCRIPTION—Vitamin B deficiency includes a number of disorders caused by inadequate or absent B vitamins: B-1 (thiamine); B-2 (riboflavin); B-3 (niacin); B-6 (pyridoxine); B-12 (cyanocobalamin). Vitamins are organic chemicals that occur in many natural foods. They are necessary for normal body function. B vitamins are water soluble, and excessive amounts cannot be stored by the body. Body parts involved: The central nervous system; heart; skin; eyes; blood.

SPECIAL CONSIDERATIONS FOR AGING
- Characteristic signs and symptoms of many disorders in older people are frequently changed or absent.
- Decreased nutrition, common among chronically ill older people, increases the risk of any disease or disorder.

SIGNS & SYMPTOMS—One or several of the following deficiencies may exist at the same time:
- B-1 deficiency (beriberi).
  Tingling or loss of sensation in the legs.
  Weakness.
  Congestive heart failure.
  Mental changes, including poor memory or psychosis.
  Lack of urinary control.
  Abdominal pain.
- B-2 deficiency.
  Cracked lips.
  Pallor.
  Sore tongue.
- B-3 deficiency (pellagra).
  Fatigue and weakness.
  Poor appetite.
  Inflamed skin that may blister, weep and split.
  Sore, burning mouth and tongue.
  Indigestion, nausea, vomiting and diarrhea.
  Mental changes, including confusion and psychosis.
- B-6 deficiency.
  Dermatitis.
  Sore mouth and tongue.
  Abdominal pain, vomiting and diarrhea.
  Convulsions.
- B-12 deficiency.
  See Pernicious Anemia in the Illnesses section.

CAUSES & RISK FACTORS—Caused by malnutrition, including malnutrition incurred from fad diets; alcoholism; gastrointestinal diseases with poor absorption; stomach surgery (B-12 deficiency only); the use of some medications, such as isoniazid (which inactivates vitamin B-6). Risk factors include:
- Improper diet.
- Prolonged illness.
- Smoking (maybe). This decreases the absorption of vitamin C and may affect other vitamins.

DOCTOR'S TREATMENT & DIAGNOSTIC TESTS
- Medical history and physical exam.
- Laboratory blood studies of vitamin levels.
- Self-care instructions focused on the older patient.
- Hospitalization for severe malnutrition or alcoholism.

HOME TREATMENT BY SELF OR CARE-GIVER

GENERAL INSTRUCTIONS—No specific instructions except those listed under other headings.

MEDICATION (ADJUSTED FOR AGING)
- Your doctor may prescribe vitamin supplements, depending on the type of deficiency. Don't take more than the prescribed amount. Excessive doses of vitamin B-6 can *cause* the same symptoms produced by a deficiency.
- *Note:* Adverse reactions and side effects may be more frequent and severe in older persons. Remind your doctor of any medicines you already take.

ACTIVITY FOR OLDER PATIENTS
- No restrictions are necessary.
- See Appendix 20 regarding physical fitness for the active older adult.

FOOD & BEVERAGE
- No special diet is required. Prepare well-balanced meals. Don't overcook food or expose it to the air for prolonged periods, as these destroy vitamins. Use fresh fruits, vegetables and meats rather than processed foods if possible.
- See Appendix 1 regarding good nutrition for people over 50.

FUTURE CONSIDERATIONS FOR THE AGING ADULT

POSSIBLE COMPLICATIONS—Permanent brain or nerve damage; severe heart disease.

PROBABLE OUTCOME—Prompt recovery if vitamin B deficiency is treated with proper nutrition and oral supplements in the early stages. Without treatment, severe malnutrition can cause permanent disability or death.

PREVENTING RECURRENCE
- Eat a well-balanced, nutritious diet.
- Take multiple-vitamin supplements if you cannot eat well.

CALL YOUR DOCTOR IF

You have symptoms of vitamin B deficiency.

VITAMIN C DEFICIENCY
(Scurvy)

BASIC INFORMATION FOR OLDER ADULTS

DESCRIPTION—Vitamin C deficiency is a disorder caused by an inadequate intake of vitamin C. Vitamin C is essential for the body to manufacture collagen, the connective tissue that helps form healthy bones, teeth and capillaries and promotes wound healing. Body parts involved: The bones; teeth; gums; capillaries.

SPECIAL CONSIDERATIONS FOR AGING
- Characteristic signs and symptoms of many disorders in older people are frequently changed or absent.
- Decreased nutrition, common among chronically ill older people, increases the risk of any disease or disorder.

SIGNS & SYMPTOMS
- Swollen, bleeding gums.
- Nosebleeds.
- Loss of teeth.
- Rough skin.
- Bleeding or bruising under the skin or in the joints.
- Weakness and fatigue.
- Mental changes, including hallucinations and bizarre behavior.
- Increased susceptibility to infection.

CAUSES & RISK FACTORS—Caused by a diet that lacks adequate vitamin C. Risk factors include:
- Improper diet, including fad diets that don't include fruits and vegetables.
- Loss of vitamin C from foods by overcooking or improper or prolonged storage.
- Hyperthyroidism.
- Fever.
- A serious injury or burn.
- Major surgery.

DOCTOR'S TREATMENT & DIAGNOSTIC TESTS
- Medical history and physical exam.
- Laboratory blood studies such as blood counts for anemia, tests for blood levels of vitamin C and bleeding and clotting tests.
- X-rays of the bones.
- Self-care instructions focused on the older patient.

HOME TREATMENT BY SELF OR CARE-GIVER

GENERAL INSTRUCTIONS—No specific instructions except those listed under other headings.

MEDICATION (ADJUSTED FOR AGING)
- Your doctor will prescribe vitamin C tablets. Don't take more than the prescribed amount. Excessive doses of vitamin C can contribute to kidney stone formation. If massive doses are suddenly decreased, vitamin C deficiency can result.
- *Note:* Adverse reactions and side effects may be more frequent and severe in older persons. Remind your doctor of any medicines you already take.

ACTIVITY FOR OLDER PATIENTS—No restrictions are necessary. See Appendix 20 regarding physical fitness for the active older adult.

FOOD & BEVERAGE
- Eat a well-balanced diet that includes foods rich in vitamin C (see Preventing Recurrence).
- See Appendix 1 regarding good nutrition for people over 50.

FUTURE CONSIDERATIONS FOR THE AGING ADULT

POSSIBLE COMPLICATIONS—Fractures or dislocations.

PROBABLE OUTCOME—Curable with vitamin C (ascorbic acid) supplements and a balanced diet that contains foods that are high in vitamin C. All symptoms and effects except tooth loss are reversible. Without treatment, vitamin C deficiency can be fatal.

PREVENTING RECURRENCE—Eat a diet that is rich in food that contain vitamin C. These include citrus fruits, tomatoes and green vegetables such as green peppers, broccoli and cabbage. Just 4 to 6 ounces of orange juice a day provides the minimum daily requirement of vitamin C.

CALL YOUR DOCTOR IF

- You have symptoms of vitamin C deficiency.
- Your symptoms don't improve in 3 weeks despite treatment.

ILLNESSES & DISORDERS

VITAMIN D DEFICIENCY

BASIC INFORMATION FOR OLDER ADULTS

DESCRIPTION—Vitamin D deficiency is a disorder produced by the insufficient intake or absorption of vitamin D, coupled with too little exposure to sunlight. This deficiency causes osteomalacia (softening of the bone). Body parts involved: The total body, but the bones are more affected than other tissues.

SPECIAL CONSIDERATIONS FOR AGING
- Characteristic signs and symptoms of many disorders in older people are frequently changed or absent.
- Decreased nutrition, common among chronically ill older people, increases the risk of any disease or disorder.

SIGNS & SYMPTOMS
- No symptoms until the late stages (sometimes).
- Bone pain.
- Muscle weakness.
- Shortening of the vertebral column and flattening of the pelvic bones.

CAUSES & RISK FACTORS
Causes include:
- Insufficient dietary intake of vitamin D (vegetarian diet).
- Poor absorption of vitamin D, causing the poor absorption of calcium and phosphorous, which are necessary for healthy bone. Vitamin D absorption is affected by chronic diseases such as pancreatitis, celiac disease, cystic fibrosis, colitis, bile duct disorders, liver disorders, kidney disease or surgery on the stomach or small bowel.
- Inadequate exposure to sunlight. This is especially likely in persons who are confined to bed or home, those who use sunscreens or those who work at night and sleep during the day.
- Poor function of the parathyroid glands (sometimes).

Risk factors include:
- Genetic factors such as black skin, which decreases the absorption of sunlight.
- The use of anticonvulsant drugs.
- Exposure to polluted air. Smog reduces the penetration of sunlight.
- Improper diet as a result of poverty, food fads, bulimia or anorexia nervosa.

DOCTOR'S TREATMENT & DIAGNOSTIC TESTS
- Medical history and physical exam.
- Laboratory blood studies of calcium, phosphorous and bone enzyme levels.
- Self-care instructions focused on the older patient.

HOME TREATMENT BY SELF OR CARE-GIVER

GENERAL INSTRUCTIONS—Sleep on a firm mattress.

MEDICATION (ADJUSTED FOR AGING)
- Your doctor may prescribe vitamin D tablets or injections.
- *Note:* Adverse reactions and side effects may be more frequent and severe in older persons. Remind your doctor of any medicines you already take.

ACTIVITY FOR OLDER PATIENTS
- Exercise whenever possible, especially in sunlight. Weight-bearing exercise, such as walking or running, is especially beneficial.
- Avoid excessive bed rest.
- Stoop—don't bend—to lift heavy objects.
- See Appendix 20 regarding physical fitness for the active older adult.

FOOD & BEVERAGE
- Increase your intake of foods that are rich in vitamin D—even if you take vitamin D supplements. Dietary sources include fortified milk, liver, eggs, margarine, green vegetables, cauliflower, tomatoes and cheese.
- See Appendix 1 regarding good nutrition for people over 50.

FUTURE CONSIDERATIONS FOR THE AGING ADULT

POSSIBLE COMPLICATIONS—Spontaneous fractures in softened bones.

PROBABLE OUTCOME—Usually curable with an adequate diet, vitamin D supplements and treatment for any underlying disease. Bone malformation cannot be reversed.

PREVENTING RECURRENCE
- Provide vitamin D supplements for yourself and your family unless you are sure your diet supplies a satisfactory amount.
- Exercise outdoors in sunlight (in moderation).
- Don't follow fad diets, which may be deficient in many nutrients, including vitamin D.

CALL YOUR DOCTOR IF

- You have symptoms of vitamin D deficiency.
- You experience pain or a suspected fracture following an injury—even a minor injury.

VITAMIN E DEFICIENCY

BASIC INFORMATION FOR OLDER ADULTS

DESCRIPTION—Vitamin E deficiency is characterized by the effects of an inadequate intake of vitamin E. Vitamin E is present in many foods, so deficiency is rare in otherwise healthy persons. Vitamin E promotes normal growth and development. It also enhances the enzyme action necessary for the body's cells to use oxygen efficiently. Body parts involved: The blood and body cells.

SPECIAL CONSIDERATIONS FOR AGING
- Characteristic signs and symptoms of many disorders in older people are frequently changed or absent.
- Decreased nutrition, common among chronically ill older people, increases the risk of any disease or disorder.

SIGNS & SYMPTOMS—Muscle weakness or cramps.

CAUSES & RISK FACTORS
Causes include:
- Malnutrition.
- Malabsorption.
The risk increases with poor nutrition.

DOCTOR'S TREATMENT & DIAGNOSTIC TESTS
- Medical history and physical exam.
- Laboratory studies to measure the blood level of vitamin E.
- Self-care instructions focused on the older patient.

OTHER—No evidence exists that vitamin E has any effect on human sexual reproduction or activity.

HOME TREATMENT BY SELF OR CARE-GIVER

GENERAL INSTRUCTIONS—No specific instructions except those listed under other headings.

MEDICATION (ADJUSTED FOR AGING)
- Your doctor may prescribe vitamin E supplements.
- *Note:* Adverse reactions and side effects may be more frequent and severe in older persons. Remind your doctor of any medicines you already take.

ACTIVITY FOR OLDER PATIENTS
- No restrictions are necessary.
- See Appendix 20 regarding physical fitness for the active older adult.

FOOD & BEVERAGE
- Eat a well-balanced diet and avoid fad reducing diets. Good sources of vitamin E include salad and cooking oil, margarine, peanuts, beef, eggs and green vegetables.
- See Appendix 1 regarding good nutrition for people over 50.

FUTURE CONSIDERATIONS FOR THE AGING ADULT

POSSIBLE COMPLICATIONS—Chronic anemia that results in fatigue.

PROBABLE OUTCOME—Curable with proper diet and vitamin E supplements.

PREVENTING RECURRENCE
- Eat a well-balanced diet.
- Take vitamin supplements if your diet is inadequate.

CALL YOUR DOCTOR IF

You have symptoms of vitamin E deficiency.

ILLNESSES & DISORDERS

BASIC INFORMATION FOR OLDER ADULTS

DESCRIPTION—Vitamin K deficiency is caused by inadequate or absent vitamin K, a fat-soluble vitamin necessary for proper blood clotting. Some vitamin K is produced in the gastrointestinal tract. Body parts involved: The liver; the blood.

SPECIAL CONSIDERATIONS FOR AGING
- Characteristic signs and symptoms of many disorders in older people are frequently changed or absent.
- Decreased nutrition, common among chronically ill older people, increases the risk of any disease or disorder.

SIGNS & SYMPTOMS
- Unusual bleeding, such as from the gums, nose or gastrointestinal tract.
- Unexplained bruising.

CAUSES & RISK FACTORS
Causes include:
- Excessive amounts of anticoagulant drugs such as warfarin or dicumarol.
- Prolonged use of antibiotics. Vitamin K is produced by intestinal bacteria that are destroyed by antibiotics.
- Gallbladder disease.
- Chronic diarrhea.
- Malabsorption disorders, such as celiac disease, pellagra, Crohn's disease, ulcerative colitis or cystic fibrosis.

The risk increases with poor nutrition, especially an unbalanced diet with inadequate amounts of vitamin K.

DOCTOR'S TREATMENT & DIAGNOSTIC TESTS
- Medical history and physical exam.
- Laboratory studies of blood clotting.
- Self-care instructions focused on the older patient.

HOME TREATMENT BY SELF OR CARE-GIVER

GENERAL INSTRUCTIONS—If you take anticoagulants, take only the prescribed amount. Have frequent blood tests to monitor prothrombin time (see Glossary) and prevent unexpected bleeding.

MEDICATION (ADJUSTED FOR AGING)
- Your doctor will prescribe vitamin K orally or by injection.
- *Note:* Adverse reactions and side effects may be more frequent and severe in older persons. Remind your doctor of any medicines you already take.

ACTIVITY FOR OLDER PATIENTS
- No restrictions are necessary.
- See Appendix 20 regarding physical fitness for the active older adult.

FOOD & BEVERAGE
- Eat a well-balanced diet that includes foods that are high in vitamin K, such as green leafy vegetables, cauliflower, tomatoes, cheese, egg yolks and liver.
- See Appendix 1 regarding good nutrition for people over 50.

FUTURE CONSIDERATIONS FOR THE AGING ADULT

POSSIBLE COMPLICATIONS—Severe or fatal hemorrhage.

PROBABLE OUTCOME—Curable with vitamin K supplements taken orally or by injection.

PREVENTING RECURRENCE—Injections of vitamin K are given to persons with gallbladder disease or malabsorption disorders to prevent deficiency. For most people, a well-balanced diet should provide all the vitamin K necessary.

CALL YOUR DOCTOR IF

You have unexplained bleeding or bruising, especially if you take anticoagulants or have gallbladder disease or a malabsorptive disorder.

VITILIGO

BASIC INFORMATION FOR OLDER ADULTS

DESCRIPTION—Vitiligo is the loss of skin pigmentation in patches. This can affect persons of any race or ethnic group. Body parts involved: The skin on the backs of the hands, the face and armpits.

SPECIAL CONSIDERATIONS FOR AGING
- Characteristic signs and symptoms of many disorders in older people are frequently changed or absent.
- The skin becomes dryer and rougher.
- The skin becomes thinner.

SIGNS & SYMPTOMS—Macules (small areas of different skin color) or patches with the following characteristics:
- They are flat and white and can't be felt with the fingers.
- They spread to form very large, irregularly shaped areas without pigmentation.
- They are usually on both sides of the body in approximately the same place.
- Their size varies from 2mm or 3mm to several centimeters in diameter.
- They don't hurt or itch.

CAUSES & RISK FACTORS—Probably caused by autoimmune disease. The pigment-producing cells (melanocytes) don't function normally, allowing the destruction of pigment. Once pigment has been destroyed, the melanocytes can't produce more pigment. The risk increases with:
- A family history of vitiligo.
- Thyroid or adrenal disease.
- Diabetes mellitus.
- Injury, especially to the head.
- Addison's disease.
- Stomach cancer.
- Pernicious anemia.

DOCTOR'S TREATMENT & DIAGNOSTIC TESTS
- Medical history and physical exam.
- Self-care instructions focused on the older patient.
- Phototherapy using a medicine and ultraviolet light.

HOME TREATMENT BY SELF OR CARE-GIVER

GENERAL INSTRUCTIONS
- If you don't choose to use oral medication (or if it is unsuccessful), cover the lesions with waterproof, opaque makeup.

- If you don't use cosmetic makeup, apply sunscreen with a skin protective factor (SPF) of 15 or greater to protect areas without pigment from sun damage.

MEDICATION (ADJUSTED FOR AGING)
- Your doctor may prescribe:
  Psoralens, which stimulates pigmentation from healthy pigment cells bordering damaged cells. The results may be disappointing, and adverse effects are frequent.
  Topical corticosteroids.
- *Note:* Adverse reactions and side effects may be more frequent and severe in older persons. Remind your doctor of any medicines you already take.

ACTIVITY FOR OLDER PATIENTS
- No restrictions are necessary.
- See Appendix 20 regarding physical fitness for the active older adult.

FOOD & BEVERAGE
- No special diet is required.
- See Appendix 1 regarding good nutrition for people over 50.

FUTURE CONSIDERATIONS FOR THE AGING ADULT

POSSIBLE COMPLICATIONS—The disorder may never disappear completely, causing permanent disfigurement. In about 30% of cases, repigmentation occurs spontaneously.

PROBABLE OUTCOME—Treatment is prolonged and often unsatisfactory. Complete and permanent repigmentation is rarely possible. Treatment consists of using an oral medication called psoralens. When discontinued, most of the pigmentation regained is usually lost. It is impossible to predict how much improvement will occur with treatment. Younger individuals (under 30) and those who obtain treatment early usually respond best. Allow 1 year to evaluate the results.

PREVENTING RECURRENCE—Cannot be prevented at present.

CALL YOUR DOCTOR IF

- You have symptoms of vitiligo.
- New, unexplained symptoms develop. The drug used in treatment may produce side effects.

VOCAL CORD NODULES
("Singer's Nodes")

BASIC INFORMATION FOR OLDER ADULTS

DESCRIPTION—Vocal cord nodules are non-malignant overgrowths of tissue on the vocal cords. Body part involved: The larynx (the voice box).

SPECIAL CONSIDERATIONS FOR AGING
- Characteristic signs and symptoms of many disorders in older people are frequently changed or absent.
- The immune system becomes less effective, opening the way for viral, bacterial and other infections; malignancies; immune disorders; and allergies.

SIGNS & SYMPTOMS—Persistent hoarseness without pain.

CAUSES & RISK FACTORS—Caused by the continued overuse of the voice by singing, shouting, yelling, lecturing or other forms of talking too loudly or too much. Risk factors include:
- Smoking.
- Occupations involving the voice, such as those of public speakers, singers, teachers, ministers or auctioneers.
- Chemical irritants.

DOCTOR'S TREATMENT & DIAGNOSTIC TESTS
- Medical history and physical exam, usually by an ear, nose and throat specialist.
- Self-care instructions focused on the older patient.
- Surgery to remove the nodules (usually). Advancing age alone is not a deterrent.
- Speech therapy (sometimes).

HOME TREATMENT BY SELF OR CARE-GIVER

GENERAL INSTRUCTIONS
- The nodules may disappear if the voice is rested for several months. If you choose this treatment rather than surgery, speak in a whisper or write notes.
- Don't smoke, and avoid smoky environments.

MEDICATION (ADJUSTED FOR AGING)
- Your doctor may prescribe a steroid spray to inhale.
- After surgery your doctor may prescribe antibiotics to prevent infection.
- You may take mild non-prescription pain relievers such as acetaminophen or aspirin if necessary.
- *Note:* Adverse reactions and side effects may be more frequent and severe in older persons. Remind your doctor of any medicines you already take.

ACTIVITY FOR OLDER PATIENTS
- Don't use your voice after surgery until your doctor determines that healing is complete.
- See Appendix 20 regarding physical fitness for the active older adult.

FOOD & BEVERAGE
- No special diet is required.
- See Appendix 1 regarding good nutrition for people over 50.

FUTURE CONSIDERATIONS FOR THE AGING ADULT

POSSIBLE COMPLICATIONS
- Without treatment, permanent hoarseness or voice alteration.
- Misdiagnosis as larynx cancer, which also begins with hoarseness.

PROBABLE OUTCOME—Curable with a simple surgical procedure.

PREVENTING RECURRENCE
- Use a voice amplifier, such as a microphone or megaphone, when performing or speaking.
- Take voice or speech lessons to learn to make your voice carry with less effort.
- Ask others to remind you when you get overexcited, especially in activities such as sporting events, so you can lower your voice.
- Don't smoke.

CALL YOUR DOCTOR IF

- You are hoarse for more than 2 weeks.
- New, unexplained symptoms develop. The drugs used in treatment may produce side effects.

WARTS
(Verruca Vulgaris)

BASIC INFORMATION FOR OLDER ADULTS

DESCRIPTION—Warts are benign tumors caused by a virus in the outer skin layer. Warts are not cancerous. They are contagious from person to person and from one area to another on the same person. Body parts involved: The skin anywhere, but especially that of the fingers, hands and arms.

SPECIAL CONSIDERATIONS FOR AGING
- The immune system becomes less effective, opening the way for for viral, bacterial and other infections; malignancies; immune disorders; and allergies.
- The responsiveness of the skin's immune system decreases.

SIGNS & SYMPTOMS—A small, raised bump on the skin with the following characteristics:
- A wart begins very small (1mm to 3mm) and grow larger.
- A wart has a rough surface and clearly defined borders.
- A wart is usually the same color as the skin, but sometimes it is darker.
- Warts often appear in clusters around a "mother wart."
- If you cut into the wart's surface, it contains small black dots or bleeding points.
- Warts are painless and don't itch.

CAUSES & RISK FACTORS—Caused by an invasion of the outer skin layer (epidermis) by the papilloma virus. This virus stimulates some cells to grow more rapidly than normal. Warts are very common. By adulthood, 90% of all people have antibodies to the virus, indicating a history of at least one wart infection.

DOCTOR'S TREATMENT & DIAGNOSTIC TESTS
- Medical history and physical exam.
- Self-care instructions focused on the older patient.
- The careful use of a medicated cream to destroy the warts. Follow the instructions on the label.
- Cryotherapy (freezing cells to destroy them). This is an office procedure that doesn't require anesthesia or cause bleeding. Freezing stings or hurts slightly during application, and the pain may increase a bit after thawing. Usually 3 to 5 weekly treatments are necessary to destroy a wart.
- Electrosurgery (using heat to destroy cells). This treatment can usually be completed in one office visit, but healing takes longer than with cryotherapy, and secondary bacterial infections and scarring are more common.

HOME TREATMENT BY SELF OR CARE-GIVER

GENERAL INSTRUCTIONS
- If you have cryotherapy, a blister (sometimes with blood) will develop at the treatment site. The roof of the blister will come off without further treatment in 10 to 14 days. You should have little or no scarring. Wash and use make-up or cosmetics as usual. If clothing irritates the blister, cover it with a small adhesive bandage. If the blister breaks, the fluid may contain active virus and spread to other areas.
- If you have electrosurgery, keep the treatment site clean with soap and water. Cover it with an adhesive bandage if you wish.

MEDICATION (ADJUSTED FOR AGING)
- Your doctor may prescribe chemicals such as mild salicylic acid to destroy the warts. If so, apply it twice a day for 4 to 6 weeks.
- *Note:* Adverse reactions and side effects may be more frequent and severe in older persons. Remind your doctor of any medicines you already take.

ACTIVITY FOR OLDER PATIENTS
- No restrictions are necessary.
- See Appendix 20 regarding physical fitness for the active older adult.

FOOD & BEVERAGE
- No special diet is required.
- See Appendix 1 regarding good nutrition for people over 50.

FUTURE CONSIDERATIONS FOR THE AGING ADULT

POSSIBLE COMPLICATIONS
- Spread of warts to other body parts.
- Secondary infection of a wart.

PROBABLE OUTCOME—20% of warts disappear spontaneously in 1 month.

PREVENTING RECURRENCE—To keep from spreading warts, don't scratch them. Warts spread readily to small cuts and scratches. Recurrences are frequent.

CALL YOUR DOCTOR IF

- You have warts and you want them removed.
- After removal by cryosurgery or electro-surgery, signs of infection appear at the treatment site.
- After treatment, fever develops.
- The warts don't disappear completely after treatment.
- Other warts appear after treatment.

BASIC INFORMATION FOR OLDER ADULTS

DESCRIPTION—Plantar warts are warts on the soles of the feet. They may occur singly or in clusters. Body part involved: The skin of the plantar surfaces (bottoms) of the feet.

SPECIAL CONSIDERATIONS FOR AGING
- The immune system becomes less effective, opening the way for viral, bacterial and other infections; malignancies; immune disorders; and allergies.
- The responsiveness of the skin's immune system decreases.

SIGNS & SYMPTOMS
- A pinhead-sized bump that grows to 2mm or 3mm. Shaving off the top reveals small black dots, pinpoint bleeding and an underlying translucent core.
- Pain on walking. The wart compresses the underlying tender tissue.

CAUSES & RISK FACTORS—Caused by infection with the human papilloma virus, which passes from person to person by direct contact. The virus invades the skin, making the infected cells reproduce faster than normal cells. Risk factors include contact with contaminated floors in swimming pools or communal showers.

DOCTOR'S TREATMENT & DIAGNOSTIC TESTS
- Medical history and physical exam.
- Self-care instructions focused on the older patient.
- Your doctor will probably pare away the overlying calloused skin and apply chemical cauterants or cryotherapy (treatment with liquid nitrogen to destroy cells).

HOME TREATMENT BY SELF OR CARE-GIVER

GENERAL INSTRUCTIONS—Insert pads or cushions in your shoes to make walking more comfortable.

MEDICATION (ADJUSTED FOR AGING)
- For minor discomfort, you may use non-prescription drugs such as acetaminophen.
- Your doctor may prescribe chemically treated plaster for you to apply. Follow the instructions carefully.
- *Note:* Adverse reactions and side effects may be more frequent and severe in older persons. Remind your doctor of any medicines you already take.

ACTIVITY FOR OLDER PATIENTS
- No restrictions are necessary. Because walking aggravates the wart, find the most comfortable way to walk without putting weight on the wart, such as walking on your heels.
- See Appendix 20 regarding physical fitness for the active older adult.

FOOD & BEVERAGE
- No special diet is required.
- See Appendix 1 regarding good nutrition for people over 50.

FUTURE CONSIDERATIONS FOR THE AGING ADULT

POSSIBLE COMPLICATIONS—None are expected.

PROBABLE OUTCOME—Usually curable in 6 to 10 weeks with treatment, but some cases are resistant to treatment. Recurrence is common.

PREVENTING RECURRENCE
- Don't touch warts on other people.
- Don't wear another person's shoes.
- Wear footwear in public locker rooms or showers.

CALL YOUR DOCTOR IF

- You have a plantar wart.
- The treated area becomes infected, with redness, heat, increased pain and tenderness.

WARTS, VENEREAL
(Condylomata Acuminata; Genital Warts; Moist Warts)

BASIC INFORMATION FOR OLDER ADULTS

DESCRIPTION—Venereal warts are warts in the genital area. These are more contagious than other warts. Body parts involved: The urethra; genitals; rectum.

SPECIAL CONSIDERATIONS FOR AGING
- The immune system becomes less effective, opening the way for viral, bacterial and other infections; malignancies; immune disorders; and allergies.
- The responsiveness of the skin's immune system decreases.
- Stress from any emotional cause—fear, worry, anxiety, sadness, loneliness or anger—affects all aspects of any illness or disorder.

SIGNS & SYMPTOMS—Venereal warts have the following characteristics:
- They appear on moist surfaces, especially the penis, entrance to the vagina and entrance to the rectum.
- They are thin, flexible, solid elevations of the skin that grow in stalks or clusters. They are taller than they are wide.
- Each wart measures 1mm to 2mm in diameter, but clusters may be quite large.
- They don't hurt or itch.

CAUSES & RISK FACTORS—Venereal warts are caused by a subtype of the same virus that causes other warts, but they are more contagious. They spread easily on the skin of the infected person and pass easily to other people. They are usually transmitted sexually, often as a result of poor hygiene. They have an incubation time of 1 to 6 months. Risk factors include:
- Poor nutrition.
- Other venereal disease.
- Multiple sexual partners.
- Crowded or unsanitary living conditions.

DOCTOR'S TREATMENT & DIAGNOSTIC TESTS
- Medical history and physical exam.
- Tests for venereal disease.
- Treatment may include the application of liquid nitrogen to the warts.
- Surgery to remove the warts.
- Self-care instructions focused on the older patient.

OTHER—Recent clinical evidence suggests that the virus that causes venereal warts may also be associated with genital malignancies.

HOME TREATMENT BY SELF OR CARE-GIVER

GENERAL INSTRUCTIONS—These warts are generally treated with chemicals: podophyllin, trichloracetic acid or liquid nitrogen. After applying any of these, wait 4 hours; then wash the treated area carefully.

MEDICATION (ADJUSTED FOR AGING)
- If your doctor prescribes podophyllin, a topical medication, apply it carefully to avoid damaging the surrounding healthy tissue. Use petroleum jelly on the surrounding tissue first. Don't apply the medicine to large areas at one time. Wash off after 4 hours. This may cause irritation or absorption of the drug. Keep podophyllin out of your eyes.
- *Note:* Adverse reactions and side effects may be more frequent and severe in older persons. Remind your doctor of any medicines you already take.

ACTIVITY FOR OLDER PATIENTS—No restrictions are necessary, except to avoid sexual relations until the warts are gone.

FOOD & BEVERAGE
- No special diet is required.
- See Appendix 1 regarding good nutrition for people over 50.

FUTURE CONSIDERATIONS FOR THE AGING ADULT

POSSIBLE COMPLICATIONS—Cancer of the cervix is more likely.

PROBABLE OUTCOME—These small warts usually cause no symptoms. If untreated, they will probably disappear eventually. However, because the virus may be associated with genital malignancy, obtain medical treatment.

PREVENTING RECURRENCE—To prevent the spread of the warts to other parts of the body or to other persons:
- Don't scratch the warts.
- Avoid sexual activity until the warts heal completely.
- Use condoms during sexual intercourse.
- Have frequent cervical smear tests.

CALL YOUR DOCTOR IF

- You have symptoms of venereal warts.
- Any of the following occurs after treatment:
  The treated area becomes infected (red, swollen, painful or tender).
  You develop a fever.
  You feel generally ill.

WHIPLASH
(Acceleration-Deceleration Cervical Injury)

BASIC INFORMATION FOR OLDER ADULTS

DESCRIPTION—Whiplash is an injury to the neck that is caused when it is forcefully whipped forward and then backward (or vice versa)—usually in an accident. Body parts involved: The muscles, ligaments, tendons, disks and nerves in the neck.

SPECIAL CONSIDERATIONS FOR AGING
- Years of weight bearing cause wear and tear on the bones, joints and ligaments.
- Stress from any emotional cause—fear, worry, anxiety, sadness, loneliness or anger—affects all aspects of any illness or disorder.

SIGNS & SYMPTOMS
- Pain or stiffness in the front and back of the neck—either immediately following or up to 24 hours after injury.
- Dizziness; headache.
- Nausea and vomiting (sometimes).

CAUSES & RISK FACTORS—Caused by injury, usually from motor vehicle accidents. Risk factors include:
- Osteoarthritis of the spine.
- Situations that make accidents more likely, such as:
  Driving in rainy, icy or snowy weather.
  "Tailgating" or other poor driving habits.
  Driving after excessive alcohol consumption or the use of mind-altering drugs.

DOCTOR'S TREATMENT & DIAGNOSTIC TESTS
- Medical history and physical exam.
- X-rays of the neck.
- Diathermy or ultrasound treatments (see Glossary).
- Surgery to remove an injured spinal disk (rare). Advancing age alone is not a deterrent.
- Self-care instructions focused on the older patient.
- Physical therapy.

HOME TREATMENT BY SELF OR CARE-GIVER

GENERAL INSTRUCTIONS
- Apply ice packs to the injured area for 10 to 20 minutes each hour during the first 24 hours.
- After 24 hours, use ice packs or heat to relieve the pain. Heat may include hot showers twice a day, in which the water beats on your neck and shoulders for 10 to 20 minutes. Between showers, apply hot soaks (see Appendix 18) to the neck or use a heat lamp several times a day for 10 to 15 minutes.
- Try to improve your posture. Pull in your chin and abdomen when sitting or standing. Sit in a firm chair and force your buttocks to touch the chair's back.

- If your symptoms are severe, buy and wear a soft, padded, fabric collar (a Thomas collar) until the pain subsides.
- Sleep without a pillow. Instead, roll a small towel to 2 inches in diameter or use a cervical pillow or a Thomas collar. Poor sleeping positions delay healing.
- If you have nerve root pressure with numbness and weakness in the hand or arm, buy or rent a cervical traction apparatus. This can be hung over a doorway. Ask your doctor for specific instructions.

MEDICATION (ADJUSTED FOR AGING)
- Your doctor may prescribe pain relievers or muscle relaxants (sometimes).
- You may use non-prescription drugs such as aspirin or acetaminophen for minor pain.
- *Note:* Adverse reactions and side effects may be more frequent and severe in older persons. Remind your doctor of any medicines you already take.

ACTIVITY FOR OLDER PATIENTS
- Depends on the severity of your symptoms. During the acute or severe stage, rest as much as possible. As your symptoms improve, resume your normal activities gradually.
- See Appendix 20 regarding physical fitness for the active older adult.

FOOD & BEVERAGE
- No special diet is required.
- See Appendix 1 regarding good nutrition for people over 50.

FUTURE CONSIDERATIONS FOR THE AGING ADULT

POSSIBLE COMPLICATIONS—Temporary numbness and weakness in the arms if the nerve roots are injured. This may persist until recovery.

PROBABLE OUTCOME—Usually curable in 1 week to 3 months with treatment.

PREVENTING RECURRENCE—Use the padded headrests in your auto. These have decreased the frequency and severity of auto whiplash injuries. Drive carefully and defensively. Don't drive after drinking or using mind-altering drugs.

CALL YOUR DOCTOR IF

- You have a painful neck injury.
- Pain, numbness, tingling or weakness develops in the arm or face.
- New, unexplained symptoms develop. The drugs used in treatment may produce side effects.

WHITE BLOOD CELLS, DISORDERS OF
(Agranulocytosis; Granulocytopenia; Leukopenia; Neutropenia)

BASIC INFORMATION FOR OLDER ADULTS

DESCRIPTION—White blood cell disorders are characterized by a reduction in the normal number of circulating white blood cells (granulocytes or neutrophils) in the bloodstream. These cells are the first line of attack for bacterial infections. Body parts involved: The blood and bone marrow.

SPECIAL CONSIDERATIONS FOR AGING— Blood cell production in the bone marrow decreases beginning at about age 70.

SIGNS & SYMPTOMS
- Fever; aching; sore throat.
- Ulcers (especially in the mouth and throat) that do not produce pus.
- Any sign of infection in someone who has had agranulocytosis in the past. This may signal a recurrence.

CAUSES & RISK FACTORS—Caused by increased destruction or impaired production of granulocytes (white blood cells). The most common reason for this is an adverse reaction to medications, including anticancer drugs, anticonvulsants, antihistamines, antithyroid drugs, arsenic, chloramphenicol, dibenzapine, gold salts, immunosuppressant drugs, indomethacin, nitrofurantoin, nitrous oxide, phenothiazines, phenylbutazone, procainamide, sulfonamides, synthetic penicillins and thiazide diuretics. Genetic factors can increase the risk.

DOCTOR'S TREATMENT & DIAGNOSTIC TESTS
- Medical history and physical exam.
- Laboratory studies of the blood and bone marrow and cultures of the blood, urine and secretions of the nose and throat.
- Hospitalization for intensive treatment during the active phase, with strict reverse isolation techniques (see Glossary) and transfusions of white blood cells (sometimes).
- Self-care instructions focused on the older patient.

HOME TREATMENT BY SELF OR CARE-GIVER

GENERAL INSTRUCTIONS—Hospitalization may be necessary during the acute phase. The following may be helpful after hospitalization:
- Be extra careful about personal cleanliness.
- Keep your mouth clean by rinsing it frequently with warm salt water (1 teaspoon salt to 8 oz. water) or gargling with hydrogen peroxide.
- Pay particular attention to oral hygiene. Brush your teeth gently with a very soft brush, avoiding irritation of the gums.

- Avoid contact with harmful materials such as cleaning chemicals, glue, insecticide, fertilizer, paint remover and others.

MEDICATION (ADJUSTED FOR AGING)
- Your doctor may:
  Prescribe intravenous and oral antibiotics if the white blood cell count is very low.
  Prescribe lithium to stimulate the bone marrow to produce more granulocytes.
  Stop prescribing any drug that is suspected of causing agranulocytosis.
- *Note:* Adverse reactions and side effects may be more frequent and severe in older persons. Remind your doctor of any medicines you already take.

ACTIVITY FOR OLDER PATIENTS
- Rest in bed during the acute stage. Resume your normal activities gradually after your symptoms subside.
- See Appendix 20 regarding physical fitness for the active older adult.

FOOD & BEVERAGE
- No restrictions are necessary.
- See Appendix 1 regarding good nutrition for people over 50.

FUTURE CONSIDERATIONS FOR THE AGING ADULT

POSSIBLE COMPLICATIONS
- Kidney damage.
- Dangerous, sometimes fatal infections (bacterial, fungal, viral or others)—even with vigorous treatment.

PROBABLE OUTCOME—Depending on the cause, usually curable with intensive treatment.

PREVENTING RECURRENCE
- Prevent recurrences by avoiding any suspect medicine or drug that may have triggered these disorders previously.
- Talk to your doctor about monitoring white blood cell counts when you take any medicine in the future.

CALL YOUR DOCTOR IF

- You have symptoms of a white blood cell disorder.
- Any of the following occurs after treatment:
  Any sign of infection, especially fever.
  Swelling of the feet and ankles.
  Painful urination or decreased urine output in 1 day.
- New, unexplained symptoms develop. The drugs used in treatment may produce side effects.

ILLNESSES & DISORDERS

571

YEAST INFECTION, SKIN
(Candidiasis of Intertriginous Skin; Moniliasis)

BASIC INFORMATION FOR OLDER ADULTS

DESCRIPTION—This disorder is characterized by a yeast infection in the skin folds or areas of adjacent skin that come in contact with each other, such as in the groin or under the breasts. This is mildly contagious from person to person and from place to place on the same person. Body parts involved: The skin of the scrotum, vagina and vaginal lips; underarm area; spaces between the fingers and toes; inner thighs; under the breasts; and over the base of the spine (sacrum).

SPECIAL CONSIDERATIONS FOR AGING
- The immune system becomes less effective, opening the way for viral, bacterial and other infections; malignancies; immune disorders; and allergies.
- The skin becomes thinner.
- The fatty layer of tissue under the skin becomes thinner.

SIGNS & SYMPTOMS—Plaques (patches or flat areas) with the following characteristics:
- They are bright red patches with poorly defined borders and are often 6cm to 12cm or larger in diameter.
- Some plaques are weeping or oozing.
- The skin of the plaque appears moist and crusted.
- Itching is usually severe.
- Smaller plaques (less than 1mm in size) sometimes surround larger plaques. They rarely form small pustules (small white blisters with pus inside).

CAUSES & RISK FACTORS
Causes include:
- Infection of the skin by a candida fungus (usually *candida albicans*). The spore form of this organism normally grows in the intestinal tract and the vagina. Signs on the skin do not begin until the yeast changes from its spore form to another growth phase, the mycelial phase. Damaged skin, moisture and warmth are all necessary for the infection to take over.
- Inadequate immunity due to disease or immunosuppressant drugs.

The risk increases with:
- The use of oral antibiotics.
- The use of steroids (oral, injectible or topical).
- Diabetes; obesity; poor nutrition.
- Excessive sweating.
- Crowded or unsanitary living conditions.

DOCTOR'S TREATMENT & DIAGNOSTIC TESTS
- Medical history and physical exam.
- Laboratory culture to identify the yeast organism.
- Self-care instructions focused on the older patient.

HOME TREATMENT BY SELF OR CARE-GIVER

GENERAL INSTRUCTIONS
- Keep the skin cool and dry. Expose the affected areas to sunlight as much as possible.
- Wear loose cotton clothing. Avoid synthetic or wool fabrics.
- Protect the skin from injury.
- If you have a vaginal infection as well as an infection of the surrounding skin, obtain treatment for the vaginitis (see Vaginitis, Monilial in the Illnesses section).

MEDICATION (ADJUSTED FOR AGING)—Your doctor may prescribe antifungal topical medications. Gently massage a small amount into the affected area 3 or 4 times a day. Use only enough to cover. Larger amounts don't help.

ACTIVITY FOR OLDER PATIENTS—No restrictions are necessary, except to avoid heat and sweating.

FOOD & BEVERAGE—No special diet.

FUTURE CONSIDERATIONS FOR THE AGING ADULT

POSSIBLE COMPLICATIONS
- Secondary bacterial infections.
- Id reactions (described in the Illnesses section).
- Blood poisoning.

PROBABLE OUTCOME—Usually curable in 2 weeks with treatment. Without treatment, healing may be slow (4 to 5 years). Recurrence is common.

PREVENTING RECURRENCE
- If you must take antibiotics, consult your doctor about eating yogurt, buttermilk or sour cream or taking acidophilus tablets. These help prevent yeast infections that may result as an adverse effect of the drugs.
- Avoid excessive sweets.
- Keep the skin cool and dry.

CALL YOUR DOCTOR IF

- You have symptoms of a yeast infection.
- Any of the following occurs during treatment:
  The infection continues to spread despite treatment.
  You develop signs of secondary bacterial infection (pain, tenderness, redness, warmth or oozing).
- New, unexplained symptoms develop. The drugs used in treatment may produce side effects.

ZINC DEFICIENCY

BASIC INFORMATION FOR OLDER ADULTS

DESCRIPTION—Zinc deficiency is an inadequate amount of zinc in the body's cells. This affects the functioning of the testes, liver and muscles and affects the structure of the bones, teeth, hair and skin. Zinc is a vital part of many enzymes that facilitate the chemical reactions necessary for normal body functions—including immune functions and skin healing. Body parts involved: All body cells.

SPECIAL CONSIDERATIONS FOR AGING
- Characteristic signs and symptoms of many disorders in older people are frequently changed or absent.
- Decreased nutrition increases the risk of infections.

SIGNS & SYMPTOMS—Two or more of the following:
- Poor appetite.
- Poor growth.
- Sensations of unpleasant tastes and odors and decreased senses of taste and smell.
- Decreased sex drive.
- Darkening of the skin all over the body.
- Sparse hair growth.
- Deformed nails.

CAUSES & RISK FACTORS
Causes include:
- Excessive consumption of substances that bind zinc and prevent its absorption from the gastrointestinal tract. These include calcium, vitamin D and phytate enzyme (found in unleavened bread).
- Surgical removal of any part of the gastrointestinal tract, especially the stomach.
- Parasite infestation of the gastrointestinal tract.

Risk factors include:
- Alcoholism. Alcohol increases the excretion of zinc.
- The use of cortisone drugs, which increase zinc excretion.
- Burns (which cause cell damage).
- Diuretic drugs.
- Cirrhosis.
- Diabetes.

DOCTOR'S TREATMENT & DIAGNOSTIC TESTS
- Medical history and physical exam.
- Laboratory blood studies of zinc levels.
- Self-care instructions focused on the older patient.

HOME TREATMENT BY SELF OR CARE-GIVER

GENERAL INSTRUCTIONS—No specific instructions except those listed under other headings.

MEDICATION (ADJUSTED FOR AGING)
- Your doctor may prescribe zinc supplements. Take them with milk or meals to prevent stomach upset.
- *Note:* Adverse reactions and side effects may be more frequent and severe in older persons. Remind your doctor of any medicines you already take.

ACTIVITY FOR OLDER PATIENTS
- No restrictions are necessary.
- See Appendix 20 regarding physical fitness for the active older adult.

FOOD & BEVERAGE
- Eat foods that are high in zinc, such as red meat.
- See Appendix 1 regarding good nutrition for people over 50.

FUTURE CONSIDERATIONS FOR THE AGING ADULT

POSSIBLE COMPLICATIONS
- Iron-deficiency anemia. Zinc is necessary for iron absorption.
- Poor wound healing.
- Liver and spleen enlargement.
- Excessive zinc replacement or overdose may interfere with the body's manufacture of necessary enzymes.

PROBABLE OUTCOME—Usually curable in 2 months with zinc supplements and the removal or treatment of the underlying causes.

PREVENTING RECURRENCE
- Adults should not drink or eat more than the recommended amounts of milk, other dairy products or unleavened bread. Maintain your calcium intake at 1500mg or less daily.
- Don't take large doses of vitamin D supplements.
- Take zinc supplements if you have had gastrointestinal surgery.
- Obtain medical treatment for parasite infections.
- Don't drink more than 1 or 2 alcoholic drinks—if any—in a day.

CALL YOUR DOCTOR IF

You have symptoms of zinc deficiency.

Surgeries

ABDOMINAL AORTIC ANEURYSM, REMOVAL OF

BASIC INFORMATION

DESCRIPTION—Removal of an abdominal aortic aneurysm (swelling, dilatation or ballooning of a blood vessel).

BODY PARTS INVOLVED—Abdominal aorta.

REASONS FOR SURGERY—To remove the risk of rupture.

SPECIAL CONSIDERATIONS FOR OLDER PATIENTS
- *Note:* Advancing age alone does not preclude surgery.
- Characteristic signs and symptoms of many surgical disorders and complications are frequently atypical, changed or absent.
- Surgical repair is complete and effective, but healing takes longer.
- More likely to experience respiratory and kidney problems, confusion and blood clots after surgery.
- Multiple medications causing various complications are more likely to be used by older patients.

SURGICAL RISK INCREASES WITH
- Smoking; obesity; stress.
- Poor nutrition; recent or chronic illness.
- Atherosclerosis; hypertension; coronary artery disease; peripheral vascular disease (see Glossary); or diabetes mellitus.
- Use of medicines such as antihypertensives; muscle relaxants; tranquilizers; sleep inducers; insulin; sedatives; beta-adrenergic blockers; cortisone.

BEFORE SURGERY

WHO OPERATES—General surgeon or vascular surgeon, usually in hospital.

DIAGNOSTIC TESTS—Blood and urine studies; x-rays of chest; ECG; sonogram; angiogram (see Glossary for all).
After surgery: Blood studies.

ANESTHESIA—Epidural spinal anesthesia or general anesthesia by inhalation and injection, with an airway tube placed in the windpipe.

DESCRIPTION OF OPERATION
- An incision is made from the breastbone to the lower abdomen.
- The abdominal muscles are separated.
- The aneurysm is located, isolated and clamped at both ends.
- The section of the artery between the clamps is cut free and removed.
- A plastic or polyester graft to fit the removed artery section is fashioned and sewn in place.

- Muscles are closed in layers. The skin is closed with sutures or clips, which usually can be removed about 1 week after surgery.

AFTER SURGERY

POSSIBLE COMPLICATIONS
- Excessive bleeding; graft infection.
- Decreased blood supply to large bowel.
- Occlusion of arteries distal to the operation site.
- Kidney failure.
- Inadvertent injury to the ureters, small intestine or branches of the aorta.

AVERAGE HOSPITAL STAY—5 to 7 days.

PROBABLE OUTCOME FOR OLDER PATIENTS—Expect complete healing without complications. Allow about 6 weeks for recovery from surgery.

GUIDE TO RECUPERATION FOR PEOPLE OVER 50
- Don't smoke. It delays healing and adds risks.
- Move legs often while resting in bed to decrease the likelihood of deep-vein blood clots.
- See Appendix 19.

MEDICATIONS & TESTS—Your doctor may prescribe:
- Pain relievers. Follow dosage schedule.
- Stool softeners to prevent constipation.
- Antibiotics to fight infection.

ACTIVITY FOR OLDER PATIENTS—Ask your doctor for personalized instructions.
Typical times for resuming:
Bathing . . . . .Immediately.
Exercise . . . . .When able.
Driving . . . . .When able.
Sexual activity . . . . .When able.
Work . . . . .Variable.

FOOD & BEVERAGE—Clear liquid diet until the gastrointestinal tract begins to function again. Then eat a well-balanced, high-protein diet to promote healing. After recovery, eat a diet low in fat, low in salt and high in fiber. See Appendices 7, 8 and 9.

CALL YOUR DOCTOR IF

- Pain, swelling, redness, drainage or bleeding increases in the surgical area.
- Signs of infection develop: headache, muscle aches, dizziness or a general ill feeling and fever.
- New symptoms occur such as nausea, vomiting, constipation or abdominal swelling.
- Your feet become cold, discolored or numb.

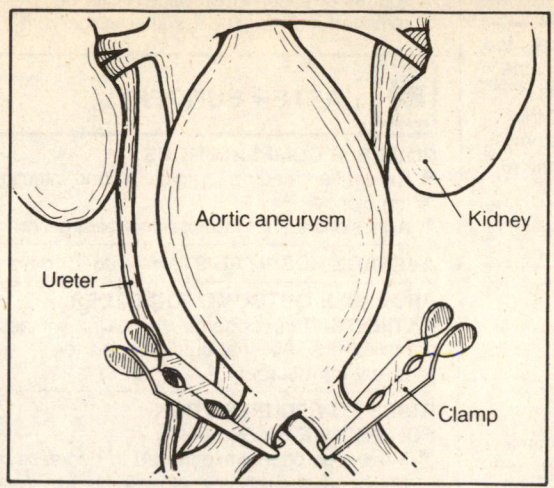

Appearance and anatomical relationships of the abdominal aortic aneurysm. Clamps applied to diseased tissue to be removed.

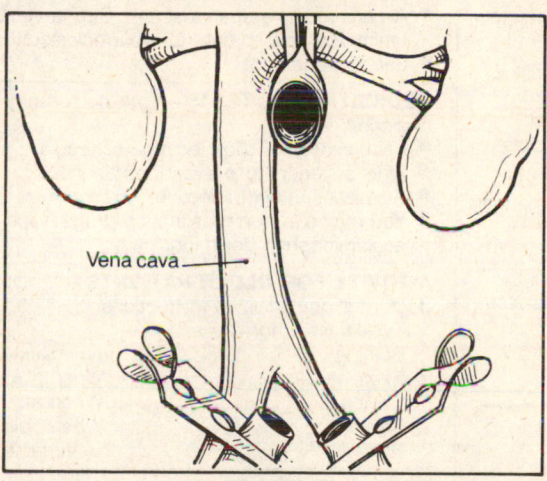

Aneurysm removed between clamped blood vessels.

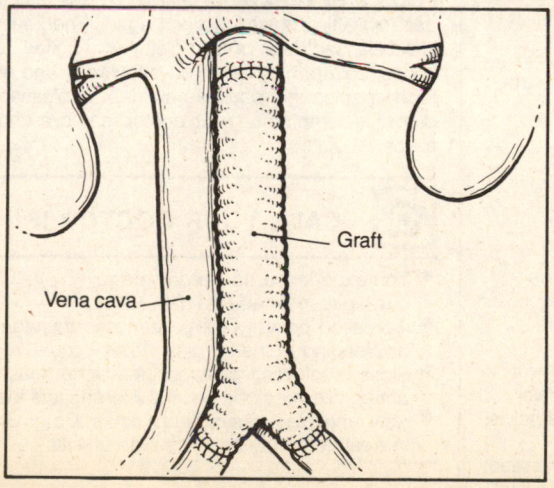

Plastic or polyester graft to fit the removed artery section is sewn into place.

SURGERIES

BASIC INFORMATION

DESCRIPTION—Removal of cancerous cells in the rectum and anus through an incision in the lower abdomen and the perineum. Enough of the anus and rectum are removed so that the intestines cannot be reconnected. A colostomy is performed at the same time so that digestive function is not disrupted.

BODY PARTS INVOLVED—Rectum; anus; sigmoid colon; perineum; abdomen.

REASONS FOR SURGERY—Cancer of the rectum.

SPECIAL CONSIDERATIONS FOR OLDER PATIENTS
- *Note:* Advancing age alone does not preclude surgery.
- Characteristic signs and symptoms of many surgical disorders and complications are frequently atypical, changed or absent.
- Surgical repair is complete and effective, but healing takes longer.
- Weakened cough reflexes increase the risk of lung and bronchial complications.
- More likely to experience respiratory and kidney problems, confusion and blood clots after surgery.

SURGICAL RISK INCREASES WITH
- Smoking; obesity; stress.
- Poor nutrition; recent or chronic illness.
- Excessive alcohol consumption.
- Use of medicines such as: antihypertensives; muscle relaxants; tranquilizers; sleep inducers; insulin; sedatives; beta-adrenergic blockers; cortisone.

BEFORE SURGERY

WHO OPERATES—Proctologist or general surgeon, usually in hospital.

DIAGNOSTIC TESTS—X-rays of lower gastro-intestinal tract; blood and urine studies; colonoscopy (see Glossary).

ANESTHESIA—General anesthesia by inhalation and injection, with an airway tube placed in the windpipe.

DESCRIPTION OF OPERATION
- An incision is made in the abdomen. The abdominal muscles are divided and the peritoneal cavity is entered. The sigmoid colon is located, isolated and divided. The nearest bowel portion is brought to the skin surface for a colostomy. The farther bowel portion is closed and placed deep in the pelvis.
- Incisions are made in the perineum.
- The rectum, anus and end of the bowel (intestine) are isolated and cut free of connective tissue.

- Tubes are left in to allow drainage. The skin edges of both incisions are closed with sutures or clips, which usually can be removed in 7 to 10 days after surgery.

AFTER SURGERY

POSSIBLE COMPLICATIONS
- Excessive bleeding; surgical wound infection.
- Impotence.
- Adhesions leading to intestinal obstruction.

AVERAGE HOSPITAL STAY—7 to 10 days.

PROBABLE OUTCOME FOR OLDER PATIENTS—Expect complete healing without complications. Allow about 3 months for recovery from surgery.

GUIDE TO RECUPERATION FOR PEOPLE OVER 50
- Move legs often while in bed to decrease the likelihood of deep-vein blood clots.
- An enterostomy specialist (see Glossary) can teach you how to care for your colostomy.
- See Appendix 19.

MEDICATIONS & TESTS—Your doctor may prescribe:
- Pain relievers. Follow dosage schedule.
- Stool softeners to prevent constipation.
- Antibiotics to fight infection.
- You may use non-prescription drugs, such as acetaminophen, for minor pain.

ACTIVITY FOR OLDER PATIENTS—Ask your doctor for personalized instructions. Typical times for resuming:

Bathing	Immediately.
Exercise	When able.
Driving	When able.
Sexual activity	When able.
Work	Variable.

FOOD & BEVERAGE—Clear liquid diet until the gastrointestinal tract functions again. Then eat a well-balanced, high-protein diet. Avoid coffee, tea, cocoa, cola drinks, alcoholic beverages and any food or spice that causes painful or unpleasant digestive symptoms. Your doctor may prescribe a special diet.

CALL YOUR DOCTOR IF

- You experience nausea, vomiting, constipation or abdominal swelling.
- Increased pain, swelling, redness, drainage or bleeding in the surgical areas occurs.
- Signs of infection develop: headache, muscle aches, dizziness or a general ill feeling and fever.
- New, unexplained symptoms occur. Drugs used in treatment may produce side effects.

ABDOMINO-PERINEAL RESECTION

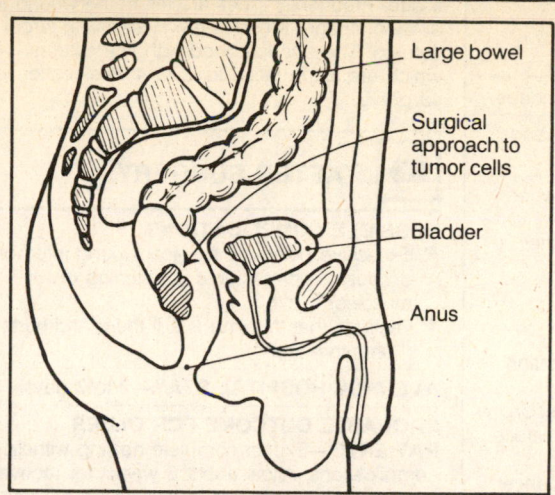

Large bowel

Surgical approach to tumor cells

Bladder

Anus

An illustration of the appearance and anatomical relationships of the large bowel with representation of a large bowel tumor.

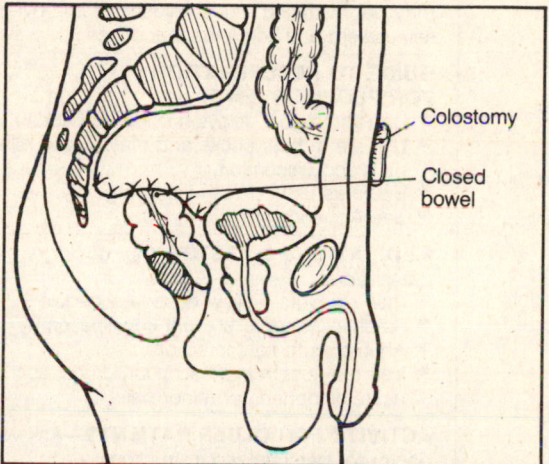

Colostomy

Closed bowel

The colostomy which protrudes through the abdominal wall and skin.
- The closed distal portion of the bowel.

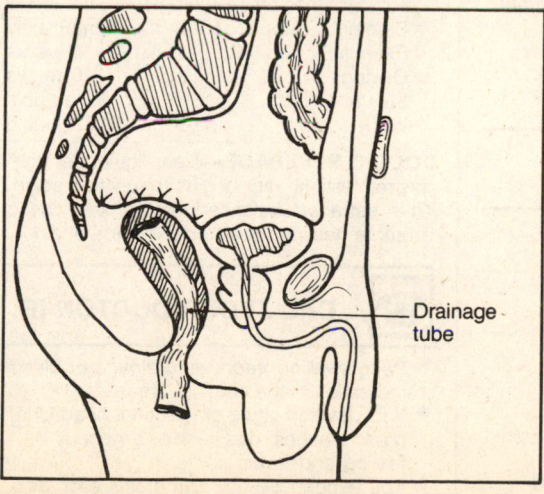

Drainage tube

Tumor removed, along with rectum, bowel and anus.
- Drainage tube left in place to be removed after healing.

SURGERIES

AMPUTATION

BASIC INFORMATION

DESCRIPTION—Removal of a limb or appendage.

BODY PARTS INVOLVED—Arms; legs; hands; feet; fingers; or toes.

REASONS FOR SURGERY—Performed when blood circulation to a part of the body is irreversibly interrupted, usually by one of the following:
- Injury to blood vessels that cannot be repaired or reconstructed.
- Hardening of the arteries.
- Impaired blood circulation as a complication of diabetes mellitus.
- Buerger's disease; Raynaud's phenomenon.
- Severe infection with gangrene; severe frostbite.
- Obstructions in the arteries.

Also performed to prevent the spread of cancer.

SPECIAL CONSIDERATIONS FOR OLDER PATIENTS
- *Note:* Advancing age alone does not preclude surgery.
- Characteristic signs and symptoms of many surgical disorders and complications are frequently atypical, changed or absent.
- Surgical repair is complete and effective, but healing takes longer.
- Nursing care needs to be more intense and skillful.
- More likely to experience respiratory and kidney problems, confusion and blood clots after surgery.

SURGICAL RISK INCREASES WITH
- Smoking; obesity; stress.
- Poor nutrition; recent or chronic illness.
- Excessive alcohol consumption.
- Coronary artery disease.
- Disease that increases coagulability of blood.
- Use of drugs such as antihypertensives; muscle relaxants; tranquilizers; sleep inducers; insulin; sedatives; narcotics; beta-adrenergic blockers; cortisone.

BEFORE SURGERY

WHO OPERATES—General surgeon or orthopedic surgeon, usually in hospital.

DIAGNOSTIC TESTS—Blood and urine studies; x-rays of part to be amputated.

ANESTHESIA—General anesthesia by inhalation and injection, with an airway tube placed in the windpipe.

DESCRIPTION OF OPERATION—An incision is made around the part to be amputated. Tissue, muscles, blood vessels, nerves and bone are severed. The bone is filed smooth, and the bone end is covered with connective tissue. Frequently tubes are left in the wound to allow drainage. Muscles are closed with large sutures. The skin is closed with fine sutures, which are left in place for 3 to 4 weeks after surgery.

AFTER SURGERY

POSSIBLE COMPLICATIONS
- Excessive bleeding, surgical wound infection or muscle contractures (shortening of muscles).
- Feelings that the limb is still there and hurts ("phantom limb").

AVERAGE HOSPITAL STAY—2 to 7 days.

PROBABLE OUTCOME FOR OLDER PATIENTS—Expect complete healing without complications. Allow about 6 weeks for recovery from surgery. A physical rehabilitation program may be frustrating, but it will lead to improved self-esteem and some independence.

GUIDE TO RECUPERATION FOR PEOPLE OVER 50
- Don't smoke. It delays healing and adds risks.
- Use warm heat packs and massage to relieve pain and discomfort.
- Bathe as usual. Wash incision gently.
- See Appendix 19.

MEDICATIONS & TESTS—Your doctor may prescribe:
- Pain relievers. Follow dosage schedule.
- Stool softeners to prevent constipation.
- Antibiotics to fight infection.
- You may use non-prescription drugs, such as acetaminophen, for minor pain.

ACTIVITY FOR OLDER PATIENTS—Ask your doctor for personalized instructions.
Typical times for resuming:
Bathing . . . . .Immediately.
Exercise . . . . .4 weeks.
Driving . . . . .6 weeks.
Sexual activity . . . . .When able.
Work . . . . .Variable.

FOOD & BEVERAGE—Clear liquid diet until the gastrointestinal tract begins to function again. Then eat a well-balanced, high-protein diet to promote healing. See Appendices 7 and 1.

CALL YOUR DOCTOR IF

- Pain, swelling, redness, drainage or bleeding increases in the surgical area.
- You develop signs of infection: headache, muscle aches, dizziness or a general ill feeling and fever.
- You experience new symptoms such as nausea, vomiting or constipation.

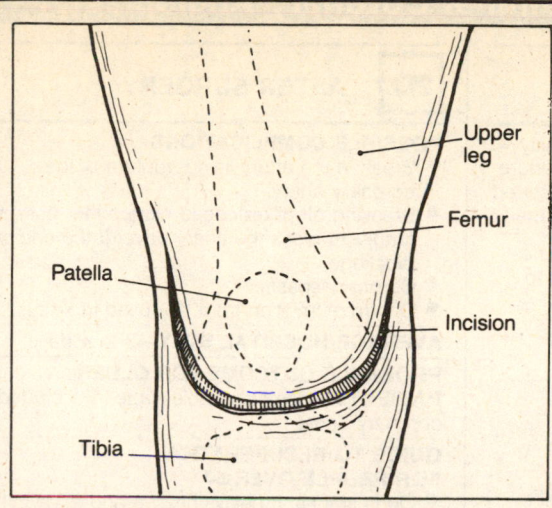

An illustration of a lower leg amputation.

Upper leg

Femur

Patella

Incision

Tibia

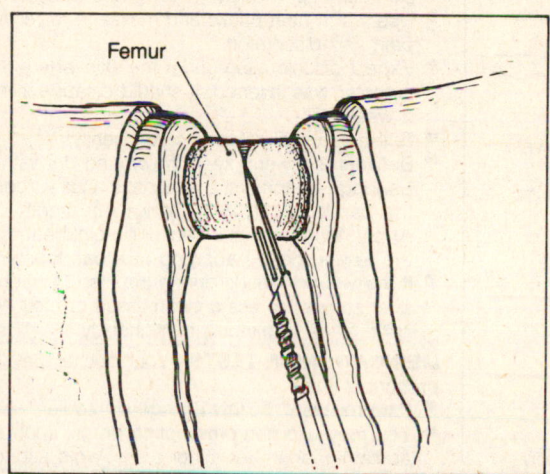

Skin, connective tissue, muscles, blood vessels, nerves, and bone are severed.

Femur

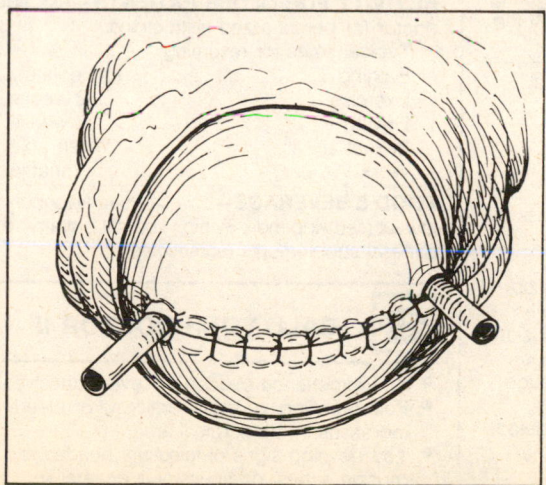

Bone end filed smooth and covered with connective tissue.

• Muscles closed with large sutures, skin closed with fine sutures.
• Drains remain in place.

SURGERIES

ANGIOPLASTY
(Percutaneous Transluminal Coronary Angioplasty)

 BASIC INFORMATION

DESCRIPTION—Angio = blood vessel; plasty = surgical shaping or alteration of. In this procedure, a catheter with an inflatable balloon tip is inserted into a blocked or partially blocked coronary artery.

BODY PARTS INVOLVED—Coronary arteries (the blood vessels that supply nourishment to the heart muscle).

REASONS FOR SURGERY—To remove a block or partial block of a coronary artery.

SPECIAL CONSIDERATIONS FOR OLDER PATIENTS
- *Note:* Advancing age alone does not preclude surgery.
- More likely to experience respiratory and kidney problems, confusion and blood clots after surgery.

SURGICAL RISK INCREASES WITH
- Stress; obesity; smoking.
- Excessive alcohol consumption.
- Use of medicines such as antihypertensives; muscle relaxants; tranquilizers; sleep inducers; insulin; sedatives; beta-adrenergic blockers; cortisone.
- Angina (for more than 1 year).
- Calcification of blood vessels.

 BEFORE SURGERY

WHO OPERATES—Cardiologist or general surgeon, usually in hospital.

DIAGNOSTIC TESTS—Heart catheterization with x-ray and fluoroscopic examinations. During surgery: x-rays after injection of dye through the catheter into various parts of the heart.

ANESTHESIA—Local, with standby general anesthesia.

DESCRIPTION OF OPERATION
- The cardiac balloon catheter is inserted into an artery in the arm or leg. Fluoroscopy provides guidance for the catheter to pass through the artery to the heart.
- The catheter is guided into the coronary artery system. Fluoroscopy allows identification of any disease in the coronary arteries.
- The catheter is passed through the occlusion, the balloon is inflated and the occlusion is compressed, allowing blood to flow through once again.
- When all examinations have been completed, the catheter balloon is withdrawn, and the artery into which it was inserted is compressed until bleeding stops.

 AFTER SURGERY

POSSIBLE COMPLICATIONS
- Break in the artery lining; rupture of the coronary artery.
- Breaking off of dislodged plaque that passes further to block the artery beyond the original blockage.
- Coronary spasm.
- Chemical irritation from dye used in x-ray.

AVERAGE HOSPITAL STAY—3 to 4 days.

PROBABLE OUTCOME FOR OLDER PATIENTS—Removal of blockage in occluded coronary artery.

GUIDE TO RECUPERATION FOR PEOPLE OVER 50
- Don't smoke. It delays healing and adds risks.
- Use warm heat packs and massage to relieve pain and discomfort.
- Expect discoloration under the skin where the catheter was inserted. It should disappear in 2 weeks.
- Bathe as usual. Wash incision gently.
- Between showers, keep the wound dry with a bandage for the first 2 or 3 days after surgery. If a bandage gets wet, change it promptly. Apply non-prescription antibiotic ointment to the wound before applying new bandages.
- If the wound bleeds during the first 24 hours after surgery, press a clean tissue or cloth to it for 10 to 15 minutes continuously.

MEDICATIONS & TESTS—Your doctor may prescribe:
- Pain relievers. Follow dosage schedule.
- You may use non-prescription drugs, such as acetaminophen, for minor pain. Avoid aspirin.

ACTIVITY FOR OLDER PATIENTS—Ask your doctor for personalized instructions.
Typical times for resuming:
Bathing . . . . Immediately.
Exercise . . . . 2 weeks.
Driving . . . . 2 weeks.
Sexual activity . . . . When able.
Work . . . . Variable.

FOOD & BEVERAGE—Low-salt (see Appendix 9), low-fat (see Appendix 8), high-fiber diet; vitamin and mineral supplements (sometimes).

 CALL YOUR DOCTOR IF

- You experience sudden or severe chest pain.
- Pain, swelling, redness, drainage or bleeding increases in the surgical area.
- You develop signs of infection: headache, muscle aches, dizziness or a general ill feeling and fever.

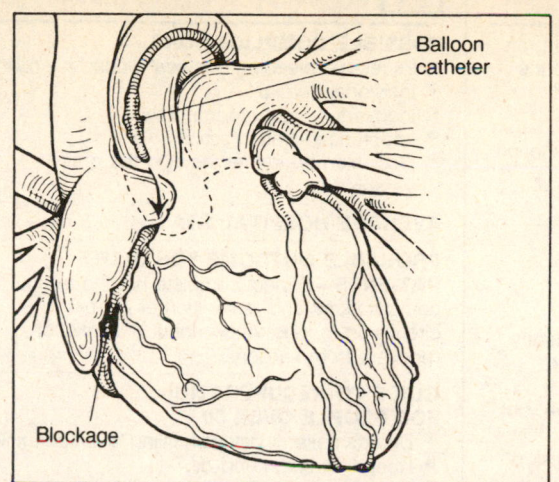

Balloon catheter

Blockage

An illustration of the cardiac balloon catheter about to enter the right coronary artery.

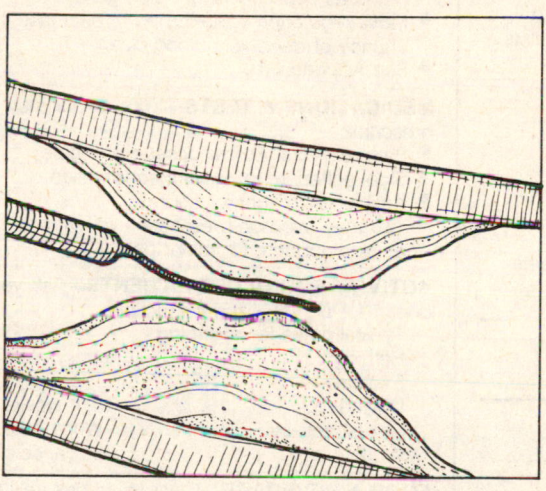

Fluoroscopy allows identification of any disease in the coronary arteries and the catheter is passed through the occlusion.

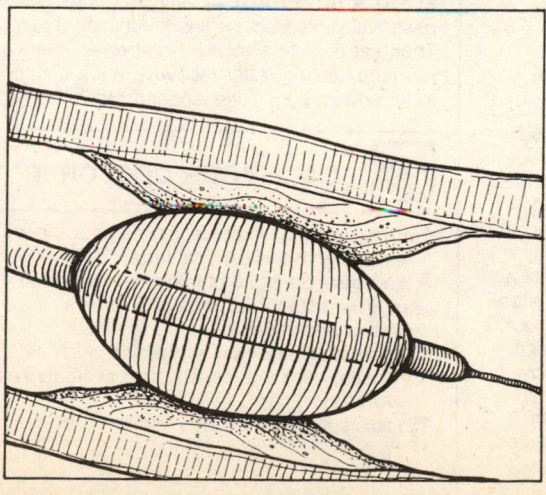

Then the balloon is inflated, the plaque is broken, and the occlusion is dilated allowing blood to flow freely once again. After all examinations have been completed, the catheter balloon is withdrawn.

SURGERIES

AORTO-ILIAC BYPASS GRAFT

BASIC INFORMATION

DESCRIPTION—Placement of an artificial graft to bypass a blood clot or artery closure in the arteries that supply blood to the abdomen, genital area and legs.

BODY PARTS INVOLVED—Aorta; iliac arteries.

REASONS FOR SURGERY—Restoration of normal blood circulation in the legs.

SPECIAL CONSIDERATIONS FOR OLDER PATIENTS
- *Note:* Advancing age alone does not preclude surgery.
- Characteristic signs and symptoms of many surgical disorders and complications are frequently atypical, changed or absent.
- Surgical repair is complete and effective, but healing takes longer.
- Decreased nutrition may increase the risk of surgical infections and complications.
- More likely to experience respiratory and kidney problems, confusion and blood clots after surgery.

SURGICAL RISK INCREASES WITH
- Excessive alcohol consumption; obesity; smoking.
- Diabetes mellitus; coronary artery disease; atherosclerosis.
- Use of drugs such as antihypertensives; muscle relaxants; tranquilizers; sleep inducers; insulin; sedatives; narcotics; beta-adrenergic blockers; cortisone.

BEFORE SURGERY

WHO OPERATES—General surgeon or vascular surgeon, usually in hospital.

DIAGNOSTIC TESTS—Blood and urine studies; arteriograms (see Glossary).

ANESTHESIA—General anesthesia by inhalation and injection, with an airway tube placed in the windpipe.

DESCRIPTION OF OPERATION—An incision is made in the abdomen. The abdominal muscles are separated to expose the abdominal organs, which are inspected for undetected disease. (Other surgeries may be performed at this time.) The aorta and iliac arteries are located and clamped to isolate the obstruction. A polyester graft is fashioned and fitted in place. One end fits in the aorta and the other two ends in the iliac arteries. The graft is sewn in place and the clamps are released. Blood can now circulate freely. The muscles of the abdomen are closed in layers. The skin is closed with sutures or clips, which usually can be removed about 1 week after surgery.

AFTER SURGERY

POSSIBLE COMPLICATIONS
- Excessive bleeding; surgical wound infection.
- Incisional hernia.
- Inadvertent injury to the ureter.
- Impotence; graft infection.
- Occlusion of arteries beyond the grafted vessels.

AVERAGE HOSPITAL STAY—6 to 8 days.

PROBABLE OUTCOME FOR OLDER PATIENTS—Expect complete healing without complications and restoration of normal circulation to legs. Allow about 6 weeks for recovery from surgery.

GUIDE TO RECUPERATION FOR PEOPLE OVER 50
- Don't smoke. It delays healing and adds risks.
- Keep feet clean and dry.
- Bathe as usual. Wash incision gently.
- Move legs often while in bed to decrease the chance of deep-vein blood clots.
- See Appendix 19.

MEDICATIONS & TESTS—Your doctor may prescribe:
- Pain relievers. Follow dosage schedule.
- Stool softeners to prevent constipation.
- Antibiotics to fight infection.
- You may use non-prescription drugs, such as acetaminophen, for minor pain.

ACTIVITY FOR OLDER PATIENTS—Ask your doctor for personalized instructions.
Typical times for resuming:
Bathing . . . . Immediately.
Exercise . . . . 4 weeks.
Driving . . . . 4 weeks.
Sexual activity . . . . When able.
Work . . . . Variable.

FOOD & BEVERAGE—Clear liquid diet until the gastrointestinal tract begins to function again. Then eat a well-balanced, high-protein diet to promote healing. After recovery, eat a diet low in fat and sodium. (See Appendices 7, 8 and 9.)

CALL YOUR DOCTOR IF

- Pain, swelling, redness, drainage or bleeding increases in the surgical area.
- You develop signs of infection: headache, muscle aches, dizziness or a general ill feeling and fever.
- You experience new symptoms, such as nausea, vomiting, constipation or abdominal swelling.
- Your feet become cold, discolored or numb.

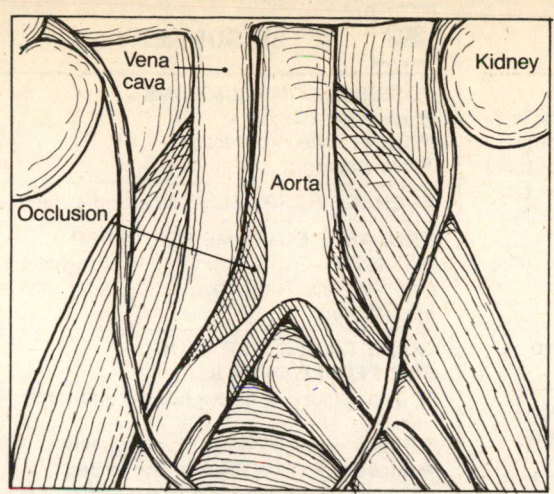

An illustration of the aorta, iliac arteries, and the occlusions to be bypassed.

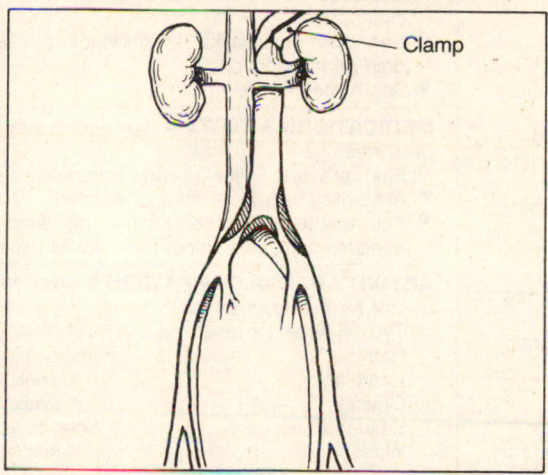

The aorta and iliac arteries are clamped to isolate the obstruction.

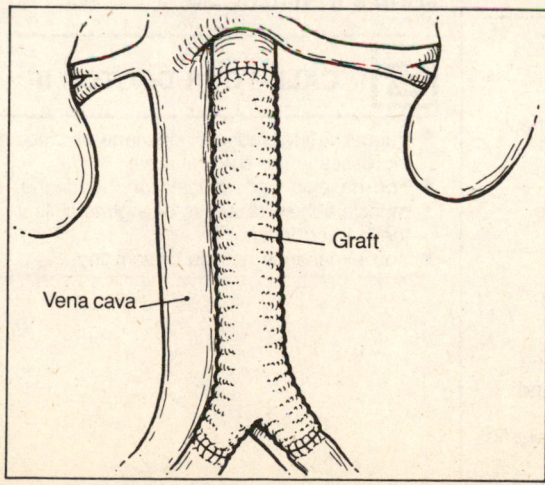

Polyester graft fitted in place. The upper end fits the aorta and the two lower ends fit the iliac arteries.

•After the graft is in place, the clamps are released. Blood can now circulate freely again.

SURGERIES

BASIC INFORMATION

DESCRIPTION—Arthro = joint; plasty = surgical shaping or alteration of. Hip arthroplasty is the surgical formulation or reformation of the hip joint. Three types may be used: cup or mold arthroplasty, total hip replacement and total hip surface replacement. Total hip replacement is explained here. In this method, a metal ball replaces the worn head of the thigh bone and a cup (often plastic) replaces the worn socket.

BODY PARTS INVOLVED—Hip joint; muscles, ligaments, bones and bursa forming the hip joint.

REASONS FOR SURGERY—Diseased or injured hip with pain and stiffness causing an altered gait and impaired quality of life.

SPECIAL CONSIDERATIONS FOR OLDER PATIENTS
- *Note:* Advancing age alone does not preclude surgery.
- Surgical repair is complete and effective, but healing takes longer.
- More likely to experience respiratory and kidney problems, confusion and blood clots after surgery.

SURGICAL RISK INCREASES WITH
- Smoking; obesity; stress.
- Poor nutrition; recent or chronic illness.
- Use of medicines such as antihypertensives; muscle relaxants; tranquilizers; sleep inducers; insulin; sedatives; beta-adrenergic blockers; cortisone.
- Excessive alcohol consumption.

 ## BEFORE SURGERY

WHO OPERATES—Orthopedist, usually in hospital.

DIAGNOSTIC TESTS—Blood and urine studies; x-rays of joint; joint expiration (to check for active infection).

ANESTHESIA—General anesthesia by inhalation and injection, with an airway tube placed in the windpipe.

DESCRIPTION OF OPERATION
- An incision is made over the affected hip.
- The head and neck of the femur are removed.
- The femoral canal is reamed to accept the metal femoral component (head, neck and stem).
- The acetabulum is reamed to accept a plastic cup.
- The ball and socket are replaced in normal position.

 ## AFTER SURGERY

POSSIBLE COMPLICATIONS
- Bleeding into joint.
- Surgical wound infection.
- Slow healing.

AVERAGE HOSPITAL STAY—2 to 4 day.

PROBABLE OUTCOME FOR OLDER PATIENTS—Expect complete healing without complications. Allow about 6 weeks for recovery from surgery.

GUIDE TO RECUPERATION FOR PEOPLE OVER 50
- Don't smoke. It delays healing and adds risks.
- Bathe as usual. Wash incision gently.
- Move legs often while resting in bed to decrease the likelihood of deep-vein blood clots.
- Use warm heat packs and massage to relieve pain and discomfort.
- See Appendix 19.

MEDICATIONS & TESTS—Your doctor may prescribe:
- Pain relievers. Follow dosage schedule.
- Antibiotics to fight infection, if needed.
- You may use non-prescription drugs, such as acetaminophen, for minor pain. Avoid aspirin.

ACTIVITY FOR OLDER PATIENTS—Ask your doctor for personalized instructions.
Typical times for resuming:
Bathing . . . . Immediately.
Exercise . . . . 4 weeks.
Driving . . . . 4 weeks.
Sexual activity . . . . When able.
Work . . . . Variable.

FOOD & BEVERAGE—No special diet.

 ## CALL YOUR DOCTOR IF

- Pain, swelling, redness, drainage or bleeding increases in the surgical area.
- You develop signs of infection: headache, muscle aches, dizziness or a general ill feeling and fever.
- You experience nausea or vomiting.

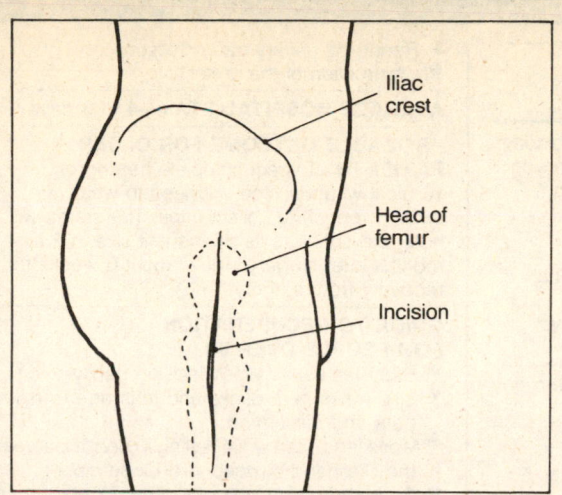

An illustration of an incison made over the affected hip showing the head of the femur which is diseased or injured.

Iliac crest

Head of femur

Incision

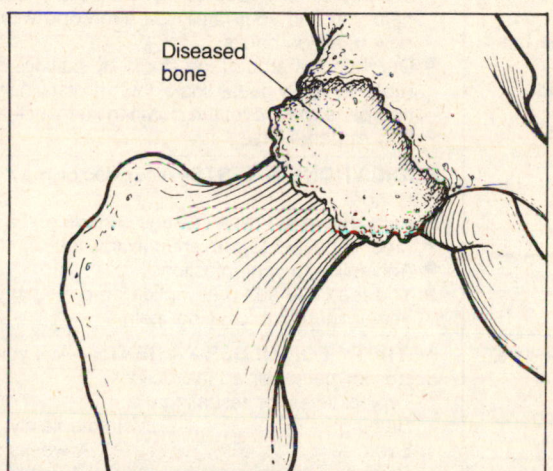

A closer view of the diseased hip joint. After the diseased bone has been removed, the artificial ball and socket are placed into normal position.

Diseased bone

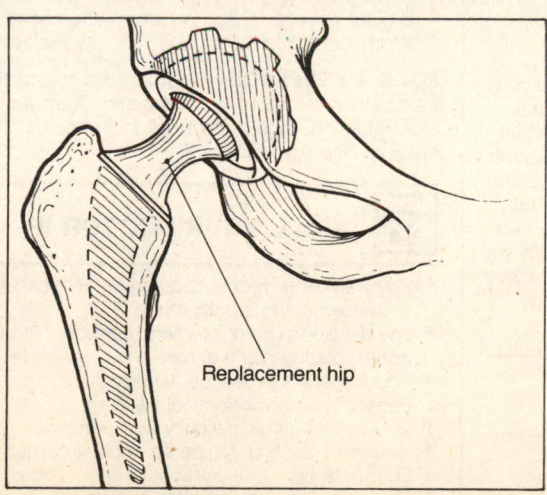

The appearance of the hip after the metal prosthesis has been inserted.

Replacement hip

SURGERIES

BASIC INFORMATION

DESCRIPTION—Removal of the urinary bladder and adjacent tissues and organs and diversion of the urinary stream to an artificial opening, which is called an "ostomy" or "stoma."

BODY PARTS INVOLVED
- Males: Bladder; prostate; urethra; seminal vesicles; small intestine.
- Females: Bladder; urethra; ureters; cervix; vagina; small intestine.

REASONS FOR SURGERY—Cancer of the bladder.

SPECIAL CONSIDERATIONS FOR OLDER PATIENTS
- *Note:* Advancing age alone does not preclude surgery.
- Surgical repair is complete and effective, but healing takes longer.
- More likely to experience respiratory and kidney problems, confusion and blood clots after surgery.

SURGICAL RISK INCREASES WITH
- Poor nutrition; recent or chronic illness.
- Repeated surgeries on the bladder.

BEFORE SURGERY

WHO OPERATES—Urologist, usually in hospital.

DIAGNOSTIC TESTS—Blood and urine studies; x-rays of kidneys and chest. During surgery: Cystoscopy (see Glossary).

ANESTHESIA—General anesthesia by inhalation and injection, with an airway tube placed in the windpipe.

DESCRIPTION OF OPERATION—An incision is made in the abdomen. The muscles are separated, and the abdominal cavity is entered. The blood supply and the ureters are cut and tied. The bladder and adjacent tissues and organs are cut free and removed. The ureters are diverted through an intestinal pouch to an opening made in the skin (the stoma). The muscles are replaced and sewn together with sutures. The skin is closed with sutures or clips, which usually can be removed about 1 week after surgery.

AFTER SURGERY

POSSIBLE COMPLICATIONS
- Excessive bleeding.
- Incisional hernia or infection.
- Impotence in males.

- Recurring urinary tract infections.
- Obstruction of the ureter.

AVERAGE HOSPITAL STAY—4 to 6 days.

PROBABLE OUTCOME FOR OLDER PATIENTS—Expect complete healing of surgical wounds. You will need to wear an external pouch to collect urine. The stoma will heal and shrink to its permanent size in 2 to 4 months after surgery. Allow about 6 weeks for recovery from surgery.

GUIDE TO RECUPERATION FOR PEOPLE OVER 50
- Bathe as usual. Wash incision gently.
- Use warm heat packs and massage to relieve pain and discomfort.
- Move legs often while resting in bed to decrease the likelihood of deep-vein blood clots.
- An enterostomy specialist (see Glossary) can help you and your family learn to cope with new urination habits.
- Dry the area around the stoma by patting, not rubbing. Apply gauze soaked with 1 part vinegar to 3 parts water over the stoma to keep it clean.
- See Appendix 19.

MEDICATIONS & TESTS—Your doctor may prescribe:
- Pain relievers. Follow dosage schedule.
- Stool softeners to prevent constipation.
- Antibiotics to fight infection.
- You may use non-prescription drugs, such as acetaminophen, for minor pain.

ACTIVITY FOR OLDER PATIENTS—Ask your doctor for personalized instructions.
Typical times for resuming:
Bathing . . . . .Immediately.
Exercise . . . . .4 weeks.
Driving . . . . .4 weeks
Sexual activity . . . . .When able.
Work . . . . .Variable.

FOOD & BEVERAGE—Clear liquid diet until the gastrointestinal tract functions again. Then eat a well-balanced, high-protein diet to promote healing. See Appendices 7 and 1.

CALL YOUR DOCTOR IF

- Pain, swelling, redness, drainage or bleeding increases in the surgical area.
- You develop signs of infection: headache, muscle aches, dizziness or a general ill feeling and fever.
- You experience nausea, vomiting, constipation or abdominal swelling.
- You have pain or difficulty with urination.
- You wish to consider penile implant surgery (if impotent).
- New, unexplained symptoms develop. Drugs used in treatment may produce side effects.

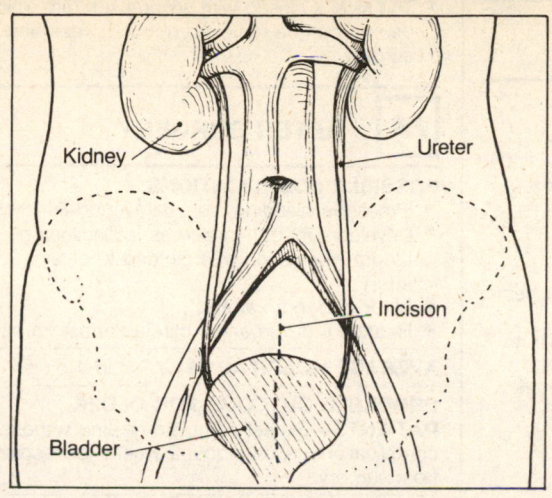

An illustration of the bladder and other parts of the urinary tract.

Kidney

Ureter

Incision

Bladder

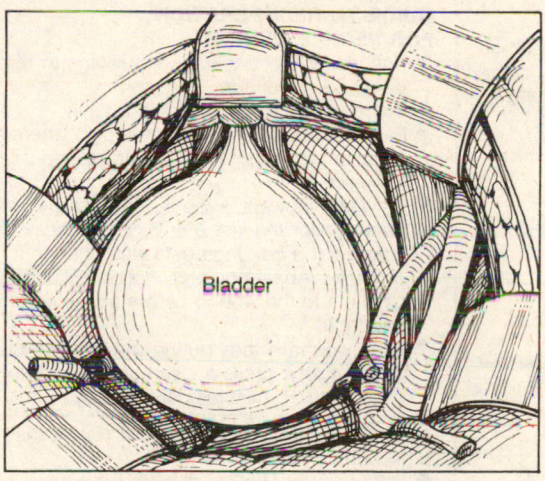

The bladder and adjacent tissues and organs are cut free and removed.

• The ureters are divided through an intestinal pouch to an opening made in the skin.

Bladder

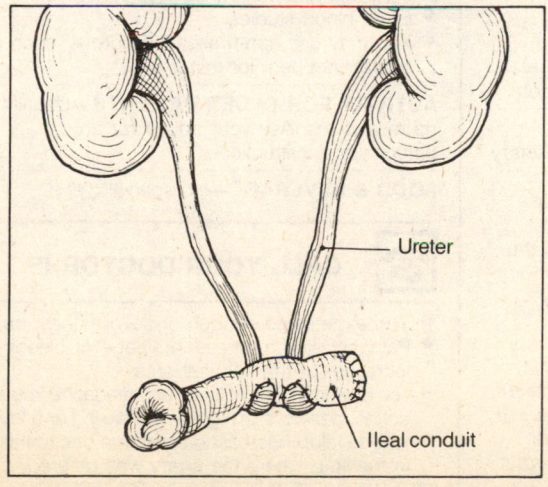

After bladder has been removed the kidneys and ureters are connected to an ileal conduit.

Ureter

Ileal conduit

SURGERIES

CARDIAC CATHETERIZATION & ANGIOCARDIOGRAPHY

BASIC INFORMATION

DESCRIPTION—Diagnostic procedures to examine functions of the heart.

BODY PARTS INVOLVED—Heart muscle and valves; coronary arteries; large artery in arm or leg.

REASONS FOR SURGERY
- Evaluation of chest pain.
- Diagnosis of a heart defect and valvular heart disease.
- Measurement of the heart muscle's ability to pump blood.
- Identification of narrowing or obstruction in the coronary arteries.

SPECIAL CONSIDERATIONS FOR OLDER PATIENTS
- *Note:* Advancing age alone does not preclude surgery.
- Weakened cough reflexes increase the risk of lung and bronchial complications.
- Characteristic signs and symptoms of many surgical disorders and complications are frequently atypical, changed or absent.

SURGICAL RISK INCREASES WITH
- Stress; obesity; smoking.
- Excessive alcohol consumption or chronic illness.

BEFORE SURGERY

WHO OPERATES—Cardiologist or general surgeon, usually in hospital.

DIAGNOSTIC TESTS—Blood and urine studies; ECG (see Glossary). During surgery: intracardiac pressures; cardiac output; cinematography; fluoroscopy; ECG (see Glossary for all).

ANESTHESIA—Local anesthesia by injection.

DESCRIPTION OF OPERATION
- The cardiac catheter is inserted into an artery in the patient's arm or leg. Fluoroscopy provides guidance for the catheter to pass through the artery to the heart.
- Blood pressure readings are taken, and the heart's ability to pump blood is tested.
- The catheter is guided into the coronary artery system. Fluoroscopy allows identification of any disease in the coronary arteries.
- When all examinations have been completed, the catheter is withdrawn, and the artery into which it was inserted is compressed until bleeding stops. If an arm artery was used, it may need to be repaired.

- The skin is closed with several sutures, which usually can be removed about 1 week after surgery.

AFTER SURGERY

POSSIBLE COMPLICATIONS
- Excessive bleeding; surgical wound infection.
- Development of hematomas (collections of blood) where skin was pierced to enter artery.
- Blood clot in an artery.
- Heartbeat disturbance; cardiac arrest (rare).

AVERAGE HOSPITAL STAY—0 to 4 days.

PROBABLE OUTCOME FOR OLDER PATIENTS—Expect complete healing without complications. Allow about 2 weeks for recovery from surgery.

GUIDE TO RECUPERATION FOR PEOPLE OVER 50
- Use warm heat packs and massage to relieve pain and discomfort.
- Bathe as usual. Wash incision gently.
- Expect discoloration under the skin where the catheter was inserted. It should disappear in 2 weeks.
- Between showers, keep the wound dry with a bandage for the first 2 or 3 days after surgery. If a bandage gets wet, change it promptly. Apply non-prescription antibiotic ointment to the wound before applying new bandages.
- If the wound bleeds during the first 24 hours after surgery, press a clean tissue or cloth to it for 10 to 15 minutes continuously.

MEDICATIONS & TESTS—Your doctor may prescribe:
- Pain relievers. Follow dosage schedule.
- ECG; blood studies.
- You may use non-prescription drugs, such as acetaminophen, for minor pain.

ACTIVITY FOR OLDER PATIENTS—Usually no restrictions. Ask your doctor for any personalized instructions.

FOOD & BEVERAGE—No special diet.

CALL YOUR DOCTOR IF

- You experience sudden or severe chest pain.
- Pain, swelling, redness, drainage or bleeding increases in the surgical area.
- You develop signs of infection: headache, muscle aches, dizziness or a general ill feeling and fever.
- You develop decreased sensation or circulation in the limb where the artery was entered.

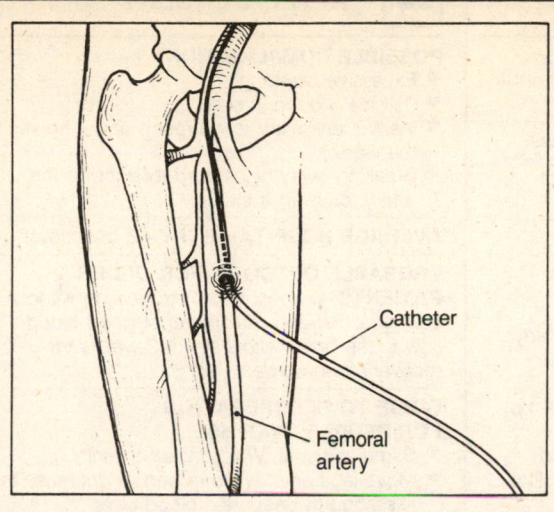

An illustration of a typical location for catheter insertion in the femoral artery of the leg. The catheter may also be placed in a large vessel in the arm.

•When the catheter is in place, accurate blood pressure measurements may be made continuously.

Catheter

Femoral artery

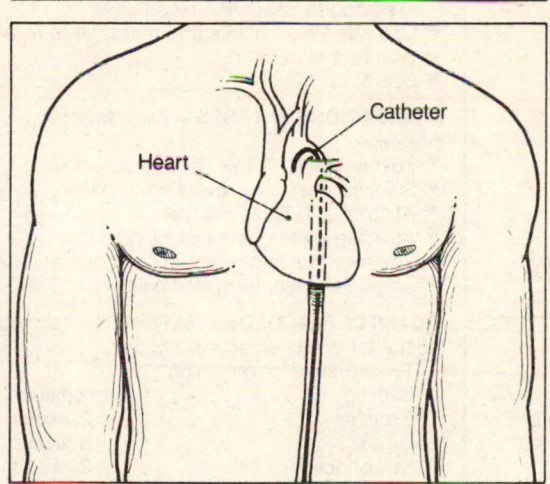

The catheter is guided into the coronary artery system. Pressure readings are made in various chambers of the heart and great blood vessels for later interpretation.

Catheter

Heart

SURGERIES

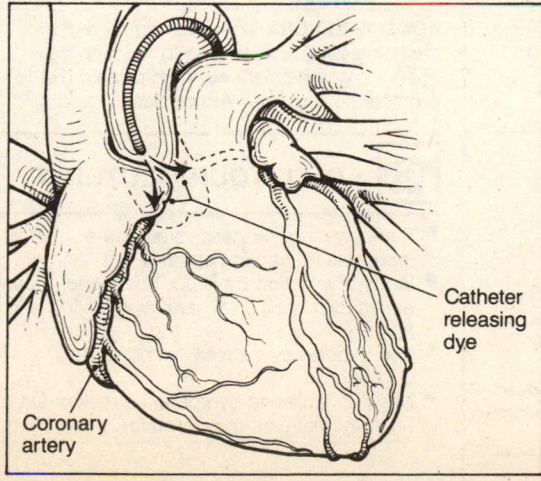

Dye is injected through the catheter to fill the coronary arteries to accurately locate any narrowings or obstructions in the coronary artery system.

•When all examinations have been completed, the catheter is withdrawn and the artery it was inserted into is compressed until bleeding stops.

Catheter releasing dye

Coronary artery

591

CAROTID ARTERY ENDARTERECTOMY

BASIC INFORMATION

DESCRIPTION—Removal of debris that has partially or totally obstructed blood supply to the brain and other parts of the head.

BODY PARTS INVOLVED—Carotid arteries.

REASONS FOR SURGERY—Prevention of stroke.

SPECIAL CONSIDERATIONS FOR OLDER PATIENTS
- *Note:* Advancing age alone does not preclude surgery.
- Characteristic signs and symptoms of many surgical disorders and complications are frequently atypical, changed or absent.
- Surgical repair is complete and effective, but healing takes longer.
- More likely to experience respiratory and kidney problems, confusion and blood clots after surgery.

SURGICAL RISK INCREASES WITH
- Smoking; obesity; stress.
- Poor nutrition; recent or chronic illness.
- Excessive alcohol consumption.
- Recent illness such as respiratory infection.
- Atherosclerosis; coronary artery disease; diabetes mellitus.
- Use of medicines such as antihypertensives; muscle relaxants; tranquilizers; sleep inducers; insulin; sedatives; beta-adrenergic blockers; cortisone.

BEFORE SURGERY

WHO OPERATES—General surgeon, neurosurgeon, cardiovascular surgeon, or peripheral vascular surgeon, usually in hospital.

DIAGNOSTIC TESTS—Blood and urine studies; ECG; arteriograms (see Glossary).

ANESTHESIA—General anesthesia by inhalation and injection, with an airway tube placed in the windpipe.

DESCRIPTION OF OPERATION
- An incision is made in the neck over the obstruction.
- The obstructed area is isolated. Sometimes a tube is grafted in to circulate blood around the obstruction.
- A small incision is made over the obstruction, which is scraped away. The opened area is patched with a graft fashioned from a vein from another part of the body.
- If the bypass tube is temporary, it is removed.
- The skin is closed with sutures or clips, which usually can be removed in 2 weeks.

AFTER SURGERY

POSSIBLE COMPLICATIONS
- Excessive bleeding.
- Surgical wound infection.
- Inadvertent injury to a branch of the nerves to the face.
- Breaking away of blood debris inside the artery, causing a stroke.

AVERAGE HOSPITAL STAY—3 to 5 days.

PROBABLE OUTCOME FOR OLDER PATIENTS—Expect complete healing without complications and restoration of good blood flow to the brain. Allow about 2 weeks for recovery from surgery.

GUIDE TO RECUPERATION FOR PEOPLE OVER 50
- Bathe as usual. Wash incision gently.
- Move legs often while in bed to decrease the likelihood of deep-vein blood clots.
- Use warm heat packs and massage to relieve pain and discomfort.
- See Appendix 19.

MEDICATIONS & TESTS—Your doctor may prescribe:
- Pain relievers. Follow dosage schedule.
- Stool softeners to prevent constipation.
- Antibiotics to fight infection.
- Anticoagulants to prevent blood clots.
- You may use non-prescription drugs, such as acetaminophen, for minor pain.

ACTIVITY FOR OLDER PATIENTS—Ask your doctor for personalized instructions.
Typical times for resuming:
Bathing . . . . .Immediately.
Exercise . . . . .2 weeks.
Driving . . . . .3 weeks.
Sexual activity . . . . .2 weeks.
Work . . . . .3 weeks.

FOOD & BEVERAGE—Clear liquid diet until the gastrointestinal tract begins to function again. Then eat a well-balanced, high-protein diet to promote healing. See Appendices 7 and 1.

CALL YOUR DOCTOR IF

- Pain, swelling, redness, drainage or bleeding increases in the surgical area.
- Signs of infection develop: headache, muscle aches, dizziness or a general ill feeling and fever.
- You experience nausea, vomiting or constipation.
- New, unexplained symptoms develop. Drugs used in treatment may produce side effects.

CAROTID ARTERY ENDARTERECTOMY

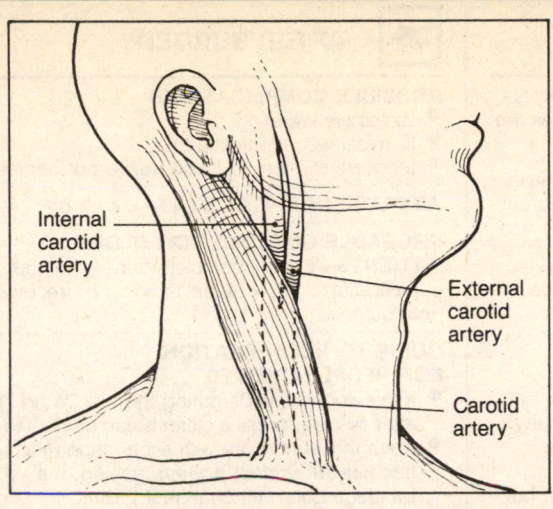

Illustration shows the anatomical locations of the carotid artery, external carotid artery, and internal carotid artery.

Internal carotid artery

External carotid artery

Carotid artery

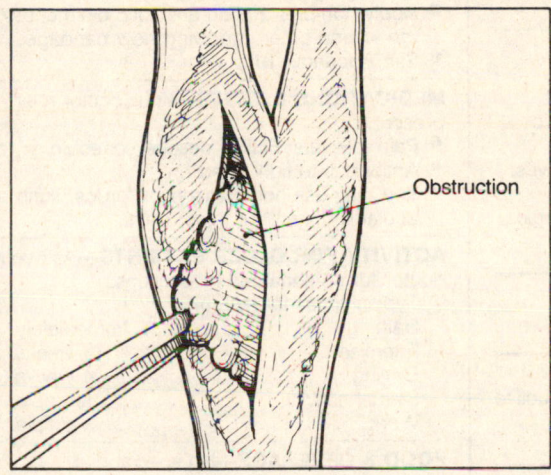

The arterial debris causing the obstruction (which was located by previous special studies) is removed.

Obstruction

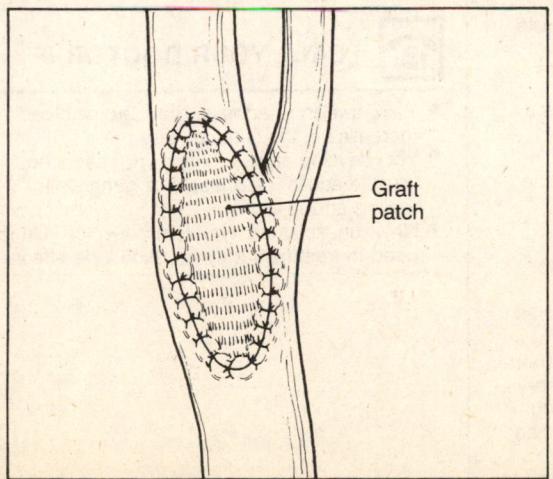

A patch is grafted in place to close the artery that has been cleared of obstruction.

Graft patch

SURGERIES

CARPAL TUNNEL SYNDROME REPAIR

 ## BASIC INFORMATION

DESCRIPTION—Cutting the transverse carpal ligament, the fibrous tissue extending across the wrist.

BODY PARTS INVOLVED—Transverse carpal ligament; median nerve and surrounding fibrous tissue; wrist joint.

REASONS FOR SURGERY—Relief of pain caused by compression of the median nerve.

SPECIAL CONSIDERATIONS FOR OLDER PATIENTS
- *Note:* Advancing age alone does not preclude surgery.
- Characteristic signs and symptoms of many surgical disorders and complications are frequently atypical, changed or absent.
- Surgical repair is complete and effective, but healing takes longer.

SURGICAL RISK INCREASES WITH
- Smoking; obesity; stress.
- Poor nutrition; recent or chronic illness.
- Excessive alcohol consumption or chronic illness.
- Use of medicines such as antihypertensives; muscle relaxants; tranquilizers; sleep inducers; insulin; sedatives; beta-adrenergic blockers; cortisone.

 ## BEFORE SURGERY

WHO OPERATES—Hand surgeon, general surgeon, orthopedist or plastic and reconstructive surgeon, usually in hospital or outpatient surgical facility.

DIAGNOSTIC TESTS—Blood and urine studies; x-rays of wrist; nerve conduction tests (see Glossary).

ANESTHESIA
- Local anesthesia by injection; sometimes a regional block.
- General anesthesia by inhalation and injection, with an airway tube placed in the windpipe.

DESCRIPTION OF OPERATION
- A tourniquet is applied above the wrist to prevent bleeding in the surgical area.
- An incision is made in the underside of the wrist.
- The transverse carpal ligament is located and cut, releasing the compressed median nerve.
- The skin is closed with fine sutures, which usually can be removed about 10 days after surgery.
- A bandage is applied, and a splint is used to hold the wrist in position.

 ## AFTER SURGERY

POSSIBLE COMPLICATIONS
- Excessive bleeding.
- Surgical wound infection.
- Inadvertent injury to blood vessels or nerves.

AVERAGE HOSPITAL STAY—0 to 1 day.

PROBABLE OUTCOME FOR OLDER PATIENTS—Expect complete healing without complications. Allow about 1 month for recovery from surgery.

GUIDE TO RECUPERATION FOR PEOPLE OVER 50
- If the wound bleeds during the first 24 hours after surgery, press a clean tissue or cloth to it.
- Keep the wound dry with a bandage until it has healed. Protect it when bathing. If a bandage gets wet, change it promptly.
- Apply non-prescription antibiotic ointment to the wound before applying new bandages.
- See Appendix 19.

MEDICATIONS & TESTS—Your doctor may prescribe:
- Pain relievers. Follow dosage schedule.
- Antibiotics to fight infection.
- You may use non-prescription drugs, such as acetaminophen, for minor pain.

ACTIVITY FOR OLDER PATIENTS—Ask your doctor for personalized instructions. Typical times for resuming:

Bathing	Immediately.
Exercise	4 weeks.
Driving	4 weeks.
Sexual activity	When able.
Work	Variable.

FOOD & BEVERAGE—No special diet.

 ## CALL YOUR DOCTOR IF

- Pain, swelling, redness, drainage or bleeding increases in the surgical area.
- You develop signs of infection: headache, muscle aches, dizziness or a general ill feeling and fever.
- New, unexplained symptoms develop. Drugs used in treatment may produce side effects.

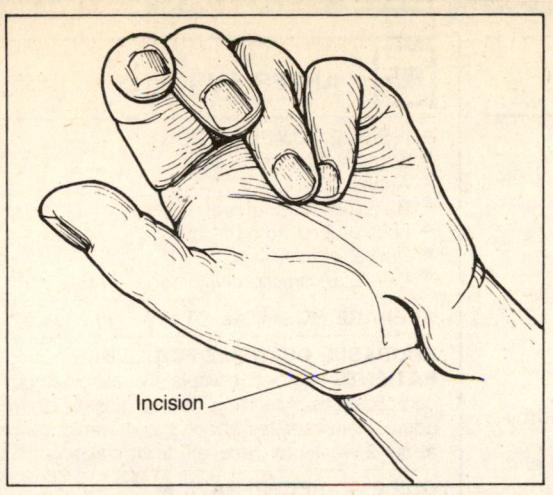

An illustration of the incision site at the wrist area where compression of the median nerve occurs.

Incision

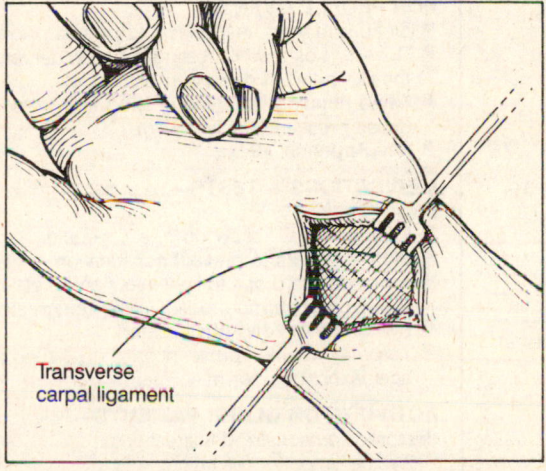

After the skin is incised, the transverse carpal ligament is exposed.

Transverse carpal ligament

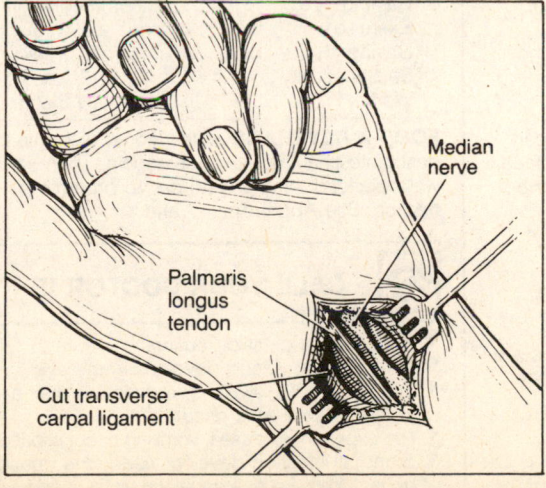

Carpal ligament is located and cut, releasing the compressed median nerve. This usually cures symptoms.

Median nerve

Palmaris longus tendon

Cut transverse carpal ligament

SURGERIES

CATARACT REMOVAL WITH INTRAOCULAR LENS REPLACEMENT

 ## BASIC INFORMATION

DESCRIPTION—Removal of cataracts.

BODY PARTS INVOLVED—Eye; cornea; lens; eyelid membrane lining.

REASONS FOR SURGERY—Restoration of normal or almost normal vision.

SPECIAL CONSIDERATIONS FOR OLDER PATIENTS
- *Note:* Advancing age alone does not preclude surgery.
- Multiple medications causing various complications are more likely to be used by older patients.
- Nursing care needs to be more intense and skillful.

SURGICAL RISK INCREASES WITH
- Smoking; obesity; stress.
- Recent illness such as upper respiratory infection.
- Chronic illness, especially diabetes mellitus.
- Use of medicines such as antihypertensives; muscle relaxants; tranquilizers; sleep inducers; insulin; sedatives; beta-adrenergic blockers; cortisone.

 ## BEFORE SURGERY

WHO OPERATES—Ophthalmologist; usually in hospital or outpatient surgical facility.

DIAGNOSTIC TESTS—Blood and urine studies; eye examinations.

ANESTHESIA
- Local anesthesia (sometimes) by injection.
- General anesthesia by inhalation and injection, with an airway tube placed in the windpipe.

DESCRIPTION OF OPERATION
- A special instrument holds the eyelids apart, and temporary sutures hold the eye in place.
- The eye is opened around the iris, and the lens is removed. Sometimes the lens is fragmented with ultrasound (see Glossary), and debris is suctioned away.
- Sometimes an artificial lens is inserted to replace the diseased lens.
- The temporary sutures are removed. Pilocarpine or atropine eye-drop solutions are placed in the eye to keep the pupil open. Bandages are applied.

 ## AFTER SURGERY

POSSIBLE COMPLICATIONS
- Surgical wound infection.
- Adhesions.
- Bleeding into the eye.
- Loss of fluid from the eye.
- Retinal detachment.
- Increased pressure within the eyeball.

AVERAGE HOSPITAL STAY—0 to 3 days.

PROBABLE OUTCOME FOR OLDER PATIENTS—Expect complete healing without complications. Adjusting to new glasses or contact lenses takes about 3 to 4 weeks. Allow about 2 weeks for recovery from surgery.

GUIDE TO RECUPERATION FOR PEOPLE OVER 50
- Sleep with your head elevated on two pillows.
- Move legs often while resting in bed to decrease the likelihood of deep-vein blood clots.
- Avoid bending, straining or lying flat. These cause pressure inside the eye.
- See Appendix 19.

MEDICATIONS & TESTS—Your doctor may prescribe:
- Pain relievers. Follow dosage schedule.
- Stool softeners to prevent constipation.
- Antibiotic eye drops to fight infection. Keep eye drops cold, but not frozen, in the refrigerator.
- Eye drops to keep pupil dilated.
- You may use non-prescription drugs, such as acetaminophen, for minor pain.

ACTIVITY FOR OLDER PATIENTS—Ask your doctor for personalized instructions.
Typical times for resuming:
Bathing . . . . .Immediately.
Exercise . . . . .2 weeks.
Driving . . . . .2 weeks.
Sexual activity . . . . .2 weeks.
Work .Variable.

FOOD & BEVERAGE—Clear liquid diet until the gastrointestinal tract functions again. Then eat a well-balanced, high-protein diet to promote healing. See Appendices 7 and 1.

 ## CALL YOUR DOCTOR IF

- Sudden loss of vision occurs.
- Sharp pain or blood develops in the eye.
- Increased pain, swelling, redness or drainage in the surgical area occurs.
- You experience nausea, vomiting or constipation.
- Signs of infection develop: headache, muscle aches, dizziness or a general ill feeling and fever.

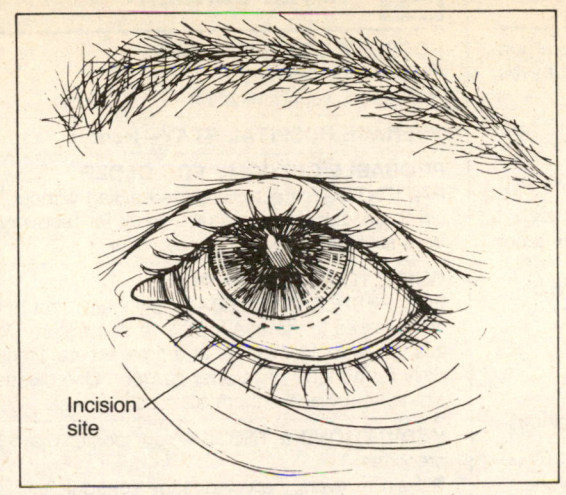

Surgical incision site below the iris.

Incision
site

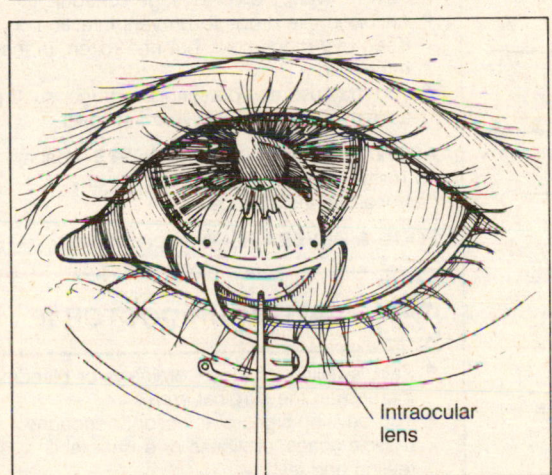

The diseased lens is removed and an
artificial intraocular lens is inserted.

Intraocular
lens

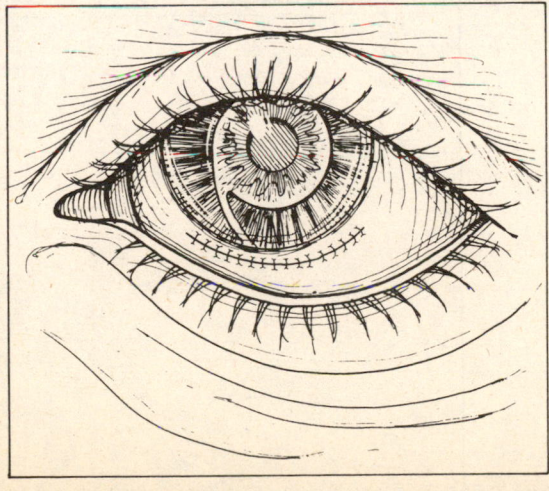

Artificial lens is in place. Incision is
closed with fine sutures.

SURGERIES

CHALAZION REMOVAL

BASIC INFORMATION

DESCRIPTION—Removal of a chalazion, a non-tender inflammation in the cartilage of the eyelid. Chalazions are caused by swelling and secretions in the meibomian glands (see Glossary).

BODY PARTS INVOLVED—Eyelids (upper or lower); meibomian glands.

REASONS FOR SURGERY—A chalazion is not cancerous or infectious. It is removed to improve appearance or to relieve pressure on an eyeball. Surgery is performed only after simpler treatment has failed.

SPECIAL CONSIDERATIONS FOR OLDER PATIENTS
Note: Advancing age alone does not preclude surgery.

SURGICAL RISK INCREASES WITH—None expected.

BEFORE SURGERY

WHO OPERATES—Ophthalmologist, usually in doctor's office or outpatient surgical facility.

DIAGNOSTIC TESTS—Complete eye examination before surgery.

ANESTHESIA—Local anesthesia by injection.

DESCRIPTION OF OPERATION
- The eyelid is turned inside out and held to expose its underside.
- The chalazion is identified.
- An incision is made on the surface of the chalazion.
- The chalazion is cut free and removed.
- The eye is bandaged.

AFTER SURGERY

POSSIBLE COMPLICATIONS
- Excessive bleeding.
- Surgical wound infection.

AVERAGE HOSPITAL STAY—None.

PROBABLE OUTCOME FOR OLDER PATIENTS—Expect complete healing without complications. Allow about 1 week for recovery from surgery. Chalazions may recur.

GUIDE TO RECUPERATION FOR PEOPLE OVER 50—Apply warm (not hot) compresses to the eye to relieve discomfort. Do this for 10 to 15 minutes at a time several times daily for about 2 days after surgery. Use clean cloths, and discard them after use.

MEDICATIONS & TESTS—Your doctor may prescribe:
- Pain relievers. Follow dosage schedule.
- Antibiotic eye drops to prevent infection. Keep eye drops cold, but not frozen, in the refrigerator.
- You may use non-prescription drugs, such as acetaminophen, to relieve minor pain.

ACTIVITY FOR OLDER PATIENTS—Usually no restrictions. Ask your doctor for any personalized instructions.

FOOD & BEVERAGE—No special diet.

CALL YOUR DOCTOR IF

- Pain, swelling, redness, drainage or bleeding increase in the surgical area.
- You develop signs of infection: headache, muscle aches, dizziness or a general ill feeling and fever.
- Your vision changes.

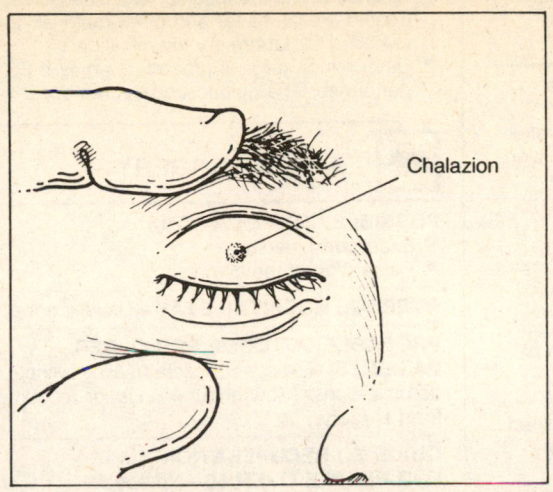

Appearance of the chalazion seen through the eyelid skin.

Chalazion

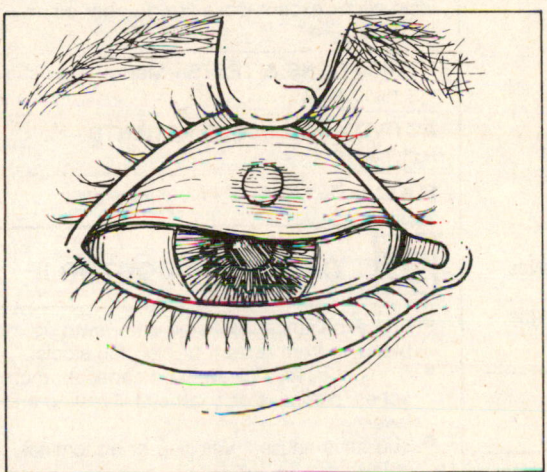

The eyelid is turned inside out and held to expose its underside. The chalazion is identified on the inverted lid.

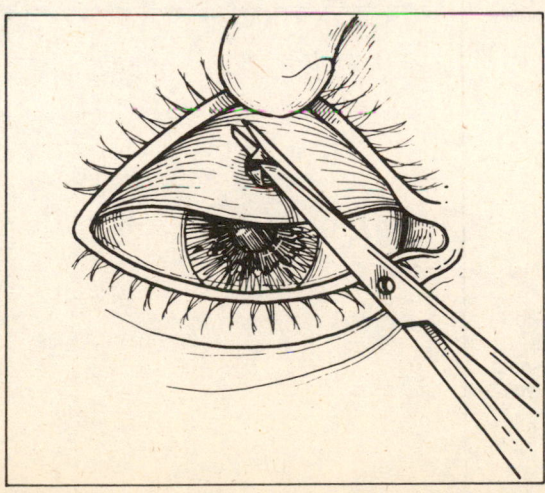

An incision made on the membranous lining of the eyelid allows the chalazion to be cut free and removed.

SURGERIES

COLONOSCOPY

BASIC INFORMATION

DESCRIPTION—Visual examination of the inside of the rectum and the colon (large intestine). Fecal matter, tissue or foreign matter usually are removed for laboratory examination. The procedure is performed with a colonoscope, a fiber optic instrument that makes examination and some surgeries simple, practical and safe.

BODY PARTS INVOLVED—Anus; rectum; colon.

REASONS FOR SURGERY—Examination of the rectum and lower intestinal tract for disorders that may include fissures; fistulas; narrowed sections of the intestine; unexplained blood in stools; benign or cancerous tumors; pre-cancerous polyps.

SPECIAL CONSIDERATIONS FOR OLDER PATIENTS
- *Note:* Advancing age alone does not preclude surgery.
- Characteristic signs and symptoms of many surgical disorders and complications are frequently atypical, changed or absent.

SURGICAL RISK INCREASES WITH
- Smoking; obesity; stress.
- Poor nutrition; recent or chronic illness.
- Use of medicines such as antihypertensives; muscle relaxants; tranquilizers; sleep inducers; insulin; sedatives; beta-adrenergic blockers; cortisone.

BEFORE SURGERY

WHO OPERATES—General surgeon, family doctor, proctologist or gastroenterologist, usually in hospital or outpatient surgical facility.

DIAGNOSTIC TESTS—Blood and urine studies; stool examinations; x-rays of lower gastrointestinal tract.

ANESTHESIA—Local anesthesia by topical application.

DESCRIPTION OF OPERATION
- The examination is best accomplished just after a normal bowel movement. If a normal bowel movement has not occurred just before examination, it may be necessary to use a suppository or delay the test until a laxative has cleared the area to be examined.
- The colonoscope is lubricated, inserted into the rectum and passed into the colon.

- Affected areas are located, examined or treated. Fecal matter and other materials are removed for laboratory examination.
- Other minor surgical procedures may be performed. The colonoscope is removed.

AFTER SURGERY

POSSIBLE COMPLICATIONS
- Excessive bleeding.
- Perforation of the colon.

AVERAGE HOSPITAL STAY—Usually none.

PROBABLE OUTCOME FOR OLDER PATIENTS—Expect complete healing without complications. Allow about 4 days for recovery from surgery.

GUIDE TO RECUPERATION FOR PEOPLE OVER 50—No special instructions except those listed under other headings.

MEDICATIONS & TESTS—Medicine is usually not necessary.

ACTIVITY FOR OLDER PATIENTS—No restrictions.

FOOD & BEVERAGE—No special diet.

CALL YOUR DOCTOR IF

- You experience increased pain, swelling, or bleeding from rectum or blood in stools.
- Signs of infection develop: headache, muscle aches, dizziness or a general ill feeling and fever.
- You have nausea, vomiting or abdominal pain.

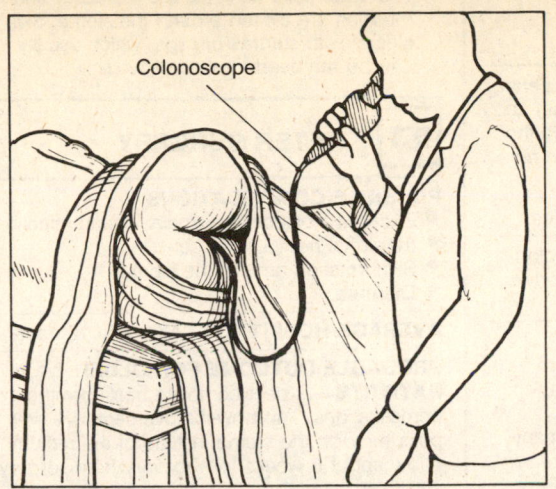

Colonoscope

An illustration of a draped patient and the colonoscope inserted into the anal opening and rectum.

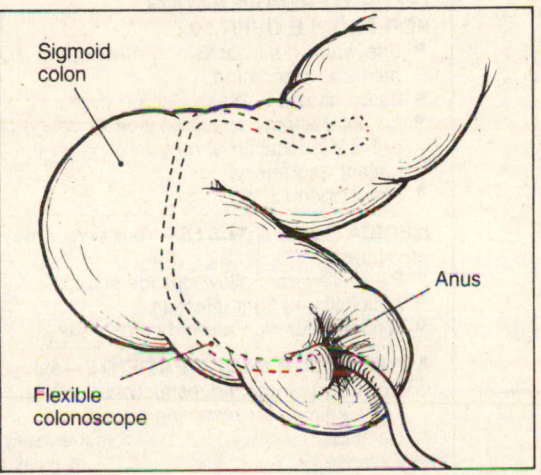

Sigmoid colon

Anus

Flexible colonoscope

The colonoscope is advanced through the rectum into the sigmoid colon.

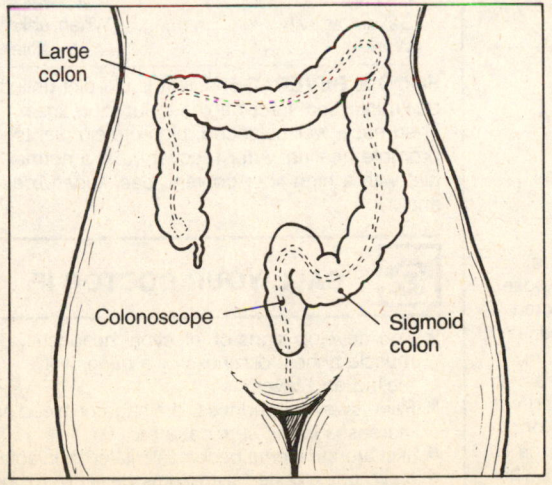

Large colon

Colonoscope

Sigmoid colon

The colonoscope is inserted to the full length of the large intestine. This procedure locates possible affected areas to be examined or treated. Fecal material may be removed for further examination and suspicious areas may be biopsied for microscopic examination.

COLOSTOMY

BASIC INFORMATION

DESCRIPTION—Creation of an artificial opening between a part of the colon (large intestine) and the surface of the body. All feces will leave the body through this opening, which is called an ostomy or stoma.

BODY PARTS INVOLVED—Large intestine.

REASONS FOR SURGERY—Diseased colon will not allow feces to pass through the body normally.

SPECIAL CONSIDERATIONS FOR OLDER PATIENTS
- *Note:* Advancing age alone does not preclude surgery.
- Characteristic signs and symptoms of many surgical disorders and complications are frequently atypical, changed or absent.
- Surgical repair is complete and effective, but healing takes longer.
- More likely to experience respiratory and kidney problems, confusion and blood clots after surgery.

SURGICAL RISK INCREASES WITH
- Smoking; obesity; stress.
- Excessive alcohol consumption.
- Poor nutrition; recent or chronic illness.
- Chronic illness of the heart, lungs, liver or gastrointestinal tract.
- Use of drugs such as antihypertensives; muscle relaxants; tranquilizers; sleep inducers; insulin; sedatives; narcotics; beta-adrenergic blockers; cortisone.

BEFORE SURGERY

WHO OPERATES—General surgeon, usually in hospital.

DIAGNOSTIC TESTS—Blood and urine studies; x-rays of kidneys, chest and gastrointestinal system; ECG (see Glossary).

ANESTHESIA—General anesthesia by inhalation and injection, with an airway tube placed in the windpipe.

DESCRIPTION OF OPERATION
- An incision is made in the abdomen. The abdominal muscles are separated to expose the abdominal organs, which are inspected for any undetected disease. Other surgeries may be performed at this time.
- The colon section that is to be opened is isolated and clamped on both sides, then cut between the clamps. The end of the colon closer to the stomach is brought out of the abdomen and clamped outside the skin. The end farther from the stomach is closed.

- The abdominal contents are replaced, and muscles are closed around the stoma. Skin is closed with sutures or clips, which usually can be removed in about 1 week.

AFTER SURGERY

POSSIBLE COMPLICATIONS
- Excessive bleeding; surgical wound infection.
- Incisional hernia.
- Skin irritation around the stoma.
- Diarrhea.

AVERAGE HOSPITAL STAY—7 to 12 days.

PROBABLE OUTCOME FOR OLDER PATIENTS—Expect complete healing without complications. The bowel movements will now pass through the stoma instead of the rectum. Allow about 6 weeks for recovery from surgery.

GUIDE TO RECUPERATION FOR PEOPLE OVER 50
- Use warm heat packs and massage to relieve pain and discomfort.
- Bathe as usual. Wash incision gently.
- An enterostomy specialist (see Glossary) can provide education and counseling for the patient and family.
- See Appendix 19.

MEDICATIONS & TESTS—Your doctor may prescribe:
- Pain relievers. Follow dosage schedule.
- Antibiotics to fight infection.
- Ointment for skin around ostomy site.

ACTIVITY FOR OLDER PATIENTS—Ask your doctor for personalized instructions.
Typical times for resuming:
Bathing . . . . Immediately.
Exercise . . . . 4 weeks.
Driving . . . . 4 weeks.
Sexual activity . . . . When able.
Work . . . . Variable.

FOOD & BEVERAGE—Clear liquid diet until the gastrointestinal tract begins to function again. Then eat a well-balanced, high-protein diet to promote healing. After recovery, eat a normal diet with a high fiber content. See Appendices 7 and 1.

📞 CALL YOUR DOCTOR IF

- You develop signs of infection: headache, muscle aches, dizziness or a general ill feeling and fever.
- Pain, swelling, redness, drainage or bleeding increases in the surgical area.
- Skin around stoma becomes irritated or infected.
- New, unexplained symptoms develop. Drugs in treatment may produce side effects.

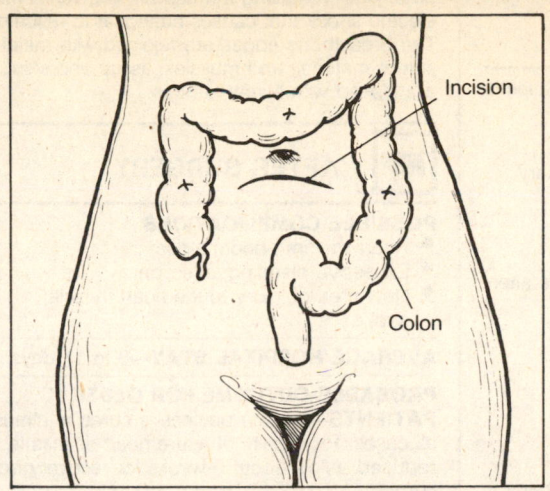

An illustration of the incision site in the left lower abdominal quadrant. The "x's" mark common areas for colon resection.

Incision

Colon

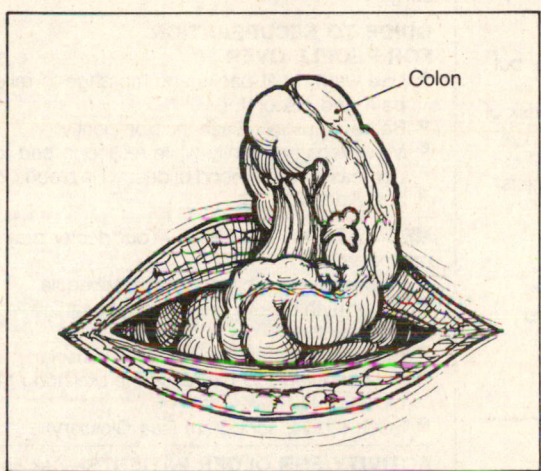

The abdominal muscle is separated to expose the abdominal organs. The colon section to be opened is isolated, clamped on both sides, then cut between the clamps.

Colon

SURGERIES

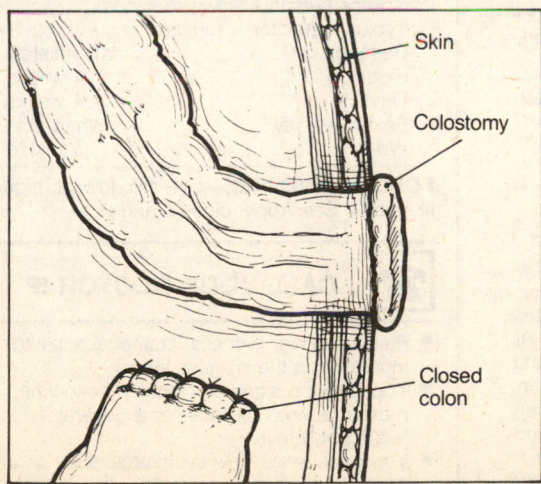

The end of the colon closer to the stomach is brought out of the abdomen and clamped outside the skin. The end farther from the stomach is closed.

• After the operation, bowel movements will emerge through the open end of the colostomy which has been sewn to the skin through an opening in the abdominal wall.

Skin

Colostomy

Closed colon

CORONARY ARTERY BYPASS GRAFT

BASIC INFORMATION

DESCRIPTION—Using a section of the patient's leg vein to bypass a partial or complete blockage in the coronary artery system.

BODY PARTS INVOLVED—Heart; coronary arteries; large veins of legs.

REASONS FOR SURGERY
- Angina pectoris.
- Restoration of blood to the heart muscle after a heart attack.
- Prevention of a possible heart attack if coronary arteries have narrowed.

SPECIAL CONSIDERATIONS FOR OLDER PATIENTS
- *Note:* Advancing age alone does not preclude surgery.
- Characteristic signs and symptoms of many surgical disorders and complications are frequently atypical, changed or absent.
- Surgical repair is complete and effective, but healing takes longer.
- Weakened cough reflexes increase the risk of lung and bronchial complications.
- More likely to experience respiratory and kidney problems, confusion and blood clots after surgery.

SURGICAL RISK INCREASES WITH
- Smoking; obesity; stress.
- Recent or chronic illness such as severe heart attack; high blood pressure; thyroid disease; diabetes mellitus.
- Chronic obstructive pulmonary disease (COPD).

BEFORE SURGERY

WHO OPERATES—Cardiovascular surgeon, usually in hospital.

DIAGNOSTIC TESTS—Blood studies; chest x-ray; cardiac catheterization; ECG; sonogram (see Glossary for all). During surgery: ECG; angiograms (see Glossary).

ANESTHESIA—General anesthesia by inhalation and injection, with an airway tube placed in the windpipe.

DESCRIPTION OF OPERATION—A section of the patient's large leg vein is removed and set aside to be used as the bypass vein graft. An incision is made through the breastbone, and the chest is spread open to expose the heart. A connection is made to a heart-lung machine. The heart is stopped with a chemical solution that temporarily paralyzes the heart muscle fibers, and the heart's temperature is reduced. The bypass vein graft is sutured in place to allow blood flow to resume beyond the blocked

area. After reheating the heart, it is given a mild electric shock that causes heartbeat to resume. The breastbone edges are rejoined with metal suture material, and muscles, tissue and skin are closed with lighter sutures.

AFTER SURGERY

POSSIBLE COMPLICATIONS
- Heart rhythm abnormalities.
- Excessive bleeding; infection.
- New area of injury to the heart muscle; stroke.

AVERAGE HOSPITAL STAY—8 to 11 days.

PROBABLE OUTCOME FOR OLDER PATIENTS—Angina pectoris is cured in almost all cases. Probability of future heart attacks is reduced. Allow about 6 weeks for recovery from surgery.

GUIDE TO RECUPERATION FOR PEOPLE OVER 50
- Use warm heat packs and massage to relieve pain and discomfort.
- Bathe as usual. Wash incision gently.
- Move legs frequently while resting in bed to decrease the likelihood of deep-vein blood clots.
- See Appendix 19.

MEDICATIONS & TESTS—Your doctor may prescribe:
- Pain relievers. Follow dosage schedule.
- Antiarrhythmics to prevent heartbeat irregularities.
- Digitalis to strengthen the heart muscle.
- Anticoagulants to decrease the likelihood of blood clots.
- ECG; x-rays; sonogram (see Glossary).

ACTIVITY FOR OLDER PATIENTS—Ask your doctor for personalized instructions.
Typical times for resuming:
Bathing . . . . Immediately.
Exercise . . . . 4 weeks.
Driving . . . . 4 weeks.
Sexual activity . . . . When able.
Work . . . . Variable.

FOOD & BEVERAGE—Low-salt, low-fat, high-fiber diet. See Appendices 8 and 9.

CALL YOUR DOCTOR IF

- Pain, swelling, redness, drainage or bleeding increases in the surgical area.
- You develop signs of infection: headache, muscle aches, dizziness or a general ill feeling and fever.
- You experience new symptoms, such as a cough, heartbeat irregularities, leg pain or constipation.

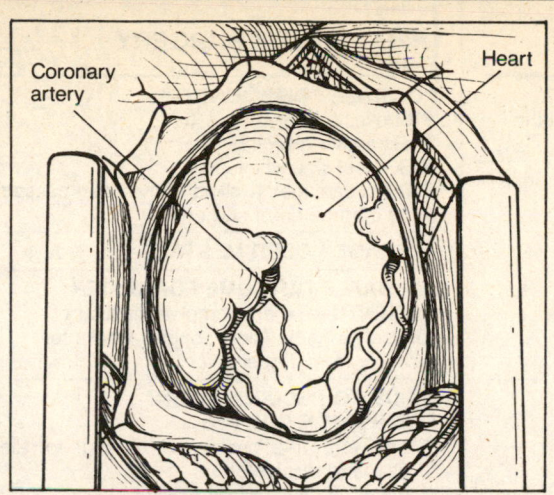

Coronary artery

Heart

An illustration of the heart showing an example of a clogged or occluded coronary artery.

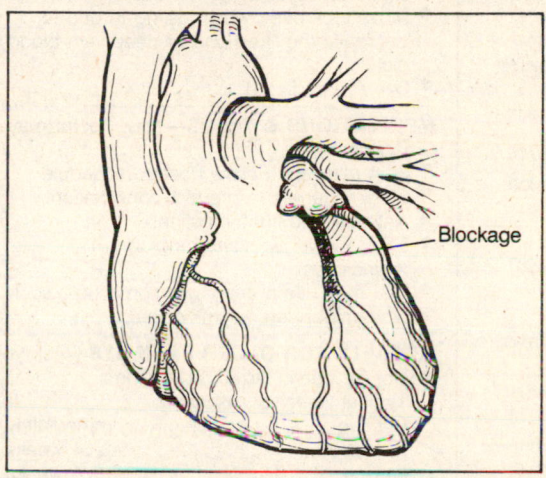

Blockage

The blocked area in this illustration is the left anterior descending coronary artery, a common site for such blockage to occur.

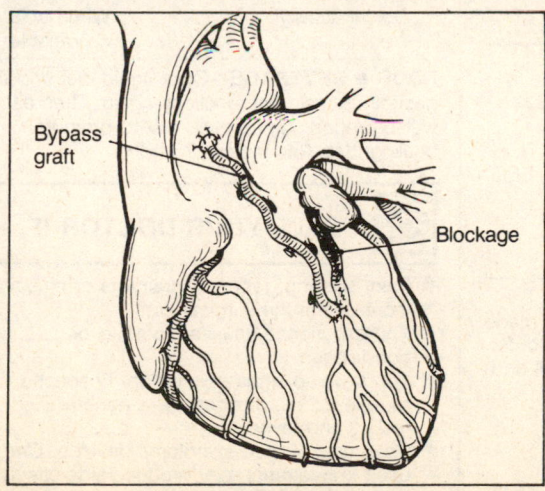

Bypass graft

Blockage

A bypass vein grafted in place allows blood flow to resume beyond the blocked area and thus restore more normal circulation to some of the damaged heart muscle.

SURGERIES

CRANIOTOMY

 BASIC INFORMATION

DESCRIPTION—Cutting through the skull (cranium) to expose and treat disorders in the brain or associated tissues.

BODY PARTS INVOLVED—Scalp; skull; brain and membrane coverings.

REASONS FOR SURGERY
- Removal of blood clots, aneurysms or tumors.
- Repair of tears in the brain's membrane coverings.
- Drainage of a brain abscess.

SPECIAL CONSIDERATIONS FOR OLDER PATIENTS
- *Note:* Advancing age alone does not preclude surgery.
- Characteristic signs and symptoms of many surgical disorders and complications are frequently atypical, changed or absent.
- Surgical repair is complete and effective, but healing takes longer.
- Nursing care needs to be more intense and skillful.
- More likely to experience respiratory and kidney problems, confusion and blood clots after surgery.

SURGICAL RISK INCREASES WITH
- Smoking; excessive alcohol consumption.
- Chronic illness; recent illness, especially upper respiratory infection.
- Use of medicines such as antihypertensives; muscle relaxants; tranquilizers; sleep inducers; insulin; sedatives; beta-adrenergic blockers; cortisone.

 BEFORE SURGERY

WHO OPERATES—Neurosurgeon, usually in hospital or emergency room.

DIAGNOSTIC TESTS—Blood and urine studies; x-rays of skull; angiogram; EEG; CT scan (see Glossary for all). During surgery: EEG.

ANESTHESIA—General anesthesia by inhalation and injection, with an airway tube placed in the windpipe.

DESCRIPTION OF OPERATION
- The entire head is shaved. An incision is made in the scalp over the area of suspected disorder.
- A flap of bone is cut away from the skull and set aside.
- The disorder is located and treated as necessary and the bone flap is replaced.
- The scalp is closed with sutures or clips, which usually can be removed about 1 week after surgery.

 AFTER SURGERY

POSSIBLE COMPLICATIONS
- Stroke; seizure.
- Excessive bleeding.
- Surgical wound infection.
- Brain damage; swelling of the brain caused by the trauma of surgery.

AVERAGE HOSPITAL STAY—7 to 9 days.

PROBABLE OUTCOME FOR OLDER PATIENTS—Expect complete healing of surgical wounds. Allow about 8 weeks for recovery from surgery.

GUIDE TO RECUPERATION FOR PEOPLE OVER 50
- Use warm heat packs and massage to relieve pain and discomfort.
- Bathe as usual. Wash incision gently.
- Move legs often while resting in bed to decrease the likelihood of deep-vein blood clots.
- See Appendix 19.

MEDICATIONS & TESTS—Your doctor may prescribe:
- Pain relievers. Follow dosage schedule.
- Stool softeners to prevent constipation.
- Antibiotics to fight infection.
- EEG; x-rays; CT scan; angiogram (sometimes).
- You may use non-prescription drugs, such as acetaminophen, for minor pain.

ACTIVITY FOR OLDER PATIENTS—Ask your doctor for personalized instructions.
Typical times for resuming:
Bathing . . . . Immediately.
Exercise . . . . 4 weeks.
Driving . . . . 4 weeks.
Sexual activity . . . . When able.
Work . . . . Variable.

FOOD & BEVERAGE—Clear liquid diet until the gastrointestinal tract functions again. Then eat a well-balanced, high-protein diet to promote healing. See Appendices 7 and 1.

 CALL YOUR DOCTOR IF

- Pain, swelling, redness, drainage or bleeding increases in the surgical area.
- You experience nausea, vomiting or constipation.
- You develop signs of infection: headache, muscle aches, dizziness or a general ill feeling and fever.
- New, unexplained symptoms develop. Drugs used in treatment may produce side effects.

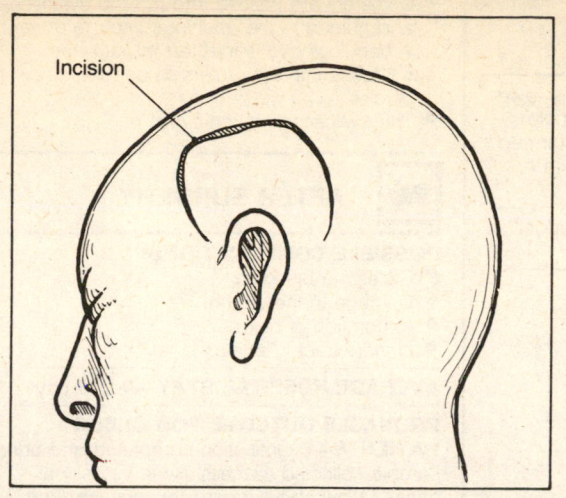

An illustration of a shaved head and a typical incision site on the scalp.

Incision

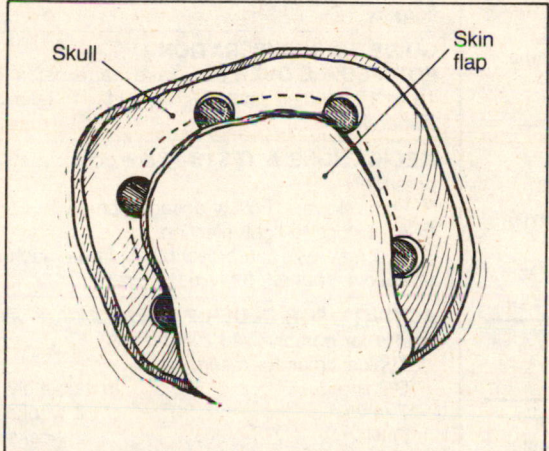

Skin over the scalp is incised, exposing the skull bone, and a flap is formed.

Skull

Skin flap

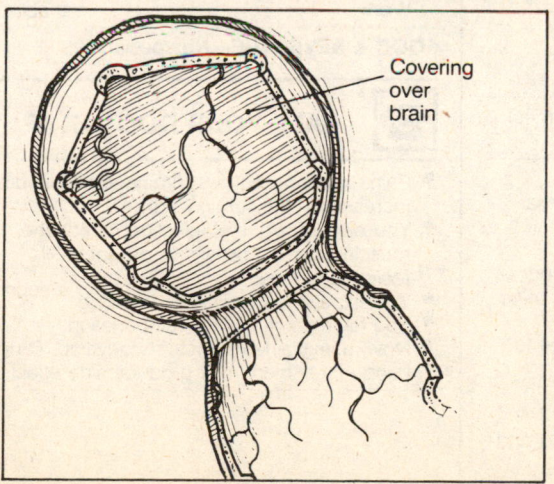

Skin and bone flap are retracted to expose the brain covering where the suspected area of pathology is located.

Covering over brain

SURGERIES

CYSTOSCOPY

BASIC INFORMATION

DESCRIPTION—Visual examination of the lower urinary tract and collection of a urine sample from the bladder. The examination is performed with a cystoscope, an optic instrument with a lighted tip.

BODY PARTS INVOLVED—Urethra; bladder; openings into the bladder.

REASONS FOR SURGERY
- Blood in the urine (hematuria).
- Inability to control urination (incontinence).
- Urinary tract infection.
- Tumors of the bladder.
- Bladder or kidney stones.
- Tightening of the urethra or the ureters.

SPECIAL CONSIDERATIONS FOR OLDER PATIENTS
- *Note:* Advancing age alone does not preclude surgery.
- Characteristic signs and symptoms of many surgical disorders and complications are frequently atypical, changed or absent.

SURGICAL RISK INCREASES WITH
- Smoking; obesity; stress.
- Recent or chronic illness.
- Use of medicines such as antihypertensives; muscle relaxants; tranquilizers; sleep inducers; insulin; sedatives; beta-adrenergic blockers; cortisone.

BEFORE SURGERY

WHO OPERATES—Urologist, usually in hospital, doctor's office or outpatient surgical facility.

DIAGNOSTIC TESTS—Blood and urine studies; x-rays of kidneys. During surgery: retrograde pyelograms (see Glossary).

ANESTHESIA—Spinal anesthesia (sometimes) by injection.

DESCRIPTION OF OPERATION
- The patient urinates before surgery so that urine remaining in the bladder can be measured.
- The cystoscope is lubricated and inserted through the urethra into the bladder. A urine sample is collected.
- Fluid is pumped through the cystoscope to inflate the bladder, which allows visual examination of the entire bladder wall.
- Bladder or kidney stones are removed if necessary. Tissue samples are gathered and lesions are treated if necessary.

- Catheters are passed through the cystoscope and guided to the openings into the ureters. A harmless dye is injected through the catheters into the ureters to perform x-ray studies.
- The cystoscope is removed.

AFTER SURGERY

POSSIBLE COMPLICATIONS
- Excessive bleeding.
- Damage to the urethra.
- Perforation of bladder.
- Urinary tract infection.

AVERAGE HOSPITAL STAY—0 to 3 days.

PROBABLE OUTCOME FOR OLDER PATIENTS—Examination completed and urine sample collected successfully in virtually all cases. Allow about 4 days for recovery from surgery.

GUIDE TO RECUPERATION FOR PEOPLE OVER 50—Take warm baths for 10 to 15 minutes several times a day to relieve discomfort.

MEDICATIONS & TESTS—Your doctor may prescribe:
- Pain relievers. Follow dosage schedule.
- Antibiotics to fight infection.
- You may use non-prescription drugs, such as acetaminophen, for minor pain.

ACTIVITY FOR OLDER PATIENTS—Ask your doctor for personalized instructions.

Typical times for resuming:
Bathing . . . . Immediately.
Exercise . . . . 2 weeks.
Driving . . . . 2 weeks.
Sexual activity . . . . 4 weeks.
Work . . . . Variable.

FOOD & BEVERAGE—No special diet.

CALL YOUR DOCTOR IF

- Pain, swelling, redness, drainage or bleeding increases in the surgical area.
- You develop signs of infection: headache, muscle aches, dizziness or a general ill feeling and fever.
- You experience nausea or vomiting.
- You have painful or difficult urination.
- New, unexplained symptoms develop. Drugs used in treatment may produce side effects.

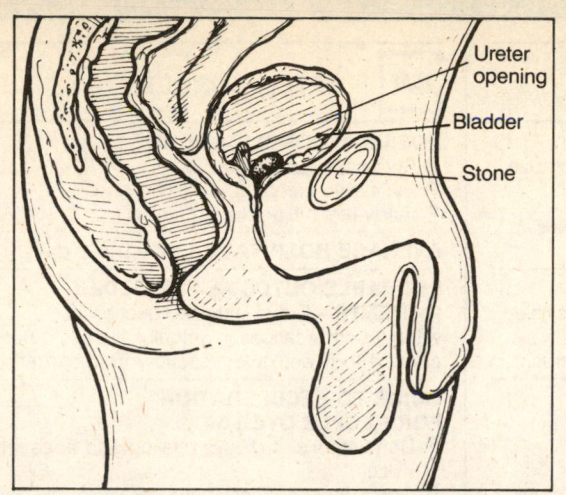

A cross-section of the male pelvis showing the urethra, bladder and openings into the bladder. A typical stone inside the bladder is illustrated.

Labels: Ureter opening, Bladder, Stone

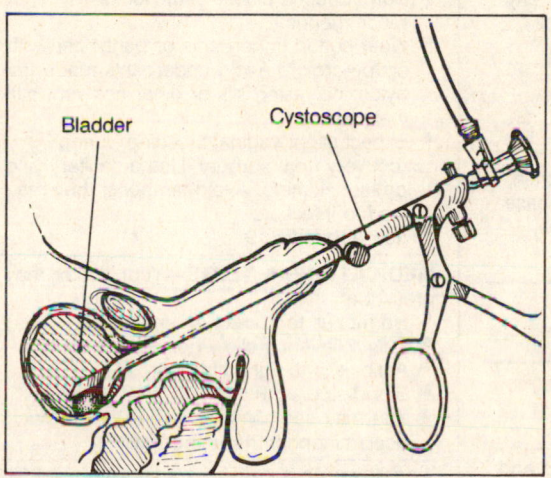

A lubricated cystoscope is inserted through the urethra into the bladder to allow removal of the stone. If needed, a catheter can be passed through the cystoscope.

Labels: Bladder, Cystoscope

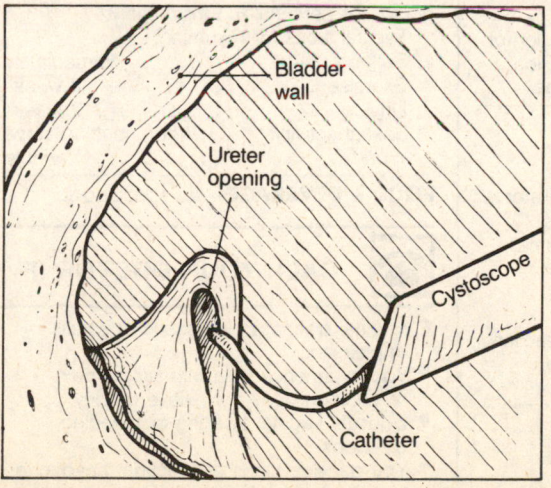

A catheter passed through the cystoscope toward the opening of the ureter. The catheter can be passed through the urethral opening to remove other stones higher in the urinary tract.

Labels: Bladder wall, Ureter opening, Cystoscope, Catheter

SURGERIES

DILATATION & CURETTAGE OF THE UTERUS (D&C)

BASIC INFORMATION

DESCRIPTION—Opening the cervix and scraping the inner wall of the uterus to remove tissue.

BODY PARTS INVOLVED—Uterus; cervix; vagina (as route for surgery).

REASONS FOR SURGERY
- Diagnosis of abnormal bleeding or possible cancer inside the uterus.
- Treatment of minor diseases of the uterus.

SPECIAL CONSIDERATIONS FOR OLDER PATIENTS
- *Note:* Advancing age alone does not preclude surgery.
- Characteristic signs and symptoms of many surgical disorders and complications are frequently atypical, changed or absent.

SURGICAL RISK INCREASES WITH
- Obesity.
- Smoking.
- Excessive alcohol consumption.
- Recent or chronic illness, including anemia, diabetes mellitus, and heart or lung disease.
- Use of drugs, such as antihypertensives; cortisone; diuretics; insulin.

BEFORE SURGERY

WHO OPERATES—Obstetrician-gynecologist, general surgeon or family doctor, usually in outpatient surgical facility or hospital.

DIAGNOSTIC TESTS—Pap smear; blood and hormonal studies.

ANESTHESIA—Local anesthesia by injection or general anesthesia by inhalation and injection, with an airway tube placed in the windpipe.

DESCRIPTION OF OPERATION
- The vagina is cleansed with an antiseptic solution.
- The cervix is carefully opened with a dilator, and a curette is inserted into the uterus.
- The curette is used to scrape away a small part of the uterine lining for laboratory analysis.
- The instruments are removed.
- Some surgeons now collect tissue by suction curettage rather than by the procedure described here.

AFTER SURGERY

POSSIBLE COMPLICATIONS
- Surgical wound infection.
- Excessive bleeding.
- Inadvertent injury to the uterus.

AVERAGE HOSPITAL STAY—1 to 2 days.

PROBABLE OUTCOME FOR OLDER PATIENTS—Tissue obtained successfully without complications in virtually all cases. Allow about 4 to 6 weeks for recovery from surgery.

GUIDE TO RECUPERATION FOR PEOPLE OVER 50
- Don't smoke. It delays healing and adds risks.
- Don't douche unless your doctor recommends it.
- Wear cotton underpants or pantyhose with a cotton crotch. Avoid underpants made from nylon, polyester, silk or other non-ventilating materials.
- Expect slight vaginal bleeding during recovery from surgery. Use a sanitary pad to protect clothing. Avoid tampons; they may lead to infection.
- See Appendix 19.

MEDICATIONS & TESTS—Your doctor may prescribe:
- Hormones to correct an imbalance.
- Pain relievers. Follow dosage schedule.
- Antibiotics to fight infection.
- Blood studies; Pap smear in 2 months.
- You may use non-prescription drugs, such as acetaminophen, for minor pain.

ACTIVITY FOR OLDER PATIENTS—Ask your doctor for personalized instructions.
Typical times for resuming:
Bathing . . . . Immediately.
Exercise . . . . 2 weeks.
Driving . . . . 2 weeks.
Sexual activity . . . . . . When spotting stops.
Work . . . . Variable.

FOOD & BEVERAGE—No special diet.

CALL YOUR DOCTOR IF

- Vaginal discharge increases or smells unpleasant.
- You experience pain that simple pain medication does not relieve quickly.
- Unusual vaginal swelling or bleeding develops.
- You develop signs of infection: headache, muscle aches, dizziness or a general ill feeling and fever.

DILATATION & CURETTAGE OF THE UTERUS (D&C)

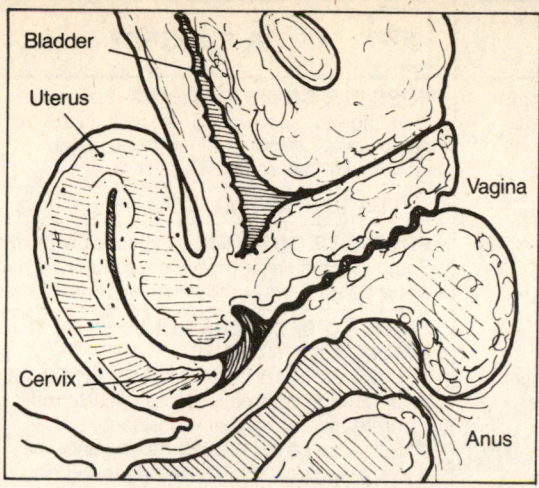

A side view of the female genital area.

Bladder

Uterus

Vagina

Cervix

Anus

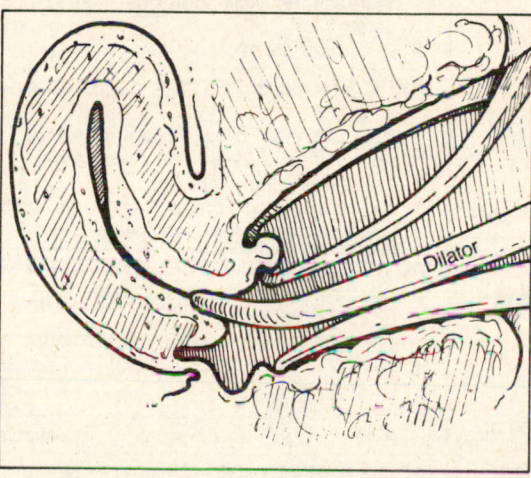

Forceps grasp the anterior portion of the cervix and a dilator is inserted into uterus.

Dilator

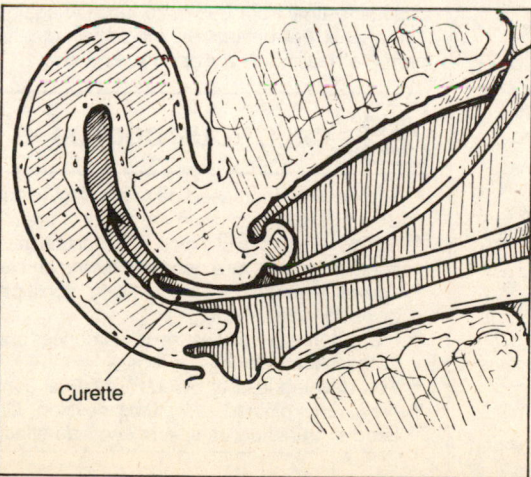

After the cervix has been dilated, a curette is passed into the cavity of the uterus. The curette is used to scrape away the uterine lining for laboratory analysis or therapeutic reasons.

Curette

SURGERIES

DISK, RUPTURED, REMOVAL OF
(Laminectomy)

 BASIC INFORMATION

DESCRIPTION—Removal of an intervertebral disk that has protruded from its normal position.

BODY PARTS INVOLVED—Spine; intervertebral disk.

REASONS FOR SURGERY—Relief of painful symptoms.

SPECIAL CONSIDERATIONS FOR OLDER PATIENTS
- *Note:* Advancing age alone does not preclude surgery.
- Characteristic signs and symptoms of many surgical disorders and complications are frequently atypical, changed or absent.
- Surgical repair is complete and effective, but healing takes longer.

SURGICAL RISK INCREASES WITH
- Stress; obesity; poor nutrition; smoking; excessive alcohol consumption.
- Chronic illness, especially back pain.
- Use of drugs such as antihypertensives; muscle relaxants; tranquilizers; sleep inducers; insulin; sedatives; beta-adrenergic blockers; cortisone.

 BEFORE SURGERY

WHO OPERATES—Neurosurgeon, orthopedist or general surgeon (sometimes), usually in hospital.

DIAGNOSTIC TESTS—Blood and urine studies; x-rays of back; myelogram; CT scan or MRI (see Glossary for all).

ANESTHESIA—General anesthesia by inhalation and injection, with an airway tube placed in the windpipe.

DESCRIPTION OF OPERATION
- An incision is made over the protruded disk.
- The arches of the spine are cut away and removed.
- The protruding disk is scooped out.
- Sometimes the vertebral bone around the affected area is joined together with normal bone. This procedure is called fusion.
- The skin is closed with sutures or clips that will be removed about 1 week after surgery.

 AFTER SURGERY

POSSIBLE COMPLICATIONS—Excessive bleeding; surgical wound infection; injury to nerve roots, which can lead to paralysis; incomplete disk removal.

AVERAGE HOSPITAL STAY—3 to 6 days.

PROBABLE OUTCOME—Expect slow healing. Some discomfort and weakness may continue. Allow about 5 weeks for recovery from surgery.

GUIDE TO RECUPERATION FOR PEOPLE OVER 50
- Use warm heat packs and massage to ease discomfort and pain. Some patients may prefer to use ice packs instead.
- Bathe as usual. Wash incision gently.
- Move legs often while resting in to bed to decrease the likelihood of deep-vein blood clots.
- See Appendix 19.

MEDICATIONS & TESTS—Your doctor may prescribe:
- Pain relievers. Follow dosage schedule.
- Stool softeners to prevent constipation.
- Antibiotics to fight infection.
- You may use non-prescription drugs, such as acetaminophen, for minor pain.

ACTIVITY FOR OLDER PATIENTS—Ask your doctor for personalized instructions.
Typical times for resuming:
Bathing . . . . Immediately.
Exercise . . . . 4 weeks.
Driving . . . . 4 weeks
Sexual activity . . . . 4 weeks
Work . . . . Variable.

FOOD & BEVERAGE—Clear liquid diet until the gastrointestinal tract begins to function again. Then eat a well-balanced, high-protein diet to promote healing. See Appendices 7 and 1.

 CALL YOUR DOCTOR IF

- You develop increased pain, swelling, redness, drainage or bleeding in the surgical area.
- You develop signs of infection: headache, muscle aches, dizziness or a general ill feeling and fever.
- You experience nausea, vomiting, constipation or abdominal swelling.
- There is a return of weakness, numbness or pain in the back, buttocks or legs.
- You develop loss of bladder or bowel control.
- New, unexplained symptoms develop. Drugs used in treatment may produce side effects.

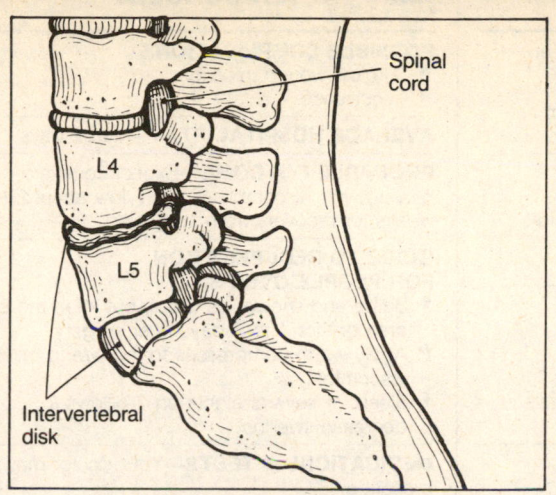

An illustration of the bony spine, the spinal cord and the protruding intervertebral disk. This example shows the disk separating the 4th and 5th lumbar vertebral bodies.

Spinal cord

L4

L5

Intervertebral disk

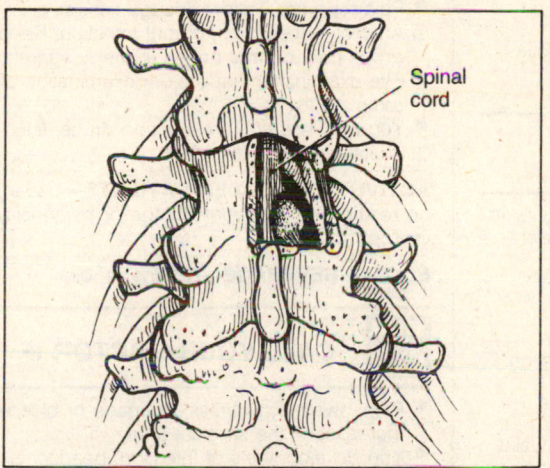

After the skin has been incised, the arches of the bone are located, cut away and removed allowing the protruding disk to be scooped out.

Spinal cord

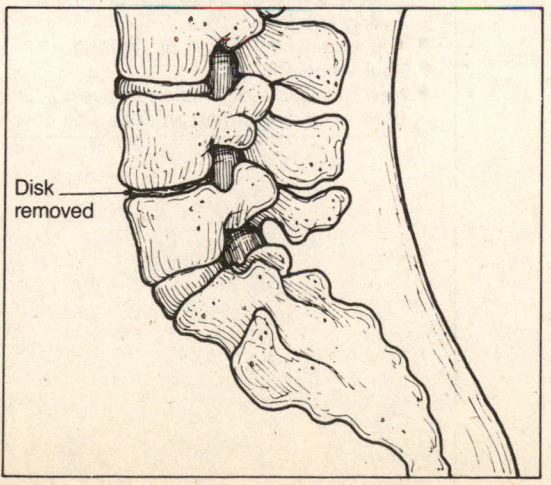

Appearance after the disk has been removed.

Disk removed

SURGERIES

ECTROPION REPAIR

BASIC INFORMATION

DESCRIPTION—Repair of an ectropion, an outward turning of the skin of the eyelid.

BODY PARTS INVOLVED—Lower eyelid usually. Sometimes involves upper eyelid.

REASONS FOR SURGERY
- Improved appearance.
- Relief of redness, irritation and discomfort.
- Reduced likelihood of infection in the membrane surrounding the eye.

SPECIAL CONSIDERATIONS FOR OLDER PATIENTS
- *Note:* Advancing age alone does not preclude surgery.
- Decreased nutrition may increase the risk of surgical infections and complications.

SURGICAL RISK INCREASES WITH
- Smoking.
- Stress.
- Recent illness.
- Excessive alcohol consumption or chronic illness.

BEFORE SURGERY

WHO OPERATES—Ophthalmologist, usually in hospital, ophthalmologist's office or outpatient surgical facility.

DIAGNOSTIC TESTS—Blood and urine studies; eye examination.

ANESTHESIA—Local anesthesia by injection.

DESCRIPTION OF OPERATION
- An incision is made in the eyelid.
- The cartilage is cut close to the outer eyelid edge. A small wedge of cartilage is cut free and removed. The cartilage is sewn back together.
- The skin is closed with sutures, which usually can be removed about 10 days after surgery.

AFTER SURGERY

POSSIBLE COMPLICATIONS
- Surgical wound infection.
- Recurrence.

AVERAGE HOSPITAL STAY—1 to 2 days.

PROBABLE OUTCOME—Expect complete healing without complications. Allow about 2 weeks for recovery from surgery.

GUIDE TO RECUPERATION FOR PEOPLE OVER 50
- Bathe and shower as usual, but keep the eye area dry for 4 to 5 days after surgery.
- Apply warm compresses to the eye to relieve discomfort.
- Sleep for several nights on 2 pillows to decrease swelling.

MEDICATIONS & TESTS—Your doctor may prescribe:
- Pain relievers. Follow dosage schedule.
- Antibiotic eye drops to fight infection. Keep drops cold but not frozen in the refrigerator.
- Eye examination; laboratory examination of removed tissue.
- You may use non-prescription drugs, such as acetaminophen, for minor pain.

ACTIVITY FOR OLDER PATIENTS—Usually no restrictions. Ask your doctor for personalized instructions.

FOOD & BEVERAGE—No special diet.

CALL YOUR DOCTOR IF

- Pain, swelling, redness, drainage or bleeding increases in the surgical area.
- You develop signs of infection: headache, muscle aches, dizziness or a general ill feeling and fever.
- You experience nausea or vomiting.
- Your vision changes.
- New, unexplained symptoms develop. Drugs used in treatment may produce side effects.

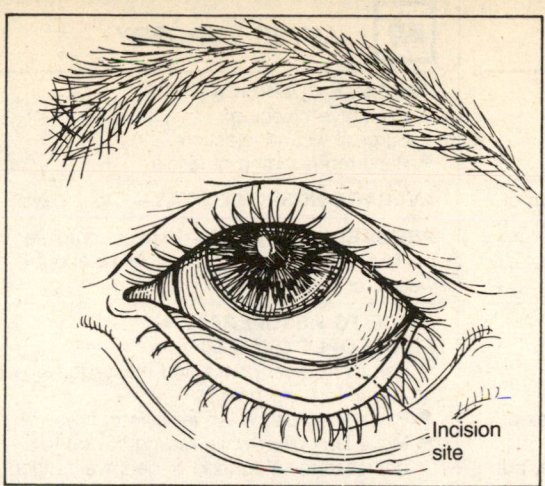

An illustration of the eye, eyelid and typical incision site for ectropion repair.

Incision site

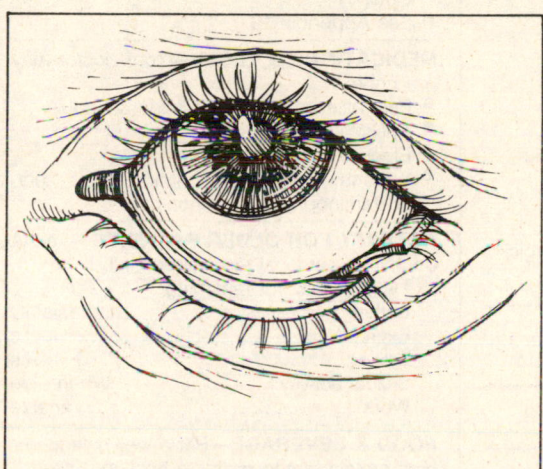

Cartilage is cut close to the outer eyelid edge. A small wedge of cartilage is cut free and removed.

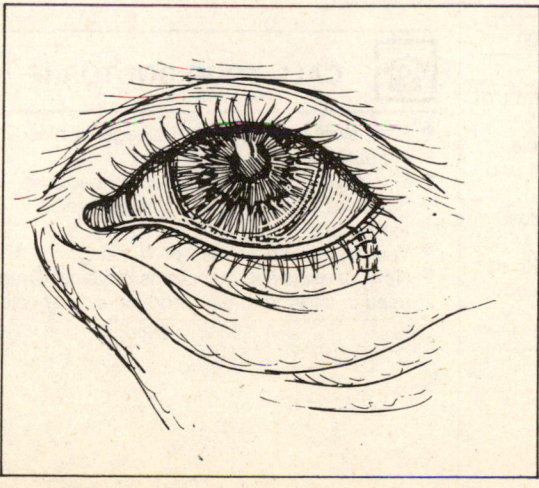

The cartilage is sewn back together and skin closed with small sutures which are usually removed about 10 days after surgery.

SURGERIES

FASCIECTOMY

BASIC INFORMATION

DESCRIPTION—Removal of fascia (fibrous tissue) in the muscles of the hand that has scarred (usually called Dupuytren's contracture) as a result of an unknown cause.

BODY PARTS INVOLVED—Fascia in palm of the hand.

REASONS FOR SURGERY—Restoration of normal function of the hand.

SPECIAL CONSIDERATIONS FOR OLDER PATIENTS
- *Note:* Advancing age alone does not preclude surgery.
- Decreased nutrition may increase the risk of surgical infections and complications.
- Surgical repair is complete and effective, but healing takes longer.

SURGICAL RISK INCREASES WITH
- Obesity.
- Smoking.
- Poor nutrition.
- Recent illness.
- Excessive alcohol consumption or chronic illness.
- Use of drugs such as antihypertensives; muscle relaxants; tranquilizers; sleep inducers; insulin; sedatives; beta-adrenergic blockers; cortisone.

BEFORE SURGERY

WHO OPERATES—Hand surgeon, usually in hospital or outpatient surgical facility.

DIAGNOSTIC TESTS—Blood and urine studies.

ANESTHESIA—Local anesthesia by injection.

DESCRIPTION OF OPERATION
- A tourniquet is applied to the patient's arm to prevent the surgical area from bleeding.
- An incision is made over the scarred fascia.
- The fascia is cut free of connective tissue and removed.
- Sometimes a skin graft is performed to close the gap left by the removed fascia.
- The tourniquet is removed. The skin is closed with sutures, which usually can be removed about 10 days after surgery.

AFTER SURGERY

POSSIBLE COMPLICATIONS
- Excessive bleeding.
- Surgical wound infection.
- Recurrent scarring of fascia.

AVERAGE HOSPITAL STAY—1 to 2 days.

PROBABLE OUTCOME—Expect complete healing without complications. Allow about 6 weeks for recovery from surgery.

GUIDE TO RECUPERATION FOR PEOPLE OVER 50
- Use warm heat packs and massage to ease discomfort and pain.
- Bathe as usual. Wash incision gently.
- Move legs often while resting in bed to decrease the likelihood of deep-vein blood clots.
- See Appendix 19.

MEDICATIONS & TESTS—Your doctor may prescribe:
- Pain relievers. Follow dosage schedule.
- Antibiotics to fight infection.
- Blood studies.
- You may use non-prescription drugs, such as acetaminophen, for minor pain.

ACTIVITY FOR OLDER PATIENTS—Ask your doctor for personalized instructions.
Typical times for resuming:
Bathing . . . . Immediately.
Exercise . . . . 2 weeks.
Driving . . . . 3 weeks.
Sexual activity . . . . When able.
Work . . . . Variable.

FOOD & BEVERAGE—Eat a well-balanced, high-protein diet to promote healing. See Appendix 1.

CALL YOUR DOCTOR IF

- Pain, swelling, redness, drainage or bleeding increases in the surgical area.
- You develop signs of infection: headache, muscle aches, dizziness or a general ill feeling and fever.
- You experience nausea or vomiting.
- New, unexplained symptoms develop. Drugs used in treatment may produce side effects.

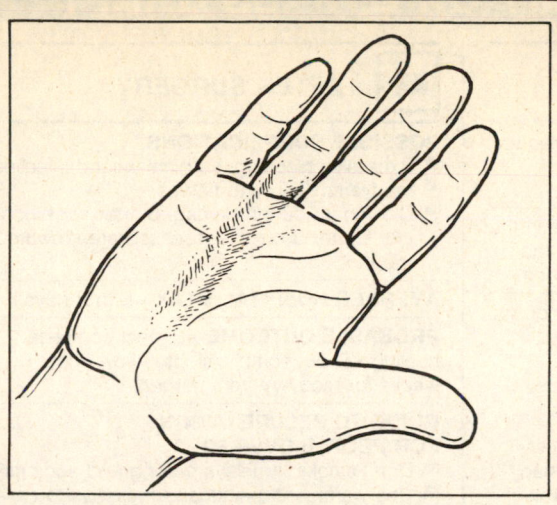

An illustration of fascia (fibrous tissue) and the hand muscles that have scarred.

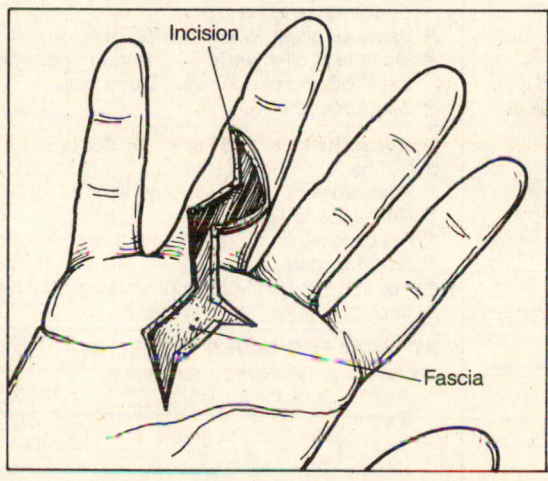

Incision

Fascia

Fascia is cut free of connective tissue and removed.

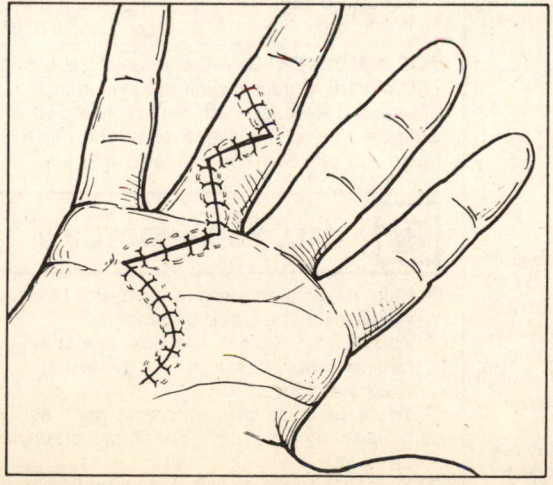

Appearance of hand after closure of surgical wound. Sometimes closure requires a skin graft to close the gap.

FEMORAL-POPLITEAL ARTERY ENDARTERECTOMY OR BYPASS GRAFT

 BASIC INFORMATION

DESCRIPTION—Removal or bypass of plaque or a blood clot that has blocked blood circulation in the leg.

BODY PARTS INVOLVED—Blood vessel in the leg that is called the femoral artery below the groin and the popliteal artery below the knee.

REASONS FOR SURGERY—Restoration of normal blood circulation in the leg and foot.

SPECIAL CONSIDERATIONS FOR OLDER PATIENTS
- *Note:* Advancing age alone does not preclude surgery.
- Characteristic signs and symptoms of many surgical disorders and complications are frequently atypical, changed or absent.
- Surgical repair is complete and effective, but healing takes longer.
- More likely to experience respiratory and kidney problems, confusion and blood clots after surgery.

SURGICAL RISK INCREASES WITH
- Obesity; smoking.
- Recent or chronic illness, especially atherosclerosis or diabetes mellitus.
- Use of drugs such as antihypertensives; muscle relaxants; tranquilizers; sleep inducers; insulin; sedatives; beta-adrenergic blockers; cortisone.

 BEFORE SURGERY

WHO OPERATES—General surgeon or vascular surgeon, usually in hospital.

DIAGNOSTIC TESTS—Blood and urine studies; arteriograms (see Glossary). During surgery: Arteriograms.

ANESTHESIA—General anesthesia by inhalation and injection, with an airway tube placed in the windpipe.

DESCRIPTION OF OPERATION
- An incision is made in the thigh and the plaque or blood clot in the artery is located. Suction is used to remove it if possible.
- If a bypass must be used, a large vein from the leg is selected and cut free. (Sometimes a plastic graft is used for a bypass graft instead of a vein.) Large tributaries of the vein are tied off.
- The graft is sewn in place above and below the blocked artery.
- The muscles and skin are closed with sutures or clips that are removed about 1 week after surgery.

 AFTER SURGERY

POSSIBLE COMPLICATIONS
- Excessive bleeding; surgical wound infection.
- Inadvertent injury to nerves.
- Clotting inside the damaged artery or blood clot further down the diseased area toward the foot.

AVERAGE HOSPITAL STAY—6 to 8 days.

PROBABLE OUTCOME—Expect complete healing without complications. Allow about 6 weeks for recovery from surgery.

GUIDE TO RECUPERATION FOR PEOPLE OVER 50
- Don't smoke. It delays healing and adds risks.
- Use warm heat packs and massage to ease discomfort and pain.
- Bathe as usual. Wash incision gently.
- Move legs often while in to bed to decrease the likelihood of deep-vein blood clots.
- See Appendix 19.

MEDICATIONS & TESTS—Your doctor may prescribe:
- Pain relievers. Follow dosage schedule.
- Antibiotics to fight infection.
- Anticoagulants to prevent blood clot formation.
- Blood studies.
- You may use non-prescription drugs, such as acetaminophen, for minor pain.

ACTIVITY FOR OLDER PATIENTS—Ask your doctor for personalized instructions.
Typical times for resuming:
Bathing . . . . Immediately.
Exercise . . . . 4 weeks.
Driving . . . . 4 weeks.
Sexual activity . . . . When able.
Work . . . . Variable.

FOOD & BEVERAGE—Clear liquid diet until the gastrointestinal tract begins to function again. Then eat a well-balanced, high-protein diet to promote healing. After recovery, eat a diet low in fat and salt. See Appendices 8 and 9.

 CALL YOUR DOCTOR IF

- Pain, swelling, redness, drainage or bleeding increases in the surgical area.
- You develop signs of infection: headache, muscle aches, dizziness or a general ill feeling and fever.
- You experience new symptoms, such as nausea, vomiting, constipation or abdominal swelling.
- Your foot becomes cold, discolored or numb or you develop pain in the calf when walking.

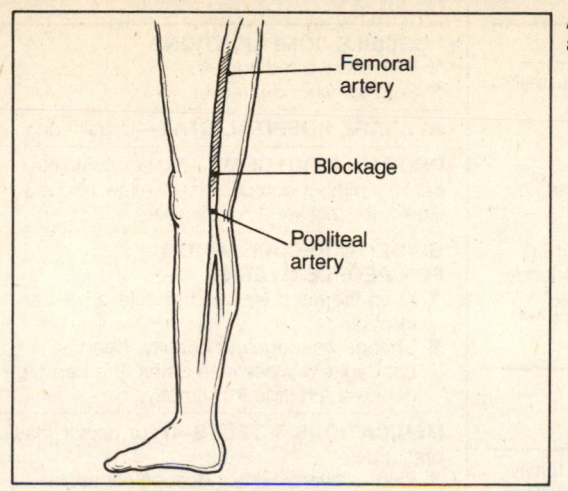

An illustration of a blocked femoral artery in the upper leg.

Femoral artery

Blockage

Popliteal artery

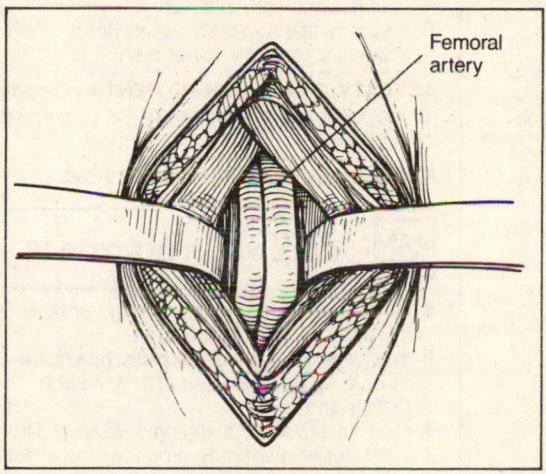

After the skin has been incised and muscles retracted, the area of blockage can be located.

Femoral artery

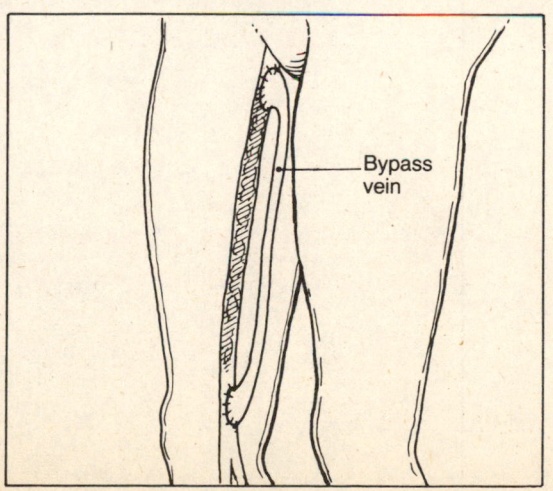

Vein used to bypass the blocked area is sewn into place allowing resumption of normal flow distal to the blockage.

Bypass vein

SURGERIES

BASIC INFORMATION

DESCRIPTION—Removal of a fingernail.

BODY PARTS INVOLVED—Fingernail, usually in the thumb or first finger.

REASONS FOR SURGERY
- Fingernail infection.
- Correction of abnormal fingernail growth.

SPECIAL CONSIDERATIONS FOR OLDER PATIENTS—Surgical repair is complete and effective, but healing takes longer.

SURGICAL RISK INCREASES WITH—None expected.

BEFORE SURGERY

WHO OPERATES—General surgeon or family doctor, usually in hospital or outpatient surgical facility.

DIAGNOSTIC TESTS—Blood and urine studies.

ANESTHESIA—Local anesthesia by injection.

DESCRIPTION OF OPERATION
- An incision is made in the skin around the fingernail.
- The fingernail is pushed up from its bed past the cuticle with a blunt instrument.
- The nail is removed and the nail bed is scraped.
- Usually the surgical wound is left open to heal from the bottom out.
- A special non-stick bandage is applied to prevent bleeding.

AFTER SURGERY

POSSIBLE COMPLICATIONS
- Excessive bleeding.
- Surgical wound infection.

AVERAGE HOSPITAL STAY—Usually none.

PROBABLE OUTCOME—Expect complete healing without complications. Allow about 3 weeks for recovery from surgery.

GUIDE TO RECUPERATION FOR PEOPLE OVER 50
- Keep the hand elevated to relieve pain and throbbing.
- Change bandages frequently. Keep bandages dry between baths. If a bandage gets wet, change it promptly.

MEDICATIONS & TESTS—Your doctor may prescribe:
- Pain relievers. Follow dosage schedule.
- Antibiotics to fight infection.
- You may use non-prescription drugs, such as acetaminophen, for minor pain.

ACTIVITY FOR OLDER PATIENTS—Usually no restrictions. Ask your doctor for personalized instructions.

FOOD & BEVERAGE—No special diet.

CALL YOUR DOCTOR IF

- Pain, swelling, redness, drainage or bleeding increases in the surgical area.
- You develop signs of infection: headache, muscle aches, dizziness or a general ill feeling and fever.
- New, unexplained symptoms develop. Drugs used in treatment may produce side effects.

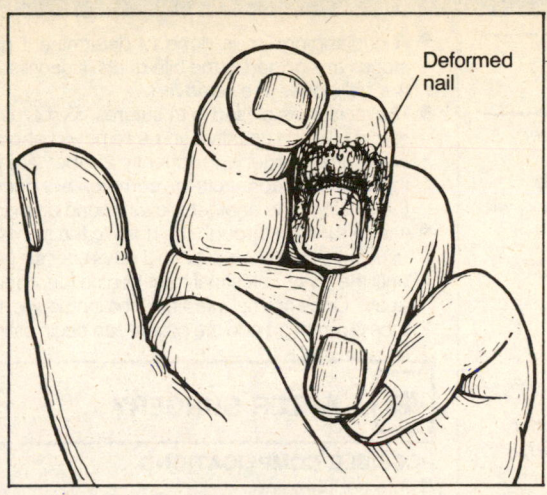

An illustration of a deformed fingernail.

Deformed nail

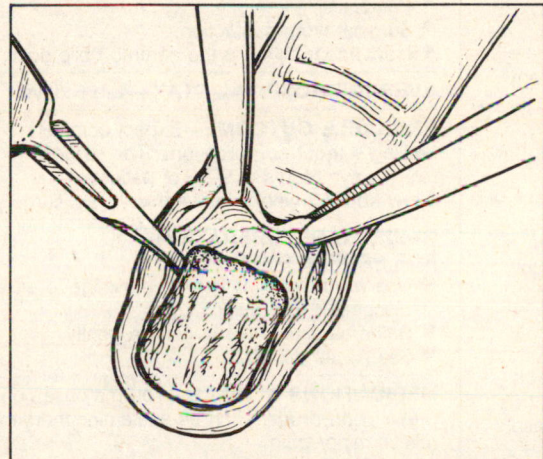

An incision is made in the skin around the fingernail.
- With a blunt instrument, the fingernail is pushed up from its bed past the cuticle.

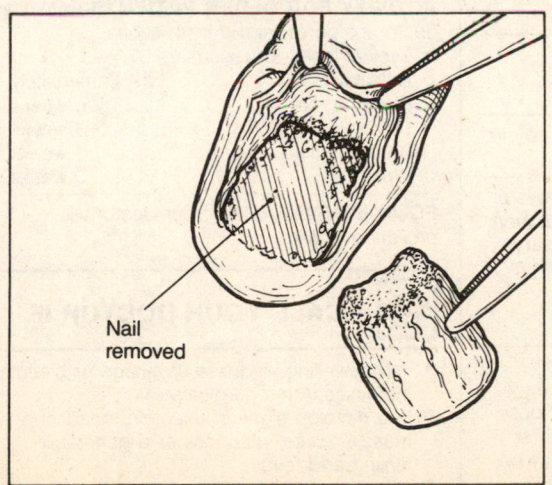

The nail is removed and the nailbed scraped.
- The surgical wound is left open to heal from the bottom out. A new fingernail usually grows to replace the old one within 6 months.

Nail removed

SURGERIES

GALLBLADDER REMOVAL
(Cholecystectomy)

BASIC INFORMATION

DESCRIPTION—Removal of the gallbladder. This information is for regular surgical procedure. There are several new methods being studied. Ask your doctor what method will work best for you.

BODY PARTS INVOLVED—Gallbladder; bile ducts.

REASONS FOR SURGERY
- Gallstones.
- Suspected gallbladder tumors.
- Chronic gallbladder infection.
- Sudden, severe infection of the gallbladder that does not respond rapidly to treatment.

SPECIAL CONSIDERATIONS FOR OLDER PATIENTS
- *Note:* Advancing age alone does not preclude surgery.
- Characteristic signs and symptoms of many surgical disorders and complications are frequently atypical, changed or absent.
- Surgical repair is complete and effective, but healing takes longer.
- Weakened cough reflexes increase the risk of lung and bronchial complications.
- More likely to experience respiratory and kidney problems, confusion and blood clots after surgery.

SURGICAL RISK INCREASES WITH
- Obesity.
- Smoking or excessive alcohol consumption.
- Recent or chronic illness, especially cirrhosis of the liver; diabetes mellitus; heart disease; calcification of the gallbladder; chronic obstructive pulmonary disease (COPD).

BEFORE SURGERY

WHO OPERATES—General surgeon, usually in hospital.

DIAGNOSTIC TESTS—Blood studies; x-rays of the gallbladder; ultrasonic screen (see Glossary). During surgery: Cholangiogram (see Glossary).

ANESTHESIA—General anesthesia by inhalation and injection, with an airway tube placed in the windpipe.

DESCRIPTION OF OPERATION
- An incision is made under the right rib cage. Abdominal muscles are separated to expose abdominal organs, which are inspected for undetected disease. Other surgeries may be performed at this time.
- The gallbladder is cut free and removed from under the liver.

- A cholangiogram is done to determine if gallstones are lodged in the bile ducts. If necessary, the gallstones are removed.
- The incision is closed with sutures, skin clips or staples, which usually can be removed about 1 week after surgery. Frequently 2 tubes are left in place. One connects the common bile duct to the outside, and another allows wound drainage.
- A tube running through the nose to the stomach usually remains at least 2 to 3 days after surgery until the gastrointestinal tract begins functioning again. Once normal intestinal function begins, the tube is removed and the patient can begin eating.

AFTER SURGERY

POSSIBLE COMPLICATIONS
- Internal bleeding.
- Peritonitis.
- Surgical wound infection.
- Inadvertent injury to the common bile duct.

AVERAGE HOSPITAL STAY—4 to 6 days.

PROBABLE OUTCOME—Expect complete healing without complications. The surgery relieves symptoms in 90% of patients. Allow about 3 weeks for recovery from surgery.

GUIDE TO RECUPERATION FOR PEOPLE OVER 50
- Use warm heat packs and massage to ease discomfort and pain.
- Bathe as usual. Wash incision gently.
- See Appendix 19.

MEDICATIONS & TESTS—You may use non-prescription drugs, such as acetaminophen, to relieve minor pain.

ACTIVITY FOR OLDER PATIENTS—Ask your doctor for personalized instructions.
Typical times for resuming:
Bathing . . . . Immediately.
Exercise . . . . 6 weeks.
Driving . . . . 3 weeks.
Sexual activity . . . . 3 weeks.
Work . . . . 6 weeks.

FOOD & BEVERAGE—Your doctor will prescribe a diet.

CALL YOUR DOCTOR IF

- Pain, swelling, redness, drainage or bleeding increases in the surgical area.
- You develop signs of infection: headache, muscle aches, dizziness or a general ill feeling and fever.
- You experience new symptoms, such as hiccups, constipation or abdominal swelling.

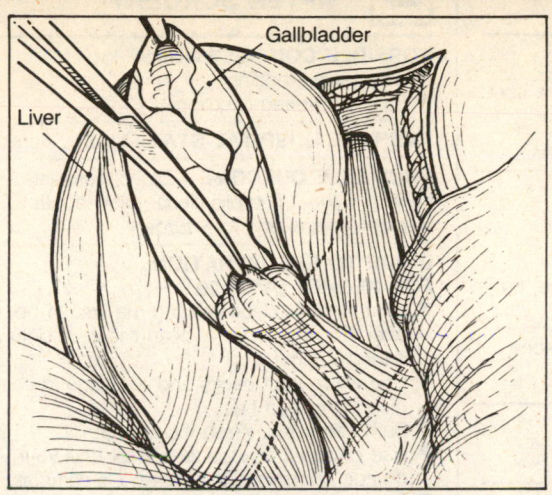

An illustration of the liver and gallbladder located just under the right ribcage. The liver must be retracted upward in order to expose the gallbladder.

Liver

Gallbladder

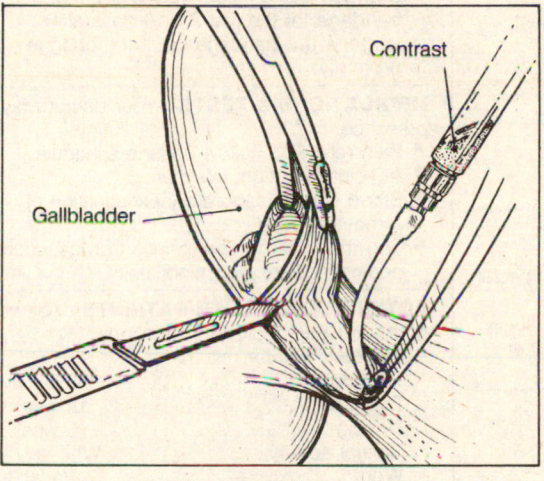

Gallbladder is cut free and removed. Catheter is inserted into bile duct to inject contrast for a cholangiography.

Contrast

Gallbladder

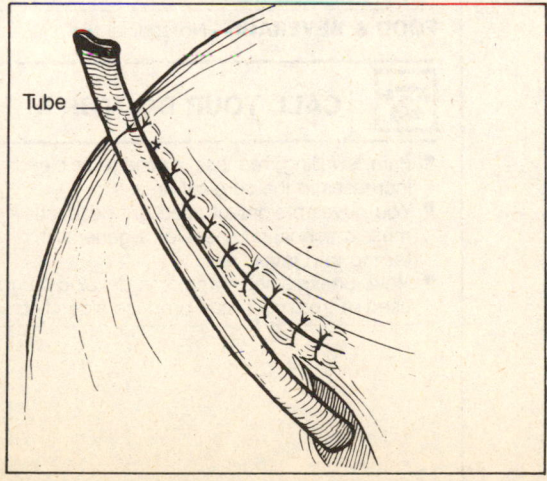

The skin is closed and a drainage tube is left in place and pulled through a stab wound in the abdomen.

Tube

SURGERIES

HEEL SPUR REMOVAL

BASIC INFORMATION

DESCRIPTION—Removal of a heel spur.

BODY PARTS INVOLVED—Bottom of the heel bone.

REASONS FOR SURGERY—Relief of pain.

SPECIAL CONSIDERATIONS FOR OLDER PATIENTS
- *Note:* Advancing age alone does not preclude surgery.
- Surgical repair is complete and effective, but healing takes longer.

SURGICAL RISK INCREASES WITH—None expected.

BEFORE SURGERY

WHO OPERATES—General surgeon, orthopedist or podiatrist, usually in outpatient surgical facility or doctor's office.

DIAGNOSTIC TESTS—Blood and urine studies; x-rays of both feet.

ANESTHESIA
- Local anesthesia by injection.
- Spinal anesthesia by injection.

DESCRIPTION OF OPERATION
- An incision is made over the spur.
- The spur is cut free and removed with special instruments.
- The skin is closed with sutures, which usually can be removed about 10 to 14 days after surgery.

AFTER SURGERY

POSSIBLE COMPLICATIONS
- Excessive bleeding.
- Surgical wound infection.

AVERAGE HOSPITAL STAY—Usually none.

PROBABLE OUTCOME—Expect complete healing without complications. Allow about 6 weeks for recovery from surgery.

GUIDE TO RECUPERATION FOR PEOPLE OVER 50
- If the wound bleeds during the first 24 hours after surgery, press a clean tissue or cloth to it for 10 minutes.
- Use warm heat packs and massage to ease discomfort and pain.
- Bathe as usual. Wash incision gently.
- Use crutches or a cane to walk until your doctor determines that healing is complete.
- Between baths, keep wound dry with a bandage for the first 2 or 3 days after surgery. If a bandage gets wet, change it promptly.

MEDICATIONS & TESTS—Your doctor may prescribe:
- Pain relievers. Follow dosage schedule.
- Antibiotics to fight infection.
- Blood studies; laboratory examination of removed tissue.
- You may use non-prescription drugs, such as acetaminophen, for minor pain.

ACTIVITY FOR OLDER PATIENTS—Ask your doctor for personalized instructions.
Typical times for resuming:
Bathing . . . . Immediately.
Exercise . . . . 12 weeks.
Driving . . . . 6 weeks.
Sexual activity . . . . When able.
Work . . . . Variable.

FOOD & BEVERAGE—No special diet.

CALL YOUR DOCTOR IF

- Pain, swelling, redness, drainage or bleeding increases in the surgical area.
- You develop signs of infection: headache, muscle aches, dizziness or a general ill feeling and fever.
- New, unexplained symptoms develop. Drugs used in treatment may produce side effects.

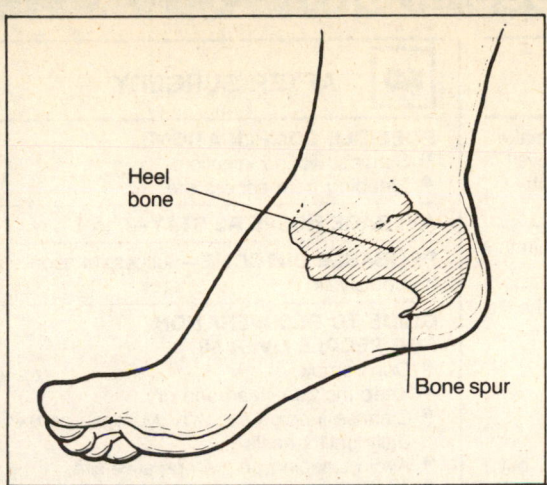

An illustration of a typical bone spur on the heelbone.

Heel bone

Bone spur

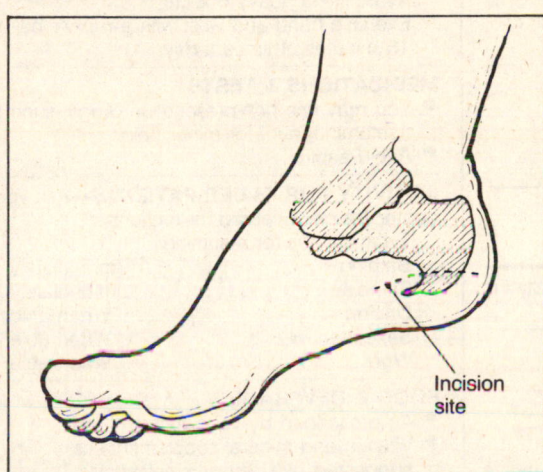

A typical incision site to enable removal of the bone spur which is cut free and removed with special instruments.

Incision site

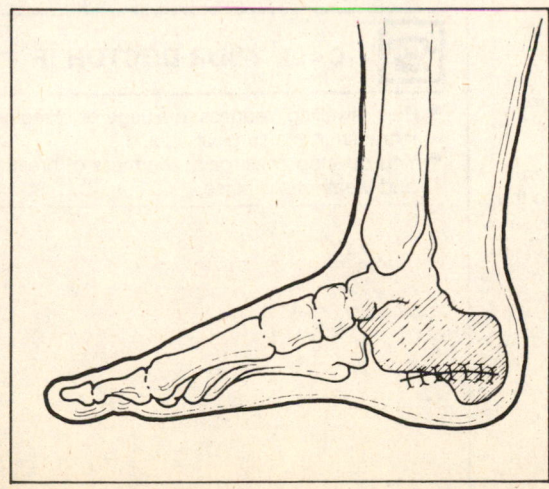

Skin is closed with sutures which can usually be removed about 10 to 14 days after surgery.

SURGERIES

HEMODIALYSIS ACCESS BY ARTERIOVENOUS SHUNT

 BASIC INFORMATION

DESCRIPTION—A surgical procedure to make it possible to perform hemodialysis to remove toxic wastes from the blood of a patient with kidney failure.

BODY PARTS INVOLVED—Artery and vein in the neck, leg or arm.

REASONS FOR SURGERY—To prolong the life of patients with kidney failure.

SPECIAL CONSIDERATIONS FOR OLDER PATIENTS
- *Note:* Advancing age alone does not preclude surgery.
- Surgical repair is complete and effective, but healing takes longer.
- Decreased nutrition may increase the risk of surgical infections and complications.

SURGICAL RISK INCREASES WITH
- Obesity.
- Smoking.
- Excessive alcohol consumption.

 BEFORE SURGERY

WHO OPERATES—General surgeon, usually in hospital or outpatient surgical facility.

DIAGNOSTIC TESTS—Blood and urine studies.

ANESTHESIA—Local.

DESCRIPTION OF OPERATION
- An incision is made on the underside of the wrist over large blood vessels.
- The surgeon inserts a 6- to 10-inch silastic cannula into an artery and another into a vein.
- The surgeon tunnels the cannulas through small incisions and connects them on the outside of the skin with teflon tubing.
- Hemodialysis can now be performed when the blood vessel lines from the dialyzer to the needles are connected to the access site.

 AFTER SURGERY

POSSIBLE COMPLICATIONS
- Surgical wound infection.
- Bleeding from access site.

AVERAGE HOSPITAL STAY—0 to 1 day.

PROBABLE OUTCOME—Successful access for hemodialysis.

GUIDE TO RECUPERATION FOR PEOPLE OVER 50
- Don't smoke.
- Keep incision clean and dry.
- Cleanse incision site with hydrogen peroxide daily until it heals.
- Avoid sleeping on the operative site.
- Avoid lifting heavy objects.
- Exercise hand and wrist with a rubber ball for 15 minutes, 4 times a day.

MEDICATIONS & TESTS
- You may use non-prescription drugs, such as acetaminophen, for minor pain.
- Avoid aspirin.

ACTIVITY FOR OLDER PATIENTS—Ask your doctor for personalized instructions.
Typical times for resuming:
Bathing . . . . Immediately.
Exercise . . . . Immediately.
Driving . . . . When able.
Sexual activity . . . . When able.
Work . . . . When able.

FOOD & BEVERAGE
- As prescribed by your doctor.
- Vitamin and mineral supplements as suggested by doctor (sometimes).

 CALL YOUR DOCTOR IF

- Pain, swelling, redness, drainage or bleeding increase in the surgical area.
- You develop chest pain, shortness of breath and weak, rapid pulse.

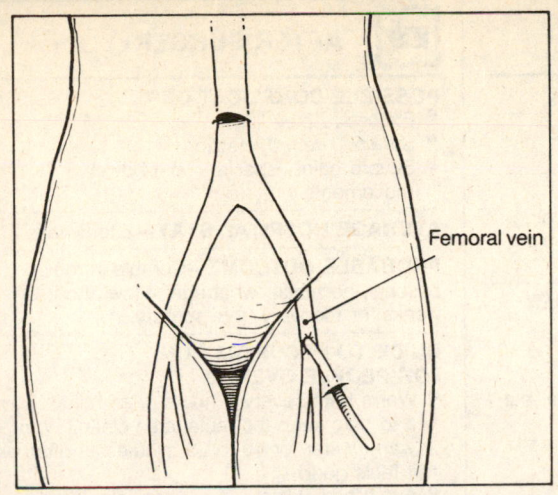

This illustration shows the femoral vein access site with silastic cannula in place.

Femoral vein

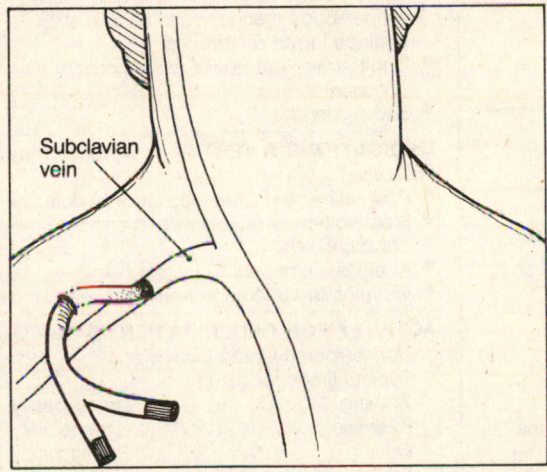

This illustrates an access site in the neck and the subclavian vein.

Subclavian vein

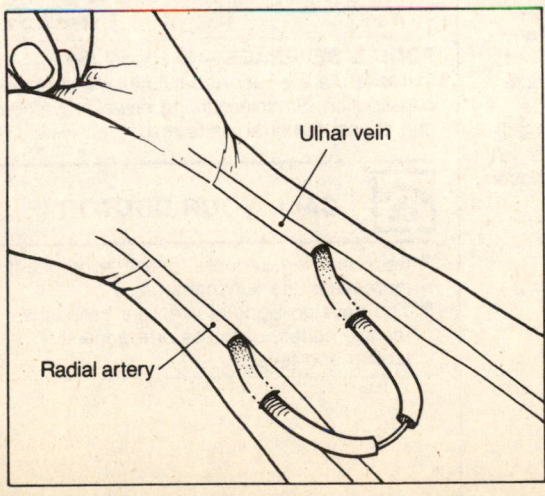

This illustrates a hemodialysis access site in the wrist.

Ulnar vein

Radial artery

SURGERIES

HEMORRHOID REMOVAL
(Hemorrhoidectomy)

 BASIC INFORMATION

DESCRIPTION—Removal of hemorrhoids.

BODY PARTS INVOLVED—Dilated veins around the anus or just inside the rectum.

REASONS FOR SURGERY
- Relief of excessive itching, pain or bleeding.
- Relief of a painful thrombosed hemorrhoid (hemorrhoid containing a blood clot).

SPECIAL CONSIDERATIONS FOR OLDER PATIENTS
- *Note:* Advancing age alone does not preclude surgery.
- Surgical repair is complete and effective, but healing takes longer.

SURGICAL RISK INCREASES WITH
- Obesity.
- Smoking.
- Poor nutrition.
- Excessive alcohol consumption.
- Chronic illness.

 BEFORE SURGERY

WHO OPERATES—Proctologist, general surgeon or family doctor, usually in doctor's office, outpatient surgical facility or hospital.

DIAGNOSTIC TESTS—Blood studies.

ANESTHESIA
- Local anesthesia by injection.
- Spinal anesthesia by injection.
- General anesthesia by inhalation and injection, with an airway tube placed in the windpipe.

DESCRIPTION OF OPERATION
- The dilated veins from around the anus and inside the rectum are cut free and removed, with care taken not to damage the sphincter muscle. Sometimes anal muscles must be dilated vigorously to expose the hemorrhoids.
- The surgical area may be sewn closed or left open, and medicated gauze is used to cover it.

 AFTER SURGERY

POSSIBLE COMPLICATIONS
- Excessive bleeding.
- Surgical wound infection.
- Severe pain, especially with bowel movements.

AVERAGE HOSPITAL STAY—2 to 3 days.

PROBABLE OUTCOME—Curable in most patients, no matter what age. Allow about 2 weeks for recovery from surgery.

GUIDE TO RECUPERATION FOR PEOPLE OVER 50
- Warm baths every 4 hours or so relieve pain and help keep the rectal area clean. Sit in warm water for 10 to 20 minutes as often as it feels good.
- Avoid heavy lifting. If not possible, learn proper body mechanics to reduce strain contributing to recurrence.
- Don't strain with bowel movements or urination.
- See Appendix 19.

MEDICATIONS & TESTS—Your doctor may prescribe:
- Pain relievers. Follow dosage schedule.
- Stool softeners or laxatives to prevent constipation.
- Analgesic ointment to relieve pain.
- Vitamins to encourage healing.

ACTIVITY FOR OLDER PATIENTS—Ask your doctor for personalized instructions.
Typical times for resuming:
Bathing . . . . Immediately.
Exercise . . . . Immediately.
Driving . . . . Immediately.
Sexual activity . . . . When able.
Work . . . . Immediately.

FOOD & BEVERAGE—No special diet. Increase dietary fiber and fluid intake to prevent constipation. Straining during bowel movements can cause hemorrhoids to recur.

 CALL YOUR DOCTOR IF

- Pain, swelling, redness, drainage or bleeding increase in the surgical area.
- You develop signs of infection: headache, muscle aches, dizziness or a general ill feeling and fever.

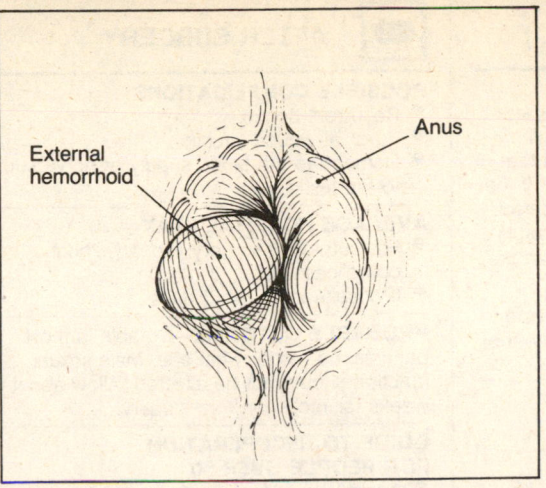

An illustration of a typical external hemorrhoid arising from inside the anus and extending through the anal opening.

Anus

External hemorrhoid

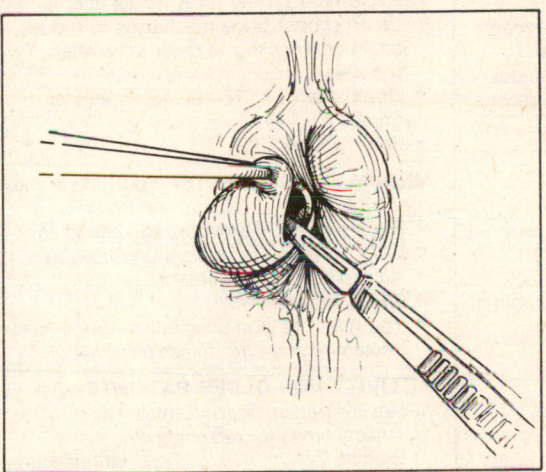

Dilated veins around the anus and inside the rectum are cut free and removed with care taken not to damage the sphincter muscles.

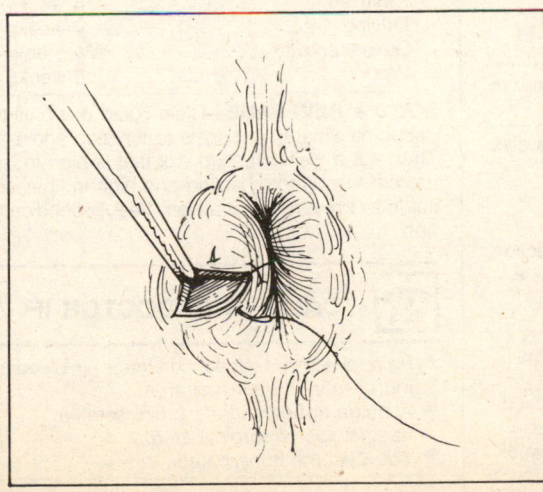

The surgical area is sewn closed or left open and medicated gauze is used to cover.

SURGERIES

HERNIA, INGUINAL, REPAIR OF
(Inguinal Herniorrhaphy)

BASIC INFORMATION

DESCRIPTION—Closing or repairing an inguinal hernia, an internal defect or weakness in the muscular layer of the abdominal wall. Sometimes an intestine protrudes through the hernia defect, causing a noticeable bulge. If the intestine becomes trapped in the hernia defect, it is called an incarcerated hernia. If the hernia defect blocks the intestine's blood supply, it is called a strangulated hernia.

BODY PARTS INVOLVED—Groin muscles and ligaments inside the lower abdomen next to the genitals; abdominal muscles.

REASONS FOR SURGERY
- Incarcerated hernia. This is a medical emergency.
- Strangulated hernia. This is a medical emergency.
- Uncomplicated hernia. Most doctors recommend operating on a hernia even if no hernia symptoms are present to prevent the serious complications of incarceration or strangulation.

SPECIAL CONSIDERATIONS FOR OLDER PATIENTS
- *Note:* Advancing age alone does not preclude surgery.
- Characteristic signs and symptoms of many surgical disorders and complications are frequently atypical, changed or absent.
- Surgical repair is complete and effective, but healing takes longer.

SURGICAL RISK INCREASES WITH
- Obesity; smoking.
- Family history of hernias.
- Excessive alcohol consumption.

BEFORE SURGERY

WHO OPERATES—General surgeon, usually in hospital or outpatient surgical facility.

DIAGNOSTIC TESTS—Blood and urine studies.

ANESTHESIA
- Spinal anesthesia by injection.
- Local anesthesia by injection.
- General anesthesia by inhalation and injection, with an airway tube placed in the windpipe.

DESCRIPTION OF OPERATION
- An incision is made in the abdomen. The abdominal muscles are separated, and the peritoneal cavity is opened.
- The hernia is located and repaired or closed. The skin is closed with sutures or staples, which usually can be removed about 1 week after surgery.

AFTER SURGERY

POSSIBLE COMPLICATIONS
- Recurrent hernia.
- Surgical wound infection.
- Damage to the blood supply or nerve supply to the testicles.

AVERAGE HOSPITAL STAY
- For outpatient surgery: None (without complications).
- If hospitalized: 2 to 3 days.

PROBABLE OUTCOME—Curable in most patients, no matter what age. Male sexual function should not be affected. Allow about 6 weeks for recovery from surgery.

GUIDE TO RECUPERATION FOR PEOPLE OVER 50
- Avoid heavy lifting for 6 weeks after surgery. Learn proper body mechanics to reduce strain contributing to recurrence after recovery.
- Don't strain with bowel movements or urination.
- See Appendix 19.

MEDICATIONS & TESTS—Your doctor may prescribe:
- Pain relievers. Follow dosage schedule.
- Stool softeners to prevent constipation.
- Antibiotics to fight infection.
- Blood studies.
- You may use non-prescription drugs, such as acetaminophen, for minor pain.

ACTIVITY FOR OLDER PATIENTS—Ask your doctor for personalized instructions.
Typical times for resuming:
Bathing . . . . Immediately.
Exercise . . . . 4 weeks.
Driving . . . . 4 weeks.
Sexual activity . . . . When able.
Work . . . . 6 weeks.

FOOD & BEVERAGE—Clear liquid diet until the gastrointestinal tract begins to function again. Then eat a well-balanced diet that is high in protein to promote healing and high in fiber and fluids to prevent constipation. See Appendices 7 and 1.

CALL YOUR DOCTOR IF

- Pain, swelling, redness, drainage or bleeding increase in the surgical area.
- A bulge appears in the groin, scrotum, vaginal lips or surgical area.
- You become constipated.

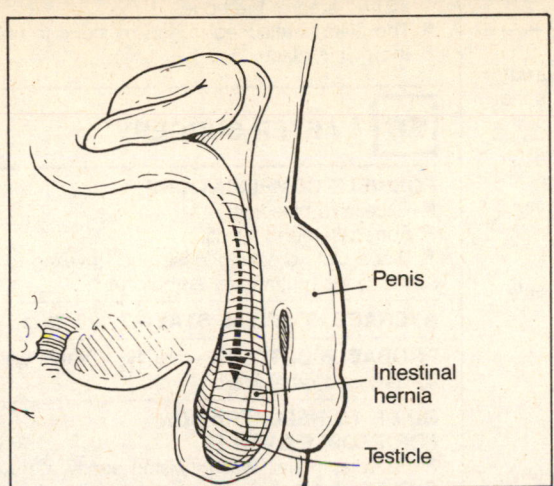

A side view of the male pelvic region.

•A typical inguinal hernia in which a loop of intestine has dropped down into the scrotum.

Penis

Intestinal hernia

Testicle

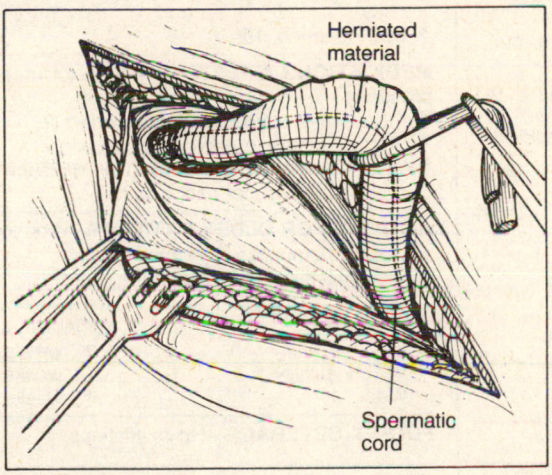

Herniated material

Spermatic cord

The hernia is located and repaired or closed being careful not to injure the spermatic cord.

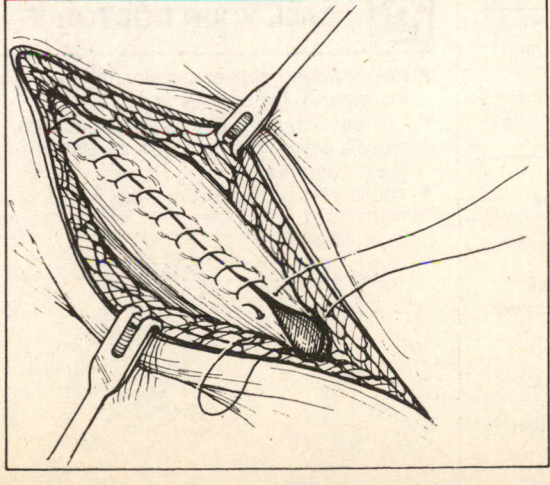

Sometimes, if the hernia is large enough to warrant more than natural tissue, a fine mesh gauze patch may be sewn in place to prevent abdominal contents from causing a recurrent hernia.

SURGERIES

HIP NAILING FOR HIP FRACTURE

BASIC INFORMATION

DESCRIPTION—A surgical procedure to reattach the broken fragments of the fractured femur (the large bone in the thigh that joins the hip bone to form the hip joint).

BODY PARTS INVOLVED—The head and neck of the femur and the acetabulum (the socket of the hip bone that receives the femur to form the hip joint).

REASONS FOR SURGERY
- To make movement of the hip joint possible again after fracture.
- To prevent prolonged bed confinement.

SPECIAL CONSIDERATIONS FOR OLDER PATIENTS
- *Note:* Advancing age alone does not preclude surgery.
- Characteristic signs and symptoms of many surgical disorders and complications are frequently atypical, changed or absent.
- Surgical repair is complete and effective, but healing takes longer.
- Weakened cough reflexes increase the risk of lung and bronchial complications.
- Decreased nutrition may increase the risk of surgical infections and complications.

SURGICAL RISK INCREASES WITH
- Obesity.
- Smoking.
- Excessive alcohol consumption.
- Heart failure.
- Kidney failure.
- Use of many different drugs. (Be sure to inform the surgeon and anesthesiologist of the medicines you take.)

BEFORE SURGERY

WHO OPERATES—General surgeon (sometimes) or orthopedic surgeon, usually in hospital.

DIAGNOSTIC TESTS—Blood and urine studies; x-rays of hip and lungs.

ANESTHESIA— General anesthesia by inhalation and injection, with an airway tube placed in the windpipe.

DESCRIPTION OF OPERATION
- After anesthesia, the area adjacent to the fractured hip is cleaned, shaven and draped.
- An incision is made at a point allowing access to the fractured parts.
- The broken fragments are realigned under direct vision.
- Plates are fitted to hold the nail to be inserted into the fractured fragments.

- The nail is hammered into the broken parts to hold them together and give strength to the injured area of the bone.
- The plate is attached to healthy bone to hold the nail in place.

AFTER SURGERY

POSSIBLE COMPLICATIONS
- Excessive bleeding.
- Surgical wound infection.
- Blood clots breaking loose and traveling to the lungs (pulmonary embolism).

AVERAGE HOSPITAL STAY—7 to 9 days.

PROBABLE OUTCOME—Usually curable with surgery and rehabilitation.

GUIDE TO RECUPERATION FOR PEOPLE OVER 50
- Bathe as usual. Wash incision gently.
- Don't smoke. It delays healing and adds risks.
- See Appendix 19.

MEDICATIONS & TESTS—Your doctor may prescribe:
- Pain relievers. Follow dosage schedule.
- Stool softeners to prevent constipation.
- You may use non-prescription drugs, such as acetaminophen, for minor pain.

ACTIVITY FOR OLDER PATIENTS—Ask your doctor for personalized instructions.
Typical times for resuming:
Bathing . . . . .Immediately.
Exercise . . . . .Immediately.
Driving . . . . .12 weeks.
Sexual activity . . . . .4 weeks.
Work . . . . .12 weeks.

FOOD & BEVERAGE—No restrictions.

CALL YOUR DOCTOR IF

- Pain, swelling, redness, drainage or bleeding increases in the surgical area.
- You develop signs of infection: headache, muscle aches, dizziness or a general ill feeling and fever.
- You experience nausea or vomiting.

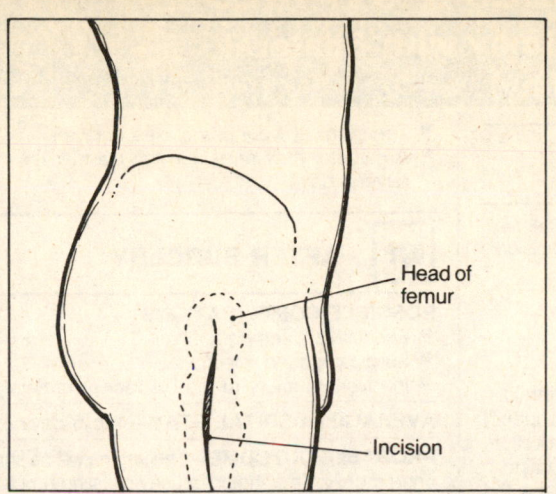

An illustration of an incision made over the affected hip showing the head of the femur which is fractured.

Head of femur

Incision

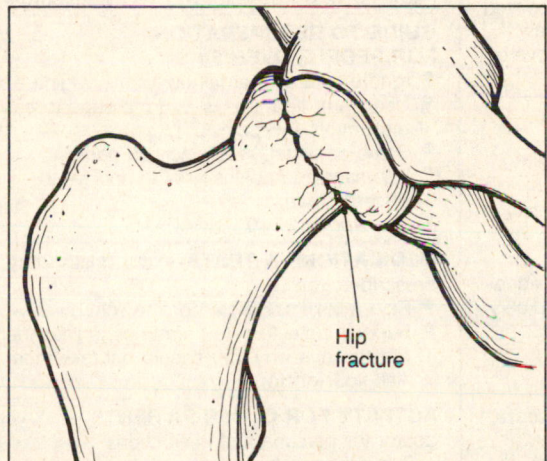

A closer view of the fractured hip.

Hip fracture

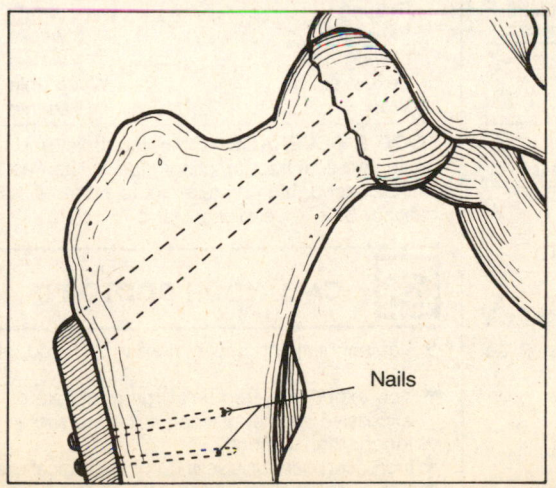

The bone is aligned with a brace and nails inserted.

Nails

HYSTERECTOMY (ABDOMINAL) WITH REMOVAL OF TUBES & OVARIES
(Abdominal Hysterectomy with Bilateral Salpingo-Oophorectomy)

 BASIC INFORMATION

DESCRIPTION—Removal of the uterus, cervix, Fallopian tubes and ovaries through an incision in the abdomen.

BODY PARTS INVOLVED—Uterus; cervix; Fallopian tubes; ovaries; vagina.

REASONS FOR SURGERY
- Uterus: Cancer or suspected cancer; fibroid tumors; chronic bleeding; prolapsed (dropped) uterus; endometriosis; chronic pelvic infection; severe menstrual pain; voluntary sterilization.
- Fallopian tubes and ovaries: Cancer or suspected cancer of the ovaries; precancerous or twisted ovarian cysts; ovarian pregnancy; ovarian abscess; damage to the ovaries from severe endometriosis.

SPECIAL CONSIDERATIONS FOR OLDER PATIENTS
- Surgical repair is complete and effective, but healing takes longer.
- Characteristic signs and symptoms of many surgical disorders and complications are frequently atypical, changed or absent.
- More likely to experience respiratory and kidney problems, confusion and blood clots after surgery.

SURGICAL RISK INCREASES WITH
- Obesity.
- Smoking.
- Iron-deficiency anemia; heart or lung disease; diabetes mellitus.
- Use of drugs such as cortisone; antihypertensives; diuretics; beta-adrenergic blockers.

 BEFORE SURGERY

WHO OPERATES—General surgeon or obstetrician-gynecologist, usually in hospital.

DIAGNOSTIC TESTS—Blood and urine studies; x-rays of abdomen and kidneys; dilatation and curettage of the uterus (D&C).

ANESTHESIA—General anesthesia by inhalation and injection, with an airway tube placed in the windpipe.

DESCRIPTION OF OPERATION
- An incision is made in the abdomen.
- The abdominal organs are examined.
- The uterus, cervix, Fallopian tubes and ovaries are cut free and removed.
- The vagina is closed with sutures at its deeper end.

- The surgical wound is closed in layers.
- A catheter may remain in the bladder for several days.

 AFTER SURGERY

POSSIBLE COMPLICATIONS
- Excessive bleeding.
- Surgical wound infection.
- Inadvertent injury to the bladder or ureters.

AVERAGE HOSPITAL STAY—4 to 6 days.

PROBABLE OUTCOME—The vagina will be shortened slightly. This should cause no lasting problem. Allow about 6 weeks for recovery from surgery.

GUIDE TO RECUPERATION FOR PEOPLE OVER 50
- Ignore sutures that fall out of the vagina.
- Use warm heat packs and massage to ease discomfort and pain.
- Bathe as usual. Wash incision gently.
- Use sanitary napkins—not tampons—to absorb blood.
- See Appendix 19.

MEDICATIONS & TESTS—Your doctor may prescribe:
- Pain relievers. Follow dosage schedule.
- Supplemental female hormones, unless there are reasons why you should not take them. Ask your doctor.

ACTIVITY FOR OLDER PATIENTS—Ask your doctor for personalized instructions.
Typical times for resuming:
Bathing . . . . Immediately.
Exercise . . . . 4 weeks.
Driving . . . . 4 weeks.
Sexual activity . . . . When able.
Work . . . . Variable.

FOOD & BEVERAGE—Clear liquid diet until the gastrointestinal tract functions again. Then eat a well-balanced, high-protein diet to promote healing. See Appendices 1 and 7.

 CALL YOUR DOCTOR IF

- Vaginal bleeding soaks more than 1 pad per hour.
- You experience frequent urge to urinate or excessive vaginal discharge that persists longer than 1 month.
- Increased pain or swelling in the surgical area.
- Signs of infection: headache, muscle aches, dizziness or a general ill feeling and fever.

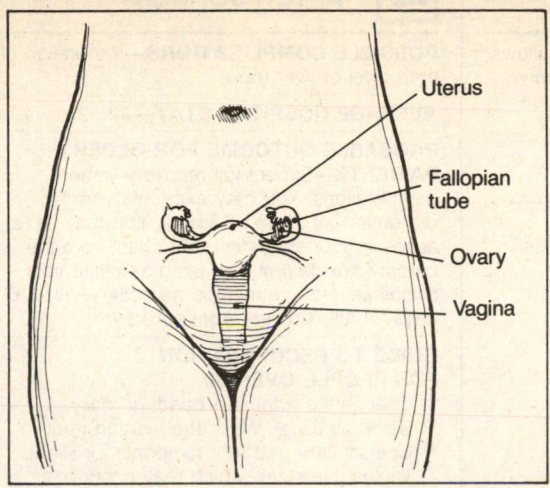

Shown are parts of the female reproductive tract including the uterus, fallopian tubes, ovaries and vagina.

Uterus

Fallopian tube

Ovary

Vagina

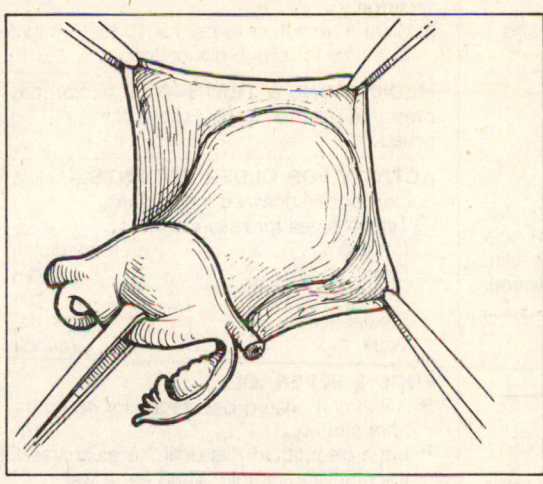

After an incision (either vertical or transverse) has been made in the lower abdomen and the muscles retracted, the uterus, cervix, fallopian tubes and ovaries are cut free and removed.

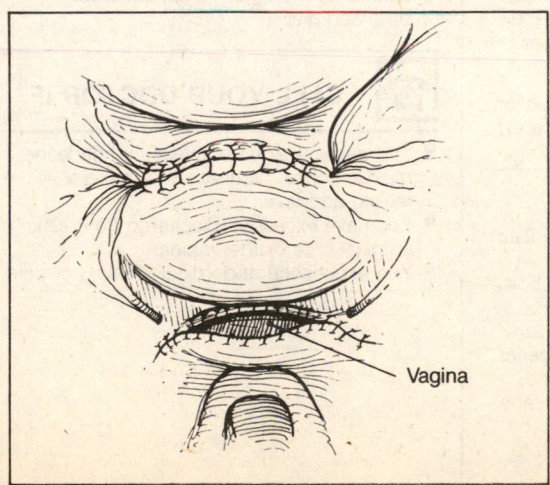

The vagina is closed with sutures.

•The abdominal wall is closed in layers and the skin is closed with sutures which usually can be removed in 10 to 14 days (not illustrated).

Vagina

LAPAROSCOPY

 BASIC INFORMATION

DESCRIPTION—This is a procedure that allows visual examination and treatments of the pelvic and abdominal organs. Surgery is performed with a laparoscope, a fiber optic instrument.

BODY PARTS INVOLVED—Abdomen and all its contents.

REASONS FOR SURGERY
- Diagnosis of reasons for infertility in women.
- Minimal endometriosis.
- Complications from pelvic disease.
- Masses or cysts in the pelvis.
- Undiagnosed pelvic pain.
- Fibroid tumors of the uterus.
- Voluntary sterilization.

SPECIAL CONSIDERATIONS FOR OLDER PATIENTS
- *Note:* Advancing age alone does not preclude surgery.
- Nursing care needs to be more intense and skillful.

SURGICAL RISK INCREASES WITH
- Obesity.
- Smoking.
- Heart or lung disease.
- Advanced pregnancy.
- Previous abdominal surgery, especially hernias.
- Use of drugs such as antihypertensives; muscle relaxants; tranquilizers; sleep inducers; insulin; sedatives; beta-adrenergic blockers; cortisone.

 BEFORE SURGERY

WHO OPERATES—General surgeon or obstetrician-gynecologist, usually in outpatient surgical facility or hospital.

DIAGNOSTIC TESTS—Blood studies. During surgery: Dye passed through Fallopian tubes.

ANESTHESIA
- General anesthesia by inhalation and injection, with an airway tube placed in the windpipe.
- Local anesthesia (sometimes).

DESCRIPTION OF OPERATION
- A small incision is made in or below the patient's navel. A needle is inserted to inflate the abdomen with carbon dioxide.
- The operating table is tilted to allow the bowel and carbon dioxide to float up toward the chest. The laparoscope is used to examine the abdomen visually or to perform surgeries if necessary. The laparoscope is removed, and the carbon dioxide is allowed to escape from the abdomen. Small sutures under the skin and an adhesive bandage are used to close the wound.

 AFTER SURGERY

POSSIBLE COMPLICATIONS—Perforation of the bowel or liver (rare).

AVERAGE HOSPITAL STAY—0 to 2 days.

PROBABLE OUTCOME FOR OLDER PATIENTS—Expect full recovery without complications. You may experience slight discomfort for 24 to 48 hours. You may have aches in your shoulders and chest from the carbon dioxide that was used to inflate your abdomen. No treatment is necessary. Allow 6 days for full recovery from surgery.

GUIDE TO RECUPERATION FOR PEOPLE OVER 50
- Change the adhesive bandage daily.
- Bathe as usual. Wash the incision gently.
- Use sanitary pad (not tampons) for slight vaginal bleeding, which may occur after surgery.
- Sit in a hot tub of water for 10 to 15 minutes at a time to relieve discomfort.

MEDICATIONS & TESTS—Your doctor may prescribe pain relievers. Follow dosage schedule.

ACTIVITY FOR OLDER PATIENTS—Ask your doctor for personalized instructions.
Typical times for resuming:
Bathing . . . . Immediately.
Exercise . . . . 1 day.
Driving . . . . 1 day.
Sexual activity . . . . 1 day.
Work . . . . Variable.

FOOD & BEVERAGE
- Avoid carbonated beverages for 48 hours after surgery.
- Eat a clear liquid diet until the gastrointestinal tract functions again. Then eat a well-balanced diet.

 CALL YOUR DOCTOR IF

- You develop signs of infection: headache, muscle aches, dizziness or a general ill feeling and fever.
- You have excessive discharge from either the surgical area or the vagina.
- You experience abdominal swelling or pain.

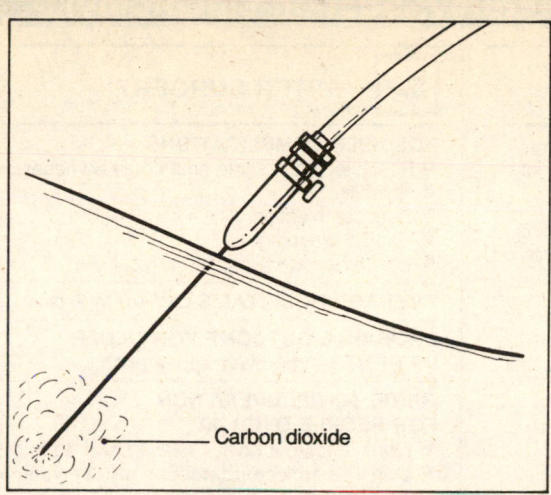

Carbon dioxide

A hollow needle is inserted through the abdominal wall to inflate the abdomen with carbon dioxide.

•The operating table is tilted to allow the bowel and carbon dioxide to flow upward toward the chest.

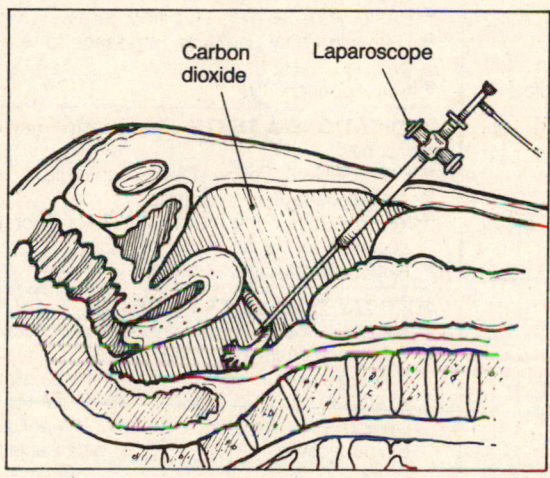

Carbon dioxide

Laparoscope

The laparoscope is inserted through the incision area to allow examination of the abdominal contents under direct vision.

SURGERIES

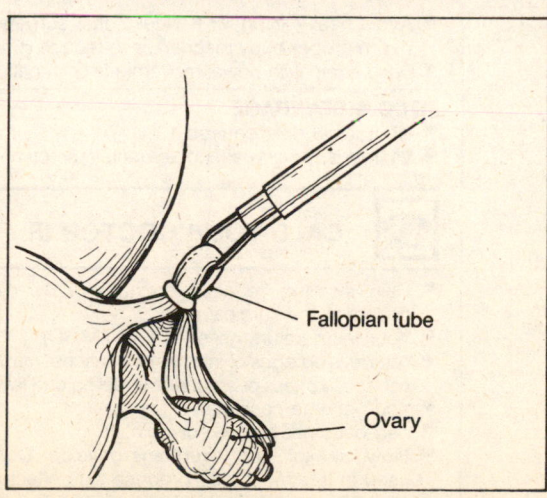

Fallopian tube

Ovary

The laparoscope may be used to provide passage of other instruments for physicians to perform surgical procedures if necessary.

•After the laparoscope is removed, carbon dioxide is allowed to escape from the abdomen. The small amount remaining will be readily absorbed by the body.
•Sutures under the skin and adhesive bandages are used to close the wound (not illustrated).

LIPOSUCTION
(Suction-Assisted Lipectomy; Suction Lipectomy)

 BASIC INFORMATION

DESCRIPTION—A surgical technique using suction equipment to permanently remove fat deposits. Surgery requires 1 to 2 hours.

BODY PARTS INVOLVED—Thighs and hips; buttocks; fat cells of the abdominal wall; chin or other small areas.

REASONS FOR SURGERY—Cosmetic improvement of fat areas that won't go away without extreme dieting that may leave the rest of the body too thin.

SPECIAL CONSIDERATIONS FOR OLDER PATIENTS
- Advancing age alone does not preclude surgery.
- Surgical repair is complete and effective, but healing takes longer.
- More likely to experience respiratory and kidney problems, confusion and blood clots after surgery.

SURGICAL RISK INCREASES WITH
- Extreme obesity.
- Smoking.
- Excessive alcohol consumption.
- History of phlebitis.

 BEFORE SURGERY

WHO OPERATES—Plastic surgeon, usually in outpatient surgical facility or hospital.

DIAGNOSTIC TESTS—Blood and urine studies.

ANESTHESIA
- Local anesthesia and sedation for small areas.
- General anesthesia by inhalation and injection, with an airway tube placed in the windpipe.

DESCRIPTION OF OPERATION
- The plastic surgeon marks areas to be operated on.
- Incisions (about 1 inch each) are made in suction areas.
- A suction tube, with one end attached to suction equipment, is pushed through the incision into the excess fat and moved back and forth repeatedly (20 to 30 times at each site).
- Each incision is stitched.

 AFTER SURGERY

POSSIBLE COMPLICATIONS
- Resuctioning in some areas may be necessary.
- Phlebitis.
- Surgical infection.
- Excess bleeding.
- Blotchy brown areas at surgical site.

AVERAGE HOSPITAL STAY—0 to 2 days.

PROBABLE OUTCOME FOR OLDER PATIENTS—Improved appearance.

GUIDE TO RECUPERATION FOR PEOPLE OVER 50
- Don't smoke. It delays healing and adds risks.
- Don't be concerned about small amounts of oozing at the surgical sites.
- Bathe as usual. Wash incision gently.
- Use warm heat packs and massage to relieve pain.
- See Appendix 19.

MEDICATIONS & TESTS—Your doctor may prescribe:
- Pain relievers. Follow dosage schedule.
- Antibiotics to fight infection.
- You may use non-prescription drugs, such as acetaminophen, for minor pain.
- Avoid aspirin.

ACTIVITY FOR OLDER PATIENTS
- Ask your doctor for personalized instructions. Typical times for resuming:
  Bathing . . . . .Immediately.
  Exercise . . . . .4 weeks.
  Driving . . . . .4 weeks.
  Sexual activity . . . . .When able.
  Work . . . . .Variable.
- Avoid heavy lifting for 6 weeks after surgery. Learn proper body mechanics to reduce strain.
- Don't strain with bowel movements or urination.

FOOD & BEVERAGE
- No special diet required.
- Vitamin and mineral supplements (sometimes).

 CALL YOUR DOCTOR IF

- Pain, swelling, redness, drainage or bleeding occurs in the surgical area.
- Your temperature rises to 101F (38.3C).
- You develop signs of infection: headache, muscle aches, dizziness or a general ill feeling and fever.
- You become constipated.
- Leg becomes swollen or painful.
- New, unexplained symptoms develop. Drugs used in treatment may produce side effects.

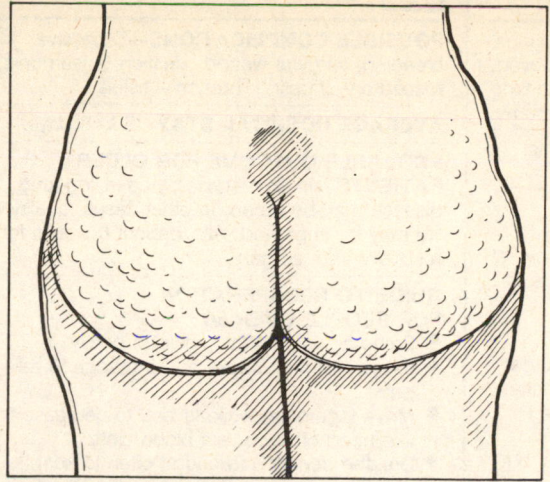

An illustration of fatty deposits under the skin in the buttocks area.

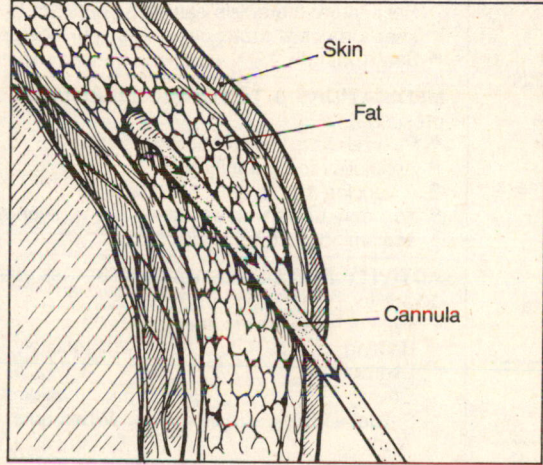

Skin

Fat

Cannula

Approximate 1" incisions are made in suction areas and a suction tube with one end attached to suction equipment is pushed through the incision into the excess fat and moved back and forth repeatedly.

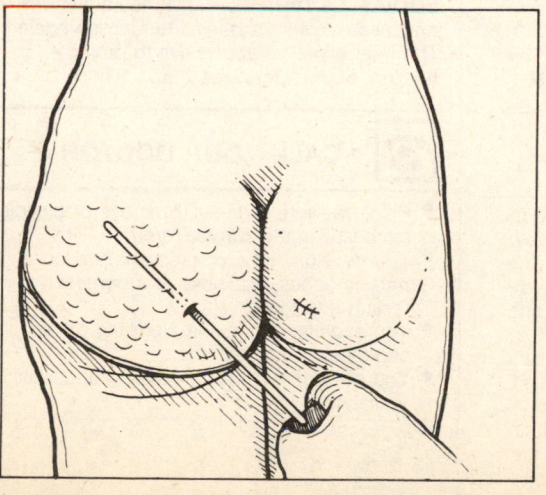

Liposuction complete on the patient's right side and progressing on the left side.

SURGERIES

LUNG RESECTION

 BASIC INFORMATION

DESCRIPTION—Removal of tissue from the lungs. If part of a lung (usually called a lobe) is removed, the surgery is called lobectomy. If the entire lung is removed, the surgery is called pneumonectomy.

BODY PARTS INVOLVED—Lung; bronchial tubes; blood vessels in chest; ribs.

REASONS FOR SURGERY
- Cancer or suspected cancer of the lung.
- Diseased lobes of the lung caused by several chronic conditions, especially bronchiectasis.

SPECIAL CONSIDERATIONS FOR OLDER PATIENTS
- Advancing age alone does not preclude surgery.
- Characteristic signs and symptoms of many surgical disorders and complications are frequently atypical, changed or absent.
- Surgical repair is complete and effective, but healing takes longer.
- Weakened cough reflexes increase the risk of lung and bronchial complications.
- More likely to experience respiratory and kidney problems, confusion and blood clots after surgery.

SURGICAL RISK INCREASES WITH
- Obesity; smoking; poor nutrition.
- Excessive alcohol consumption; chronic illness.
- Recent illness, especially upper respiratory infection.
- Use of drugs such as antihypertensives; muscle relaxants; tranquilizers; sleep inducers; insulin; sedatives; narcotics; beta-adrenergic blockers; cortisone.

 BEFORE SURGERY

WHO OPERATES—Thoracic surgeon, usually in hospital.

DIAGNOSTIC TESTS—Blood and urine studies; x-rays of chest; ECG (see Glossary). During surgery: ECG monitor.

ANESTHESIA—General anesthesia by inhalation and injection, with an airway tube placed in the windpipe.

DESCRIPTION OF OPERATION—An incision is made in the chest. Sometimes a rib is removed for better exposure to the lungs. The blood supply to the diseased area is isolated and tied off. The diseased area is located and examined. The growth, the lobe in which it appears or the entire lung is cut free and removed. A tube is inserted to drain fluid and air from the surgical area. The muscles are reconstructed with strong sutures. The skin is closed with sutures or clips, which usually can be removed about 1 week after surgery.

 AFTER SURGERY

POSSIBLE COMPLICATIONS—Excessive bleeding; surgical wound infection; pneumonia; respiratory crippling; bronchial fistula.

AVERAGE HOSPITAL STAY—6 to 8 days.

PROBABLE OUTCOME FOR OLDER PATIENTS—In some cases, underlying lung disease may be cured. In other cases, quality of life may be improved. Allow about 6 weeks for recovery from surgery.

GUIDE TO RECUPERATION FOR PEOPLE OVER 50
- Bathe as usual. Wash incision gently.
- Use warm heat packs and massage to relieve pain.
- Move legs often while in bed to decrease the likelihood of deep-vein blood clots.
- Breathe deeply and cough often to keep secretions from pooling inside the lungs. Respiratory therapists can help you learn to keep bronchial tubes clear. Ask your doctor.
- See Appendix 19.

MEDICATIONS & TESTS—Your doctor may prescribe:
- Pain relievers. Follow dosage schedule.
- Antibiotics to fight infection.
- A vaccine to prevent pneumonia.
- You may use non-prescription drugs, such as acetaminophen, for minor pain.

ACTIVITY FOR OLDER PATIENTS—Ask your doctor for personalized instructions.
Typical times for resuming:
Bathing . . . . Immediately.
Exercise . . . . 4 weeks.
Driving . . . . 4 weeks.
Sexual activity . . . . When able.
Work . . . . Variable.

FOOD & BEVERAGE—Clear liquid diet until the gastrointestinal tract begins to function again. Then eat a well-balanced diet to promote healing. See Appendices 7 and 1.

 CALL YOUR DOCTOR IF

- Pain, swelling, redness, drainage or bleeding increases in the surgical area.
- You develop signs of infection: headache, muscle aches, dizziness or a general ill feeling and fever.
- You experience nausea, vomiting or shortness of breath.
- You develop a "bubbly" feeling under skin of your chest.

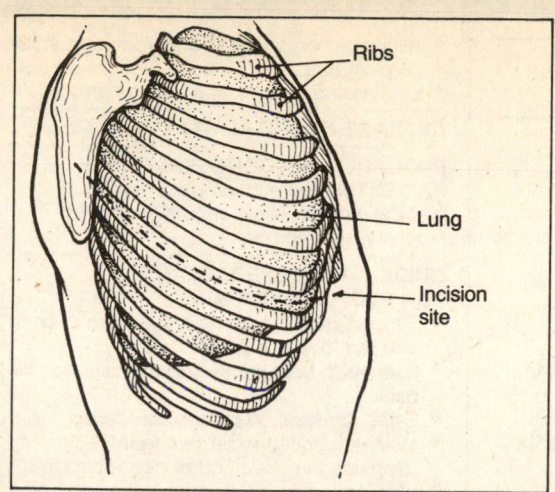

An illustration showing the usual incision site across the chest.

Ribs

Lung

Incision site

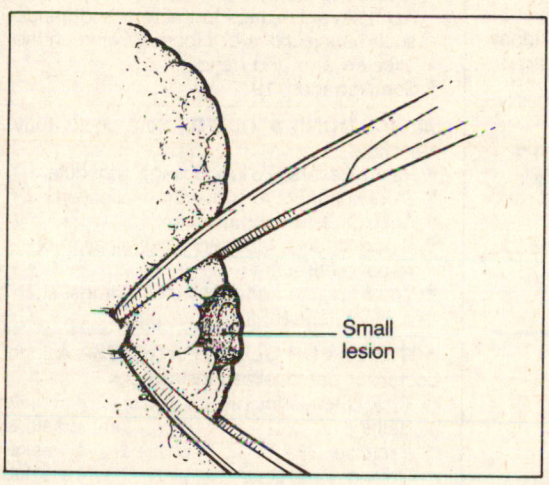

The diseased area on the lung is located and examined. The tumor, the lobe in which it appears, or the entire lung may be cut free and removed.

Small lesion

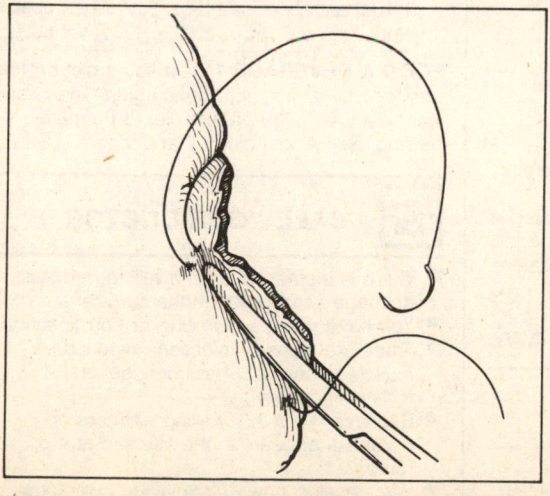

Muscles of the chest wall are reconstructed with strong sutures. A tube is usually left in place to drain fluid and air from the surgical area and to help the lung reinflate following surgery.

SURGERIES

MASTECTOMY, MODIFIED RADICAL
(Total Mastectomy)

BASIC INFORMATION

DESCRIPTION—Removal of the breast.

BODY PARTS INVOLVED—Breast; lymph glands (sometimes).

REASONS FOR SURGERY—Cancer of the breast.

SPECIAL CONSIDERATIONS FOR OLDER PATIENTS
- *Note:* Advancing age alone does not preclude surgery.
- Characteristic signs and symptoms of many surgical disorders and complications are frequently atypical, changed or absent.
- Surgical repair is complete and effective, but healing takes longer.
- Weakened cough reflexes increase the risk of lung and bronchial complications.
- More likely to experience respiratory and kidney problems, confusion and blood clots after surgery.

SURGICAL RISK INCREASES WITH—Obesity or poor nutrition; smoking; stress; recent or chronic illness; use of drugs such as antihypertensives, muscle relaxants, tranquilizers, sleep inducers, insulin, sedatives, beta-adrenergic blockers, excessive alcohol or cortisone.

BEFORE SURGERY

WHO OPERATES—General surgeon or oncological surgeon, usually in hospital.

DIAGNOSTIC TESTS
- Blood and urine studies; mammogram; needle biopsy (see Glossary for all).
- During surgery: Laboratory examination of removed tissue by frozen section.

ANESTHESIA—General anesthesia by inhalation and injection, with an airway tube placed in the windpipe.

DESCRIPTION OF OPERATION
- An incision is made encompassing the entire breast.
- The underlying tissue is cut free and removed in one piece with the lymph glands from the armpit. Bleeding is controlled with ties and electrocauterization. A tube is inserted for drainage.
- The skin is closed with sutures or clips, which usually can be removed about 1 week after surgery.

AFTER SURGERY

POSSIBLE COMPLICATIONS
- Excessive bleeding; surgical wound infection.
- Depression.

- Accumulation of blood under the skin in the surgical area.
- Limited shoulder motion; nerve damage.

AVERAGE HOSPITAL STAY—3 to 4 days.

PROBABLE OUTCOME FOR OLDER PATIENTS—Expect complete healing of the surgical wound. Allow about 6 weeks for recovery from surgery.

GUIDE TO RECUPERATION FOR PEOPLE OVER 50
- Support groups can help you learn to cope with the loss of a breast.
- Use warm heat packs and massage to relieve pain.
- Bathe as usual. Wash incision gently.
- Move legs often while resting in bed to decrease the likelihood of deep-vein clots.
- Wear long sleeves to protect the arm and hand. Avoid injuries to the arm and hand, such as injections or blood drawing, in the affected arm and hand.
- See Appendix 19.

MEDICATIONS & TESTS—Your doctor may prescribe:
- Pain relievers. Follow dosage schedule.
- Stool softeners to prevent constipation.
- Antibiotics to fight infection.
- Blood studies; laboratory examination of removed tissue.
- You may use non-prescription drugs, such as acetaminophen, for minor pain.

ACTIVITY FOR OLDER PATIENTS—Ask your doctor for personalized instructions.
Typical times for resuming:
Bathing . . . . Immediately.
Exercise . . . . 4 weeks.
Driving . . . . 4 weeks.
Sexual activity . . . . When able.
Work . . . . Variable.

FOOD & BEVERAGE—Clear liquid diet until the gastrointestinal tract functions again. Then eat a well-balanced, high-protein diet to promote healing. See Appendices 7 and 1.

CALL YOUR DOCTOR IF

- There is increased pain, swelling, redness, drainage or bleeding in the surgical area.
- You have nausea, vomiting or constipation.
- There are signs of infection: headache, muscle aches, dizziness or a general ill feeling and fever.
- Redness, warmth, swelling, stiffness or hardness appears in the affected arm or hand.
- You develop new, unexplained symptoms.

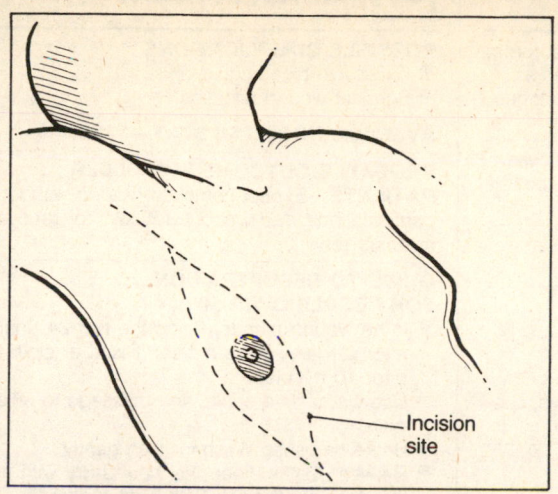

The usual site and elliptical form of the incison to remove the breast and underlying tissue.

Incision site

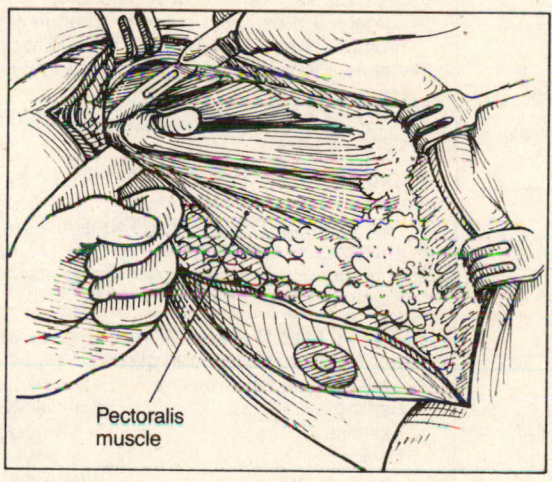

Underlying tissues (breast tissue, muscles, blood vessels, nerves, lymph vessels) are cut free and removed in 1 block with lymph glands from the armpit.

Pectoralis muscle

SURGERIES

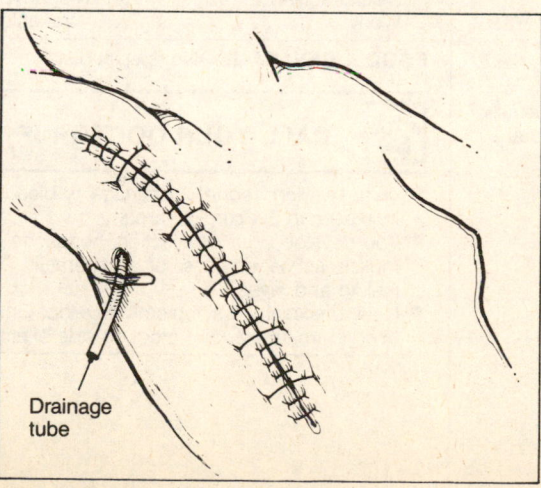

A tube is inserted for drainage. The tissues under the skin are closed with large, absorbable sutures. The skin is closed with sutures or clips which usually can be removed about 1 week after surgery.

Drainage tube

MORTON'S NEUROMA, REMOVAL OF

 BASIC INFORMATION

DESCRIPTION—Removal of Morton's neuroma, a small benign tumor in the nerve that serves the toes. Its cause is unknown, and it produces severe pain.

BODY PARTS INVOLVED—The area between the 2nd and 3rd toes or the 3rd and 4th toes. It may occur in either or both feet.

REASONS FOR SURGERY—Relief of pain caused by the neuroma.

SPECIAL CONSIDERATIONS FOR OLDER PATIENTS
- Advancing age alone does not preclude surgery.
- Surgical repair is complete and effective, but healing takes longer.

SURGICAL RISK INCREASES WITH
- Obesity.
- Smoking.
- Poor nutrition.
- Recent or chronic illness.
- Use of drugs such as antihypertensives; muscle relaxants; tranquilizers; sleep inducers; insulin; sedatives; beta-adrenergic blockers; cortisone.

 BEFORE SURGERY

WHO OPERATES—General surgeon or podiatrist, usually in hospital, outpatient surgical facility, doctor's office or emergency room.

DIAGNOSTIC TESTS—Blood and urine studies; x-rays of the foot.

ANESTHESIA—Local anesthesia by injection.

DESCRIPTION OF OPERATION
- A tourniquet is wrapped around the leg to prevent the surgical area from bleeding.
- The neuroma is located, cut free from surrounding tissue and removed.
- The skin is closed with sutures, which usually can be removed about 10 to 14 days after surgery. The tourniquet is removed.

 AFTER SURGERY

POSSIBLE COMPLICATIONS
- Excessive bleeding.
- Surgical wound infection.

AVERAGE HOSPITAL STAY—1 day.

PROBABLE OUTCOME FOR OLDER PATIENTS—Expect complete healing without complications. Allow about 3 weeks for recovery from surgery.

GUIDE TO RECUPERATION FOR PEOPLE OVER 50
- If the wound bleeds during the first 24 hours after surgery, press a clean tissue or cloth to it for 10 minutes.
- Use warm heat packs and massage to relieve pain.
- Bathe as usual. Wash incision gently.
- Between baths, keep the wound dry with a bandage for the first 2 or 3 days after surgery. If a bandage gets wet, change it promptly. Apply non-prescription antibiotic ointment to the wound before applying new bandages.
- Keep the foot elevated as much as possible during recovery.

MEDICATIONS & TESTS—Your doctor may prescribe:
- Pain relievers. Follow dosage schedule.
- Antibiotics to fight infection.
- You may use non-prescription drugs, such as acetaminophen, for minor pain.

ACTIVITY FOR OLDER PATIENTS—Ask your doctor for personalized instructions.
Typical times for resuming:
Bathing . . . . Immediately.
Exercise . . . . 4 weeks.
Driving . . . . 4 weeks.
Sexual activity . . . . When able.
Work . . . . Variable.

FOOD & BEVERAGE—No special diet.

 CALL YOUR DOCTOR IF

- Pain, swelling, redness, drainage or bleeding increases in the surgical area.
- You develop signs of infection: headache, muscle aches, dizziness or a general ill feeling and fever.
- New, unexplained symptoms develop. Drugs used in treatment may produce side effects.

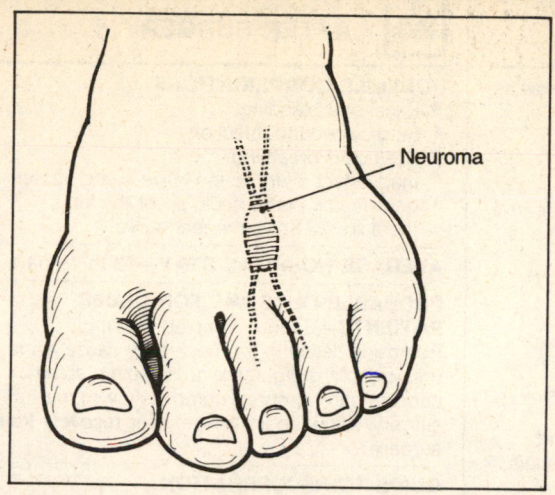

A typical location between the 3rd and 4th toes for a Morton's neuroma (a small benign tumor of nerve tissue).

Neuroma

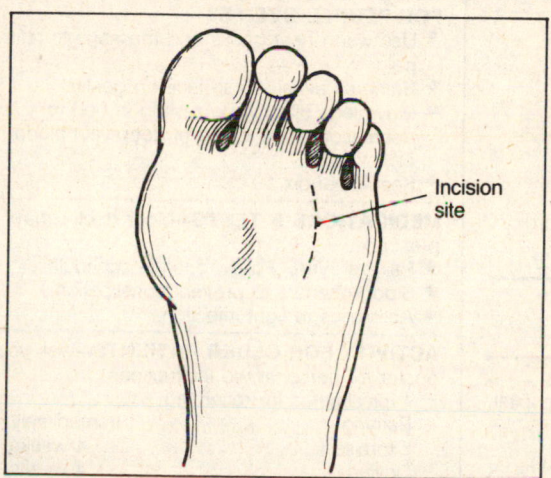

After a tourniquet has been wrapped around the leg to prevent the surgical area from bleeding, an incision through the skin is made.

Incision site

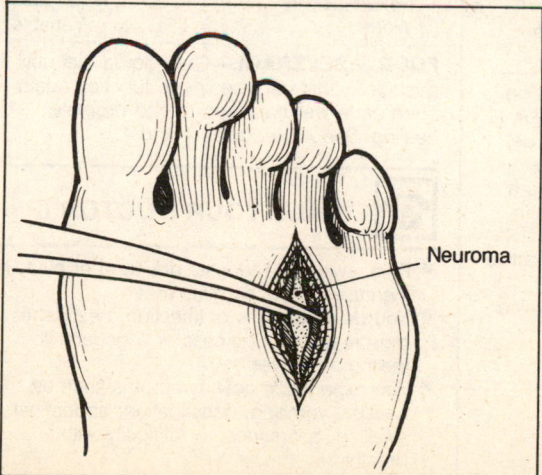

The neuroma is located, cut free from the surrounding tissue and removed.

•After removal, skin is closed with sutures which usually can be removed about 10 to 14 days after surgery (not illustrated).
•The tourniquet is removed to allow normal circulation to the leg and foot (not illustrated).

Neuroma

SURGERIES

NECK, RADICAL DISSECTION OF

BASIC INFORMATION

DESCRIPTION—Removal of cancerous growths in the tissues in the neck.

BODY PARTS INVOLVED—Neck muscles; lymph glands; windpipe.

REASONS FOR SURGERY—Cancer in the oral cavity or neck, which will spread to other parts of the body if not removed.

SPECIAL CONSIDERATIONS FOR OLDER PATIENTS
- Advancing age alone does not preclude surgery.
- Surgical repair is complete and effective, but healing takes longer.
- More likely to experience respiratory and kidney problems, confusion and blood clots after surgery.

SURGICAL RISK INCREASES WITH
- Obesity; smoking.
- Poor nutrition.
- Recent or chronic illness, especially respiratory illness.
- Excessive alcohol consumption.
- Use of drugs such as antihypertensives; muscle relaxants; tranquilizers; sleep inducers; insulin; sedatives; beta-adrenergic blockers; cortisone.

BEFORE SURGERY

WHO OPERATES—Ear, nose and throat specialist or general surgeon, usually in hospital.

DIAGNOSTIC TESTS—Blood and urine studies; x-rays of chest; ECG (see Glossary).

ANESTHESIA—General anesthesia by inhalation and injection, with an airway tube placed in the windpipe.

DESCRIPTION OF OPERATION—An incision shaped like an ''H'' is made in the neck. Skin flaps are separated from the underlying tissue. The lymph glands, muscles and connective tissue are cut free and removed. Sometimes a tracheostomy is performed (see description in the Surgeries section). Tubes are left in the surgical area to drain secretions. The connective tissue is closed, and the skin is closed with sutures or clips, which usually can be removed about 1 week after surgery.

AFTER SURGERY

POSSIBLE COMPLICATIONS
- Excessive bleeding.
- Surgical wound infection.
- Restricted breathing.
- Inadvertent injury to the large blood vessels and nerves in the neck, tip of the lung, thoracic duct or laryngeal nerve.

AVERAGE HOSPITAL STAY—13 to 15 days.

PROBABLE OUTCOME FOR OLDER PATIENTS—Expect complete healing. Removing tissue in the neck may cause some unavoidable disfigurement. However, some cancers can be cured completely with this surgery. Allow about 4 weeks for recovery from surgery.

GUIDE TO RECUPERATION FOR PEOPLE OVER 50
- Use warm heat packs and massage to relieve pain.
- Bathe as usual. Wash incision gently.
- Move legs often while resting in bed to decrease the likelihood of deep-vein blood clots.
- See Appendix 19.

MEDICATIONS & TESTS—Your doctor may prescribe:
- Pain relievers. Follow dosage schedule.
- Stool softeners to prevent constipation.
- Antibiotics to fight infection.

ACTIVITY FOR OLDER PATIENTS—Ask your doctor for personalized instructions.
Typical times for resuming:
Bathing . . . . Immediately.
Exercise . . . . 4 weeks.
Driving . . . . 4 weeks.
Sexual activity . . . . When able.
Work . . . . Variable.

FOOD & BEVERAGE—Clear liquid diet until the gastrointestinal tract begins to function again. Then eat a well-balanced diet to promote healing. See Appendices 7 and 1.

CALL YOUR DOCTOR IF

- Pain, swelling, redness, drainage or bleeding increases in the surgical area.
- You develop signs of infection: headache, muscle aches, dizziness or a general ill feeling and fever.
- You experience new symptoms such as nausea, vomiting, constipation, abdominal swelling, hoarseness or difficulty with breathing.

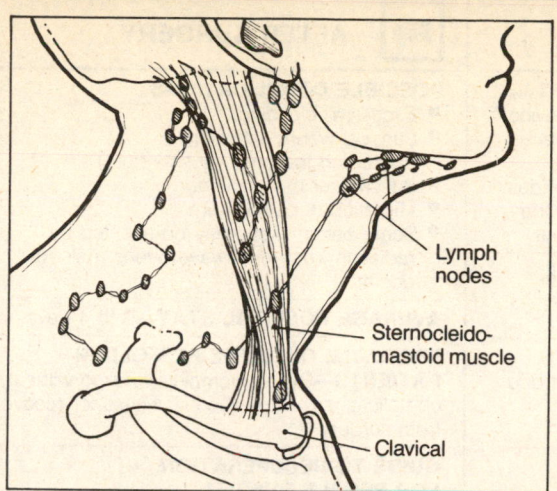

The lymph nodes, muscle and bone in the neck.

Lymph nodes

Sternocleido-mastoid muscle

Clavical

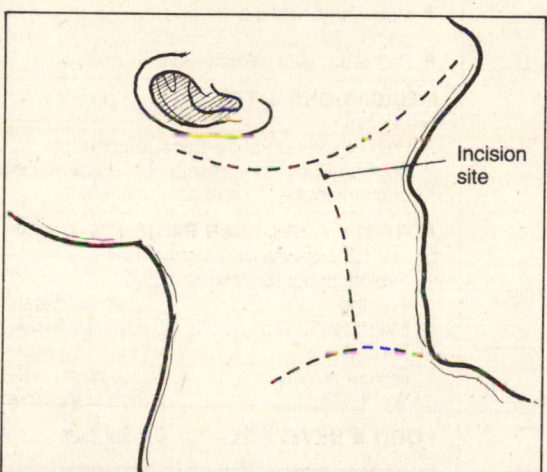

An illustration of the usual incision sites for radical neck dissection.

Incision site

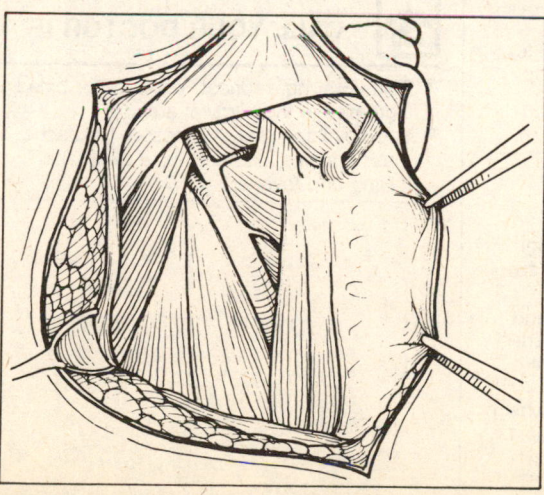

The lymph glands, muscles and connective tissue are cut free and removed.

- Sometimes a tracheostomy is performed to allow free passage of air following surgery.
- Tubes are left in the surgical area to drain secretions (not illustrated).
- The connective tissues are closed and the skin is closed with sutures or clips which usually can be removed about 1 week after surgery (not illustrated).

SURGERIES

PACEMAKER INSERTION

 BASIC INFORMATION

DESCRIPTION—Insertion of a pacemaker into the chest. A pacemaker is an electronic device consisting of an electrode connected to the heart muscle and a regulatory device and power source implanted in the skin. It provides regular, mild electric shocks that stimulate the heart muscle and maintain normal heartbeat.

BODY PARTS INVOLVED—Veins in neck; tissue under the skin below the collarbone; heart.

REASONS FOR SURGERY
- Regulation of heartbeat that has slowed due to heart disease.
- Prevention of heart block.

SPECIAL CONSIDERATIONS FOR OLDER PATIENTS
- Advancing age alone does not preclude surgery.
- Surgical repair is complete and effective, but healing takes longer.

SURGICAL RISK INCREASES WITH
- Stress.
- Obesity.
- Smoking.
- Excessive alcohol consumption.
- Use of drugs such as antihypertensives; muscle relaxants; tranquilizers; sleep inducers; insulin; sedatives; beta-adrenergic blockers; cortisone.

 BEFORE SURGERY

WHO OPERATES—Cardiovascular surgeon, usually in outpatient surgical facility or hospital.

DIAGNOSTIC TESTS—Blood and urine studies; x-rays of chest; ECG (see Glossary for all). During surgery: ECG monitor; fluoroscopy (see Glossary for both).

ANESTHESIA—Local anesthesia by injection.

DESCRIPTION OF OPERATION
- Small incisions are made below the collarbone and in the vein under the collarbone. An electrode is passed through the vein into the heart. The implantation site is confirmed.
- The electrode is attached to the power and regulating units. The entire device is inserted under the skin into a pouch created from tissue under the collarbone.
- The skin is closed with suture material, which usually can be removed about 1 week after surgery.

 AFTER SURGERY

POSSIBLE COMPLICATIONS
- Excessive bleeding.
- Surgical wound infection.
- Rupture in the heart muscle (rare).
- Pacemaker malfunction.
- Migration of pacing wire.
- Some pacemakers may be affected by radiation from microwave ovens. Ask your doctor.

AVERAGE HOSPITAL STAY—0 to 4 days.

PROBABLE OUTCOME FOR OLDER PATIENTS—Expect complete healing without complications. Allow about 2 weeks for recovery from surgery.

GUIDE TO RECUPERATION FOR PEOPLE OVER 50
- Use warm heat packs and massage to relieve pain.
- Bathe as usual. Wash incision gently.

MEDICATIONS & TESTS—Your doctor may prescribe:
- Pain relievers. Follow dosage schedule.
- You may use non-prescription drugs, such as acetaminophen, for minor pain.

ACTIVITY FOR OLDER PATIENTS—Ask your doctor for personalized instructions.
Typical times for resuming:
Bathing . . . . Immediately.
Exercise . . . . Variable.
Driving . . . . 1 week
Sexual activity . . . . When able.
Work . . . . Variable.

FOOD & BEVERAGE—No special diet.

 CALL YOUR DOCTOR IF

- Pain, swelling, redness, drainage or bleeding increases in the surgical area.
- You develop signs of infection: headache, muscle aches, dizziness or a general ill feeling and fever.

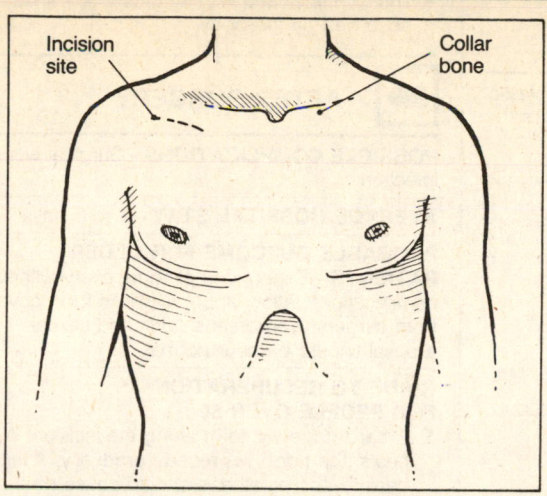

An illustration of the chest, collarbone and incison site generally used for pacemaker insertion.

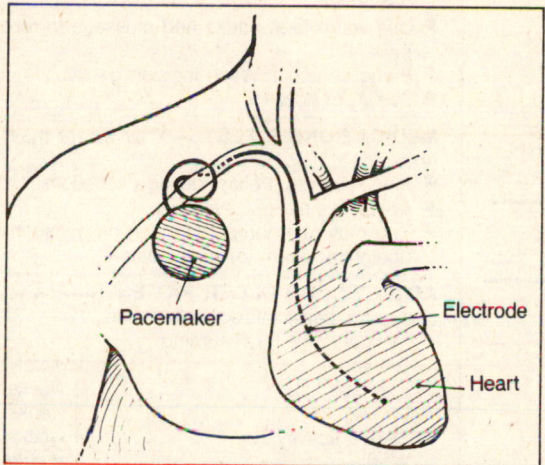

An electrode is passed through a vein at the incision site which ends inside the heart cavity.

• The electrode is attached to the power and regulating units. The entire device is inserted under the skin into a pouch created from tissue under the collarbone.

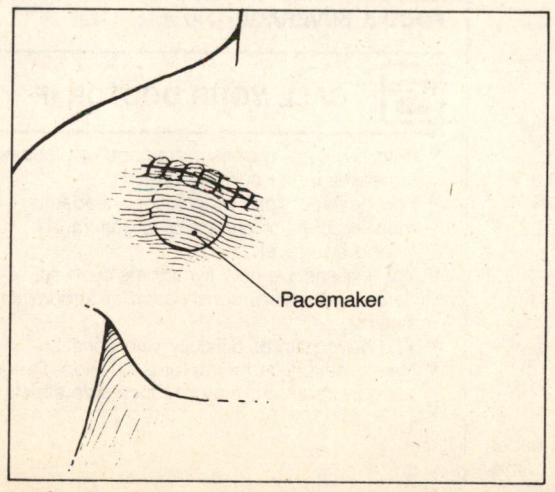

The pacemaker in place. The skin has been closed with sutures which usually can be removed about 1 week after surgery.

SURGERIES

PENILE IMPLANT

BASIC INFORMATION

DESCRIPTION—Insertion of semi-flexible plastic bars or an inflatable prosthesis into the penis. The former produces a permanent, partial erection. The latter can be inflated at will.

BODY PARTS INVOLVED—Penis.

REASONS FOR SURGERY—Impotence.

SPECIAL CONSIDERATIONS FOR OLDER PATIENTS
- Advancing age alone does not preclude surgery.
- Surgical repair is complete and effective, but healing takes longer.

SURGICAL RISK INCREASES WITH
- Obesity.
- Smoking.
- Stress.
- Poor nutrition.
- Recent or chronic illness.
- Excessive alcohol consumption.
- Use of drugs such as antihypertensives; muscle relaxants; tranquilizers; sleep inducers; insulin; sedatives; beta-adrenergic blockers; cortisone.

BEFORE SURGERY

WHO OPERATES—Urologist, usually in hospital.

DIAGNOSTIC TESTS—Blood and urine studies.

ANESTHESIA
- Spinal anesthesia by injection.
- General anesthesia by inhalation and injection, with an airway tube placed in the windpipe.

DESCRIPTION OF OPERATION
Plastic Implant:
- An incision is made in the underside of the penis.
- The tissues on both sides of the urethra are expanded to allow placement of the implants.
- An implant is placed on each side of the urethra.
- The skin is closed with sutures that will be absorbed by the body.

Inflatable Prosthesis:
- An incision is made in the top side of the penis.
- The penile tissue is stretched to allow placement of the prosthesis. The fluid reservoir for the prosthesis is implanted under the skin above the bladder at the base of the pelvis. The prosthesis can be inflated by applying pressure on the reservoir.

- The skin is closed with sutures that will be absorbed by the body.

AFTER SURGERY

POSSIBLE COMPLICATIONS—Surgical wound infection.

AVERAGE HOSPITAL STAY—1 to 3 days.

PROBABLE OUTCOME FOR OLDER PATIENTS—Expect complete recovery without complications. Allow about 4 weeks for recovery from surgery. Penile sensations and sexual arousal should be near normal.

GUIDE TO RECUPERATION FOR PEOPLE OVER 50
- A hard ridge will form along the incision. As it heals, the ridge will recede gradually. After healing, the prosthesis should cause no discomfort.
- Use warm heat packs and massage to relieve pain.
- Bathe as usual. Wash incision gently.
- See Appendix 19.

MEDICATIONS & TESTS—Your doctor may prescribe:
- Pain relievers. Follow dosage schedule.
- Antibiotics to fight infection.
- You may use non-prescription drugs, such as acetaminophen, for minor pain.

ACTIVITY FOR OLDER PATIENTS—Ask your doctor for personalized instructions.
Typical times for resuming:
```
Bathing . . . . . . . . . . . . . . . . . . . .Immediately.
Exercise . . . . . . . . . . . . . . . . . . .2 weeks.
Driving . . . . . . . . . . . . . . . . . . . .2 weeks.
Sexual activity . . . . . . . . . . . . . . .4 weeks.
Work . . . . . . . . . . . . . . . . . . . . . .Variable.
```

FOOD & BEVERAGE—No special diet.

CALL YOUR DOCTOR IF

- Pain, swelling, redness, drainage or bleeding increases in the surgical area.
- You develop signs of infection: headache, muscle aches, dizziness or a general ill feeling and fever.
- You experience new symptoms such as nausea, vomiting, constipation or abdominal swelling.
- You have pain or difficulty with urination.
- New, unexplained symptoms develop. Drugs used in treatment may produce side effects.

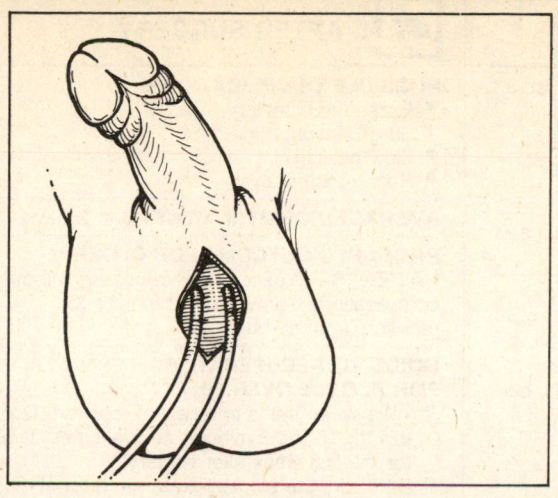

The incision for a penile implant which maybe either semi-rigid or an inflatable prosthesis. These drawings illustrate the inflatable form only. The equipment is different for a semi-rigid prosthesis but the principles and techniques for insertion are similar for both procedures.

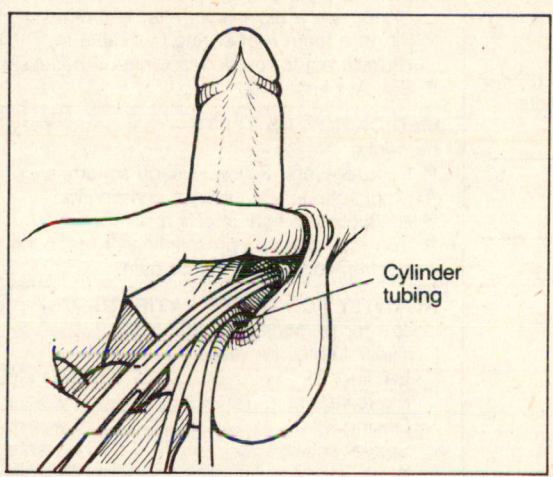

After an incision has been made on the underside of the penis, the tissues on both sides of the urethra are expanded to allow placement of the implants.

Cylinder tubing

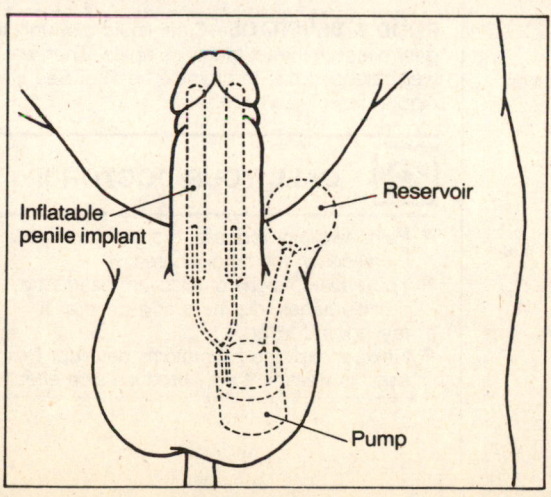

Implants in place, surgical incision closed with absorbable sutures.

Inflatable penile implant

Reservoir

Pump

PILONIDAL CYST REMOVAL

BASIC INFORMATION

DESCRIPTION—Removal of a pilonidal cyst, a cyst that contains elements found in the skin, including hair, sweat and glands.

BODY PARTS INVOLVED—Area over the tailbone.

REASONS FOR SURGERY—Relief of pain and prevention of the spread of infection.

SPECIAL CONSIDERATIONS FOR OLDER PATIENTS
- Decreased nutrition may increase the risk of surgical infections and complications.
- Surgical repair is complete and effective, but healing takes longer.

SURGICAL RISK INCREASES WITH
- Obesity.
- Smoking.
- Recent or chronic illness.
- Use of drugs such as antihypertensives; muscle relaxants; tranquilizers; sleeping pills; insulin; sedatives; beta-adrenergic blockers; cortisone.

BEFORE SURGERY

WHO OPERATES—General surgeon or proctologist, usually in hospital or outpatient surgical facility.

DIAGNOSTIC TESTS—Blood and urine studies; sigmoidoscopy (see Glossary).

ANESTHESIA
- Local anesthesia by injection.
- General anesthesia by inhalation and injection, with an airway tube placed in the windpipe.

DESCRIPTION OF OPERATION
- The cyst and its cavities (also called sinuses) over the tailbone are identified with probes. An incision is made in the cyst.
- The cyst and all affected sinuses are removed.
- Bleeding is controlled with sutures or electrocauterization.
- The skin is usually left open to heal from the bottom out.

AFTER SURGERY

POSSIBLE COMPLICATIONS
- Excessive bleeding.
- Surgical wound infection.
- Slow healing.
- Recurrence of cyst.

AVERAGE HOSPITAL STAY—0 to 2 days.

PROBABLE OUTCOME FOR OLDER PATIENTS—Expect complete healing without complications. Allow about 2 months for recovery from surgery.

GUIDE TO RECUPERATION FOR PEOPLE OVER 50
- Take warm baths to relieve discomfort. Do this for 15 to 20 minutes several times daily for the first week after surgery.
- Don't dry the surgical area with a towel. Drip dry or use a blow dryer after bathing.
- Sit on a foam rubber ring (available in drugstores) to relieve discomfort if necessary.
- See Appendix 19.

MEDICATIONS & TESTS—Your doctor may prescribe:
- Pain relievers. Follow dosage schedule.
- Stool softeners to prevent constipation.
- Antibiotics to fight infection.
- You may use non-prescription drugs, such as acetaminophen, for minor pain.

ACTIVITY FOR OLDER PATIENTS—Ask your doctor for personalized instructions.
Typical times for resuming:
Bathing . . . . Immediately.
Exercise . . . . 2 weeks.
Driving . . . . 4 weeks.
Sexual activity . . . . When able.
Work . . . . Variable.

FOOD & BEVERAGE—Clear liquid diet until the gastrointestinal tract functions again. Then eat a well-balanced diet to promote healing. See Appendices 7 and 1.

CALL YOUR DOCTOR IF

- Pain, swelling, redness, drainage or bleeding increases in the surgical area.
- You develop signs of infection: headache, muscle aches, dizziness or a general ill feeling and fever.
- New, unexplained symptoms develop. Drugs used in treatment may produce side effects.

PILONIDAL CYST REMOVAL

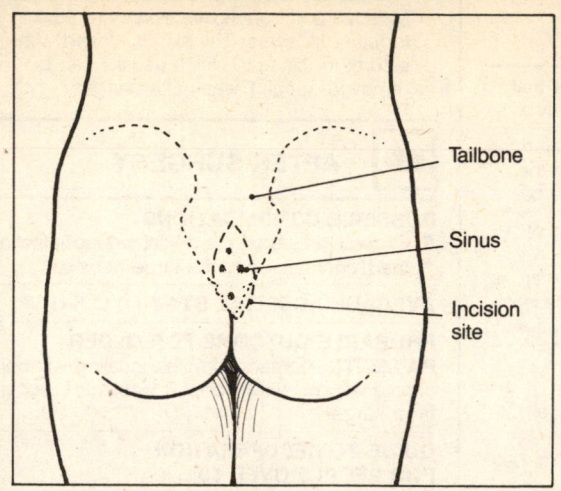

An illustration of several sinuses that begin inside the lumen of the rectum and extend out through the skin.

Tailbone

Sinus

Incision site

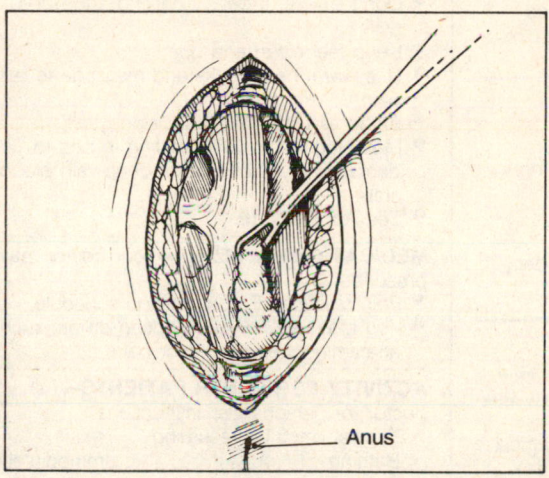

The cyst and all affected sinuses are identified and removed.

Anus

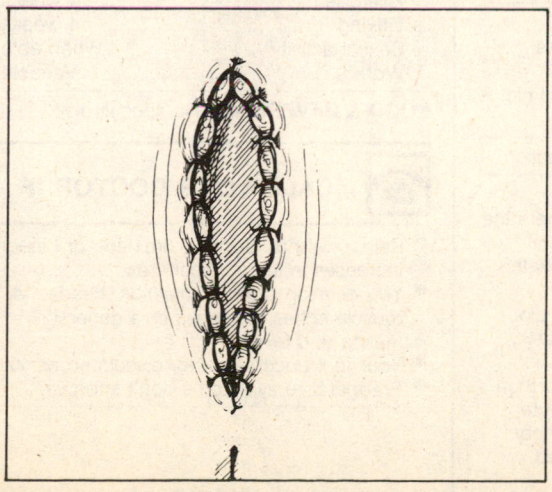

The skin is usually left open to heal slowly from the bottom. Some surgeons close the skin over the operative site at the time of surgery.

SURGERIES

653

POPLITEAL ARTERY EMBOLECTOMY

BASIC INFORMATION

DESCRIPTION—Removal of a blood clot that has blocked blood supply to the leg and foot.

BODY PARTS INVOLVED—Blood vessel in the leg that is called the femoral artery below the groin and the popliteal artery behind the knee.

REASONS FOR SURGERY—Restoration of normal blood circulation in the legs. Re-establishing blood flow can restore muscular function, prevent gangrene and enable patients to return to normal or almost normal activities.

SPECIAL CONSIDERATIONS FOR OLDER PATIENTS
- Advancing age alone does not preclude surgery.
- Surgical repair is complete and effective, but healing takes longer.
- More likely to experience respiratory and kidney problems, confusion and blood clots after surgery.

SURGICAL RISK INCREASES WITH
- Obesity.
- Smoking.
- Rheumatic heart disease or coronary artery disease.
- Use of drugs such as antihypertensives; muscle relaxants; tranquilizers; sleep inducers; insulin; sedatives; narcotics; beta-adrenergic blockers; cortisone.

BEFORE SURGERY

WHO OPERATES—General surgeon or vascular surgeon, usually in outpatient surgical facility or hospital.

DIAGNOSTIC TESTS
- Before surgery: Blood and urine studies; arteriogram (see Glossary).
- During surgery: Arteriogram after blood clot is removed.

ANESTHESIA—Spinal anesthesia by injection.

DESCRIPTION OF OPERATION
- An incision is made over the artery where the clot is lodged.
- The artery is clamped above and below the blood clot.
- The artery is opened above the blood clot.
- A special catheter is passed into the artery beyond the blood clot. The catheter is expanded with air beyond the clot and then withdrawn, forcing the clot out of the artery.
- An anticoagulant is injected into the artery, and normal blood circulation is restored.

- The clamps are removed from the arteries. Muscles and connective tissue are sewn together in layers. The skin is closed with sutures or clamps, which usually can be removed about 1 week after surgery.

AFTER SURGERY

POSSIBLE COMPLICATIONS
- Excessive bleeding; surgical wound infection.
- Inadvertent injury to the large nerves.

AVERAGE HOSPITAL STAY—0 to 6 days.

PROBABLE OUTCOME FOR OLDER PATIENTS—Expect complete healing without complications. Allow about 3 weeks for recovery from surgery.

GUIDE TO RECUPERATION FOR PEOPLE OVER 50
- Don't smoke. It delays healing and adds risks.
- Keep feet clean and dry.
- Use warm heat packs and massage to relieve pain.
- Bathe as usual. Wash incision gently.
- Move legs often while resting in bed to decrease the likelihood of deep-vein blood clots.
- See Appendix 19.

MEDICATIONS & TESTS—Your doctor may prescribe:
- Pain relievers. Follow dosage schedule.
- You may use non-prescription drugs, such as acetaminophen, for minor pain.

ACTIVITY FOR OLDER PATIENTS—Ask your doctor for personalized instructions.
Typical times for resuming:
Bathing . . . . Immediately.
Exercise . . . . 4 weeks.
Driving . . . . 4 weeks.
Sexual activity . . . . When able.
Work . . . . Variable.

FOOD & BEVERAGE—No special diet.

CALL YOUR DOCTOR IF

- Pain, swelling, redness, drainage or bleeding increases in the surgical area.
- You develop signs of infection: headache, muscle aches, dizziness or a general ill feeling and fever.
- Your foot becomes cold, discolored or numb.
- Preoperative symptoms don't improve.

POPLITEAL ARTERY EMBOLECTOMY

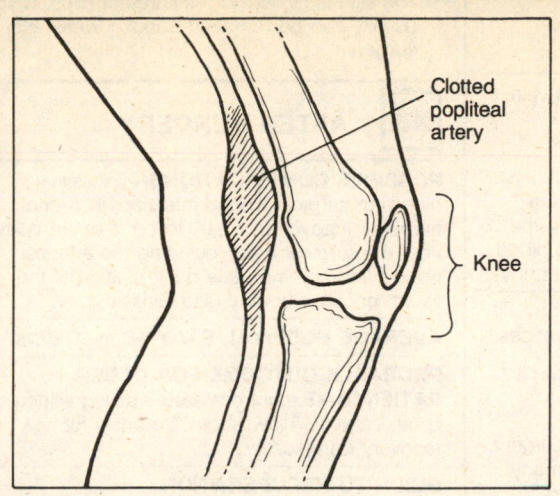

Clotted popliteal artery

Knee

An illustration of a clot in the popliteal artery extending behind the knee.

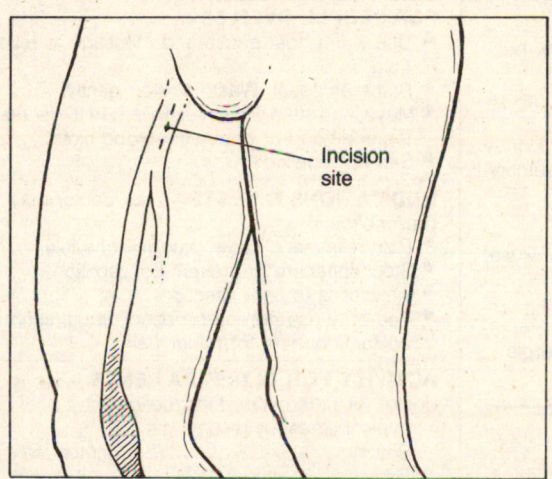

Incision site

An incision for the introduction of a special catheter is made inside the upper thigh at the inguinal level.

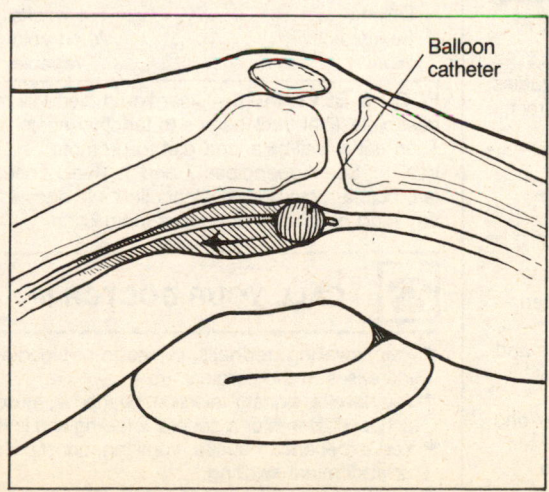

Balloon catheter

A special catheter is passed into the artery beyond the blood clot. It is expanded with air and then withdrawn, forcing the clots out of the artery.

•After the clot has been removed, muscles and connective tissues are sewn together in layers. The skin is closed with sutures or clamps.

PORTACAVAL SHUNT

BASIC INFORMATION

DESCRIPTION—Connection of the portal vein with the vena cava to release backed-up pressure in the venous system (veins) that drains the intestinal tract.

BODY PARTS INVOLVED—Portal vein (the large vein that drains the liver); vena cava (the largest vein in the body that drains all the blood from the intestines and the lower part of the body).

REASONS FOR SURGERY—Treatment or prevention of bleeding from esophageal varices (large veins in the lower esophagus).

SPECIAL CONSIDERATIONS FOR OLDER PATIENTS
- Advancing age alone does not preclude surgery.
- Characteristic signs and symptoms of many surgical disorders and complications are frequently atypical, changed or absent.
- Surgical repair is complete and effective, but healing takes longer.
- Weakened cough reflexes increase the risk of lung and bronchial complications.
- More likely to experience respiratory and kidney problems, confusion and blood clots after surgery.

SURGICAL RISK INCREASES WITH
- Obesity; smoking; poor nutrition.
- Recent or chronic illness, particularly liver disease.
- Excessive alcohol consumption.
- Use of drugs such as antihypertensives; muscle relaxants; tranquilizers; sleep inducers; insulin; sedatives; beta-adrenergic blockers; cortisone.

BEFORE SURGERY

WHO OPERATES—General surgeon or vascular surgeon, usually in hospital.

DIAGNOSTIC TESTS—Blood and urine studies; x-rays of chest and upper gastrointestinal tract; ECG; esophagoscopy (see Glossary).

ANESTHESIA—General anesthesia by inhalation and injection, with an airway tube placed in the windpipe.

DESCRIPTION OF OPERATION
- An incision is made in the abdomen.
- The portal vein and vena cava are located and isolated.
- The portal vein is clamped in two places and divided between the clamps. A "window" is cut into the vena cava. One end of the severed portal vein is tied, and the other end is sewn into the window in the vena cava. This allows blood from the portal vein to drain directly into the vena cava.
- The abdominal cavity is closed, and the muscle layers are reconstructed with sutures.

- The skin is closed with sutures or clips, which usually can be removed about 1 week after surgery.

AFTER SURGERY

POSSIBLE COMPLICATIONS—Excessive bleeding; surgical wound infection; incisional hernia or inadvertent injury to parts of the body near the surgical area, including the arteries, nerves and common bile duct; clotting of the shunt; encephalopathy (see Glossary).

AVERAGE HOSPITAL STAY—6 to 10 days.

PROBABLE OUTCOME FOR OLDER PATIENTS—Expect complete healing without complications. Allow about 2 months for recovery from surgery.

GUIDE TO RECUPERATION FOR PEOPLE OVER 50
- Use warm heat packs and massage to relieve pain.
- Bathe as usual. Wash incision gently.
- Move legs often while resting in bed to decrease the likelihood of deep-vein blood clots.
- See Appendix 19.

MEDICATIONS & TESTS—Your doctor may prescribe:
- Pain relievers. Follow dosage schedule.
- Stool softeners to prevent constipation.
- Antibiotics to fight infection.
- You may use non-prescription drugs, such as acetaminophen, for minor pain.

ACTIVITY FOR OLDER PATIENTS—Ask your doctor for personalized instructions.
Typical times for resuming:
Bathing . . . . Immediately.
Exercise . . . . 4 weeks.
Driving . . . . 4 weeks.
Sexual activity . . . . When able.
Work . . . . Variable.

FOOD & BEVERAGE—Clear liquid diet until the gastrointestinal tract begins to function again. Then eat a well-balanced diet to promote healing. See Appendices 7 and 1. Avoid coffee, tea, cocoa, cola drinks, alcoholic beverages and any food or spice that causes indigestion.

CALL YOUR DOCTOR IF

- Pain, swelling, redness, drainage or bleeding increases in the surgical area.
- You develop signs of infection: headache, muscle aches, dizziness or a general ill feeling and fever.
- You experience nausea, vomiting, constipation or abdominal swelling.
- You vomit blood or have black, tarry stools.

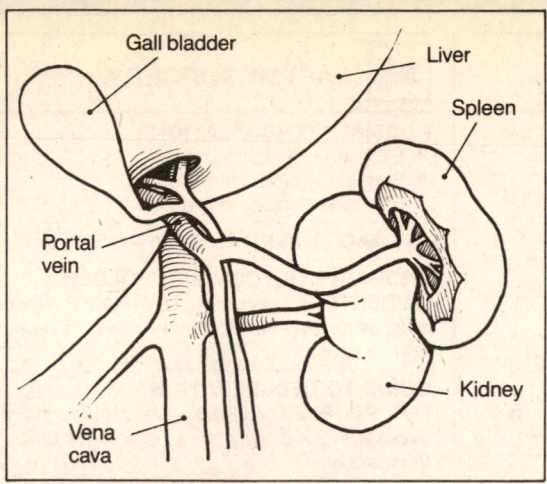

An illustration of the liver, gallbladder, bile ducts leading from the gallbladder and abdominal blood vessels that supply the liver.

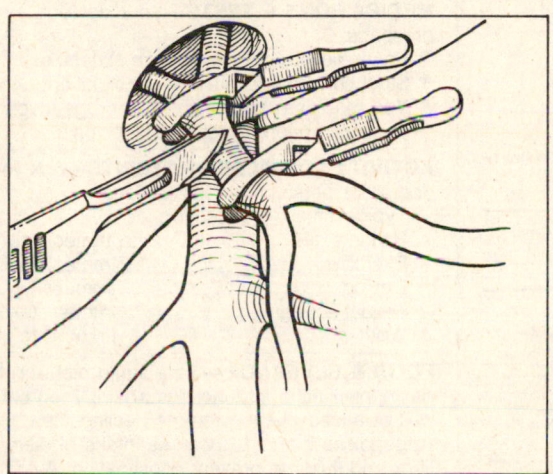

After the abdomen has been opened and muscles retracted, the portal vein and vena cava are located and isolated.

•The portal vein is clamped in 2 places and divided between the clamps.

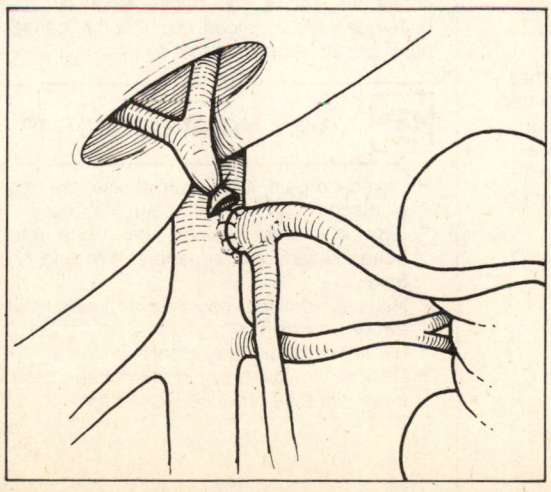

A window is cut into the vena cava.

•One end of the severed portal vein is tied and the other end is sewn into the window in the vena cava. This allows blood from the portal vein to drain directly into the cava vena.

SURGERIES

RECTAL OR COLON POLYP, REMOVAL OF
(Polypectomy)

 BASIC INFORMATION

DESCRIPTION—Removal of a polyp from the membrane lining inside the rectum or colon.

BODY PARTS INVOLVED—Membrane lining of the rectum and colon.

REASONS FOR SURGERY—Removal of a possible source of cancer.

SPECIAL CONSIDERATIONS FOR OLDER PATIENTS
- Advancing age alone does not preclude surgery.
- Surgical repair is complete and effective, but healing takes longer.

SURGICAL RISK INCREASES WITH
- Obesity.
- Smoking.
- Poor nutrition.
- Recent or chronic illness.
- Use of drugs such as antihypertensives; muscle relaxants; tranquilizers; sleep inducers; insulin; sedatives; beta-adrenergic blockers; cortisone.

 BEFORE SURGERY

WHO OPERATES—General surgeon or proctologist, usually in hospital or outpatient surgical facility.

DIAGNOSTIC TESTS—Blood and urine studies; x-rays of lower gastrointestinal tract; colonoscopy (see Glossary).

ANESTHESIA—Intravenous sedative and narcotic pain killer.

DESCRIPTION OF OPERATION
- Surgery is preceded by medicated enemas.
- A colonoscope or sigmoidoscope is inserted through the rectum into the sigmoid colon. The polyp is located and removed with a wire snare, ultrasound or a laser beam.
- Bleeding is controlled with electric current or pressure applied with gauze soaked in epinephrine (see Glossary).

 AFTER SURGERY

POSSIBLE COMPLICATIONS
- Excessive bleeding.
- Surgical wound infection.
- Inadvertent injury to the colon.

AVERAGE HOSPITAL STAY—0 to 1 day.

PROBABLE OUTCOME FOR OLDER PATIENTS—Expect complete healing without complications. Allow about 12 days for recovery from surgery.

GUIDE TO RECUPERATION FOR PEOPLE OVER 50—Watch for signs of excessive bleeding, such as bloody or black, tarry stools.

MEDICATIONS & TESTS—Your doctor may prescribe:
- Pain relievers. Follow dosage schedule.
- Stool softeners to prevent constipation.
- You may use non-prescription drugs, such as acetaminophen, to relieve minor pain.

ACTIVITY FOR OLDER PATIENTS—Ask your doctor for personalized instructions.
Typical times for resuming:
Bathing . . . . .Immediately.
Exercise . . . . .Immediately.
Driving. . . . . .Immediately.
Sexual activity . . . . .Immediately.
Work .Immediately.

FOOD & BEVERAGE—Clear liquid diet until the gastrointestinal tract functions again. Then eat a well-balanced diet to promote healing. See Appendices 7 and 1. Increase intake of dietary fiber and fluids to prevent constipation. Avoid coffee, tea, cocoa, cola drinks, alcoholic beverages and any food or spice that causes painful or irritating digestive symptoms.

 CALL YOUR DOCTOR IF

- Increased pain, swelling, redness, drainage or bleeding occurs in the surgical area.
- Signs of infection develop: headache, muscle aches, dizziness or a general ill feeling and fever.
- Nausea, vomiting, constipation, abdominal swelling or pain.
- Bloody or black, tarry stools.
- New, unexplained symptoms. Drugs used in treatment may produce side effects.

RECTAL OR COLON-POLYP, REMOVAL OF
(Polypectomy)

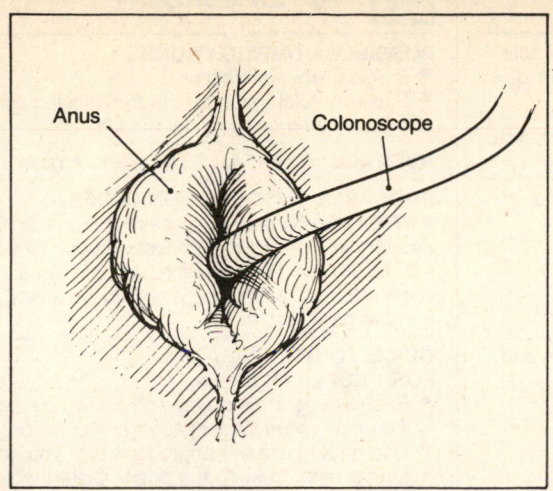

Anus

Colonoscope

An illustration of a flexible colono-scope inserted into the anus.

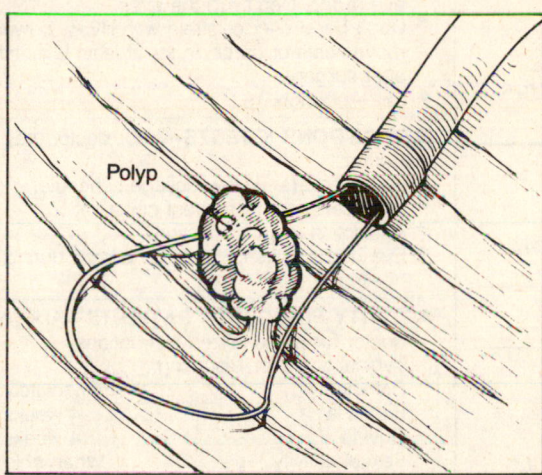

Polyp

The colonoscope or sigmoidoscope is advanced to reach the sigmoid colon where polyps (when present) are usually located.

•The polyp is removed with a wire snare, ultrasound or a laser beam.

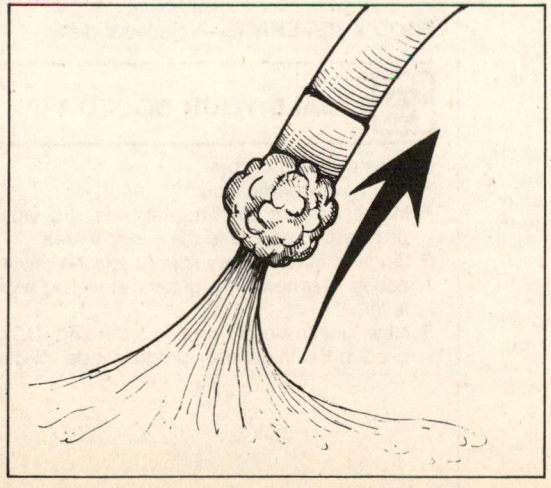

After the polyp has been removed, bleeding of the remaining stump is controlled with electric current.

RETINAL DETACHMENT REPAIR

 BASIC INFORMATION

DESCRIPTION—Reattachment of a retina that has become separated from the remainder of the eye.

BODY PARTS INVOLVED—The eye and all its parts.

REASONS FOR SURGERY—Prevention of vision loss.

SPECIAL CONSIDERATIONS FOR OLDER PATIENTS
- Advancing age alone does not preclude surgery.
- Nursing care needs to be more intense and skillful.

SURGICAL RISK INCREASES WITH
- Obesity; smoking; excessive alcohol consumption.
- Poor nutrition.
- Recent or chronic illness.
- Use of drugs such as antihypertensives; muscle relaxants; tranquilizers; sleep inducers; insulin; sedatives; beta-adrenergic blockers; cortisone.

 BEFORE SURGERY

WHO OPERATES—Ophthalmologist, usually in hospital or outpatient surgical facility.

DIAGNOSTIC TESTS—Complete eye examination; blood and urine studies.

ANESTHESIA
- Local anesthesia by injection or topical application.
- General anesthesia by inhalation and injection, with an airway tube placed in the windpipe.

DESCRIPTION OF OPERATION
- Sometimes tears or holes in the retina are repaired with laser beams that coagulate the eye tissue and cause it to readjust to its normal position.
- Otherwise the membrane lining the eye is cut. A cryosurgical probe is placed around the detached retina. The probe applies extreme cold, causing eye tissue to coagulate and to adhere to its normal position.
- If a cornea transplant is required, it is performed.
- The membrane around the eye is closed with fine sutures, which usually can be removed about 1 week after surgery.

 AFTER SURGERY

POSSIBLE COMPLICATIONS
- Surgical wound infection.
- Partial or total vision loss in the affected eye from recurrence of retinal detachment.

AVERAGE HOSPITAL STAY—3 to 4 days.

PROBABLE OUTCOME FOR OLDER PATIENTS—Surgery is successful in preserving eyesight in over 90% of patients. About 10% will require another operation, which is usually successful. Allow about 2 weeks for recovery from surgery.

GUIDE TO RECUPERATION FOR PEOPLE OVER 50
- Rest with your head elevated on two pillows. You may move your head in any direction.
- Use dark glasses in bright light until you no longer need to keep the pupils dilated with eye drops. Don't rub the eyes.
- Don't bend over or strain with lifting, bowel movements or urination for at least 6 months after surgery.
- See Appendix 19.

MEDICATIONS & TESTS—Your doctor may prescribe:
- Pain relievers. Follow dosage schedule.
- Stool softeners to prevent constipation.
- Antibiotics to fight infection.
- Eye drops to keep the pupil dilated during healing.

ACTIVITY FOR OLDER PATIENTS—Ask your doctor for personalized instructions.
Typical times for resuming:
Bathing . . . . Immediately.
Exercise . . . . 4 weeks.
Driving . . . . 4 weeks.
Sexual activity . . . . When able.
Work . . . . Variable.

FOOD & BEVERAGE—No special diet.

 CALL YOUR DOCTOR IF

- Loss of vision occurs.
- You have constipation.
- Increased pain, swelling, redness, drainage or bleeding occurs in the surgical area.
- Signs of infection develop: headache, muscle aches, dizziness or a general ill feeling and fever.
- New, unexplained symptoms develop. Drugs used in treatment may produce side effects.

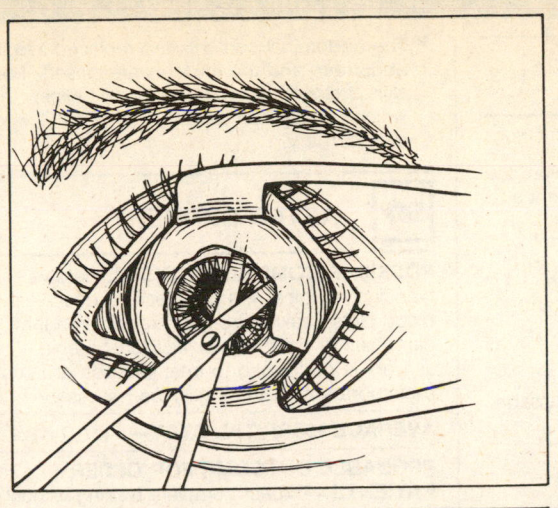

An illustration of the relationship of parts of the eye.

•Scissors cutting the conjunctiva (the membrane lining the eye).

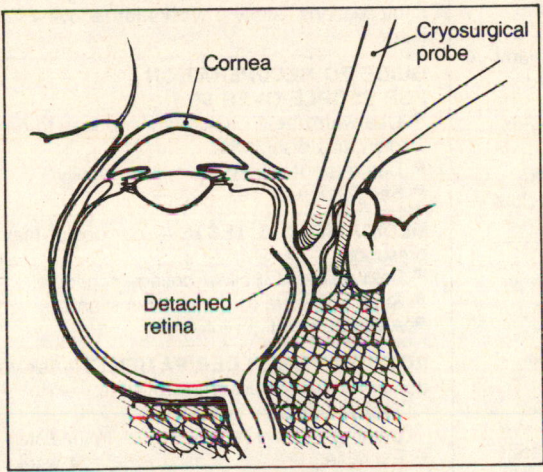

Cornea

Cryosurgical probe

Detached retina

Cyrosurgical probe is placed around the detached retina. The probe applies extreme cold causing eye tissue to coagulate and adhere to its normal position.

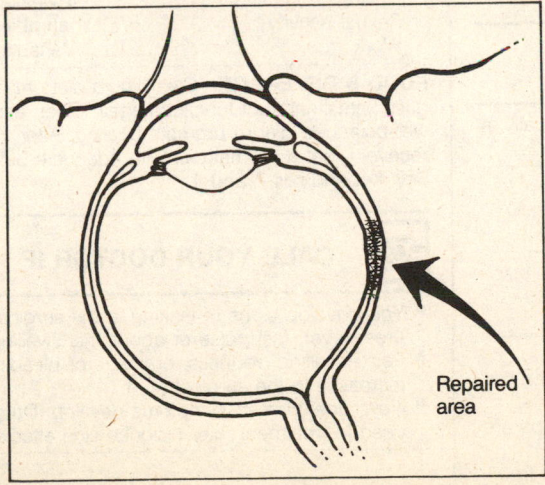

Repaired area

The retina returned to normal position after the detached retina has been secured in its proper position.

SURGERIES

SIGMOID COLON REMOVAL
(Sigmoid Colectomy)

BASIC INFORMATION

DESCRIPTION—Removal of the sigmoid colon.

BODY PARTS INVOLVED—Sigmoid colon, the part of the large intestine (colon) that extends from the descending colon to the rectum.

REASONS FOR SURGERY
- Diverticulitis with bleeding and infection.
- Diverticulitis with ruptured diverticulae and peritonitis from infection caused by perforations.
- Cancer or precancerous polyps.
- Obstruction in the colon that blocks passage of feces.

SPECIAL CONSIDERATIONS FOR OLDER PATIENTS
- Advancing age alone does not preclude surgery.
- Characteristic signs and symptoms of many surgical disorders and complications are frequently atypical, changed or absent.
- Surgical repair is complete and effective, but healing takes longer.
- More likely to experience respiratory and kidney problems, confusion and blood clots after surgery.

SURGICAL RISK INCREASES WITH
- Obesity; smoking; stress; poor nutrition.
- Excessive alcohol consumption; chronic illness.
- Recent illness such as acute diverticulitis.
- Family history of diverticular disease.
- Use of drugs such as antihypertensives; muscle relaxants; tranquilizers; sleep inducers; insulin; beta-adrenergic blockers; cortisone.

BEFORE SURGERY

WHO OPERATES—General surgeon, usually in hospital.

DIAGNOSTIC TESTS—Blood and urine studies; x-rays of upper and lower gastrointestinal tract; ECG (see Glossary).

ANESTHESIA—General anesthesia by inhalation and injection, with an airway tube placed in the windpipe.

DESCRIPTION OF OPERATION
- An incision is made in the abdomen, and the abdominal muscles are opened.
- The sigmoid colon is isolated and clamps are placed at each end.
- All of the diseased sigmoid colon is cut free and removed. The two healthy ends are brought back together and joined.

- The abdominal contents are replaced into the abdomen, and the muscles are closed. The skin is closed with sutures or skin clips, which usually can be removed about 1 week after surgery.

AFTER SURGERY

POSSIBLE COMPLICATIONS—Excessive bleeding; surgical wound infection; deep-vein blood clots; leaking from the repair area that can result in peritonitis or incisional hernia. If surgery is performed to treat infection or tumor, a temporary colostomy may be necessary.

AVERAGE HOSPITAL STAY—7 to 10 days.

PROBABLE OUTCOME FOR OLDER PATIENTS—Expect complete healing without complications. Allow 8 weeks for recovery from surgery.

GUIDE TO RECUPERATION FOR PEOPLE OVER 50
- Use warm heat packs and massage to relieve pain and discomfort.
- Bathe as usual. Wash incision gently.
- See Appendix 19.

MEDICATIONS & TESTS—Your doctor may prescribe:
- Pain relievers. Follow dosage schedule.
- Stool softeners to prevent constipation.
- Antibiotics to fight infection.

ACTIVITY FOR OLDER PATIENTS—Ask your doctor for personalized instructions.
Typical times for resuming:
Bathing . . . . Immediately.
Exercise . . . . 4 weeks.
Driving . . . . 4 weeks.
Sexual activity . . . . When able.
Work . . . . Variable.

FOOD & BEVERAGE—Clear liquid diet until the gastrointestinal tract functions again. Then eat a well-balanced diet to promote healing. After recovery, eat a normal diet with adequate bulk. See Appendices 7 and 1.

CALL YOUR DOCTOR IF

- You develop signs of leaking in the surgical area: fever, fast pulse or abdominal swelling.
- Pain, swelling, redness, drainage or bleeding increases in the surgical area.
- New, unexplained symptoms develop. Drugs used in treatment may produce side effects.

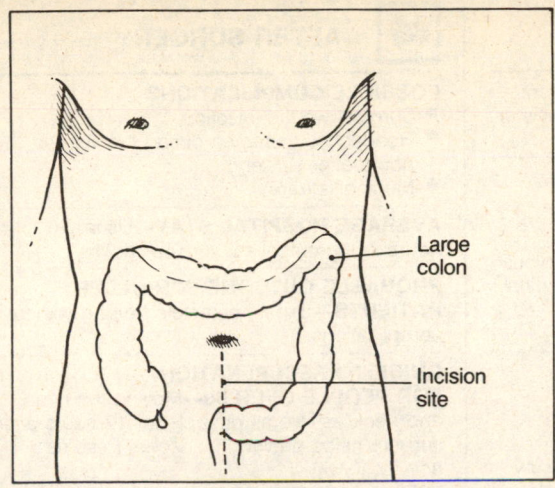

An illustration of the large intestine, sigmoid colon and the usual incision site for this surgical procedure.

Large colon

Incision site

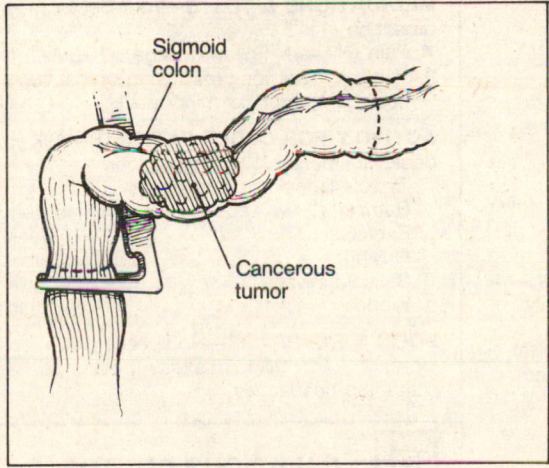

The sigmoid colon is isolated and clamps are placed at each end.
- All of the diseased sigmoid colon is cut free and removed.

Sigmoid colon

Cancerous tumor

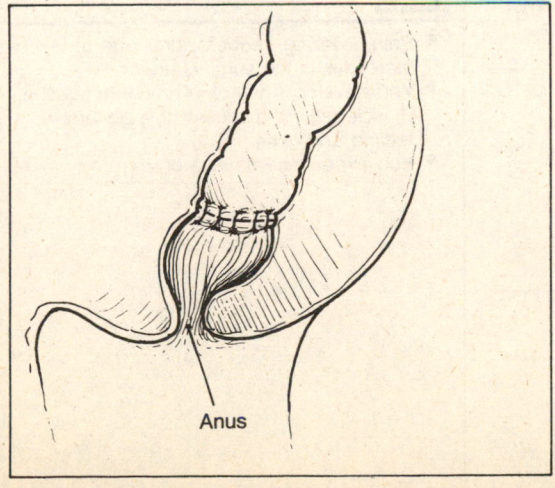

The two healthy ends of the colon are repositioned and joined whenever possible.

Anus

SURGERIES

SPINAL TAP
(Lumbar Puncture)

 BASIC INFORMATION

DESCRIPTION—Removal of spinal fluid from the spinal canal, either for laboratory analysis or prior to surgery with spinal anesthesia.

BODY PARTS INVOLVED—Skin; muscles; covering of spinal cord (meninges).

REASONS FOR SURGERY
- Diagnosis of disorders of the central nervous system that may involve the brain, the spinal cord or their coverings.
- Injection of spinal anesthesia.

SPECIAL CONSIDERATIONS FOR OLDER PATIENTS
- Advancing age alone does not preclude surgery.
- Characteristic signs and symptoms of many surgical disorders and complications are frequently atypical, changed or absent.

SURGICAL RISK INCREASES WITH
- Recent or chronic illness.
- Excessive alcohol consumption.
- Increased intracranial pressure due to any cause.
- Central nervous system infection.

 BEFORE SURGERY

WHO OPERATES—General surgeon, family doctor, neurologist, neurosurgeon, anesthesiologist or internist, usually in hospital, outpatient surgical facility or emergency room.

DIAGNOSTIC TESTS
- Blood and urine studies.
- During surgery: Spinal fluid pressure measured with a manometer (see Glossary).
- After surgery: Laboratory examination of removed fluid.

ANESTHESIA—Local anesthesia by injection.

DESCRIPTION OF OPERATION
- The patient is positioned on his side with the knees drawn as close to the chest as possible.
- A hollow needle is inserted in the back between the 2nd and 3rd lumbar vertebrae.
- The spinal canal is penetrated with the needle. Fluid pressure is measured and then fluid is removed.
- The surgical wound will heal by itself.

 AFTER SURGERY

POSSIBLE COMPLICATIONS
- Surgical wound infection.
- Headaches (common during the first 24 hours after surgery).
- Meningitis (rare).

AVERAGE HOSPITAL STAY—Usually 6 to 24 hours in the outpatient surgical facility.

PROBABLE OUTCOME FOR OLDER PATIENTS—Expect complete healing without complications.

GUIDE TO RECUPERATION FOR PEOPLE OVER 50—Moving the head and neck as little as possible for 12 hours after surgery helps prevent headache. Resume activity slowly.

MEDICATIONS & TESTS—Your doctor may prescribe:
- Pain relievers. Follow dosage schedule.
- You may use non-prescription drugs, such as acetaminophen, for minor pain.

ACTIVITY FOR OLDER PATIENTS—Ask your doctor for personalized instructions.
Typical times for resuming:
Bathing . . . . Immediately.
Exercise . . . . 1 week.
Driving . . . . Immediately.
Sexual activity . . . . When able.
Work . . . . Variable.

FOOD & BEVERAGE—No special diet. Increase fluid intake. This may prevent post-spinal tap headaches.

 CALL YOUR DOCTOR IF

- Pain, swelling, redness, drainage or bleeding increases in the surgical area.
- You develop signs of infection: headache, muscle aches, dizziness or a general ill feeling and fever.
- You experience nausea or vomiting.

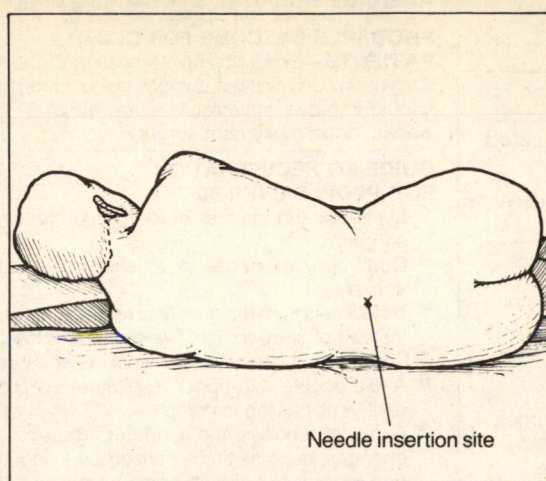

An illustration of a typical needle insertion site and the mid-spine.

Needle insertion site

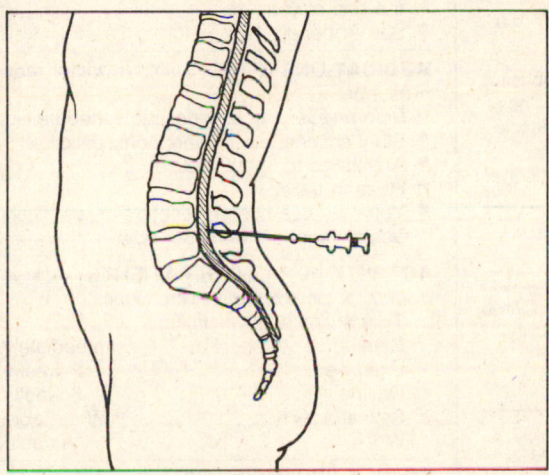

The needle is inserted between sinus processes of the bone into the cavity of the spinal canal which surrounds the spine and is filled with fluid.

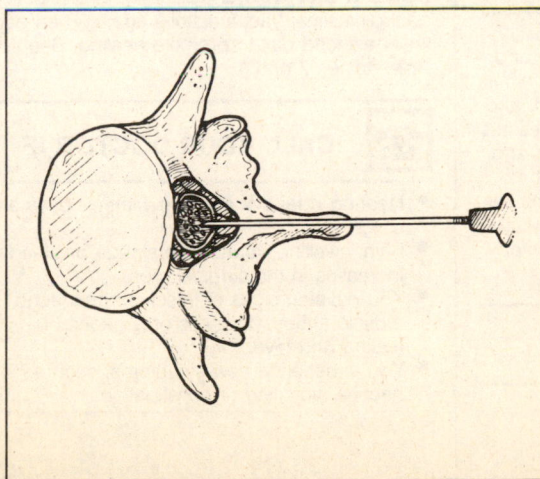

The spinal canal is penetrated with the needle. The fluid pressure is measured, then fluid is removed for laboratory examination.

SURGERIES

STAPES REMOVAL
(Stapedectomy)

BASIC INFORMATION

DESCRIPTION—Removal of the stapes, one of the bones in the middle ear that transmit sound waves to the inner ear. The stapes is also called the stirrup.

BODY PARTS INVOLVED—External ear canal; eardrum; middle ear; stapes.

REASONS FOR SURGERY—Improvement of hearing ability or prevention of continued hearing loss, usually due to otosclerosis. Surgery is done on one ear at a time.

SPECIAL CONSIDERATIONS FOR OLDER PATIENTS
- Advancing age alone does not preclude surgery.
- Characteristic signs and symptoms of many surgical disorders and complications are frequently atypical, changed or absent.
- Surgical repair is complete and effective, but healing takes longer.

SURGICAL RISK INCREASES WITH—Obesity; smoking; poor nutrition; recent or chronic illness; use of drugs such as antihypertensives, muscle relaxants, tranquilizers, sleeping pills, insulin, sedatives, beta-adrenergic blockers or cortisone.

BEFORE SURGERY

WHO OPERATES—Ear, nose and throat specialist, usually in hospital or outpatient surgical facility.

DIAGNOSTIC TESTS—Blood and urine studies; hearing tests.

ANESTHESIA—General anesthesia by inhalation and injection, with an airway tube placed in the windpipe.

DESCRIPTION OF OPERATION
- The operating microscope is positioned, and an incision is made in the middle ear.
- The small bones in the ear are identified, and the stapes is isolated and removed. Sometimes a prosthesis made of stainless steel wire and cellulose sponge is inserted to replace it.
- Blood and fluid are suctioned gently from the ear.
- The wound is closed with fine sutures, which usually can be removed about 1 week after surgery.

AFTER SURGERY

POSSIBLE COMPLICATIONS
- Excessive bleeding.
- Surgical wound infection.
- Hearing worsens or is lost (rare).

AVERAGE HOSPITAL STAY—1 to 2 days.

PROBABLE OUTCOME FOR OLDER PATIENTS—Expect complete healing of the surgical wound without complications. Hearing should improve immediately. Allow about 3 weeks for recovery from surgery.

GUIDE TO RECUPERATION FOR PEOPLE OVER 50
- Lie flat during the first 24 to 48 hours after surgery.
- Don't blow your nose for at least 1 week after surgery.
- Protect ears from moisture or cold. Take tub baths instead of showers for 2 weeks after surgery.
- Don't strain, bend or lift for 3 weeks after surgery.
- Avoid people with upper respiratory infections until your healing is complete.
- Avoid loud noises and sudden pressure changes, such as those caused by flying in non-pressurized aircraft or scuba diving, for the rest of your life.
- See Appendix 19.

MEDICATIONS & TESTS—Your doctor may prescribe:
- Pain relievers. Follow dosage schedule.
- Stool softeners to prevent constipation.
- Antibiotics to fight infection.
- Hearing tests.
- You may use non-prescription drugs, such as acetaminophen, for minor pain.

ACTIVITY FOR OLDER PATIENTS—Ask your doctor for personalized instructions.
Typical times for resuming:
Bathing . . . . Immediately.
Exercise . . . . 2 weeks.
Driving . . . . 3 weeks.
Sexual activity . . . . When able.
Work . . . . Variable.

FOOD & BEVERAGE—Clear liquid diet until the gastrointestinal tract functions again. Then eat a well-balanced diet to promote healing. See Appendices 7 and 1.

CALL YOUR DOCTOR IF

- Hearing does not improve within 2 days after surgery.
- Pain, swelling, redness, drainage or bleeding increases in the surgical area.
- You develop signs of infection: headache, muscle aches, dizziness or a general ill feeling and fever.
- You experience new symptoms, such as nausea, vomiting or constipation.

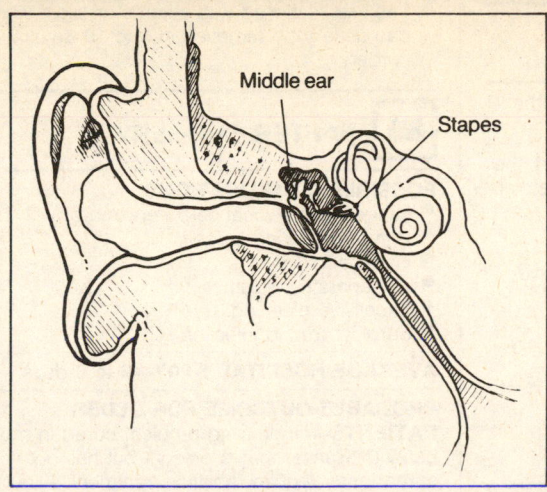

An illustration of the outer ear, middle ear and the stapes (one of the bones in the middle ear that transmits sound waves to the inner ear). The stapes is also called the stirrup.

Middle ear

Stapes

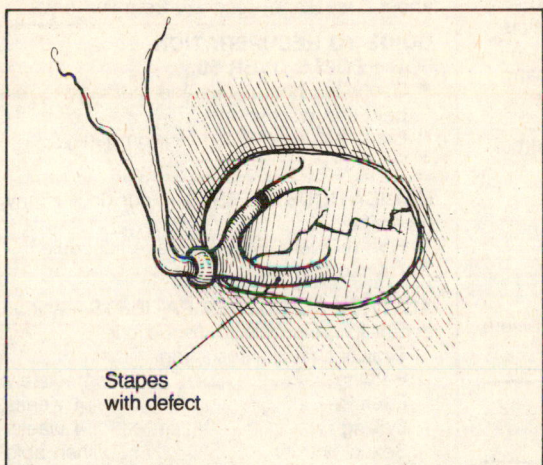

Appearance of the middle ear structure as seen through an operating microscope. Small bones in the ear are identified and the stapes is isolated and removed.

Stapes
with defect

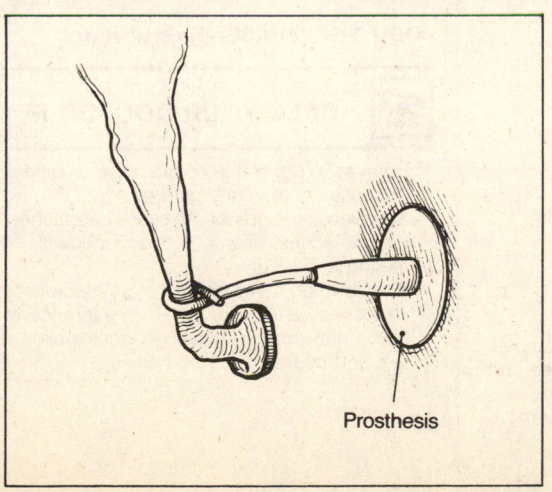

Sometimes a prosthesis made of stainless steel wire and cellulose sponge is inserted to replace the defected stapes.

Prosthesis

THYROID GLAND REMOVAL
(Thyroidectomy)

BASIC INFORMATION

DESCRIPTION—Removal of part or all of the thyroid gland.

BODY PARTS INVOLVED—Thyroid gland, the organ in the neck below the Adam's apple that controls the body's metabolism.

REASONS FOR SURGERY
- Benign or cancerous tumors of the thyroid.
- Thyroglossal cysts (see Glossary).
- To treat thyrotoxicosis (excess thyroid hormone).
- Goiter that causes swallowing difficulties.

SPECIAL CONSIDERATIONS FOR OLDER PATIENTS
- Advancing age alone does not preclude surgery.
- More likely to experience respiratory and kidney problems, confusion and blood clots after surgery.
- Characteristic signs and symptoms of many surgical disorders and complications are frequently atypical, changed or absent.
- Surgical repair is complete and effective, but healing takes longer.

SURGICAL RISK INCREASES WITH
- Obesity.
- Smoking.
- Poor nutrition.
- Untreated hyperthyroidism.

Use of antithyroid medication and iodides before surgery decreases risk. Ask your doctor.

BEFORE SURGERY

WHO OPERATES—General surgeon.

WHERE PERFORMED—Hospital.

DIAGNOSTIC TESTS—Blood studies; sonograms; CT scan; needle biopsy; radioactive-iodine uptake and scan (see Glossary).

ANESTHESIA—General anesthesia by inhalation and injection, with an airway tube placed in the windpipe.

DESCRIPTION OF OPERATION
- An incision is made in the neck following natural skin lines.
- Blood supply to the thyroid gland is clamped.
- All or part of the thyroid gland is cut free and removed, and a drain is left in place. In certain cases, some normal thyroid gland tissue is left intact.

- The skin is closed with sutures or clips, which can usually be removed in 2 to 10 days after surgery.

AFTER SURGERY

POSSIBLE COMPLICATIONS
- Hoarseness if vocal cord nerves are damaged during surgery.
- Hypothyroidism.
- Hypoparathyroidism.
- Excessive bleeding.
- Surgical wound infection.

AVERAGE HOSPITAL STAY—6 to 8 days.

PROBABLE OUTCOME FOR OLDER PATIENTS—Underlying problem cured in most patients. Cancer that is present but has not spread may require radiation treatment. Allow about 6 weeks for recovery from surgery.

GUIDE TO RECUPERATION FOR PEOPLE OVER 50
- Use warm heat packs and massage to relieve pain and discomfort.
- Bathe as usual. Wash incision gently.
- See Appendix 19.

MEDICATIONS & TESTS—Your doctor may prescribe:
- Pain relievers. Follow dosage schedule.
- Thyroid hormones.

ACTIVITY FOR OLDER PATIENTS—Ask your doctor for personalized instructions.
Typical times for resuming:
Bathing . . . . Immediately.
Exercise . . . . 4 weeks.
Driving . . . . 4 weeks.
Sexual activity . . . . When able.
Work . . . . Variable.

FOOD & BEVERAGE—No special diet.

CALL YOUR DOCTOR IF

- Pain, swelling, redness, drainage or bleeding increases in the surgical area.
- You develop signs of infection: headache, muscle aches, dizziness or a general ill feeling and fever.
- You develop symptoms of hypothyroidism: excessive weakness, fatigue, intolerance of cold, menstrual irregularities, constipation or dry and coarse skin and hair.

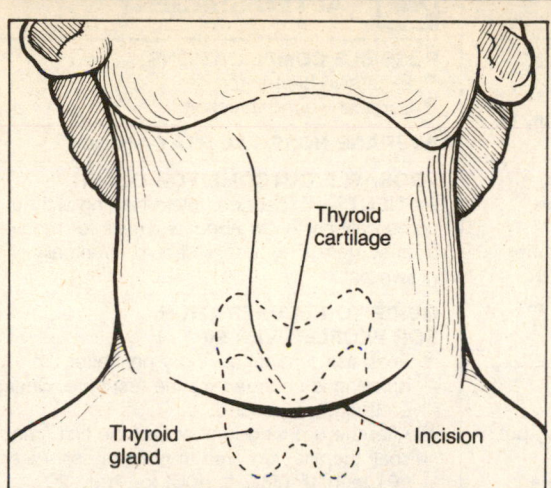

An illustration of structures in the neck and the typical incision site for thyroid gland removal.

Thyroid cartilage

Thyroid gland

Incision

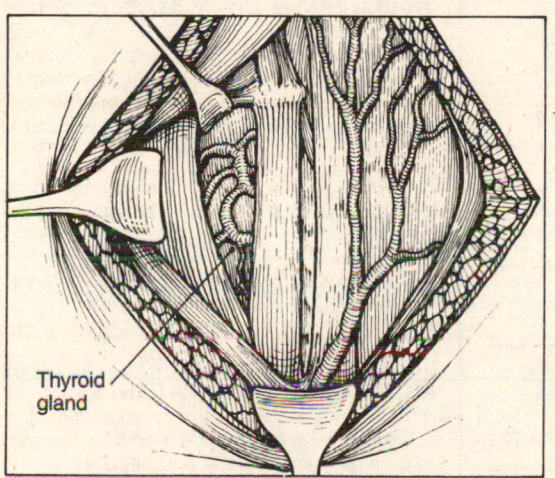

Muscles and connective tissue are retracted revealing the thyroid gland.

Thyroid gland

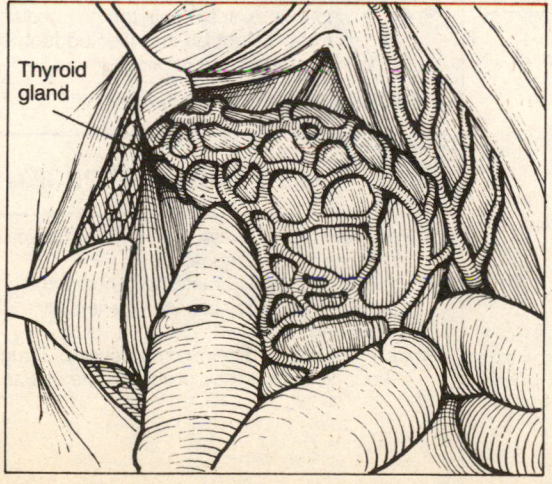

The blood supply to the thyroid gland is clamped and all or part of the gland is cut free and removed.

•The remaining tissue is replaced in its normal position. The skin is closed with sutures or clips (not illustrated).

Thyroid gland

SURGERIES

TOENAIL REMOVAL

 BASIC INFORMATION

DESCRIPTION—Removal of part or all of a toenail.

BODY PARTS INVOLVED—Toenail, usually in the big toe.

REASONS FOR SURGERY
- Relief of painful symptoms of an ingrown toenail, with or without an infection.
- Toenails may be removed for reasons other than ingrown toenail, including injury with part of the toenail torn away; splinters that cannot be removed without removing the toenail; warts under the nail.

SPECIAL CONSIDERATIONS FOR OLDER PATIENTS
- Surgical repair is complete and effective, but healing takes longer.
- Nursing care needs to be more intense and skillful.

SURGICAL RISK INCREASES WITH
- Illnesses such as diabetes mellitus; arterial occlusive disease with poor circulation to the feet; other infections of the foot; excessive alcohol consumption.
- Use of drugs such as antihypertensives; muscle relaxants; tranquilizers; sleep inducers; insulin; beta-adrenergic blockers; cortisone.

 BEFORE SURGERY

WHO OPERATES—General surgeon, family doctor, dermatologist or podiatrist, usually in doctor's office or outpatient surgical facility.

DIAGNOSTIC TESTS—None required.

ANESTHESIA—Local anesthesia by injection.

DESCRIPTION OF OPERATION
- A section of skin is cut on the affected side of the toe.
- Part or all of the nail is pulled up along its bed and cut free of its underlying tissue.
- The nail bed along the affected side is scraped.
- A special non-stick bandage is applied tightly to prevent bleeding. Usually no sutures are needed.

 AFTER SURGERY

POSSIBLE COMPLICATIONS
- Excessive bleeding.
- Surgical wound infection.

AVERAGE HOSPITAL STAY—None.

PROBABLE OUTCOME FOR OLDER PATIENTS—Expect complete healing without complications. Allow about 3 weeks for recovery from surgery. The toenail should eventually grown back.

GUIDE TO RECUPERATION FOR PEOPLE OVER 50
- Keep the surgical area dry until after the dressing is changed for the first time. Change dressings as needed.
- After the dressing is changed the first time, soak the affected area in plain or salt water at 101 to 104F (38.3 to 40C) for 10 to 20 minutes several times a day to reduce pain and swelling.
- Avoid shoes that fit tightly, especially those with narrow toes. Wear white cotton socks.
- To prevent a recurrence when the toenail grows back, cut it straight across instead of rounding off at the corners.
- See Appendix 19.

MEDICATIONS & TESTS—Your doctor may prescribe:
- Pain relievers. Follow dosage schedule.
- Antibiotics or antifungal medication to fight infection.
- You may use non-prescription drugs, such as acetaminophen, for minor pain.

ACTIVITY FOR OLDER PATIENTS
- Activity instructions will vary according to your general health, age, need for nursing care, physical therapy and need for mechanical aids.
- Avoid vigorous exercise until the nail heals. Don't put any weight on the affected foot for 24 hours, then resume walking gradually.

FOOD & BEVERAGE—No special diet.

 CALL YOUR DOCTOR IF

- Pain, swelling, redness, drainage or bleeding increases in the surgical area.
- You develop signs of infection: headache, muscle aches, dizziness or a general ill feeling and fever.
- New, unexplained symptoms develop. Drugs used in treatment may produce side effects.

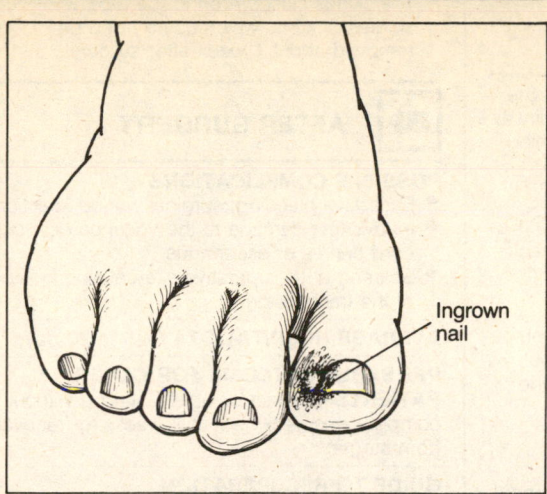

An ingrown toenail in the great toe.

Ingrown
nail

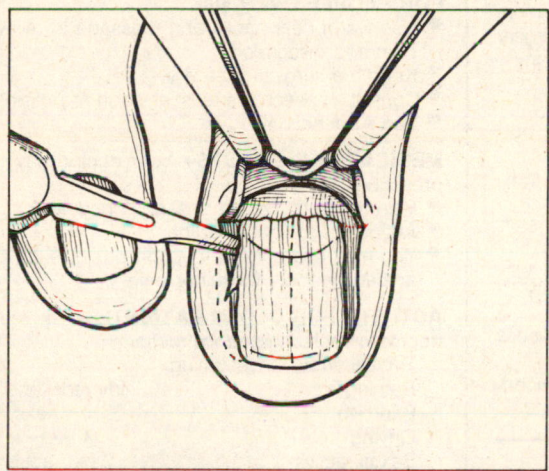

A section of the skin is cut on the affected side of the toe.

•Part or all of the nail is pulled up along its bed and cut free of its underlying tissue.

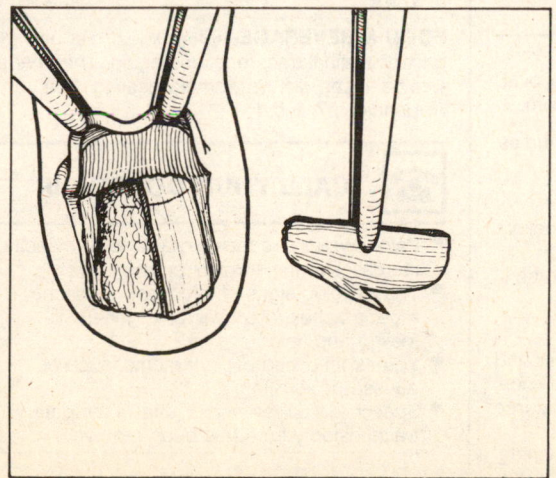

The toenail is removed and the nailbed along the affected side is scraped to prevent recurrence, if possible. The nailbed hardens slowly. A new nail usually grows to replace the removed one.

SURGERIES

TRACHEOSTOMY

BASIC INFORMATION

DESCRIPTION—Creation of an opening in the windpipe (trachea) that will function as an airway either temporarily or permanently. The opening bypasses obstructions that prevent air from being inhaled.

BODY PARTS INVOLVED—Windpipe; muscles, blood vessels and nerves in the neck.

REASONS FOR SURGERY
- Restoration of normal breathing.
- Control of secretions from the nose and throat, particularly in people who are unconscious.
- Creation of an open airway in patients who require prolonged breathing assistance.

SPECIAL CONSIDERATIONS FOR OLDER PATIENTS
- Advancing age alone does not preclude surgery.
- More likely to experience respiratory and kidney problems, confusion and blood clots after surgery.
- Characteristic signs and symptoms of many surgical disorders and complications are frequently atypical, changed or absent.
- Surgical repair is complete and effective, but healing takes longer.
- Nursing care needs to be more intense and skillful.

SURGICAL RISK INCREASES WITH
- Obesity; smoking; poor nutrition.
- Recent illness, especially upper respiratory infection.
- Excessive alcohol consumption or chronic illness.
- Use of drugs such as antihypertensives; muscle relaxants; tranquilizers; sleep inducers; insulin; beta-adrenergic blockers; cortisone.

BEFORE SURGERY

WHO OPERATES—Ear, nose and throat specialist or general surgeon, usually in hospital, outpatient surgical facility or emergency room.

DIAGNOSTIC TESTS—Blood and urine studies and x-rays of chest.

ANESTHESIA
- Local anesthesia (in emergencies) by injection.
- General anesthesia (when time allows) by inhalation and injection, with an airway tube placed in the windpipe.

DESCRIPTION OF OPERATION
- An incision is made in the neck. The muscles and connective tissue around the windpipe are divided.
- A section at the front of the windpipe is cut free and removed.
- A tracheostomy tube is fitted into the opening in the windpipe to function as an airway. The patient will breathe through this tube as long as it is in place.

- The skin is closed around the tube with sutures or clips, which usually can be removed about 1 week after surgery.

AFTER SURGERY

POSSIBLE COMPLICATIONS
- Excessive bleeding; surgical wound infection.
- Inadvertent damage to the vocal cords, vocal-cord nerves or esophagus.
- Scarring at the operative site causing closure of the tracheostomy.

AVERAGE HOSPITAL STAY—5 to 20 days.

PROBABLE OUTCOME FOR OLDER PATIENTS—Expect complete healing without complications. Allow about 2 weeks for recovery from surgery.

GUIDE TO RECUPERATION FOR PEOPLE OVER 50
- Use warm heat packs and massage to relieve pain and discomfort.
- Keep the surgical area dry.
- Consult a speech therapist as soon as possible.
- See Appendix 19.

MEDICATIONS & TESTS—Your doctor may prescribe:
- Pain relievers. Follow dosage schedule.
- Antibiotics to fight infection.
- You may use non-prescription drugs, such as acetaminophen, for minor pain.

ACTIVITY FOR OLDER PATIENTS—Ask your doctor for personalized instructions.
Typical times for resuming:
Bathing . . . . Immediately.
Exercise . . . . 4 weeks.
Driving . . . . 4 weeks.
Sexual activity . . . . When able.
Work . . . . Variable.

FOOD & BEVERAGE—Clear liquid diet until the gastrointestinal tract functions again. Then eat a well-balanced diet to promote healing. See Appendices 7 and 1.

CALL YOUR DOCTOR IF

- Pain, swelling, redness, drainage or bleeding increases in the surgical area.
- You develop signs of infection: headache, muscle aches, dizziness or a general ill feeling and fever.
- You experience new symptoms, such as nausea or vomiting.
- Speech difficulties persist after a temporary tracheostomy tube has been removed.

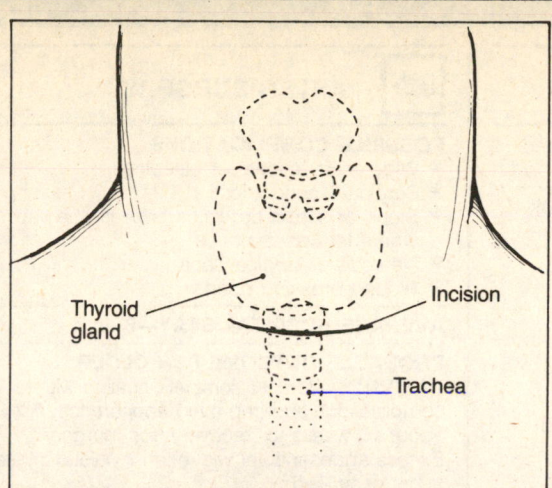

An illustration of structures in the neck and the usual incision site through the skin.

Thyroid gland

Incision

Trachea

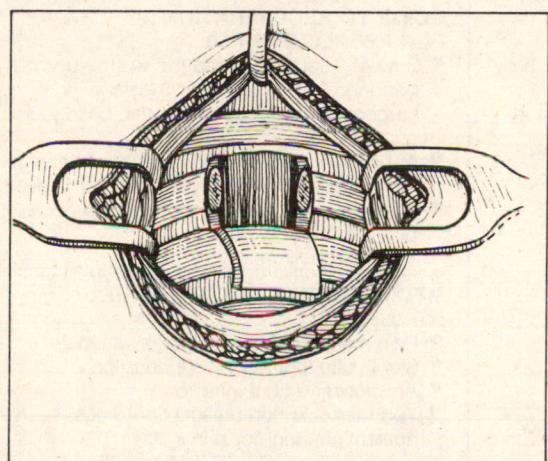

A section at the front of the windpipe is incised and widened.

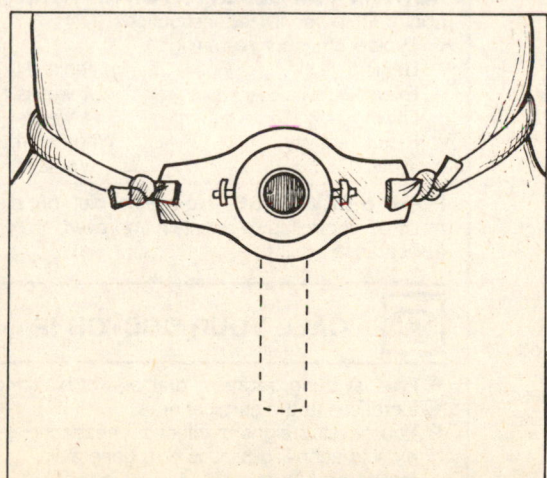

A tracheostomy tube is fitted into the opening in the windpipe to function as an airway. As long as the tracheostomy tube is in place and open, the patient will breathe through it instead of through the mouth or nose.

SURGERIES

TUMMY TUCK
(Abdominoplasty)

BASIC INFORMATION

DESCRIPTION—Removal of excess skin and fat from the abdomen.

BODY PARTS INVOLVED—Fat between skin and muscles in abdomen; skin.

REASONS FOR SURGERY—Improved appearance.

SPECIAL CONSIDERATIONS FOR OLDER PATIENTS
- Advancing age alone does not preclude surgery.
- More likely to experience respiratory and kidney problems, confusion and blood clots after surgery.
- Characteristic signs and symptoms of many surgical disorders and complications are frequently atypical, changed or absent.
- Surgical repair is complete and effective, but healing takes longer.
- Nursing care needs to be more intense and skillful.

SURGICAL RISK INCREASES WITH
- Stress; smoking; excessive alcohol consumption.
- Poor nutrition.
- Previous abdominal surgery.
- Recent or chronic illness.

BEFORE SURGERY

WHO OPERATES—Plastic and reconstructive surgeon, usually in hospital.

DIAGNOSTIC TESTS—Blood and urine studies.

ANESTHESIA—General anesthesia by inhalation and injection, with an airway tube placed in the windpipe.

DESCRIPTION OF OPERATION
- A large, elliptical incision is made in the abdomen.
- Excessive skin and the underlying apron of excess fat are cut free and removed.
- Drains are left under the operative site to prevent accumulation of blood and fluid from tissue drainage.
- Both edges of the skin are gently stretched and carefully sewn together with sutures.
- Sutures can usually be removed in 10 to 14 days.

AFTER SURGERY

POSSIBLE COMPLICATIONS
- Wide scars; excessive bleeding.
- Surgical wound infection.
- Blood or serum collection beneath the flap where fat was removed.
- Necrosis of surgical flaps.
- Wound breaking open.

AVERAGE HOSPITAL STAY—6 days.

PROBABLE OUTCOME FOR OLDER PATIENTS—Expect complete healing without complications and improved appearance. Allow about 10 weeks for recovery from surgery. Excess abdominal fat will return if caloric intake is not controlled.

GUIDE TO RECUPERATION FOR PEOPLE OVER 50
- Between showers, keep the wound dry with a bandage for the first 2 or 3 days after surgery. If a bandage gets wet, change it promptly.
- Apply non-prescription antibiotic ointment to the wound before applying new bandages.
- Use warm heat packs and massage to relieve pain and discomfort.
- See Appendix 19.

MEDICATIONS & TESTS—Your doctor may prescribe:
- Pain relievers. Follow dosage schedule.
- Stool softeners to prevent constipation.
- Antibiotics to fight infection.
- You may use non-prescription drugs, such as acetaminophen, for minor pain.

ACTIVITY FOR OLDER PATIENTS—Ask your doctor for personalized instructions.
Typical times for resuming:
Bathing . . . . Immediately.
Exercise . . . . 4 weeks.
Driving . . . . 4 weeks.
Sexual activity . . . . When able.
Work . . . . Variable.

FOOD & BEVERAGE—No special diet, but diet must be controlled to maintain improved appearance.

CALL YOUR DOCTOR IF

- Pain, swelling, redness, drainage or bleeding increases in the surgical area.
- You develop signs of infection: headache, muscle aches, dizziness or a general ill feeling and fever.
- You experience nausea, vomiting, constipation or abdominal swelling.

TUMMY TUCK
(Abdominoplasty)

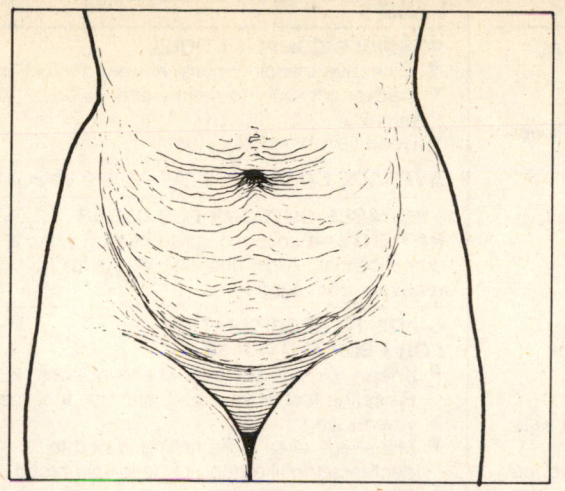

An illustration of typical distribution of excess skin and fat in the lower abdomen.

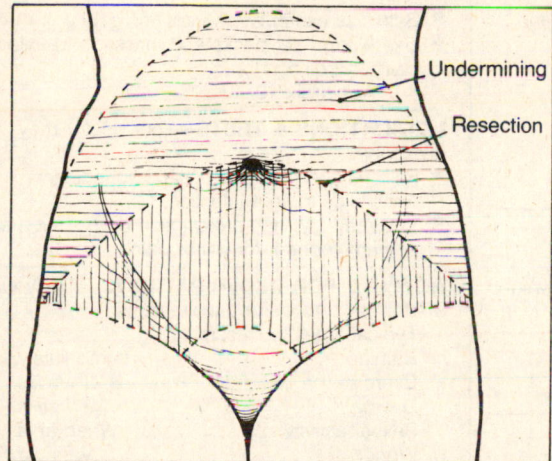

A large elliptical incision is made in the lower abdomen.

- Excessive skin and the underlying apron of excess fat are cut and removed.

Undermining

Resection

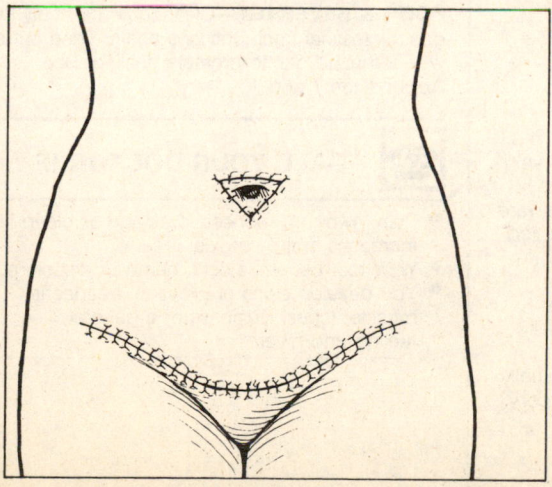

Drains are usually left under the operative site to prevent accumulation of blood and fluid from tissue drainage.

- Both edges of the skin are gently stretched and carefully sewn together with sutures, which can usually be removed in 10 to 14 days.

VARICOSE VEIN REMOVAL

 BASIC INFORMATION

DESCRIPTION—Removal of varicose veins.

BODY PARTS INVOLVED—Diseased veins in the legs, usually in the greater and lesser saphenous veins, the largest veins in the lower body.

REASONS FOR SURGERY
- Improvement of blood circulation in the legs and feet.
- Relief of painful symptoms.

SPECIAL CONSIDERATIONS FOR OLDER PATIENTS
- Advancing age alone does not preclude surgery.
- More likely to experience respiratory and kidney problems, confusion and blood clots after surgery.
- Surgical repair is complete and effective, but healing takes longer.
- Nursing care needs to be more intense and skillful.

SURGICAL RISK INCREASES WITH
- Family history of varicose veins.
- Stress; obesity; smoking.
- Excessive alcohol consumption.
- Poor nutrition.

 BEFORE SURGERY

WHO OPERATES—General surgeon, usually in outpatient surgical facility or hospital.

DIAGNOSTIC TESTS—Blood and urine studies.

ANESTHESIA—General anesthesia by inhalation and injection, with an airway tube placed in the windpipe.

DESCRIPTION OF OPERATION
- An incision is made over the top of the saphenous-femoral vein system (see Glossary).
- The large, diseased veins are identified. The upper and lower ends of each diseased vein are cut and tied. An instrument is passed beginning at the ankle and extending upward through the inside of the entire vein and tied. The entire vein is stripped.
- After the main veins have been removed, smaller veins are identified, incisions are made and the smaller veins are individually tied and removed.
- The skin is closed with sutures, which usually can be removed about 1 week after surgery.
- The legs are wrapped snugly in elastic bandages.

 AFTER SURGERY

POSSIBLE COMPLICATIONS
- Excessive bleeding; surgical wound infection.
- Inadvertent injury to nearby arteries or nerves.
- Deep-vein blood clots (rare).

AVERAGE HOSPITAL STAY—1 to 3 days.

PROBABLE OUTCOME FOR OLDER PATIENTS—Expect complete healing without complications. Allow about 11 weeks for recovery from surgery.

GUIDE TO RECUPERATION FOR PEOPLE OVER 50
- Keep your legs elevated whenever possible. Raise the foot of your bed, and use foot rests when sitting.
- Move legs often while resting in bed to decrease the likelihood of deep-vein blood clots.
- Bathe as usual. Wash incisions gently.
- Use warm heat packs and massage to relieve pain and discomfort.
- See Appendix 19.

MEDICATIONS & TESTS—Your doctor may prescribe:
- Pain relievers. Follow dosage schedule.
- Antibiotics to fight infection.
- You may use non-prescription drugs, such as acetaminophen, for minor pain.

ACTIVITY FOR OLDER PATIENTS—Ask your doctor for personalized instructions.
Typical times for resuming:
Bathing . . . . Immediately.
Exercise . . . . 3 weeks.
Driving . . . . 3 weeks.
Sexual activity . . . . When able.
Work . . . . Variable.

FOOD & BEVERAGE—Clear liquid diet until the gastrointestinal tract functions again. Then eat a well-balanced diet to promote healing. See Appendices 7 and 1.

 CALL YOUR DOCTOR IF

- Pain, swelling, redness, drainage or bleeding increases in the surgical area.
- Your foot becomes cold, numb or discolored.
- You develop signs of infection: headache, muscle aches, dizziness or a general ill feeling and fever.

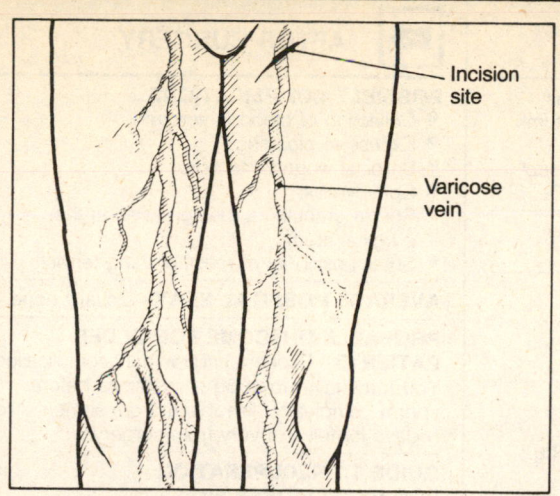

An illustration of diseased veins in the legs, usually the greater and lesser saphonous veins, the largest veins in the lower extremities.

Incision site

Varicose vein

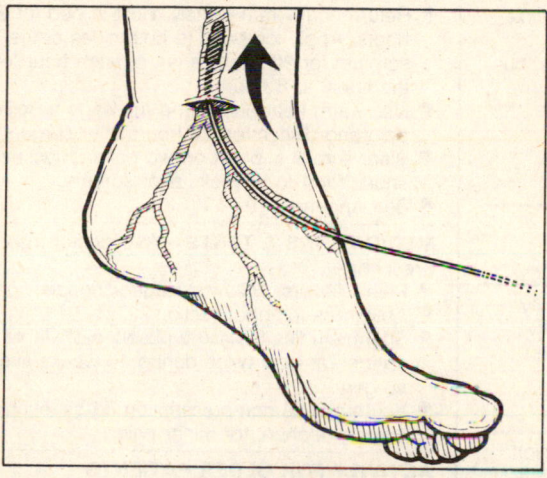

The large diseased veins are identified.

•The upper and lower ends of each diseased vein are cut and tied and an instrument is passed through the inside of the entire vein and tied.

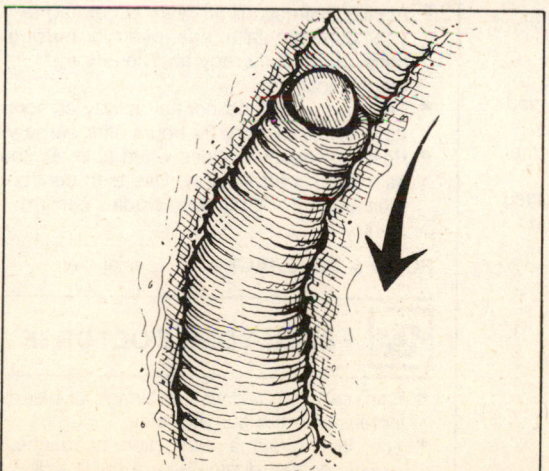

The entire vein is stripped.

•After the main veins have been removed, smaller veins are identified, incisions are made into the skin and smaller veins are tied individually and removed.
•After surgery, the legs are wrapped snugly in elastic bandages.

SURGERIES

VASECTOMY

BASIC INFORMATION

DESCRIPTION—Cutting and tying the vas deferens (sperm channels inside the scrotum). The surgery stops the flow of sperm and provides a safe, effective form of birth control without affecting sexual desire or ability.

BODY PARTS INVOLVED—Scrotum; vas deferens.

REASONS FOR SURGERY
- Voluntary sterilization.
- Recurrent epididymitis when caused by chronic prostate infection.

SPECIAL CONSIDERATIONS FOR OLDER PATIENTS
- Advancing age alone does not preclude surgery.
- More likely to experience respiratory and kidney problems, confusion and blood clots after surgery.
- Surgical repair is complete and effective, but healing takes longer.

SURGICAL RISK INCREASES WITH
- Emotional instability.
- Recent illness, especially one with fever.

BEFORE SURGERY

WHO OPERATES—General surgeon, family doctor, urologist or plastic and reconstructive surgeon, usually in doctor's office, outpatient surgical facility or hospital.

DIAGNOSTIC TESTS—Sperm studies.

ANESTHESIA—Local anesthesia by injection.

DESCRIPTION OF OPERATION
- The scrotum is shaved at home before surgery.
- Incisions are made on both sides of the scrotum. The vas deferens is identified, tied in two places and cut between the ties.
- The divided vas deferens is returned to the scrotum.
- The edges of incised skin are reconstructed with fine sutures, which usually fall out in about 7 days.

AFTER SURGERY

POSSIBLE COMPLICATIONS
- Collection of blood in scrotum.
- Excessive bleeding.
- Surgical wound infection.
- Epididymitis.
- Sperm granuloma (benign lump in the surgical area).
- Small possibility of reestablishing fertility.

AVERAGE HOSPITAL STAY—Usually none.

PROBABLE OUTCOME FOR OLDER PATIENTS—Expect sterility without complications. You may have up to 30 ejaculations before sperm completely disappears from semen. Allow 6 days for full recovery from surgery.

GUIDE TO RECUPERATION FOR PEOPLE OVER 50
- Return home immediately. Rest in bed for 24 hours. Apply ice bags to both sides of the scrotum for 20 minutes out of each hour for the first 6 to 8 hours.
- Use warm heat packs and massage to relieve pain and discomfort 24 hours after surgery.
- Wear scrotal support or two pairs of jockey shorts for 4 to 6 weeks after surgery.
- See Appendix 19.

MEDICATIONS & TESTS—Your doctor may prescribe:
- Pain relievers. Follow dosage schedule.
- Antibiotics to fight infection.
- Sperm studies to assure absence of viable sperm—at least twice during 10 weeks after surgery.
- You may use non-prescription drugs, such as acetaminophen, for minor pain.

ACTIVITY FOR OLDER PATIENTS
- Activity instructions will vary according to your general health, age, need for nursing care, physical therapy and need for mechanical aids.
- Return to work and normal activity as soon as possible (usually 24 hours after surgery).
- Resume sexual relations when able, as soon as 1 week after surgery. Use birth control measures until laboratory studies confirm sterility.

FOOD & BEVERAGE—No special diet.

CALL YOUR DOCTOR IF

- Pain, swelling, redness, drainage or bleeding increases in the surgical area.
- You develop signs of infection: headache, muscle aches, dizziness or a general ill feeling and fever.

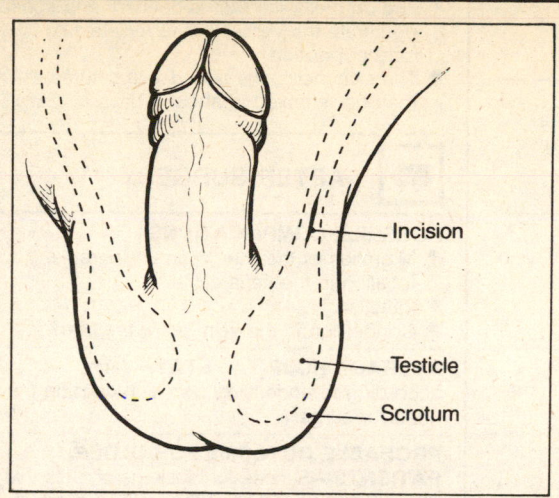

The penis, scrotum and testicles showing a typical incision site for a vasectomy.

Incision

Testicle

Scrotum

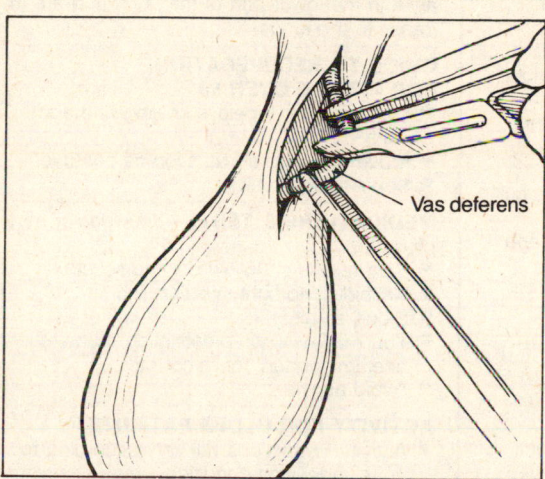

The vas deferens is identified, tied in 2 places and cut between the ties.

Vas deferens

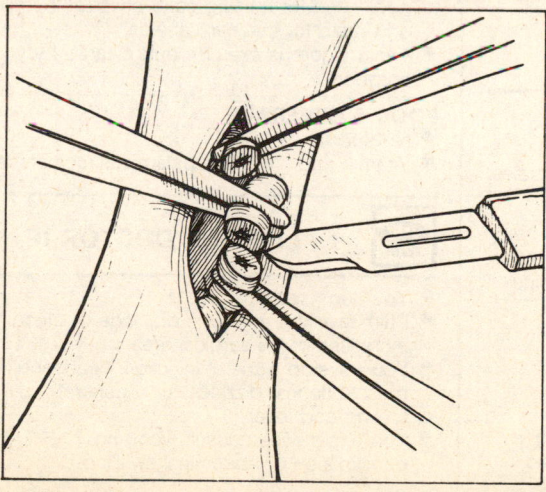

The divided vas deferens is returned to the scrotum and the edges of incised skin are reconstructed with fine sutures which usually fall out in about 7 days (not illustrated).

SURGERIES

VENA CAVA FILTER INSERTION

BASIC INFORMATION

DESCRIPTION—Insertion of an umbrella-shaped filtering device into the inferior vena cava (large vein in the illustration). The filter prevents passage of blood clots without interrupting blood flow.

BODY PARTS INVOLVED
- Jugular vein (large neck vein) or femoral vein (large leg vein).
- The inferior vena cava.

REASONS FOR SURGERY—Repeated blood clots from the veins of the pelvis or legs traveling through the vena cava to lodge in the lungs, thereby threatening life.

SPECIAL CONSIDERATIONS FOR OLDER PATIENTS
- Advancing age alone does not preclude surgery.
- More likely to experience respiratory and kidney problems, confusion and blood clots after surgery.
- Characteristic signs and symptoms of many surgical disorders and complications are frequently atypical, changed or absent.
- Surgical repair is complete and effective, but healing takes longer.
- Nursing care needs to be more intense and skillful.

SURGICAL RISK INCREASES WITH
- Obesity.
- Smoking.
- Excessive alcohol consumption.
- Use of drugs such as antihypertensives; muscle relaxants; tranquilizers; sleep inducers; insulin; beta-adrenergic blockers; cortisone.

BEFORE SURGERY

WHO OPERATES—General or vascular surgeon, usually in hospital.

DIAGNOSTIC TESTS—Blood and urine studies.

ANESTHESIA
- Local anesthesia.
- General anesthesia by inhalation and injection, with an airway tube placed in the windpipe.

DESCRIPTION OF OPERATION
- The filter is prepared according to manufacturer's instructions.
- Skin in groin is incised and the right femoral vein is isolated.
- The filter is inserted into a small opening in the vein and threaded under fluoroscopic guidance to the appropriate place in the inferior vena cava.
- The umbrella-like filter is opened, and spokes penetrate the vessel wall to maintain its correct position.
- The skin incision is closed with sutures which may be removed in about 7 days.

AFTER SURGERY

POSSIBLE COMPLICATIONS
- Migration of the filter to an undesirable location in the vena cava.
- Infection.
- Congestion in the vein below the filter.

AVERAGE HOSPITAL STAY—Varies according to underlying condition causing the need for surgery.

PROBABLE OUTCOME FOR OLDER PATIENTS—Successful blockage of clots that arise in the lower part of the body and are in transit to the lungs.

GUIDE TO RECUPERATION FOR PEOPLE OVER 50
- Don't smoke. It delays healing and adds risks.
- Move legs actively as soon as possible.
- See Appendix 19.

MEDICATIONS & TESTS—Your doctor may prescribe:
- Pain relievers. Follow dosage schedule.
- Antibiotics to fight infection.
- Blood studies.
- You may use non-prescription drugs, such as acetaminophen, for minor pain.
- Avoid aspirin.

ACTIVITY FOR OLDER PATIENTS
- Activity instructions will vary according to your underlying condition, general health, age, need for nursing care, physical therapy and need for mechanical aids.
- Avoid vigorous exercise until cleared by your surgeon.

FOOD & BEVERAGE
- No special diet.
- Vitamin and mineral supplements (sometimes).

CALL YOUR DOCTOR IF

- Your legs swell.
- Pain, swelling, redness, drainage or bleeding increases in the surgical area.
- You develop signs of infection: headache, muscle aches, dizziness or a general ill feeling and fever.
- You experience nausea, vomiting, constipation or abdominal swelling.

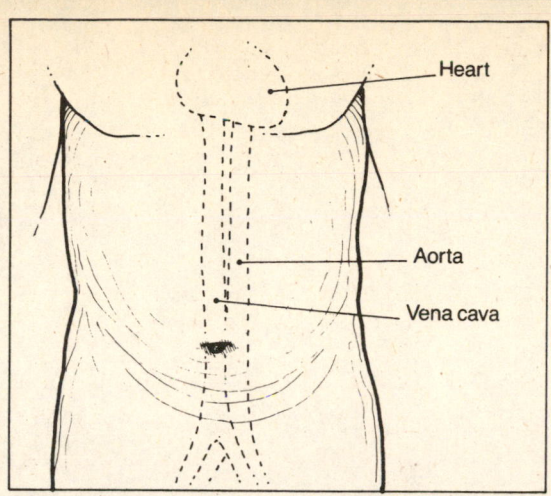

An illustration showing the anatomical position of the aorta, heart, and vena cava, a very large vein that returns blood to the right side of the heart.

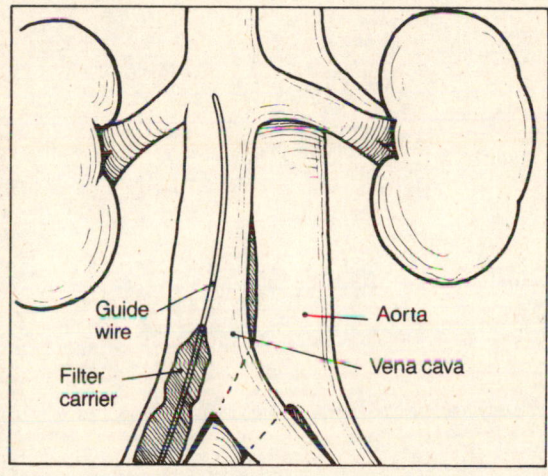

This illustration shows the filter being placed in position in the vena cava by using a guide wire.

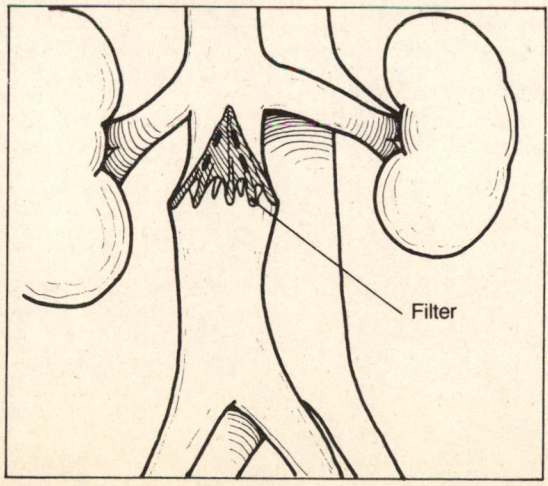

The vena cava as seen after it has had the filter inserted.

SURGERIES

Medications

ACETAMINOPHEN

BRAND & GENERIC NAMES

Acetaminophen is a popular pain-killer and is contained in many combination drugs, such as cough and cold medicines, muscle relaxants, headache compounds, sinus medications and others. The complete list of brand names is too extensive to list here. Look carefully in any combination medicine to see if acetaminophen is an ingredient. Popular brand names include Anacin, CoTylenol (M), Datril, Excedrin (M), Panadol, Parafon-forte (M), Percocet-5 (M), Sine-Off, Sinutab (M), Tempra, Triaminicin, Tylenol, Tylenol with codeine (M) and Vicodin (M). (The (M) means it is a mixture or combination drug.) Additional brand names are available.

 ## USES

- Treatment of mild to moderate pain and fever.
- Acetaminophen does not relieve redness, stiffness or swelling of joints or tissue inflammation. Use aspirin or other non-steroidal anti-inflammatory drugs for inflammation.

 ## POSSIBLE ADVERSE REACTIONS OR SIDE EFFECTS

If any of the following occurs, consult a doctor:
- Light-headedness.
- Trembling.
- Fatigue.
- Rash.
- Itch.
- Hives.
- Sore throat.
- Fever.
- Unexplained bleeding or bruising.
- Blood in urine.
- Painful or frequent urination.
- Jaundice (yellow eyes; yellow skin; dark urine).
- Decreased urine output.

 ## WARNINGS & PRECAUTIONS

- Before you start, consult your doctor if you have kidney disease or liver damage.
- Don't take if you are allergic to acetaminophen.
- If your symptoms don't improve after 2 days, call your doctor.
- See Appendix 21.

 ## AGE-RELATED FACTORS

- Toxic effects are more likely.
- Older patients are more likely to have age-related kidney or liver function impairment. This may lead to the need for reduction of the usual dosage.
- Possible increased risk of gastrointestinal bleeding or ulcers.

 ## POSSIBLE INTERACTIONS WITH OTHER DRUGS

- If you are using or taking any other drug (prescription or non-prescription), ask your doctor or pharmacist if there are possible interactions.
- Acetaminophen cannot safely be taken with some drugs.
- Acetaminophen taken with some drugs may require dosage adjustment.

Do not drink alcoholic beverages or use cocaine, marijuana or tobacco while taking this medicine. These may decrease the effectiveness of the medicine or cause uncomfortable or dangerous adverse reactions.

 ## OVERDOSE

SYMPTOMS
Stomach upset; irritability; sweating; convulsions; coma.

WHAT TO DO
- Dial 911 (emergency) or 0 (operator) for an ambulance or medical help. Then give first aid immediately.
- If patient is unconscious and not breathing, give mouth-to-mouth breathing. If there is no heartbeat, use cardiac massage and mouth-to-mouth breathing (CPR). Don't try to make patient vomit. If you can't get help quickly, take patient to nearest emergency facility.

ANALGESICS (Narcotic)

BRAND & GENERIC NAMES

All narcotics may be habit-forming and lead to addiction. Codeine and hydrocodone are included in combination with other ingredients in many brand-name cough and cold preparations, analgesics and muscle relaxants. Commonly prescribed brand names (start with a Capital) and generic names (all CAPITALS) include Apap with codeine (M), PAP BUPRENORPHINE, BUTORPHANOL, CODEINE, Darvon, Demerol, Dilaudid, Doloine, Hycodane, HYDROCODONE, HYDROMORPHONE, LEVORPHANOL, MEPERI-DINE, METHADONE, MORPHINE, NALBUPHINE, OPIUM, OXYCODONE, OXYMORPHONE, Pantapon, Paveral, Percocet-5 (M), PENTAZOCINE, PROPOXYPHENE, Talwin and Vicodin (M). (The (M) means it is a mixture or combination drug.) Additional brand names are available.

 ## USES

- Relieves pain.
- Suppresses cough (codeine and hydrocodone).
- Relieves diarrhea.

 ## POSSIBLE ADVERSE REACTIONS OR SIDE EFFECTS

If any of the following occurs, consult a doctor:
- Hives.
- Rash.
- Intense itching.
- Faintness soon after a dose.
- Dizziness.
- Flushed face.
- Unusual tiredness.
- Severe constipation.
- Abdominal pain.
- Vomiting.
- Nausea.
- Facial swelling.
- Slow heartbeat.
- Irregular breathing.
- Hallucinations.
- Disorientation.
- Depression.
- Blurred vision.
- Decreased mental performance.
- Anxiety.
- Insomnia.
- Weakness and faintness when arising from bed or chair.
- Euphoria.

 ## WARNINGS & PRECAUTIONS

- All narcotics are habit-forming and must be prescribed by a doctor before you can purchase them or refill a prescription.

- Don't take if you have taken any MAO inhibitor (see Glossary) in previous 2 weeks.
- Before taking this medicine, consult your doctor if you have brain disease, head injury, colitis, convulsions (seizures), history of emphysema, asthma or other chronic lung disease, enlarged prostate or problems with urination, gallbladder disease or gallstones, heart disease, kidney disease, liver disease or underactive thyroid.
- Don't drive or try risky physical activity until you know how drug affects you.
- See Appendix 21.

 ## AGE-RELATED FACTORS

- Side effects and adverse reactions are more likely to occur with advancing age, especially breathing difficulty.
- May contribute to increased dental problems with gums, cavities and yeast infections.
- Lower-than-standard doses and longer intervals between doses may be required.
- Your doctor or care-giver should carefully monitor your response to this drug.

 ## POSSIBLE INTERACTIONS WITH OTHER DRUGS

- If you are using or taking any other drug (prescription or non-prescription), ask your doctor or pharmacist if there are possible interactions.
- Analgesics (narcotic) cannot safely be taken with some drugs.
- Analgesics (narcotic) taken with some drugs may require dosage adjustment.

Do not drink alcoholic beverages or use cocaine, marijuana or tobacco while taking this medicine. These may decrease the effectiveness of the medicine or cause uncomfortable or dangerous adverse reactions.

 ## OVERDOSE

SYMPTOMS
Deep sleep; slow breathing; slow pulse; respiratory arrest; flushed warm skin; constricted pupils.

WHAT TO DO
- Dial 911 (emergency) or 0 (operator) for an ambulance or medical help. Then give first aid immediately.
- If patient is unconscious and not breathing, give mouth-to-mouth breathing. If there is no heartbeat, use cardiac massage and mouth-to-mouth breathing (CPR). Don't try to make patient vomit. If you can't get help quickly, take patient to nearest emergency facility.

ANGIOTENSIN-CONVERTING ENZYME (ACE) INHIBITORS

BRAND & GENERIC NAMES

Commonly prescribed brand names (start with a Capital) and generic names (all CAPITALS) include CAPTOPRIL, Capoten, ENALAPRIL, LISINOPRIL, Prinivil, Vasotec and Zestril.

 ## USES

- Treats high blood pressure.
- Treats congestive heart failure.

 ## POSSIBLE ADVERSE REACTIONS OR SIDE EFFECTS

If any of the following occurs, consult a doctor:
- Hives.
- Rash.
- Intense itching.
- Faintness soon after a dose.
- Difficulty breathing.
- Loss of taste.
- Swelling of mouth, face, hands or feet.
- Dizziness.
- Chest pain.
- Fast or irregular heartbeat.
- Coughing.
- Sore throat.
- Cloudy urine.
- Fever.
- Chills.
- Nausea.
- Vomiting.
- Indigestion.
- Abdominal pain.

 ## WARNINGS & PRECAUTIONS

- Avoid heavy exercise in hot weather.
- Before taking this medicine, consult your doctor if you have diabetes mellitus (sugar diabetes), heart disease, blood vessel disease, kidney disease, liver disease, systemic lupus erythematosus or have recently had a heart attack, stroke or kidney transplant.
- Don't drive or try risky physical activity until you know how drug affects you.
- See Appendix 21.

 ## AGE-RELATED FACTORS

- Older patients are more likely to have age-related kidney or liver function impairment. This may lead to the need for reduction of the usual dosage.
- Aging does not affect expected results.
- Your doctor or care-giver should carefully monitor your response to this drug.

 ## POSSIBLE INTERACTIONS WITH OTHER DRUGS

- If you are using or taking any other drug (prescription or non-prescription), ask your doctor or pharmacist if there are possible interactions.
- Angiotensin-converting enzyme inhibitors cannot safely be taken with some drugs.
- Angiotensin-converting enzyme inhibitors taken with some drugs may require dosage adjustment.

Do not drink alcoholic beverages or use cocaine, marijuana or tobacco while taking this medicine. These may decrease the effectiveness of the medicine or cause uncomfortable or dangerous adverse reactions.

 ## OVERDOSE

SYMPTOMS
Fever; chills; sore throat; fainting; convulsions; coma.

WHAT TO DO
- Dial 911 (emergency) or 0 (operator) for an ambulance or medical help. Then give first aid immediately.
- If patient is unconscious and not breathing, give mouth-to-mouth breathing. If there is no heartbeat, use cardiac massage and mouth-to-mouth breathing (CPR). Don't try to make patient vomit. If you can't get help quickly, take patient to nearest emergency facility.

ANTACIDS

BRAND & GENERIC NAMES

Most brands are sold as non-prescription medicines. The complete list of brand names is too extensive to list here.

 ## USES

- Neutralizes stomach acidity.
- Treats peptic ulcers of stomach and duodenum.
- Reduces reflux of stomach acid into esophagus.
- Some have a laxative effect (check label).

 ## POSSIBLE ADVERSE REACTIONS OR SIDE EFFECTS

If any of the following occurs, consult a doctor:
- Constipation.
- Appetite loss.
- Lower abdominal pain and swelling.
- Bone pain.
- Muscle weakness.
- Swollen wrists or ankles.
- Difficult or painful urination.
- Unusual tiredness or weakness.

 ## WARNINGS & PRECAUTIONS

- If you have a tendency to retain fluid, take only low-sodium antacids. These can be purchased without prescription.
- Antacids may interfere with absorption of many medicines.
- If you have kidney disease, don't take antacids that contain magnesium or sodium bicarbonate.
- Before taking this medicine, consult your doctor if you have Alzheimer's disease, appendicitis, bone fractures, colitis, colostomy, constipation (severe and continuing), diarrhea (chronic), swelling of feet or lower legs, heart disease, hemorrhoids, ileostomy, inflamed bowel, intestinal blockage, intestinal or rectal bleeding (of unknown cause), kidney disease, liver disease, sarcoidosis or underactive parathyroid gland.
- See Appendix 21.

 ## AGE-RELATED FACTORS

Avoid aluminum-containing antacids. Aluminum may be one of the contributing causes of Alzheimer's disease. In addition, some forms of bone disease may be aggravated by reduced absorption of fluoride, which may be caused by chronic use of aluminum-containing antacids.

 ## POSSIBLE INTERACTIONS WITH OTHER DRUGS

- If you are using or taking any other drug (prescription or non-prescription), ask your doctor or pharmacist if there are possible interactions.
- Antacids cannot safely be taken with some drugs.
- Antacids taken with some drugs may require dosage adjustment.

Do not drink alcoholic beverages or use cocaine, marijuana or tobacco while taking this medicine. These may decrease the effectiveness of the medicine or cause uncomfortable or dangerous adverse reactions.

 ## OVERDOSE

SYMPTOMS
Weakness; fatigue; dizziness confusion.

WHAT TO DO
Overdose unlikely to threaten life. If person takes much larger amount than prescribed, call doctor, poison control center or hospital emergency room for instructions.

MEDICATIONS

ANTIANXIETY MEDICATIONS
(Minor Tranquilizers)

BRAND & GENERIC NAMES

Commonly prescribed brand names (start with a Capital) and generic names (all CAPITALS) include APRAZOLAM, Ativan, Barbidonna (M), Barbita, Bronkotab (M), CHLORDIAZEPOXIDE, CLONAZEPAM, Clonopin, Deprol (M), DIAZEPAM, Donnatal (M), Equagesic (M), Equanil, Inderal, Inderal-LA, Inderide (M), Inderide-LA (M), Librax (M), Librium, Limbritol (M), LORAZEPAM, Luminal, MEPROBAMATE, Micrainin (M), Milprem (M), Miltown, OXAZEPAM, OXPRENOLOL, Pathibamate (M), PBR-12, PHENOBARBITAL, PROPRANOLOL, Quadrinal (M), Serax, Slow-Transicor, Solfoton, Transicor, Valium, Valrelease and Xanax. (The (M) means it is a mixture or combination drug.) Additional brand names are available.

 ## USES

- Reduces anxiety.
- Helps induce sleep.
- Relaxes muscles.

 ## POSSIBLE ADVERSE REACTIONS OR SIDE EFFECTS

If any of the following occurs, consult a doctor:
- Clumsiness.
- Drowsiness.
- Dizziness.
- Hallucinations.
- Confusion.
- Depression.
- Irritability.
- Rash.
- Itching.
- Vision changes.
- Constipation.
- Diarrhea.
- Nausea.
- Vomiting.
- Difficult urination.
- Vivid dreams.
- Slow heartbeat.
- Breathing difficulty.
- Mouth and throat ulcers.
- Yellow skin and eyes (jaundice).
- Decreased sex drive.

 ## WARNINGS & PRECAUTIONS

- These medications may be habit-forming.
- Don't discontinue abruptly.
- Alcohol use while taking these medications is particularly dangerous.

- Before taking this medicine, consult your doctor if you have brain problems, any chronic lung disease, epilepsy, kidney disease, liver disease, depression, porphyria or myasthenia gravis.
- See Appendix 21.
- Don't drive or try risky physical activity until you know how drug affects you.

 ## AGE-RELATED FACTORS

- Older patients are more likely to have age-related kidney or liver function impairment. This may lead to the need for reduction of the usual dosage.
- Side effects and adverse reactions are more likely to occur with advancing age.
- Doses should be the smallest effective dose to prevent ataxia (unsteady gait), oversedation, dizziness or slow heartbeat.
- Your doctor or care-giver should carefully monitor your response to this drug.

 ## POSSIBLE INTERACTIONS WITH OTHER DRUGS

- If you are using or taking any other drug (prescription or non-prescription), ask your doctor or pharmacist if there are possible interactions.
- Antianxiety medications cannot safely be taken with some drugs.
- Antianxiety medications taken with some drugs may require dosage adjustment.

Do not drink alcoholic beverages or use cocaine, marijuana or tobacco while taking this medicine. These may decrease the effectiveness of the medicine or cause uncomfortable or dangerous adverse reactions.

 ## OVERDOSE

SYMPTOMS
Drowsiness; weakness; tremor; stupor; coma.

WHAT TO DO
- Dial 911 (emergency) or 0 (operator) for an ambulance or medical help. Then give first aid immediately.
- If patient is unconscious and not breathing, give mouth-to-mouth breathing. If there is no heartbeat, use cardiac massage and mouth-to-mouth breathing (CPR). Don't try to make patient vomit. If you can't get help quickly, take patient to nearest emergency facility.

ANTIARRHYTHMICS

BRAND & GENERIC NAMES

Commonly prescribed brand names (start with a Capital) and generic names (all CAPITALS) include BETA BLOCKERS (see separate entry), CALCIUM CHANNEL BLOCKERS (see separate entry), Cardioquin, DISOPYRAMIDE, Duraquin, Isordil, ISOSORBIDE DINITRATE, LIDOCAINE, NITROGLYCERIN, Normodyne, Norpace, PROCAINAMIDE, Procan SR, Pronestyl, Quinaglute, QUINIDINE, Quinora, Timpotic, Xylocaine, Xylocaine with epinephrine (M). (The (M) means it is a mixture or combination drug.) Additional brand names are available.

USES

Controls heartbeat irregularities.

POSSIBLE ADVERSE REACTIONS OR SIDE EFFECTS

If any of the following occurs, consult a doctor:
- Shortness of breath.
- Agitation.
- Nervousness.
- Dizziness.
- Drowsiness.
- Bloating.
- Constipation.
- Appetite loss.
- Abdominal pain.
- Blurred vision.
- Warm, flushed skin.
- Dry mouth.
- Frequent or difficult urination.
- Light-headedness.
- Dry skin.
- Headache.
- Insomnia.
- Weakness.
- Confusion.
- Fever.
- Hives.
- Rash.
- Intense itching.
- Faintness soon after a dose.
- Bitter taste.
- Diarrhea.
- Nausea.
- Vomiting.
- Ringing in ears.
- Unusual bleeding or bruising.
- Difficulty or pain on swallowing.
- Joint pain.
- Jaundice (yellow eyes; yellow skin; dark urine).
- Hepatitis.
- Tiredness.
- Unusually fast or slow heartbeat.
- Wheezing.
- Cough.
- Numbness or tingling in hands and feet.
- Swollen feet, ankles or legs.
- Depression.
- Psychosis.
- Vivid dreams.
- Hair loss.
- Hallucinations.
- Sore throat.
- Convulsions.

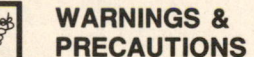

WARNINGS & PRECAUTIONS

- If your diet contains large amounts of fiber, such as bran, tell your doctor.
- Before taking this medicine, consult your doctor if you have diabetes mellitus (sugar diabetes), difficult urination, enlarged prostate, glaucoma (history of), kidney disease, liver disease, myasthenia gravis, asthma, systemic lupus erythematosus (history of), lung disease (severe), heart problems or rheumatic fever.
- Don't drive or try risky physical activity until you know how drug affects you.
- See Appendix 21.

AGE-RELATED FACTORS

- Older patients are more likely to have age-related kidney or liver function impairment. This may lead to the need for reduction of the usual dosage.
- Side effects and adverse reactions are more likely to occur with advancing age.
- Your doctor or care-giver should carefully monitor your response to this drug.

POSSIBLE INTERACTIONS WITH OTHER DRUGS

- If you are using or taking any other drug (prescription or non-prescription), ask your doctor or pharmacist if there are possible interactions.
- Antiarrhythmics cannot safely be taken with some drugs.
- Antiarrhythmics taken with some drugs may require dosage adjustment.

Do not drink alcoholic beverages or use cocaine, marijuana or tobacco while taking this medicine. These may decrease the effectiveness of the medicine or cause uncomfortable or dangerous adverse reactions.

OVERDOSE

SYMPTOMS
Dilated pupils; rapid pulse; rapid breathing; dizziness; fever; hallucinations; confusion; slurred speech; agitation; flushed face; convulsions; coma; cramps; weakness; drowsiness; weak pulse; faint feeling; lethargy; breathing difficulty; fainting; seizures; cardiac arrest.

WHAT TO DO
- Dial 911 (emergency) or 0 (operator) for an ambulance or medical help. Then give first aid immediately.
- If patient is unconscious and not breathing, give mouth-to-mouth breathing. If there is no heartbeat, use cardiac massage and mouth-to-mouth breathing (CPR). Don't try to make patient vomit. If you can't get help quickly, take patient to nearest emergency facility.

MEDICATIONS

ANTIBACTERIAL MEDICATIONS (Ophthalmic)

BRAND & GENERIC NAMES

Commonly prescribed brand names (start with a Capital) and generic names (all CAPITALS) include Achromycin, Ak-Sulf, Bleph, Blephamide (M), Cetamide, CHLORAMPHENICOL (Ophthalmic), Chloromycetin, Chloroptic, E-Mycin, Econochlor, ERYTHROMYCIN (Ophthalmic), Genoptic, Gentacidin, GENTAMYCIN (Ophthalmic), GRAMICIDIN (Ophthalmic), Ilotycin, Metimyd (M), Neosporin (Ophthalmic) (M), Ophthochlor (Ophthalmic), Ophthocort (M), Panmycin, Robitet, Sodium Sulamyd, Sulfacet-R (M), SULFACETAMIDE (Ophthalmic), Sultrin (M), Sumycin, TETRACYCLINE (Ophthalmic), Topicycline and Vasocidin (M). (The (M) means it is a mixture or combination drug.) Additional brand names are available.

 ## USES

Treats bacterial infection of the eye, such as bacterial conjunctivitis (pinkeye).

 ## POSSIBLE ADVERSE REACTIONS OR SIDE EFFECTS

If ointment causes blurred vision for a few minutes, consult a doctor.

 ## WARNINGS & PRECAUTIONS

- You may have increased sensitivity to sun and light.
- Notify doctor if symptoms fail to improve in 2 to 4 days.
- Keep medicine cool, but don't freeze.
- Prolonged use may cause sensitivity reaction.
- Follow doctor's instructions or package insert for proper use of this drug.
- See Appendix 21.

 ## AGE-RELATED FACTORS

None.

 ## POSSIBLE INTERACTIONS WITH OTHER DRUGS

None expected.

 ## OVERDOSE

None expected.

ANTIBACTERIAL MEDICATIONS (Topical)

BRAND & GENERIC NAMES

Commonly prescribed brand names (start with a Capital) and generic names (all CAPITALS) include BACITRACIN (Topical), Bactine (M), CETRIMIDE (Topical), CHLORHEXIDINE (Topical), CLINDAMYCIN (Topical), COLISTIN (Topical), Coly-Mycin S (M), Cortisporin (M), Foile (M), GRAMICIDIN (Topical), Myciguent, Mycitracin (M), Mycolog (M), Neo-Synalar (M), NEOMYCIN (Topical), Neosporin (M), POTASSIUM PERMANGANATE, SILVER SULFADIAZINE (Topical), Spectrocin (M), TETRACYCLINE (Topical) and Triple Antibiotic Ointment (M). (The (M) means it is a mixture or combination drug.) Additional brand names are available.

USES

Treats skin infections that may accompany burns, superficial boils, insect bites or stings, skin ulcers or minor surgical wounds.

POSSIBLE ADVERSE REACTIONS OR SIDE EFFECTS

If new skin irritations appear after starting treatment, consult your doctor.

WARNINGS & PRECAUTIONS

- Heat and moisture can cause breakdown of medicine.
- Keep medicine cool, but don't freeze.
- Follow instructions in package insert.
- See Appendix 21.

AGE-RELATED FACTORS

None.

POSSIBLE INTERACTIONS WITH OTHER DRUGS

Consult a doctor or pharmacist before applying medication if you use any other topical or oral medications with the same name as this product or if you are using any other topical medication on the same area of skin.

OVERDOSE

None expected.

MEDICATIONS

ANTIBIOTICS (Antibacterials)

BRAND & GENERIC NAMES

Commonly prescribed generic names include AMOXICILLIN, AMPICILLIN, BACITRACIN, CEFACLOR, CEFAZOLIN, CEFOXITAN, CEPHALAOTHIN, CEPHALEXIN, CHLORAMPHENICOL, CIPROFLOXACIN, CLISTIN, CLOXACILLIN, DOXYCYCLINE, GENTAMYCIN, GRAMICIDIN, NALDIXIC ACID, NEOMYCIN, NETILMICIN, PENICILLIN G, PENICILLIN V, STREPTOMYCIN, SULFACETAMIDE, SULFASUXIZOLE, TETRACYCLINE and TOBRAMYCIN. Additional brand names are available.

 ## USES

Treats bacterial infections.

 ## POSSIBLE ADVERSE REACTIONS OR SIDE EFFECTS

If any of the following occurs, consult a doctor:
- Nausea.
- Vomiting.
- Diarrhea.
- Yeast infections.
- Skin rashes.
- Fever.
- Painful or swelling joints.
- Wheezing.
- Unexpected bleeding.

 ## WARNINGS & PRECAUTIONS

- Don't take at same time as antacid.
- Some antibiotics cause yeast infections of the gastrointestinal tract and reproductive organs.
- Many antibiotics, particularly penicillin, and many derivatives cause allergic reactions (rashes; fever; swelling; wheezing). Get medical help quickly if this occurs.
- If there are no side effects, complete entire course of medicine.
- Before taking this medicine, consult your doctor if you have kidney disease, liver disease, colitis.
- You may have increased sensitivity to sun and light.
- See Appendix 21.

 ## AGE-RELATED FACTORS

- Older patients are more likely to have age-related kidney or liver function impairment. This may lead to the need for reduction of the usual dosage.
- Toxic effects are more likely.
- Your doctor or care-giver should carefully monitor your response to this drug.

 ## POSSIBLE INTERACTIONS WITH OTHER DRUGS

- If you are using or taking any other drug (prescription or non-prescription), ask your doctor or pharmacist if there are possible interactions.
- Antibiotics cannot safely be taken with some drugs.
- Antibiotics taken with some drugs may require dosage adjustment.

Do not drink alcoholic beverages or use cocaine, marijuana or tobacco while taking this medicine. These may decrease the effectiveness of the medicine or cause uncomfortable or dangerous adverse reactions.

 ## OVERDOSE

SYMPTOMS
Diarrhea; nausea; vomiting.

WHAT TO DO
Overdose unlikely to threaten life. Call doctor, poison control center or hospital emergency room for instructions.

ANTICANCER MEDICATIONS

BRAND & GENERIC NAMES

Commonly prescribed generic names include BUSULFAN, CARMUSTINE, CHLORAMBUCIL, CYCLOPHOSPHAMIDE, CYTABRINE, FLOXURIDINE, FLUOROURACIL, HYDROXYUREA, IFOSFAMIDE, LEUCOVORIN, LOMUSTINE, MECHLORETHAMINE, MELPHALAN, MERCAPTOPURINE, METHOTREXATE, THIOGUANINE, THIOTEPA and URACIL MUSTARD. Additional brand names are available.

USES

Treats cancer.

POSSIBLE ADVERSE REACTIONS OR SIDE EFFECTS

If any of the following occurs, consult a doctor:
- Nausea.
- Vomiting.
- Hair loss.
- Sore throat.
- Fever or chills.
- Mouth sores.
- Confusion.
- Convulsions (seizures).
- Cough.
- Diarrhea.
- Fast or irregular heartbeat.
- Pain at place of injection.
- Painful urination.
- Reddening of skin.
- Shortness of breath.
- Abdominal pain.
- Swelling of feet and lower legs.
- Unusual bleeding or bruising.
- Wheezing.
- Agitation.
- Awkwardness.
- Back pain.
- Darkening or redness of skin (after x-ray treatment).
- Dark or red urine.
- Dizziness.
- Drowsiness.
- Frequent urination.
- Headache.
- Jaw pain.
- Joint pain.
- Slurred speech.
- Unusual thirst.
- Unusual tiredness or weakness.
- Yellow eyes or skin (jaundice).
- Acne.
- Bloating.
- Boils.
- Darkening of soles, palms or nails.
- Flushing or redness of face.
- Itchy skin.
- Loss of appetite.
- Pale skin.
- Rash.
- Colored bumps on fingertips, elbows or palms.
- Sweating.

WARNINGS & PRECAUTIONS

- Have frequent blood cell counts to detect anemia or low white cell counts.
- Avoid contact with people with infections, if possible.
- See Appendix 21.

AGE-RELATED FACTORS

- Side effects and adverse reactions are more likely to occur with advancing age.
- Your doctor or care-giver should carefully monitor your response to this drug.

POSSIBLE INTERACTIONS WITH OTHER DRUGS

- If you are using or taking any other drug (prescription or non-prescription), ask your doctor or pharmacist if there are possible interactions.
- Anticancer drugs cannot safely be taken with some drugs.
- Anticancer drugs taken with some drugs may require dosage adjustment.

Do not drink alcoholic beverages or use cocaine, marijuana or tobacco while taking this medicine. These may decrease the effectiveness of the medicine or cause uncomfortable or dangerous adverse reactions.

OVERDOSE

SYMPTOMS
Combination of any of the above adverse reactions.

WHAT TO DO
- Dial 911 (emergency) or 0 (operator) for an ambulance or medical help. Then give first aid immediately.
- If patient is unconscious and not breathing, give mouth-to-mouth breathing. If there is no heartbeat, use cardiac massage and mouth-to-mouth breathing (CPR). Don't try to make patient vomit. If you can't get help quickly, take patient to nearest emergency facility.

ANTICOAGULANTS (Thrombolytics)

BRAND & GENERIC NAMES

Commonly prescribed brand names (start with a Capital) and generic names (all CAPITALS) include Calciprine, Coumadin, DICUMAROL, DIPYRIDAMOLE, Embolex, HEPARIN, Hepin Liquaemin, Lipo, Panwarfin, Persantine and WARFARIN. Additional brand names are available.

USES

- Prevents blood from clotting in blood vessels.
- Treats abnormal clotting inside blood vessels.

POSSIBLE ADVERSE REACTIONS OR SIDE EFFECTS

If any of the following occurs, consult a doctor:
- Bloating.
- Gas.
- Black stools.
- Bloody vomit.
- Coughing up blood.
- Rash.
- Hives.
- Itching.
- Blurred vision.
- Sore throat.
- Easy bruising.
- Bleeding.
- Cloudy or red urine.
- Back pain.
- Jaundice (yellow eyes, yellow skin, dark urine).
- Fever.
- Chills.
- Fatigue.
- Weakness.
- Diarrhea.
- Cramps.
- Nausea.
- Vomiting.
- Swollen feet or legs.
- Hair loss.
- Skin starts dying.
- Dizziness.
- Headache.
- Mouth sores.

WARNINGS & PRECAUTIONS

- Carry notification (a card, necklace or bracelet) to state you take anticoagulants.
- Don't discontinue medication abruptly.
- Before taking this medicine, consult your doctor if you have recently had any of the following conditions or medical procedures: falls or blows to the body or head, fever lasting more than a couple of days, medical or dental surgery, severe or continuing diarrhea, spinal anesthesia or x-ray (radiation) treatment.
- See Appendix 21.

AGE-RELATED FACTORS

- Side effects and adverse reactions are more likely to occur with advancing age.
- Your doctor or care-giver should carefully monitor your response to this drug.
- Dosage may need to be reduced as you get older.

POSSIBLE INTERACTIONS WITH OTHER DRUGS

Consult a doctor first if you take any medication (prescription, non-prescription, herbs, vitamins or minerals).

Do not drink alcoholic beverages or use cocaine, marijuana or tobacco while taking this medicine. These may decrease the effectiveness of the medicine or cause uncomfortable or dangerous adverse reactions.

OVERDOSE

SYMPTOMS
Bloody vomit; bloody or black stools; red urine.

WHAT TO DO
- Dial 911 (emergency) or 0 (operator) for an ambulance or medical help. Then give first aid immediately.
- If patient is unconscious and not breathing, give mouth-to-mouth breathing. If there is no heartbeat, use cardiac massage and mouth-to-mouth breathing (CPR). Don't try to make patient vomit. If you can't get help quickly, take patient to nearest emergency facility.

ANTICONVULSANTS

BRAND & GENERIC NAMES

Commonly prescribed brand names (start with a Capital) and generic names (all CAPITALS) include Barbita, CARBAMAZIPINE, CLONAZEPAM, Clonopin, Depakene, Depakote, DIAZEPAM, Dilantin, Dilantin with Phenobarbital (M), Dyphenylan, ETHOSUXIMIDE, Luminal, Myidone, Mysoline, PBR-12, PHENOBARBITAL, PHENYTOIN, PRIMIDONE, Solfoton, Tegretol, Valium, VALPROIC ACID, Valrelease and Zarontin. (The (M) means it is a mixture or combination drug.) Additional brand names are available.

 ## USES

Prevents epileptic seizures.

 ## POSSIBLE ADVERSE REACTIONS OR SIDE EFFECTS

If any of the following occurs, consult a doctor:
- Enlarged, tender, receding or bleeding gums.
- Nausea.
- Vomiting.
- Constipation (mild).
- Dizziness.
- Sleeplessness.
- Hallucinations.
- Confusion.
- Slurred speech.
- Staggering.
- Rash.
- Change in vision.
- Headache.
- Diarrhea.
- Drowsiness.
- Muscle twitching.
- Increased body and facial hair.
- Sore throat.
- Fever.
- Abdominal pain.
- Unusual bleeding or bruising.
- Swollen lymph glands.
- Jaundice (yellow eyes; yellow skin; dark urine).

 ## WARNINGS & PRECAUTIONS

- Many people will need to take anticonvulsants for their entire life.
- Don't stop using anticonvulsants abruptly.
- Don't drink alcohol while taking this medication.
- Before taking this medicine, consult your doctor if you have blood disease, intermittent porphyria, kidney disease (severe), liver disease, diseases of the eye or optic nerve, alcoholism (active), diabetes mellitus (sugar diabetes), heart disease or thyroid disease.

- Don't drive or try risky physical activity until you know how drug affects you.
- You may have increased sensitivity to sun and light.
- See Appendix 21.

 ## AGE-RELATED FACTORS

- Older patients are more likely to have age-related kidney or liver function impairment. This may lead to the need for reduction of the usual dosage.
- Side effects and adverse reactions are more likely to occur with advancing age.
- Your doctor or care-giver should carefully monitor your response to this drug.

 ## POSSIBLE INTERACTIONS WITH OTHER DRUGS

- If you are using or taking any other drug (prescription or non-prescription), ask your doctor or pharmacist if there are possible interactions.
- Anticonvulsants cannot safely be taken with some drugs.
- Anticonvulsants taken with some drugs may require dosage adjustment.

Do not drink alcoholic beverages or use cocaine, marijuana or tobacco while taking this medicine. These may decrease the effectiveness of the medicine or cause uncomfortable or dangerous adverse reactions.

 ## OVERDOSE

SYMPTOMS
Jerky eye movements; staggering; slurred speech; imbalance; drowsiness; blood pressure drop; slow, shallow breathing; coma.

WHAT TO DO
- Dial 911 (emergency) or 0 (operator) for an ambulance or medical help. Then give first aid immediately.
- If patient is unconscious and not breathing, give mouth-to-mouth breathing. If there is no heartbeat, use cardiac massage and mouth-to-mouth breathing (CPR). Don't try to make patient vomit. If you can't get help quickly, take patient to nearest emergency facility.

ANTIDEPRESSANT MEDICATIONS (FLUOXETINE)

BRAND & GENERIC NAMES

Commonly prescribed brand names (start with a Capital) and generic names (all CAPITALS) include FLUOXETINE and Prozac.

 USES

Treats mental depression, particularly in people who do not tolerate other antidepressant medicines such as tricyclic antidepressants.

 POSSIBLE ADVERSE REACTIONS OR SIDE EFFECTS

If any of the following occurs, consult a doctor:
- Rash.
- Itchy skin.
- Breathing difficulty.
- Chest pain.
- Diarrhea.
- Nervousness.
- Drowsiness.
- Headache.
- Increased sweating.
- Weight loss.
- Chills; fever; joint or muscle pain.
- Enlarged lymph glands.
- Blurred vision.
- Unusual excitability.
- Convulsions.
- Fast heartbeat.
- Abdominal pain.
- Nausea and vomiting.
- Constipation.
- Cough.

 WARNINGS & PRECAUTIONS

- Don't take if you have severe liver or kidney disease.
- Don't take without consulting your doctor if you have a history of seizure disorders.

 AGE-RELATED FACTORS

- Side effects and adverse reactions are more likely to occur with advancing age.
- Lower-than-standard doses and longer intervals between doses may be required.
- Your doctor or care-giver should carefully monitor your response to this drug.

 POSSIBLE INTERACTIONS WITH OTHER DRUGS

- If you are using or taking any other drug (prescription or non-prescription), ask your doctor or pharmacist if there are possible interactions.
- Don't drive or engage in risky physical activity until you see how this medicine affects you.
- Don't discontinue taking this drug without consulting your doctor. Dose may require gradual reduction if you have taken drug for a long time. Doses of other drugs may also require adjustment.

Do not drink alcoholic beverages or use cocaine, marijuana or tobacco while taking this medicine. These may decrease the effectiveness of the medicine or cause uncomfortable or dangerous adverse reactions.

 OVERDOSE

SYMPTOMS
Confusion.

WHAT TO DO
- Dial 911 (emergency) or 0 (operator) for an ambulance or medical help. Then give first aid immediately.
- If patient is unconscious and not breathing, give mouth-to-mouth breathing. If there is no heartbeat, use cardiac massage and mouth-to-mouth breathing (CPR). Don't try to make patient vomit. If you can't get help quickly, take patient to nearest emergency facility.

ANTIDEPRESSANTS, TRICYCLIC

BRAND & GENERIC NAMES

Commonly prescribed brand names (start with a Capital) and generic names (all CAPITALS) include Adepin, Amitril, AMITRIPTYLINE, AMOXAPINE, Ascendin, Desyrel, DOXEPIN, Elavil, Etrafon, IMIPRAMINE, Janimine, Limbitrol, Ludiomil, MAPROTILINE, MONOAMINE OXIDASE INHIBITORS (see separate entry under MAO Inhibitors), NORTRIPTYLINE, Pamelor, Sinequan, SK-Pramine, Tofranil, TRAZADONE and Triavil. Additional brand names are available.

 ## USES

- Gradually relieves, but doesn't cure, symptoms of depression.
- Pain relief (sometimes).
- Relieves inflammation of sensory nerves in arms, legs, hands and feet (sometimes).

 ## POSSIBLE ADVERSE REACTIONS OR SIDE EFFECTS

If any of the following occurs, consult a doctor:

- Seizures.
- Tremor.
- Headache.
- Dry mouth.
- Unpleasant taste.
- Constipation.
- Diarrhea.
- Nausea.
- Indigestion.
- Fatigue.
- Drowsiness.
- Nervousness.
- Anxiety.
- Excessive sweating.
- Insomnia.
- Sweet tooth.
- Hallucinations.
- Shakiness.
- Dizziness.
- Fainting.
- Blurred vision.
- Eye pain.
- Vomiting.
- Irregular heartbeat.
- Slow pulse.
- Inflamed tongue.
- Abdominal pain.
- Jaundice (yellow eyes; yellow skin; dark urine).
- Hair loss.
- Rash.
- Fever.
- Chills.
- Joint pain.
- Palpitations.
- Hiccups.
- Visual changes.
- Difficult or frequent urination.
- Decreased sex drive.
- Muscle aches.
- Abnormal dreams.
- Nasal congestion.
- Weakness and faintness when arising from bed or chair.
- Back pain.
- Itchy skin.
- Sore throat.
- Involuntary movements of jaw, lips and tongue.
- Confusion.
- Swollen breasts in males.
- Decreased potassium (by blood test).

 ## WARNINGS & PRECAUTIONS

- Before taking this medicine, consult your doctor if you have alcoholism (active), asthma, manic-depressive illness, blood disorders, convulsions (seizures), difficult urination, enlarged prostate, glaucoma, increased eye pressure, heart disease, liver disease, overactive thyroid, schizophrenia or stomach or intestinal problems.
- Don't drive or try risky physical activity until you know how drug affects you.
- You may have increased sensitivity to sun and light.
- See Appendix 21.

 ## AGE-RELATED FACTORS

- Toxic effects are more likely.
- Older patients are more likely to have age-related kidney or liver function impairment. This may lead to the need for reduction of the usual dosage.
- Males more likely to experience urinary retention.
- Your doctor or care-giver should carefully monitor your response to this drug.
- In the presence of heart disease, adverse reactions are even more likely.

 ## POSSIBLE INTERACTIONS WITH OTHER DRUGS

- If you are taking any other drug (prescription or non-prescription), ask your doctor or pharmacist if there are possible interactions.
- Tricyclic antidepressants cannot safely be taken with some drugs.
- Tricyclic antidepressants taken with some drugs may require dosage adjustment.

Do not drink alcoholic beverages or use cocaine, marijuana or tobacco while taking this medicine. These may decrease the effectiveness of the medicine or cause uncomfortable or dangerous adverse reactions.

 ## OVERDOSE

SYMPTOMS

Hallucinations; respiratory failure; fever; cardiac arrhythmias; convulsions; coma.

WHAT TO DO

- Dial 911 (emergency) or 0 (operator) for an ambulance or medical help. Then give first aid immediately.
- If patient is unconscious and not breathing, give mouth-to-mouth breathing. If there is no heartbeat, use cardiac massage and mouth-to-mouth breathing (CPR). Don't try to make patient vomit. If you can't get help quickly, take patient to nearest emergency facility.

ANTIDIABETICS, ORAL (Hypoglycemics, Oral)

BRAND & GENERIC NAMES

Commonly prescribed brand names (start with a Capital) and generic names (all CAPITALS) include ACETOHEXAMIDE, CHLORPROPAMIDE, Dia Beta, Diabenese, Dymelor, GLIPIZIDE, Glucotrol, GLYBURIDE, Micronase, Orimide, Orinase, TOLAZAMIDE, TOLBUTAMIDE and Tolinase. Additional brand names are available.

USES

Treats diabetes in adults who can't control blood sugar by diet, weight loss and exercise.

POSSIBLE ADVERSE REACTIONS OR SIDE EFFECTS

If any of the following occurs, consult a doctor:
- Low blood sugar (hunger; anxiety; cold sweats; rapid pulse).
- Dizziness.
- Diarrhea.
- Appetite loss.
- Nausea.
- Stomach pain.
- Heartburn.
- Fatigue.
- Itching.
- Rash.
- Ringing in ears.
- Sore throat.
- Fever.
- Unusual bleeding or bruising.
- Jaundice (yellow eyes; yellow skin; dark urine).

WARNINGS & PRECAUTIONS

- Before taking this medicine, consult your doctor if you have allergy to sulfa, adrenal disease, infection (severe), kidney disease, liver disease, pituitary disease, thyroid disease or heart disease.
- You may have increased sensitivity to sun and light.
- See Appendix 21.

AGE-RELATED FACTORS

- Older patients are more likely to have age-related kidney or liver function impairment. This may lead to the need for reduction of the usual dosage.
- Your doctor or care-giver should carefully monitor your response to this drug.

POSSIBLE INTERACTIONS WITH OTHER DRUGS

- If you are taking any other drug (prescription or non-prescription), ask your doctor or pharmacist if there are possible interactions.
- Antidiabetics cannot safely be taken with some drugs.
- Antidiabetics taken with some drugs may require dosage adjustment.

Do not drink alcoholic beverages or use cocaine, marijuana or tobacco while taking this medicine. These may decrease the effectiveness of the medicine or cause uncomfortable or dangerous adverse reactions.

OVERDOSE

SYMPTOMS
Excessive hunger; nausea; anxiety; cool skin; cold sweats; drowsiness; rapid heartbeat; weakness; unconsciousness; coma.

WHAT TO DO
- Dial 911 (emergency) or 0 (operator) for an ambulance or medical help. Then give first aid immediately.
- If patient is unconscious and not breathing, give mouth-to-mouth breathing. If there is no heartbeat, use cardiac massage and mouth-to-mouth breathing (CPR). Don't try to make patient vomit. If you can't get help quickly, take patient to nearest emergency facility.

ANTIDIARRHEALS

BRAND & GENERIC NAMES

Commonly prescribed brand names (start with a Capital) and generic names (all CAPITALS) include Antispas, Band O Suprettes (M), BELLADONNA, Bellergal (M), Bentyl, CODEINE, Cologel, DICYCLOMINE, DIPHENOXYLATE WITH ATROPINE, Effersyllium, Empirin with Codeine, Fiberall (M), Hydrocil, Imodium, KAOLIN, Kaopectate, Konsyl, Lomotil, LOPERAMIDE, Metamucil, METHYLCELLULOSE, Murocel (M), Neoquess, Perdiem (M), Phenaphen with Codeine, PSYLLIUM and Wyanoids (M). (The (M) means it is a mixture or combination drug.) Additional brand names are available.

 ## USES

Relieves diarrhea. Some preparations (with kaolin, chalk or charcoal) absorb extra fluid; others slow contractions of bowel muscle to retard diarrhea.

 ## POSSIBLE ADVERSE REACTIONS OR SIDE EFFECTS

If any of the following occurs, consult a doctor:
- Hives.
- Rash.
- Intense itching.
- Faintness soon after a dose.
- Dry mouth.
- Swollen gums.
- Rapid heartbeat.
- Dizziness.
- Depression.
- Drowsiness.
- Itching.
- Blurred vision.
- Decreased urination.
- Restlessness.
- Flush.
- Fever.
- Headache.
- Stomach pain.
- Nausea.
- Vomiting.
- Bloating.
- Constipation.
- Numbness of hands or feet.

 ## WARNINGS & PRECAUTIONS

- Don't use for prolonged periods. They may cause constipation.
- Before taking this medicine, consult your doctor if you have alcoholism, colitis, intestinal disease, emphysema, asthma, bronchitis, chronic lung disease, enlarged prostate, gallbladder disease, gallstones, heart disease, irregular heartbeat, kidney disease, liver disease, underactive thyroid, hiatal hernia, high blood pressure, myasthenia gravis, urinary tract blockage or difficult urination.
- See Appendix 21.

 ## AGE-RELATED FACTORS

Side effects and adverse reactions are more likely to occur with advancing age.

 ## POSSIBLE INTERACTIONS WITH OTHER DRUGS

- If you are taking any other drug (prescription or non-prescription), ask your doctor or pharmacist if there are possible interactions.
- Antidiarrheals cannot safely be taken with some drugs.
- Antidiarrheals taken with some drugs may require dosage adjustment.

Do not drink alcoholic beverages or use cocaine, marijuana or tobacco while taking this medicine. These may decrease the effectiveness of the medicine or cause uncomfortable or dangerous adverse reactions.

 ## OVERDOSE

SYMPTOMS
Excitement; constricted pupils; shallow breathing; coma.

WHAT TO DO
- Dial 911 (emergency) or 0 (operator) for an ambulance or medical help. Then give first aid immediately.
- If patient is unconscious and not breathing, give mouth-to-mouth breathing. If there is no heartbeat, use cardiac massage and mouth-to-mouth breathing (CPR). Don't try to make patient vomit. If you can't get help quickly, take patient to nearest emergency facility.

ANTIEMETICS

BRAND & GENERIC NAMES

Commonly prescribed brand names (start with a Capital) and generic names (all CAPITALS) include Anergan, ANTIHISTAMINES (see separate entry), Antivert, Bonine, Combid (M), Compazine, DIMENHYDRINATE, Dramamine, Etrafon (M), FLUPHENAZINE, MECLIZINE, METOCLOPRAMIDE, PERPHENAZINE, Phenazine, Pro-Iso, PROCHLOPERAZINE, PROMAZINE, PROMETHAZINE, Prorex, Reglan, Ru-Vert-M, Sparine, Triavil (M) and Trilafon. (The (M) means it is a mixture or combination drug.) Additional brand names are available.

USES

- Treats nausea and vomiting.
- Some, such as Antivert (MECLIZINE), prevent motion sickness.

POSSIBLE ADVERSE REACTIONS OR SIDE EFFECTS

If any of the following occurs, consult a doctor:
- Drowsiness.
- Headache.
- Diarrhea.
- Constipation.
- Fast heartbeat.
- Dry mouth, nose or throat.
- Rash.
- Hives.
- Restlessness.
- Excitement.
- Insomnia.
- Blurred vision.
- Frequent or difficult urination.
- Appetite loss.
- Nausea.

WARNINGS & PRECAUTIONS

- Don't take if cause of nausea or vomiting is unknown.
- Before taking this medicine, consult your doctor if you have alcoholism (active), blood disease, breast cancer, difficult urination, enlarged prostate, glaucoma, heart disease, blood vessel disease, liver disease, lung disease, Parkinson's disease, seizure disorders or stomach ulcers.
- Don't drive or try risky physical activity until you know how drug affects you.
- See Appendix 21.

AGE-RELATED FACTORS

- Older patients are more likely to have age-related kidney or liver function impairment. This may lead to the need for reduction of the usual dosage.
- Side effects and adverse reactions are more likely to occur with advancing age.
- Males more likely to experience urinary retention.
- Your doctor or care-giver should carefully monitor your response to this drug.

POSSIBLE INTERACTIONS WITH OTHER DRUGS

- If you are taking any other drug (prescription or non-prescription), ask your doctor or pharmacist if there are possible interactions.
- Antiemetics cannot safely be taken with some drugs.
- Antiemetics taken with some drugs may require dosage adjustment.

Do not drink alcoholic beverages or use cocaine, marijuana or tobacco while taking this medicine. These may decrease the effectiveness of the medicine or cause uncomfortable or dangerous adverse reactions.

OVERDOSE

SYMPTOMS
Drowsiness; confusion; lack of coordination; stupor; coma; weak pulse; shallow breathing; hallucinations.

WHAT TO DO
- Dial 911 (emergency) or 0 (operator) for an ambulance or medical help. Then give first aid immediately.
- If patient is unconscious and not breathing, give mouth-to-mouth breathing. If there is no heartbeat, use cardiac massage and mouth-to-mouth breathing (CPR). Don't try to make patient vomit. If you can't get help quickly, take patient to nearest emergency facility.

ANTIFUNGAL MEDICATIONS (Topical)

BRAND & GENERIC NAMES

Commonly prescribed brand names (start with a Capital) and generic names (all CAPITALS) include AMPHOTERICIN B (Topical), CICLOPIROX (Topical), CLOTRIMAZOLE (Topical), ECONAZOLE (Topical), Fungizone, KETOCONAZOLE (Topical), Loprox, Lotrimin, Micatin, MICONAZOLE (Topical), Mycelex (Topical), Mycostatin (Topical), Nilstat (Topical), Nizoral (Topical), NYSTATIN (Topical), Nystex (Topical), Spectazole, Tinactin (Topical), TOLNAFTATE (Topical) and Zeasorb-AF. Additional brand names are available.

 ## USES

Fights fungal infections, such as ringworm of the scalp, athelete's foot, jock itch, "sun fungus," nail fungus and others.

 ## POSSIBLE ADVERSE REACTIONS OR SIDE EFFECTS

If itching, redness or swelling of treated skin appears after treatment starts, consult a doctor.

 ## WARNINGS & PRECAUTIONS

- Avoid contact with the eyes.
- Heat and moisture can cause breakdown of medicine.
- Keep medicine cool, but don't freeze.
- Store medicine away from heat and sunlight.
- Don't use on other family members without consulting doctor.
- If using for jock itch, don't wear tight underwear.
- If using for athelete's foot, dry feet carefully after bathing and wear clean cotton socks with sandals or well-ventilated shoes.
- See Appendix 21.
- You may have increased sensitivity to sun and light.

 ## AGE-RELATED FACTORS

Side effects and adverse reactions are more likely to occur with advancing age.

 ## POSSIBLE INTERACTIONS WITH OTHER DRUGS

Consult your doctor or pharmacist if you use any other topical medicine on the infected skin.

 ## OVERDOSE

None expected.

BRAND & GENERIC NAMES

Commonly prescribed brand names (start with a Capital) and generic names (all CAPITALS) include BUTOCONAZOLE (Vaginal), Canesten (Vaginal), CLOTRIMAZOLE (Vaginal), ECONAZOLE (Vaginal), Ecostatin (Vaginal), GENETIAN VIOLET (Vaginal), Gyne-Lotrimin, MICONAZOLE (Vaginal), Monistat (Vaginal), Mycelex-G (Vaginal), Mycostatin (Vaginal), Nadostine (Vaginal), Nilstat (Vaginal), NYSTATIN (Vaginal), Terazol 3 and TERCONAZOLE (Vaginal). Additional brand names are available.

 ## USES

Treats fungal (yeast) infections of the vagina.

 ## POSSIBLE ADVERSE REACTIONS OR SIDE EFFECTS

If any of the following occurs after treatment is started, consult a doctor:
* Burning.
* Itching.
* Swelling of labia.
* Rash.
* Hives.
* Irritation of sex partner's genitals.

 ## WARNINGS & PRECAUTIONS

* Keep the genital area clean. Use plain unscented soap.
* Take showers rather than tub baths.
* Wear cotton briefs or pantyhose with a cotton crotch. Avoid briefs made of non-ventilating materials. Wear freshly laundered underwear.
* Don't sit around in wet clothing—especially a wet bathing suit.
* Taking antibiotics may cause yeast infections. Ask your doctor about eating yogurt, sour cream or buttermilk or taking acidophilus tablets as a preventive if you must take antibiotics in the future.
* After urination or bowel movements, cleanse by wiping or washing from front to back (vagina to anus).
* Don't douche unless your doctor recommends it.
* If urinating causes burning, urinate through a tubular device (such as a toilet paper roll or a plastic cup with the end cut out) or pour cup of warm water over genital area as you urinate.
* See Appendix 21.

 ## AGE-RELATED FACTORS

Irritation of sensitive vaginal lining may be more likely with advancing age.

 ## POSSIBLE INTERACTIONS WITH OTHER DRUGS

Consult your doctor or pharmacist if you use any other topical vaginal medication.

 ## OVERDOSE

None expected.

ANTIGLAUCOMA EYEDROPS

BRAND & GENERIC NAMES

Commonly prescribed brand names (start with a Capital) and generic names (all CAPITALS) include ACETAZOLAMIDE, Adsorbocarpine, Ak-Zol, Blocadren, Dazamide, Diamox, E-Pilo (M), Isopto P-ES (M), Isopto Carpine, Ocusert Pilo, Pilocarpine HS, TIMOLOL and Timoptic. (The (M) means it is a mixture or combination drug.) Additional brand names are available.

USES

Treats glaucoma (open-angle; secondary; angle-closure during or after eye surgery).

POSSIBLE ADVERSE REACTIONS OR SIDE EFFECTS

If any of the following occurs, consult a doctor:
- Headache.
- Stinging, burning, watery eyes.
- Eye pain.
- Changes in vision.
- Blurred vision.
- Faintness.
- Increased sweating.
- Irregular or fast heartbeat.
- Paleness.

WARNINGS & PRECAUTIONS

- Don't drive or try risky physical activity until you know how drug affects you.
- Before taking this medicine, consult your doctor if you have other eye disease, Parkinson's disease, heart disease, asthma, myasthenia gravis, stomach problems, urinary problems, overactive thyroid or high blood pressure.
- Follow doctor's instructions or package insert information on how to use the drops or ointment.
- Keep container tightly closed.
- Keep medicine cool, but don't freeze.
- Wash hands immediately after using.
- See Appendix 21.

AGE-RELATED FACTORS

Side effects and adverse reactions more likely to occur with advancing age.

POSSIBLE INTERACTIONS WITH OTHER DRUGS

- If you are taking any other drug (prescription or non-prescription), ask your doctor or pharmacist if there are possible interactions.
- Antiglaucoma eyedrops cannot safely be used with some drugs.
- Antiglaucoma eyedrops used with some drugs may require dosage adjustment.

OVERDOSE

None expected.

ANTIHISTAMINES

BRAND & GENERIC NAMES

Commonly prescribed brand names (start with a Capital) and generic names (all CAPITALS) include Actidil, Actifed, Aller-Chlor, Allerfin, Allermine, Atarax, AZATADINE, Benadryl, Benadryl Decongestant, Bendylate, Benylin, Bromphen, BROMPHINERAMINE, Chlor-Trimeton, CHLORPHENIRAMINE, CLEMASTINE, Deconamine (M), DIMENHYDRINATE, Dimetane, DIPHENHYDRAMINE, Drixoral, Durrax, Histex, HYDROXYZINE, MECLIZINE, Myidil, Naldecon (M), Optimine, Ornade (M), PROMETHAZINE, Rynatan (M), Seldane, Tavist-D, Teldin, Temaril, TERFENADINE, TRIMEPRAZINE, Trinalin (M), Triphed, TRIPOLIDINE, Tussi-Organidin (M), Valdrene, Vistaril. (The (M) means it is a mixture or combination drug.) Additional brand names are available.

USES

- Reduces allergic symptoms, such as hay fever, hives, rash or itching.
- Prevents motion sickness, nausea and vomiting.
- Aids sleep.

POSSIBLE ADVERSE REACTIONS OR SIDE EFFECTS

If any of the following occurs, consult a doctor:
- Drowsiness.
- Dizziness.
- Dry mouth, nose or throat.
- Nausea.
- Vision changes.
- Less tolerance for contact lenses.
- Difficult urination.
- Appetite loss.
- Nightmares.
- Agitation.
- Irritability.
- Sore throat.
- Fever.
- Rapid heartbeat.
- Unusual bleeding or bruising.
- Fatigue.
- Weakness.

WARNINGS & PRECAUTIONS

- Before taking this medicine, consult your doctor if you have asthma attacks, enlarged prostate, glaucoma, urinary tract blockage or difficult urination.
- Don't drive or try risky physical activity until you know how drug affects you.

- You may have increased sensitivity to sun and light.
- See Appendix 21.

AGE-RELATED FACTORS

- Dizziness, sedation, confusion, dry mouth, urinary retention, and a drop in blood pressure more likely with advancing age.
- Older patients are more likely to have age-related kidney or liver function impairment. This may lead to the need for reduction of the usual dosage.
- Other side effects and other adverse reactions are more likely to occur with advancing age, except for TERFENADINE, ASTEMIZOLE AND LORATIDINE.

POSSIBLE INTERACTIONS WITH OTHER DRUGS

- If you are taking any other drug (prescription or non-prescription), ask your doctor or pharmacist if there are possible interactions.
- Antihistamines cannot safely be taken with some drugs.
- Antihistamines taken with some drugs may require dosage adjustment.

Do not drink alcoholic beverages or use cocaine, marijuana or tobacco while taking this medicine. These may decrease the effectiveness of the medicine or cause uncomfortable or dangerous adverse reactions.

OVERDOSE

SYMPTOMS
Convulsions; red face; hallucinations; coma.

WHAT TO DO
- Dial 911 (emergency) or 0 (operator) for an ambulance or medical help. Then give first aid immediately.
- If patient is unconscious and not breathing, give mouth-to-mouth breathing. If there is no heartbeat, use cardiac massage and mouth-to-mouth breathing (CPR). Don't try to make patient vomit. If you can't get help quickly, take patient to nearest emergency facility.

ANTIHYPERTENSIVES
(High Blood Pressure Medicine)

BRAND & GENERIC NAMES

Commonly prescribed brand names (start with a Capital) and generic names (all CAPITALS) include Aldeclor (M), Aldomet, Aldoril (M), ANGIOTENSIN-CONVERTING ENZYME INHIBITORS (see separate entry), Apresazide (M), Apresoline (M), BETA-ADRENERGIC BLOCKERS (see separate entry), CALCIUM CHANNEL BLOCKERS (see separate entry), Catapres, CLONIDINE, Combipres (M), DIURETICS (see separtate entry), GUANETHIDINE, HYDRALAZINE, Ismelin, METHYLDOPA, Minipres, PRAZOSIN, Ser-Ap-Es (M) and Unipres. (The (M) means it is a mixture or combination drug.) Additional brand names are available.

USES

- Treats high blood pressure. Note: ACE inhibitors, beta-adrenergic blockers, calcium channel blockers and diuretics are also used to treat high blood pressure.
- Prevents vascular headache (CLONIDINE).
- Treats congestive heart failure.

POSSIBLE ADVERSE REACTIONS OR SIDE EFFECTS

If any of the following occurs, consult a doctor:
- Chest pain.
- Irregular or fast heartbeat.
- Weak pulse.
- Nausea.
- Vomiting.
- Headache.
- Diarrhea.
- Appetite loss.
- Frequent urination.
- Dry mouth.
- Thirst.
- Rash.
- Black, bloody or tarry stool.
- Red or flushed face.
- Sore throat.
- Fever.
- Mouth sores.
- Constipation.
- Swollen lymph glands.
- Blurred vision.
- Dizziness.
- Confusion.
- Watery eyes.
- Joint pain.
- Weight gain.
- Weight loss.
- Jaundice (yellow eyes; yellow skin; dark urine).

WARNINGS & PRECAUTIONS

- May cause lupus (an arthritis-like illness).
- Possible psychosis.
- May cause numbness and tingling in hands or feet.

- Before taking this medicine, consult your doctor if you have angina, heart disease, blood vessel disease, irritated or scraped skin (when using transdermal skin patch system), kidney disease, mental depression (history of), Raynaud's syndrome, systemic lupus erythematosus, Parkinson's disease, diabetes, gout or pancreatitis.
- Don't drive or try risky physical activity until you know how drug affects you.
- See Appendix 21.

AGE-RELATED FACTORS

- Older patients are more likely to have age-related kidney or liver function impairment. This may lead to the need for reduction of the usual dosage.
- Side effects and adverse reactions are more likely to occur with advancing age.

POSSIBLE INTERACTIONS WITH OTHER DRUGS

- If you are taking any other drug (prescription or non-prescription), ask your doctor or pharmacist if there are possible interactions.
- Antihypertensives cannot safely be taken with some drugs.
- Antihypertensives taken with some drugs may require dosage adjustment.

Do not drink alcoholic beverages or use cocaine, marijuana or tobacco while taking this medicine. These may decrease the effectiveness of the medicine or cause uncomfortable or dangerous adverse reactions.

OVERDOSE

SYMPTOMS
Severe cramps; drowsiness; weak pulse; rapid and weak heartbeat; fainting; extreme weakness; cold, sweaty skin; coma.

WHAT TO DO
- Dial 911 (emergency) or 0 (operator) for an ambulance or medical help. Then give first aid immediately.
- If patient is unconscious and not breathing, give mouth-to-mouth breathing. If there is no heartbeat, use cardiac massage and mouth-to-mouth breathing (CPR). Don't try to make patient vomit. If you can't get help quickly, take patient to nearest emergency facility.

ANTIPARKINSONISM MEDICATIONS

BRAND & GENERIC NAMES

Commonly prescribed brand names (start with a Capital) and generic names (all CAPITALS) include AMANTADINE, Artane, BENZTROPINE, BROMOCRIPTINE, Cogentin, Disipal, Dopar, Flexoject, Kermadrin, Larodopa, LEVODOPA, Marflex, Norflex, Norgesic (M), ORPHENADRINE, Parlodel, PROCYCLIDINE, SELEGILINE, Sinemet (M), Symmetrel, Tremin, Trihexane, TRIHEXYPHENIDYL and X-Otag. Additional brand names are available.

USES

Controls Parkinson's disease symptoms such as rigidity, tremor and unsteady gait.

POSSIBLE ADVERSE REACTIONS OR SIDE EFFECTS

If any of the following occurs, consult a doctor:
- Mood changes.
- Uncontrollable body movements.
- Diarrhea.
- Dry mouth.
- Body odor.
- Fainting.
- Severe dizziness.
- Headache.
- Insomnia.
- Nightmares.
- Rash.
- Itch.
- Nausea and vomiting.
- Irregular heartbeat.
- Flushed face.
- Blurred vision.
- Muscle twitching.
- Discolored or dark urine.
- Difficult urination.
- Constipation.
- Tiredness.
- Upper abdominal pain.

WARNINGS & PRECAUTIONS

- Don't take if you are allergic to levodopa or carbidopa.
- Before taking this medicine, consult your doctor if you have diabetes, epilepsy, high blood pressure, heart disease, lung disease, liver disease, kidney disease, peptic ulcer or malignant melanoma; if you have taken MAO inhibitors (see Glossary) in the last 2 weeks; or if you plan to have surgery (including dental) within 2 months.
- See Appendix 21.

AGE-RELATED FACTORS

- Older patients are more likely to have age-related kidney or liver function impairment. This may lead to the need for reduction of the usual dosage.
- Toxic effects are more likely.
- Males more likely to experience urinary retention.

POSSIBLE INTERACTIONS WITH OTHER DRUGS

- If you are taking any other drug (prescription or non-prescription), ask your doctor or pharmacist if there are possible interactions.
- Antiparkinsonism medicines cannot safely be taken with some drugs.
- Antiparkinsonism medicines taken with some drugs may require dosage adjustment.

Do not drink alcoholic beverages or use cocaine, marijuana or tobacco while taking this medicine. These may decrease the effectiveness of the medicine or cause uncomfortable or dangerous adverse reactions.

OVERDOSE

SYMPTOMS
Muscles twitch; spastic eyelid closure; nausea; vomiting; diarrhea; irregular and rapid pulse; weakness; fainting; confusion; agitation; hallucination; coma.

WHAT TO DO
- Dial 911 (emergency) or 0 (operator) for an ambulance or medical help. Then give first aid immediately.
- If patient is unconscious and not breathing, give mouth-to-mouth breathing. If there is no heartbeat, use cardiac massage and mouth-to-mouth breathing (CPR). Don't try to make patient vomit. If you can't get help quickly, take patient to nearest emergency facility.

ANTIPSYCHOTICS

BRAND & GENERIC NAMES

Commonly prescribed brand names (start with a Capital) and generic names (all CAPITALS) include CHLORPROMAZINE, Combid (M), Compazine, Eskalith, Etrafon (M), FLUPHENAZINE, Haldol, HALOPERIDOL, Lithane, LITHIUM, Lithobid, Lithonate, Lithotabs, Mellaril, Permitil, PERPHENAZINE, Prochlor-Iso, PROCHLORPERAZINE, Prolixin, THIORIDAZINE, Thorazine, Triavil (M) and Trilafon. (The (M) means it is a mixture or combination drug.) Additional brand names are available.

 ## USES

- Stops nausea and vomiting.
- Reduces anxiety and agitation.

 ## POSSIBLE ADVERSE REACTIONS OR SIDE EFFECTS

If any of the following occurs, consult a doctor:
- Muscle spasms of face and neck.
- Unsteady gait.
- Restlessness.
- Tremor.
- Drowsiness.
- Decreased sweating.
- Dry mouth.
- Runny nose.
- Constipation.
- Fainting.
- Rash.
- Difficult urination.
- Diminished sex drive.
- Swollen breasts.
- Change in vision.
- Sore throat.
- Fever.
- Jaundice (yellow eyes; yellow skin; dark urine).

 ## WARNINGS & PRECAUTIONS

- Before taking this medicine, consult your doctor if you have alcoholism (active), blood disease, breast cancer, difficult urination, enlarged prostate, glaucoma, heart disease, blood vessel disease, liver disease, lung disease, Parkinson's disease, seizure disorders or ulcers of the stomach or duodenum.
- Don't drive or try risky physical activity until you know how drug affects you.
- See Appendix 21.

 ## AGE-RELATED FACTORS

- Older patients are more likely to have age-related kidney or liver function impairment. This may lead to the need for reduction of the usual dosage.
- Side effects and adverse reactions are more likely to occur with advancing age.
- Males more likely to experience urinary retention.
- Your doctor or care-giver should carefully monitor your response to this drug.

 ## POSSIBLE INTERACTIONS WITH OTHER DRUGS

- If you are taking any other drug (prescription or non-prescription), ask your doctor or pharmacist if there are possible interactions.
- Antipsychotics cannot safely be taken with some drugs.
- Antipsychotics taken with some drugs may require dosage adjustment.

Do not drink alcoholic beverages or use cocaine, marijuana or tobacco while taking this medicine. These may decrease the effectiveness of the medicine or cause uncomfortable or dangerous adverse reactions.

 ## OVERDOSE

SYMPTOMS
Stupor; convulsions; coma.

WHAT TO DO
- Dial 911 (emergency) or 0 (operator) for an ambulance or medical help. Then give first aid immediately.
- If patient is unconscious and not breathing, give mouth-to-mouth breathing. If there is no heartbeat, use cardiac massage and mouth-to-mouth breathing (CPR). Don't try to make patient vomit. If you can't get help quickly, take patient to nearest emergency facility.

MEDICATIONS

ANTISPASMODICS

BRAND & GENERIC NAMES

Commonly prescribed brand names (start with a Capital) and generic names (all CAPITALS) include Antispas, Band O Supprettes (M), BELLADONNA, Bellergal (M), Bentyl, Butibel (M), DICYCLOMINE, Neoquess (M), SCOPOLAMINE and Wyanoids (M). (The (M) means it is a mixture or combination drug.) There are numerous antispasmodic combination drugs with belladonna and one of the barbiturates as the active ingredients. The list of those brand names is too extensive to include here.

USES

- Reduces spasms of digestive tract, bladder and urethra.
- Treats ulcers of stomach and duodenum.

POSSIBLE ADVERSE REACTIONS OR SIDE EFFECTS

If any of the following occurs, consult a doctor:
- Confusion.
- Delirium.
- Rapid heartbeat.
- Nausea.
- Vomiting.
- Decreased sweating.
- Constipation.
- Dryness in ears, nose or throat.
- Headache.
- Difficult or painful urination.
- Rash.
- Hives.
- Abdominal pain.
- Blurred vision.
- Fever.

WARNINGS & PRECAUTIONS

- Before taking this medicine, consult your doctor if you have bleeding problems (severe), colitis (severe), dry mouth (severe and continuing), enlarged prostate, fever, glaucoma, heart disease, hiatal hernia, high blood pressure (hypertension), intestinal blockage, other intestinal problems, kidney disease, liver disease, lung disease (chronic), myasthenia gravis, overactive thyroid, urinary tract blockage, difficult urination, allergy to anticholinergic drugs (see Glossary), stomach bloating, angina, chronic bronchitis, asthma or peptic ulcer.
- Don't drive or try risky physical activity until you know how drug affects you.
- See Appendix 21.

AGE-RELATED FACTORS

- Side effects and adverse reactions are more likely to occur with advancing age.
- Males more likely to experience urinary retention.
- Older patients are more likely to have age-related kidney or liver function impairment. This may lead to the need for reduction of the usual dosage.

POSSIBLE INTERACTIONS WITH OTHER DRUGS

- If you are taking any other drug (prescription or non-prescription), ask your doctor or pharmacist if there are possible interactions.
- Antispasmodics cannot safely be taken with some drugs.
- Antispasmodics taken with some drugs may require dosage adjustment.

Do not drink alcoholic beverages or use cocaine, marijuana or tobacco while taking this medicine. These may decrease the effectiveness of the medicine or cause uncomfortable or dangerous adverse reactions.

OVERDOSE

SYMPTOMS
Dilated pupils; rapid pulse; rapid breathing; dizziness; fever; hallucinations; confusion; slurred speech; agitation; flushed face; convulsions; coma.

WHAT TO DO
- Dial 911 (emergency) or 0 (operator) for an ambulance or medical help. Then give first aid immediately.
- If patient is unconscious and not breathing, give mouth-to-mouth breathing. If there is no heartbeat, use cardiac massage and mouth-to-mouth breathing (CPR). Don't try to make patient vomit. If you can't get help quickly, take patient to nearest emergency facility.

ANTIULCER MEDICATIONS

BRAND & GENERIC NAMES

Commonly prescribed brand names (start with a Capital) and generic names (all CAPITALS) include Carafate, CIMETIDINE, FAMOTIDINE, Pepcid, RANITIDINE, SUCRALFATE, Tagamet and Zantac.

USES

- Relieves symptoms of ulcers.
- Helps heal ulcers in stomach, esophagus and duodenum.
- Frequently used with antacids.

POSSIBLE ADVERSE REACTIONS OR SIDE EFFECTS

If any of the following occurs, consult a doctor:
- Diarrhea.
- Jaundice.
- Dizziness.
- Headache.
- Diminished sex drive.
- Male breast swelling and soreness.
- Hair loss.
- Confusion.
- Skin rash.
- Heartbeat irregularities.
- Muscle cramps or pain.
- Weakness.
- Numbness in hands and feet.

WARNINGS & PRECAUTIONS

- Don't take if you know that you are allergic to any antiulcer drugs.
- Don't take if you also take aspirin. Aspirin may irritate the stomach.

AGE-RELATED FACTORS

- Side effects and adverse reactions are more likely to occur with advancing age.
- May contribute to increased dental problems with gums, cavities and yeast infections.
- Lower-than-standard doses and longer intervals between doses may be required.
- Your doctor or care-giver should carefully monitor your response to this drug.

POSSIBLE INTERACTIONS WITH OTHER DRUGS

- If you are taking any other drug (prescription or non-prescription), ask your doctor or pharmacist if there are possible interactions.
- Don't drive or engage in risky physical activity until you see how this medicine affects you.
- Prolonged use may cause liver damage.

Do not drink alcoholic beverages or use cocaine, marijuana or tobacco while taking this medicine. These may decrease the effectiveness of the medicine or cause uncomfortable or dangerous adverse reactions.

OVERDOSE

SYMPTOMS

Confusion; slurred speech; breathing difficulty; rapid heartbeat; delirium.

WHAT TO DO

- Dial 911 (emergency) or 0 (operator) for an ambulance or medical help. Then give first aid immediately.
- If patient is unconscious and not breathing, give mouth-to-mouth breathing. If there is no heartbeat, use cardiac massage and mouth-to-mouth breathing (CPR). Don't try to make patient vomit. If you can't get help quickly, take patient to nearest emergency facility.

ANTIVIRAL MEDICATIONS

BRAND & GENERIC NAMES

Commonly prescribed brand names (start with a Capital) and generic names (all CAPITALS) include ACYCLOVIR, AMANTADINE, Retrovir, Symadine, Symmetrel, ZIDOVUDINE (AZT) and Zovirax. Additional brand names are available.

 USES

- Treats viral infections (herpes and others).
- Protects against some viral illnesses, such as influenza.
- AMANTADINE also used in treatment of Parkinson's disease.
- Retrovir (ZIDOVUDINE) is used in treatment of infection from the human immunodeficiency virus (HIV).

 POSSIBLE ADVERSE REACTIONS OR SIDE EFFECTS

If any of the following occurs, consult a doctor:
- Hallucinations.
- Confusion.
- Light-headedness.
- Dizziness.
- Headache.
- Purple skin blotches.
- Appetite loss.
- Nausea.
- Dry mouth.
- Fainting.
- Slurred speech.
- Difficult or painful urination.
- Rash.
- Uncontrollable rolling of eyes.
- Irregular heartbeat.
- Blurred vision.
- Sore throat.
- Fever.
- Vomiting.
- Constipation.

 WARNINGS & PRECAUTIONS

- Before taking this medicine, consult your doctor if you have ever had a stroke or transient ischemic attack (TIA), eczema (recurring), epilepsy or other seizures (history of), heart disease, circulation problems, kidney disease, liver disease, mental or emotional illness, nerve disease, stomach or intestinal ulcers or swelling of feet and ankles.
- Protect the liquid medication from freezing.
- See Appendix 21.

 AGE-RELATED FACTORS

- Older patients are more likely to have age-related kidney or liver function impairment. This may lead to the need for reduction of the usual dosage.
- Males more likely to experience urinary retention.

 POSSIBLE INTERACTIONS WITH OTHER DRUGS

- If you are taking any other drug (prescription or non-prescription), ask your doctor or pharmacist if there are possible interactions.
- Antivirals cannot safely be taken with some drugs.
- Antivirals taken with some drugs may require dosage adjustment.

Do not drink alcoholic beverages or use cocaine, marijuana or tobacco while taking this medicine. These may decrease the effectiveness of the medicine or cause uncomfortable or dangerous adverse reactions.

 OVERDOSE

SYMPTOMS
Heart rhythm disturbances; blood-pressure drop; convulsions; toxic psychosis.

WHAT TO DO
- Dial 911 (emergency) or 0 (operator) for an ambulance or medical help. Then give first aid immediately.
- If patient is unconscious and not breathing, give mouth-to-mouth breathing. If there is no heartbeat, use cardiac massage and mouth-to-mouth breathing (CPR). Don't try to make patient vomit. If you can't get help quickly, take patient to nearest emergency facility.

ANTIVIRAL MEDICATIONS (Ophthalmic)

BRAND & GENERIC NAMES

Commonly prescribed brand names (start with a Capital) and generic names (all CAPITALS) include Herplex Liquifilm, IDOXURIDINE (Ophthalmic), Stoxil, TRIFLURIDINE and Viropic. Additional brand names are available.

USES

Treats viral infections of the eye.

POSSIBLE ADVERSE REACTIONS OR SIDE EFFECTS

If any of the following occurs, consult a doctor:
- Burning or stinging in the eye.
- Eye irritations not present before treatment.

WARNINGS & PRECAUTIONS

- You may have increased sensitivity to sun and light.
- Notify doctor if symptoms fail to improve in 2 to 4 days.
- Keep medicine cool, but don't freeze.
- Prolonged use may cause sensitivity reaction.
- Follow doctor's instructions or package insert for proper use of this drug.
- See Appendix 21.

AGE-RELATED FACTORS

None.

POSSIBLE INTERACTIONS WITH OTHER DRUGS

Consult your doctor or pharmacist if you are using any other eye medication.

OVERDOSE

None expected.

MEDICATIONS

BRAND & GENERIC NAMES

Commonly prescribed brand names (start with a Capital) and generic names (all CAPITALS) include ACYCLOVIR (Topical) and Zovirax.

 ## USES

Relieves pain and discomfort and helps heal the sores of herpes simplex.

 ## POSSIBLE ADVERSE REACTIONS OR SIDE EFFECTS

If any of the following occurs, consult a doctor:
- Burning or stinging.
- Skin irritations not present before treatment.

 ## WARNINGS & PRECAUTIONS

- Women who use this medicine should have Pap test (see Glossary) at least once a year.
- Keep skin area being treated clean and dry.
- Wear loose-fitting clothing.
- Avoid sexual activity if either partner has active symptoms of herpes.
- See Appendix 21.

 ## AGE-RELATED FACTORS

None.

 ## POSSIBLE INTERACTIONS WITH OTHER DRUGS

None expected.

 ## OVERDOSE

None expected.

ASPIRIN (Salicylates)

BRAND & GENERIC NAMES

In addition to use for pain, aspirin is very frequently used in combination with other ingredients, such as antihistamines, cough suppressants, narcotics, expectorants, muscle relaxants and others. There are over 200 brand names of medicine that contain aspirin as one of the ingredients—too many to be listed here. Some of the well-known brand names are as follows Ascriptin, Aspergum, Bayer, Bufferin (M), Easprin, Ecotrin, Empirin (M), Fiorinal with Codeine (M), Fiorinal (M), Percodan (M), St. Joseph's and Zorprin. (The (M) means it is a mixture or combination drug.)

USES

- Reduces pain, fever and inflammation.
- Relieves swelling, stiffness and joint pain of arthritis or rheumatism.
- Prevents blood clots that may cause heart attack.

POSSIBLE ADVERSE REACTIONS OR SIDE EFFECTS

If any of the following occurs, consult a doctor:
- Black or bloody vomit.
- Blood in urine.
- Difficulty breathing.
- Hives.
- Intense itching.
- Rash.
- Faintness soon after a dose.
- Nausea or vomiting.
- Heartburn.
- Indigestion.
- Ringing in ears.
- Black stools.
- Unexplained fever.
- Diminished vision.
- Shortness of breath.
- Wheezing.
- Jaundice (yellow eyes; yellow skin; dark urine).
- Mental confusion.
- Drowsiness.

WARNINGS & PRECAUTIONS

- Don't take at same time as antacids or tetracyclines. Space doses at least 3 hours apart.
- Avoid taking if you are sensitive to aspirin or if aspirin has a strong vinegar-like odor, which means it has decomposed.

- Before taking this medicine, consult your doctor if you have asthma, gout, nasal polyps, or a history of peptic or duodenal ulcers or other bleeding disorder or if you are on a sodium-restricted diet.
- You may have increased sensitivity to sun and light.
- See Appendix 21.

AGE-RELATED FACTORS

- Toxic effects are more likely.
- Possible increased risk of gastrointestinal bleeding or ulcers. If these side effects occur, analgesics are more likely to cause serious consequences in older people.

POSSIBLE INTERACTIONS WITH OTHER DRUGS

- If you are taking any other drug (prescription or non-prescription), ask your doctor or pharmacist if there are possible interactions.
- Aspirin and salicylates cannot safely be taken with some drugs.
- Aspirin and salicylates taken with some drugs may require dosage adjustment.

Do not drink alcoholic beverages or use cocaine, marijuana or tobacco while taking this medicine. These may decrease the effectiveness of the medicine or cause uncomfortable or dangerous adverse reactions.

OVERDOSE

SYMPTOMS
Ringing in ears; nausea; vomiting; dizziness; fever; deep and rapid breathing; hallucinations; convulsions; coma.

WHAT TO DO
- Dial 911 (emergency) or 0 (operator) for an ambulance or medical help. Then give first aid immediately.
- If patient is unconscious and not breathing, give mouth-to-mouth breathing. If there is no heartbeat, use cardiac massage and mouth-to-mouth breathing (CPR). Don't try to make patient vomit. If you can't get help quickly, take patient to nearest emergency facility.

BARBITURATES

BRAND & GENERIC NAMES

Except for PHENOBARBITAL (still used in seizure disorders), barbiturates are seldom prescribed as a single-ingredient medicine. There are other more effective and safer sedatives. However, there are many combination drugs that have barbiturates as an active component. They are especially popular in combination with belladonna and belladonna-like drugs when used as antispasmodics (which reduce excess movement in the intestinal tract). Generic names include AMOBARBITAL, APROBARBITAL, BUTABARBITAL, MEPHOBARBITAL, METHABARBITAL, PHENOBARBITAL, PENTOBARBITAL, SECOBARBITAL, and TALBUTAL. Additional brand names are available.

 ## USES

- Aid sleep.
- Reduce anxiety or nervous tension. (Low dose and occasional use only. Barbiturates have mostly been supplanted by other medications for this use.)

 ## POSSIBLE ADVERSE REACTIONS OR SIDE EFFECTS

If any of the following occurs, consult a doctor:
- Hives.
- Rash.
- Intense itching.
- Faintness soon after a dose.
- Dizziness.
- Drowsiness.
- Hangover effect.
- Face or lip swelling.
- Swollen eyelids.
- Sore throat.
- Fever.
- Depression.
- Confusion.
- Slurred speech.
- Diarrhea.
- Nausea.
- Vomiting.
- Joint or muscle pain.
- Agitation.
- Slow heartbeat.
- Difficult breathing.
- Jaundice (yellow eyes; yellow skin; dark urine).
- Unexplained bleeding or bruising.

 ## WARNINGS & PRECAUTIONS

- Great potential for abuse. Other medicines are preferable for insomnia.
- Before taking this medicine, consult your doctor if you have anemia (severe), asthma (history of), emphysema, chronic lung disease, diabetes mellitus (sugar diabetes), kidney disease, mental depression, overactive thyroid, pain, porphyria (or history of) or underactive adrenal gland.
- Don't drive or try risky physical activity until you know how drug affects you.
- You may have increased sensitivity to sun and light.
- See Appendix 21.

 ## AGE-RELATED FACTORS

- Dizziness, sedation, confusion, dry mouth, urinary retention and a drop in blood pressure more likely with advancing age.
- Side effects and adverse reactions are more likely to occur with advancing age.

 ## POSSIBLE INTERACTIONS WITH OTHER DRUGS

- If you are taking any other drug (prescription or non-prescription), ask your doctor or pharmacist if there are possible interactions.
- Barbiturates cannot safely be taken with some drugs.
- Barbiturates taken with some drugs may require dosage adjustment.

Do not drink alcoholic beverages or use cocaine, marijuana or tobacco while taking this medicine. These may decrease the effectiveness of the medicine or cause uncomfortable or dangerous adverse reactions.

 ## OVERDOSE

SYMPTOMS
Deep sleep; weak pulse; coma.

WHAT TO DO
- Dial 911 (emergency) or 0 (operator) for an ambulance or medical help. Then give first aid immediately.
- If patient is unconscious and not breathing, give mouth-to-mouth breathing. If there is no heartbeat, use cardiac massage and mouth-to-mouth breathing (CPR). Don't try to make patient vomit. If you can't get help quickly, take patient to nearest emergency facility.

BETA-ADRENERGIC BLOCKERS

BRAND & GENERIC NAMES

Commonly prescribed brand names (start with a Capital) and generic names (all CAPITALS) include ACEBUTOLOL, Apo-Metaprolol, Apo-Propranolol, Apo-Timol, ATENOLOL, Betaloc, BETAXOLOL, Blocadren, CARTEOLOL, Cartrol, Colgard, Detensol, Inderal, Inderide (M), Inderide LA (M), Kerlone, LABETALOL, Levatol, Lopressor, METOPROLOL, Monitan, NADOLOL, Normodyne, Novometoprol, Novopranolol, OXPRENOLOL, PENBUTOLOL, PINDOLOL, PROPRANOLOL, Sectral, Slow-Transicor, Sotacor, SOTALOL, Syn-Nadolol, Syn-Pindolol, Tenoretic (M), Tenormin, Timoliode (M), TIMOLOL, Trandate, Transicor and Visken. Additional brand names are available.

USES

- Reduces angina attacks.
- Stabilizes irregular heartbeat.
- Lowers blood pressure.
- Reduces frequency of migraine headaches. (Does not relieve headache pain).
- Other uses prescribed by your doctor.

POSSIBLE ADVERSE REACTIONS OR SIDE EFFECTS

If any of the following occurs, consult a doctor:
- Pulse slower than 50 beats per minute.
- Drowsiness.
- Fatigue.
- Numbness or tingling of fingers or toes.
- Dizziness.
- Diarrhea.
- Nausea.
- Weakness.
- Cold hands or feet.
- Dry mouth or skin.
- Hallucinations.
- Nightmares.
- Insomnia.
- Headache.
- Difficult breathing.
- Joint pain.
- Anxiety.
- Confusion.
- Reduced alertness.
- Depression.
- Impotence.
- Constipation.
- Rash.
- Sore throat.
- Fever.
- Unusual bleeding and bruising.
- Dry, burning eyes.

WARNINGS & PRECAUTIONS

- May mask symptoms of hypoglycemia (low blood sugar) if you have diabetes.
- Before taking this medicine, consult your doctor if you have allergy, history of asthma, eczema, hay fever, hives, bradycardia (unusually slow heartbeat), bronchitis, diabetes mellitus (sugar diabetes), emphysema, heart or blood vessel disease, kidney disease, liver disease, mental depression, myasthenia gravis (a muscle disease), overactive thyroid, pheochromocytoma or psoriasis.
- Don't drive or try risky physical activity until you know how drug affects you.
- See Appendix 21.

AGE-RELATED FACTORS

- Older patients are more likely to have age-related kidney or liver function impairment. This may lead to the need for reduction of the usual dosage.
- Your doctor or care-giver should carefully monitor your response to this drug.

POSSIBLE INTERACTIONS WITH OTHER DRUGS

- If you are taking any other drug (prescription or non-prescription), ask your doctor or pharmacist if there are possible interactions.
- Beta blockers cannot safely be taken with some drugs.
- Beta blockers taken with some drugs may require dosage adjustment.

Do not drink alcoholic beverages or use cocaine, marijuana or tobacco while taking this medicine. These may decrease the effectiveness of the medicine or cause uncomfortable or dangerous adverse reactions.

OVERDOSE

SYMPTOMS
Weakness; slow or weak pulse; blood pressure drop; fainting; difficulty breathing; convulsions; cold and sweaty skin.

WHAT TO DO
- Dial 911 (emergency) or 0 (operator) for an ambulance or medical help. Then give first aid immediately.
- If patient is unconscious and not breathing, give mouth-to-mouth breathing. If there is no heartbeat, use cardiac massage and mouth-to-mouth breathing (CPR). Don't try to make patient vomit. If you can't get help quickly, take patient to nearest emergency facility.

BRONCHODILATORS

BRAND & GENERIC NAMES

Commonly prescribed brand names (start with a Capital) and generic names (all CAPITALS) include Adrenalin, Aerolone, ALBUTEROL, Alupent, AMINOPHYLLINE, Asmacol (M), ATROPINE, Brethaire, Brethine, Bricanyl, Bronkolixir (M), Dainite KI (M), EPHEDRINE, EPINEPHRINE, ISOPROTERENOL, Isuprel, Marax (M), Medihaler, Metaprel, METAPROTERENOL, Micronefrin, Phyllocontin, Primatene, Proventil, Quadrinal (M), Quibron (M), Slo-Bid, Slo-Phyllin, Somophyllin, Sus-Phrine, Tedral (M), TERBUTALINE, Theo-Dur, Theo-Organidin (M), THEOPHYLLINE, Vaponefrin and Ventolin. (The (M) means it is a mixture or combination drug.) Additional brand names are available.

 USES

- Opens bronchial tubes in lungs when narrowed by muscle spasms.
- Treats asthma symptoms.
- Note: Some used as tablets, others as sprays or liquid rectal enemas.

 POSSIBLE ADVERSE REACTIONS OR SIDE EFFECTS

If any of the following occurs, consult a doctor:
- Headache.
- Irritability.
- Nervousness.
- Nausea.
- Restlessness.
- Insomnia.
- Vomiting.
- Stomach pain.
- Rash or hives.
- Flushed face.
- Diarrhea.
- Appetite loss.
- Rapid breathing.
- Irregular heartbeat.
- Dizziness or light-headedness.
- Frequent urination.

 WARNINGS & PRECAUTIONS

- Before taking this medicine, consult your doctor if you have active alcoholism, diarrhea, enlarged prostate, fever, fibrocystic breast disease, heart disease, high blood pressure, irritation or infection of the rectum or lower colon (for AMINOPHYLLINE rectal enema only), kidney disease, liver disease, overactive thyroid, respiratory infections such as influenza (flu), stomach ulcer (history of) or other stomach problems, brain damage, convulsions (seizures), diabetes mellitus (sugar diabetes), mental disease or Parkinson's disease.
- See Appendix 21.

 AGE-RELATED FACTORS

Aging does not affect expected results.

 POSSIBLE INTERACTIONS WITH OTHER DRUGS

- If you are taking any other drug (prescription or non-prescription), ask your doctor or pharmacist if there are possible interactions.
- Bronchodilators cannot safely be taken with some drugs.
- Bronchodilators taken with some drugs may require dosage adjustment.

Do not drink alcoholic beverages or use cocaine, marijuana or tobacco while taking this medicine. These may decrease the effectiveness of the medicine or cause uncomfortable or dangerous adverse reactions.

 OVERDOSE

SYMPTOMS
Restlessness; irritability; confusion; delirium; convulsions; rapid pulse; coma.

WHAT TO DO
- Dial 911 (emergency) or 0 (operator) for an ambulance or medical help. Then give first aid immediately.
- If patient is unconscious and not breathing, give mouth-to-mouth breathing. If there is no heartbeat, use cardiac massage and mouth-to-mouth breathing (CPR). Don't try to make patient vomit. If you can't get help quickly, take patient to nearest emergency facility.

CALCIUM CHANNEL BLOCKERS

BRAND & GENERIC NAMES

Commonly prescribed brand names (start with a Capital) and generic names (all CAPITALS) include Calan, Cardizem, DILTIAZEM, Isoptin, NIFEDIPINE, Procardia and VERAPAMIL. Additional brand names are available.

 ## USES

- Prevents angina attacks.
- Stabilizes irregular heartbeat.
- Treats high blood pressure.

 ## POSSIBLE ADVERSE REACTIONS OR SIDE EFFECTS

If any of the following occurs, consult a doctor:
- Unusually fast or unusually slow heartbeat.
- Wheezing.
- Cough.
- Shortness of breath.
- Dizziness.
- Numbness or tingling in hands and feet.
- Swollen feet, ankles or legs.
- Difficult urination.
- Nausea.
- Constipation.
- Fainting.
- Depression.
- Psychosis.
- Rash.
- Jaundice (yellow eyes; yellow skin; dark urine).
- Headache.
- Insomnia.
- Vivid dreams.
- Hair loss.

 ## WARNINGS & PRECAUTIONS

- Before taking this medicine, consult your doctor if you have kidney disease, liver disease or other heart or blood vessel disorders.
- See Appendix 21.

 ## AGE-RELATED FACTORS

Older patients are more likely to have age-related kidney or liver function impairment. This may lead to the need for reduction of the usual dosage.

 ## POSSIBLE INTERACTIONS WITH OTHER DRUGS

- If you are taking any other drug (prescription or non-prescription), ask your doctor or pharmacist if there are possible interactions.
- Calcium channel blockers cannot safely be taken with some drugs.
- Calcium channel blockers taken with some drugs may require dosage adjustment.

Do not drink alcoholic beverages or use cocaine, marijuana or tobacco while taking this medicine. These may decrease the effectiveness of the medicine or cause uncomfortable or dangerous adverse reactions.

 ## OVERDOSE

SYMPTOMS
Unusually fast or unusually slow heartbeat; loss of consciousness; cardiac arrest.

WHAT TO DO
- Dial 911 (emergency) or 0 (operator) for an ambulance or medical help. Then give first aid immediately.
- If patient is unconscious and not breathing, give mouth-to-mouth breathing. If there is no heartbeat, use cardiac massage and mouth-to-mouth breathing (CPR). Don't try to make patient vomit. If you can't get help quickly, take patient to nearest emergency facility.

MEDICATIONS

CARBONIC ANHYDRASE INHIBITORS

BRAND & GENERIC NAMES

Commonly prescribed brand names (start with a Capital) and generic names (all CAPITALS) include Acetazolam, ACETAZALOMIDE, Ak-Zol, Apo-Acetazolamide, Daranide, Dazamide, Diamox, DICHLORPHENAMIDE, METHAZOLAMIDE and Naptazane.

USES

- Decreases pressure in eye in glaucoma.
- Treats epileptic seizures.
- Treatment of body fluid retention.
- Treats altitude illness symptoms.

POSSIBLE ADVERSE REACTIONS OR SIDE EFFECTS

If any of the following occurs, consult a doctor:
- Convulsions.
- Back pain.
- Sedation.
- Fatigue.
- Weakness.
- Tingling or burning in feet or hands.
- Headache.
- Mood changes.
- Nervousness.
- Clumsiness.
- Trembling.
- Confusion.
- Hives.
- Rash.
- Itch.
- Sores.
- Ringing in ears.
- Hoarseness.
- Dry mouth.
- Thirst.
- Sore throat.
- Fever.
- Appetite change.
- Nausea.
- Vomiting.
- Black, tarry stool.
- Breathing difficulty.
- Irregular or weak heartbeat.
- Easy bleeding or bruising.
- Muscle cramps.
- Painful or frequent urination.
- Blood in urine.
- Depression.

WARNINGS & PRECAUTIONS

- May increase sugar levels in blood and urine. Diabetics may need insulin adjustment.
- Before taking this medicine, consult your doctor if you have diabetes mellitus (sugar diabetes), emphysema or other chronic lung disease, gout, kidney disease or stones, liver disease, low blood levels of potassium or sodium or underactive adrenal gland (Addison's disease).
- Don't drive or try risky physical activity until you know how drug affects you.
- You may have increased sensitivity to sun and light.
- See Appendix 21.

AGE-RELATED FACTORS

- Older patients are more likely to have age-related kidney or liver function impairment. This may lead to the need for reduction of the usual dosage.
- Aging does not affect expected results.

POSSIBLE INTERACTIONS WITH OTHER DRUGS

- If you are taking any other drug (prescription or non-prescription), ask your doctor or pharmacist if there are possible interactions.
- Carbonic anhydrase inhibitors cannot safely be taken with some drugs.
- Carbonic anhydrase inhibitors taken with some drugs may require dosage adjustment.

Do not drink alcoholic beverages or use cocaine, marijuana or tobacco while taking this medicine. These may decrease the effectiveness of the medicine or cause uncomfortable or dangerous adverse reactions.

OVERDOSE

SYMPTOMS
Drowsiness; confusion; excitement; nausea; vomiting; numbness in hands and feet; coma.

WHAT TO DO
- Dial 911 (emergency) or 0 (operator) for an ambulance or medical help. Then give first aid immediately.
- If patient is unconscious and not breathing, give mouth-to-mouth breathing. If there is no heartbeat, use cardiac massage and mouth-to-mouth breathing (CPR). Don't try to make patient vomit. If you can't get help quickly, take patient to nearest emergency facility.

CORTICOSTEROIDS
(Steroidal Anti-Inflammatories)

BRAND & GENERIC NAMES

Commonly prescribed brand names (start with a Capital) and generic names (all CAPITALS) include Ak-Tate, Ak-Trol, Anusol HC (M), Aristocort, Aristospan, BECLOMETHASONE, Beclovent, Beconase, BETAMETHASONE, Blephamide (M), Celestone, Colymycin S (Otic) (M), Cortaid, Cortenema, CORTISONE, Cortisporin (Otic) (M), Cortone, CoSol-HC (M), Dalalone, Decadron, Deltasone, Dexacidin, DEXAMETHASONE, Diprolene, FLUOCINOLONE, Fluonid, Fluosyn, HYDROCORTISONE, Hytone, Kenalog, Lotrisone (M), Maxidex, Maxitrol, Medrol, Mepred, METHYLPREDNISOLONE, Meticorten, Myco-Triacet (M), Mycolog (M), Neo-Synalar (M), Nutracort, Orasone, Poly-Pred (M), Pred-5, PREDNISOLONE, PREDNISONE, Solu Cortef, Synalar HP, Synalar, Synemol, TRIAMCINOLONE, Uticort, Valisone, Vancenase, Vanceril and Westcort (M). (The (M) means it is a mixture or combination drug.) Additional brand names are available.

USES

- Reduces inflammation caused by many different medical problems.
- Treatment of some allergic diseases, blood disorders, kidney diseases, asthma and emphysema.
- Replaces corticosteroid deficiencies.

POSSIBLE ADVERSE REACTIONS OR SIDE EFFECTS

If any of the following occurs, consult a doctor:
- Hives.
- Rash.
- Intense itching.
- Faintness soon after a dose.
- Poor wound healing.
- Thirst.
- Indigestion.
- Nausea.
- Vomiting.
- Black, bloody or tarry stool.
- Blurred vision.
- Halos around lights.
- Sore throat.
- Fever.
- Muscle cramps.
- Swollen legs or feet.
- Mood change.
- Fatigue.
- Insomnia.
- Weakness.
- Restlessness.
- Frequent urination.
- Weight gain.
- Round face.
- TB recurrence.
- Irregular heartbeat.
- Joint pain.
- Acute psychosis.
- Hair loss.
- Severe upper abdominal pain.
- Numbness or tingling in hands or feet.
- Convulsions.
- Pain in calf of leg.
- Hallucinations.

WARNINGS & PRECAUTIONS

- Avoid immunizations (vaccinations) if possible while taking this drug.
- Before taking this medicine, consult your doctor if you have bone disease, colitis, diabetes mellitus (sugar diabetes), diverticulitis, fungus infection or any other infection, glaucoma, heart disease, herpes simplex infection of the eye, high blood pressure, high cholesterol levels, kidney disease (especially if you are receiving dialysis) or kidney stones, liver disease, myasthenia gravis, over-active thyroid, stomach ulcer or other stomach or intestine problems, systemic lupus erythematosus, tuberculosis (active TB, nonactive TB, or past history of) or underactive thyroid.
- See Appendix 21.

AGE-RELATED FACTORS

- More likely to develop high blood pressure and osteoporosis (bone disease) with advancing age.
- Your doctor or care-giver should carefully monitor your response to this drug.

POSSIBLE INTERACTIONS WITH OTHER DRUGS

- If you are taking any other drug (prescription or non-prescription), ask your doctor or pharmacist if there are possible interactions.
- Corticosteroids cannot safely be taken with some drugs.
- Corticosteroids taken with some drugs may require dosage adjustment.

Do not drink alcoholic beverages or use cocaine, marijuana or tobacco while taking this medicine. These may decrease the effectiveness of the medicine or cause uncomfortable or dangerous adverse reactions.

OVERDOSE

SYMPTOMS
Headache; convulsions; heart failure.

WHAT TO DO
- Dial 911 (emergency) or 0 (operator) for an ambulance or medical help. Then give first aid immediately.
- If patient is unconscious and not breathing, give mouth-to-mouth breathing. If there is no heartbeat, use cardiac massage and mouth-to-mouth breathing (CPR). Don't try to make patient vomit. If you can't get help quickly, take patient to nearest emergency facility.

COUGH & COLD COMBINATION MEDICATIONS

BRAND & GENERIC NAMES

Most of the cough and cold remedies are combination drugs that can be purchased without a prescription. The complete list of brand names is too extensive to list here. Whatever brand you buy, read the package label and follow those instructions carefully.

 USES

- Antihistamine: Relieves allergy symptoms, such as dripping nose; watery eyes; sneezing.
- Decongestant: Clears nasal congestion.
- Antitussive: Relieves coughing.
- Expectorant: Loosens mucus in the lungs.
- Analgesic: Relieves aches and pains of common cold.
- *Note:* Some have codeine or other narcotics that carry significant dangers.

 POSSIBLE ADVERSE REACTIONS OR SIDE EFFECTS

Not all of these symptoms have been reported for each ingredient, but they have all been reported for at least one of them. If any of the following occurs, consult a doctor:

- Hives.
- Itching.
- Shortness of breath.
- Cold skin.
- Confusion.
- Hearing loss.
- Vision problems.
- Nervousness.
- Unusual thirst.
- Flapping movement of hands.
- Pinpoint eye pupils.
- Slow heartbeat.
- Irregular heartbeat.
- Increased sweating.
- Hallucinations.
- Weakness.
- Appetite loss.
- Abdominal pain.
- Bloody urine.
- Dizziness.
- Upper abdominal swelling.
- Constipation.
- Nightmares.
- Drowsiness.
- Rash.
- Diarrhea.
- Nausea or vomiting.
- Nose and throat dryness.

 WARNINGS & PRECAUTIONS

- Before taking this medicine, consult your doctor if you have asthma, liver disease, anemia, gout, hemophilia, peptic ulcers, colitis, brain disease, seizures, diabetes, enlarged prostate, glaucoma, heart disease, kidney disease or thyroid disease.
- Read all label instructions carefully.
- Don't take medicines containing acetaminophen if you have a history of alcoholism.

- Hot weather may require reduced dosage.
- Don't drive or try risky physical activity until you know how drug affects you.
- See Appendix 21.

 AGE-RELATED FACTORS

- Side effects and adverse reactions are more likely to occur with advancing age.
- Possible increased risk of gastrointestinal bleeding or ulcers. If these side effects occur, analgesics are more likely to cause serious consequences in older people.
- Dizziness, sedation, confusion, dry mouth, urinary retention and a drop in blood pressure more likely with advancing age.

 POSSIBLE INTERACTIONS WITH OTHER DRUGS

- If you are taking any other drug (prescription or non-prescription), ask your doctor or pharmacist if there are possible interactions.
- Cough and cold combinations cannot safely be taken with some drugs.
- Cough and cold combinations taken with some drugs may require dosage adjustment.

Do not drink alcoholic beverages or use cocaine, marijuana or tobacco while taking this medicine. These may decrease the effectiveness of the medicine or cause uncomfortable or dangerous adverse reactions.

 OVERDOSE

SYMPTOMS
Uncontrollable movements; stupor; seizures; coma.

WHAT TO DO
- Dial 911 (emergency) or 0 (operator) for an ambulance or medical help. Then give first aid immediately.
- If patient is unconscious and not breathing, give mouth-to-mouth breathing. If there is no heartbeat, use cardiac massage and mouth-to-mouth breathing (CPR). Don't try to make patient vomit. If you can't get help quickly, take patient to nearest emergency facility.

DIGITALIS PREPARATIONS

BRAND & GENERIC NAMES

Commonly prescribed brand names (start with a Capital) and generic names (all CAPITALS) include Cedilanid, Cedilanid-D, Crystodigin, DIGITOXIN, DIGOXIN, DESLANOSIDE, Lanoxicaps, Lanoxin and Novodigoxin.

USES

- Strengthens weak heart muscle contractions to prevent congestive heart failure.
- Treats or corrects irregular heartbeat.

POSSIBLE ADVERSE REACTIONS OR SIDE EFFECTS

If any of the following occurs, consult a doctor:
- Appetite loss.
- Diarrhea.
- Drowsiness.
- Lethargy.
- Disorientation.
- Rash.
- Hives.
- Heartbeat irregularities.
- Depression.
- Psychosis.
- Double or yellow-green vision.
- Enlarged, sensitive male breasts.
- Tiredness.
- Weakness.

WARNINGS & PRECAUTIONS

- Don't take if you are allergic to any digitalis preparations or if your heartbeat is slower than 50 beats per minute.
- Before you start, consult your doctor if you have kidney or liver disease or thyroid disorder or if you have surgery (including dental) scheduled in the next two months.
- Wear a Medical Alert tag or carry I.D. showing that you take this drug.
- See Appendix 21.

AGE-RELATED FACTORS

- Side effects and adverse reactions are more likely to occur with advancing age.
- Older patients are more likely to have age-related kidney or liver function impairment. This may lead to the need for reduction of the usual dosage.

POSSIBLE INTERACTIONS WITH OTHER DRUGS

- If you are taking any other drug (prescription or non-prescription), ask your doctor or pharmacist if there are possible interactions.
- Digitalis preparations cannot safely be taken with some drugs.
- Digitalis preparations taken with some drugs may require dosage adjustment.

Do not drink alcoholic beverages or use cocaine, marijuana or tobacco while taking this medicine. These may decrease the effectiveness of the medicine or cause uncomfortable or dangerous adverse reactions.

OVERDOSE

SYMPTOMS
Nausea; appetite loss; abdominal pain; diarrhea; extreme tiredness or weakness; very slow heartbeat (less than 50 per minute); blurred vision; white halos around objects; fainting; headache.

WHAT TO DO
- Dial 911 (emergency) or 0 (operator) for an ambulance or medical help. Then give first aid immediately.
- If patient is unconscious and not breathing, give mouth-to-mouth breathing. If there is no heartbeat; use cardiac massage and mouth-to-mouth breathing (CPR). Don't try to make patient vomit. If you can't get help quickly, take patient to nearest emergency facility.

DIURETICS (Water Pills)

BRAND & GENERIC NAMES

Commonly prescribed brand names (start with a Capital) and generic names (all CAPITALS) include Aldactone, Alatone, Alazide (M), Aldactazine (M), Aldoclor (M), Aldoril (M), AMILORIDE, BUMETANIDE, Bumex, Cemi-Regroton (M), CHLOROTHIAZIDE, CHLORTHALIDONE, Combipres (M), Diulo, Diupre (M), Diuril, Dyazide (M), Dyrenium, Esidrix, FUROSEMIDE, HYDROCHLORTHIAZIDE, Hydrodiuril, Hydromal, Hygroton, INDAPAMIDE, Lasix, Lozol, Maxazide (M), METOLAZONE, Midamor, Moduretic (M), Oretic, Regroton (M), Spiromazide (M), SPIRONOLACTONE, Spirozide (M), Tenoretic (M), Thalidone, Thiuretic, TRIAMTERENE and Zaroxolyn. (The (M) means it is a mixture or combination drug.) Additional brand names are available.

USES

- Controls, but doesn't cure, high blood pressure and congestive heart failure.
- Reduces fluid retention (edema).

POSSIBLE ADVERSE REACTIONS OR SIDE EFFECTS

If any of the following occurs, consult a doctor:
- Blurred vision.
- Severe abdominal pain.
- Nausea.
- Vomiting.
- Irregular heartbeat.
- Weak pulse.
- Dizziness.
- Mood change.
- Headache.
- Weakness.
- Tiredness.
- Weight changes.
- Dry mouth.
- Thirst.
- Rash or hives.
- Sore throat.
- Fever.
- Jaundice (yellow eyes; yellow skin; dark urine).

WARNINGS & PRECAUTIONS

- Hot weather and fever may cause dehydration and drop in blood pressure. Dose may require temporary adjustment.
- Weigh daily and report any unexpected weight decreases to your doctor.
- May cause rise in uric acid leading to gout.

- May cause blood sugar rise in diabetics.
- You may have increased sensitivity to sun and light.
- Before taking this medicine, consult your doctor if you have gout, liver, pancreas or kidney disorder; frequent laboratory studies of blood to monitor potassium level; diabetes mellitus (sugar diabetes); diarrhea; hearing problems or lupus erythematosus (history of) or if you have recently had a heart attack or are allergic to any thiazide diuretic drug or sulfa drug.
- See Appendix 21.

AGE-RELATED FACTORS

- Older patients are more likely to have age-related kidney or liver function impairment. This may lead to the need for reduction of the usual dosage.
- Side effects and adverse reactions are more likely to occur with advancing age.

POSSIBLE INTERACTIONS WITH OTHER DRUGS

- If you are taking any other drug (prescription or non-prescription), ask your doctor or pharmacist if there are possible interactions.
- Diuretics cannot safely be taken with some drugs.
- Diuretics taken with some drugs may require dosage adjustment.

Do not drink alcoholic beverages or use cocaine, marijuana or tobacco while taking this medicine. These may decrease the effectiveness of the medicine or cause uncomfortable or dangerous adverse reactions.

OVERDOSE

SYMPTOMS
Cramps; weakness; drowsiness; weak pulse; coma.

WHAT TO DO
- Dial 911 (emergency) or 0 (operator) for an ambulance or medical help. Then give first aid immediately.
- If patient is unconscious and not breathing, give mouth-to-mouth breathing. If there is no heartbeat, use cardiac massage and mouth-to-mouth breathing (CPR). Don't try to make patient vomit. If you can't get help quickly, take patient to nearest emergency facility.

HORMONES, FEMALE (Estrogens)

BRAND & GENERIC NAMES

Commonly prescribed brand names (start with a Capital) and generic names (all CAPITALS) include Amen, CONJUGATED ESTROGENS, Curretab, DIETHYLSTILBESTROL (DES), Estinyl, Estraderm, ESTRADIOL, ETHINYL ESTRADIOL, Feminone, HYDROXYPROGESTERONE, Lo/Ovral, MEDROXYPROGESTERONE, Megace, MEGESTROL, Nordette, NORGESTREL, NORETHINDRONE, NORETHINDRONE ACETATE, Ortho-Novum, Ovral (M), Ovrette, Premarin with Methyltestosterone (M), Premarin, Progens, PROGESTERONE, Provera, Stilbestrol, Stilphostrol and Triphasil. (The (M) means it is a mixture or combination drug.) Additional brand names are available.

 ## USES

- Treatment for symptoms of menopause.
- Replacement for female hormonal deficiency.
- Treatment for cancer of the prostate in males.

 ## POSSIBLE ADVERSE REACTIONS OR SIDE EFFECTS

If any of the following occurs, consult a doctor:
- Stomach cramps.
- Appetite loss.
- Nausea.
- Diarrhea.
- Swollen feet and ankles.
- Tender, swollen breasts.
- Rash.
- Stomach or side pain.
- Depression.
- Dizziness.
- Headache.
- Irritability.
- Vomiting.
- Breast lumps.
- Brown blotches on skin.
- Hair loss.
- Vaginal discharge or bleeding.
- Changes in sex drive.
- Jaundice (yellow eyes; yellow skin; dark urine).
- Intolerance of contact lenses.

 ## WARNINGS & PRECAUTIONS

- Before taking this medicine, consult your doctor if you have asthma, blood clots (or history of), cancer (or history of), vaginal bleeding, diabetes mellitus (sugar diabetes), epilepsy, heart or circulation disease, high blood cholesterol, kidney disease, liver or gallbladder disease, mental depression (or history of), migraine headaches, stroke (or history of) or bone disease.
- You may have increased sensitivity to sun and light.
- See Appendix 21.

 ## AGE-RELATED FACTORS

- Aging does not affect expected results.
- Your doctor or care-giver should carefully monitor your response to this drug.

 ## POSSIBLE INTERACTIONS WITH OTHER DRUGS

- If you are taking any other drug (prescription or non-prescription), ask your doctor or pharmacist if there are possible interactions.
- Female hormones cannot safely be taken with some drugs.
- Female hormones taken with some drugs may require dosage adjustment.

Do not drink alcoholic beverages or use cocaine, marijuana or tobacco while taking this medicine. These may decrease the effectiveness of the medicine or cause uncomfortable or dangerous adverse reactions.

 ## OVERDOSE

SYMPTOMS
Nausea; vomiting; fluid retention; breast enlargement and discomfort; abnormal vaginal bleeding.

WHAT TO DO
Overdose unlikely to threaten life. If person takes much larger amount than prescribed, call doctor, poison control center or hospital emergency room for instructions.

MEDICATIONS

HORMONES, MALE (Androgens)

BRAND & GENERIC NAMES

Commonly prescribed brand names (start with a Capital) and generic names (all CAPITALS) include Deca-Durabolin, Deladumone, Delatestryl, Durabolin, NANDROLONE, TESTOSTERONE and Testred. Additional brand names are available.

 USES

- Corrects male hormone deficiency.
- Reduces male menopause symptoms (loss of sex drive; depression; anxiety).
- Decreases calcium loss of osteoporosis (softened bones).
- Blocks growth of breast cancer cells in females.
- Stimulates weight gain after illness or injury or for chronically underweight persons.

 POSSIBLE ADVERSE REACTIONS OR SIDE EFFECTS

If any of the following occurs, consult a doctor:
- Intense itching.
- Weakness.
- Loss of consciousness.
- Acne or oily skin in females.
- Deep voice.
- Enlarged clitoris.
- Frequent erections.
- Swollen breasts in men.
- Sore mouth.
- Higher sex drive.
- Jaundice (yellow eyes; yellow skin; dark urine).
- Depression or confusion.
- Flushed face.
- Rash or itch.
- Nausea.
- Vomiting.
- Diarrhea.
- Swollen feet or legs.
- Vaginal bleeding.
- Hives.
- Black stool.
- Sore throat.
- Fever.
- Abdominal pain.

 WARNINGS & PRECAUTIONS

- Don't take in hopes of enhancing athletic performance.
- Before taking this medicine, consult your doctor if you have breast cancer (in males), diabetes mellitus (sugar diabetes), edema (swelling of face, hands, feet or lower legs), enlarged prostate, heart or blood vessel disease, kidney disease, liver disease or prostate cancer.
- See Appendix 21.

 AGE-RELATED FACTORS

- Aging does not affect expected results.
- Your doctor or care-giver should carefully monitor your response to this drug.

 POSSIBLE INTERACTIONS WITH OTHER DRUGS

- If you are taking any other drug (prescription or non-prescription), ask your doctor or pharmacist if there are possible interactions.
- Male hormones cannot safely be taken with some drugs.
- Male hormones taken with some drugs may require dosage adjustment.

Do not drink alcoholic beverages or use cocaine, marijuana or tobacco while taking this medicine. These may decrease the effectiveness of the medicine or cause uncomfortable or dangerous adverse reactions.

 OVERDOSE

SYMPTOMS
None expected.

WHAT TO DO
Overdose unlikely to threaten life. If person takes much larger amount than prescribed, call doctor, poison control center or hospital emergency room for instructions.

IMMUNOSUPPRESSIVES

BRAND & GENERIC NAMES

Commonly prescribed brand names (start with a Capital) and generic names (all CAPITALS) include AZATHIOPRINE, CHLORAMBUCIL, CYCLOPHOSPHAMIDE, CYCLOSPORINE, Cytoxan, Folex, Imuran, Leukeran, MERCAPTOPURINE, METHOTREXATE, Mexate, Mexate AQ, Neosar, Procytox, Purinethol and Sandimmune.

USES

- Suppresses the immune response in patients who have transplants of the heart, lung, kidney, liver or pancreas.
- Cyclosporine treats rejection as well as helps prevent it.

POSSIBLE ADVERSE REACTIONS OR SIDE EFFECTS

If any of the following occurs, consult a doctor:
- Seizures.
- Wheezing with shortness of breath.
- Gum inflammation.
- Blood in urine.
- Jaundice (yellow eyes; yellow skin; dark urine).
- Increased hair growth.
- Fever.
- Chills.
- Sore throat.
- Shortness of breath.
- Frequent urination.
- Confusion.
- Irregular heartbeat.
- Numbness of hands and feet.
- Nervousness.
- Weakness.
- Face flushing.
- Severe abdominal pain.
- Headache.

WARNINGS & PRECAUTIONS

- Request regular laboratory studies to measure levels of potassium; evaluate liver and kidney function; check blood pressure (CYCLOSPORINE sometimes causes hypertension).
- Don't store liquid solution in the refrigerator.
- Mix CYCLOSPORINE with milk, chocolate milk or orange juice in glass container.
- Avoid any immunizations except those specifically recommended by your doctor.
- Maintain good dental hygiene.

- Before taking this medicine, consult your doctor if you have chickenpox (including recent exposure), herpes zoster (shingles) infection, intestine problems, kidney disease or liver disease.
- See Appendix 21.

AGE-RELATED FACTORS

- Older patients are more likely to have age-related kidney or liver function impairment. This may lead to the need for reduction of the usual dosage.
- Side effects and adverse reactions are more likely to occur with advancing age.

POSSIBLE INTERACTIONS WITH OTHER DRUGS

- If you are taking any other drug (prescription or non-prescription), ask your doctor or pharmacist if there are possible interactions.
- Immunosuppressives cannot safely be taken with some drugs.
- Immunosuppressives taken with some drugs may require dosage adjustment.

Do not drink alcoholic beverages or use cocaine, marijuana or tobacco while taking this medicine. These may decrease the effectiveness of the medicine or cause uncomfortable or dangerous adverse reactions.

OVERDOSE

SYMPTOMS
Irregular heartbeat; seizures; coma.

WHAT TO DO
- Dial 911 (emergency) or 0 (operator) for an ambulance or medical help. Then give first aid immediately.
- If patient is unconscious and not breathing, give mouth-to-mouth breathing. If there is no heartbeat, use cardiac massage and mouth-to-mouth breathing (CPR). Don't try to make patient vomit. If you can't get help quickly, take patient to nearest emergency facility.

MEDICATIONS

LAXATIVES

BRAND & GENERIC NAMES

Commonly prescribed brand names (start with a Capital) and generic names (all CAPITALS) include BISACODYL, Cephulac, Chronoluc, Clysodrast (M), Ducolax, Effer-syllium, Ex-Lax, Feenamint, Fiberall (M), Fleet Bisocodyl, Hydrocil, Konsyl, LACTULOSE, Metamucil, METHYLCELLULOSE, MINERAL OIL, Naturacil, Perdiem (M), PHENOLPHTHALEIN, PSYLLIUM and SENNA. (The (M) means it is a mixture or combination drug.) Additional brand names are available.

 ## USES

Temporary relief of constipation.

 ## POSSIBLE ADVERSE REACTIONS OR SIDE EFFECTS

If any of the following occurs, consult a doctor:
* Difficult breathing or wheezing.
* Abdominal swelling and pain.
* Skin rash or itching.
* Swallowing difficulty (feeling of lump in throat).
* Confusion.
* Dizziness or light-headedness.
* Irregular heartbeat.
* Muscle cramps.
* Unusual tiredness or weakness.
* Confusion.
* Changes in urine color.
* Throat irritation.
* Diarrhea.
* Gas.
* Increased thirst.
* Belching.
* Nausea.

 ## WARNINGS & PRECAUTIONS

* Before taking this medicine, consult your doctor if you have appendicitis, colostomy, diabetes mellitus (sugar diabetes), heart disease, high blood pressure, ileostomy, intestinal blockage, kidney disease, laxative habit, rectal bleeding of unknown cause or swallowing difficulty.
* See Appendix 21.

 ## AGE-RELATED FACTORS

* Older patients are more likely to have age-related kidney or liver function impairment. This may lead to the need for reduction of the usual dosage.
* Lower doses and longer intervals between doses may be required.
* Beware of habitual use.

 ## POSSIBLE INTERACTIONS WITH OTHER DRUGS

* If you are taking any other drug (prescription or non-prescription), ask your doctor or pharmacist if there are possible interactions.
* Laxatives cannot safely be taken with some drugs.
* Laxatives taken with some drugs may require dosage adjustment.

Do not drink alcoholic beverages or use cocaine, marijuana or tobacco while taking this medicine. These may decrease the effectiveness of the medicine or cause uncomfortable or dangerous adverse reactions.

 ## OVERDOSE

SYMPTOMS
Explosive diarrhea; weakness.

WHAT TO DO
Discontinue medicine. If diarrhea doesn't improve in 24 hours seek medical attention.

MAO INHIBITORS
(Monoamine Oxidase Inhibitors)

BRAND & GENERIC NAMES

Commonly prescribed brand names (start with a Capital) and generic names (all CAPITALS) include ISOCARBOXAZID, Marplan, Nardil, Parnate, PHENELZINE and TRANYLCYPROMINE. Additional brand names are available.

 USES

Treatment for depression.

 POSSIBLE ADVERSE REACTIONS OR SIDE EFFECTS

If any of the following occurs, consult a doctor:
- Fatigue.
- Weakness.
- Dizziness when changing position.
- Restlessness.
- Tremors.
- Dry mouth.
- Constipation.
- Difficult urination.
- Fainting.
- Severe headache.
- Chest pain.
- Hallucinations.
- Insomnia.
- Nightmares.
- Diarrhea.
- Rapid or pounding heartbeat.
- Swollen feet or legs.
- Joint pain.
- Diminished sex drive.
- Rash.
- Nausea.
- Vomiting.
- Stiff neck.
- Jaundice (yellow eyes; yellow skin; dark urine).
- Fever.
- Increased sweating.

 WARNINGS & PRECAUTIONS

- Before taking this medicine, consult your doctor if you have active alcoholism, angina (chest pain), asthma or bronchitis, diabetes mellitus (sugar diabetes), epilepsy, headaches (severe or frequent), heart or blood vessel disease, high blood pressure, kidney disease, liver disease, mental illness (history of), overactive thyroid, Parkinson's disease or Pheochromocytoma (PCC) or if you have recently had a stroke or heart attack.
- Don't drive or try risky physical activity until you know how drug affects you.
- See Appendix 21.

 AGE-RELATED FACTORS

- Dizziness, sedation, confusion, dry mouth, urinary retention and a drop in blood pressure more likely with advancing age.
- Your doctor or care-giver should carefully monitor your response to this drug.

 POSSIBLE INTERACTIONS WITH OTHER DRUGS

- If you are taking any other drug (prescription or non-prescription), ask your doctor or pharmacist if there are possible interactions.
- MAO inhibitors cannot safely be taken with some drugs.
- MAO inhibitors taken with some drugs may require dosage adjustment.

Do not drink alcoholic beverages or use cocaine, marijuana or tobacco while taking this medicine. These may decrease the effectiveness of the medicine or cause uncomfortable or dangerous adverse reactions.

 OVERDOSE

SYMPTOMS
Restlessness; agitation; excitement; fever; convulsions; coma.

WHAT TO DO
- Dial 911 (emergency) or 0 (operator) for an ambulance or medical help. Then give first aid immediately.
- If patient is unconscious and not breathing, give mouth-to-mouth breathing. If there is no heartbeat, use cardiac massage and mouth-to-mouth breathing (CPR). Don't try to make patient vomit. If you can't get help quickly, take patient to nearest emergency facility.

MEDICATIONS

MUSCLE RELAXANTS

BRAND & GENERIC NAMES

Commonly prescribed brand names (start with a Capital) and generic names (all CAPITALS) include BACLOFEN, CARISOPRODOL, CHLORZOXAZONE, CYCLOBENZAPRINE, Dantrium, DANTROLENE, Delaxin, DIAZEPAM, Disipal, Flexiril, Flexoject, Lioresal, Marbaxin, Marflex, METHOCARBAMOL, Norgesic (M), ORPHENADRINE, Paraflex, Parafon Forte (M), Rela, Robaxin, Robaxisal (M), Soma, Soma Compound (M), Soprodol, Valium, Valrelease and X-Otag. (The (M) means it is a mixture or combination drug.) Additional brand names are available.

 ## USES

Adjunctive treatment to rest, analgesics and physical therapy for muscle spasms.

 ## POSSIBLE ADVERSE REACTIONS OR SIDE EFFECTS

If any of the following occurs, consult a doctor:
- Drowsiness.
- Fainting.
- Dizziness.
- Orange or red-purple urine.
- Agitation.
- Constipation or diarrhea.
- Nausea.
- Cramps.
- Vomiting.
- Wheezing.
- Shortness of breath.
- Black, tarry or bloody stool.
- Rash.
- Hives.
- Itch.
- Sore throat.
- Fever.
- Jaundice (yellow eyes; yellow skin; dark urine).
- Tiredness.
- Weakness.

 ## WARNINGS & PRECAUTIONS

- Before taking this medicine, consult your doctor if you have history of allergies, epilepsy, kidney disease, liver disease or porphyria.
- Don't drive or try risky physical activity until you know how drug affects you.
- See Appendix 21.

 ## AGE-RELATED FACTORS

- Older patients are more likely to have age-related kidney or liver function impairment. This may lead to the need for reduction of the usual dosage.
- Side effects and adverse reactions are more likely to occur with advancing age.
- Your doctor or care-giver should carefully monitor your response to this drug.

 ## POSSIBLE INTERACTIONS WITH OTHER DRUGS

- If you are taking any other drug (prescription or non-prescription), ask your doctor or pharmacist if there are possible interactions.
- Muscle relaxants cannot safely be taken with some drugs.
- Muscle relaxants taken with some drugs may require dosage adjustment.

Do not drink alcoholic beverages or use cocaine, marijuana or tobacco while taking this medicine. These may decrease the effectiveness of the medicine or cause uncomfortable or dangerous adverse reactions.

 ## OVERDOSE

SYMPTOMS
Nausea; vomiting; diarrhea; headache. May progress to severe weakness; difficult breathing; sensation of paralysis; coma.

WHAT TO DO
- Dial 911 (emergency) or 0 (operator) for an ambulance or medical help. Then give first aid immediately.
- If patient is unconscious and not breathing, give mouth-to-mouth breathing. If there is no heartbeat, use cardiac massage and mouth-to-mouth breathing (CPR). Don't try to make patient vomit. If you can't get help quickly, take patient to nearest emergency facility.

NON-STEROIDAL ANTI-INFLAMMATORY AGENTS

BRAND & GENERIC NAMES

Commonly prescribed brand names (start with a Capital) and generic names (all CAPITALS) include Advil, Anaprox, Azolid, Butazolidin, Clinoril, DIFLUNISAL, Dolobid, Feldene, FENOPROFEN, IBUPROFEN, Indocin, INDOMETHACIN, KETO-PROFEN, MECLOFENAMATE, Meclomen, MEFENAMIC ACID, Motrin, Nalfon, Naprosyn, NAPROXYN, Nuprin, Orudis, PHENYLBUTAZONE, PIROXICAM, Ponstel, Rufen, SULINDAC, Tolectin and TOLMETIN. Additional brand names are available.

 ## USES

Reduces redness, heat, pain and swelling associated with inflammation due to infections and many non-infective conditions such as gout, arthritis, injuries and others.

 ## POSSIBLE ADVERSE REACTIONS OR SIDE EFFECTS

If any of the following occurs, consult a doctor:
- Hives.
- Rash.
- Intense itching.
- Faintness soon after a dose (anaphylaxis in aspirin-sensitive persons).
- Dizziness.
- Nausea.
- Pain.
- Headache.
- Depression.
- Drowsiness.
- Ringing in ears.
- Constipation or diarrhea.
- Vomiting.
- Swollen feet and legs.
- Convulsions.
- Confusion.
- Blurred vision.
- Black, bloody or tarry stool.
- Difficult breathing.
- Tightness in chest.
- Rapid heartbeat.
- Unusual bleeding or bruising.
- Blood in urine.
- Jaundice (yellow eyes; yellow skin; dark urine).
- Severe abdominal pain.
- Psychosis.
- Frequent, painful or difficult urination.
- Fatigue.
- Weakness.
- Rectal pain or irritation (with suppository).
- May worsen Parkinsonism and epilepsy.
- Swollen breasts in males.
- Impotence.

 ## WARNINGS & PRECAUTIONS

- Before taking this medicine, consult your doctor if you have low blood pressure, asthma, liver disease, recent head injury, abdominal pain, vomiting, ulcers in the stomach or duodenum, any bleeding disorder, anemia, colitis, diabetes mellitus (sugar diabetes), epilepsy, fluid retention (swelling of feet or lower legs), heart disease, hepatitis, mental illness, Parkinson's disease, polymyalgia rheumatica, rectal irritation or bleeding, systemic lupus erythematosus, temporal arteritis, ulcers or sores or white spots in mouth.
- You may have increased sensitivity to sun and light.
- Don't drive or try risky physical activity until you know how drug affects you.
- See Appendix 21.

 ## AGE-RELATED FACTORS

- Possible increased risk of gastrointestinal bleeding or ulcers. If these side effects occur, analgesics are more likely to cause serious consequences in older people.
- Older patients are more likely to have age-related kidney or liver function impairment. This may lead to the need for reduction of the usual dosage.
- Toxic effects are more likely.
- Your doctor or care-giver should carefully monitor your response to this drug.

 ## POSSIBLE INTERACTIONS WITH OTHER DRUGS

- If you are taking any other drug (prescription or non-prescription), ask your doctor or pharmacist if there are possible interactions.
- Non-steroidal anti-inflammatories cannot safely be taken with some drugs.
- Non-steroidal anti-inflammatories taken with some drugs may require dosage adjustment.

Do not drink alcoholic beverages or use cocaine, marijuana or tobacco while taking this medicine. These may decrease the effectiveness of the medicine or cause uncomfortable or dangerous adverse reactions.

 ## OVERDOSE

SYMPTOMS
Confusion; agitation; incoherence; convulsions; possible hemorrhage from stomach or intestine; coma.

WHAT TO DO
- Dial 911 (emergency) or 0 (operator) for an ambulance or medical help. Then give first aid immediately.
- If patient is unconscious and not breathing, give mouth-to-mouth breathing. If there is no heartbeat, use cardiac massage and mouth-to-mouth breathing (CPR). Don't try to make patient vomit. If you can't get help quickly, take patient to nearest emergency facility.

MEDICATIONS

SEDATIVES, NIGHT-TIME (Sleeping Aids)

BRAND & GENERIC NAMES

Commonly prescribed brand names (start with a Capital) and generic names (all CAPITALS) include ANTIDEPRESSANTS (see separate entry), ANTIHISTAMINES (see separate entry), CHLORAL HYDRATE, Dalmane, FLURAZEPAM, Halcion, Restoril, SECOBARBITAL, Seconal, TEMAZEPAM, TRIAZOLAM and Tuinal (M). (The (M) means a mixture or combination drug.) Additional brand names are available.

USES

- Treatment for insomnia.
- Some of the same medicines used as aids to sleep are also used as daytime antianxiety medicines, allergy medicines, or anti-depression medicines. When used as a night-time sedative alone, the dosage schedule and amount may be quite different. Secobarbital and other barbiturates are rarely prescribed for insomnia during the past few years because the other drugs are usually just as effective and are not as likely to have the same degree of adverse reactions or side effects.

POSSIBLE ADVERSE REACTIONS OR SIDE EFFECTS

If any of the following occurs, consult a doctor:
- Clumsiness.
- Daytime drowsiness.
- Dizziness.
- Hallucinations.
- Confusion.
- Depression.
- Irritability.
- Rash.
- Itch.
- Change in vision.
- Constipation or diarrhea.
- Nausea and vomiting.
- Painful or difficult urination.
- Slow heartbeat.
- Difficult breathing.
- Mouth or throat ulcers.
- Jaundice (yellow eyes; yellow skin; dark urine).

WARNINGS & PRECAUTIONS

- Don't take if you are allergic to any barbiturate, benzodiazepine, antihistamine or antidepressant.
- Don't take if you have myasthenia gravis or if you are an active or recovering alcoholic.
- Don't take if you have liver, kidney or lung disease.
- Consult your doctor if you have diabetes, epilepsy or porphyria.

AGE-RELATED FACTORS

- Side effects and adverse reactions are more likely to occur with advancing age. Much more likely to develop agitation, rage or "hangover effect."
- Lower-than-standard doses and longer intervals between doses may be required.
- Your doctor or care-giver should carefully monitor your response to this drug.

POSSIBLE INTERACTIONS WITH OTHER DRUGS

- If you are taking any other drug (prescription or non-prescription), ask your doctor or pharmacist if there are possible interactions. Some interactions may be very dangerous.
- Don't drive or try risky physical activity until you see how this drug affects you.
- Don't discontinue taking this drug without consulting your doctor. Dose may require gradual reduction if you have taken drug for a long time. Doses of other drugs may also require adjustment.

Do not drink alcoholic beverages or use cocaine, marijuana or tobacco while taking this medicine. These may decrease the effectiveness of the medicine or cause uncomfortable or dangerous adverse reactions.

OVERDOSE

SYMPTOMS
Drowsiness; weakness; tremor; stupor; coma.

WHAT TO DO
- Dial 911 (emergency) or 0 (operator) for an ambulance or medical help. Then give first aid immediately.
- If patient is unconscious and not breathing, give mouth-to-mouth breathing. If there is no heartbeat, use cardiac massage and mouth-to-mouth breathing (CPR). Don't try to make patient vomit. If you can't get help quickly, take patient to nearest emergency facility.

THYROID HORMONES

BRAND & GENERIC NAMES

Commonly prescribed brand names (start with a Capital) and generic names (all CAPITALS) include Cyronine, Cytomel, Levothyroid, LEVOTHYROXINE, LIOTHYRONINE and Synthroid. Additional brand names are available.

 ## USES

Replacement for thyroid hormone deficiency.

 ## POSSIBLE ADVERSE REACTIONS OR SIDE EFFECTS

If any of the following occurs, consult a doctor:
- Tremor.
- Headache.
- Irritability.
- Insomnia.
- Appetite change.
- Diarrhea.
- Leg cramps.
- Fever.
- Heat sensitivity.
- Unusual sweating.
- Weight loss.
- Hives.
- Rash.
- Vomiting.
- Chest pain.
- Rapid and irregular heartbeat.
- Shortness of breath.

 ## WARNINGS & PRECAUTIONS

- Do not take to help lose weight.
- Before taking this medicine, consult your doctor if you have diabetes mellitus (sugar diabetes), hardening of the arteries, heart disease, high blood pressure, overactive thyroid (history of), underactive adrenal gland, underactive pituitary gland or asthma.
- See Appendix 21.

 ## AGE-RELATED FACTORS

- Aging does not affect expected results.
- Your doctor or care-giver should carefully monitor your response to this drug.

 ## POSSIBLE INTERACTIONS WITH OTHER DRUGS

- If you are taking any other drug (prescription or non-prescription), ask your doctor or pharmacist if there are possible interactions.
- Thyroid hormones cannot safely be taken with some drugs.
- Thyroid hormones taken with some drugs may require dosage adjustment.

Do not drink alcoholic beverages or use cocaine, marijuana or tobacco while taking this medicine. These may decrease the effectiveness of the medicine or cause uncomfortable or dangerous adverse reactions.

 ## OVERDOSE

SYMPTOMS
Heart palpitations; nervousness; sweating; hand tremors; insomnia; rapid and irregular pulse; headache; irritability; diarrhea; weight loss; muscle cramps.

WHAT TO DO
Overdose unlikely to threaten life. If person takes much larger amount than prescribed, call doctor, poison control center or hospital emergency room for instructions.

MEDICATIONS

VASODILATORS (Antianginals)

BRAND & GENERIC NAMES

Commonly prescribed brand names (start with a Capital) and generic names (all CAPITALS) include ACE INHIBITORS (see separate entry), CALCIUM CHANNEL BLOCKERS (see separate entry), Dilatrate-SR, GUANETHIDINE, Ismelin, Iso-Bid, Isordil, ISOSORBIDE DINITRATE, Minipress, Minizide (M), Nitro-bid, NITROGLYCERIN, Nitrostat, PRAZOSIN, Sorbitrate and Transderm-Nitro. (The (M) means it is a mixture or combination drug.)

 USES

- Helps increase oxygen supply to heart muscle.
- Treats and prevents angina.
- Treats heart failure and some circulatory disorders.

 POSSIBLE ADVERSE REACTIONS OR SIDE EFFECTS

If any of the following occurs, consult a doctor:
- Headache.
- Flushed face and neck.
- Dry mouth.
- Nausea.
- Vomiting.
- Rapid heartbeat.
- Fainting.
- Restlessness.
- Blurred vision.
- Rash.
- Severe irritation and peeling of skin (if administered by patch).

 WARNINGS & PRECAUTIONS

- Before taking this medicine, consult your doctor if you have anemia (severe), glaucoma, intestinal problems, kidney disease, liver disease or overactive thyroid.
- See Appendix 21.

 AGE-RELATED FACTORS

- Older patients are more likely to have age-related kidney or liver function impairment. This may lead to the need for reduction of the usual dosage.
- Dizziness, sedation, confusion, dry mouth, urinary retention and a drop in blood pressure more likely with advancing age.

 POSSIBLE INTERACTIONS WITH OTHER DRUGS

- If you are taking any other drug (prescription or non-prescription), ask your doctor or pharmacist if there are possible interactions.
- Vasodilators cannot safely be taken with some drugs.
- Vasodilators taken with some drugs may require dosage adjustment.

Do not drink alcoholic beverages or use cocaine, marijuana or tobacco while taking this medicine. These may decrease the effectiveness of the medicine or cause uncomfortable or dangerous adverse reactions.

 OVERDOSE

SYMPTOMS
Dizziness; blue fingernails and lips; fainting; shortness of breath; weak, fast heartbeat; convulsions.

WHAT TO DO
- Dial 911 (emergency) or 0 (operator) for an ambulance or medical help. Then give first aid immediately.
- If patient is unconscious and not breathing, give mouth-to-mouth breathing. If there is no heartbeat, use cardiac massage and mouth-to-mouth breathing (CPR). Don't try to make patient vomit. If you can't get help quickly, take patient to nearest emergency facility.

Appendices

Good Nutrition for People over 50

The basic recommendations given here are for all people whose conditions do not require dietary treatment. For lots of reasons, older adults are more likely to veer from these guidelines than younger people. However, maintaining good nutrition remains one of the most important aspects of healthy aging. Your diet should follow the basic principles of the Dietary Guidelines for Americans, which have been developed by the U.S. Department of Agriculture and the U.S. Department of Health and Human Services:

- Eat a variety of foods.
- Maintain a desirable weight.
- Avoid too much fat, saturated fat and cholesterol.
- Eat foods with adequate starch and fiber.
- Avoid too much sodium.
- If you drink alcoholic beverages, do so in moderation.

SPECIAL NUTRITIONAL CONSIDERATIONS

- **Fiber**—Most dietetic experts recommend a diet with increased fiber (roughage) to promote normal bowel function. Increased roughage also protects against diverticulosis, some forms of intestinal cancer and perhaps even atherosclerosis, thus protecting against heart attack and stroke. Foods that are high in roughage (fiber) include whole grains, fresh vegetables, fresh fruits and bran.

- **Fat**—Your daily fat intake should not exceed 30% of the total calories you ingest. A low-fat diet (see Appendix 8) will help control obesity and decrease the likelihood of atherosclerosis.

- **Refined Sugar**—For optimal health, reduce your intake of refined sugars, such as those in candy. Eat unrefined sugars such as those found in fresh fruits, vegetables, potatoes and whole-grain breads and cereals.

- **Salt**—Reduce your salt intake to 3 to 4 grams (usually in the form of table salt) a day. See Appendix 9 for suggestions.

BASIC DIET SUGGESTIONS

Since metabolism is decreased in persons over 50, you probably will not require as many calories per day as younger people. Eat every 5 hours or so. Do not let more than 14 hours pass between an evening meal and breakfast.

The recommended daily caloric intake for persons over 50 who are of normal weight and capable of normal activity is 1,800 to 2,100 calories for men and 1,500 to 1,800 calories for women.

A pattern for daily food choices includes:

Breads, Cereals & Other Grain Products—6 to 11 servings from:

1 slice bread
1/2 hamburger bun or English muffin
1 small roll, biscuit or muffin
1/2 cup cooked cereal, rice or pasta
1 ounce of ready-to-eat breakfast cereal

Fruits—2 to 4 servings from:

1 apple, banana or orange
1/2 grapefruit
1 melon wedge
3/4 cup fruit juice
1/2 cup berries
1/2 cup cooked or canned fruit
1/4 cup dried fruit

Vegetables—3 to 5 servings from:

1/2 cup cooked vegetables
1/2 cup raw vegetables
1 cup leafy raw vegetables

Meat, Poultry, Fish & Substitutes—2 to 3 servings from:

5 to 7 ounces per day cooked lean meat, poultry or fish
Count 1 egg, 1/2 cup cooked beans or peas or 2 tablespoons peanut butter as 1 ounce of meat.

Milk, Cheese & Yogurt—2 servings from:

1 cup milk
8 ounces yogurt
1-1/2 ounces natural cheese
2 ounces processed cheese

Fats, Sweets & Alcoholic Beverages—Avoid too many sweets or fats. If you drink alcoholic beverages, do so in moderation.

SAMPLE MENU

The sample menu that follows adds up to 2,000 calories, and 30% of the calories come from fat:

Breakfast

1 cup cornflakes with blueberries
1 cup 1% milk
1 slice rye toast with 1 teaspoon margarine
1 cup orange juice
Black coffee or tea

Snack

Toasted bagel with 1 teaspoon margarine

Lunch

1 tuna salad sandwich (3 ounces tuna salad) on whole wheat bread with lettuce and tomato
1 graham cracker
Tea with lemon

Snack

1 apple

Dinner

3 ounces broiled lean ground beef with ketchup
1 baked potato with low-fat yogurt and chives
3/4 cup steamed broccoli with 1 teaspoon margarine
Tossed salad with 1 tablespoon oil and vinegar dressing
1 cup 1% milk
1 small piece homemade gingerbread

Vitamins, Minerals and Dietary Supplements

BASIC GUIDELINES

Everyone consumes vitamins, minerals and other supplements in some form. Most people rely on their diets to supply all their needs. Others take pills, capsules, powders, tonics or injections frequently on the advice of knowledgeable professionals. Some are prompted by advertising or recommendations from friends to try certain products that imply they will cure disease, improve one's sex life, prevent illnesses and prolong life. Health professionals want consumers to take the proper nutrients if they need them, but not to abuse them. Megadoses (doses from 10 to 20 times the recommended amount) can be dangerous. The Recommended Dietary Allowance (RDA) established by the National Research Council, which is part of the National Academy of Sciences, represents the best currently available assessment of safe and adequate intakes. It is important to know that vitamins, minerals and supplements are chemicals with pharmacologic properties because they can cause a change in the body's physiology or internal anatomy.

CONSIDERATIONS FOR OLDER ADULTS

In most cases, the nutrients needed each day are provided by the foods consumed in a well-balanced diet.

The diets of some older people may not provide the basic requirements of vitamins and minerals due to reduced calorie intake.

Preparing nutritional meals is not always easy or feasible. People living alone often do not take the time to prepare complete meals. Certain medications can interfere with the body's ability to use the vitamins and minerals present in foods.

Digestive problems and difficulty in chewing are more prevalent in older people.

Certain medical conditions may require the restriction of some foods in the diet that normally meet one's nutritional needs. In these cases supplements may be important.

Doctors may advise the use of vitamins or minerals by patients who have diseases such as osteoporosis (brittle bones), who are heavy users of alcohol or tobacco or who are anticipating or recovering from surgery.

Medical studies show that vitamin D levels in older people are often low. This may be a result of aging, lack of exposure to sunshine (sunscreen can block absorption) or inadequate intake of dairy products.

Institutions (nursing homes or other care facilities) may serve meals that do not appeal to everyone.

WHAT TO DO

To determine if your nutritional needs are being met, talk to your doctor or a registered dietitian about the foods you eat, the medicines you currently take and your state of health. They can help you decide whether to take dietary supplements.

Do not be misled by television commercials or magazine ads that make unrealistic promises about food supplements. Some supplements may pass right through the body and be excreted by the kidneys and therefore be of no value.

Avoid megadoses of any product. They can cause side effects as other medicines do and can sometimes cause permanent damage to bones or liver, and some, like iron supplements, can build to harmful levels in the liver and other organs.

People often take a "one-a-day" vitamin pill as a healthy guarantee, and there is normally no harm in doing so. It may provide a feeling of well-being that makes it worthwhile.

Read the labels on food packages to determine the nutritional value of the contents.

WHO CAN HELP

Be an informed consumer. Check at your local library for books on nutrition or supplements. Discuss nutrition, your diet and the need for supplements with your doctor.

Cholesterol

WHAT IS CHOLESTEROL?

Cholesterol, a fat or lipid, is a white, waxy substance that is an essential element in the body. The liver manufactures all the cholesterol the body needs. Consuming foods that contain cholesterol adds to the level already produced by the body. The cholesterol manufactured is either the "good" kind, high-density lipoprotein (HDL), or the "bad" kind, low-density lipoprotein (LDL). You should pay attention to the amount of cholesterol and the total fat you consume each day.

Cholesterol testing usually involves the determination of total cholesterol levels. If levels are high, retesting to verify results and also to determine the levels of HDL and LDL is recommended before you make any stringent dietary changes.

CONSIDERATIONS FOR OLDER ADULTS

Excess cholesterol may accumulate in the coronary arteries as atherosclerotic plaque, causing the arteries to narrow. This reduces or blocks the blood flow, and a heart attack may result.

High levels of cholesterol in men over age 50 increases the risk of future heart disease. Studies on women have been few, but it is safe to assume that women run similar risks.

Other risk factors that influence heart disease include smoking, a family history of heart disease, a sedentary lifestyle and poor nutrition. It is never too late to change your habits and reduce your cholesterol level.

Know your cholesterol level. Bring it down if the cholesterol level is above 240 mg/dl (240 milligrams of cholesterol per deciliter of blood).

WHAT TO DO

Get your cholesterol level checked, preferably in a doctor's office or at a location where it is done by health professionals. Mass cholesterol screenings done at supermarkets or malls have proven not to be reliable.

If your cholesterol level is over 200 mg/dl you should get a second test to confirm the results. Also get an analysis of the HDL and LDL levels.

Treatment for an excessive cholesterol level will depend on the presence or absence of several factors: cholesterol levels that are borderline (200 to 239 mg/dl) or high (240mg/dl or over), smoking, a family history of heart disease, high blood pressure, chronic illness, male or female sex, obesity, low concentration of the "good" cholesterol (HDL) and the general state of your health.

If you have a very high level of "bad" cholesterol (LDL), drug treatment may be recommended. There are several drugs available, and they all have significant side effects. Be sure your doctor discusses all of these with you.

For the majority of people with high cholesterol levels, a change in dietary habits is one of the cornerstones of treatment. Understand and know what products contain cholesterol and how dietary fat is involved.

There is some controversy among health experts as to the importance of cholesterol and the problems it causes. But everyone agrees that reducing one's total fat intake can do no harm. Try to keep your total fat consumption below 25 grams per day.

WHO CAN HELP

Your doctor should be the best source of advice and supervision for you about your diet. He or she will counsel you and determine the best course of action.

You may be referred to a dietician by your doctor, or you may seek assistance from a dietician directly.

There is a vast amount of printed material available about cholesterol. It has become one of the most written-about heath issues in the last few years. Most of this literature is available without cost, including material from the federal government. Check with your local library or health-care facility.

Read the labels of the products you buy. The advertising may promote the fact that a product has very little or no cholesterol, but the product may still have a high percentage of saturated fat. The consumption of saturated fat will inevitably raise the cholesterol level of your blood.

APPENDIX 4

Milk-Restricted Diet

This diet is used for the treatment of lactose intolerance and milk allergy.

Lactose intolerance is caused by a deficiency of the enzyme lactase, which breaks down lactose, the form of sugar found in milk. Some adults with lactase deficiency can tolerate small amounts of milk products, especially when they are consumed with a meal or other foods. This contributes valuable calcium to the diet. The diet should be individualized, depending on what you can tolerate.

Lactose-reduced milk is available, or you can purchase milk that has the lactase added. You may also purchase the lactase enzyme from a drug store over the counter and add it to milk to break down the lactose.

Milk allergy is a reaction caused by hypersensitivity to the protein found in milk, which can frequently cause an allergic reaction. Some people who are allergic to milk in one form may be able to use milk that has been boiled, evaporated or dried because these processes change the protein.

Milk is an important source of calcium, protein, vitamins A and D and riboflavin. Foods that are rich in these nutrients should be selected when milk has been excluded from your diet. Talk to your doctor about the use of calcium and vitamin D supplements.

Be a label reader. Know the ingredients by the technical names that are milk products: caseinate, casein, curds, dry milk solids, nonfat dry milk and whey.

SAMPLE MILK-RESTRICTED MENU

BREAKFAST	LUNCH	DINNER
Orange juice	Vegetable bouillon	Beef noodle soup
Oatmeal	Beef stew	Pork chops
Poached egg	Peas	Baked potato
Toast	Lettuce/vinegar & oil	Carrots
Margarine	Rhubarb pie	Fruit salad
Milk Substitute	Iced tea	Black coffee

Gluten-Restricted Diet

There may be a need to eliminate the consumption of gluten because of an intolerance that causes gastrointestinal problems. Gluten, a protein substance, is found in wheat, barley, rye, oats and buckwheat. The proteins found in corn, rice, soybean and tapioca flours and those in potato, arrowroot and corn starches contain no gluten.

Some people are allergic just to wheat gluten and need to omit only wheat flour, wheat starches and combinations containing wheat from their diets.

Read product labels carefully to determine if gluten is an ingredient. Look for terms such as bran, all-purpose flour, wheat flour, farina, graham flour, malt, wheat germ, whole wheat flour, wheat starch, barley, oats, rye and buckwheat.

For substitution, use soy, rice, corn, potato and tapioca flours. Homemade baked products using substitutes will not have the same consistency as those made with wheat flour. The batter may be thinner or thicker, and the finished items will be heavier, smaller in volume and more crumbly. They tend to dry out more quickly, so wrap them tightly. For long storage, put them in the freezer.

To thicken sauces and gravies, use nonwheat flour and starches. Rice flour is good for this use as it will not affect color or taste. Use the same amount as you would of wheat flour.

Allergy Diet

Many people suffer allergic reactions after eating certain foods. This diet is used to prevent or reduce those reactions by eliminating the offending foods.

FOODS	ALLOWED	OMITTED
Highly Seasoned Foods		Highly seasoned foods.
Beverages	Tea; carbonated beverages; cereal beverages.	Coffee; cola beverages; chocolate-flavored beverages.
Meats	Any except those in the omitted column; cottage cheese.	Highly seasoned meats such as cold cuts; fresh pork; fish; shellfish; eggs*; other cheeses; peanut butter; corned beef; cheese spreads.
Fats	Any except those in the omitted column.	Cream cheese; nuts; salad dressings made with eggs or cheese.
Milk	Milk; milk drinks.	Chocolate milk; eggnog; hot cocoa.
Breads	Any except those in the omitted column.	Commercially prepared mixes; any bread made with eggs or nuts; cornbread.
Vegetables	Any except those in the omitted column.	Tomatoes; tomato products (puree, sauce, ketchup, etc.).
Fruits	Any except those in the omitted column.	Fresh or frozen apples; cherries; berries+. Fresh, frozen, dried or cooked bananas; grapes; mangoes; papayas; pineapple; rhubarb; raisins.
Soups	Any except those in the omitted column.	Any made with corn, tomatoes or shellfish.
Desserts	Any except those in the omitted column.	Any made with chocolate, cocoa, eggs, nuts or omitted fruits; commercially prepared mixes.
Sweets	Any except those in the omitted column.	Jelly, jam or marmalade made with omitted fruits; candy with chocolate, eggs, nuts or omitted fruits.
Miscellaneous	Salt, spices, herbs except those omitted; vinegar; pickles; gravy; white sauce.	Garlic; strong spices; chocolate; cocoa.

*Eggs in all forms should be avoided when the diet is used for children. Adults, however, may have small amounts of cooked eggs, such as those found in most desserts. The allergic protein in eggs is denatured by cooking.

+Cooking denatures some allergens. Therefore, cooked apples, cherries and berries may be consumed. Other fruits may be extremely allergenic in some patients, and cooking does not denature the allergens.

(Adapted from The Mayo Clinic Diet Manual, Fourth and Fifth Editions. Philadelpha: W.B. Saunders Company, 1981.)

Liquid Diet

This diet is for patients who cannot chew or swallow solid foods. It is a modified form of the normal diet with changes in consistency or texture. The diet as outlined will satisfy the daily nutrient needs (except for iron and thiamine) recommended by the National Research Council, which is part of the National Academy of Sciences.

FOOD GROUPS	FOODS ALLOWED
Milk Group 4 or more 8-ounce cups milk	Whole milk; skim milk; buttermilk. Milk drinks such as eggnog, milkshakes and malted milk. Substitutes for 1 cup milk: 3 to 4 tablespoons dry milk. 4 ounces evaporated milk. 1 pint ice cream without fruit or nuts. Milk may be used in other foods, such as puddings, custards and strained cream soups.
Meat Group 2 or more servings or substitutes	Finely strained meats (about 2 tblsp. per serving) added to strained soups or broths. Substitute for 1 serving of meat: 2 eggs (in eggnog or soft custard). Commercially prepared strained meats and egg yolks.
Vegetable-Fruit Group 4 or more servings	**Sources of Vitamin C (1 Daily):** Strained grapefruit, orange, tangerine or tomato juices. **Sources of Vitamin A (1 Every Other Day):** Strained apricots, carrots, spinach or winter squash. **Other Fruits and Vegetables:** All other strained fruits and fruit juices. Other mild-flavored strained vegetables (fresh or canned) added to strained soups.
Bread-Cereal Group 4 or more servings	Strained cooked cereals. Cereals may be thinned with extra milk.
Fats	Cream; butter; margarine; oils.
Sweets and Desserts	Sugar; honey; molasses; corn syrup; ice cream; sherbet; ices; fruit whips or gelatin without nuts, seeds or whole fruits; soft-custard or rennet desserts.
Soups and Sauces	Strained soups.
Beverages	Any beverages such as coffee, tea, cocoa or carbonated drinks.
Miscellaneous	Salt and seasonings as tolerated.

(Adapted from *The Arizona Diet Manual*, by the Diet Therapy Section of the Arizona Dietetic Association, Inc., Revised 1985.)

Low-Fat Diet

Most diet experts agree that Americans eat too much fat. A low-fat diet can help prevent obesity and the dangers it causes to health. Use the diet suggestions below for general good health or for dietary treatment of your condition as recommended by your doctor.

FOODS	ALLOWED	OMITTED
Beverages	Coffee; tea; carbonated beverages.	No restrictions.
Breads and Cereals	4 servings or more a day of whole-grain or enriched cereals; white, whole wheat, rye or French bread; plain rolls; saltines; graham crackers; wheat crackers; corn or flour tortillas.	Biscuits, cornbread, pancakes and waffles unless made with allowed vegetable oils, egg white and skim milk or buttermilk; doughnuts; commercial coffee cakes; cheese crackers; pretzels; rusks.
Desserts	Angel food cake; cakes and cookies made with skim milk, oil and egg whites; fruit (preferred); fruit pie and cobblers (of pastry made with allowed oils); fruit whips; fruit meringues; gelatin desserts; puddings and custards made with skim milk; sherbet; fruit ices.	Desserts containing butter or margarine, chocolate, cream, egg yolk (unless from day's allowance), shortening or whole milk (such as ice cream and regular puddings); commercial cakes, cookies and pastries.
Eggs	Egg whites as desired, but limit egg yolks to no more than 3 per week, including those used in cooking; low-cholesterol egg substitutes.	
Fats (Use sparingly)	Corn oil; cottonseed oil; safflower oil; soybean oil; non-hydrogenated vegetable oil margarine; sunflower seed oil; commercial mayonnaise and salad dressings; peanut oil; olive oil.	All visible fat on meats; butter; chocolate; coconut oil; cream; lard; hydrogenated (hardened) fats; margarine (except that made with non-hydrogenated vegetable oil); bacon drippings.
Fruits	2 servings or more a day.	Avocado.
Meats and Meat Substitutes	5 ounces daily of lean meat, fish or poultry (trim all visible fat from meat before cooking and broil, boil or roast on a rack or barbecue using only sauce without fat); low-fat cottage cheese; sapsago cheese; mozarella cheese; specially prepared low-cholesterol cheeses; mature shelled beans and peas (for second entree when possible); nuts (particularly peanuts and walnuts if caloric allowance permits); tripe; beef or veal liver once a month.	Liver; duck; goose; bacon; salt pork; sausage; lunch meat; frankfurters; brisket; shortribs; club, porterhouse and T-bone steaks; prime rib roasts; cheese (except those allowed); any fish prepared with fats other than allowed oils; cashew nuts.
Milk	1-1/2 pints a day of skim milk or buttermilk; cocoa prepared with skim milk.	Whole milk; evaporated milk; Bulgarian buttermilk; beverages containing chocolate (note: cocoa is allowed); ice cream; ice milk; eggs; cream.

FOODS	ALLOWED	OMITTED
Miscellaneous	Herbs; ketchup; mustard; pickles; spices; gravies made from pan drippings skimmed free of fat (let stand in refrigerator until fat forms); popcorn cooked in oil or non-hydrogenated vegetable oil margarine; olives (use sparingly).	Coconut; buttered popcorn.
Potato or Substitute	White or sweet potato; brown or restored rice; corn; hominy; enriched grits; macaroni or noodles; dried beans and peas.	Fried potatoes and potato chips (unless cooked in oil).
Soups	Meat and chicken soups (soups should be cooled and fat removed from the top before reheating and serving); fat-free broth and bouillon; soups made with skim milk and allowed vegetable oil margarine.	Any soup made with butter, ordinary margarine or whole milk; most canned soups.
Sweets	Gumdrops; hard candy; homemade candies made without cream, whole milk, chocolate or butter; honey; jam; jelly; jelly beans; marshmallows; mints made with allowed ingredients; molasses; syrup; sugar.	Candies containing fats such as butter, chocolate, cocoa butter, coconut or cream.
Vegetables	2 servings or more of any vegetable. Do not cook vegetables with meat; season with non-hydrogenated vegetable oil margarine.	Any vegetables prepared with butter, ordinary margarine, cream, salt pork or bacon grease.

(Adapted from *The Arizona Diet Manual*, by the Diet Therapy Section of the Arizona Dietetic Association, Inc., Revised 1985.)

Low-Salt Diet

This is a normal diet from which are omitted only certain foods that have excessive salt or sodium. Avoid canned and prepared frozen foods. Read all labels carefully.

FOODS	ALLOWED	OMITTED
Beverages	All tea, coffee and milk.	No restrictions.
Bread and Cereals	Regular bread and cereals.	Crackers with salted tops; pretzels; salted popcorn.
Desserts	All, in moderation.	No restrictions.
Fats	All except those in the omitted column.	Bacon and bacon fat; salt pork; olives; prepared meats.
Fruits	All.	No restrictions.
Meat and Meat Substitutes	Meat; fish; poultry; eggs; cottage cheese; dried beans and peas; all cheeses except those omitted; cured meats and fish may be consumed once a week.	Any meat, fish or poultry that is smoked, brine-cured or salted, including bacon; bologna; chipped beef; corned beef; frankfurters; luncheon meats; ham; kosher meats; salt pork, sausages; salted or smoked fish such as herring, sardines, anchovies or salted codfish; processed cheese; cheese spreads; or cheese such as Roquefort or Camembert.
Potatoes and Substitutes	All except potato chips.	Potato chips.
Seasonings and Flavorings	A small amount of salt or other seasoning may be used in cooking.	Salt at the table; ketchup; pickles; relishes; soy sauce.
Soups	Cream soups; canned soups.	Bouillon cubes; prepared soup bases and canned soups containing smoked or salty meats.
Vegetables	All except those in the omitted column.	Sauerkraut and other vegetables prepared in brine.

(Adapted from *The Arizona Diet Manual*, by the Diet Therapy Section of the Arizona Dietetic Association, Inc., Revised 1985.)

Weight-Reduction Diet

This is a simple "exchange list" diet for individuals who want to lose weight. The diet provides 1,000 to 1,200 calories per day. If meals are chosen from a variety of foods, this diet will meet the adult Recommended Dietary Allowance (RDA). A diet of less than 1,000 calories per day may not meet requirements for vitamins and minerals.

Plan your meals by selecting items from the Breakfast, Lunch and Dinner columns of the Daily Portions from Food Lists. For example, breakfast allows you two different fruit portions (or two portions of the same fruit). Select two portions from the Fruit List. You may also have one portion from the Starch List for breakfast, and so on. The amounts of each portion are indicated in each food list.

Portions can be interchanged among breakfast, lunch and dinner as long as the total for the day doesn't exceed those indicated. For example, you can eat all your fruits for breakfast you want, but don't exceed 4 portions for the day.

Before starting any diet, ask your doctor for specific recommendations.

DAILY PORTIONS FROM FOOD LISTS
(See Food Lists below)

BREAKFAST	LUNCH	DINNER
2 Fruits	2 Meats	3 Meats
1 Starch	1 Vegetable	1 Fat
1/2 Milk	1 Fat	1 Starch
1 Fat	2 Starches	2 Vegetables
	1/2 Milk	1 Fruit
	1 Fruit	

FREE ITEMS: You may have these as desired.

Beverages: coffee; tea; sugar-free beverages.
Pickles, except sweet pickles.
Bouillon and consommes.
All spices, herbs, flavorings and artificial sweeteners.
Ketchup, mustard, soy sauce, vinegars and Worcestershire sauce.

FOOD LISTS

FRUIT LIST: A portion is 1 small piece or 1/2 cup unless listed.

Apple, apple juice or sauce	Fruit Cocktail	Plums (2)
Apricots (2)	Grapefruit or juice	Prunes (2)
Apricots, dried (2)	Grapes (12)	Prune juice (1/4 cup)
Banana	Grape juice	Raspberries
Blackberries	Lemon	Raisins (2 tblsp.)
Blueberries	Orange or	Rhubarb
Cantaloupe	orange juice	Strawberries (10)
Cherries	Peach	Tangerine
Dates (2)	Pear	Watermelon (1 cup)
	Pineapple	

VEGETABLE LIST: A portion is 1 cup raw or 1/2 cup cooked. Some vegetables are shown in the Starch List.

Artichoke	Celery	Parsley
Asparagus	Cucumber	Peppers
Beans, sprouts, green or wax	Eggplant	Peas
Beets	Endive	Pumpkin
Broccoli	Greens	Radish
Brussels sprouts	Lettuce	Rutabaga
Cabbage or sauerkraut	Mixed vegetables	Spinach
Cauliflower	Mushrooms	Squash
Carrot	Okra	Tomato
	Onions	Turnips

STARCH LIST

Angel food cake (1 oz.)
Bagel (1/2)
Beans, canned (1/2 cup)
Biscuit (1)
Bread (1 slice)
Bun (1/2)
Cereal (1/2 cup)
Corn (1/3 cup)

Cornbread (1 in. cube)
Cornstarch (2 tblsp.)
English muffin (1/2)
Flour (2-1/2 tblsp.)
Graham crackers (2)
Jello (1/2 cup)
Pancakes (1)
Pastas (1/2 cup)

Popcorn, fat-free (3 cups)
Potato, white (1/2 cup)
Potato, sweet (1/3 cup)
Pretzels (5 small)
Rice (1/2 cup)
Saltines (5)
Taco shell (1)
Tortilla (one 6-inch)

MEAT OR MEAT SUBSTITUTE: A portion is 1 ounce or 1/4 cup or as listed.

Beef (lean cuts)
Cheese (skim milk types)
Cold cuts or frankfurters
Cottage cheese (1/3 cup)

Eggs (3 per week)
Fish (all types)
Lamb (leg, roasted)
Peanut butter (1 tblsp.)

Poultry or game hen
Pork (chops; ham; roast)
Shellfish
Soybeans, cooked (1/3 cup)
Veal

FAT LIST

Bacon, crisp (1 slice)
Cheese, cream (1 tblsp.)
Coconut (1 tblsp.)
Cream, light (2 tblsp.)

Gravy (2 tblsp.)
Margarine (1 tsp.)
Mayonnaise (1 tsp.)
Nuts (6 to 10)

Oils (1 tsp.)
Olives (5 small)
Salad dressings (1 tblsp.)
Seeds (1 tblsp.)

MILK

Skim milk (1 cup)

Buttermilk (1 cup)

Yogurt (2/3 cup)

- Purchase fruits fresh, fresh frozen or canned unsweetened or in natural juices. All juices should be unsweetened.
- Vegetable and fruit portions are for the edible amounts of the items.
- Allowed amounts of meats are *after* cooking; amounts shown are for edible parts only (excluding bones). Be sure to trim all extra fat away from meat prior to cooking. Remove skin from all poultry. Roasting or broiling of meats is preferred.

Soft Diet

This diet is used frequently as a transition between a liquid diet and a regular diet. Usually this diet is used during recovery from surgery, especially dental surgery.

FOODS	ALLOWED	OMITTED
Beverages	Milk; cocoa; tea; coffee; fruit juices; carbonated beverages; decaffeinated coffee; cereal beverages.	No restrictions.
Cereals and Breads	Eat 4 or more servings daily of the following: dry or cooked refined cereals such as creamed wheat, farina, oatmeal, hominy grits, rice or cornmeal; cornflakes; puffed rice or puffed wheat; plain or toasted white or wheat-blend breads; saltines; flour tortillas.	All whole-grain breads; all hot breads including cornbread, pancakes, fried breads and sweet rolls; all whole-grain cereals except oatmeal.
Condiments	Salt and pepper in moderation; cinnamon; nutmeg; paprika; flavoring extracts.	All others, including chili and garlic.
Desserts	Simple desserts such as custard, gelatin, plain ice cream and sherberts; simple cakes and cookies; allowed fruits.	Rich pastries; any dessert containing dates, nuts, raisins or coconut.
Fats	Butter, cream, margarine and crisp bacon in moderation; mayonnaise.	Lard; pork fat; highly spiced salad dressings.
Fruits	Drink 1 serving of citrus juice daily; eat 2 or more servings of other fruits such as ripe avocado or banana; sectioned citrus fruit without membrane; fruit juices; cooked or canned apples, pears, peaches, white cherries, apricots, pineapple or fruit cocktail.	All fruits containing seeds and skins; all raw fruits except those allowed.
Meat, Fish Poultry, Eggs	Eat 2 or more 3-ounce servings daily of broiled, roasted, baked or stewed tender lean beef, mutton, lamb, veal, chicken, turkey, liver, pork, ham, bacon or whitefish; canned tuna, salmon or oysters; cottage cheese or other mild cheese used in cooking; poached, soft-cooked, hard-cooked, creamed or scrambled eggs.	All fried meat, fish or fowl; fried eggs; all strong-flavored cheese.
Milk	2 or more cups daily for adults; 3 to 4 cups daily for children.	No restrictions.
Potatoes or Substitutes	White or sweet potatoes; rice; noodles; spaghetti; macaroni.	Fried potatoes; potato chips or corn chips.
Soups	Broths or creamed soups made with allowed vegetables, strained tomatoes or creamed corn.	All soups not made with allowed vegetables; highly seasoned soups.
Sweets	Sugar; syrup; jelly; honey; plain hard candies; molasses.	Rich candies; jam with seeds.
Vegetables	Vegetable juices; cooked vegetables with low fiber content such as young peas, asparagus tips, carrots, beets, green beans, spinach, squash, cooked tomatoes or wax beans.	All gas-forming vegetables such as corn, radishes, Brussels sprouts, onions, dried beans and peas, broccoli, cabbage, parsnips, turnips, chili peppers or hominy.

(Adapted from *The Arizona Diet Manual*, by the Diet Therapy Section of the Arizona Dietetic Association, Inc., Revised 1985.)

Extending Your Life

The following suggestions represent the conclusions of a group of researchers headed by Drs. Belloc and Breslow of the University of California at Los Angeles, who studied the physical health status and health practices of thousands of older adults to find out why they had lived so long.

Their conclusions scientifically validate what we have known all along. To live a long time we should eat well, sleep well, not smoke, exercise, maintain a normal weight, love and be loved and stay active in our families and communities. Simple as these guidelines seem, you must accept them, review them and follow them if you desire to maintain optimum health and stay at your highest level of physical fitness, mental alertness and creativity.

Here are some suggestions for healthy living based on the results of the study:

GET ENOUGH SLEEP

Get the right amount of sleep (an average of 8 hours for men, 7 for women) each night. The right amount must also be coupled with the right *quality* of sleep. Consider these suggestions for good sleep:

- **Use the bedroom for sleep and intimacy only**—Avoid taking business or private worries to bed with you. Avoid getting caught up in suspenseful reading or television while relaxing in bed. If you toss and turn on occasion and can't get to sleep, go to another room and do something productive.
- **Learn relaxation techniques**—Try meditation or breathing exercises or alternate by tensing and relaxing muscles. Use one or more of these techniques, followed by a warm bath, before going to bed at night.

EAT A GOOD BREAKFAST

Don't skip breakfast! Failing to eat because you "don't have time" or ill-advisedly reducing the calories you consume per day can lead to poor health. The scientific evidence for this recommendation is convincing.

EAT THREE MEALS A DAY AT REGULAR TIMES

Regular meals keep the metabolic and digestive systems functioning at their most efficient levels. If you get hungry between meals, don't resort to fatty, salty or refined sugar snacks. Instead, eat fruit, raw vegetables or whole-grain snacks.

EXERCISE REGULARLY

Exercise that you enjoy is most likely to be successful and continued. See Appendix 20 for recommendations.

CONTROL YOUR WEIGHT

Even small amounts of excessive weight can shorten your life! Extreme obesity is associated with many physical and mental disorders. If you need to reduce, do so (see Appendix 10 for a weight-reduction diet). If your weight is ideal, work to keep it that way.

DRINK ALCOHOL MODERATELY—OR NOT AT ALL

Alcohol abuse can cause serious diseases, reduce your lifespan and make your life miserable. Moderate consumption can be defined as drinking no more than 3 ounces of alcohol in any form on any day.

DON'T SMOKE

There is overwhelming evidence that smoking damages the human body and shortens life. Cigarette smoking is a risk factor for many illnesses, particularly lung cancer, chronic lung disease, hardening of the arteries and heart disease. Anyone who smokes is at greater risk of problems with anesthesia during surgery.

DON'T ABUSE DRUGS

Evidence is mounting about the cumulative ill effects of drug abuse. Common sense dictates avoiding them if you want to stay mentally and physically healthy.

APPENDIX 13

Stress & Nervousness

Changes in lifestyle and disruptions in your normal routine can bring about stress. Some of the common causes of stress are:

- The recent death of a loved one—a spouse, child or friend.
- The loss of anything valuable to you.
- Injury or severe illness.
- Getting fired or changing jobs.
- A recent move to a new home.
- Sexual difficulties between you and your partner.
- Business or financial reverses or taking on a large debt, such as purchasing a new home.
- Regular conflict between you and a family member, close friend or business associate.
- Constant fatigue brought about by inadequate rest, sleep or recreation.

STRESS-RELATED DISORDERS

A certain amount of stress is not always bad. It varies from person to person how much stress one can handle easily. Sometimes stress can push us on to greater achievement. But excessive stress can be self-defeating. Too much stress can also lead to any of the following disorders:

- Mental and emotional upheavals.
- Skin eruptions, such as eczema and neurodermatitis.
- Digestive system problems, including peptic ulcers, colitis and irritable colon.
- Endocrine disorders, including overactive thyroid, adrenal or pituitary gland overactivity or underactivity, impotence and premature ejaculation in men or orgasmic dysfunction in women.
- Lung disorders associated with spasms of the bronchial tubes, such as asthma.
- Pain syndromes, such as chronic or recurrent disabling headaches or back pain.
- Eating disorders, either overeating or loss of appetite.

Many doctors believe that stress has a role in almost any disorder. Practically no one doubts that stress can complicate an illness by preventing normal recovery, prolonging pain and sustaining disability.

TIPS FOR REDUCING STRESS

The following techniques will help you reduce the amount of stress in your life if you practice them regularly:

- **Meditate**—Learn a meditation technique and practice it regularly—daily if possible. There are many methods available. Most of them include "tuning in to" and giving complete attention to a word, sound, sentence or concept that you silently repeat to yourself. Don't try to banish other thoughts that enter your mind during your period of concentration, but don't focus on them enough to stop you from meditating. The purpose of meditation is to empty your mind of all disturbing thoughts for a given period of time to encourage mental relaxation. Mental relaxation, in turn, will help reduce stress.
- **Learn to relax your body**—Take a short period of time away from any stressful situation you encounter during a day. Practice a muscle-tensing and muscle-relaxing technique. Close your eyes, and take a series of deep breaths. Then start with the muscle groups in your face. Consciously tense them and hold the contraction for a few seconds. Then consciously relax them. Continue through all major muscle groups in your body: your neck, shoulders, hands, abdomen, back and legs. When you become skillful, you can use this technique to produce relaxation quickly any time you need to and in almost any environment.
- **Exercise**—Adopt an exercise program (see Appendix 20). People in good physical condition are less likely to suffer the negative effects of stress, anxiety or depression.
- **Don't take your problems to bed with you**—At the end of the day, spend a few minutes reviewing your entire day's experiences, event by event, as if you're replaying a tape. Release all negative emotions you have harbored (anger, feelings of insecurity or anxiety). Relish all good energy or emotion (loving thoughts or good feelings about your work or yourself). Reach a decision about unfinished events, and release mental or muscular tension. Now you're ready for a relaxing and emotionally healing sleep.

PSYCHOSOMATIC ILLNESS

We can't separate our bodies from our minds or our spirits. Most departures from good health have some connection with these elements of ourselves.

Psychosomatic illness is a term used to describe an illness in which factors other than physical ones are dominant. They may also play an important part in complications. Such illnesses are real—not imagined, as many people think. The links between body, mind and spirit may be poorly defined at times, but they are provable by accepted scientific methods.

Although medical researchers are beginning to understand the basic mechanisms, we still have much to learn about psychosomatic illness. One group of researchers believes that mental, emotional or spiritual stress can trigger almost any illness in a person who is genetically predisposed to that illness. Such illnesses include asthma, cancer, digestive disturbances and heart disease. All these and others are more common in certain families and are more likely to complicate normal aging.

Yet all persons with the same genetic makeup do not succumb to the same illnesses. Here are some simple suggestions to help you improve, prevent or cope with psychosomatic illness:

- Define and resolve all personal conflicts. Define and confront areas of personal conflict in your spiritual, emotional, occupational, civic or recreational involvements. If you can't resolve these conflicts alone, seek help from family members, friends or competent counselors.
- Be moderate in all your activities.
- Seek a balanced life of work, intellectual and physical challenges, recreation, intimacy, reflection and rest.
- Be of good humor whenever possible.
- Be a friend.
- Give and receive love.
- Keep a positive outlook on life. Considerate, respectful and loving attitudes toward yourself and others are powerful allies.

Breast Self-Examination

WHY YOU SHOULD EXAMINE YOUR BREASTS MONTHLY

Most breast cancer is first discovered by women themselves. Since breast cancer found early and treated promptly has an excellent chance for cure, learning how to examine your breasts properly can help save your life. Use the simple 3-step breast self-examination (BSE) procedure described below.

WHEN TO EXAMINE YOUR BREASTS

After menopause, check your breasts on the first day of each month. Breast cancer is more common after menopause than before menopause. Doing a monthly self-exam will give you peace of mind, and seeing your doctor once a year will reassure you there is nothing wrong.

THREE-STEP BREAST SELF-EXAM

1. In the Shower

Examine your breasts during a bath or shower, as your hands glide more easily over your skin when it's wet. With your fingers flat, move your hand gently over every part of each breast. Use your right hand to examine your left breast, your left hand for your right breast. Check for any lump, hard knot or thickening.

2. In Front of a Mirror

Inspect your breasts with your arms at your sides. Next, raise your arms high overhead. Look for any changes in the contour of each breast, such as a swelling, dimpling of the skin or changes in the nipple.

3. Lying Down on Your Back

To examine your right breast, put a pillow or folded towel under your right shoulder. Place your right hand under your head to distribute the breast tissue more evenly on your chest.

With your hand, fingers flat, press gently in small circular motions around an imaginary clock face. Begin at the top outermost part of your right breast for 12 o'clock, then move to 1 o'clock, and so on around the circle back to 12. A ridge of firm tissue in the lower curve of each breast is normal. Then move in an inch toward the nipple, and keep circling to examine every part of your breast, including the nipple. This requires at least three more circles.

Now slowly repeat the procedure on your left breast with a pillow under your left shoulder and your left hand under your head. Notice how your breast structure feels.

Finally, squeeze the nipple of each breast gently between your thumb and index finger. Any discharge, clear or bloody, should be reported to your doctor immediately.

WHAT TO DO IF YOU FIND A LUMP OR THICKENING

If you discover a lump, dimple or discharge during a self-exam, it is important to see your doctor as soon as possible. Don't be frightened. Most breast lumps or changes are not cancer, but only your doctor can make the diagnosis.

(Courtesy of the American Cancer Society)

APPENDIX 15

Back Care

EXERCISES TO DO WHEN YOU ARE EXPERIENCING BACK PAIN
While lying on your back in bed:

- Bring one knee up to your chest. Lower it slowly, but do not straighten the leg. Relax. Repeat with each leg 10 times.
- Bring both knees slowly up to your chest. Tighten your abdominal muscles and press your back flat against the bed. Hold your knees to your chest 20 seconds, then lower your legs slowly. Relax. Repeat 5 times. This exercise gently stretches shortened muscles of your lower back while strengthening your abdominal muscles.
- Clasp your knees and bring them up to your chest, at the same time coming to a sitting position. Rock back and forth.

EXERCISES TO DO AFTER YOUR BACK PAIN HAS LEFT
Use these inconspicuous exercises whenever you have a spare moment during the day, both to reduce tension and to improve the tone of important muscle groups:

- Rotate your shoulders forward and backward.
- Turn your head slowly side to side.
- Turn your head down and to the right as if stretching to see your right armpit. Stretch your neck slowly up, around and down, switching to gaze at your left armpit. Repeat, starting on the left side.
- Slowly touch your left ear to your left shoulder, then your right ear to your right shoulder. Raise both shoulders to touch your ears, then drop them as far down as possible.
- At any pause in the day (such as waiting for an elevator or traffic light), pull in your abdominal muscles, tighten and hold them for the count of 8 without breathing. Relax slowly. Increase the count gradually after the first week, and practice breathing normally with your abdomen flat and contracted. Do this while sitting, standing and walking.

HOW TO PREVENT RECURRENT BACK PAIN
- Never bend from your waist only. Bend both your hips and your knees.
- Never lift a heavy object higher than your waist.
- Always turn and face the object you wish to lift.
- Avoid carrying unbalanced loads. Hold heavy objects close to your body.
- Never carry anything heavier than you can easily manage.
- Never lift or move heavy furniture alone. Get help from someone who knows the principles of leverage.
- Avoid sudden movements that "overload" your muscles. Learn to move deliberately, swinging your legs from your hips.
- Train yourself to use your abdominal muscles to flatten your lower abdomen. In time, this muscle contraction will become a habit.
- For good posture, concentrate on strengthening "nature's corset," the muscles of your abdomen and buttocks.
- For proper bed posture, a firm mattress is essential. If you have a soft mattress, put a 3/4-inch piece of plywood under it. Lie and sleep on your side with your knees flexed.
- Learn to keep your head in line with your spine when standing, sitting and lying in bed.
- Don't sit in soft chairs and deep couches. During prolonged sitting, cross your legs to rest your back.
- Use a rocking chair. Rocking rests your back.
- Avoid exercise that arches or overstrains your lower back, such as backward bends, forward bends or touching your toes with your knees straight.

Immunizations, Checkups & Screening Exams

RECOMMENDED IMMUNIZATIONS:

IMMUNIZATION	FREQUENCY	COMMENTS
Tetanus and diphtheria	Every 10 years	Repeat at the time of any dirty injury.
Pneumococcus	At least once	Protects against pneumococcal pneumonia.
Influenza	Once each year	The dosage is determined annually and is provided to your doctor or health department by the Centers for Disease Control in Atlanta.

Vaccines are also available to protect against hepatitis, rabies, typhoid fever and other diseases. These vaccines are given only under special circumstances. Ask your doctor, health department or travel agent about vaccinations and preventive medications (such as malaria protection) required or recommended before travel in another country. Inquire several months before your expected departure if possible.

CHECKUPS

After age 50, you should have a thorough physical examination every 2-1/2 years to every 5 years. Schedules will depend on your state of health and your primary doctor's recommendation. After you reach age 75, an annual physical examination is suggested.

SCREENING EXAMS

There are special health screening exams that should be done more frequently, such as mammograms to detect breast cancer in women and exams for men to check for prostate problems. Preventive measures are the best way to head off health problems. You and your doctor need to establish a specific set of guidelines for you to follow. There is no one set of rules that can apply to everyone about what screening exams to take and when. Your medical history, current health status and risk factors (smoking, overweight, etc.) will determine what exams are appropriate and how often to obtain them.

SCREENING EXAMS TO CONSIDER	FREQUENCY
Blood count	Every 1 to 3 years.
Blood glucose	Every 5 to 10 years.
Blood in stool	Annually.
Breast exam/mammogram	Annually.
Cholesterol	Every 3 to 5 years.
Colon (sigmoidoscopy)	Every 3 to 5 years.
Eyes/glaucoma	Every 1 to 2 years.
Hearing	Every 3 to 5 years.
Pap smear	Heed doctor's recommendation.
Prostate	Annually.
Urinalysis	Every 3 to 5 years.

Care of Casts

A cast is used to help immobilize an injured part of the body after a fracture or other injury.

A cast is usually applied by placing a splint along the injured part and then wrapping it with gauze saturated with plaster of Paris. Before the injury heals, it may be necessary to change the cast one or more times. The time that the cast remains in place depends on how much time is needed for healing. Some casts are needed for only two weeks. Others remain in place for several months.

X-rays through the cast will determine that there is satisfactory alignment of the bones involved and later will demonstrate evidence of healing or non-healing.

CARE OF THE CAST

Do not allow pressure on any part of the cast until it is completely dry. The time required for drying varies, depending on the thickness of the cast, the temperature and the humidity. Drying can require 24 hours or longer.

If the cast accidentally gets wet and a soft area appears, return to the doctor's office, emergency room or outpatient surgical facility for repairs.

CARE OF THE PATIENT IN A CAST

Whenever possible, raise the part enclosed in the cast. This decreases the likelihood of swelling of the tissues underneath the cast. Prop a leg cast on a pillow when your are in bed and on a footstool or chair when your are sitting. Prop an arm cast on a pillow placed on your chest.

No matter how carefully the injured tissues are handled and no matter how expertly the cast is applied, it is still possible for swelling to occur under the cast. If this happens, one or more of the following symptoms will probably become noticeable:

1. Severe and persistent pain.
2. Change in the color of the tissues beyond the cast, such as a change to blue or gray under the nails of the fingers or toes.
3. Coldness of the tissues beyond the cast when the rest of the body is warm.
4. Numbness or complete loss of feeling in the skin beyond the cast.
5. Swelling of the tissue to a greater extent than was present before the cast was applied.

If any of the above signs or symptoms occurs, contact your doctor or an emergency room as soon as possible for treatment.

Soaks

Soaks are used to treat symptoms or diseases of the skin.

Soaks can surround a scraped, injured or denuded part of the skin with fluid. Fluid frequently calms nerve endings that transmit pain and itching sensations. Soaks also soften and dissolve crusts (such as scabs) and remove material that may invite secondary bacterial infection or cause fluid to collect and damage the skin.

WRAPPED SOAKS

Moisten and wring out strips of cotton cloth just enough so they are not dripping wet. Wrap the strips around the affected area. Keep the strips moist, and keep them applied for at least 30 minutes at a time.

Repeat the soaks several times a day.

IMMERSION SOAKS

Use a bathtub, sitz bath or foot pan with enough lukewarm or cool water to cover the affected area. Use soaks 30 to 40 minutes at a time, and repeat them several times a day. Use swirling water such as that in a whirlpool or spa if possible.

Water temperature is not critical for any kind of soak, but in general cool water relieves itching and warm water relieves pain.

Chronic skin ulcers may require several weeks of soaks. Patients with other skin problems should use soaks for only 2 to 3 days. Otherwise, the skin may become dehydrated and the underlying problem will worsen.

APPENDICES

Recovery from Surgery

To achieve maximum recovery from surgery in the shortest period of time and to prevent complications, several goals need to be accomplished. The medical professionals involved concern themselves with your recovery from the procedure itself, the prevention of complications, restoring lost functioning, helping you adapt to changes that must be made and helping your family to adjust. There are many different components within these goals, and each one needs to be adapted to each individual's needs.

LOCATIONS FOR RECOVERY AND REHABILITATION

Your actual rehabilitation will begin in the hospital where the surgery takes place. Activities can begin while you are still in bed. Sitting up and moving around are simple starts.

Locations for further rehabilitation include your own home, a family member's home, a nursing home or a rehabilitation facility. Determinants will be the degree of your functional disability, whether you need full-time help by a care-giver, the rehabilitation requirements, your financial capabilities and Medicare coverage.

PSYCHOLOGICAL (EMOTIONAL AND MENTAL) CONSIDERATIONS

Your healing can be hampered or delayed by your fear of pain, fear of disability or fear of lost function and postoperative depression. Do everything possible to keep a positive attitude about recovery. Optimism and perseverance can be your greatest allies. Remember that aging alone is never a contraindication for surgery and that even very old people regularly come through the total experience successfully. Age is not a deterrent to rehabilitation, either, but recovery may take longer and be more frustrating for older persons.

PHYSIOLOGICAL (PHYSICAL AND CHEMICAL) CONSIDERATIONS

In the Hospital

- Cough and deep breathing exercises prevent pneumonia and/or the collapse of small segments of the lung, promote mental alertness, improve circulation, encourage better kidney function, prevent clots in your leg veins, quicken the recovery of normal bowel function, increase the rate of metabolism and prevent the loss of muscle tone.

  Force yourself to cough at least every two hours after surgery to help keep your lungs free of secretions. Lie in a comfortable position and splint the incision with a pillow if the incision is in your chest or abdomen. Your nurse will coach you through these basic steps:

  Take a deep, slow breath.
  Expand your chest as much as you can.
  Breathe out through your mouth.
  Cough at least two or three times every two hours—more if possible. Repeat the deep-breathing exercises several times each hour.

- To reduce incisional pain, use bed siderails for support when you move around; place one hand above and one below your incision or place a small pillow over the incision when you move.
- Do leg exercises to reduce the chance of blood clots forming in the veins and prevent muscle atrophy. Move your legs frequently from a flat position by bending your knees and flexing your thighs every 15 minutes or so. Between flexing, alternate contracting and relaxing the calf muscles as you lie in bed. Do this as often as your strength will allow.

At Home

- Use elastic stockings unless your surgeon directs otherwise. These will help reduce the possibility of blood clots in the veins of your legs.
- Observe the incision daily for evidence of increased warmth, redness or swelling. Any of these symptoms may represent an infection and require a call to your surgeon.
- Unless directed otherwise, wash over the incision whenever you wish, being sure to use clean water and cloths. If possible, use showers instead of tub baths.
- Keep the incision clean and dry between washings.
- Discard dressings in a plastic bag.
- Wash your hands carefully each time before attending to the incision or dressings.
- Become and stay as active as possible to avoid pressure sores. These have a tendency to be more common in older people because of less subcutaneous fat, poor capillary circulation and lower blood volume.

- Make sure you have specific instructions about your activity and exercise level. Don't hesitate to talk to your surgeon about sex, driving, returning to work, or any other concerns.
- Follow the medication instructions exactly.
- Request specific instructions about your diet and meal plans.
- Report to your doctor any new or dramatic changes that may occur, such as bleeding or discharge from the incision, an abrupt worsening of incisional pain, fever, diarrhea or vomiting.

Rehabilitation

The elements of rehabilitation will vary from one surgical procedure to another, but the basic elements of rehabilitation are approximately the same. Your doctor may refer you to other medical professionals for assistance. Physical therapists, speech therapists, visiting nurses and social workers are available to provide the services required or train you or a family member to perform them. Here is a list of important rehabilitation modalities and facts about some of them:

- **Heat**—When heat is applied to any part of the body, it dilates the small blood vessels in the area, increasing the blood flow. The increased blood supply nourishes the tissues and hastens healing. Heat also reduces pain at the site of the operation and reduces muscle spasms.

  Heat can be applied in several ways: hot compresses, wet packs, heat lamps, heating pads, whirlpool baths or hot tubs, ultrasound and diathermy. Your doctor or therapist should prescribe the best program for you and provide guidance throughout your rehabilitation program. You will need instructions about when to start, how long to apply heat during each treatment, and how long to continue with heat treatments. These factors are determined by many variables, such as your age and previous medical history, the site and extent of your surgery, your expected healing rate and others.
- **Massage**—Gentle massage is useful for treating soreness in muscles that is brought on by required bed rest. It is also useful in preventing bed sores. Massage consists of the gentle or firm stroking of muscle groups. The strokes should be directed toward the heart. The appropriate amount of pressure and length of massage must be determined by the person receiving the massage. Massage that induces pain is too hard.

  When properly administered, massage has several benefits. It can reduce fluid accumulation and swelling around the site of an operation and can stimulate circulation through the veins and lymphatic vessels. However, overzealous massage can aggravate discomfort and increase bleeding.
- **Exercise**—Many operations, such as open reduction of bone fractures, amputations, and many others, require rehabilitation of muscle groups as a very important part of recovery. These exercises should be prescribed by your surgeon or physical therapist. They include range-of-motion exercises, passive exercises, muscle-strengthening exercises and exercises to improve your endurance and coordination.
- **Electricity**—This may be used with special equipment by trained personnel to stimulate muscles that you are unable to contract voluntarily. Ten to twenty contractions per session are usually sufficient. Transcutaneous electrical nerve and muscle stimulation (TENS) has been used by some to reduce chronic pain.
- **Traction**—This is frequently prescribed following operations to reduce fractures of the spine.
- **Orthotic Devices**—There are a great number of these available, including specially constructed orthopedic shoes, canes, crutches and walkers, leg braces, neck braces, corsets, wheelchairs and others. Your doctor, nurse or pharmacist may direct you to the places where these are available in your community.
- **Speech Therapy**—Following surgical procedures on the throat or brain, your speech may be temporarily impaired. Speech pathologists and speech therapists may give you guidance and coaching to help you develop the motor skills necessary to regain speech.

Physical Fitness for the Active Older Adult

People of all ages benefit from regular exercise. Many persons aged 50 and older exercise regularly and stay as physically fit as their general health allows. These persons grow older with a style and vigor far surpassing that of their sedentary contemporaries.

CONSIDERATIONS FOR OLDER ADULTS

More people reach age 65 and older who are physically fit than those who are not. Those who remain physically active continue to have more stamina than their inactive counterparts.

Although exercise probably does not retard the aging process, it reduces the likelihood of untimely death from medical problems that are caused in part by a sedentary lifestyle. These include coronary artery disease, high blood pressure, stroke, kidney disease, chronic lung disease and depression.

THE BENEFITS OF AEROBIC EXERCISE

Aerobic exercise is the most effective way to achieve physical and psychological benefits. Aerobic exercise is physical activity that uses major muscle groups of the body and is sustained for 20 minutes or more.

Proper aerobic benefit is derived from exercise that is sufficient to accelerate your heart rate to a prescribed level and keep it there a certain length of time. For maximum benefit, 3 to 5 aerobic exercise sessions a week are necessary. The best forms of aerobic exercise include brisk walking, swimming, low-impact aerobic exercises, bike riding, rope jumping and rowing. Sports such as bowling, tennis or golf have good recreational effects, but they do not require enough effort to reach sustained aerobic levels.

Persons over 50 receive the same benefits from aerobic exercise as do younger persons—even if they choose the less strenuous forms of exercise. Following is an explanation of the effects of aerobic exercise on the body.

Exercise & the Cardiovascular System

Older persons are most at risk for cardiovascular problems. Exercise benefits the cardiovascular system by increasing the number of circulating red blood cells (thus providing more oxygen and better nourishment to all body cells), increasing blood flow during exercise, increasing the enzymes necessary to change glucose into usable energy by body cells and increasing the high-density lipoproteins in the circulating blood, thereby protecting against hardening of the arteries, which is responsible for heart attacks, strokes and chronic kidney failure.

Exercise & Circulation to the Brain & Other Body Parts

Exercise in a healthy person produces an increase in an enzyme that helps prevent the deposit of fibrin (a clotting factor in the blood) in blood vessels to the brain and other body parts. Fibrin deposits on the lining of the blood vessels narrow the arteries and decrease the blood supply to the cells supplied by the affected blood vessels. Narrowed arteries and decreased blood flow can result in stroke, heart attack and lack of sufficient blood supply to the kidneys and legs, causing kidney failure.

Exercise & the Lungs

Regular exercise can increase maximum breathing capacity, improving or preventing chronic lung disease.

Exercise & the Musculoskeletal System

Regular, adequate exercise helps maintain the normal size and contour of muscles and bones. The combination of exercise and adequate calcium intake is an important factor in preventing osteoporosis (softening of the bones), a common disorder in women past menopause. (In addition to exercise and calcium, estrogen replacement in women may also be necessary to prevent osteoporosis). Exercise promotes healthy new bone formation in all age groups. This new bone protects against bone fractures that commonly occur in older people of both sexes.

Exercise & the Mind

Exercise helps rid the body of undesirable levels of catecholamines (breakdown products of adrenalin, which is released by the body as a reaction to physical or mental stress). Many studies have shown that regular exercise has a positive influence on one's sense of well-being and self-esteem.

An exercise program can also be very beneficial in relieving depression; it is now commonly prescribed as part of therapy.

Exercise and Sexuality

Men who remain physically active maintain a higher level of testosterone than their sedentary contemporaries. People who exercise regularly are generally healthier emotionally, have a better self-image and enjoy increased muscular strength. These factors are all important in meaningful sexual relationships.

People who are fit—no matter what their age—are more sexually attractive to others.

WHO CAN HELP

Regular exercise has proved to be of great benefit in minimizing the negative effects of aging. If you have not remained physically fit, discuss a fitness program with your doctor. Follow his or her suggestions about what you can safely do.

An Exercise Prescription

After obtaining a medical history and performing a physical examination, your doctor may address four components of your exercise "prescription":

1. Type of Exercise—Popular ones include brisk walking, swimming, bike riding and lowimpact aerobics.

2. Frequency of Exercise—It's best to start at about three exercise sessions per week, then increase gradually to four, five or more.

3. Duration of Exercise—The ideal duration is 30 minutes of continuous activity. It's best to begin with 10 or 15 minutes and increase as your tolerance for exercise improves.

4. Intensity of Exercise—This component varies greatly depending on your age, sex and medical condition. If your doctor prescribes an exercise program, he or she will give specific instructions that uniquely apply to you after your physical checkup.

Recruit a spouse or a friend to exercise with. Companionship makes exercise fun!

Safe Use of Medications

Some suggestions for the wise and safe use of medications apply to all medicines and are particularly important to older patients. Your doctor and dentist must have complete information to prescribe drugs wisely for you. Before prescriptions are given, always give the following information to your physician, dentist or other health-care professional:

- **Your Complete Medical History**—Tell the important facts of your medical history dealing with medicines. Include allergic reactions, side effects or adverse reactions you have experienced in the past. Describe the allergic problems you have, such as hay fever, asthma, eye watering and itching, throat irritation and reactions to food. People who have allergies to common substances are more likely to develop side effects or adverse reactions to drugs.
- **Medications You Are Taking Now**—List all prescription and non-prescription drugs and carry the list with you for each medical appointment. Don't forget common ones such as laxatives; vitamin or mineral supplements; skin, rectal or vaginal medicines; antacids; antihistamines; cold and cough remedies; aspirin and aspirin-containing pain pills; motion sickness remedies; weight-loss aids; salt and sugar substitutes; caffeine (in coffee, tea, cola drinks and cocoa); sleeping pills; or "tonics."

WHAT YOU SHOULD KNOW BEFORE TAKING ANY MEDICATION

- The generic names and brand names of all the medicines you take. Write them down to help you remember. If a drug is a mixture of two or more generic ingredients, learn the names of each.
- The uses for each medicine you take.
- How to take each medicine—for example, with or without water or with food.
- When to take each medicine.
- What to do if you forget a dose.
- How each drug works in your body.
- The time lapse before the drug works.
- Symptoms of and treatment for overdose.
- Possible adverse reactions and side effects and what to do if they occur.
- Interactions with other drugs and other substances such as alcohol, food, beverages, cocaine, marijuana and tobacco. When mixed with some medicines, these substances can sometimes cause life-threatening interactions.
- All warnings and precautions that apply to special circumstances, such as:
  1. Reasons not to take the drug in the presence of some medical conditions. These reasons are called *contraindications*.
  2. Implications for prolonged use, exposure to sun and sunlight, driving, piloting aircraft, hazardous work and flying in airplanes.
  3. Instructions for discontinuing the drug.

All this information, written in simple, easy-to-understand language, can be found in my book *Complete Guide to Prescription and Non-Prescription Drugs,* which is published by Perigee Books.

CONSIDERATIONS FOR OLDER ADULTS

There are special considerations regarding the use of medications by older adults. The following statements will summarize them. Bear them in mind, and talk to your doctor about how any of them may apply to you.

Reduced elimination capabilities due to decreasing kidney function may result in higher concentrations of drugs in the bloodstream and may require some modification of the usual dosage, such as lower doses and longer intervals between doses.

In older people who take aspirin and other non-steroidal anti-inflammatory medicines (such as ibuprofen and others), there is an increased risk of gastrointestinal bleeding or ulcers. If these side effects occur, they are more likely to cause serious consequences in older people than in younger adults, particularly gastrointestinal bleeding.

Monitoring a patient's response is more important in older patients. Adverse reactions and side effects are not only more likely to occur, but they may also be more difficult to evaluate and treat.

Narcotics, antihistamines, sleeping aids, sedatives, tranquilizers, and muscle-relaxing drugs are more likely to cause both mental and physical depression in older persons.

Avoid *aluminum-containing* antacids. Aluminum, according to some studies, may be one of the contributing causes of Alzheimer's disease. In addition, some forms of bone disease may be aggravated by the reduced absorption of fluoride, which may be caused by chronic use of aluminum-containing antacids.

Atropine-like drugs, including many antihistamines, antispasmodics and others, are more likely to cause dizziness, sedation, confusion, dry mouth and a drop in blood pressure in older patients.

Aging patients are twice as susceptible to adverse drug reactions as younger patients.

Older patients apparently need more medicines, as they take nearly three times as many drugs as younger people.

Older patients are more vulnerable to medication problems because of body composition, reduced elimination capabilities due to decreasing kidney function, and slowed metabolism.

Drug levels become higher with standard doses because total body weight declines and lean body mass relative to total weight and total body water declines.

Changes in the aging brain reduce cognitive skills, so elderly patients may not recognize changes brought about by medication side effects.

PRECAUTIONS FOR THE USE OF MEDICATIONS

- Use memory aids to help you remember dose times.
- Ask for a drug in its simplest dosage form.
- Make sure labels are easily readable.
- Inform any physician about all the drugs you take (over-the-counter drugs included) to prevent double treatment or dangerous interactions.
- Put your glasses on before taking medicines.
- Discuss plans with your doctor for any elective surgery, including dental surgery.
- Tell your doctor about any new or unexpected symptoms you develop while taking a medicine. You may need to change medicines or have a dosage adjustment.
- Store all medicines out of children's reach. Keep drugs in a cool, dry place, such as a kitchen cabinet or bedroom. Avoid medicine cabinets in bathrooms, as they get too moist and warm at times. Keep medicine in its original container, tightly closed. Don't remove the label! If directions call for refrigeration, keep the medicine cool, but don't freeze it.
- Study any information you can find about the specific drugs you take. An excellent reference is *Complete Guide to Prescription and Non-Prescription Drugs,* which is published by Perigree Books.
- Don't save expired drugs.
- Don't take a drug that was prescribed for you long ago without asking your doctor.
- Don't keep pills at your bedside.
- Don't keep similar-looking drug containers grouped together.
- Don't hesitate to ask questions about a drug. Your doctor, nurse and pharmacist will be able to provide more information if they are familiar with you and your past medical history, especially regarding medicines.
- Don't take medicine in the dark! It is always possible to take the wrong one. Recheck the label before each drug use.
- Don't save leftover oral or injectable medicine to use later. Discard it before or on the expiration date shown on the container. Dispose of it safely to protect children and pets.
- Don't take any drug prescribed for someone else.

Abuse of the Elderly

Elder abuse is a newly recognized problem involving the abuse or mistreatment of an elderly person (usually over age 65). The abuse can be mild to severe and may present itself in various forms:

- **Physical abuse** such as hitting, slapping or shoving.
- **Verbal abuse** such as the use of harsh words, swearing at the person or being silent.
- **Psychological abuse** that triggers emotional stress.
- **Financial abuse** including the mishandling of money or possessions.

Those who abuse may be spouses, children, other family members or hired care-givers. Most often the abuse will be detected by a third party. Abusers are not likely to talk about it, and victims are often fearful or ashamed.

CONSIDERATIONS FOR OLDER ADULTS

It is estimated that 10% of the people over the age of 65 may experience abuse.

Abuse takes place in all economic groups. Victims include males as well as females.

Victims are usually dependent on others for some or all of their daily care needs. The victim may be competent or incompetent.

Stress and frustration of the care-giver may cause the abuse. Violence and abuse may be a part of the total family history.

Mistreatment and abuse are difficult for others to detect. The victim may feel ashamed to speak up about it.

The abuse may be accidental because of misunderstanding on the part of the care-giver, e.g., how to give medications.

WHAT TO DO

Be sure that any person caring for an elderly patient is emotionally and mentally competent to handle the task. Sometimes adult children who live with parents do so because of a history of mental illness, drug abuse or other psychiatric disorder, and this could create a potential for abuse.

Ideally the abuser will recognize his or her problem and seek help. Or the victim may seek outside assistance.

Some states have laws permitting the investigation of suspected cases. However, state laws vary on how suspected cases may be investigated. Even though this type of abuse is nearly as prevalent as child abuse, fewer dollars are spent on protective services for the elderly.

It takes the efforts of all the parties involved to work out solutions to the problem. Too frequently, though, the victim is not competent and cannot help to change an aggravating behavior.

Make sure care-givers get some time away from everyday responsibilities. People in care-giving positions should schedule time off for themselves to enjoy and should not feel guilty about doing so.

WHO CAN HELP

If you are aware of possible mistreatment or abuse, seek help from the authorities, social service agencies, other family members or your doctor.

Special services for the elderly can be found in many communities. The patient, care-giver or family member may check with one of these organizations to seek assistance.

Assistive Devices

People with various degrees of functional impairment find that the use of assistive devices enables them to improve their lifestyle and lessen their dependence on others. Assistive devices may range from the very simple, such as a magnifying glass to aid in reading, to the complex, such as a specially designed wheelchair for a paraplegic.

CONSIDERATIONS FOR THE OLDER ADULT

The chance of incurring a chronic illness or disability increases with aging.

Even with general good health, the muscles become less flexible, aches and pains seem to come more often, the eyesight worsens, hearing ability decreases and stability while walking or standing might need assistance.

Older people use more prescribed medications, which in turn cause side effects such as dizziness, lightheadedness or weakness.

WHAT TO DO

Recognize that you have a functional deficit. You may realize this for yourself, or a family member or friend may point it out. If it appears that medication is the cause, talk to your doctor about changing dosage levels or trying an equally effective drug.

Try not to get depressed because you need help in performing a task or because your hearing needs assistance or you need a cane to help you walk. Functioning well is more important than appearance or pride.

Assistive devices exist for just about any known problem. Manufacturers develop new and improved products continuously. If there doesn't seem to be a solution for your immediate need, keep looking.

You may want to rent the assistive device to start. This way you can see how it works for you. It's a good idea to rent when the need for the device is temporary while you recover from an injury or from surgery.

Medicare may cover up to 80% of the cost for some prescribed assistive devices.

Learn the proper technique for using the assistive device, and persevere in practicing it. A physical therapist may provide training and follow-up. Keep a positive attitude, and don't give up out of frustration or anger. Maybe it is not the right solution for you, but give it a fair trial.

Make sure that the use of an assistive device does not worsen other health problems or create new ones. A cane that aids walking but is the wrong length may cause arm muscle weakness or increase your discomfort while walking.

WHO CAN HELP

Your doctor is the best source for information and guidance. Referral to a physical therapist for special help and training may also be desirable.

If you have a chronic illness, consult organizations such as the Arthritis Foundation for specific recommendations about assistive devices.

Check with a local medical supply store or drugstore that carries medical equipment.

Look for mail order catalogs that provide medical equipment. General catalogs often have simpler assistive devices that you can order.

Cancer Facts

Cancer is a disease in which cells grow in an abnormal way. If left untreated, the cells continue to grow and eventually invade and destroy normal tissue. There are a number of treatments that may be used to cure cancer or to delay its devastating effects.

Common cancers in people over 50 are cancers of the lung, breast, colon and rectum; prostate (men); uterus, ovary, and cervix (women); and skin.

SYMPTOMS OF COMMON CANCERS

Lung
- A persistent cough that won't go away.
- Coughing up blood.
- Shortness of breath.

Breast
- Rapid change in breast size.
- Discharge from the nipple.
- Lump in the breast.

Colon and Rectum
- Bleeding from the rectum.
- Blood in the stool that appears either bright red or black (tarry).
- Changes in bowel habits, such as chronic diarrhea, persistent constipation or a persistent change in the caliber of the stool.

Prostate (Men)
- Difficulty or pain while urinating.
- A need to urinate often, especially at night after retiring.
- Difficulty in initiating urination.
- A feeling of incomplete emptying of the bladder.
- Persistent change in the caliber of the urinary stream.

Uterus, Ovary or Cervix (Women)
- Vaginal bleeding after menopause.
- Unusual vaginal discharge.
- Abdominal enlargement.
- Pain during sexual intercourse.

Skin
- A sore that does not heal.
- A change in the size, shape or color of a wart or mole. Look particularly for black or purple enlargements with irregular borders.
- The sudden appearance of a mole.

WHAT TO DO

If you have one or more of the symptoms listed above, contact your doctor as soon as possible. Remember that pain is not a usual early warning sign of cancer. Don't fail to mention symptoms to your doctor just because you think they are unimportant or "normal" for your age.

Even if you don't have symptoms, there are tests that can be performed periodically that may detect cancer before symptoms begin. Some of them are as follows:

- **Guaiac Test**—One or more stool samples can be checked for blood or traces of blood. There are simple kits available from the pharmacy or from your doctor that make it possible to do the test yourself in privacy and mail it to your doctor or to a laboratory.
- **Rectal Exam**—Performed by a physician or physician's assistant with a gloved finger inserted into the rectum. It may be uncomfortable for you, but only for a short time. This test can detect prostate tumors in men and rectal tumors in women or men.

- **Sigmoidoscopy or Procto-Sigmoidoscopy**—An examination of the rectum and part of the colon with a metal instrument containing a system of lights to allow direct visualization of rectal or colon tumors.
- **Pelvic Examinations and Pap (Papanicolaou) Smears**—Performed by a doctor or assistant to check the female reproductive organs. The Pap smear is a painless test which involves removing cells from the cervix and examining them through a microscope.
- **Breast Examination and Mammography**—The best examinations may very well be done by yourself. (See Appendix 14 on breast self-examination). Self-exams should be coupled with mammograms and periodic examinations by a physician to check for thickening, lumps, or discharge from the nipple. Mammograms (x-rays of the breasts) can detect tumors even before they can be felt. Take advantage of this technique every 1 or 2 years.

A positive test on any of the above does not necessarily mean that you have cancer, but it may indicate the need for more testing. Biopsy may be the next step. A biopsy is a surgical procedure in which a small piece of suspected tissue is removed for staining and microscopic examination for malignant cells.

WHO CAN HELP

- If tests show that you have cancer, treatment should begin right away. Treatment may consist of surgery, radiation treatment or chemotherapy.
- To ensure that you will be comfortable with your decision to have a particular treatment, you may wish to seek the opinion of more than one doctor. This is always your prerogative. Don't hesitate to exercise it.
- A federal agency, the Cancer Information Service, is available to answer your cancer-related questions. Call (800) 422-6237. Spanish-speaking staff members are available in California, Georgia, Illinois, New Jersey, New York City and Texas.

Care-Giving

Care-giving is a term describing the task of providing some or all of the daily needs of another person. The person cared for may live independently or in the same house as the care-giver.

CONSIDERATIONS FOR OLDER ADULTS

People are living longer and often require help in some aspects of their daily lives.

Adult children who themselves are considered senior citizens often find themselves as care-givers for parents who live into their 80s and 90s.

In many instances, institutional care is not affordable, nor is it desirable.

It is expected in a great number of families that the grown children will care for the aging parents when that time arrives.

Women live longer then men and will usually be available to care for their ailing spouses.

Since women normally outlive men, they are the ones most likely to need the assistance of a care-giver.

WHAT TO DO

Lead as healthy a lifestyle as possible in order to prevent or delay any need for care-giver help for yourself.

Make plans with adult children ahead of the time that any care might be needed so everyone will know the expectations and preferences of each other.

Recognize that being a care-giver is stressful. New burdens, responsibilities, resentment and lack of a social life are just some of the problems. These feelings are normal.

Understand that natural roles may be reversed. A wife now takes care of a husband who has always been the "strong" one, or a child is now taking the parenting role.

Don't make hasty permanent decisions (such as selling a home) in a moment of crisis. They can cause serious problems later on.

If you are the care-giver, learn all you can about the illness or problem of the person you give care to. In particular, learn about the medications the person is taking, be dependable, encourage the older person to be as independent as possible and be alert to the emotional needs of both of you.

If the cared-for person lives alone, make sure he or she prepares and eats regular meals. A surprising number of older people forget to eat. Make arrangements for a telephone call once a day to make sure that everything is going satisfactorily.

WHO CAN HELP

Family members are the main source of help and support.

Other sources of help include the family doctor, minister, social worker and special health-care organizations for the elderly.

The care-giver's friends are important. They can provide support, encouragement and someone to talk to.

The patient's friends are important, too. They can sometimes relieve the care-giver during visits and talk over "old times" with the patient and may be more willing and able (timewise) to sit and listen.

Support groups exist for care-givers. Joining one may be helpful.

Day-care centers for adults are available. They can be a benefit both to the care-giver and the patient.

Dental Care

Preventive health care includes many elements—exercise, nutritious meals and prompt medical treatment when necessary. It also includes regular dental care, both in the home and in the dentist's office.

CONSIDERATIONS FOR OLDER ADULTS

Tooth loss and the need for dentures is no longer a certainty. Advances in dental health have changed that.

Too often, older people—especially those who wear dentures—feel they no longer need dental check-ups. And because the idea of preventive dental care dates back only to the 1950s, most people over 65 were not trained at an early age to be concerned with preventive care of the teeth. If you haven't learned the basic elements of good oral hygiene, now is the time to start.

WHAT TO DO

Cleaning Your Teeth

The most important part of good dental care is knowing how to clean your teeth. Brush them on all sides with short strokes using a soft-bristle brush and any free-style brushing stroke that is comfortable. Pay special attention to the gum line. Brushing your tongue and the roof of your mouth will help remove germs and prevent bad breath. It is best to brush after every meal, but brushing thoroughly at least once a day, preferably at bedtime, is a must. See your dentist if brushing results in repeated bleeding or pain.

Even though brushing is the most important means of removing film and food particles from the mouth, there are many places a toothbrush cannot reach. To remove germs and pieces of food from between the teeth and near the gum line, dentists recommend daily flossing with dental floss. A dentist or dental hygienist can instruct you in its proper use.

There are several good products available that can provide additional protection against decay and probably against plaque, a sticky, colorless film that forms on the teeth and contains harmful germs. These products contain stannous fluoride. Look for one that has the seal of approval from the American Dental Association, and use it according to directions.

Some people with arthritis or other conditions that limit motion may find it hard to hold a toothbrush. To overcome this, the brush handle can be attached to your hand with a wide elastic band or may be enlarged by attaching it to a sponge, styrofoam ball, or similar object. Those with limited shoulder movement might find brushing easier if the handle of the brush is lengthened by attaching a long piece of wood or plastic. Electric toothbrushes and water pics are of benefit to many.

Preventing Periodontal Disease

Careful daily brushing can help remove plaque. If the plaque is not removed every day, it hardens into calculus (tartar), a substance that can be removed only by a dentist or dental hygienist. The buildup of plaque and calculus can lead to periodontal (gum) disease, in which the normally pink gums begin to redden, swell and occasionally bleed.

If untreated, periodontal disease will get worse, and pockets of infection will form between the teeth and gums. As the infection spreads, the gums recede. Eventually, the structures that hold the teeth in place are destroyed, the bone socket enlarges, and the tooth loosens and is lost. A regular program of complete oral hygiene can prevent gum disease and tooth decay in most people.

Caring for Dentures

If you have dentures, you should keep them clean and free from deposits that can cause permanent staining, bad breath, and gum irritation. Once a day, brush all surfaces of the dentures with a denture-care product. Remove your dentures from your mouth for at least 6 or 8 hours each day and place them in water (but never in hot water) or a denture-cleansing solution. It is also helpful to rinse your mouth with a warm salt-water solution in the morning, after meals and at bedtime.

Partial dentures should be cared for in the same way as full dentures. Because germs tend to collect under the clasps of partial dentures, it is especially important that this area be cleaned thoroughly.

Dentures will seem awkward at first. When learning to eat with dentures, you should select soft, non-sticky food. Cut your food into small pieces and chew it slowly using both sides of your mouth. Dentures tend to make your mouth less sensitive to hot foods and liquids and less able to detect the presence of harmful objects such as bones. If problems in eating, talking, or simply wearing dentures continue after the first few weeks, your dentist can make proper adjustments.

After a number of years, dentures might have to be relined or even replaced. Do not attempt to repair dentures at home, as this can damage the dentures and be harmful to the tissues of the mouth.

The Importance of Dental Check-Ups

Even with good home oral hygiene, it is important to have yearly dental check-ups. Many dentists give regular fluoride treatments to adult patients to help prevent tooth decay.

Dental check-ups not only help maintain a healthy mouth, but they are necessary for the early discovery of oral cancer and other diseases. Mouth cancer often goes unnoticed in its early and curable stages. This is true in part because many older people do not visit their dentists often enough and because pain is not an early symptom of the disease. If you notice any red or white spots or sores in your mouth that bleed or do not go away within 2 weeks, be sure to have them checked by a dentist.

It is essential to take care of dental problems before undergoing major surgery. The results of a complicated and successful heart operation, for example, could be endangered if certain bacteria— which are always present in the mouth—get into the bloodstream and lodge on the heart valves. Likewise, there are several chronic medical problems, particularly heart problems, which require prophylactic antibiotics before any kind of dental procedure, including prophylactic cleaning, etc. Be sure to talk to your doctor or dentist about this need.

WHO CAN HELP

If you have no regular dentist, check with personnel of the local dental society. They can provide you a list of names to consider. Your friends or family doctor may help with recommendations also.

Driving

Driving an automobile is an activity that is taken for granted by most people once a driver's license is obtained. The reflex actions, skills, physical dexterity and mental alertness that are used in driving are performed almost automatically once you are behind the wheel of a car. But these capabilities and other aspects of driving can change with age.

CONSIDERATIONS FOR OLDER ADULTS

Vision changes occur with aging. The eyes take longer to focus, peripheral vision may decrease and night-time driving becomes a strain.

Arthritis and other illnesses cause pain, stiffness and loss of movement in the neck, shoulders or back that limits one's ability to look behind or to the side while driving.

Reflex time is slower (sometimes due to medications) and may delay one's response to emergency traffic situations or even to a yellow light.

Older drivers tend to drive slower, which unknowingly causes frustration in other drivers who then become impatient and take unnecessary risks.

Older persons may lack knowledge about traffic or safety regulations.

WHAT TO DO

Don't drink alcoholic beverages and then drive.

Get in the habit of always using a seat belt.

Continually assess your ability to drive. Take into consideration your physical, mental and emotional health.

Keep up with the driving laws and regulations in your state by reviewing the current driver's manual.

Get eye examinations annually. Be sure eyeglasses or contact lenses have up-to-date prescription lenses.

Know the possible side effects of any medications you take. When starting a new medication, don't drive until you see how you react to it.

If your body movements are limited, ask your doctor about flexibility exercises. Get an extra-large rearview mirror and be sure to have a mirror on the right side of the vehicle.

If you are driving an unfamiliar vehicle, such as a rental, get the seat adjusted and mirrors aligned before you start the motor. Know the location of light switches and windshield wipers. Practice driving in the parking lot until you feel comfortable with the mechanics of steering, acceleration and breaks. Know how to get to your destination. If it is an unfamiliar location, call for directions before starting.

Ask a friend or family member to ride with you specifically to assess your driving abilities. Have him or her point out your weak areas as well as your strong points.

Recognize the reality that at some time you will need to give up driving. This will be one of the most profound losses you will experience.

WHO CAN HELP

Discuss concerns about your driving abilities with your family.

The American Association of Retired Persons sponsors an 8-hour defensive driving course for people over 50. Check to see if it is available in your area.

The National Safety Council has a 6-hour course for seniors called "Coaching the Mature Driver." It may qualify you for an insurance discount. Check with your local or state chapter.

Ask your doctor how the medicines you take or an illness might affect your driving abilities.

Start looking for alternative modes of transportation and give some of them a trial. Public transportation is provided in most larger cities, and special transportation services for the elderly are available in some.

Exercise for People with Heart Disease & Chronic Lung Disease

Some persons suffer from serious disease that can last many years. Each case must be evaluated on an individual basis, but many of these persons can benefit from regular exercise. Exercise can play a vital role in improving their sense of well-being. In a few instances, it may help retard the progress of the disease. Two of the most serious and common forms of chronic disease are heart disease and chronic obstructive pulmonary (lung) disease.

HEART DISEASE & EXERCISE

The most common types of heart disease are coronary artery disease and hardening of the arteries (atherosclerosis or arteriosclerosis). Three important risk factors for developing heart disease are hypertension (high blood pressure), obesity and a sedentary lifestyle. Exercise plays an important role in controlling hypertension and obesity, making it significant in the treatment of heart disease.

Cardiovascular Benefits of Exercise
The known benefits of cardiovascular fitness include:

- Increased blood supply to the heart.
- Decreased oxygen demand.
- Increased blood flow through the coronary arteries.
- Increased efficiency of heart muscle function.
- Indirect evidence of decreased electrical irritability of the heart, lessening the chance that abnormal or life-threatening heartbeat irregularities will occur.
- Indirect evidence of delayed development of hardening of the arteries.

These benefits are possible for men and women in all age groups, but the most positive evidence of benefit is in men over 40.

Exercise after Heart Disease Is Diagnosed
Many medical centers throughout the world have developed rehabilitation centers for patients who have had heart attacks. The American College of Sports Medicine has established guidelines and certification programs for exercise leaders who are trained in cardiac rehabilitation techniques. These centers prescribe exercise after a thorough evaluation and supervise the exercise carefully with monitors.

Following a heart attack, cardiac patients can frequently benefit from enrolling in one of these programs at a YMCA, a college or university physical education department or a cardiac rehabilitation center. It is unsafe for a recent cardiac patient to try to develop an exercise program at home.

A specialized facility, under the supervision of trained professionals, can monitor your responses to an individually designed exercise program. Repeated studies have shown that such careful programs have brought quicker recovery, earlier return to work, an enhanced feeling of well-being and less likelihood of developing a subsequent heart attack. Ask your physician for a referral.

CHRONIC OBSTRUCTIVE PULMONARY DISEASE & EXERCISE

Chronic obstructive pulmonary disease (COPD) is any long-term lung disorder that is characterized by gradually increasing breathing difficulty. Some underlying diseases that produce COPD include chronic bronchitis, bronchiectasis, emphysema, asthma and other disorders associated with spasms of the bronchial tubes.

Supervised exercise and activity can enhance breathing function and improve your sense of well-being. However, exercise programs for people with this disorder must be individualized. A physical therapist or doctor can teach you how to increase your breathing ability and capacity.

Breathing retraining begins with exercises using forced expiration against pursed lips and other techniques to teach you to use the diaphragm and accessory muscles of the chest wall. When breathing rehabilitation reaches an acceptable level, a program of walking can increase breathing capacity and general health. See your doctor for detailed instructions.

Eye Problems

Poor eyesight is not inevitable with age. Some physical changes occur during the normal aging process that can cause a gradual decline in vision, but most older people maintain good eyesight into their 80s and beyond.

CONSIDERATIONS FOR OLDER ADULTS

Older people generally need brighter light for such tasks as reading, cooking or driving a car. Incandescent light bulbs (regular household bulbs) are better than fluorescent lights (tubular overhead lights) for older eyes.

Certain eye disorders and diseases occur more frequently in old age, but a great deal can be done to prevent or correct these conditions.

COMMON EYE PROBLEMS

- **Presbyopia (prez-bee-oh'pe-uh)** is a gradual decline in the ability to focus on close objects or to see small print. It is common after the age of 40. People with this condition often hold reading materials at arm's length, and some may have headaches or "tired eyes" while reading or doing other close work. There is no known prevention of presbyopia, but the focusing problem can be easily compensated for with glasses or contact lenses.
- **Floaters** are tiny spots or specks that float across the field of vision. Most people notice them in well-lighted rooms or outdoors on a bright day. Although floaters are normal and are usually harmless, they may be a warning of certain eye problems, especially if they are associated with light flashes. If you notice a sudden change in the type or number of spots or flashes, call your doctor.
- **Dry eyes** occur when the tear glands produce too few tears. The result is itching and burning or even reduced vision. An eye specialist can prescribe special eyedrop solutions ("artificial tears") to correct the problem.
- **Excessive tears** may be a sign of increased sensitivity to light, wind, or temperature changes. In these cases, protective measures (such as sunglasses) may solve the problem. Tearing may also indicate more serious problems, such as an eye infection or a blocked tear duct, both of which can be treated and corrected.

COMMON EYE DISEASES

- **Cataracts** are cloudy or opaque areas in part or all of the transparent lens located inside the eye. Normally the lens is clear and allows light to pass through. When a cataract forms, light cannot easily pass through the lens, and this affects vision. Cataracts usually develop gradually, without pain, redness or tearing in the eye. Some remain small and do not seriously affect vision. If a cataract becomes larger or denser, however, it can be surgically removed.

  Cataract surgery (in which the clouded lens is removed) is a safe procedure that is almost always successful. Cataract patients should discuss with their doctors the risks and benefits of this elective procedure. After surgery, vision is restored by using special eyeglasses or contact lenses or by having an intraocular lens implant (a plastic lens that is implanted in the eye during surgery).
- **Glaucoma** occurs when there is too much fluid pressure in the eye that is causing internal eye damage and gradually destroys vision. The underlying cause of glaucoma is often not known, but with early diagnosis and treatment it can usually be controlled and blindness prevented. Treatment consists of special eyedrops, oral medications, laser treatments or in some cases surgery.

  Glaucoma seldom produces early symptoms, and usually there is no pain from increased pressure. For these reasons, it is important for eye specialists to test for the disease during routine eye examinations in those over 50.
- **Retinal disorders** are the leading cause of blindness in the United States. The retina is a thin lining on the back of the eye made up of nerves that receive visual images and pass them on to the brain. Retinal disorders include senile macular degeneration, diabetic retinopathy and retinal detachment.

  Senile macular degeneration is a condition in which the macula (a specialized part of the retina responsible for sharp central and reading vision) loses its ability to function efficiently. The first signs may include blurring of reading matter, distortion or loss of central vision (for example, a dark spot in the center of the field of vision) and distortion of vertical lines. Early detection of macular degeneration is important since some cases may be treated successfully with laser treatments.

Diabetic retinopathy is one of the possible complications of diabetes and occurs when the small blood vessels that nourish the retina fail to do so properly. In the early stages of the condition, the blood vessels may leak fluid, which distorts vision. In the later stages, new vessels may grow and release blood into the center of the eye, resulting in serious loss of vision.

Retinal detachment is a separation between the inner and outer layers of the retina. Detached retinas can usually be surgically re-attached with good or partial restoration of vision. New surgical and laser treatments are being used today with increasing success.

WHAT TO DO

Health-Care Options

Have regular health check-ups to detect such treatable diseases as high blood pressure and diabetes, both of which may cause eye problems.

Have a complete eye examination every 1 to 3 years since many eye diseases have no early noticeable symptoms. The examination should include a vision (and glasses) evaluation, eye muscle check, check for glaucoma and thorough internal and external eye health exams.

Seek more frequent eye health care if you have diabetes or a family history of eye disease. Make arrangements for care immediately if you experience signs such as loss or dimness of vision, eye pain, excessive discharge from the eye, double vision or redness or swelling of the eye or eyelid.

Aids for Low Vision

Many people with visual impairments can be helped by using low-vision aids. These are special devices that provide more power than regular eyeglasses. Low-vision aids include telescopic glasses, light-filtering lenses and magnifying glasses, along with a variety of electronic devices. Some are designed to be hand-held; others rest directly on reading materials. Partially sighted individuals often notice surprising improvements with the use of these aids.

WHO CAN HELP

Eye-care professionals including ophthalmologists, optometrists and opticians will be your source for help for eye problems. An **ophthalmologist** is recommended for major eye disorders and in most states is the only one permitted to prescribe medications. An **optometrist** performs eye exams and can diagnose eye disorders, while an **optician** is one who fills lens prescriptions and does the fitting of eyeglasses or contact lens. See the Resources and Additional Reading sections for suggestions on obtaining further information.

Falls

Accidental falls occur due to tripping, bumping, collapsing, toppling or tumbling off of something; rolling out of bed; or slipping.

CONSIDERATIONS FOR OLDER ADULTS

Approximately one-third of people over age 65 have falls, the most common form of accident in the aging population.

Older people are particularly prone to falling in showers or tubs or on stairs.

Complications from falls include fractures, bruises and burns.

Complications from fall injuries may lead to other serious medical problems because of immobility during recovery. One of the most significant complications is the possibility of blood clots from an injury site breaking loose and lodging in the lungs (pulmonary embolism).

People living in nursing homes suffer more falls than those at home, most likely because that group has increased disabilities.

Once a person experiences a fall, the fear of falling again may curtail his or her activities, bringing on some depression and loneliness.

People over age 50 take more medications. Many of these can cause disabling side effects such as dizziness and impaired reflexes.

Eyesight and hearing capabilities decrease with age, and muscles become weaker.

Some chronic illnesses cause gait impairment.

Osteoporosis (brittle and weakened bones), common in older women, leads to serious fractures when accidents occur.

WHAT TO DO

Don't ignore falls, even if you are not injured. They may be symptoms of an impending illness. Call your doctor.

If any new medication is prescribed, be particularly careful about your activities until you see how the dosage affects you.

Be sure your eyeglasses are properly fitted and the lenses are correct for your visual problem.

Wear properly fitted footwear, and take care of your feet. Talk to your doctor about ways to prevent fragile or brittle bones. Estrogen replacement therapy helps many postmenopausal women.

Maintain as high a fitness level as your health permits.

Fall-proof your home to the extent possible: Have adequate lighting with accessible light switches; use a nightlight; keep electrical and telephone cords out of walkways; have handrails for the bath, shower and stairways; don't have slippery area rugs on floors; take castors off furniture; have railings on your bed; install a high toilet seat; put kitchen supplies and other storage items on shelves that are between hip and eye level to reduce your reaching or bending; and use chairs with armrests.

WHO CAN HELP

Ask your doctor for recommendations. He or she knows your state of health and can help determine to what extent you need to change your lifestyle.

Have a family member walk through your home with you to watch how you perform activities and help you decide if any hazards exist.

Helpful illustrated publications are available about safety for older adults. Check your public library, a local council for the aging or other organizations that provide social services.

If you live alone and are prone to falls, consider a personal emergency response system (PERS), sometimes called Lifeline. With the push of a button, emergency help can be obtained.

APPENDICES

Finding a Personal Physician

Finding the best possible medical care, a difficult task at any time of life, becomes more difficult just as you begin to need it most—after you have reached age 60 or 70.

While most older people are basically healthy and report themselves in good to excellent health, many tend to under-report specific health problems and mistakenly think they are caused by "old age" rather than disease. Yet old age does affect people's health, mainly by causing them to react differently to various diseases and drugs (see Considerations for Older Adults, below).

The older person needs a doctor who is aware of special needs and problems. But finding such a person may be difficult because doctors in the United States do not routinely receive special training in the care of older persons, relying mainly upon personal experience. Only recently has geriatrics—the study of the care of the aged—begun to be included in medical school curricula. Geriatrics is not a separate medical specialty like pediatrics or cardiology.

Another problem is that many older people who have been treated by the same doctor for years lose their family doctors to retirement or death.

The health care of older people should improve soon, however. The over-65 age group is expected to constitute 20 percent of the population by the year 2030 (versus 11 percent today and 4 percent in 1900). As the number of older persons increases, so should the number of medical students and practicing physicians studying geriatrics.

CONSIDERATIONS FOR OLDER ADULTS

Some diseases may have different signs in older people. For example, a heart attack may occur in an older person without chest pains, and appendicitis may occur without the same abdominal tenderness that a younger person usually experiences.

An older person may have several health problems and take several medications at the same time. These often interact and cause a confusing array of symptoms and reactions that need to be considered in deciding upon the proper medical treatment.

Drugs act differently in older people than in the young, making unusual reactions from drugs more likely with increasing age.

WHAT TO DO

The following checklist may help you in finding a new doctor or dentist or in evaluating your present one:

- Are you comfortable with your doctor? Can you openly discuss your feelings and talk about personal concerns such as sexual and emotional problems?
- Do you believe your doctor will stand by you, no matter how difficult your problems become?
- Does your doctor listen to you and answer all your questions about the causes and treatment of your physical problems? Or is he or she vague, impatient or unwilling to answer?
- Does your doctor take a thorough "history" on you and ask about past physical and emotional problems, your family medical history, drugs you are taking and other matters affecting your health?
- Does your doctor seem to automatically prescribe drugs rather than dealing with the real causes of your medical problems?
- Does your doctor attribute your problems to "old age"?
- Does your doctor have an associate to whom you can turn should your doctor retire or die?

Unfortunately, some doctors still equate aging with inevitable mental and physical decline. Remember that you are a consumer and are entitled to ask questions when selecting a doctor and to expect reasonable, satisfying answers, not age-worn cliches.

A good doctor-patient relationship is based upon mutual respect and open communication. The doctor should give you an active role in deciding when to seek medical attention, whether to accept the doctor's advice and when to seek a second opinion from another doctor. You, the patient, owe your physician cooperation and honesty, and you owe yourself a continuing interest in seeking the best medical care.

WHO CAN HELP

As a start towards finding a doctor who has a special interest in treating older people, you can contact your county medical society or state agency on aging. Other possible sources of information include local referral services, medical schools, or university medical centers.

Talk to friends who are in your age group about their doctors, and ask if they would recommend them.

Foot Care

Feet can take quite a beating in life. The main causes are poor posture, ill-fitting shoes, overweight and lack of exercise. Women suffer more foot problems than men, most likely due to years of wearing high-heeled shoes and shoes with pointed toes.

CONSIDERATIONS FOR OLDER ADULTS

This is the time of life that years of foot abuse may finally catch up with a person.

A side effect of some medications is swelling of the feet and ankles. Because older people take more medications, the risk of developing these symptoms is higher.

Some aspects of aging, such as thinning skin, poor circulation and muscle atrophy, all affect the feet as well as other body parts.

Chronic illnesses, more prevalent in older people, can cause some foot problems.

DAILY CARE OF THE FEET

Shoes

Start with well-fitting, comfortable shoes. Carefully break them in gradually, about 1 hour a day. For working around the house or walking outside, wear lightweight, flexible jogging or walking shoes or a leather walking shoe with a soft crepe sole. If you live in a wet and tropical climate, try wearing sandals to protect your feet and keep them dry.

Socks

Wear cotton or wool socks instead of socks made from mixtures containing polyesters. Use cotton bed socks if you need extra warmth at night while sleeping.

Exercise

Walk regularly for increasingly longer times. Walking is universally one of the very best exercises to help you stay physically fit. You can do it no matter where you live. Stop walking when your feet feel sore.

While Traveling

When sitting for any period of time while you are flying or riding in an auto, bus or train, get up from your seat and walk frequently. At other times, whenever possible, elevate your feet during rest periods.

Foot Hygiene

Wash your feet daily with soap and warm water. Dry them thoroughly and gently, especially between the toes. Powder your feet frequently with talcum. Remove your shoes for short periods of time during your normal day when you can. After bathing and drying the feet thoroughly, rub toilet lanolin into the skin of the feet to keep the skin soft and free from scales and dryness. Do not rub so vigorously that the feet become tender.

Do not cut corns or calluses or try to remove them with patent or other medicines. (See Corns and Calluses in the Illnesses section). If your toes overlap or are pushed close together, separate them with lamb's wool or cotton. Don't wear garters or sit with your legs crossed. Either will decrease the circulation to your feet. Don't go barefoot in wet, tropical climates.

FOOT PROBLEMS

Blisters

Clean the area, being careful not to puncture the blister. Protect tender areas with moleskin, adhesive tape or gauze. If the blister ruptures, apply an antibiotic ointment from your medical kit. Reduce your walking for several days to speed healing.

Toenail Problems

Keep your toenails relatively short, but exercise care when clipping them. If your toenails are brittle and dry, apply lanolin generously around the nails for a few nights after soaking. Read the information under Toenails, Ingrown, in the Illnesses section.

Heel Spurs

Heel spurs (plantar fasciitis) are frequently problems among active walkers and travelers. A heel spur is caused by a partial or complete tear in the fascia (the fibrous connective tissue of the bottom of the foot). It is characterized by pain just under the heel bone. Causes include inadequate arch supports, poorly fitting shoes or shoes with soles that are too stiff, sudden turns or stops and weak ankles. Rest is the only satisfactory treatment. See Heel Spur in the Illnesses section.

WHO CAN HELP

For further information concerning feet, read the following sections in the Illnesses section:

ATHLETE'S FOOT
CORNS AND CALLUSES
HEEL SPUR
SPRAINS & STRAINS
TOENAIL, INGROWN
WARTS, PLANTAR

Discuss foot problems with your doctor. Ask specifically if your medications or a chronic illness you have cause the symptoms.
See a podiatrist, a specialist in the field of medicine that deals with the care of the foot.

Health History & Medical Records

The health history or medical records maintained by your personal doctor usually provide the pertinent information required for him or her to render you the best medical care possible. These records include information on your past medical history, current treatment, medications currently prescribed and recommendations for maintaining good health and fitness.

Work with your doctor or nurse to assemble a similar record for yourself to keep with you at all times. Having the record provides several benefits. It can provide an important tool to help you be an effective, active member of your health-care team. More and more patients are recognizing that they are important participants in making decisions about their treatments, medications and surgical options.

CONSIDERATIONS FOR OLDER ADULTS

Having a record at home will assure you that important information about medications, doctor's instructions and facts about chronic disorders is always available to you or to your care-giver. Don't rely on memory alone.

Keeping your own records will help you in communicating with your doctor or other health-care providers.

WHAT TO DO

Use a loose-leaf notebook to store the information. Arrange the information in the way you find most practical. There are many different ways to set up the file. Pre-printed forms are also available for this purpose.

Include information that may seem basic, but would be necessary if someone else needed to know. This can include names of doctors and dentists, insurance company identification numbers, your blood type and special allergies (to foods, medications, insects, plants, etc.). List medications you currently take, both brand and generic names, why they were prescribed, the dosage, what pharmacy filled the prescription and how long they are to be taken. Add to the file any written instructions given to you by the doctor or pharmacist about each drug. Put in notes about any side effects you experience.

Write down information about any chronic disorders you have and the prescribed treatments. Add information from other resources about your disorders, such as magazine articles or handouts the doctor gave you.

Make notes about other illnesses or ailments that occur, even if you don't go to the doctor for treatment, such as colds or diarrhea. If you do see the doctor, write down the treatment recommended. Always include dates and other pertinent data.

Keep information about medical tests in the file, such as cholesterol levels and blood pressure readings. Record the dates when you had x-rays or special chemical studies.

Try to reconstruct your past medical history (from childhood on), including illnesses, surgeries, vaccinations, hospital stays, injuries and emotional upsets. Write down information about your family history if you know it. Information of this type is less important as you grow older, but it still can prove useful. It can be of importance to children and grandchildren as well.

WHO CAN HELP

Your doctor will be the best source of current and ongoing information. Make notes following each appointment. Ask for written instructions or handouts that you can take home. Get copies of the results of medical tests. In some states, you also have the legal right to see your medical records. If not, many doctors are willing to let you see them if you ask.

Go to your local library to find information about medical problems you have. Make copies of pages you think will be useful. Most libraries have copy machines available. Ask the information librarian for help in locating resources if you are unable to locate any.

APPENDICES

Hearing Impairment

In the world of the hearing impaired, words in a conversation may be misunderstood, musical notes may be missed and a ringing doorbell may go unanswered. Hearing impairment ranges from difficulty understanding words or certain sounds to total deafness.

Because of fear, misinformation or pride, people sometimes will not admit to themselves or others that they have hearing problems. Hearing impairments may be caused by exposure to very loud noises over a long period of time, viral infections, heart conditions or strokes, head injuries, certain drugs, tumors, excessive earwax and age-related changes in the ear mechanisms.

Signs of hearing loss include difficulty understanding words or thinking that another person's speech sounds mumbled, constantly hearing a hissing or ringing and deriving no enjoyment from movies and television because one can't hear the words.

CONSIDERATIONS FOR OLDER ADULTS

It is estimated that 30% of people aged 64 to 74 have some hearing loss, as do 50% of those over 75. Older people may withdraw socially, may feel that other people are mumbling or not speaking up and may be labeled as confused.

WHAT TO DO

Help is available in the form of surgery, treatment with medicines, special training and the use of a hearing aid or some form of alternate listening device.

If a hearing aid is recommended for you, be an informed consumer. There are many different models on the market. Consider the device itself, the service provided, plus counseling and training about its use. The most expensive device may not necessarily be the best one for you. Take advantage of any free trial period (usually 30 days) to try the aid out.

Help people with hearing problems by speaking slightly louder than normal, but don't shout. Stand 3 to 6 feet away from them, and make sure they can see your face. Don't speak directly into a person's ear, and if something isn't understood, rephrase it in short, concise sentences. Don't speak to a third person as if the hearing-impaired person is not in the room.

WHO CAN HELP

See your doctor for treatment or referral to a hearing specialist. Audiological testing involves simple, painless tests to determine how well the eardrum and inner ear function.

Look at medical supply stores or catalogs that carry products for the hard of hearing to see if there are devices that will be useful to you. There are special telecommunication devices, doorbells that make lights go on in the house, smoke alarms that flash and portable amplifying units that fit in a pocket and can be used at concerts, plays or movies.

Home Heath Care, Long-Term

Home health care is a growing area and offers one of the viable options for people who face major decisions regarding optimal care for themselves or family members. In the past, an older person with certain chronic disorders, a severe disability, a critical illness or a neurological problem often required the care provided in a hospital or nursing home. Today, though, due to advanced technology and improvements in outpatient care, these people can be cared for at home (their own homes or the homes of family members). The need to reduce health-care costs has been one of the contributing factors, but in addition, people seem to recover faster and live longer if they are at home.

CONSIDERATIONS FOR OLDER ADULTS

Life expectancy is increasing. People 85 and over are the fastest growing age group. But many in the older age groups require health-care help now or will need it in the future.

Costs are usually less if care can be given at home, which is a plus for many older adults on fixed incomes. The quality of life in the home environment is perceived to be better than that in a nursing home, and home care allows you to maintain some control of your life.

About 60% of older adults who need care move in with their children. Money concerns, love or even guilt may prompt this action. You may be able to live alone and still get the care you need.

WHAT TO DO

There are numerous home health-care options. Following is a brief list of ones to consider for your particular circumstances.

- **Overall Management of the Home Care**—This is provided by public health organizations, private home health-care agencies, social services agencies or hospitals or nursing homes. Check to see if they are licensed by the state, have references you can check and are Medicare-certified.
- **Special Services**—These include services by nurses to provide training, assessment, wound care and injections; physical therapists to help with exercises and therapy; occupational therapists who assess and teach changes needed in daily living routines; speech therapists to assist people in overcoming speech problems; and social workers to help with emotional, housing or financial difficulties.
- **Medical Equipment**—Such equipment includes cardiopulmonary monitors, equipment for intravenous medications and tube feeding, dialysis machines, ventilators and oxygen tanks, hospital beds, walkers, special chairs, portable toilets, wheelchairs and many more. It is usually best to rent equipment first and purchase it later once the device has proven useful. Other high-tech equipment for use at home is becoming more readily available.
- **Other Services**—These provide assistance with meals, transportation, day care and chores such as cleaning.

WHO CAN HELP

Talk to family members and friends to get advice.
Discuss your needs with your doctor, hospital social worker or discharge planner.
Your church or a social organization you belong to may offer assistance in some form.
Contact your local health department or visiting nurse association.

Imaging Procedures & Tests

There are many types of imaging now available. The choice of the type for you for any particular problem will depend on many considerations that you and your doctor should discuss, including cost, time required, safety, etc. Don't hesitate to ask questions of anyone providing health care for you.

The body imaging procedures represent some of the most useful and important diagnostic techniques available in modern medicine. They produce images of body structures that are impossible to see otherwise. The forms of imaging are described below.

X-RAYS (PLAIN FILMS)

X-rays have been used since the turn of the 20th century. They revolutionized the whole field of medical diagnostics by making it possible for the first time to view bones, lungs, other organs and internal tissues without opening the body. X-rays pass through some tissues unobstructed and are blocked by denser tissues, casting shadows that project onto a fluoroscopic screen or photographic film. Plain x-rays (also called radiograms) remain a most frequently used diagnostic tool, despite many advances and variations discussed below.

X-RAYS WITH CONTRAST MEDIA

Some soft tissues show on x-rays so poorly that radiologists use contrasting substances that are opaque to x-rays in order to make these tissues more visible. The contrast chemicals may be:

- **Barium,** which is used mostly for examination of the gastrointestinal tract.
- **Iodine derivatives** that are swallowed in tablet or liquid form and are used for gallbladder studies called cholecystography.
- **Special chemicals** that are introduced into the bronchial tubes and lungs through a bronchoscope for a study called bronchography.
- **Iodine derivatives** that are injected into arteries or veins for studies of the arteries and veins called angiography or venography.
- **Iodine derivatives** that are injected into a vein and travel to the kidney, are excreted there, and in their passage demonstrate the structure of the urinary tract.

Contrast media are injected into other organs and tissues for even more types of studies.

SCANNING

Scanning procedures which were introduced in the 1970s have further enhanced our diagnostic capabilities with procedures that bring more clarity without increased risk. Scanning procedures include ultrasound, computer enhancement, magnetic resonance imaging (MRI), CT scanning, positron emission tomography and radionuclide scanning.

- **Ultrasound** was the first of the modern scanning procedures, representing a completely non-invasive form of imaging that can render valuable information. High-frequency sound waves pass through the body and are recorded by a transducer that is placed on the skin. Structures of different density reflect the sound waves to make patterns of echoes which an electronic monitor records on a screen. Ultrasonography may be used in the diagnosis of many diseased organs and is the diagnostic procedure of choice for studies of the gallbladder, kidney, female genital tract and others.
- **Computerized tomography scanning (CT scanning)** is also called CAT (computerized axial tomography) scanning or "whole-body scanning." The patient lies on a large table that moves up and down to allow accurate positioning of the machine. With this technique, x-rays pass through the body at differing angles. The computer records these as cross-sectional images (slices) of the tissues examined.

  CT scanning makes remarkably clear pictures and has replaced many of the imaging techniques formerly used for diagnosing diseases of the brain, spinal cord and other tissues. This testing requires only a modest and safe exposure to x-rays. With special techniques the images can be manipulated to provide three-dimensional views. The CT scanning equipment is costly, and the examinations are expensive. (Present costs range from $800 to $1200.)

- **Magnetic resonance imaging (MRI)** is expensive, but the information obtained may be priceless. With this technique, the patient lies inside a large, hollow, cylindrical tube in a very strong magnetic field while radio-frequency waves pass through tissues. Magnetic coils detect changes in the alignment of protons of the body's hydrogen atoms when they are subjected to short bursts of the powerful magnetic field. Hydrogen protons in the cells rearrange themselves under these conditions.

  The computer analyzes the changes and makes possible the clear visualization of tissues. MRI allows the construction of images in any plane, providing precise diagnostic information on tumors and other abnormalities of the brain, other structures of the nervous system, the eye, ear, joints, heart, major blood vessels and other organs and tissues. There are no known risks or side effects.

  Note: CT scanning and MRI scanning are both completely harmless. Good studies require cooperation on the part of the patient, for they require 20-60 minutes of lying motionless in a relatively confined area. Some patients find this quite difficult, particularly if they are subject to claustrophobia. The information obtained is definitely worth the effort. If you are particularly wary about the environment necessary for the tests, the radiologist or your physician may ease your discomfort with a mild sedative or temporary tranquilizer.

- **Positron emission tomography (PET scanning)** gives information not only about structure, but also about the function of tissues of the central nervous system. Short-lived radioisotopes are introduced into tissues from which gamma waves are emitted. The gamma rays are analyzed by computer and sometimes yield precise information not available from any other study at present.

- **Radionuclide scanning** yields information about structure and function. Radioactive substances are selectively injected into the blood stream, and a gamma camera records uptake by various organs to give three-dimensional images. Computers analyze the results. One of the common uses of this type of study is called MUGGA, a test to measure the efficiency of the left ventricle of the heart in ejecting the blood pumped into it.

Injuries, Treatment of

RICE is an acronym (a word coined from first letters of words) for the most important elements—*rest, ice, compression and elevation*—in the first aid treatment of many injuries. Use the word *RICE* to jog your memory when you are faced with such injuries as contusions, sprains, strains, dislocations or uncomplicated fractures.

REST

Stop using the injured part and rest it as soon as you realize an injury has taken place. Continued exercise or other activity could cause further injury, delay healing, increase pain and stimulate bleeding. Use crutches to avoid bearing weight on an injured foot, ankle, knee or leg. Use splints for injuries of the hand, wrist, elbow or arm. After medical treatment, the injured part may require immobilization with splints or a cast to keep the area at rest until it heals.

ICE

Ice helps stop internal bleeding from injured blood vessels and capillaries. Sudden cold causes small blood vessels to contract. This contraction of the blood vessels decreases the amount of blood that can collect around the wound. The more blood that collects, the longer the healing time. Ice can be safely applied in several ways using the following instructions:

- For injuries to small areas, such as a finger, toe, foot or wrist, immerse the injured area in a bucket of ice water. Use ice cubes to keep the water cold as the ice dissolves.
- For injuries to larger areas, use ice packs. Avoid placing the ice directly on the skin. Before applying the ice, place a towel, cloth, or one or two layers of an elasticized compression bandage on the skin to be iced. To make the ice pack, put ice chips or ice cubes in a plastic bag or wrap them in a thin towel. Place the ice pack over the cloth. The pack may sit directly on the injured part, or it may be wrapped in place.
- Ice the injured area for about 30 minutes, no matter what form of ice treatment you are using.
- Remove the ice to allow the skin to warm for 15 minutes.
- Reapply the ice.
- Repeat the icing and warming cycles for 3 hours, as well as following the instructions below for compression and elevation. If pain and swelling persist after 3 hours, consult your doctor (if you have not already done so). Your doctor may change the icing schedule after the first 3 hours. Regular ice treatment is often discontinued after 24 to 48 hours. At that point, heat is often more comfortable.

COMPRESSION

Compression decreases swelling by slowing bleeding and limiting the accumulation of blood and plasma near the injury site. Without compression, fluid from adjacent normal tissue seeps into the injury area. The more blood and fluid that accumulates around an injury, the slower the healing. Following are instructions for safely applying compression to an injury:

- Use an elasticized bandage (Ace bandage) for compression if possible. If you do not have one available, any kind of cloth will suffice for a short time.
- Wrap the injured part firmly, wrapping over the ice also. Begin wrapping below the injury site and extend the wrap above the injury site. Be careful not to compress the area so tightly that the blood supply is impaired. Signs of blood supply deprivation include pain, numbness, cramping and blue or dusky-colored nails. Remove the compression bandage immediately if any of these symptoms appear. Leave the bandage off until all signs of impaired circulation disappear. Then rewrap the area—less tightly this time.

ELEVATION

Elevating the injured part above the level of the heart is another way to decrease swelling and pain at the injury site. Elevate the iced, compressed area in whatever way is most convenient. Prop an injured leg on solid objects or pillows. Elevate an injured arm by lying down and placing pillows under the arm or placing the pillows on the chest with the arm folded across the pillows. The whole upper part of the body may be elevated gently using pillows or a reclining chair or by raising the top of the bed on blocks.

Injuries, Recovery & Rehabilitation

Rehabilitation, when applied to injuries from exercising, falls or other accidents, means the restoration of health. Traditionally this has meant exercising muscles to restore their strength, endurance and normal range of motion. A broader interpretation includes other methods and techniques that facilitate the healing process.

CONSIDERATIONS FOR OLDER ADULTS

Age has no bearing on whether or not rehabilitation is appropriate following an injury. There are so many degrees of rehabilitaion available today that there will always be some steps that can be taken in an effort to restore any lost function.

WHAT TO DO

Physical agents such as heat, cold, massage and electric current can be used in conjunction with exercise programs—and sometimes medications—to hasten rehabilitation. The first three can often be used at home under the supervision of a doctor, physical therapist or trainer. These trained professionals can oversee your progress, shifting from one type of exercise to another when advisable.

The different methods are explained in greater detail below. Electrical current can only be used with specialized equipment in a clinical setting, but it is very effective in muscle retraining and restoration of strength.

Heat

When heat is applied to an injury, it dilates (enlarges) the small blood vessels in the area, increasing the blood flow. The increased blood supply nourishes the tissues and hastens healing. Heat also reduces pain in an injured area and reduces muscle spasms. But heat increases the chance that small capillaries will leak blood and plasma into soft tissues around the injury.

While dilation of the blood vessels and increased blood flow are desirable in healing, capillary leakage is undesirable. It leads to greater fluid accumulation and swelling, which retards the healing process. To be beneficial, heat should not be applied until the capillaries have had a chance to seal and stop leaking. This usually requires 24 to 48 hours following injury if ice, compression and elevation were used immediately.

Depending on the type of injury, heat can be applied in several ways: hot compresses, hydrocollator packs (see Glossary), heat lamps, heating pads, whirlpool baths or hot tubs, ultrasound or diathermy (seldom used now; see Glossary).

Your doctor or therapist must prescribe the best program for you and provide supervision and guidance throughout your rehabilitation program. You will need instructions about when to start, how long to apply heat during each treatment and how long to continue with heat treatments. These factors are determined by many variables, such as the type and extent of the injury and your previous medical history and healing rate.

Cold (Cryotherapy)

During the past several years, cold treatment has been used increasingly in first aid and in the rehabilitation of athletic injuries. Localized cold treatments provide these important benefits:

- Reduction and control of swelling (edema).
- Facilitation of active or passive joint motion, allowing a return to exercise sooner than is possible without cryotherapy. Ice is applied before exercise during the healing phase.
- Reduction of pain and muscle spasms. Because ice can be applied prior to exercise, reducing pain and muscle spasms, muscle and joint movements can start sooner without interfering with the healing process. A thin margin of safety regarding when exercise should start and continue makes clinical supervision necessary during rehabilitation.

Ice can be applied using ice packs, ice compresses or ice massage. Ice massage is particularly helpful for sore muscles or muscles in spasm. Techniques of ice massage are as follows:

- Fill a large Styrofoam cup with water and freeze it.
- Tear a small amount of foam from the top of the cup so that the ice protrudes.
- Massage firmly over the injured area in a circle about the size of a softball.
- Do this for 15 minutes at a time 3 or 4 times a day and before workouts or competition.

APPENDIX 38 (continued)

Massage

Gentle massage is useful for treating sore muscles. It consists of gentle or firm stroking of the injured area. The strokes should be directed toward the heart. The appropriate amount of pressure and the length of the massage should be determined by the person receiving the massage. Massage that increases pain is too hard.

When properly administered, massage can reduce fluid accumulation and swelling around an injury. It will stimulate circulation through the veins and lymphatic vessels. However, *overzealous* massage can aggravate an injury and increase bleeding.

WHO CAN HELP

Your doctor will be the team leader in arranging for rehabilitaion. He or she will determine your needs, refer you to the other medical professionals for therapy and training and follow up to make sure that the quality and quantity of the care you receive is appropriate.

Insurance, Medical

TYPES OF MEDICAL INSURANCE

Health insurance may be provided by a number of private companies or by the federal government through Medicare and Medicaid.

- **Medicare** is the federal program designed to help with the medical expenses of those 65 and older and of persons with some chronic disabilities or severe kidney disease. Medicare is divided into two parts: Part A and Part B. Part A automatically begins at age 65. Part B must be applied for. (See What To Do, below, for further information.) You may obtain full information about Medicare from your local Social Security office.
- **Medicaid** is a state-sponsored program using help from federal funds. This program is designed to help newly poor older persons as well as the chronically needy. Full information is available in all state social services departments.
- **Private medical insurance** is a wise purchase. Your local Social Security office will provide a pamphlet titled *Guide to Health Insurance for People with Medicare*. If you have private insurance and become eligible for Medicare or Medicaid, do not cancel your private insurance until you gain experience with the repayment performance of the agencies.

WHAT TO DO

Medicare

When you first become eligible for Part B (which is offered at a monthly premium to cover doctors' services, physical therapy and rehabilitation), you should take advantage of its provisions if you can. If you refuse it when it is first offered, it becomes much more expensive if it is added at a later date. You may obtain full information about Medicare from your local Social Security office.

Medicaid

If you may be eligible, apply for aid through the appropriate state health agency. When you go for your first appointment to determine your eligibility, be sure to take along a relative or friend for the interview. And be sure to carry with you all the documentation that the agency will require. The requirements vary from state to state, and the application process may be grueling.

Private Insurance

If you have private insurance and become eligible for Medicare or Medicaid, do not cancel your private insurance until you gain experience with the repayment performance of the agencies. Actual coverage frequently will turn out to be something other than what you may have expected.

Long-Term Health Insurance

Seventy or so insurance companies offer long-term health insurance that covers some nursing home expenses and some home health care. Look into these policies vary carefully. Zealous sales agents sometimes misrepresent the services, coverage and limitations that the policies provide. Before you buy read the policy, not just a brochure.

WHO CAN HELP

Medicare—The local Social Security office.
Medicaid—State social services departments.
Private health insurance—Contact local agencies.

Living Will

A living will is a written statement, signed by you, that specifies what treatments and life-support measures you will want or not want if you become incapacitated due to terminal illness, an accident or complications following surgery. Living wills allow your family and medical professionals to know what your desires would be if these events should occur. Recent court cases in which families have tried to obtain legal permission to discontinue life-support systems for comatose patients have pointed out the need for a way to let all those concerned know ahead of time what you would want if you were the patient involved. A living will is the best answer.

CONSIDERATIONS FOR OLDER ADULTS

Older patients are more likely to have terminal illnesses that may leave them unconscious for very long periods.

Family members should know what your feelings are about life-support measures but may be reluctant to initiate a discussion that involves dying.

You should be the one making the decisions instead of leaving it up to family members, doctors, hospital administrators or possibly the courts.

Recognize that certain disorders such as Alzheimer's disease or stroke may be incapacitating, but are not covered by a living will because they are not life-threatening.

WHAT TO DO

Decide whether you want to execute a living will.

Because there are many different aspects to consider, it is best to obtain a pre-printed form to fill out. You will want to be specific about your wishes. Just stating that no "heroic" measures should be taken is insufficient and leaves too much to interpretation.

Documents are available free of charge from the Society for the Right to Die, 250 W. 57th St., New York, NY 10107. Send a self-addressed envelope that is stamped with two first-class stamps.

Another type of living will form called the Medical Directive is available for $1 from the Harvard Medical School Health Letter, 164 Longwood Ave., 4th Floor, Boston, MA 02115. Send a self-addressed stamped envelope.

Your living will should name a proxy and an alternate. This is someone who can be the spokesperson regarding your medical care. Usually this will be a close family member. Be sure this person will respect your wishes and defend them if necessary to other family members, doctors, hospitals or courts.

If you want stronger protection, you can execute a health-care power of attorney. This is a legally binding document that empowers a designated person to make health-care decisions for you. This form is an addition to the living will.

Keep a copy of the living will at home, and provide copies to your proxy and alternate as well as your doctor.

WHO CAN HELP

Talk to your family about your plans and what your specific desires are, and together decide who your proxy will be.

Discuss all aspects of the living will with your doctor. Make an appointment that will give you and your doctor time to discuss it. Send a copy of the living will ahead of time if appropriate.

An attorney is usually not needed to help you fill out the living will form, but one may be consulted if you have concerns or unanswered questions.

Your state health department or a department on aging can give you information about laws in the state where you live.

Check at your library for books on aging or books specifically about living wills that can provide additional information.

Loss

Loss can encompass many areas of one's life. The loss may involve another human being, a pet, a job, your driver's license, your home, your health, your independence, and on and on. The response to a loss will be different for each individual, and there is no right or wrong way to handle the feelings evoked. The loss of a beloved pet may be as grievous to one person as the loss of a spouse is to another. No other person can know exactly how you feel your pain. Temporary feelings of despair, hopelessness, depression, numbness, guilt, irritability and anger are all quite normal and should be expected.

CONSIDERATIONS FOR OLDER ADULTS

It is natural to expect loss as you get older. Death is going to occur among family members, friends and acquaintances.

Losses may come in clusters. A serious illness that causes loss of health may also bring financial loss, loss of independence and the loss of your home.

WHAT TO DO

Talk to someone. Don't keep your feelings to yourself. Even if you think the other person might not understand your grief, talking about it will be a step toward recovery. You may even want to talk into a tape recorder to express your feelings.

Write in a journal about your feelings. This helps you get them sorted out and understood.

Recognize that there are phases in recovering from loss that people go through, but because individuals are so different, there is no set schedule or timing as to when each phase will occur. It may take a year or more to cope healthily with the loss of a loved one, but time does heal.

Look for new interests and challenges in your life. Let others help you. Don't ever just quit living and retire to your rocking chair.

If your recovery is prolonged or your grief is too intense, seek professional help. You don't want to lose your health. Lack of sleep, poor eating habits, the use of tranquilizers, excessive alcohol consumption and loneliness can lead to other serious health problems. People really can die of a broken heart.

WHO CAN HELP

Family members and friends are your best support. Rely on them; don't feel that you are imposing or that you must always be the strong one. Let your adult children fill the parent role temporarily.

Talk to your minister.

Get help from a professional therapist.

Join a self-help group. Groups such as Widow to Widow are made up of people who have been through similar losses and can be wonderful listeners and an excellent source of support.

APPENDIX 42

Medic Alert & Emergency Alert Products

DESCRIPTION

- **Medic Alert** is a personal identification tag, usually a bracelet, neck chain or wallet card, that states special medical information about you. This can include information about chronic illnesses or other health disorders, allergies and what medications you are currently taking. This information can be life-saving in some emergency situations when you may be unable to speak for yourself.
- **Emergency Alert** is for people who live alone and may need emergency help. This device sends out a radio signal through your telephone and places a call for help to a monitoring location. The device is referred to as a PERS (personal emergency response system).

CONSIDERATIONS FOR OLDER ADULT

- **Medic Alert**—Older people are more likely to have chronic illnesses or to be taking one or more medications that someone may need to be aware of, or an accident or injury may confuse an older person and limit the amount of information a doctor or health professional can obtain.
- **Emergency Alert**—This device allows a person to remain independent while assuring both the user and the family that help can be quickly obtained with just the push of a button.

WHAT TO DO

Contact one of the organizations listed below to obtain information about these products.

WHO CAN HELP

Medic Alert Products

Apex Medical Corporation, (800) 328-2935, has bracelets, necklaces or keychains showing a person's medical problem along with a wallet card that goes into more detail.

The Medic Alert Corporation, (800) IDALERT, has bracelets and necklaces engraved with its symbol and your primary medical problem. It also has a 24-hour hotline that will give further details about your medical record.

National Medi-Card Systems, (800) 266-1787, can provide a wallet-sized card with information on your medical history, immunization record, insurance and more.

Emergency Alert Devices

Check with local or state health departments, special organizations for the aging or non-profit health organizations. Write to the American Association of Retired Persons (obtain the address from the Resources section) for its booklet titled *Meeting the Need for Security and Independence with PERS*.

Medical Fraud & Health Quackery

If a medical cure sounds too good to be true, it probably is. You may read an advertisement, hear a pitchman expound or have a friend tell you of some miraculous new medical discovery. Most of these "sure cures" are frauds. The impact of fraud affects all ages, but older people form the largest group of victims. The Subcommittee on Health and Long-Term Care of the U.S. House of Representatives conducted a 4-year investigation on quackery. The conclusions are that quackery represents a $10 billion scandal and that 60% of all victims of health fraud are older persons, although older people comprise only 12% of the U.S. population.

CONSIDERATIONS FOR OLDER ADULTS

Most people who succumb to health fraud and quackery are desperate for some offer of hope. Older people have more chronic illness than others (such as high blood pressure, diabetes, arthritis and cancer). Accordingly they are likely targets for medical fraud. The three largest areas for health quackery are aging, arthritis and cancer.

Aging

There are many useless products that promise to reverse the aging process or relieve conditions associated with old age. Beware of cosmetics purported to erase wrinkles or enhance virility. A healthy lifestyle will help delay many conditions associated with aging, but no preparation or device can stop it.

Cancer

This is not a single disease, but a complicated problem that may affect many body systems. Cancer accounts for one-fifth of all deaths in the United States. Cancer occurs more often in older people than in younger patients. Quacks—those who sell unproven remedies—have been around for generations. They are still here and find fertile grounds for profit in cancer victims. They prey on older people's fears and lack of information by offering treatments that have no proven value. Among these are drastic diets that not only are of no proven value in treating cancer, but are dangerously low in protein or other nutrients. Equally dishonest is the practice of selling worthless drugs such as Laetrile.

Proven treatments for cancer include surgery, radiation and chemotherapy. The progress using these methods makes it possible for 50% of cancer victims to survive for 5 or more years. This rate might be higher if all patients promptly consulted qualified doctors instead of losing valuable treatment time on worthless and costly remedies.

Arthritis

This is another favorite field for quackery. Arthritis "remedies" are especially easy to fall for because the symptoms of arthritis tend to recede or disappear for periods of time for unknown reasons. Persons with arthritis then associate the remedy they happen to be using with relief from symptoms. Unapproved "extracts," metallic devices or adornments, herbal remedies and other forms of hoaxes not only delay appropriate treatment, but also may themselves be harmful. For most forms of arthritis there is no known cure at present, but treatments are available through qualified medical resources that can help reduce your pain and improve your flexibility. These include drugs, heat, a balance of rest and exercise and in some cases surgical implants.

WHAT TO DO

Stay alert to signs of quackery. Carefully question what you see or hear in advertisements. Find out about health products before you buy them. Check out door-to-door sales efforts through a local agency such as the Better Business Bureau.

Beware of these common ploys of dishonest promoters:

- Promises of quick or painless cures.
- Promoting products made from "secret" formulas, especially those available only by mail or from only one merchant.
- Presenting testimonials or case histories from random "satisfied" patients.
- Advertising a product as being effective for a wide variety of human ailments.
- Claiming to understand the cause or cure for diseases such as arthritis or cancer that are not yet understood by competent scientists.

WHO CAN HELP

The Council of Better Business Bureaus and the Food and Drug Administration have produced two brochures that are available to the public free. Send one self-addressed envelope for each brochure to:

Council of Better Business Bureaus
1515 Wilson Blvd.
Arlington, VA 2209
(Attn: Standards and Practices)

Ask for *Tips on Medical Quackery* and/or *Arthritis: Quackery and Unproven Remedies.*

Report any mail you think represents fraud or quackery to:

The United States Postal Service
Postal Inspection Service
Office of Criminal Investigation
Washington, D.C. 20260-2166

Refer to your local telephone directory for professional organizations concerned with specific diseases, such as the American Cancer Society or the Arthritis Foundation, for help and information.

Nursing Home, How To Choose

Nursing homes vary greatly in accommodations, size and the manner in which they provide services. The majority are run for profit, with the balance run by nonprofit organizations or government agencies. To qualify for Medicare and Medicaid certification, a nursing home will be required to provide 24-hour nursing coverage and a wide range of services. There are many factors involved in selecting a home, and the decision should not be rushed. Take your time, check out what is available and select the one that will provide the best possible care.

CONSIDERATIONS FOR OLDER ADULTS

People are living longer because of medical advances, but these advances do not necessarily allow for independent living. Some degree of care frequently may be needed.

Hospitals, primarily because of reimbursement procedures, may sometimes release patients before they are really able to care for themselves at home. A nursing home stay may be required for a period of time.

Older adults are more likely to incur the problems that lead to nursing home admission: behavior difficulties, bone fractures, confusion, frequent falls, incontinence, stroke and inability to care for oneself.

WHAT TO DO

Get recommendations for nursing homes from knowledgeable people or local referral services.

Check with your state health department to review the data about the homes in the federal government publication *Medicare/Medicaid Nursing Home Information*. It provides an evaluation of the care, conditions and other aspects of more than 16,000 facilities in the U.S.

Once your list is narrowed down, plan on visiting each home.

Make a list ahead of time of those areas of the home that you want to visually observe or need to discuss with the administrator. Include physical appearance of the accommodations, safety features, appearance of the residents, what medical and nursing staff members the organization provides, food and nutrition quality, the rehabilitation services offered, activities for patients, spiritual services and, of course, the costs.

Recognize that it will be difficult to assess everything completely on one visit, but if you can talk to current residents, they may be the best source of information. Find out if they basically like the home and would recommend it.

WHO CAN HELP

A hospital-based social worker deals daily with decisions of this type and is a good source of recommendations.

Friends who have gone through the same process for themselves can provide guidance.

Human services agencies, such as the United Way, can provide help.

Your doctor or minister may have suggestions.

Look at the yellow pages in your telephone directory.

Retirement

Retirement from one's primary occupation is desired by many, resisted by others, forced upon a few because of health or job loss and occasionally feared by both the retiree and the retiree's spouse. Retirement involves income adjustments and changes in social activities and feelings of self-worth. Because of the difficulty of making the transition for some people, their physical and mental health can be affected.

CONSIDERATIONS FOR OLDER ADULTS

This is the age at which retirement usually occurs.

Stories abound about people who retired and died shortly thereafter. This might happen to those who retired due to illness or disability, but it is not likely to occur in people who are in general good health.

WHAT TO DO

Planning is the key to making retirement successful and not letting it lead to problems that will affect your health and well-being.

Start as early as possible in life to plan for retirement. Discuss all aspects with your spouse, consider options, make plans, review your finances and think as if you will live to 100 or more. Life is certainly not over.

Make health and fitness a priority in your planning. This may be a time to consider giving up smoking, cutting down on alcohol consumption and taking up an exercise program such as walking. You will no longer have the excuse of job stress or lack of time for not making these changes a part of your life.

Stay active no matter what it is that you do. This is probably the number-one factor in maintaining mental health. Some people thrive, getting a part-time job or doing volunteer work.

WHO CAN HELP

Talk to other retirees. They will have gone through many of the adjustments you are facing and can suggest ways to ease the transition.

Discuss your plans with adult children.

Take advantage of any counselling your employer may offer about retirement.

Get information about retirement planning from your library or write to the American Association of Retired Persons (address is in the Resources Section).

Get private counseling if you find that adjusting to retirement is causing anxiety, stress, increased alcohol use or interpersonal problems with your spouse.

Salt & Sodium Use

Salt is a necessary part of life, not only because it flavors and protects foods, but because our bodies need sodium, which is present in salt. Sodium helps to maintain blood volume, regulate water balance, transmit nerve impulses and perform other vital functions.

Unfortunately, many people consume far too much salt. Table salt consists of 40% sodium and 60% chloride. One teaspoon of salt has 2 grams of sodium. The Food and Nutrition Board of the National Academy of Sciences believes that an adequate and safe level of sodium each day is 1.1 to 3.3 grams. Most Americans now consume between 2.3 and 6.9 grams daily.

CONSIDERATIONS FOR OLDER ADULTS

As people grow older, their sensitivity to flavors and smells usually decreases. Because of this, there may be a desire for more salt to combat the flat taste of foods.

Older people in particular should be cautious about using too much salt. The main reason for caution is that the overuse of sodium is one factor that is associated with high blood pressure. High blood pressure, in turn, can lead to heart disease, stroke and kidney failure. Blood pressure rises with age, and all of these disorders are much more common among older persons.

WHAT TO DO

If your doctor has suggested that you cut back on salt, there are several steps you can take. It is easy to change a few habits that will reduce your level of sodium without changing your diet drastically.

Learn which foods in general contain less sodium. Fresh foods usually have less sodium than processed ones. Fresh meats, for example, are lower in sodium than processed ones such as lunch meats, bacon, hot dogs, sausage and ham, all of which have sodium added to flavor and preserve them. Likewise, most fresh vegetables are naturally low in sodium. Canned vegetables and vegetable juices usually have salt added, but some new lines are canned without it. Plain frozen vegetables without sauces are generally low in sodium. Fresh, frozen and canned fruits and fruit juices are low in sodium.

Commercially prepared foods such as soups, frozen dinners and other convenience items have salt added in their preparation. Some of these are available with substantially less sodium, so check the labels. Snacks such as potato chips, pretzels, corn chips, popcorn, crackers and nuts normally have a great deal of salt added and are best used sparingly.

When grocery shopping, look for low-sodium and sodium-free items. Many food manufacturers list the sodium content of their products on the labels. (Foods labeled ''salt-free,'' ''sodium-free,'' low-salt,'' or ''low-sodium'' must have this information.) If sodium is one of the first three ingredients listed, the product is high in sodium.

When cooking meals at home, try to gradually reduce the amount of salt you use each day. And remember that adding salt is not the only way to flavor foods. You can also use lemon, pepper, herbs, spices, onion and garlic powders (not salts), powdered mustard, small amounts of sugar, finely chopped garlic and fresh grated horseradish. Experiment with flavorings you haven't used before.

At the table, taste your food before adding salt. If you think the food needs some, add only a small amount. Ketchup, mustard, relish, salad dressings, sauces, brines and dips contain sodium. As your use of salt goes down, it may be tempting to use more of these. But go easy on them. Pickles and olives are also prepared with a considerable amount of sodium.

Before using a salt substitute, ask your doctor about it. These preparations usually contain potassium, which can be harmful to people with some medical conditions, but helpful to others, particularly those who take thiazide diuretics for high blood pressure.

When eating out, choose items that are less likely to have large amounts of salt added. Some restaurants will prepare low-sodium meals if asked to do so.

Restricting the amount of sodium in the diet helps lower high blood pressure in many individuals who already have the disease. It can also increase the effectiveness of drug treatment, making a lower dosage possible.

WHO CAN HELP

Talk to your doctor about your salt intake. If a decrease is recommended, follow the guidelines suggested above.

Many books on the subject of cooking with less salt are now available in libraries and stores. Newspapers and magazines often offer low-salt recipes.

APPENDICES

APPENDIX 47

Senility

Senility—something which most of us fear in old age—is not a normal sign of growing old; in fact, it is not even a disease. Rather, senility is the word commonly used to describe a large number of conditions with an equally large number of causes, many of which respond to prompt treatment.

SYMPTOMS & OF SENILITY

The symptoms of what is popularly called "senility" include serious forgetfulness, confusion and certain other changes in personality and behavior. While doctors and patients alike used to routinely dismiss these symptoms as incurable effects of old age, they are not necessarily. Nor are small memory lapses in old age a sign of senility. Slight confusion or occasional forgetfulness throughout life may only signify an overload of facts in the brain's storehouse of information.

Mental decline in old age might be called dementia, organic brain disorder, chronic brain syndrome, arteriosclerosis, cerebral atrophy or pseudodementia. The important thing to remember is that some of the problems which are generally referred to under the medical description of senile dementia can be treated and cured, while at this time others can only be treated without hope of restoring lost brain function. Thus a complete, careful investigation of the source of the symptoms is necessary.

CONSIDERATIONS FOR OLDER ADULTS

The two most common incurable forms of mental impairment in old age are *multi-infarct dementia* and *Alzheimer's disease* (also called *senile dementia of the Alzheimer type* or SDAT).

Multi-infarct dementia is caused by a series of minor strokes which result in widespread death of brain tissue. This condition accounts for about 20% of the irreversible cases of mental impairment.

In Alzheimer's disease, changes in the nerve cells of the outer layer of the brain result in the death of a large number of cells. Some 50% to 60% of all elderly persons with mental impairment have Alzheimer's disease.

Some 100 reversible conditions may mimic these disorders. A minor head injury, high fever, brain tumor, poor nutrition or adverse drug reactions, for example, can temporarily upset the normal activity of extremely sensitive brain cells. If left untreated, such medical emergencies can result in permanent damage to the brain, and possibly even death.

In much the same way, emotional problems can be mistakenly confused with irreversible brain disease. Depression, loss of self-esteem, loneliness, anxiety and boredom can become more common as elderly persons face retirement, the deaths of relatives and friends and other such crises—often at the same time.

WHAT TO DO

Persons who are suspected of having Alzheimer's disease or multi-infarct dementia should have thorough physical, neurological and psychiatric evaluations. These include a complete medical exam, as well as tests of the patient's mental state and highly specific tests such as a brain scan. A brain scan is useful in that it can rule out a curable disorder. A brain scan may also show signs of normal age-related changes in the brain, such as shrinkage, which are not necessarily a sign of disease.

The patient plays an important role in the diagnosis by giving information on past medical history, the use of drugs—both prescription and over-the-counter—diet, and general health. Because part of the medical exam depends upon how much a patient is able to remember about past events, the doctor may also ask a close relative for information.

The best treatment comes only after a complete medical examination by one who does not dismiss complaints as "just old age." If there is a diagnosis of a curable disease, the doctor will know how to treat it or will have ready access to the best resources or specialists.

If the diagnosis is one of the irreversible disorders, there is still much that can be done to treat the patient and to help the family cope. The careful use of drugs can lessen agitation, anxiety and depression and can improve sleeping patterns if this is needed. Proper nutrition is particularly important, although special diets or supplements are usually not necessary. The person should be encouraged to maintain daily routines, physical activities and social contacts and should not be discouraged from trying new things. Often stimulating the individual—by supplying information on the time of day, place of residence and what is going on in the immediate environment and in world events—encourages the use of skills and information which remain. This, in turn, may keep brain activity from failing at a more rapid pace.

Providing memory aids helps people help themselves in day-to-day living. Such aids can include a very visible calendar, a list of daily activities, written notes about simple safety measures and directions to and labeling of commonly used items.

WHO CAN HELP

Any patient with an irreversible mental disorder should be under the care of a doctor. This may be a neurologist, a psychiatrist or a family doctor or internist who is willing to devote the time and interest required to closely watch treatment, to treat the physical and emotional problems that may complicate the course of the disease and, of course, to answer the many questions that the patient and family may ask.

See the Resources and Additional Reading sections for suggestions about further information.

Sexuality

Most older people want—and are able to lead—an active, satisfying sex life. With age, women do not ordinarily lose their physical capacity for orgasm, nor do men lose their capacity for erection and ejaculation. There is, however, a gradual slowing of response, especially in men, a process currently considered part of "normal" aging, but perhaps eventually treatable or even reversible.

A pattern of regular sexual activity (which may include masturbation) helps to preserve sexual ability. When problems occur, they should not be viewed as inevitable, but rather as the result of disease, disability, drug reactions or emotional upset—and as requiring medical care.

CONSIDERATIONS FOR OLDER ADULTS

Women generally experience little serious loss of sexual capacity due to age alone. Those changes that do occur—mainly in the shape, flexibility and lubrication of the vagina—can usually be traced directly to lowered levels of the hormone estrogen during and after menopause. Women who have severe problems are sometimes treated with estrogen.

Older men often notice more distinct changes in sexual functioning, although these vary greatly from man to man. It may take somewhat longer to attain an erection than when young (usually a matter of a few minutes more after stimulation). The erection may not be quite as firm or as large as in earlier years. There can be a shorter sensation that an ejaculation is about to occur. The loss of erection following orgasm may be more rapid, followed by a longer period of time before an erection is again possible.

A common emotional problem in older men is the fear of impotence. It is important to remember that all men are impotent at times due to fatigue, tension, illness or the consumption of alcohol. Usually potency returns by itself, but if a man is too worried he may continue to be impotent due to his fears alone.

Sexual Activity & Disease

The incidence of illness and disability increases with age. Although they can affect sexuality in later life, even the most serious diseases rarely warrant stopping sexual activity.

Heart disease, especially if a heart attack has occurred, leads many older people to give up sex altogether for fear of causing another attack. Yet the risk of death during sexual intercourse is very low. Although a doctor's advice is needed, sex usually can and should be resumed an average of 12 to 16 weeks after a heart attack, depending on one's physical conditioning. An active sex life may in fact decrease the risk of a future attack.

Diabetes is one of the few diseases that can cause impotence (a loss of the ability to achieve and maintain an erection hard enough for sexual intercourse). Once diabetes is diagnosed and controlled, however, potency may be restored. But when impotence persists in well-controlled diabetes, it may be permanent.

Stroke rarely damages physical aspects of sexual functioning, and it is unlikely that sexual exertion will cause another stroke. Using different positions or medical devices that assist body functions can help make up for any weakness or paralysis that may have occurred.

Joint pain due to rheumatoid arthritis can limit sexual activity. Surgery and drugs can relieve these problems, but in some cases the medicines used can decrease sexual desire. Exercise, rest, warm baths and changes in position and timing of sexual activity (such as avoiding evening and early morning hours, when pain is more likely) can be helpful.

Sexual Activity after Hysterectomy or Prostatectomy

If performed correctly, hysterectomy (womb removal) does not harm sexual functioning. Those women who believe they have been damaged by a hysterectomy—or men who consider their partners "less feminine" after this surgery—should seek counseling. The same is true of mastectomy (breast removal), since the loss of a breast can be quite upsetting because of the changes in physical appearance. Programs such as Reach to Recovery (sponsored by the American Cancer Society) are valuable to women in making an adjustment, as are a carefully fitted artificial breast and, in some cases, reconstructive surgery.

Prostatectomy (removal of the male prostate gland) rarely affects potency. Only the "perineal" approach, which is sometimes used in the surgical treatment of cancer or in other extreme situations, is likely to result in impotence. Except for a lack of seminal fluid, sexual capacity and enjoyment after a prostatectomy should return to the pre-surgery level.

The excessive use of alcohol, which reduces potency in men and delays orgasm in women, is probably the most widespread drug-related cause of sexual problems. Tranquilizers, antidepressants, and certain drugs for high blood pressure can cause impotence; other drugs can lead to failure to ejaculate in men and reduced sexual desire in women. Such effects are reversed when the medication is stopped. A doctor can often prescribe a drug with less sexual effect if he or she realizes that this is important to the patient.

WHAT TO DO

Public acceptance of sexuality in later life is gradually increasing. We can expect the day when the special aspects of sexuality in old age will become generally understood and when diagnosis and treatment of sexual problems will be refined to a much greater degree. Until then, follow the simple suggestions made in this section. The following should also be considered:

- Limit your alcohol use or abstain completely.
- To aid intercourse, use lubricants such as water-soluble lubricating jelly or baby oil. However, baby oil and other petroleum products should *not* be used with condoms.
- Seek counseling if appropriate and available.
- Don't insist on climaxes for yourself or your partner. Satisfying sexual experiences don't always require orgasms.
- For a man who can't achieve and maintain an erection, a penile prosthetic implant might be appropriate.

WHO CAN HELP

Older couples may have the same problems that affect people of any age. In addition, reactions to physical changes with age, retirement, other shifts in lifestyle and illness can cause sexual difficulties—and can usually be helped by counseling.

Talk to your doctor about your problems. It may be that medications are the cause and the dosages can be adjusted.

Skin Care

Consumers spend millions of dollars each year on wrinkle creams, skin bleaches to fade "age spots," oils and other cosmetics in order to keep their skin looking young. At the same time, they spend not only money but countless hours trying to tan their skin in the belief that a tan will make them look healthy and more attractive. Unfortunately, most people do not realize that long periods of exposure to the sun are the major reason their skin looks wrinkled before old age.

People often believe that a tanned person is healthier. While this is not true as far as the skin itself is concerned, limited exposure to the sun is one way to provide the body with vitamin D, which is necessary to maintain and repair bone. However, vitamin D is present in most American diets since it is added to dairy products such as milk, butter and margarine and is found in eggs and cod liver oil.

CONSIDERATIONS FOR OLDER ADULTS

Signs of aging rarely appear in protected skin until sometime after age 50, and even then aging progresses very slowly.

Ultraviolet (UV) radiation from the sun causes long-term damage to the skin even if the skin does not appear to burn. A suntan may prevent further sunburn, but it does not protect the skin from sun damage, which may not be visible for many years. The sun's rays damage the elastic fibers beneath the skin's surface. Dark patches or "age spots" may appear on sun-exposed skin with age. In addition to thickened, leathery-looking skin, lines and wrinkles around the eyes, on the upper lip and on the neck and hands usually result from prolonged exposure to the sun.

Sunlamps also deliver a strong dose of UV radiation. Dermatologists (doctors who specialize in treating skin problems) agree that sunlamps and tanning salons produce skin damage and warn that they must be used with great caution.

Mild to severe itching resulting from dry skin is one of the most common and uncomfortable characteristics of aging skin. Dry skin can appear after exposure to soaps, irritating cleaning products (disinfectants, cleansers, etc.) and dry air in overheated rooms (often called "winter itch"). It is important for an older person to use lotions to prevent severe itching because the scratching that often follows can lead to infection or long-term skin irritation.

The body's immune system, its defense against disease, is less efficient as we grow older. The skin, which becomes more fragile with age, wounds more easily and is more prone to infection. Because the skin reacts more slowly to irritants, an older person may not realize that the skin can be damaged by a strong chemical or a hot substance.

WHAT TO DO

Once the skin shows signs of aging, the damage cannot be reversed, but further damage can be prevented. An estimated 300,000 cases of skin cancer each year result from overexposure to the sun over a period of years. Skin cancer is easily cured in most cases when it is detected early. However, it often recurs if prolonged exposure to the sun continues.

Protecting Yourself from the Sun

The best way to guard against the harmful effects of overexposure to the sun's rays is to take protective measures. Sunbathing in the early morning or late afternoon is less damaging to the skin than in the middle of the day. People whose work requires them to be outside all day, such as farmers and sailors, should be especially careful to protect their skin from the sun. The face and neck can be somewhat protected by hats. The best protection is to apply a sunscreen to all skin that is not covered by clothing. Sunscreens are oils, creams, gels or lotions that absorb or scatter UV light. It is important to note the rating, called the skin protection factor (SPF), that appears on the label of a sunscreen product. The higher the number, the more protection the sunscreen provides. An SPF of 8 to 15 is recommended for maximum protection, although even a product with a 15 rating will allow some tanning to take place. To be effective, sunscreens should be applied at least 1/2 hour before exposure to the sun, and they must be reapplied after swimming or perspiring.

Preventing Dryness

To prevent dryness, wear rubber gloves when washing dishes and when using strong cleaning agents or other chemicals, use mild soaps and use petroleum jelly or other moisturizers as often as necessary, especially after bathing.

Wear soft clothing and avoid strong washing detergents. Some fabric softeners can also cause skin irritation and itching.

Take care to prevent injury by not using water that is too hot, by wearing gloves when cleaning and by avoiding the use of harsh products even if no reaction appears on the skin immediately.

The abrupt onset of generalized itching can be a sign of certain diseases. If it persists after taking preventive measures to avoid dry skin, check with your doctor.

There are many different kinds of moisturizers available, ranging from heavy creams to light non-greasy lotions. Although they vary greatly in price, the most expensive product is not necessarily the best. Many dermatologists recommend moisturizers that contain petrolatum or lanolin. Highly perfumed products should be avoided.

WHO CAN HELP

Many age-related skin changes as well as most skin cancers are surgically correctable. Anyone over age 50 who has had skin cancer should see a dermatologist annually.

Sleep Problems

Sleep problems are symptoms, not diseases. They may fall into three categories:

- Difficulty falling asleep.
- Early morning awakening.
- Frequent awakening at night.

Sleep problems may have both physical and emotional components. They may be of two types:

- Transient, as with temporary insomnia associated with time zone changes, a change in work shifts and times of stress or grief. Almost everyone has experienced sleep problems of this sort.
- Chronic, the type that may be caused by a host of disorders.

CONSIDERATIONS FOR OLDER ADULTS

Although many writers claim that older people do not require as much sleep as they once did, this claim has not been proven, nor does it apply to everyone.

In general, older people probably do not sleep as well as younger people.

It may require longer to fall asleep, there may be more frequent wakeful periods in the night, and there may be more early awakening. Most older people adapt well. Some find these changes troubling.

WHAT TO DO

Limit or eliminate your use of alcohol, caffeine, nicotine, marijuana and cocaine. Beware of many prescription and non-prescription drugs, particularly appetite suppressants. They are sleep robbers. Prescription-type sleep aids can be a mixed blessing. They should never be taken for more than a few days at a time, as tolerance develops and sleep patterns may be made worse. It is very easy for one to become addicted. Non-prescription drugs that contain an antihistamine can cause muscle incoordination, memory loss and decreased alertness.

If possible, confine times of worry and worrisome encounters to early evening or earlier.

Slow the pace of your activities as evening approaches.

Maintain regular times for retiring and arising. Avoid prolonged periods of sleep beyond 7 or 8 hours without getting up and moving around a lot.

Exercise daily, but avoid vigorous exercise close to bedtime.

Use relaxation, meditation and imaging techniques and/or prayer. Try not to relive unpleasant experiences from your past. Don't review the day's annoyances and mistakes. Don't fret about possible problems. By any means possible attempt to relax, but don't try to force sleep. Any restful mental attitude will favor normal sleep.

Get up out of bed if you are unable to get to sleep within 20-30 minutes. Use your bed only for sleep (and sex). Use other rooms in the house for other activities.

Try a warm bath just before bedtime. It can help relax tense muscles.

Make your sleep environment optimal. Consider clean linens, a superior mattress and pillow, a cool temperature, subdued or absent light, eye shades and ear plugs.

If your inadequate night-time sleep requires a day-time nap, take it early in the day. Afternoon or evening naps can interfere with a normal night's rest.

Warm milk helps many. A light snack also may promote sleep. Avoid making the evening meal close to bedtime or extra large.

WHO CAN HELP

Your doctor may prescribe safe and effective medicines that act as sleep aids to be used under appropriate circumstances. These should never be used for more than a few days at a time, and then only when necessary.

Sleep centers can provide evaluation and recommend treatment for more serious sleep problems, such as apnea, sleep-related myoclonus and others. To receive a roster of accredited sleep disorder centers and clinics, write to:

The Association of Professional Sleep Societies
604 2nd St. SW
Rochester, MN 55902

Smoking

Cigarette smoke affects a smoker's lungs and air passages, causing irritation, inflammation and excessive production of mucus. These smoking effects can result in a chronic cough and, in more severe cases, the lung disease known as chronic bronchitis. Long-term lung damage can lead to emphysema, which prevents normal breathing.

SMOKING & CARDIOVASCULAR DISEASE

Smoking, high blood pressure and high blood cholesterol (a fatty substance in the blood) are major factors that contribute to coronary heart disease. A person with high blood pressure or high cholesterol who also smokes has a much greater risk of heart attack than a person who has only one of these risk factors.

When a person stops smoking, the benefits to the heart and circulatory system begin right away. The risk of heart attack, stroke and other circulatory diseases drops. The circulation of blood to the hands and feet improves. Although quitting smoking won't reverse chronic lung damage, it may slow the disease and help retain existing lung function.

SMOKING & LUNG DISEASE

Smoking causes several types of cancer, including those of the lungs, mouth, larynx and esophagus. It also plays a role in cancers of the pancreas, kidney and bladder. A smoker's risk of cancer depends in part on the number of cigarettes smoked, the number of years of smoking and how deeply the smoke is inhaled. After a smoker quits, the risk of smoking-related cancer begins to decline, and within a decade the risk is reduced to that of the non-smoker.

Smokers have a higher risk than non-smokers of getting influenza, pneumonia and other respiratory conditions such as colds. Influenza and pneumonia can be life-threatening in older people. One woman in four over age 60 develops osteoporosis, a bone-thinning disorder that leads to fractures. There is some evidence that cigarette smoking may increase the risk of developing this disabling condition.

INVOLUNTARY SMOKING

Involuntary smoking (exposure to another's smoke) is a growing concern among non-smokers who are worried about the effects of second-hand tobacco smoke on their health. This should be an especially important concern if the husband or wife of a smoker has asthma, another lung condition or heart disease. In addition, there is increasing evidence that smoke in the home is a particular health hazard for babies and young children.

Involuntary smoking by non-smokers has been linked to a higher incidence of bronchitis, pneumonia, asthma and middle ear infections in children. This is a good reason for a parent or grandparent to consider quitting or to avoid smoking while in the presence of young children and infants. Several studies even suggest that involuntary smoking increases the non-smoker's risk of cancer.

CONSIDERATIONS FOR OLDER ADULTS

At any age there are many reasons to stop smoking. Some of the benefits for older people include:

- Reduced risk of cancer and lung disease.
- Healthier heart and lungs.
- Improved blood circulation.
- Better health for non-smoking family members, particularly children.

Smoking doesn't just cut a few years off the end of each smoker's life: it prematurely kills hundreds of thousands of people and seriously disables millions of others. It's never too late to stop.

WHAT TO DO

There are many ways to stop smoking. No single method works for everyone, so each person must try to find what works best. Most people stop on their own, but others need help from doctors, clinics or organized groups. Some studies have found that older people who take part in programs to stop smoking have higher success rates than younger ones do.

Withdrawal symptoms reported by some people who quit smoking include anxiety, restlessness, drowsiness, difficulty concentrating and digestive problems. Many people have no withdrawal symptoms at all.

When prescribing medication or nicotine gum, many doctors also recommend joining an organized support group or using self-help materials to assist the patient in quitting smoking. Nicotine chewing gum is not recommended for people who have certain forms of heart disease. Denture wearers may find it difficult to chew.

WHO CAN HELP

Your doctor knows your health status and is in the best position to give you recommendations and ideas to stop smoking.

Organizations and clinics offering stop-smoking programs are listed in the phone book under "Smokers' Treatment and Information Centers."

See the Resources and Additional Reading sections for suggestions for further information.

Surgery & Second Opinions

Before you agree to undergo surgery, above all be sure that an operation is necessary and that the benefits outweigh the risks. Most people for whom elective (non-emergency) surgery is recommended are given time to think the matter over and review other options. Deciding whether or not to have an operation is difficult for anyone, but especially for older persons.

CONSIDERATIONS FOR OLDER ADULTS

Normal changes that occur with age and diseases which are more common in later life, particularly heart ailments, may make surgery more risky for older people. Although the following suggestions apply to anyone who is considering surgery, they are particularly important for the elderly.

WHAT TO DO

Begin by seeing your family doctor to find out about your illness and treatment choices. An internist, general practitioner or family practitioner is likely to give equal attention to surgical and non-surgical approaches to treatment. Consult a surgeon once you and your doctor have decided that surgery is a promising method of treatment.

Check the Surgeon's Qualifications

When choosing a surgeon, it is useful to find out if he or she has been certified by a surgical board (such as the American Board of Orthopaedic Surgery or the American Board of Colon and Rectal Surgery). Surgeons who are board-certified have had a number of years of training in dealing with certain diseases and have passed the examinations for their specialties. Don't hesitate to call the doctor's office and ask for this information. Your state or local medical society and the hospital where the surgeon operates should also be able to verify his or her qualifications.

Another way of checking a surgeon's qualifications is to see if he or she is a Fellow of the American College of Surgeons. The letters FACS after the surgeon's name indicate that he or she has passed an evaluation of surgical training and skills as well as ethical fitness.

Try to choose an experienced surgeon who operates on a regular basis (several times a week).

Get a Second Opinion

If time permits, seek the advice of another qualified doctor. Getting a second opinion is a common medical practice that most doctors encourage. Don't be afraid to tell your surgeon that you want another opinion and would like your medical records forwarded to the second doctor. This can save time, money and possible discomfort since tests you have already had may not need to be repeated if the second doctor has the results.

Ask the Right Questions

Before undergoing a surgical procedure, you will be asked to sign a statement giving consent for the operation. It is important that you discuss all of your concerns about your condition and the operation with your surgeon before you sign this statement. In most cases, the surgeon will volunteer a great deal of information, but don't hesitate to ask any questions you still have. The following list might be helpful:

- What are the chances of survival without the operation?
- What are the chances of survival with the operation?
- Are there other forms of treatment that could be tried before surgery?
- What are the risks of surgery?
- How long will the recovery period be, and what is involved?
- How much will the operation cost? Will my insurance cover all of the costs, including special tests?
- Who will administer the anesthesia? Has the doctor or nurse-anesthetist had experience treating older persons?

WHO CAN HELP

To find a specialist in your area who can give you a second opinion, ask your doctor or call the government's toll-free number, (800) 638-6833. In Maryland, call (800) 492-6603.

See the Resources and Additional Reading sections for suggestions for further information.

Terminal Illness & Hospice Care

Death may not be unwelcome to someone with a long-term illness that he or she knows is terminal. The person can recognize that death means the end of a full life and the end to any pain and suffering. The person who is dying needs care, but not necessarily the acute type of care provided in hospitals. The patient and the family have emotional, psychological and physical needs still to be met.

The hospice movement grew out of these needs by finding ways to help people cope with dying in a more humane manner. The hospice goal is to keep the dying person free of pain and, at the same time, to provide the family and loved ones with emotional support.

Hospice care may be given in the patient's home, or the hospice may have its own special wing in a hospital or its own separate facility.

The hospice services provided at the patient's home can include the services of a visiting nurse, a social worker and other staff personnel. They will help in providing or finding special equipment that may be needed, such as oxygen and feeding tubes.

CONSIDERATIONS FOR OLDER ADULTS

Aging brings more likelihood of developing certain types of cancers and other terminal illnesses.

Suffering and pain can usually be alleviated more readily in a hospice environment than in a hospital setting.

Family members will know that the patient is as comfortable as possible and will be allowed to die with dignity.

The dying patient is often concerned about being a burden to the family, about the welfare of his or her spouse and about experiencing a painful death. Hospice care can help alleviate these concerns.

WHAT TO DO

The patient, along with his or her spouse, family members and personal doctor, can together decide if regular hospital care, a nursing home or hospice care will be best.

Insurance coverage may influence the decision. Medicare may cover only a portion of hospice care, and the hospice needs to be Medicare-certified.

WHO CAN HELP

A hospital-based social worker or discharge planner is a good source of information and referral.

Hospices may be listed in your local telephone directory.

Contact the local chapter of The American Cancer Society for help and guidance.

Check your local library for books on dying and hospice care.

Travel & Health

Travel may consist of a short weekend trip or a journey of several months to foreign countries. It can bring great joy for many people, but it can quickly turn into a nightmare if an unexpected illness or other health problem happens to you or a traveling companion. Chronic health problems, disabilities or other aspects of aging should not deter you from enjoying the benefits of travel. Preparation and prevention can help prevent some health problems and lessen the impact of others.

CONSIDERATIONS FOR OLDER ADULTS

Susceptibility to infections increases with aging. Traveling often involves being in crowded places, such as airports, where infectious people abound.

Older adults have an increased sensitivity to environmental factors (altitude, heat and cold).

There are more pronounced symptoms of jet lag, such as fatigue, lack of appetite, headaches, irritability or upset stomach.

Any chronic medical problem you have may worsen. Qualified medical help may not always be readily available.

WHAT TO DO

Know the physical demands involved in making the trip and get yourself in as good shape as possible before you go.

Have a medical and dental check before you embark on a lengthy trip within the U.S. and prior to any foreign travel. Discuss the trip with your doctor and together decide on any special needs you may have. Recommended immunizations and any additional ones required for your trip should be current.

Carry a supply of prescription medicines to last the entire trip. Don't pack the whole supply. Keep some on your person or carry them in a purse, camera bag or briefcase. Always keep medicines in their original prescription containers (this is particularly important for foreign travel). Carry written prescriptions, too. This will help you obtain more if you need it and will sometimes help you get through customs in some countries.

Medicare will not cover medical expenses outside the U.S. Check other insurance you have to see if it does, and if not purchase special travel insurance.

If you are traveling to a non-English-speaking country, get the names of doctors there who do speak English.

Plan your schedule so that you will have time to recover from jet lag symptoms.

Follow all food and water safety guidelines for the areas you visit.

Have a personal medical kit with you. Include aspirin or acetaminophen, diarrhea medicine, motion sickness pills, sunscreen, insect repellent, bandages, antiseptic sprays or ointments, cotton balls and other items that you think might be useful. If you have a special health problem or allergy, wear or carry a Medic Alert information tag.

WHO CAN HELP

Get a copy of the brochure titled *Health Information for International Travel*, which is published by the U.S. government. Write the Government Printing Office, Washington, DC 20402. The cost is $5.00.

For information about English-speaking doctors in foreign countries, write to the International Association for Medical Assistance to Travelers (IAMAT), 736 Center St., Lewiston, NY, 20402. A small donation may be required.

The American Association of Retired Persons (AARP) has various publications available concerning travel. Write that organization at 1909 K St. NW, Washington, DC 20049.

The federal government has a variety of publications available about travel. Write to the Consumer Information Center, P.O. Box 100, Pueblo, CO 81002, for a current catalog.

Your local or state health department is a good source of information. If you will be traveling within the U.S., consider contacting the health department at your destination for specific information about the location.

For current information about health problems and immunization requirements in foreign countries, call the Centers for Disease Control (CDC) at (404) 332-4555 for recorded messages.

GLOSSARY

A

Abdominal Aorta—Section of the aorta that passes through the abdomen to supply blood to the lower part of the body.

Abscess—Swollen, inflamed, tender area of infection containing pus.

Accident Proneness—Tendency of some persons to have more accidents than normal. It may be due to a risk factor such as poor vision, but unconscious factors are often the cause.

Acetaminophen—Non-prescription medication used to relieve minor pain and to reduce fever. Its analgesic effects are similar to those of aspirin, but it does not reduce inflammation or swelling. It is less irritating to the stomach than aspirin.

Achalasia—Condition of the esophagus that disrupts normal swallowing.

Acupuncture—Method of anesthesia and treatment of pain developed by the Chinese. Needles are inserted through the skin to stimulate precise areas.

Acute—Beginning suddenly; also severe, but of short duration.

Addiction—Intense craving for substances such as alcohol, tobacco or narcotics or a compulsive behavior such as gambling.

Adenoids—Infection-fighting tissue (part of the lymphatic system) in the upper throat near the tonsils.

Adenoids, Enlarged—Adenoids that have swollen and impaired speech.

Adenovirus—Group of viruses that cause certain respiratory and eye infections.

Adhesions—Small strands of fibrous tissue that cause organs in the abdomen and pelvis to cling together abnormally, creating a risk of intestinal obstruction.

Adrenal Glands—Two glands attached to the kidneys. Each has an outer layer (cortex) that produces steroid hormones and an inner layer (medulla) that produces adrenalin.

Adrenalin—Hormone produced by the adrenal glands that increases heart rate and prepares the body for crisis. Also called epinephrine.

Aging—The process or the effects of growing mature or older.

Airways—Tubular passages that air passes through to the lungs: the trachea (windpipe), bronchi and bronchioles.

Allergy—A hypersensitive state caused by exposure to an allergen (an allergy-producing substance of any sort—chemical or physical). Allergic reactions may be immediate or delayed. The most common allergies include asthma, hay fever (seasonal rhinitis), allergic conjunctivitis, allergic sinusitis, skin allergies (atopy), food allergies (milk, strawberries or eggs) and drug allergies. Heredity seems to play a part in developing allergies.

Allergy Skin Test—Test in which small amounts of allergens are placed on the skin in a patch test or introduced just below the skin or into the skin with a needle. Redness, swelling and itching at the site of the test represents sensitivity to that allergen.

Alveoli—Lung cells at the ends of the airways where oxygen enters the blood and waste gases leave the blood.

Ambulatory Medical Center—A health-care facility for patients who do not require prolonged bed rest or hospitalization.

Amphetamine Drugs—Habit-forming drugs that stimulate the brain and central nervous system, increase blood pressure, reduce nasal stuffiness or suppress appetite.

Amyloid Deposits—Abnormal protein material deposited in tissues, usually caused by diseases. These deposits cause impairment of certain organs.

Analgesics—Medications that relieve pain.

Anemia—Condition in which red blood cells or hemoglobin (the oxygen-carrying substance in the blood) is inadequate.

Anesthesia, General—Inhaled gases or injected anesthetics that cause temporary loss of consciousness and inability to feel pain.

Anesthesia, Local—Injected medication that temporarily prevents pain.

Anesthesia, Local (Nerve Block)—Local anesthetic injected near the nerves of the surgical area.

Aneurysm—Abnormal swelling or ballooning of a blood vessel.

Angina—Pain or pressure beneath the breastbone caused by inadequate blood supply to the heart.

Angiogram, Angiography—Study of arteries and veins by injecting material into them that x-rays can outline.

Anoscopy—Visual examination of the anus by means of a short tube called an anoscope, an optical instrument with lenses and a lighted tip.

Antacid—Medicine taken orally that reduces or neutralizes stomach acid.

Antiarrhythmics—Medications used to treat heartbeat irregularities (arrhythmias).

Antibiotics—Medications that attack germs and fight infection.

Antibiotics, Cephalosporin—Class of antibiotics related to penicillin that is capable of destroying more kinds of germs than penicillin.

Antibiotics, Erythromycin—Class of antibiotics that destroys germs similar to those destroyed by penicillin. Often used to treat infections in patients who are allergic to penicillin.

Antibodies—Proteins created in blood and body tissue by the immune system to neutralize or destroy sources of disease.

Anticancer Drugs—Medications that weaken or destroy cancerous tissues without harming healthy tissues.

Anticholinergic Drugs—Medications that reduce nerve impulses in the parasympathetic nervous system. They control some activities of the gastrointestinal system, heart, bladder and other organs.

Anticoagulants—Medications that slow or delay blood clotting.

Anticonvulsants—Medications that control seizures (convulsions), pain or conditions in which the brain or nerves are overly sensitive.

Antidepressants—Medications that help control depression.

Antiemetic Drugs—Medications that prevent or stop nausea and vomiting.

Antifungal Drugs—Medications used to treat fungus diseases.

Antigens—Germs or other sources of disease that antibodies (produced by the immune system) neutralize or destroy.

Antihelminthic or Anthelmintic Drugs—Medications used to treat worms in the intestines.

Antihistamines—Medications used to treat allergies.

Antihyperlipidemic Drugs—Medications that reduce fat (cholesterol) in the blood. They help prevent blood vessel disease.

Antihypertensives—Medications used to reduce blood pressure.

Anti-Inflammatory Drugs—Medications used to control inflammation not caused by infection.

Antimalarial Drugs—Medications used to prevent or treat malaria.

Antimetabolite Drugs—Medications used to treat some cancers and autoimmune diseases.

Antimicrobial Drugs—See Antibiotics.

Antinuclear Antibody—Substance that appears in the blood, indicating the presence of an autoimmune disease.

Antiparkinsonian Drugs—Medications used to treat Parkinson's disease.

Antiprotozoal Drugs—Medications used to treat infestations of single-celled parasites (protozoa).

Antipruritic Drugs—Medications that reduce itching.

Antispasmodic Drugs—Medications that improve digestion and relieve intestinal cramps.

Antistreptococcal Titer—Blood test that measures the body's response to infection by streptococcal bacteria.

Antithyroid Drugs—Medications used to counter the effects of an overactive thyroid gland.

Antiviral Drugs—Medications used to treat infections caused by viruses.

Anus—A muscular band at the end of the rectum that opens and expands to allow the passage of feces.

Anxiety—Uncomfortable feeling that something unpleasant or dangerous will happen.

Aorta—The body's largest blood vessel, arising from the top of the heart. It carries blood from the heart to all parts of the body.

Aphrodisiac—Substance claimed to increase sexual arousal or pleasure.

Appendage—Body part that has a minor role (or no role at all) in normal body function. For example, the appendix is an appendage to the colon that seems to have no function.

Arteriogram, Arteriography—Study of arteries by injecting material into them that x-rays can outline.

Artery—Blood vessel that carries blood from the heart to the body.

Arthrograms—X-rays of the joints taken with an arthroscope.

Arthroscope—Slender optical instrument with a lighted tip that allows direct visual examination of some joints. It can also be used to correct some defects in joints.

Artificial Limbs—Mechanical substitutions for amputated arms or legs.

Ascending Colon—First part of the large colon (intestine) extending from the lower end of the small intestine.

Aspiration—1) Removal of accumulated pus or fluid with a needle. 2) Accidental inhalation of objects or fluids into the lungs.

Astigmatism—Visual impairment caused by abnormal eye shape.

Asymmetrical—Uneven in size, shape or position.

Atria—Small chambers in the heart that pump blood into the ventricles. Also called auricles.

Atropine—Medication used to treat diseases of the eye, heart, gastrointestinal system and nervous system.

Audiogram, Audiometry—Test of hearing ability.

Autoantibody—An antibody which unexplainably acts against the cells and tissues of one's own body. The disease produced by a reaction to an autoantibody is termed hypersensitivity. Included in this category are rheumatoid arthritis, insulin-dependent diabetes mellitus and lupus erythematosus.

Autoimmune Disorder, Autoimmunity—Disease in which a person's immune system attacks its own tissues.

Autoimmune Assays (ANA Tests)—Blood tests to identify autoimmune disease.

Autonomic Nervous System—Part of the nervous system that controls organs that function involuntarily, such as the heart, lungs, digestive system and blood vessels.

B

Bacteria—One-celled micro-organisms that can sometimes cause disease.

Balloon Angioplasty—Treatment for obstructed arteries, especially those supplying blood to the heart and brain. A small uninflated balloon is passed up the artery to the obstruction and then expanded to release the obstruction.

Barium Enema X-Rays—Examination of the colon by filling it with a barium solution that is detected by x-rays.

Bartholin's Glands—Small glands in the lips of the vagina that secrete a lubricating fluid, especially during sexual arousal.

Belladonna—Medication derived from a plant used to treat some diseases of the gastrointestinal system. It is similar to atropine.

Benign—1) Tumor or growth that is neither cancerous nor located where it might impair normal function. 2) Harmless.

Beta-Adrenergic Blockers (Beta Blockers)—Medications that reduce heart or blood vessel overactivity to improve blood circulation. Also used to prevent migraine headaches, high blood pressure and angina.

Bile—A digestive juice produced in the liver and stored in the gallbladder. Bile empties into the small intestine for digestive processes.

Bile Duct—A small tube that allows bile to pass from the gallbladder into the intestines.

Bilirubin—A yellowish, red blood cell waste product in bile that the blood carries to the liver. It contributes to urine's yellowish color and can cause jaundice if it builds up in the blood.

Biofeedback—The process of providing visual or auditory evidence to a person of the status of various body functions that are not usually considered to be under voluntary control. Example: The sounding of a tone when blood pressure is at a desirable level so that one may exert control over the function.

Biopsy—Removal of a small amount of tissue or fluid for laboratory examination that aids in diagnosis.

Biopsy Needle—Instrument often used to perform a biopsy.

Bladder—An organ that holds fluids such as urine (urinary bladder) or bile (gallbladder).

Blood Cells, Red—Microscopic cells in the blood that carry oxygen to tissues of the body. One drop of blood contains about 200 million red cells.

Blood Cells, White—Microscopic cells in the blood that help fight infection by destroying germs. One drop of blood contains about 400,000 white cells.

Blood Chemistries—Tests that measure chemicals in the blood.

Blood Count—A count of red and white blood cells to aid in diagnosis of many diseases.

Blood Platelets—See Platelet Count.

Blood Studies—Examination of a blood sample to measure white blood cells, red blood cells, hemoglobin, hematocrit and chemical substances. See Blood Chemistries.

Blood Vessels—Arteries, veins and capillaries; the tubes in which blood circulates through the body.

Bone Bank—Facility where human bone is stored and made available for transplantation.

Bone Spurs—Abnormal and sometimes painful protrusions of bone with sharp points near joints or tendons.

Bronchial Tubes (Bronchi)—Hollow air passageways that branch from the windpipe (trachea) into the lungs. They carry oxygen into the lungs and pass waste gases (mostly carbon dioxide) out of the body.

Bronchioles—Small air passageways that serve the same purpose as bronchial tubes. Bronchioles are the smallest parts of the respiratory system.

Bronchodilator Drugs—Medications used to treat diseases of the bronchi that cause shortness of breath, such as asthma. The medicines help constricted tubes to relax.

Bronchogram—A test to diagnose lung diseases by placing a material in the lung that x-rays can outline.

Bronchoscope—An optical instrument with a lighted tip that is passed into the windpipe, then into the bronchi.

Bronchoscopy—A test using a bronchoscope to study the bronchial tubes and allow the withdrawal of material from the bronchial tubes for diagnosis.

Bruising—Discoloration under the skin caused by injury or bleeding.

C

Caffeine Intoxication—A clinical syndrome brought on by ingesting caffeine that is characterized by any of the following symptoms: panic attacks; chronic nervousness and irritability; digestive disturbances including heartburn; indigestion and ulcers; migraine-like headache attacks; decreased blood sugar; increased blood pressure.

Calcification—A process in which calcium from the blood is deposited abnormally into tissues due to injury, infection or aging. Often it is part of healing and not a sign of active disease.

Calcium Channel Blocker Drugs—Medications used to treat angina, hypertension and heartbeat irregularities.

Cancerous Growths—Extensions of cancerous tissues that invade nearby healthy tissues.

Cancers—Destructive tumors that can arise in almost all parts of the body. Cancer can destroy nearby healthy tissue and may spread to distant organs.

Capillaries—Microscopic vessels that supply all body cells and tissues with blood.

Carbohydrates, Complex—Starches, sugars, cellulose and gums. Complex carbohydrates are those contained in whole grains, fresh fruits and fresh vegetables. These are considered more nutritious than simple carbohydrates.

Carbohydrates, Simple—Refined carbohydrates (sugars) that have lower molecular weights than complex carbohydrates. They produce a quick rise in blood sugar levels. Most nutrition counselors recommend that daily diets contain minimal amounts of refined sugars. So-called "junk foods" are frequently very high in simple carbohydrates.

Cardiac Catheter—A slender tube that is inserted into an artery or vein and then passed into the heart. It is used to examine the heart and nearby blood vessels by injecting material into the heart that x-rays can detect.

Cardiac Catheterization—Studying heart function with a cardiac catheter.

Cardiac Monitoring—A special procedure in which a patient is connected to electronic sensors that transmit signals to an observation station. By this method a trained observer can detect life-threatening changes in the electric system of the heart.

Cardiopulmonary Resuscitation (CPR)—Emergency treatment for a patient whose heart has stopped (cardiac arrest).

Cardiovascular—Relating to the heart and blood vessels.

Cardiovascular Surgeon—Doctor specially trained to operate on the heart and blood vessels.

Cardiovascular System—System that supplies the body with blood. It consists of the heart and blood vessels (arteries, capillaries and veins).

Carotid Arteries—Large arteries that supply much of the blood to the brain.

Cartilage—Rubbery, dense connective tissue that permits smooth movement of joints. It also helps shape flexible parts of the nose and external ear.

Caruncle—Small, red protrusion of tissue near a body opening. The most common caruncles arise from the urethra or cervix.

CAT (or CT) Scan (Computerized Axial Tomography)—A computerized x-ray procedure that provides exceptionally clear images of parts of the body. It aids in the diagnosis of diseases that cannot be diagnosed by ordinary x-ray methods.

Catheter—A hollow tube used to introduce fluids into the body or to drain fluids away.

Catheterization—The insertion of a hollow tube into a body cavity for the purpose of introducing fluid or removing fluid. The most common use for a catheter is to be passed into the bladder to remove urine.

Caudal Anesthesia—Form of local (low spinal) anesthesia used to reduce pain during surgery on pelvic areas. Also called "saddle block" anesthesia.

Cauterant—Chemical used to destroy abnormal or diseased cells on the skin.

Cautery—Destroying small areas of diseased tissue by burning with an electric needle or laser beam, freezing with low-temperature instruments or using a chemical that destroys tissue.

Cecum—The part of the intestinal tract at the beginning of the large colon (intestine).

Central Nervous System—System that controls the body's voluntary acts. It consists of the brain and spinal cord.

Cervical Spine—Bones in the neck at the top of the spinal column.

Cervix—Lower third of the uterus, which protrudes into the vagina.

Chancre—Hard, slightly ulcerated, painless lesion that forms where syphilis enters the body, usually on the genital lips or penis.

Chemocautery—Destruction of abnormal tissue by means of acids, caustics or poisons.

Chemotherapy—Treatment of cancer by injecting medications that kill cancer cells without harming healthy tissue. It is used to treat cancers that cannot be completely cured or treated with surgery or radiation.

Chiggers—Small red biting insects. Also called "red bugs."

Chiropractor—Practitioner of the chiropractic treatment of disease, which involves massage and manipulations that chiropractors claim restore normal body functions.

Chokes—Severe breathing difficulties experienced by scuba divers and others who go from high to normal air pressure too rapidly. Bubbles of nitrogen develop in the blood stream and obstruct blood supply to vital organs, sometimes resulting in severe injury or death.

Cholangiogram, Cholangiography—X-ray procedure to diagnose diseases of the bile system (liver, gallbladder and bile ducts). Special medications are used to make the bile system visible on x-rays.

Cholera—Acute, severe, infectious disease causing extreme diarrhea and dehydration.

Choroiditis—Inflammation of the part of the eye that supports the retina and supplies blood to it.

Chromosomes—Structures inside the nucleus of living cells which contain hereditary information. Defects in chromosomes cause many birth defects and inherited diseases.

Chronic—Long-term; continuing. Chronic illnesses are usually not curable, but they can often be prevented from worsening. Symptoms usually can be controlled.

Cinematography—Form of motion-picture photography used to record a fast-moving series of x-ray images.

Circulatory System—System that provides blood to the body, consisting of the heart, arteries, veins and lymphatic system.

Clinician—Health-care professional who has direct contact with patients. The word literally means "someone who is at the patient's bedside."

Clips—See Skin Clips.

Clot Retraction Test—Measurement of the time necessary for a tube of blood to form a clot. Abnormal results often indicate a defect in blood platelets, cells important in blood coagulation.

Clotting—Activity of the blood and blood vessels that cause blood to form a jellylike clot, usually near an injury. Clotting helps stop bleeding. The body's clotting mechanism is slowed or reduced ("thinning the blood") with anticoagulants to treat certain diseases.

Coagulation—See Clotting.

Cocaine—Medication applied directly to mucous membranes to control pain in the nose and throat. Used illegally as a mind-altering drug, it is addicting and dangerous.

Colic, Colicky—A pain that recurs in a regular pattern every few seconds or minutes.

Collagen—A gelatinous protein from which body tissues are formed.

Colon—The last major portion of the gastrointestinal tract, where waste material is formed into feces and held for elimination. It is also known as the large intestine.

Colonoscopy—Method of diagnosing diseases of the colon by visual examination of the inside of the colon through a flexible colonoscope, a fiber optic instrument with a lighted tip.

Color Blindness—Inability to recognize red and green, which appear to be gray. It is usually hereditary.

Colposcopy—Visual examination of the cervix by means of a colposcope, a slender optical instrument with a lighted tip.

Complication—Undesirable event during disease or treatment that causes further symptoms and delay in recovery.

Compress—A cloth, sometimes soaked in warm water or coated with medication. It is applied to the skin to relieve discomfort.

Compression—Application of pressure to the surface of the body, usually to stop bleeding.

Compulsion, Compulsive—Intense, irrational urge to perform some action.

Condom—A thin sheath, usually of rubber, applied to the penis before sexual intercourse. It is used to prevent disease of the genitals and as a contraceptive.

Congenital Defect—Abnormality of the body that is present at birth. Congenital defects may be inherited or caused by conditions occurring while the fetus grows in the uterus.

Conization of the Cervix—Removal of a cone of tissue from the cervix. Laboratory examination of the removed tissue identifies possible cancer.

Conjunctiva—The mucous membrane lining the outermost surface of the eye ("white of the eye").

Connective Tissue—Body's supporting framework of tissue consisting of strands of collagen, elastic fibers and simple cells.

Contact Lenses—Small plastic lenses worn on the eyes to correct nearsightedness, farsightedness or astigmatism.

Contagious—Disease or condition that spreads from one person to another.

Convalescence—Recovery from an illness or surgery.

COPD (Chronic Obstructive Pulmonary Disease)—Several usually incurable lung diseases associated with gradually increasing breathing difficulty.

Copious—Large in amount.

Cornea—Clear thickened surface of the eye through which light passes. It has no blood supply and can be transplanted without danger of rejection.

Coronary—Referring to the blood vessels supplying the heart. Sometimes it refers to a heart attack resulting from coronary artery obstruction.

Coronary Care Unit (CCU)—Area of a hospital equipped to care for patients who have suffered heart attacks or other life-threatening heart conditions.

Cortisone Drugs—Medications similar to natural hormones produced by the central core of the adrenal glands.

Cosmetic Surgery—Surgery to improve appearance.

Coxsackie Viruses—Group of viruses causing infections such as poliomyelitis, aseptic meningitis, herpangina and myocarditis.

CPR—See Cardiopulmonary Resuscitation.

Cranium—Bones that make up the skull.

Creatinine—A chemical substance made in the human body that is cleared through urine excretion from the kidney when the kidney function is normal.

Cryosurgery—Destruction of abnormal tissue by applying freezing temperatures, usually with liquid nitrogen.

Cryotherapy—The use of cold (below -200F) temperatures in treatment.

CT Scan—See CAT Scan.

Culdocentesis—Piercing of the space deep in the vagina under the cervix to obtain fluid. Laboratory examination of the removed fluid aids in diagnosis of pelvic disorders.

Culdoscopy—Visual examination of the female pelvic organs by means of a slender instrument brought into the pelvic cavity by penetrating through the space deep in the vagina under the cervix.

Culture—Identification of bacteria, fungi and viruses. Material (pus, blood or urine) from an infected area is collected, placed on nutrient material and kept warm (usually in an incubator) until the infecting agent has grown. The resulting growth is examined with a microscope.

Curettage—Scraping process frequently used to obtain tissue from the lining of the uterus for laboratory examination. Laboratory examination of the removed tissue aids in diagnosis.

Curette—Instrument with a sharp end used to scrape tissue from the inner lining of the uterus and to scrape away skin lesions.

Cyst—Sac or cavity filled with fluid or diseased matter.

Cyst Aspiration—Removal of cyst contents for examination or drainage for relief of symptoms.

Cystoscopy—Visual examination of the inside of the urinary bladder by means of a cystoscope, a slender optical instrument with a lighted tip.

Cytomegalovirus (CMV)—A form of herpes virus that can infect man and other mammals. The infection causes the production of large cells which have strange matter included in their nuclei.

Cytotoxic Drugs—Medications used to destroy cancerous cells with minimal harm to healthy cells.

D

DC Cardioversion—A procedure using DC electrical current to convert abnormal heart rhythms back to normal rhythms. The procedure requires special equipment and experienced operators to perform it safely. The procedure is usually performed in emergency situations during heart attacks or in a hospital environment where the patient can be safely anesthetized for a very short period of time.

D&C (Dilatation and Curettage)—A surgical procedure in which the cervix is dilated and the inner lining of the womb is scraped with a curette to remove tissue.

Debilitating—Causing a general weakening or deterioration in health.

Defibrillation, Cardiac—Application of an electric current to the chest over the heart to interrupt fibrillation, a disturbance of heartbeat.

Dehydration—Loss of essential fluids from the tissues and blood of the body.

Dependence—Condition in which a person requires substances such as narcotics or alcohol to remain comfortable. If the substances are not used, withdrawal symptoms develop.

Dermatome—Area of the skin to which feeling (sensation) is provided by a nerve to the spinal cord.

Descending Colon—The part of the colon in the left side of the abdomen that stores feces until they are passed from the body.

Diabetic Retinopathy—Degeneration of the retina that develops in patients with diabetes mellitus. It may cause vision impairment or blindness.

Diagnosis—Identification of disease. A complete diagnosis names the part of the body affected, the disease process (such as inflammation, cancer or allergy) and the cause of disease.

Dialysis—Removal of natural wastes from the bloodstream. It is used to treat patients with kidney failure.

Diaphragm—Thin, broad sheet of muscle separating the chest cavity from the abdominal cavity.

Diathermy—Treatment in which mild heat is generated within the body by high-frequency radio waves.

Digestive System—Organs in which food is processed for absorption into the blood stream. The major digestive organs are the mouth, esophagus, stomach, duodenum, small bowel (small intestine), colon (large intestine) and rectum. The liver, gallbladder and pancreas are also considered parts of the digestive system.

Digitalis—A drug used to treat congestive heart failure and some other heart diseases.

Dilate, Dilatation—To widen, expand or open up.

Dilatation and Curettage—See D&C.

Dilator—Instrument used to widen organs that have narrowed because of disease.

Discomfort—Unpleasant physical or mental sensation.

Disease—Adverse change in health; sickness or ailment. A disease can be defined by the body part involved (for example, the heart or liver), by the abnormality present (cancer, infection, allergy, degeneration, etc.) or by its cause (bacteria, poisons, injury, etc.).

Disk—See Intervertebral Disk.

Disorder—See Disease.

Diuretics—Medications that force the kidneys to excrete more urine, sodium and potassium than normal, which helps eliminate excessive body fluid.

Diverticulum—Small pouch or sac that develops in the wall of tubular organs such as the esophagus or colon.

Dizziness—Sensation of faintness, lightheadedness or spinning (vertigo).

Donor—Person who gives to someone else. In transplantation surgery, the donor gives up an organ (such as a kidney) to be transplanted into the recipient.

Doppler Sonography—See Sonogram; this is one of several methods of sonography.

Dormant—Sleeping or inactive state of living things. Also an inactive state of a disease.

Drainage—Passage of fluids out of the body through an opening or incision.

Duodenum—First 12 inches of the small intestine.

Dupuytren's Contracture—Chronic condition in which scar tissue forms in the palms. In severe cases, it can impair use of the fingers.

Dysphagia—Difficulty in swallowing. Causes include stroke, Parkinson's and other neurological diseases, tumors in the throat and larynx, bony spurs in the spine, weak esophagus muscles and achalasia (failure of smooth muscle fibers to relax). Treatment consists of dilating the esophagus with an inflatable bulb or the use of drugs (smooth muscle-relaxing drugs) to dispel the spasm of the lower part of the esophagus.

E

Ear Canal—Passageway extending from the outer ear inward to the eardrum.

Ear, Nose and Throat (ENT) Specialist—A physician specially trained to treat diseases of the ears, nose and throat.

ECG (Electrocardiography)—Method of diagnosing heart diseases by measuring electrical activity of the heart with an electrocardiograph. The record produced is called an electrocardiogram.

Echocardiogram, Echocardiography—Study of the heart by examining sound waves created by an instrument placed on the chest. The waves reflected from the heart form an image (echocardiogram) on a monitor, aiding in the diagnosis of heart diseases.

Echography—Any test that uses ultrasound waves to study human disease.

Edema—Accumulation of fluid under the skin, in the lungs or elsewhere.

EEG (Electroencephalography)—Studying the brain by measuring electric activity ("brain waves") with an electroencephalograph. The record produced is the electroencephalogram.

EKG—See ECG.

Electrocardiogram, Electrocardiography—See ECG.

Electrocautery—Destruction of tissue by heat applied with a controlled electric current.

Electroconvulsive Therapy (ECT)—A therapeutic maneuver in which an electric shock is used to induce a seizure in an attempt to treat psychiatric illness. Muscle-relaxing drugs are used to prevent injury to muscles and bones prior to the shock. This form of treatment is used almost exclusively for severe depression.

Electroencephalogram, Electroencephalography—See EEG.

Electrolyte—A chemical that is dissolved in the blood and all other body fluids. Electrolytes play an essential role in all body functions. The major electrolytes are sodium, potassium, chloride, calcium, phosphorus, magnesium and carbon dioxide. Electrolytes come from food. They are regulated mostly by the kidneys and lungs.

Electrolyte Measurement—Laboratory test on blood or urine to identify and measure the electrolytes present.

Electrolyte Supplements—Electrolytes taken to correct or to prevent body fluid or electrolyte imbalance.

Electromyography, Electromyogram—Study of nerve and muscle disorders by recording electrical activity of muscles with an electromyograph. The record produced is the electromyogram.

Endemic—Disease that is constantly present in a community or group of people. Endemic disease may affect only a few people at any one time.

Endocrine System—System of organs that secrete hormones into the blood to regulate basic functions of cells and tissues. The endocrine organs are the anterior and posterior pituitary glands, thyroid and parathyroid glands, pancreas, adrenal glands, ovaries (in women) and testicles (in men).

Endocrinologist—Doctor specially trained in diagnosis and treatment of endocrine disorders.

Endoscopy—Method of diagnosing diseases in hollow organs. An endoscope (an optical instrument with a lighted tip) is inserted into the organ, which allows visual examination of the cavity. Used in the abdomen, pelvis, lumen of the bronchial tubes, or intestines.

Endotracheal Tube—Tube temporarily placed in the trachea (windpipe) of patients who are unable to breathe normally because of disease or surgery.

Enteric—Relating to the small intestine. Enteric-coated medicine is coated with a hard shell that dissolves when it reaches the small intestine.

Enterostomy—Surgically created artificial opening for elimination of feces. An enterostomy nurse or enterostomy specialist is a professional who teaches patients how to care for the artificial opening.

Enzymes—Proteins manufactured by the body that regulate the rate of essential life processes (metabolism).

Epinephrine—See Adrenalin.

Episcleritis—Inflammation of tissues on the sclera (the white of the eye).

Epithelial Horn—Thick, rough lesion protruding from the skin. It may become cancerous if not removed.

Epstein-Barr Virus Infection—A group of chronic symptoms including malaise, chronic fatigue, slight elevation of body temperature and other non-specific symptoms. This diagnosis is usually made only after excluding other illnesses that can be determined with diagnostic laboratory tests. There is no specific treatment. Antiviral drugs don't help. Epstein-Barr virus is the causative agent for infectious mononucleosis—an entirely different disease.

Equine Virus—Virus that causes a serious form of encephalitis in horses and man.

Ergot—Medication derived from a fungus that grows on rye plant. It is used to treat migraine headache.

Esophageal Varices—Enlarged veins on the lining of the esophagus. They are subject to severe bleeding and often appear in patients with severe liver disease.

Esophagoscopy—Method of diagnosing diseases of the esophagus by means of an esophagoscope, an optical instrument with lenses and a lighted tip.

Esophagus—Muscular tube connecting the throat and stomach.

Estrogen—Female sex hormone, primarily secreted by the ovaries. It can also be produced synthetically for use in estrogen replacement therapy.

Estrogen Receptor Value—Used in the study of breast cancer cells to determine the best treatment.

Etiology—Cause or causes of a disease.

Eustachian Tubes—Slender passages between the throat and the middle ear that maintain normal air pressure in the middle ear.

Exercise, Passive—Exercise in which someone other than the patient moves muscle groups through their range of motion. The patient exerts no effort or energy.

Excise—To remove by cutting out.

Exploratory Laparotomy—Means of diagnosing abdominal disease by surgically opening the abdomen and examining its contents.

Extremities—Arms and legs.

Eye Bank—Facility where living corneas are stored and made available for transplantation.

F

Fallopian Tubes—Organs of the female reproductive tract through which an egg (ovum) passes from the ovary to the uterus. Tying these tubes (tubal ligation) accomplishes sterility.

Familial Polyposis—Inherited condition in which the lining of the intestines contains many polyps, some of which may become cancerous.

Family History—Information about illnesses that tend to occur within a family. This information is used to determine the likelihood of diseases occurring in other members of the family.

Farsightedness—See Hypermetropia.

Fascia—Sheet or band of tough, fibrous tissue that covers muscles and other body organs.

Fecal—Relating to feces, waste products eliminated through the lower intestinal tract.

Fecal-Oral—Pathway by which some fecal germs gain entry into the bloodstream. Sewage in drinking water, hand-to-mouth transmission after bowel movements or sexual contact can cause infection.

Feces—Body waste formed of undigested food that has passed through the gastro-intestinal system to the colon. Feces are produced and stored in the colon until they are eliminated.

Fever—Above-normal body temperature. Normal mouth temperature is 98.6F (37C). Normal rectal temperature is 99.6F (37.6C).

Fiber—A non-nutritious ingredient of many complex carbohydrates. Fiber increases bulk in the diet. Many nutritionists recommend including ample fiber in the diet. Experimental studies and clinical studies show that people who eat high-fiber diets are less likely to develop colon cancer, diverticulitis, atherosclerosis and gallbladder disease.

Fiber Optics—System of transmitting light and images through thread-like strands of glass. Fiber optic instruments make some examinations and surgical procedures simple, safe and effective.

Fibrin—Protein formed by the action of blood clotting on fibrinogen.

Fibrinogen—Protein in the blood needed for blood clotting.

Fibrositis—Inflammatory conditions affecting connective tissue of muscles, joints, ligaments and tendons.

First Molars—First permanent flat teeth used for grinding food, which appear at about age 6 to 7.

Fissure—Break in the skin or inner lining of organs.

Fistula—Abnormal passage between two organs or between the body and the outside.

Flank—Area on the side of the body below the ribs and above the hip.

Fleas—Tiny biting insects. Most cause minor skin irritation; some carry and transmit serious diseases such as plague and typhus.

Fluorescein Dye Test—Method of diagnosis using fluorescein, a dye, to study tissues and germs. When these dyed tissues are exposed to ultraviolet light, they glow. Substances to which the dye does not cling do not glow.

Fluorescent Antibody Studies—Tests used to study some allergic and infectious conditions. When antibodies created by these conditions are present in the blood, they can be made to glow by using a dye and a microscope with ultraviolet light.

Fluoroscopy—Method of x-ray diagnosis in which moving organs (such as the heart or intestinal tract) can be studied in action.

Foley Catheter—Slender, flexible tube used to drain urine from the bladders of patients who are unable to urinate normally.

Forceps—Instrument with two blades and handles. It is used to grasp tissue, body parts or sterile materials. Also used to deliver babies when progress of labor is slow.

Fracture—Break; usually used to refer to a bone or tooth.

Frei Test—Test used to make a precise diagnosis of lymphogranuloma, a sexually transmitted disease.

Friedreich's Ataxia—Rare, inherited nervous system disease that causes loss of balance and coordination, awkward walking, speech difficulty and tremors.

Frozen Section—A study in a pathology laboratory of fresh tissue that was removed during surgery. The purpose is to determine if a suspicious area is or is not cancerous.

Fungus—Mold or yeast that may infect skin, internal surfaces (mouth and vagina) or tissues.

Fungus Infection—Infection caused by fungus.

Fusiform Bacteria—Bacteria shaped like slender rods.

G

Gallbladder—Small organ under the liver that stores bile. For digestion, the gallbladder contracts to empty bile into the intestines.

Gamma Globulin—Protein in the blood manufactured by the immune system to help destroy or neutralize infection-causing germs. Gamma globulin that is derived and concentrated from the blood of other humans is used to help create temporary immunity to some diseases.

Gammaglobulinemia—Extremely low levels in the blood of gamma globulin brought about by a disease of the immune system. The deficiency causes increased susceptibility to many infections by bacteria, viruses and fungi. Also called hypogammaglobulinemia.

Gangrene—Death of tissue, usually due to partial or total loss of blood supply.

Gastrectomy—Removal of part or all of the stomach.

Gastroenterologist—Doctor who specializes in the diagnosis and treatment of diseases of the gastrointestinal system.

Gastrointestinal Series (Upper GI Series)—X-rays of the upper digestive system (esophagus, stomach and duodenum).

Gastrointestinal Tract—See Digestive System.

Gastroscopy—Visual examination of the inside of the stomach by means of a gastroscope, an optical instrument with a lighted tip.

Gene—Basic unit of protein molecules in chromosomes of cells. Genes transmit inherited characteristics such as eye color, blood type, gender or body shape. Defective genes cause many kinds of birth defects and inborn diseases.

Gene, Dominant or Recessive—A dominant gene, if present in either the mother's egg or the father's sperm, will transmit its characteristics to the newborn child. Recessive genes must be present in both parents before their characteristics will be transmitted.

General Surgeon—A doctor specially trained to perform operations.

Genetic Counseling—Counseling to help couples decide whether to have children or not when there is a risk of genetic disease being transmitted to the child.

Genetics—Science of determining inherited factors that result in the unique make-up of every human being; also the science that traces the appearance patterns to genetic (inherited) disease.

Genitourinary Tract—Body system that forms, stores and eliminates urine. Also has a role in male and female reproductive functions. Organs include the kidneys, ureters, bladder, urethra, uterus, Fallopian tubes, ovaries, vagina, cervix, penis, scrotum and testicles.

Germs—Organisms that cause infection such as bacteria, viruses or fungi.

Glucagon—Hormone secreted by the pancreas that increases blood sugar. A synthetic form is sometimes used as emergency treatment for patients with diabetes who have temporarily low blood sugar.

Glucose—Major form of sugar in the blood, stored primarily in the liver. It provides energy to most tissues, organs and systems.

Glucose Tolerance Test—Method of diagnosing diabetes mellitus or functional hypoglycemia. The patient drinks a measured amount of glucose (sugar). The blood and urine are tested at measured intervals for glucose content.

Gluten—Protein found in wheat and other foods that cannot be digested by some persons because of genetic disease. A gluten-free diet allows persons with the disorder to digest food and grow normally.

Gonads—Parts of the reproductive system that produce and release female eggs (ovaries) or male sperm (testes).

Gynecologist—Doctor specially trained to treat diseases of the female reproductive system.

H

H₂ Blocker Drugs—Class of antihistamines that reduce the production of stomach acid for treatment of peptic ulcers.

Halitosis—Bad breath. This usually results from smoking, poor oral or dental hygiene, certain foods (garlic or onions) or drinking alcoholic beverages. Less common, but more serious causes, include sinusitis with post-nasal drip, nasal infections, mouth infections or chronic lung diseases. In these instances, the underlying cause needs to be treated. Mouth washes provide only temporary treatment.

Hallucinogens—Substances that produce hallucinations, apparent sights, sounds or other experiences that do not actually exist.

Hand Surgeon—Surgeon specially trained to treat hand diseases, injuries, infections and arthritic conditions.

Hangover—Unpleasant aftereffects of excessive consumption of alcoholic beverages. Symptoms include irritability, headache and nausea. Sometimes the same feelings result from using certain medications.

Hashimoto's Thyroiditis—One of several kinds of inflammation of the thyroid gland.

HDL Cholesterol—This is the abbreviation for high-density lipoprotein. HDL molecules are desirable kinds of fat molecules, whereas low-density lipoprotein (LDL) molecules are considered to increase the risk of heart attacks. Total cholesterol contains both types. For complete information, measuring the HDL and LDL provides much more useful data than measuring total cholesterol alone.

Heart Catheterization—See Cardiac Catheterization.

Heart Murmur—See Murmur.

Heart Tumors—Rare tumors that grow in the heart wall or in the heart chambers, interfering with normal heart function.

Heart-Lung Machine—Complex mechanical device that provides artificial function of a patient's heart and lungs for a short time during open heart surgery and heart or lung transplantation.

Hematocrit—Blood test used to detect anemia and other blood disorders. It is expressed as the percentage of blood made up of red blood cells; the remainder of the blood is made up of serum or plasma. The normal hematocrit range is approximately 35 to 45, but it varies with age and sex.

Hematologist—Doctor specially trained to diagnose and treat diseases of the blood and blood-forming organs.

Hemochromatosis—Disease in which excessive iron accumulates in the liver, pancreas and skin, resulting in liver disease, diabetes mellitus and a bronzed skin color.

Hemoglobin, Hemoglobin Range—1) Component that carries oxygen to body tissues. 2) Blood test used to detect anemia and other blood disorders, expressed in grams per 100 cubic centimeters. The normal hemoglobin range is approximately 12 to 18 grams per 100 cubic centimeters and varies according to age and sex.

High-Density Lipoprotein—See HDL Cholesterol.

Histamine—Chemical in body tissues that dilates the smallest blood vessels, constricts the muscle around the bronchial tubes, stimulates stomach secretions and produces an allergic response.

Holter Monitor—Instrument that detects heartbeat rhythm abnormalities for 24 hours or longer. The device is portable for patients to carry wherever they go.

Hormones—Powerful substances manufactured by the endocrine glands and carried by the blood to body tissues and organs. Hormones determine the growth and structure of many organs (such as during growth and maturation) and also control many vital body functions.

Host—Person or animal with an infection that has been received from another person, animal or plant or the environment.

HSV-1 (Herpes Simplex Virus-1)—The virus that causes cold sores.

HSV-2 (Herpes Simplex Virus-2)—The virus that cause herpes infection of the genital area.

Hygiene—Personal self-care and cleanliness that reduces the risk of infections and diseases.

Hyoid Bone—V-shaped bone located just above the larynx.

Hyperalimentation—Method of supplying total nutritional needs of patients who are unable to eat normally. The method (usually intravenous or by tube through the nose into the stomach) provides nutrients containing essential proteins, fats, carbohydrates and vitamins.

Hyperbaric Chamber—Large, sealed room in which air pressure can be raised above normal levels. It is used primarily to treat patients with either decompression sickness or severe burns (sometimes).

Hypercalcemia—Presence of excessive calcium in the blood, occasionally a sign of malignancy.

Hyperlipoproteinemia—Condition in which excessive lipoproteins (cholesterol and other fatty materials) accumulate in the blood.

Hypermetropia—Seeing distant objects clearly while nearby objects appear blurred; also called farsightedness.

Hypersensitivity—Extreme sensitivity to any agent (drugs, pollens, chemicals, etc.) that causes allergic reactions. Some reactions can be life-threatening, but most are less serious.

Hypnotics—Medications that produce sleep.

Hypochondriasis—Mental illness in which a person is convinced that serious disease is present, despite examination that proves otherwise. The symptoms of the imagined disease seem real to the patient (often called a hypochondriac).

Hypogammaglobulinemia—An immunologically deficient state characterized by an abnormally low level of all classes of gamma globulin in the blood.

Hypoplastic Anemia (Aplastic Anemia)—Group of anemias that decrease blood-producing bone marrow. This can be life-threatening.

Hypothalamus—Part of the brain that regulates body functions such as temperature, blood pressure, appetite and thirst.

Hysteria—1) Condition in which a person becomes anxious and excitable and experiences impaired sensory and motor abilities. Sometimes hysterical persons simulate conditions of diseases such as deafness or blindness. 2) Outbreak of uncontrolled emotions, such as fits of laughing or crying.

Hysterosalpingogram—A study of the uterus and Fallopian tubes done by injecting material into the uterus that x-rays can detect. The x-ray image is the hysterosalpingogram.

Hysteroscope—An instrument with a lens system and lighted tip used in direct visual examination of the cervix and the cavity of the uterus.

I

I-131 Uptake—Measurement of thyroid activity with radioactive iodine and radiation emission counters.

Ice Water Test (Also called water-caloric test)—Tests the status or function of the inner ear mechanism that controls the sense of balance. The examiner introduces water into the ear canal so it hits the eardrum directly for 30 seconds. The response is recorded on an electronystagmograph. The water may be ice cold or at temperatures that may range from 86 degrees Fahrenheit to 111.2 Fahrenheit.

Id Reaction—An allergic manifestation causing itching blisters on the hands and feet. The underlying allergy is a reaction to an infection somewhere else in the body, such as athelete's foot.

Idiopathic—Caused by unknown factors.

Ileum—Part of the small intestine just above the large intestine (colon).

Ileus—Condition of the small intestine in which either an obstruction or paralysis prevents material from passing through the intestine.

Iliac Arteries—Large arteries in the inner pelvis that supply blood to the legs.

Immune, Immunity—Resistance or protection against infection by the body's natural defenses. A person may be immune to one kind of infection but not immune to another. Some infections, such as measles, chickenpox or mumps, cause the body to become permanently immune to that infection.

Immune System—Body's system of defense against infection.

Immunization—Producing immunity by giving a vaccine (orally or by injection) of germs that have been altered so they cannot produce significant disease. The vaccine causes the body's immune system to produce antibodies that create immunity.

Immunosuppressants—Drugs used in immuno-suppression treatment to weaken the immune system and to inhibit immune response.

Immunosuppression—Prevention of the body from forming a normal immune response. It is used to treat diseases (especially when organs must be transplanted) where certain antibodies must be inactivated.

Impotence—Male's inability to achieve or to sustain an erection or to ejaculate sperm during sexual intercourse.

Incise, Incision—To cut open or cut into.

Incubation Period—The time between exposure to an infecting germ and the appearance of symptoms indicating an infection. Also describes the period of bacterial growth in laboratory cultures.

Infection, Infectious—Disease caused by germs (bacteria, viruses or fungi) that enter the body and cause inflammation or other processes that have an adverse effect on health.

Inflammation, Inflammatory Process—Process by which the body attempts to overcome illness-producing causes such as germs, injuries such as burns, or diseases such as arthritis. The process causes increased body heat (fever or local warmth), swelling, pain and tenderness. If the inflammation is near the skin, redness results.

Inhalation—Breathing air into the lungs.

Inherited Characteristic—Body characteristic that is transmitted from one generation to the next by chromosomes in the mother's egg and father's sperm. Some inherited characteristics such as brown eyes are normal; others such as Down's syndrome are disorders.

Inoculation—Injection of infected material such as pus into a nutrient medium where the germs will grow or incubate. They are then stained and analyzed through a microscope. Also describes any kind of immunization.

Insufflation Test—See Rubin's Insufflation Test.

Insulin—Hormone produced by the pancreas that helps regulate sugar in the blood and helps produce energy.

Intensive Care Unit (ICU)—Area of a hospital where patients who are seriously ill or recovering from serious surgery are given more care than is available in other hospital units. As soon as the condition improves, the patient is transferred from the ICU to a regular hospital unit.

Intermittent—Happening only occasionally or under certain conditions.

Internist—Doctor specially trained in non-surgical diagnosis and treatment of diseases in adults.

Intervertebral Disk—Cartilage that connects adjacent vertebrae in the spinal column.

Intestinal Tract—All parts of the gastrointestinal tract except the mouth, esophagus and stomach. The intestinal tract organs are the duodenum, small bowel, ileum, cecum, appendix, ascending colon, transverse colon, descending colon, sigmoid colon, rectum and anus.

Intestine, Large—Last major portion of the gastrointestinal tract located just under the small intestine. It is also called the colon or large bowel. It processes waste material into feces, which are stored until eliminated from the body.

Intestine, Small—Longest section of the gastrointestinal tract, located just under the stomach and duodenum. It absorbs digested food into the bloodstream and passes waste material into the large intestine.

Intravenous—Within the vein. Fluids, medications and nutrients that cannot be taken orally are given intravenously by a needle placed in a large vein near the surface of the skin.

Intravenous Pyelogram (IVP)—See Pyelogram, Intravenous.

IQ (Intelligence Quotient)—Supposedly a measure of a person's intelligence, rather than what one has learned. Recent research on intelligence raises questions about the accuracy and meaning of the IQ test.

Iridectomy—Surgery performed to treat some kinds of glaucoma.

Irrigation—Flooding with water or other liquid. It is used frequently to clean wounds or areas of the body that will undergo surgery.

Isolation, Reverse Isolation—Procedures to prevent the spread of infection in a hospital. Isolation protects the hospital staff and visitors from contracting a contagious disease from a patient. Reverse isolation protects a patient who is susceptible to infection because of immunosuppression from contracting infection from the hospital staff or visitors.

J

Jaundice—Yellow skin and whites of the eyes, dark urine and light stools, which are symptoms of diseases of the liver and blood.

Joint—Structure that enables two or more bones to move easily in relation to each other. A joint consists of ligaments and cartilage that hold bones together.

Joint Capsule—Tough, fibrous tissue that surrounds a joint.

Joint Replacement—Replacement of diseased joints with mechanical joints. The wrist, hip and knee joints are among the most common joints replaced.

K

Ketoacidosis—Serious complication of diabetes mellitus in which the body produces acids that cause fluid and electrolyte disorders, dehydration and sometimes coma.

L

Laceration—Wound with jagged edges.

Laparoscopy—Exploratory examination of the organs inside the abdominal cavity with a laparoscope, an optical instrument with a lighted tip. The laparoscope is inserted into the abdomen through a small incision. Visual examination can then be made of many abdominal organs.

Laparotomy—Exploratory surgery in the abdomen that is performed to diagnose and sometimes treat abdominal disease.

Laryngeal Nerve—Nerve located in the neck that controls the vocal cords and enables a person to speak.

Larynx—Structure of muscle and cartilage in the upper neck. It contains the vocal cords. Air passes through the larynx into the windpipe and then into the lungs. The "Adam's apple" is part of the larynx.

Laser Therapy—Using a laser beam to treat many diseases. Sharply focused laser light creates intense heat and is valuable in cutting tissue, destroying unwanted tissue and joining tissue together. It is most often used to treat retinal detachment, endometriosis or atherosclerosis.

Latent—Present but inactive; something that exists in an undeveloped form.

Laxatives—Medications used to treat constipation.

Lesion—General term for injury or damage to an organ or tissue.

Lethargy—Fatigue or lack of usual physical or mental energy.

Libido—Sexual desire.

Life Cycle—Growth and development from birth to death.

Ligaments—Strong, flexible cords of tissue near joints that hold bones together and permit bone motion.

Lipoproteins (High-Density and Low-Density)—Components of the fluid in blood that are measured to help predict the likelihood of atherosclerosis (hardening of the arteries).

Liquid Nitrogen—Nitrogen that has been cooled until it becomes a liquid. It is used most often in cryosurgery.

Lithotripsy—A complicated procedure that requires special equipment in a special environment that uses ultrasound waves to dissolve or dislodge stones in the gallbladder or urinary tract.

Local Anesthesia—See Anesthesia, Local.

LDL Cholesterol—The type of cholesterol (low-density lipoprotein) that accumulates and causes blockage in the blood vessels. Low-density lipoproteins are considered to increase risk of heart attacks. For complete information, measuring the HDL (high-density lipoprotein) and LDL provides much more useful data than measuring total cholesterol alone.

Low-Density Lipoprotein—See LDL Cholesterol.

Low-Residue Diet—Diet consisting of foods that are digested almost entirely, leaving minimal material to form feces.

Low Spinal Anesthesia—Also called "saddle block" or caudal anesthesia. An injection into the lower spinal canal provides anesthesia to the lower body.

Lower GI Series—See Barium Enema X-Rays.

Lumbar Puncture (Spinal Tap)—A diagnostic procedure in which a needle is inserted between 2 bones (vertebrae) of the lower spine to collect spinal fluid for laboratory examination.

Lumbar Spine—Lower part of the spine, from the lowest ribs to the bottom of the spine.

Lymph (or Lymphatic) System—Lymph channels and lymph glands considered as a single body system.

Lymph Channels—Tubes of tissue that carry lymph fluid away from tissues and back to the bloodstream. Lymph fluid is composed of proteins and water, varying in composition in different parts of the body.

Lymph Glands—Small collections of tissue (nodes) located along lymph channels in areas such as the elbow, armpit or groin. When infection is present, nearby lymph glands enlarge, become tender and destroy germs that enter lymph channels. Lymph glands also manufacture antibodies to help fight infection.

Lymphangiogram, Lymphangiography—Diagnostic method of studying the lymphatic system by injecting a material into the lymph channels that x-rays can detect. The image on x-ray film is the lymphangiogram.

Lymphatic Leukemia—Class of leukemias involving primarily lymphatic cells.

Lymphocytes—One of several types of white blood cells that help fight infection.

Lymphosarcoma—Class of cancers of the lymphatic system.

M

Macular Degeneration of the Eye—Condition of the macula (area on the retina that provides detailed vision) in which impaired blood supply causes gradual vision loss.

Macule—General term for any discolored spot or patch on the skin, such as a freckle.

Malignant—Capable of causing great harm, including death. It usually refers to cancerous growth.

Mammogram, Mammography—Diagnostic method of studying the female breast by an x-ray technique that detects cancerous growths while they are still treatable. The image on x-ray film is the mammogram.

Manic-Depressive Illness—Mental illness in which behavior alternates between unrealistic enthusiasm and deep depression.

Manometer—An instrument to measure the pressure or tension of liquids or gases in the blood or cerebrospinal fluid.

MAO Inhibitors—See Monoamine Oxidase Inhibitors.

Marfan Syndrome—A congenital disorder characterized by abnormally long fingers and toes, eye disorders, heart disorders and other deformities.

Marijuana—Mood-altering substance that is usually taken into the body by smoking. It is derived from Indian hemp or cannabis leaves, stems and seed pods.

Marrow—Core of many bones, where most of the body's blood cells are produced.

Mastoiditis—Infection of the mastoid (bony area just behind the ear).

Mediators—Substances that help nerve impulses travel from one cell to the next.

Medic Alert—Non-profit agency that maintains a medical record system. Subscribers receive a bracelet or pendant that states their medical condition and provides a toll-free number for more information. The service can save the life of a person with a major medical condition who may not be able to provide a medical history. For information write Medic Alert Foundation, P.O. Box 1009, Turlock, CA 95381.

Medical History—Essential facts about past and present medical conditions. Knowing your medical history enables your doctor to plan the best possible health care. Carry a card stating essential health details in your purse or wallet, and consider joining the Medic Alert program (see above).

Meibomian Glands—Small glands on the inner eyelid. They secrete a fluid that helps the eyelids move easily over the surface of the eye.

Membrane—Thin tissue lining a body cavity, covering an internal organ or dividing a space.

Meninges—Three-layered membrane covering the brain.

Mental System (Mind)—Functions of the brain that provide the abilities to perceive surroundings; to have emotions, imagination, memory and will; and to process information.

Metastases—Cancerous cells or infectious germs that spread from their original location to other parts of the body.

Metatarsal Bones—Bones in the middle of the foot.

Mole—Skin lesion, often dark brown or black.

Monoamine Oxidase (MAO) Inhibitors—Medications used to treat some forms of depression.

Motor Nerve—Nerve that transmits the stimulus that causes muscles to contract.

MRI (Magnetic Resonance Imaging)—A diagnostic procedure in which the patient while lying down is surrounded by electromagnets. The machine exposes the patient to short bursts of powerful magnetic fields and radio waves. The patient's tissues respond by emitting signals which can be detected and analyzed by computer techniques.

Mucous Membrane—Thin tissue lining internal cavities (nose, mouth and vagina) and tubular systems (respiratory and gastrointestinal) that produce mucus.

Mucus—Slippery liquid produced by the lining of internal cavities and tubular systems to protect tissue.

Murmur—Sound of blood rushing through the heart and blood vessels, which is detected by a stethoscope. Some murmurs are innocent, meaning they are not caused by disease. Other murmurs arise from heart disease or partial obstruction in the arteries.

Muscle—Tissue that contracts, often with considerable force, when stimulated by the motor nerve impulses.

Muscle Relaxants—Medications that relieve muscle spasms. They also can have significant side effects.

Muscle Tumors—Benign or cancerous tumors arising from muscle tissue.

Musculoskeletal System—The system of bones, muscles, ligaments and tendons that enable the body to move.

Myelogram—Special x-ray of the spinal canal and spinal cord requiring a spinal tap and injection of dye that is visible on x-ray film. Myelograms frequently are used to identify the location of ruptured disks.

Myoma—Tumor of the muscle.

Myopia—Disease of the eye in which close objects are clearly visible while distant objects are blurred. Also called nearsightedness.

N

Narcotics—Medications used to control severe pain. Narcotics should be used only when necessary because of their serious side effects: addiction; reduced breathing; nausea and vomiting; low blood pressure; reduced cough reflex; constipation.

Naso-Gastric Tube—Slender tube passed through the nose into the stomach. It is used to drain away stomach secretions or to feed patients who are unable to eat normally.

Naturopathy—Health-care system relying on diet, sunshine, exercises, herbs and other non-medicinal treatment.

Nausea—Unpleasant sensation of being about to vomit.

Nearsightedness—See Myopia.

Nebulizer—Device for administering medications used to treat asthma and similar conditions. It converts medication into a fine mist that is inhaled deeply into the lungs.

Nerve-Block Local Anesthesia—See Anesthesia, Local (Nerve Block).

Nerve Conduction Test—Diagnostic test that measures the rate at which an electrical impulse moves along a nerve. It is used to diagnose disorders of the peripheral nerves and muscle.

Nervous Breakdown—Non-technical term for mental illness that is serious enough to interfere with daily activities.

Neuritis—Inflammation of a nerve.

Neurological—Relating to the body's nervous system.

Neurologist—Doctor specially trained to diagnose and treat diseases of the nervous system.

Neuroma—Tumor arising from nerve tissue.

Neuromuscular System—Nerves and muscles acting together as a system to control body movements.

Neurosis—Mental illness in which anxiety is controlled by avoidance, blaming others, developing bodily complaints or other mechanisms.

Neurosurgeon—Doctor specially trained to diagnose and surgically treat diseases of the brain, spinal cord and nerves.

NMR (Nuclear Magnetic Resonance)—This is an imaging technique also called MRI (Magnetic Resonance Imaging).

Nodes—See Lymph Glands.

Nodule—Small, rounded lump or firm swelling underneath the skin.

Non-Steroidal Anti-Inflammatory Drugs—Medications that control inflammation other than that caused by infection. Usually used to treat conditions of the joints and muscles and pain such as headache. "Non-steroidal" means they are not steroid hormones such as cortisone, prednisone, dextramethasone and others.

Nurse Practitioner (NP)—Registered nurse with additional medical training who can diagnose and treat common illness. Nurse practitioners usually work closely with doctors, although in some states the practitioner can prescribe medicine and work independently of a physician.

Nutrient—Food or material containing elements needed to promote growth and development or to support life.

O

Obsessions—Unpleasant, frightening, senseless thoughts that won't go away despite reasoning.

Obstetrician-Gynecologist—Doctor specially trained to treat diseases of the female reproductive system.

Obstructive Pulmonary Disease—See COPD (Chronic Obstructive Pulmonary Disease).

Occlusion—Closing or obstruction. Usually used to describe a blockage in a blood vessel. In dentistry, it means the way the teeth come together when the mouth is closed.

Oncologist—Doctor specially trained to diagnose and treat cancer.

Operative Death Rate—Percentage of patients who die as a result of a certain surgery. It provides general measure of the risk of a surgery.

Ophthalmologist—Doctor specially trained to diagnose and treat diseases of the eyes.

Optic Neuritis—Inflammation of the nerve that conducts vision impulses from the eye to the brain.

Oral—Relating to the mouth.

Oral-Fecal—See Fecal-Oral.

Organic—Conditions or diseases resulting from changes in body organs that can be measured or seen. Organic diseases are distinct from functional diseases in which no change can be observed in an organ that is not functioning normally.

Organic Psychosis—Mental illness that results from disease in the brain.

Orthodontia—Straightening of the teeth by applying temporary braces.

Orthopedic Surgeon (Orthopedist)—Doctor specially trained to diagnose and treat diseases of the muscles, bones and joints using surgical or mechanical means. A rheumatologist is an internist who diagnoses and treats similar conditions primarily with medications and other non-surgical means.

Osteogenesis Imperfecta—Inherited condition in which the bones are brittle and easily broken.

Otorhinolaryngologist or Otolaryngologist—See Ear, Nose and Throat Specialist.

Ovary—Female sexual gland where, prior to menopause, eggs matured and ripened for fertilization.

P

Pain—Unpleasant sensation arising from stimulation of sensory nerves located in almost every part of the body. Disease, injury and strenuous activity can all cause pain.

Palate—Roof of the mouth, consisting of a bony front portion (hard palate) and a soft back portion (soft palate).

Palpitations—Irregular rapid heartbeat that is noticeable to the patient.

Pancreas—Organ located on the back abdominal wall that produces and secretes digestive juices into the small intestine. It also produces and secretes insulin into the bloodstream to regulate the level of sugar and other nutrients.

Pap Smear—Test done to detect cancer of the cervix in an early and treatable stage.

Papule—Small, raised skin lesion. Papules may be red, brown, yellow, white or skin-colored. They may be flat-topped, pointed or dome-shaped.

Paranoia—Mental illness in which a person believes that he or she is being talked about or plotted against.

Parasite—Organism that lives within, upon or at the expense of another living organism. Human parasites include disease-causing agents such as amoebas or worms that infect the digestive system or fungi that live on the skin.

Parasympathetic Nervous System—System of nerves that controls digestion, heartbeat, and relaxation or contraction of small muscles.

Parathyroid Glands—Small glands that control calcium levels in the blood and bones. They are located within or next to the thyroid glands at the base of the neck.

Passive Exercises—Exercises in which a therapist moves the arms and legs of a patient while the patient relaxes. These exercises keep the joints limber until the patient is able to move without assistance.

Patency—Blood vessels or any hollow organs that clog or become blocked are said to lose their patency.

Pathological—Relating to an abnormal condition.

Pathological Examination—Laboratory study of abnormal tissue to establish or confirm a diagnosis.

Pediculicide—Medication that cures body lice (pediculosis). Usually applied to the skin.

Pelvic Examination—Examination of a woman's reproductive organs to detect diseases.

Pelvic Ultrasonography—Examination of a woman's reproductive organs that uses high-frequency sound waves to create an image. It is used to diagnose disease of the pelvic organs.

Pelvis—Lower part of the trunk of the body.

Penis—Male organ used for urination and sexual intercourse.

Perforation—Abnormal hole or opening.

Perforation, Intestinal—Complication of conditions such as ulcers, cancers or injury to the digestive system. When this occurs, intestinal contents enter the abdominal cavity, causing severe inflammation.

Perfusionist—Medical technician who controls the heart-lung machine to sustain a patient's life during open-heart and lung-transplant surgery.

Perineum—Area between the vulva and anus in females and between the scrotum and anus in males.

Peripheral Nervous System—Nerves that connect to all parts of the body and carry information via electrical impulses to and from the brain and spinal cord.

Peripheral Vascular System—Network of arteries, veins and lymphatic channels supplying the head, arms and legs.

Perirectal—Skin and underlying tissue around the rectum.

Peristalsis—Rhythmic movements of hollow muscular organs (such as the intestines) that move contents (such as digestive materials) in one direction.

Peritoneal Cavity—Space enclosed by the peritoneum.

Peritoneum—Very thin, two-layered tissue. One layer lines the outer surface of all the abdominal organs. The other layer lines the abdominal wall.

Peritonsillar Abscess—Abscess forming in the back of the throat near the tonsils.

Pessary—Small ring-shaped device that is inserted into the vagina to help maintain the uterus in a normal position.

pH Balance—Measure of blood's acidity or alkalinity. The pH is controlled by body fluids and electrolytes. Body tissues cannot function normally if the pH varies from a limited range.

PET (Positive Emission Tomography)—A diagnostic technique which detects positrons (positively charged particles) emitted by labeled substances introduced into the body. The result is a three-dimensional image that reflect the chemical activity of the tissues being studied. PET scanning is particularly valuable for investigating the brain.

Phenothiazine Drugs—Medications used to slow and regulate mental system activity. Usually used to treat anxiety and other mental conditions; also useful in producing sleep.

Phlebotomy—Removing blood from the blood vessels. This was once believed to cure many diseases; today it is done to remove blood for diagnostic testing.

Phobia—Fear that cannot be overcome by reason.

Phototherapy—The treatment of disease by exposure to light.

Physical Therapy—Treatment of diseases of the bone, muscular and nervous systems to help restore normal function after disease or injury.

Physician's Assistant (PA)—Someone trained to do some of the simpler tasks ordinarily performed by a doctor. The PA works under the direction of the doctor.

Pilocarpine—Medication used principally in eye drops to treat glaucoma.

Pituitary Gland—Small endocrine gland at the base of the brain that controls growth and regulates other endocrine glands.

Plaque—1) Small raised area of abnormal material on a surface such as the skin or lining of a blood vessel. 2) Mixture of bacteria and calcium deposited on the teeth that can cause cavities and gum diseases.

Plasma—Liquid part of blood that remains when blood cells are removed.

Plasmapheresis—The removal of blood and separation of plasma by rapid centrifugation followed by reinjection of the packed red blood cells suspended in a saline or other suitable medium.

Plastic and Reconstructive Surgeon (Plastic Surgeon)—Doctor specially trained to perform plastic and reconstructive surgery.

Plastic and Reconstructive Surgery—Special surgery to repair and change body parts to improve function or appearance. The face, hands, breasts and skin are the areas most frequently treated.

Platelet Count—Platelets are blood cells (much smaller than red or white blood cells) that assist in the blood-clotting process. A drop of blood contains about 12.5 million platelets. A platelet count determines if the number of platelets is normal.

Pleura—Thin tissue lining the lungs and chest cavity. Inflammation of the pleura (pleurisy) is a painful condition caused by lung diseases.

Pleural Effusion (Pleural Fluid Effusion)—Fluid that collects around the lungs, usually caused by inflammation of the lungs and pleura or congestive heart failure.

Podiatrist—Health-care professional trained in the medical and surgical treatment of foot diseases.

Polyp—A growth, often on a stalk arising from dry mucous membranes, such as in the nose, cervix or colon.

Portal Vein System—Vein system that drains blood from the gastrointestinal system. The smaller veins empty into the portal vein, which transports blood into the liver.

Postoperative—Period of recuperation and return to normal health after surgery.

Postural Drainage—Exercises and body positions that promote drainage of fluid and secretions that collect in the lungs and airways.

Potassium—Electrolyte present in all body cells, blood and body fluids. Potassium is important in maintaining normal heart contractions and the strength and contractions of all muscles. Foods high in potassium include dried apricots and peaches; whole-grain cereals; plain cocoa, dried lentils and peas; bananas; and molasses.

Precancerous—Characteristic of a growth that has the potential to become cancerous.

Predisposition—Tendency. For example, a person who gets many infections has a predisposition to infection.

Presbyopia—Form of nearsightedness that normally accompanies aging.

Primary Disorder—Basic disease that may result in complications. Diabetes mellitus, for example, is a primary disorder that often causes secondary complications involving the kidneys, blood vessels and eyes.

Proctoscope, Proctoscopy—Method of examining the rectum and lower part of the colon with a proctoscope, an optical instrument with a lighted tip.

Prolapse—Pushing or falling out of a part or an organ from its normal position.

Prolapsed (Dropped) Uterus—Uterus that has moved from its normal position because of loose pelvic muscles and ligaments. In severe cases, it can protrude completely outside the vagina.

Prophylaxis—Measures taken to prevent an illness.

Prophylaxis, Dental—Regular care (including cleaning) of the teeth and gums that helps prevent tooth decay and gum inflammation.

Prostaglandins—Natural substances found in semen, menstrual fluid and many body tissues. They are involved in basic body functions such as inflammation, immune response and activities of the lungs, heart, kidneys, uterus and digestive system.

Prostate (Prostate Gland)—Male sex gland located at the base of the urinary bladder. It produces a fluid that is added to sperm to produce semen.

Prosthesis—Artificial device used as a substitute for a missing or badly functioning part of the body.

Prothrombin Time—Test to measure one of the components of the body's blood-clotting mechanism. It is used to diagnose clotting diseases and to control blood thinning (anticoagulation) in treatment of some diseases of the heart and blood vessels.

Provocative Stress Test—A test in which a possible allergen is intentionally administered to determine its allergenicity.

Psychiatrist—Doctor specially trained to diagnose and treat mental illnesses.

Psychoanalysis—Treatment of some mental illness that involves a detailed understanding of how past events in a person's life may have resulted in mental disturbances.

Psychologist—Health-care professional specially trained to diagnose and treat some kinds of mental illness.

Psychopathy—Psychological or mental illness.

Psychosis—Mental illness characterized by deranged personality, loss of contact with reality and possible delusions, hallucinations or illusions.

Psychosocial—Influences of society on growth and development.

Psychosomatic Illness—Illness in which thoughts and emotions play an important role.

Psychotherapist—Professional specially trained to diagnose and treat some mental illnesses.

Pubic Bone—One of the bones of the pelvis that is located above the genitals in both sexes.

Pulmonary—Relating to the lungs and breathing.

Pulmonary Hypertension—Increased pressure in the blood vessels of the lungs.

Pulse—Heartbeat (contraction of the heart) as felt in an artery. Heart rate is often measured by counting the pulse felt in the artery in the wrist.

Pus—Thick fluid, usually green or yellow, that forms to fight local infection. Pus often collects in an enclosed sac, an abscess, at the site of an infection.

Pyelogram, Intravenous—Method of studying the kidneys and urinary tract by injecting into the bloodstream a medication that x-rays can detect.

Pyelogram, Retrograde—Method of studying the kidneys that is similar to an intravenous pyelogram, but in which the medication detected by x-rays is placed in the urinary system by a catheter inserted through the bladder into the ureters.

Pyelography—See Pyelogram.

R

Radiation Therapy or Treatment—Use of high-energy waves (generated by special x-ray machines, cobalt machines and other devices) to treat some forms of cancer. Radiation destroys cancerous tissue but does little harm to healthy tissue.

Radioactive Chromium Studies—Diagnostic method used to measure total blood in the body.

Radioactive Iodine Uptake and Scan—See Thyroid Scan.

Radioactive Studies—See Radioisotope Studies.

Radioactive Technetium 99 Scan—Radioisotope scan method used to diagnose some disorders of the heart, liver, spleen and other organs.

Radio-Immunoassay—Highly sensitive, specific assay method that uses the competition between radio-labeled and unlabeled substances in an antigen-antibody reaction to determine the concentration of the unlabeled substance. Can be used to determine the concentration of any substance against which antibodies can be produced.

Radioisotope—Radioactive form of chemicals normally present in the body.

Radioisotope Scan—Scan of radioisotopes given orally or intravenously to a patient that become concentrated in organs such as the heart, lungs or brain. Instruments measure the radiation given off by the radioisotopes and create a photographic image of the organ being studied.

Radioisotope Studies—Radioisotopes are chemical elements that give off radiation. A radioisotope of a chemical element normally present in the body (such as carbon), if injected into the body, will mix with the non-isotopes. The body doesn't know the difference, but radiation from the isotopes can be detected with special instruments. Determining where radioisotopes go in the body allows the diagnosis of diseases that cannot be detected otherwise.

Radioisotope Therapy—Treatment of some cancers with radioisotopes.

Radiologist—Doctor specially trained to use x-rays and other kinds of radiation in diagnosis and treatment.

Rebound Phenomenon—A reversed response to the withdrawal of a stimulus. A common rebound phenomenon occurs when nose drops, which decrease congestion, wear off. The nasal congestion that develops on the rebound is greater than that which existed before the drops were administered.

Recovery Room—Specially equipped and staffed area of a hospital for observing and caring for patients who have just undergone surgery. Postoperative patients usually remain in the recovery room until they are awake and their vital signs (blood pressure, pulse and respiration) are satisfactory.

Rectum—End of the large intestine, which is located in the pelvis below the sigmoid colon and above the anus.

Regeneration—Ability of some parts of the body to grow back to normal after being damaged.

Regurgitate—To vomit.

Relapse—Stage of illness in which the patient gets worse after having improved.

Remission—Stage of a chronic illness when the patient's condition improves.

Renal Dialysis—Mechanical and chemical method of removing normal wastes from the body of a patient whose kidneys cannot function adequately. It is also used to remove harmful poison or a drug overdose from the bloodstream.

Reproductive Organs, Female—Organs of a woman's body that enabled her to become pregnant and deliver a baby. The major organs are the vagina, uterus, Fallopian tubes and ovaries.

Reproductive Organs, Male—Organs of a man's body that enable him to produce sperm and impregnate a woman. The major organs are the penis, testicles, seminal vesicles and prostate gland.

Reproductive System—Body system enabling impregnation and delivery of a baby. It also provides characteristic male or female appearance.

Resect—Surgical removal of a part of the body.

Retina—Light-sensitive part of the eye at the back of the eyeball on which the lens focuses images. The retina converts the image to impulses that go to the brain.

Retinal Vein Occlusion—Condition in which a clot forms in the vein supplying the retina with blood.

Retroviruses—Group of viruses that cause AIDS (Acquired Immunodeficiency Syndrome) and some types of lymphoma and leukemia.

Reverse Isolation Technique—A nursing procedure in which the people visiting a patient must practice sterile precautions.

Rh Negative Blood—A subtype of red blood cells. Blood subtypes are inherited. The major subtypes are types A, B, O and Rh negative.

Rheumatologist—A specialist in internal medicine who specializes in the medical diagnosis and treatment of rheumatic and arthritic disorders.

Rinne Test—Test using a tuning fork to diagnose hearing disorders.

S

Sacroiliac Region—Area of the lower back where the spine meets the pelvic bone.

Saline—Salt-containing solution similar to normal body fluid that is given intravenously to help correct fluid and electrolyte imbalances.

Salivary Glands—Glands located inside the mouth around the jaw that secrete saliva into the mouth.

Saphenous-Femoral Vein System—Network of large veins in the legs that helps return blood from the leg to the inferior vena cava, then to the heart.

Scale, Scaling—Flakes of dried skin which form as whitish skin lesions.

Schizophrenia—Mental illness characterized by a distorted sense of reality, bizarre behavior and fragmentation of the personality.

Sciatic Nerve—Large nerve that begins at the base of the spine and passes through the buttocks down the back side of the thigh and down the leg.

Sciatica—Painful condition resulting from irritation of the sciatic nerve.

Scleritis—Inflammation of the sclera (the white of the eye).

Scoliosis—Curvature of the spine.

Scopolamine—Medication used to treat hyperactive or spastic conditions of the digestive system and to prevent motion sickness.

Scrotum—Organ of the male reproductive system that contains the testicles, blood vessels and the vas deferens.

Scurvy—Disease of bones, gums and blood vessels caused by a deficiency of vitamin C.

Secondary Infection—Infection that results from some other problem. It may occur after surgery or develop during antibiotic treatment of another infection.

Sedative—Medication used to produce relaxation or sleep.

Sedative-Hypnotics—Class of medications that help relieve anxiety and promote sleep.

Sedimentation Rate—Blood test measuring the rate at which blood settles in a test tube. It identifies infection, inflammation or tissue damage.

Self-Care—Treatment that patients can administer for themselves.

Seminal Vesicles—Small sacs next to the prostate that help make and store seminal fluid and contract to eject semen.

Senile Dementia—Permanent loss of mental functions of older persons resulting from conditions such as Alzheimer's disease and atherosclerosis (hardening of the arteries).

Sensitivity Studies (Antibiotics)—Laboratory method of determining which antibiotic will most likely be successful in treating infections caused by bacteria.

Sensory—Having the ability to feel or experience sensations such as sound, light or pain.

Septic—Infected.

Serological Tests—Tests of serum (blood without cells) used to diagnose a variety of diseases, especially infections and autoimmune conditions.

Serum—Liquid portion of the blood that remains after blood cells and blood clots have been removed.

Serum Alkaline Phosphatase—Material present in excessive amounts in the blood of patients with some bone and liver diseases.

Serum Electrolytes—See Electrolytes.

Sesamoid Bones—Small oval-shaped bones in the tendons of the hands and feet.

Sexual Dysfunction—Inability to participate in sexual relations that are satisfactory for both partners.

Shave Biopsy—Procedure to diagnose skin disorders in which a thin layer of tissue from under a skin lesion is shaved away for laboratory examination.

Shock—Condition in which the blood pressure falls below the level needed to supply blood to the body. Signs and symptoms include weakness, paleness, rapid heartbeat, dry mouth, cold sweat and feelings of doom.

Sick-Sinus Syndrome—Form of heart rhythm disorder (arrhythmia).

Sigmoid Colon—Lower part of the large colon (intestine) located in the pelvis just above the rectum.

Sigmoidoscope, Sigmoidoscopy—See Proctoscope, Proctoscopy.

Signs—Evidence of disease that can be observed and measured, in contrast to symptoms, which only patients can experience. For example, blood pressure measurement or red tonsils are signs; headache or nausea are symptoms.

Silicone—Artificial compound used by plastic and reconstructive surgeons to reshape parts of the body, such as the breast.

Silver Nitrate—Chemical used for cautery.

Skin Clips—Small U-shaped metal strips used instead of stitches to close skin that has been incised during surgery.

Skin Test for Allergy—Diagnostic method used to determine whether a particular substance is causing allergic reactions. The test is carried out by introducing a small amount of the suspected material, such as pollen or dust, under the skin or on the skin. If inflammation results, the patient is allergic to the material.

Sleep Inducers—Medications used to produce sleep.

Sleep Study Laboratory—Laboratory where persons are studied with sensitive instruments while asleep. Information from sleep study aids in the diagnosis of sleep disorders.

Slow Viruses—Group of viruses that infect the brain but do not cause disease until many years afterward.

Soaks—Applications of moisture—either plain water or water with dissolved medicines—to an inflamed area of the skin.

Soft Palate—Fleshy part of the roof of the mouth close to the throat.

Sonogram, Sonography—Diagnostic method in which high-frequency (ultrasound) sound waves are transmitted into the body. Their reflections create images of body organs.

Spasmodic—Sudden intermittent symptoms or intermittent muscle spasms.

Spastic, Spasticity—A description of muscles that are continuously contracting and in a state of excessive tension.

Speculum—Instrument used to examine the interior of openings such as the vagina, nose, ear or rectum.

Sperm—Male reproductive cells manufactured in the testicles and ejaculated in semen.

Spherocytosis—Abnormally shaped red blood cells caused by some anemias. These cells are sphere-shaped, in contrast to the doughnut shape of normal red blood cells.

Spikes, Temperature—High but brief episodes of fever.

Spina Bifida—Congenital (inherited) disorder in which the base of the spine remains open, sometimes exposing the spinal cord and nerves.

Spinal Anesthesia—Method to provide anesthesia to the lower body by injecting an anesthetic into the fluid in the space that surrounds the lower spinal cord.

Spirometry—Test of lung (pulmonary) function.

Spleen—A large organ in the upper left abdomen that is located close to the left side of the stomach. It is the largest structure of the lymph system. The spleen causes disintegration of old red blood cells and serves as an important reservoir of blood.

Splenic Vein Thrombosis—Clot in the major vein that carries blood away from the spleen.

Splints—Rigid supports, made of metal, plastic or plaster, used to immobilize an injured or inflamed part of the body. Splints are used temporarily in the case of injury, following some surgical procedures on joints or ligaments, or occasionally in the case of arthritis.

Spore—Microscopic seed form of fungi. Spores are extremely hardy and survive extremes of temperature. If they enter the body of a susceptible person, they can cause fungal disease.

Sputum—Secretion of the lungs that is coughed up in large amounts in some lung diseases.

Staphylococcus—Bacteria which frequently cause boils, abscesses, pneumonias, bone infections and infections in other tissues or organs.

Staples—Small U-shaped metal wires used in place of stitches to close incised skin after some surgeries, especially in the digestive system. Also used to close off some portions of the stomach during operations for extreme obesity.

Sterilized—1) Made completely free of all germs, usually by steam heat, toxic gas or chemicals. All instruments used in surgeries are sterilized, as is most other medical equipment. 2) Made unable to conceive children.

Steroids—Medications which resemble hormones produced by the cortex of the adrenal glands, ovaries and testicles.

Stethoscope—Instrument used to listen to the sounds produced by the heart, lungs and blood vessels.

Stimulant Drugs—Medications that increase the activity of the brain and nervous system.

Stomatitis—Inflammation of the mouth.

Stool—Feces.

Streptococcus—Bacteria that cause illnesses such as laryngitis, cellulitis of the skin, pneumonia, meningitis and others. If not treated, streptococcal infections may also cause serious heart and kidney diseases as complications that appear after the original infection has cleared.

Sublingual Salivary Glands—Small glands near the base of the tongue that secrete saliva into the mouth.

Submaxillary Salivary Glands—Small glands near the jaw that secrete saliva into the mouth.

Sulfonamides (Sulfa Drugs)—Class of drugs used to fight infections.

Sulfonurea Drugs—Medications taken orally to treat some forms of diabetes mellitus.

Surgical Suite—Group of rooms used to perform surgery. In addition to operating rooms, where surgery takes place, there are supply areas, a recovery room, administrative rooms and a lounge where the staff can rest between surgeries.

Suture—Thread-like material used to hold tissues or skin edges together.

Symmetry, Symmetrical—Refers to the arrangement of the body in pairs, such as two arms, legs, kidneys, lungs, etc.

Sympathomimetics—Medications similar to adrenalin in their actions.

Symptoms—Effects of disease that only the patient can experience, such as pain, nausea, dizziness, anxiety, depression and others.

Synovial Membranes—Delicate tissues that line the inside of joints.

Systemic—Conditions that affect most or all of the body, in contrast to conditions that affect only a limited area. For example, diabetes mellitus is a systemic condition; an abscess is a local condition.

T

Tartar—Hard deposit that forms on the teeth and causes inflammation of the gums.

Temperature Spike—See Spikes, Temperature.

Temporomandibular Joint—Joint that joins the jaw to the other head bones.

Tenderness—Condition that causes pain when pressure is applied.

Tendon—Tough cord of tissue at the end of muscles that attach to bone. Tendons transmit the force of muscle contraction to cause movement.

Testes or Testicles—Male sex glands that produce sex hormones and sperm.

Therapeutic Trial—Form of diagnosis and treatment where medication is used even though the diagnosis is not firmly established. If the patient improves after treatment with a medication that is known to be useful in treating a specific condition, the improvement suggests that the specific disease was present. Therapeutic trials are somewhat risky and are used only when other forms of diagnosis and treatment have failed.

Therapist—Health-care professional specially trained to provide therapy.

Thermogram, Thermography—Method of diagnosis that measures body heat. The area being studied is scanned by a heat-sensitive instrument capable of producing an image (thermogram) of areas of increased heat. They are useful in studying female breast tumors and some blood vessel conditions.

Thiazide Diuretics—Class of medications that promote excretion of excess fluids by the kidneys.

Thomas Collar—A soft, flexible collar made from cloth that fits around the neck to provide support for people who have painful injuries or arthritis in this region.

Thoracic Duct—The largest channel of the lymphatic system through which lymph fluid enters the vena cava.

Thoracic Spine—That part of the spinal column below the neck and above the back. Ribs attach to the thoracic spine.

Thoracic Surgeon—A surgeon who specializes in surgical treatment of disorders of the organs in the thorax (chest), including the lungs, pericardium, heart, pleura (covering of lungs), bronchial tubes and large blood vessels.

Thrombocytopenia—Reduced platelets in the blood stream. Platelets are small white blood cells that play an important part in blood clotting.

Thyroglossal Duct—Small passageway, normally closed, located in the upper neck. It extends from the back of the tongue to just above the larynx. If an abnormally open duct becomes filled with fluid, a thyroglossal cyst results.

Thyroid Cartilage—Semihard cartilage which forms the larynx (also called the voice box or Adam's apple).

Thyroid Gland—Endocrine gland located in the lower neck next to the trachea that produces hormones that regulate the rate at which all body cells function. Thyroid hormones are also essential for normal growth and development.

Thyroid Scan—Method of examination of the thyroid gland in which a small amount of radioactive iodine introduced into the body collects in the thyroid gland. An instrument passed over the thyroid produces an image of the gland based on the concentration of the radioactive iodine.

Ticks—Small biting insects that may cause inflammation of the skin or serious infections such as Rocky Mountain spotted fever.

Tics—Brief, uncontrollable muscle spasms.

Tissue—Building blocks of body organs; living cells all of one type.

Tonsils—Lymphatic tissues located at the entrance of the throat that help fight infection.

Topical—Medications applied to the skin, conjunctiva, or mucous membranes of the mouth, nose, vagina or rectum.

Tourniquet—Cord or band wrapped around an arm or leg tightly enough to stop blood circulation temporarily.

Toxic, Toxicity—Harmful; capable of causing body damage.

Toxin—Poison. Usually refers to the chemicals produced by some living organisms that harm the human body.

Traction—Method of treating some conditions of bones, muscles, and ligaments by exerting a steady pull on the affected parts. Some bone fractures and back pain due to a ruptured disk are treated this way.

Tranquilizer—Medication used to help diminish anxiety and to produce calmness.

Tranquilizers, Benzodiazepine—Class of tranquilizers commonly used to treat anxiety, nervousness or tension.

Transfuse—To give a patient blood that is necessary in the treatment of some conditions.

Transfusion—Process of introducing blood through a needle placed in the patient's vein.

Transfusion Reaction—Undesirable symptom or condition resulting from a blood transfusion.

Transmission, Transmit—Passing a disease to another person.

Transplant—Living organ (such as a kidney, cornea, heart, bone marrow or skin) that is removed from one person (donor) and placed in the body of another (recipient).

Transverse Colon—Middle part of the colon (intestine), lying horizontally in the middle or upper abdomen.

Trauma—Force that injures or damages any part of the body.

Tricyclic Antidepressant Drugs (Tricyclics)—Class of medications used to treat depression.

Tube Feeding—Providing nutrients through a small tube that is placed in the stomach of a patient who is unable to eat. The tube may pass through the nose to the stomach or be inserted through an incision in the stomach.

Tuberous Sclerosis—Rare inherited condition of the skin, nervous system and other organs of the body.

Tumor—Literally, a swelling; usually used to refer to a benign or cancerous growth.

U

Ulceration—Wearing away of the surface or lining of an organ, exposing underlying tissue. Ulceration of the lining of the stomach exposes blood vessels, which may bleed. Ulceration may erode through the wall of an organ (perforation). Ulceration frequently affects the skin if it is rubbed excessively or if diseased.

Ultrasonography—See Sonography.

Ultrasound Treatment—Method of treatment in which high-energy sound waves are focused on the affected area, producing mild heat that helps relieve inflammation. It is especially useful in the treatment of muscular symptoms.

Underlying—Beneath, below or more basic. Thus, losing weight may result from an underlying condition such as diabetes mellitus or cancer.

Upper Gastrointestinal (GI) Series—X-ray examination of the esophagus, stomach and duodenum accomplished by having the patient swallow a barium solution that x-rays can detect.

Upper Respiratory System—Upper part of the breathing system consisting of the nose, throat, larynx, trachea and bronchial tubes.

Uremia—A serious condition associated with kidney failure in which body wastes build up in the blood and body tissues.

Ureters—Slender muscular tubes that carry urine from the kidneys to the urinary bladder, where it is stored until it is eliminated from the body.

Urethra—Tubular passageway extending from the urinary bladder to the outside of the body.

Urethrocystoscopy—Examination of the inside of the urethra and bladder by means of a hollow instrument fitted with a system of mirrors and lights.

Uric Acid—Chemical normally produced in the body from metabolism or breakdown of protein and eliminated in the urine. If the level of uric acid rises in the body as a result of disease, gout or kidney stones may result.

Urinalysis—Laboratory test performed on a urine sample that helps diagnose diseases of the kidney and other parts of the body.

Urinary Bladder—Muscular sac in the lower abdomen that stores urine brought to it from the kidneys by the ureters. The bladder stores urine until it can be eliminated through the urethra by contractions of the bladder muscles.

Urinary Studies—Laboratory or x-ray tests of the urinary tract.

Urinary Tract—Organs that produce, store and eliminate urine. The organs are the kidneys, ureters, urinary bladder and urethra.

Urine Culture—A laboratory procedure to grow bacteria from a sample of urine. The results of the culture can guide the doctor in choosing the antibiotic drug to treat urinary tract infections.

Uterus—Organ of the female reproductive system.

Uveitis—Inflammation of the parts of the eyes that make up the iris (the colored tissue encircling the clear center, the pupil).

Uvula—Soft tissue hanging down from the soft palate at the back of the throat.

V

Vaccination—Method of providing protection against disease (immunity) by giving a patient a small amount of the disease-causing germ that is weakened, killed or otherwise modified so that it cannot itself cause disease. See Immunization.

Vaccine—Medication used to provide immunity by vaccination. Vaccines are given mostly by injection or by mouth.

Vagus Nerve—Long cranial nerve arising in the base of the brain and passing to the chest and abdomen. It helps regulate heart rate, breathing, swallowing, digestion and many other body functions.

Varicose—Swollen and twisting, usually used to describe varicose veins.

Varicose Ulcers—Ulcers in the skin caused by poor blood supply to skin tissue. The poor blood supply is resultant in this case from disability-causing varicose veins.

Vas Deferens—Tube that carries sperm manufactured by the testicles toward the prostate gland and seminal vesicles.

Vasculitis—Inflammation of blood vessels, the basis of many illnesses.

Vasoconstrictor Drugs—Medications that cause blood vessels to contract, tighten or become smaller.

Vasodilator Drugs—Medications that cause small arteries to widen, providing more blood to an area of the body where the blood vessels are constricted by spasm, narrowed or obstructed.

Vector—1) An imaginary line that represents both direction and quantity that is used to study electrocardiograms (ECGs). 2) An agent that transmits infectious germs from one organism to another.

Veins—Blood vessels that return blood from body organs to the heart and lungs. Veins are much thinner than arteries. Veins carry blood at a much lower pressure than do arteries.

Vena Cava—Largest vein in the body. It collects blood from the venous system and carries it to the heart.

Venereal—Related to sexual intercourse or sexual contact. Venereal diseases such as genital herpes, gonorrhea or syphilis are now usually referred to as "sexually transmitted diseases."

Venous System—Network of veins that extend from all body organs and transport blood back to the heart.

Ventricles—Chambers containing fluid. The ventricles of the heart pump blood; ventricles of the brain contain cerebrospinal fluid.

Ventricular Aneurysm—Ballooning of the wall of the heart resulting from a weakening of the heart muscle, a complication of scarring from a previous heart attack.

Vertebrae—Bones of the spine that form the vertebral column (backbone).

Vertebral Column—The spine; the bones of the back.

Visual Field Testing—A test in which the patient sits upright in a chair about 3-1/2 feet from a tangent screen. The patient fixes his or her vision on the central target of the tangent screen and answers questions of the examiner when questioned about being able to see objects displayed at various points on the screen. The test is useful in determining the presence or absence of such things as brain tumors, retinal detachment, blood clots in the blood vessels of the eye and other significant problems.

Virulent—Extremely dangerous or harmful. Virulent bacteria are ones capable of causing diseases.

Viruses—Small germs responsible for a variety of infectious illnesses. Viruses are not alive until they enter cells of the body, where they grow and reproduce, causing viral illnesses.

Visual Acuity—Clarity with which objects are seen.

Vitamins—Chemical substances found in food that are necessary for healthy body growth, function and tissue repair.

Vitreous—Clear fluid that fills much of the eye.

Vocal Cords—Two narrow bands of fibrous and muscular tissue in the larynx that vibrate to create the sounds of the voice.

Volvulus—Twisting of loops of intestines, which become closed off (obstructed) and may lose their blood supply.

W

Warts—Small, often hard and rough skin growths caused by viruses that infect the skin.

Wasting of Body or Muscles—Severe loss of body tissues (other than surplus fat), especially muscles and vital organs, resulting in weakness, susceptibility to infection, bone fractures and sometimes death.

Weber Test—Hearing test performed with a tuning fork.

Wheezes—High-pitched sounds and whistles produced in the lungs where secretions have partially blocked air passages.

Whirlpool Treatment—Method of treating minor blood vessel and musculoskeletal diseases by immersion in a pool where jets of warm water enter and swirl under high pressure.

X

Xeroradiogram—Method of x-ray diagnosis, usually of the female breast, which uses a process similar to that used to produce photocopies.

X-Rays—High energy, invisible waves that are capable of penetrating the body and creating shadows on photographic film. The shadows provide images of the body tissues through which the x-rays pass.

Z

Zoster—"Girdle," used to describe a form of virus infection (herpes zoster or shingles) that often produces bands of inflammation across the chest or abdomen.

RESOURCES FOR ADDITIONAL INFORMATION

Many national organizations listed below have local chapters. Check your telephone directory for addresses and telephone numbers. There are other resources and self-help groups not listed due to space limitations. If you don't find the particular one that fills your needs, check your library, call a local social services referral agency or try one of the resources listed under HEALTH INFORMATION, GENERAL in this list.

ACCIDENT PREVENTION

The National Safety Council
444 N. Michigan Ave.
Chicago, IL 60611
(312) 527-4800

AGING

American Geriatric Society
10 Columbus Circle
New York, NY 10019
(212) 308-1414

The Gerontological Society of America
1835 K St. NW
Washington, DC 20006
(202) 842-1275

National Council on the Aging
600 Maryland Ave. SW
Washington, DC 20024
(202) 479-1200

National Council of Senior Citizens, Inc.
925 15th St. NW
Washington, DC 20005
(202) 347-8800

National Institution on Aging
Information Center
P.O. Box 8057
Gaithersburg, MD 20898
(301) 495-3455

ACQUIRED IMMUNODEFICIENCY SYNDROME (AIDS)

AIDS Information Hotline
Public Health Service
(800) 342-AIDS

National AIDS Information Clearinghouse
P.O. Box 6003
Rockville, MD 20850
(800) 458-8666

ALCOHOLISM

Al-Anon Family Group Headquarters
1372 Broadway
New York, NY 10018
(212) 481-6565
(800) 356-9996

Alcoholics Anonymous World Services
P.O. Box 459
Grand Central Station
New York, NY 10163
(212) 686-1100

National Council on Alcoholism
733 Third Ave.
New York, NY 10017
(212) 986-4433
(800) NCA-CALL

National Clearinghouse
for Alcoholism Information
P.O. Box 2345
Rockville MD, 20852
(301) 468-2600

ALLERGIES & ASTHMA

American Academy of Allergy &
Immunology
611 E. Wells St.
Milwaukee, WI 53202
(800) 822-2762

Asthma & Allergy Foundation of America
1717 Massachusetts Ave. NW
Washington, DC 20036
(800) 822-2762

American Lung Association
1740 Broadway
New York, NY 10019
(212) 315-8700

ALZHEIMER'S DISEASE

Alzheimer's Disease Education and
Referral Service
P.O. Box 8250
Silver Spring, MD 20907
(301) 495-3311

Alzheimer's Disease &
Related Disorders Association
70 East Lake St., Dept. X
Chicago, IL 60601
(800) 621-0379
(800) 572-6037 (IL only)

Alzheimer Society of Canada
491 Lawrence Ave. West
Toronto, Ontario M5M 1C7 Canada
(416) 789-0503

AMPUTATION

National Amputation Foundation, Inc.
12-45 150th St.
Whitestone, NY 11357
(718) 767-0596

AMYOTROPHIC LATERAL SCLEROSIS

Amyotrophic Lateral Sclerosis Association
21021 Ventura Blvd., Suite 315
P.O. Box 5951
Woodland Hills, CA 91364
(800) 782-4747

National ALS Foundation, Inc.
185 Madison Ave.
New York, NY 10016
(212) 679-4016

ARTHRITIS

Arthritis Foundation (AF)
1314 Spring St. NW
Atlanta, GA 30309
(404) 872-7100

National Institute of Arthritis &
  Metabolic Diseases
Bldg. 31
9000 Rockville Pike
Bethesda, MD 20205

BURNS

National Institute of Burn Medicine
909 E. Ann St.
Ann Arbor, MI 48104
(313) 769-9000

CANCER

American Cancer Society (ACS)
1599 Clifton Rd. NE
Atlanta, GA 30329
(404) 320-3333
(800) 227-2345

National Cancer Institute
Building 31, Room 10A18
9000 Rockville Pike
Bethesda, MD 20205
(800) 4CANCER

CARE-GIVER HELP

American Association of Retired Persons
  (AARP)
Care-Giver Information
601 E St. NW
Washington, DC 20049

Aging Network Services, Inc.
4400 East-West Highway, #907
Bethesda, MD 20814
(800) 477-4ANS

Alzheimer's Disease &
  Related Disorders Association
70 East Lake St., Dept. X
Chicago, IL 60601
(800) 621-0379
(800) 572-6037 (IL only)

Children of Aging Parents
2761 Trenton Rd.
Levittown, PA 19056
(215) 945-6900

Family Service America
Dept. FC
11700 West Lake Park Dr.
Milwaukee, WI 53224

CHOLESTEROL

National Cholesterol Education Program
National Heart, Lung & Blood Institute
C-200
National Institutes of Health
Bethesda, MD 20892

DEATH OF SPOUSE

American Association of Retired Persons
  (AARP)
Widowed Persons Service
601 E St. NW
Washington, DC 20049

DENTAL PROBLEMS

American Academy of Periodontology
  (Gum Disease)
Dept. GH
211 E. Chicago Ave., Suite 1400
Chicago, IL 60611

American Dental Association
211 E. Chicago Ave.
Chicago, IL 60611
(312) 440-2500

DEPRESSION

National Foundation for Depressive Illness
245 7th Ave.
New York, NY 10001
(800) 248-4344

DIABETES

American Diabetes Association (ADA)
1660 Duke St.
Alexandria, VA 22314
(800) 232-3472

National Institute of Arthritis, Diabetes,
  Digestive & Kidney Disorders
Bldg. 31, Room 9A04
National Institutes of Health
Bethesda, MD 20892

DIGESTIVE DISEASES

National Digestive Disease Clearinghouse
1255 23rd St. NW, Suite 275
Washington, DC 20037
(202) 296-1138

National Institute of Arthritis, Diabetes,
  Digestive & Kidney Disorders
Bldg. 31, Room 9A04
National Institutes of Health
Bethesda, MD 20892

DIZZINESS

American Academy of Otolaryngology, Inc.
One Prince St.
Alexandria, VA 22314

DRUGS

American Pharmaceutical Association
2215 Constitution Ave. NW
Washington, DC 20037
(202) 628-4410

Food & Drug Administration
Consumer Affair Branch
5600 Fisher's Lane
Rockville, MD 20857
(301) 295-8012

EMPLOYMENT

American Association of Retired Persons
  (AARP)
601 E St. NW
Washington, DC 20049

Association for Employment Services
  for the Elderly
National Council On Aging
1828 L St.
Washington, DC 20036

ENDOCRINE DISORDERS

(Thyroid, Parathyroid, Pituitary, Sex Glands
& Adrenals)

National Institute of Metabolic Disease
9650 Rockville Pike
Bethesda, MD 20205

EYE PROBLEMS & BLINDNESS

American Council of the Blind
1211 Connecticut Ave. NW
Washington, DC 20036
(800) 424-8666

American Foundation for the Blind (AFB)
15 W. 16th St.
New York, NY 10011
(212) 620-2000

American Ophthalmology Association
655 Beach St.
San Francisco, CA 94105

American Optometric Association
Communication Division
243 N. Lindbergh Rd.
St. Louis. MO 63141

American Printing House for the Blind
P.O. Box 6085
Louisville, KY 40206
(502) 895-2405

Better Vision Institute, Inc.
230 Park Ave.
New York, NY 10017
(212) 687-1731

Eye Bank Association of America
6560 Fannin, Level 9
Houston, TX 77030
(713) 798-6126

Guiding Eyes for the Blind, Inc.
611 Granite Springs Rd.
Yorktown Heights, NY 10598
(914) 245-4024

National Eye Care Project
P.O. Box 9688
San Francisco, CA 94101
(800) 222-EYES

New Eyes for the Needy
549 Milburn Ave.
Short Hills, NJ 07078
(201) 376-4903

National Library Service for the
  Blind & Physically Handicapped
The Library of Congress
1291 Taylor Ave. NW
Washington, DC 20542
(800) 424-8567

National Society to Prevent Blindness
79 Madison Ave.
New York, NY 10016

FITNESS & EXERCISE

President's Council on Physical
  Fitness & Sports
450 5th St. NW, Suite 7103
Washington, DC 20001
(202) 272-3421

National Institute on Aging/Exercise
Bldg. 31, Room 5C35
National Institutes of Health
Bethesda, MD 20892

FOOD SAFETY

Food and Drug Administration
Consumer Affair Branch
5600 Fisher's Lane
Rockville, MD 20857
(301) 295-8012

FOOT DISORDERS

American Podiatry Association
20 Chevy Chase Circle NW
Washington, DC 20015

FUNERALS

The Continental Association of Funeral &
  Memorial Societies
2001 S Street NW, Suite 530
Washington, DC 20036

HANDICAPS & DISABILITIES

Disabled American Veterans
P.O. Box 14301
Cincinnati, OH 45214

Goodwill Industries of America
9200 Wisconsin Ave.
Bethesda, MD 20814
(301) 530-6500

Information Center for Individuals
  with Disabilities, Inc.
27-43 Wormwood St.
Boston, MA 02210
(617) 727-5540

Institute for the Crippled & Disabled
400 First Ave.
New York, NY 10010

National Center for Law &
  the Handicapped, Inc.
1235 N. Eddy St.
South Bend, IN 46617

National Easter Seal Society
70 E. Lake St.
Chicago, IL 60601
(312) 243-8400
(800) 221-6827

National Rehabilation Center
8455 Colesville Rd., Suite 935
Silver Springs, MD 20910
(800) 346-2742

HEADACHE

National Headache Foundation
5252 North Western Ave.
Chicago, IL 60625
(800) 843-2256
(800) 523-8858 (IL only)

HEALTH INFORMATION, GENERAL

American Red Cross
17th & D St. NW
Washington, DC 20013
(202) 737-8300

Center for Consumer Health Education
1900 Association Dr.
Reston, VA 22091
(703) 476-3400

National Health Institute Clearinghouse
P.O. Box 1133
Washington, DC 20013
(800) 336-4797
(In Virginia, call collect (703) 522-2590)

National Self-Help Clearinghouse
33 West 42nd St., Room 1227
New York, NY 10036
(212) 887-5280

U.S. Committee for the World Health
  Organization (USA-WHO)
777 United Nations Plaza, 9A
New York, NY 10017
(212) 986-8451

HEARING OR SPEECH IMPAIRMENT

Alexander Graham Bell Association
  for the Deaf
3417 Volta Place NW
Washington, DC 20007
(202) 337-5220

American Hearing Society
919 18th St. NW
Washington, DC 20006

American Speech-Language-Hearing
  Association
10801 Rockville Pike, Dept. AP
Rockville, MD 20852
(301) 897-5700

Deafness Research Foundation
9 E. 38th St., 7th Floor
New York, NY 10016
(800) 535-3323

Dial a Hearing Test
P.O. Box 1880
Media, PA 19063
(800) 222-3277
(800) 345-3277 (PA only)

National Association of the Deaf
814 Thayer Ave.
Silver Spring, MD 20910
(301) 587-1788

National Association for Hearing
  & Speech Action
10801 Rockville Pike
Rockville, MD 20852
(800) 638-8255

Self Help for Hard of Hearing People, Inc.
P.O. Box 34889
Bethesda, MD 20817
(301) 469-7222

HEART DISEASE & BLOOD VESSEL
DISEASE

American Heart Association
7320 Greenville Ave.
Dallas, TX 75231
(214) 373-6300

National Stroke Association
300 E. Hampden, Suite 240
Englewood, CO 80110
(303) 839-1992

HERPES, GENITAL

Herpes Resource Center
Box 100
Palo Alto, CA 94302

HOME CARE

American Association of Homes
  for the Aging
1129 20th St. NW
Washington, DC 20036
(202) 296-5960

Home Health Services & Staffing Association
815 Connecticut Ave. NW
Washington, DC 20006
(202) 331-4437

National Association for Home Care
519 C St. NE
Stanton Park
Washington, DC 20002
(202) 547-7424

National Health Information Clearinghouse
P.O. Box 1133
Washington, DC 20013
(800) 336-4797
(In Virginia, call collect (703) 522-2590)

HOSPICE CARE

American Cancer Society
1599 Clifton Rd. NE
Atlanta, GA 30329
(404) 320-3333
(800) 227-2345

Cancer Care, Inc.
1180 Avenue of the Americas
New York, NY 10036
(212) 221-3300

Hospice Education Institute
5 Essex Square, Suite 3-B
Essex, CT 06426
(800) 331-1620

The National Hospice Association
1901 North Moore, Suite 901
Arlington, VA 22209
(703) 243-5900
(800) 658-8898

HYPERTENSION

Citizens for the Treatment of
  High Blood Pressure, Inc.
1140 Connecticut Ave. NW, Suite 604
Washington, DC 20036
(202) 296-7747

National High Blood Pressure
Information Center
120/80
National Institutes of Health
Bethesda, MD 20892

HYPOGLYCEMIA

Adrenal Metabolic Research Society
  of the Hypoglycemia Foundation, Inc.
153 Pawling Ave.
Troy, NY 12180
(518) 272-7154

HYSTERECTOMY

Center for Climacteric Studies
University of Florida
901 NW 8th Ave., Suite B1
Gainesville, FL 32601
(904) 392-3184

Hysterectomy Education Resources (HERS)
422 Bryn Mawr Ave.
Bala Cynwyd, PA 19004
(215) 667-7757

ILEITIS & COLITIS

National Foundation for Ileitis & Colitis
444 Park Avenue South
New York, NY 10016
(800) 343-3637

INCONTINENCE

Help for Incontinent People (HIP)
P.O. Box 544
Union, SC 29379
(803) 585-8789

Simon Foundation
Box 835X
Wilmette, IL 60091
(800) 237-4666

INFECTIOUS DISEASES

Centers for Disease Control (CDC)
1600 Clifton Rd. NE
Atlanta, GA 30333
(404) 329-3311

KIDNEY DISEASE

National Kidney Foundation
30 E. 33rd St.
New York, NY 10016
(212) 889-2210
(800) 622-9010

LEUKEMIA

Leukemia Society of America, Inc.
733 3rd Ave.
New York, NY 10017
(212) 573-8484

LIVING WILLS

Society for the Right to Die
250 W. 57th St.
New York, NY 10107
(212) 246-6973

LUNG DISEASE

American Lung Association
1740 Broadway
P.O. Box 596
New York, NY 10019
(212) 315-8700

National Heart, Lung & Blood Institute
  Information Center
National Institutes of Health
Bethesda, MD 20892

LUPUS ERYTHEMATOSUS

American Lupus Society
23751 Madison St.
Torrance, CA 90505
(213) 542-8891

Lupus Foundation of America
1717 Massachusetts Ave. NW, Suite 203
Washington, DC 20036
(800) 558-0121

MEDICAL ALERT

Medic Alert Foundation International
P.O. Box 1009
Turlock, CA 95380
(209) 668-3333

MENTAL HEALTH

American Mental Health Foundation
Two East 86th St.
New York, NY 10028
(212) 737-9027

Community Guidance Service
120 W. 58th St.
New York, NY 10019

Institute for the Development
  of Emotional and Life Skills
P. O. Box 391
State College, PA 16801
(814) 237-4805

National Mental Health Association
1021 Prince St.
Arlington, VA 22314
(703) 358-5150

Recovery, Inc.
116 S. Michigan Ave.
Chicago, IL 60603

MYASTHENIA GRAVIS

Myasthenia Gravis Foundation
53 W. Jackson Blvd., Suite 1352
Chicago, IL 60604
(800) 541-5454

NURSING HOME INFORMATION

American Nursing Home Association
American Health Care Association
1825 Connecticut Ave. NW
Washington, DC 20036
(202) 797-0657

National Citizens' Coalition for
  Nursing Home Reform
1425 16th St. NW, Room 12
Washington, DC 20036
(202) 797-0657

National Council of Senior Citizens
925 15th St. NW
Washington, DC 20005
(202) 347-8800

NUTRITION

American Dietetic Association
430 North Michigan Ave.
Chicago, IL 60611
(312) 280-5000

U.S. Department of Agriculture
Human Nutrition Information Services
Room 325A
6505 Belcrest Rd.
Hyattsville, MD 20782

OSTEOPOROSIS

National Osteoporosis Foundation
1625 I St. NW, Suite 1011
Washington, DC 20006
(202) 223-2226

OSTOMY

International Association for
  Enterostomal Therapy
505 N. Tustin Ave., Suite 282
Santa Ana, CA 92705
(714) 972-1720

United Ostomy Association, Inc.
2001 W. Beverly Blvd.
Los Angeles, CA 90057
(213) 413-5510

PARKINSON'S DISEASE

American Parkinson Disease Association
116 John St., Suite 417
New York, NY 10038
(212) 732-9550
(800) 223-2732

National Parkinson Foundation (NPF)
1501 NW 9th Ave.
Miami, FL 33136
(800) 327-4545
(800) 433-7022 (FL only)

Parkinson's Educational Program
1800 Park Newport, #302
Newport Beach, CA 92600
(800) 344-7872

United Parkinson Foundation (UPF)
220 S. State St.
Chicago, IL 60604
(312) 922-9734

PLASTIC SURGERY

American Academy of Facial Plastic &
  Reconstructive Surgery
70 West Hubbard St., Suite 202
Chicago, IL 60601
(312) 644-2623

American Society of Plastic &
  Reconstructive Surgeons
444 E. Algonquin Rd.
Arlington Heights, IL 60005
(800) 635-0635

PSORIASIS

National Psoriasis Foundation
6415 S. W. Canyon Court, Suite 200
Portland, OR 97221
(503) 297-1545

SCLERODERMA

United Scleroderma Foundation
305 W. Beach St.
P.O. Box 399
Watsonville, CA 95077
(408) 728-2202

SEXUALITY

American Association of Sex Educators,
   Counselors and Therapists (AASECT)
11 Dupont Circle NW, Suite 220
Washington, DC 20036

American Social Health Association
260 Sheridan Ave.
Palo Alto, CA 94306
(415) 327-6465

Sex Information and Education
   Council of the U. S. (SIECUS)
80 Fifth Ave., Suite 801
New York, NY 10011
(212) 929-2300

SEXUALLY TRANSMITTED DISEASES

American Social Health Association
260 Sheridan Ave.
Palo Alto, CA 94306
(415) 327-6465

VD National Hotline
(800) 227-8922
(800) 982-5883 (CA only)

SKIN DISORDERS

American Academy of Dermatology
1567 Maple Ave.
Evanston, IL 60201
(312) 869-3954

Skin Cancer Foundation
245 5th Ave., Suite 2402
New York, NY 10016
(212) 725-5176

SLEEP DISORDERS

American Sleep Disorders Association
604 2nd St. SW
Rochester, MN 55902

SMOKING

American Cancer Society (ACS)
1599 Clifton Rd. NE
Atlanta, GA 30329
(404) 320-3333
(800) 227-2345

American Heart Association
7320 Greenville Ave.
Dallas, TX 75231
(214) 373-6300

American Lung Association
1740 Broadway
P.O. Box 596
New York, NY 10019
(212) 315-8700

Smokenders
37 N. 3rd St.
Easton, PA 18042

SPINAL INJURY

National Spinal Cord Injury Association
600 W. Cummings Park, Suite 2000
Woburn, MA 01801
(800) 962-9629

STROKE

American Heart Association
7320 Greenville Ave.
Dallas, TX 75231
(214) 373-6300

National Stroke Association
300 E. Hampden, Suite 240
Englewood, CO 80110
(303) 839-1992

SURGERY

American College of Surgeons
Office of Public Education
55 E. Erie St.
Chicago, IL 60611

National Second Opinion for Surgery
   Program Hotline
200 Independence Ave. SW
Washington, DC 20201
(800) 638-6833
(In MD call (800) 492-6603)

TRAVEL & HEALTH

The International Association for
  Medical Assistance to Travelers
736 Center St.
Lewiston, NY 20402
(716) 754-4883

International SOS Assistance
P.O. Box 11568
Philadelphia, PA 10116
(800) 523-8930
(215) 244-1500 (PA only)

VOLUNTEER PROGRAMS

ACTION
806 Connecticut Ave. NW
Washington, DC 20525
(800) 424-8580

WOMEN'S HEALTH

Boston Women's Healthbook Collective
465 Mt. Auburn St.
Watertown, MA 02172
(617) 924-0271

Health Works for Women
1545 Divisadero
San Francisco, CA 94115
(415) 931-7170

Women's Sports Foundation
342 Madison Ave., Suite 728
New York, NY 10173
(800) 342-3988

SUGGESTED READING FOR ADDITIONAL INFORMATION

If you don't find your particular topic in this list, check at the local library. There are books available on almost any health or illness subject that you may be interested in.

AGING

Bonner, Joseph, and William Harris. *Healthy Aging: New Directions in Health, Biology and Medicine.* Claremont, CA: Hunter House, 1988.

Hallowell, Christopher. *Growing Old, Staying Young.* New York: Morrow, 1985.

Earle, Richard, et al. *Your Vitality Quotient: The Clinically Proven Program That Can Reduce Your Body Age and Increase Your Zest for Life.* New York: Warner Books, 1989.

Line, Francis R. *Super Seniors; Their Stories and Secrets.* Wide Horizon Press, 1989.

Linkletter, Art. *Old Age is Not for Sissies.* New York: Penquin, 1989.

AIDS

Fettner, Ann Giudici. *The Truth About A.I.D.S.: Evolution of an Epidemic.* New York: Rinehart & Winston, 1984.

Kassler, Jeanne. *Gay Men's Health: A Guide to the AID Syndrome and Other Sexually Transmitted Diseases.* New York: Harper & Row, 1983.

Kübler-Ross, Elisabeth. *AIDS.* New York: MacMillan, 1989.

ALCOHOLISM

Beasley, Joseph, M.D. *How to Defeat Alcoholism.* New York: Random House, 1989.

Elkin, Michael. *Families Under the Influence: Changing Alcoholic Patterns.* New York: Norton, 1990.

Mumey, Jack. *The Joy of Being Sober: A Book For Recovering Alcoholics—and Those Who Love Them.* Chicago: Contemporary Books, 1984.

ALLERGIES

Bachman, Judy L., Ph.D. *Allegy Environment Guidebook.* New York: Perigee, 1990.

Edelson, Edward. *Allergies.* New York: Chelsea House, 1989.

ALZHEIMER'S DISEASE

Carroll, David L. *When Your Loved One Has Alzheimer's: A Caregiver's Guide.* New York: Harper & Row, 1990.

Danforth, Art. *Living With Alzheimer's—Ruth's Story.* Falls Church, VA: Prestige, 1985.

Heston, Leonaro L. *Dementia: A Practical Guide to Alzheimer's Disease and Related Illnesses.* New York: W. H. Freeman, 1983.

Wirsig, Woodrow. *"I Love You, Too."* Boston: Little, Brown & Co., 1990.

ARTHRITIS

Fries, James F. *Arthritis: A Comprehensive Guide.* Reading, MA: Addison-Wesley, 1990.

Kantrowitz, Fred G., M.D. *Taking Control of Arthritis.* New York: Harper Collins, 1990.

McCarty, Daniel J., ed. *Arthritis and Allied Conditions: A Textbook of Rheumatology,* 10th ed. Philadelphia: Lea & Febiger, 1989.

ASTHMA

Berland, Theodore. *Living With Your Allergies and Asthma.* New York: St. Martin's, 1983.

Lane, Donald J., and Anthony Storr. *Asthma: The Facts.* New York: Oxford University Press, 1987.

Weinstein, Allan M., M.D. *Asthma.* New York: McGraw-Hill, 1987.

BACK PAIN

Sarno, John. *Mind Over Back Pain.* New York: Berkley, 1987.

White, Augustus A., M.D. *Your Aching Back: A Doctor's Guide to Relief.* New York: Simon & Schuster, 1990.

BLADDER AND INCONTINENCE DISORDERS

Chalker, Rebecca & Kristine W. Whitmore, M.D. *Overcoming Bladder Disorders.* New York: Harper Collins, 1990.

BLOOD DISORDERS

Beck, William S., ed. *Hematology.* 3rd ed. Cambridge, MA: MIT Press, 1981.

Callender, Sheila T. *Blood Disorders: The Facts.* New York: Oxford University Press, 1985.

BREAST PROBLEMS

Gross, Amy, and Dee Ito. *Women Talk About Breast Surgery.* New York: Crown, 1990.

Love, Susan M., M.D., and Karen Lindsey. *Dr. Susan Love's Breast Book.* Reading, MA: Addison-Wesley, 1990.

BREATHING DISORDERS

Haas, Francois, and Shelia Sperber Haas. *The Chronic Bronchitis & Emphysema Handbook.* New York: Wiley, 1990.

Shayevitz, Myra, and Berton Shayevitz. *Living Well With Emphysema & Bronchitis: A Handbook for Everyone With Chronic Obstructive Pulmonary Disease.* New York: Doubleday, 1985.

CANCER

The American Cancer Society Cancer Book. New York: Doubleday, 1986.

Dreher, Henry. *Your Defense Against Cancer.* New York: Harper & Row, 1989.

Levitt, Paul. *The Cancer Reference Book: Direct and Clear Answers to Everyone's Questions,* rev. ed. New York: Facts on File, 1983.

Meyer, John A., M.D. *Lung Cancer Chronicles.* New Brunswick, NJ: Rutgers University Press, 1990.

Morra, Marion, and Eve Potts *Choices: Realistic Alternatives in Cancer Treatment.* rev. ed. New York: Avon Books, 1990.

Williams, Chris and Sue. *Cancer: A Patient's Guide.* New York: Wiley, 1986.

CARE-GIVERS

Brister, C. W. *Caring for the Caregivers.* Nashville, TN: Broadman, 1985.

MacLean, Helene. *Caring for Your Parents.* New York: Doubleday, 1987.

Pierskalla, Carol, and Jane D. Heald. *Help for Families of the Aging: Caregivers Can Express Love and Set Limits.* Support Source, 1988.

COLD, COMMON

Castleman, Michael, *Cold Cures.* New York: Ballantine, 1987.

CROHN'S & ILEITIS

Scala, James. *Eating Right for a Bad Gut: The Complete Nutritional Guide to Ileitis, Colitis, Crohn's Disease and Inflammatory Bowel Disease.* NAL Books, 1990.

DEPRESSION

Fieve, Ronald R., M.D. *Moodswing.* New York: William Morrow, 1989.

Hales, Dianne. *Depression.* New York: Chelsea House, 1989.

DIABETES

Bierman, June, and Barbara Toohey. *The Diabetic's Book: All Your Questions Answered.* rev. ed. New York: St. Martin's, 1990.

Lowe, Ernest, and Gary Arsham, M.D. *Diabetes: A Guide to Living Well.* Wayzata, MN: Diabetes Center, 1989.

DRUG ABUSE

O'Brien, Robert, ed. *Encyclopedia of Drug Abuse.* New York: Facts on File, 1984.

DRUGS, GENERAL INFORMATION

Griffith, H. Winter. *Complete Guide to Prescription & Non-Prescription Drugs,* rev. ed. New York: Perigee, 1991.

Long, James W. *Essential Guide to Prescription Drugs: What You Need to Know for Safe Drug Use,* rev. ed. New York: Harper & Row, 1991.

Physician's Desk Reference. Oradell, NJ: Medical Economics, 1991.

EMERGENCY CARE

American Medical Association. *The American Medical Association's Handbook of First Aid and Emergency Care.* New York: Random House, 1987.

EPILEPSY

Richard, Adrienne, and Joel Reiter. *Epilepsy: A New Approach.* New York: Prentice-Hall, 1990.

Sands, Harry, ed. *Epilepsy: The Mental Health Professional Guide.* New York: Brunner-Mazel, 1982.

EXERCISE

Balboa, Deena, and David Balboa. *Walk for Life: The Lifetime Walking Program for a Healthy Body & Mind.* New York: Perigee, 1990.

Berland, Theodore. *Fitness for Life: Exercises for People Over Fifty.* Washington, DC: American Association for Retired People, 1987.

Yanker, Gary, and Kathy Burton. *Walking Medicine: The Lifetime Guide to Preventive and Rehabilitative Exercise Walking.* New York: McGraw-Hill, 1990.

EYE CARE

Brians, Charlene, and Michelle Moss. *Eye Book.* New York: VHI Library, 1983.

Samez, Jane. *Vision.* New York: Chelsea House, 1990.

Zinn, Walter J. *The Complete Guide to Eyecare, Eyeglasses and Contact Lenses,* rev. ed. Hollywood, FL: Frederick Fell Publishing, 1987.

FOOT CARE

Levine, Dr. Susan M. *My Feet Are Killing Me.* New York: McGraw-Hill, 1987.

GENERAL

The American Medical Association. *Home Medical Advisor.* New York: Random, 1988.

Dorland's Medical Dictionary. New York: Harper & Row, 1990.

Merck Manual of Diagnosis and Therapy, 17th ed. Rahway, NJ: Merck, 1990.

Mosby's Medical and Nursing Dictionary. St. Louis, MO: Mosby, 1989.

Rakel, Robert E., ed. *Conn's Current Therapy.* Philadelphia: W. B. Saunders Co., 1991.

HEADACHE

Saper, Joel R., and Kenneth R. Magee. *Freedom From Headaches: A Personal Guide For Understanding and Treating Headache, Face and Neck Pain.* New York: Simon & Schuster, 1986.

Murphy, Wendy. *Dealing With Headaches.* Alexandria, VA: Time-Life, 1982.

HEART DISEASE

Amsterdam, Ezra A. *Take Care of Your Heart*. New York: Facts on File, 1984.

Gordon, Neil, and Larry W. Gibbons. *The Cooper Clinic Cardiac Rehabilitation Program: Featuring the Unique Heart Points System*. New York: Simon & Schuster, 1990.

Ornish, Dean, M.D. *Dr. Dean Ornish's Program for Reversing Heart Disease*. New York: Random, 1990.

Warren, James V., M.D., and Genell J. Subak-Sharpe. *Surviving Your Heart Attack*. New York: Doubleday, 1987.

HYPERTENSION

Moser, Marvin, M.D. *Lower Your Blood Pressure and Live Longer*. New York: Villard Books, 1989.

Sorrentino, Sandy, M.D., Ph.D., and Carl Hausman. *Coping with High Blood Pressure*. New York: Dembner Books, 1986.

INSURANCE

Inlander, Charles B., and Charles K. McKay. *Medicare Made Easy*. Reading, MA: Addison-Wesley, 1989.

IRRITABLE BOWEL SYNDROME

Shimberg, Elaine Fantele. *Relief From IBS: Irritable Bowel Syndrome*. New York: Evans, 1988.

KIDNEY DISEASE

Cameron, Stewart. *Kidney Disease: The Facts*. New York: Oxford University Press, 1986.

LIVING ALONE

Brothers, Joyce. *Widowed*. New York: Simon & Schuster, 1990.

Deits, Bob. *Life After Loss*. Tucson, AZ: Fisher Books, 1988.

LONG-TERM CARE

Goldsmith, Seth. *Choosing a Nursing Home*. New York: Prentice-Hall, 1990.

Matthews, Joseph L. *Elder Care: Choosing and Financing Long-Term Care*. New York: Nolo Press, 1990.

LUPUS ERYTHEMATOSUS, SYSTEMIC

Aladjem, Henrietta. *In Search of the Sun*. New York: Scribner's, 1988.

Blau, Sheldon Paul. *Lupus: The Body Against Itself*, rev. ed. New York: Doubleday, 1984.

MENTAL HEALTH

Wender, Paul H. *Mind, Mood and Medicine: A Guide to the New Biopsychiatry.* New York: New American Library, 1982.

Gold, Mark S., M.D. *The Good News About Panic, Anxiety and Phobias.* New York: Villard Books, 1989.

MULTIPLE SCLEROSIS

Soll, Robert W., M.D., Ph.D., and Penelope B. Grenoble, Ph.D. *Multiple Sclerosis: Something Can Be Done and You Can Do It.* Chicago: Contemporary Books, 1984.

MUSCLE PROBLEMS

Davidson, Paul. *Chronic Muscle Pain Syndrome.* New York: Random, 1989.

NUTRITION

Griffith, H. Winter. *Complete Guide to Vitamins.* Tucson, AZ: Fisher Books, 1988.

Herbert, Victor, M.D., and Genell J. Subac-Sharpe. *The Mt. Sinai School of Medicine Complete Book of Nutrition.* New York: St. Martin's, 1990.

Kirschman, John D. *Nutrition Almanac,* 3rd ed. New York: McGraw-Hill, 1989.

Mayer, Jean, and Jeanne P. Goldber. *Dr. Jean Mayer's Diet and Nutrition Guide.* New York: Pharos, 1990.

OBESITY

Mirkin, Gabe. *Getting Thin: All About Fat—How You Get It, How You Lose It, How You Keep It Off For Good.* Boston, MA: Little, Brown & Co., 1986.

OSTOMY

Mullen, Barbara Dorr, and Kerry Anne McGinn, R.N. *The Ostomy Book.* Palo Alto, CA: Bull, 1980.

PAIN

Lewis, George, M.D., and Sandra Horn. *Drug Free Pain Relief.* Rochester, NY: Thorson's, 1987.

Sternbach, Dr. Richard. *Mastering Pain—A Twelve-Step Program for Coping With Chronic Pain.* New York: Putnam, 1987.

PARKINSON'S DISEASE

Duvoisin, Roger C. *Parkinson's Disease: A Guide for Patient and Family,* 2nd ed. Mahonoy City, PA: Raven, 1984.

PLASTIC SURGERY

Cirillo, Dennis P. *The Complete Book of Cosmetic Facial Surgery.* New York: Simon & Schuster, 1988.

Morgan, Elizabeth, M.D. *Complete Book of Cosmetic Surgery*. New York: Warner, 1988.

POISONING

Dreisbach, Robert H. *Handbook of Poisoning: Prevention, Diagnosis and Treatment*, 12th ed. Los Altos, CA: Appleton & Lange, 1987.

Hyams, Jay. *Poisons*. Springhouse, PA: Springhouse Books, 1986.

PROSTATE

Greenberger, Monroe E., M.D., and Mary-Ellen Siegel, M.S.W. *What Every Man Should Know About Prostate*. New York: Walker & Co., 1983.

RETIREMENT

Palder, Edward. *The Retirement Sourcebook: Your Complete Guide to Healthy, Leisure and Consumer Information*. Kensington, MD: Woodbine House, 1989.

SEXUAL DYSFUNCTION

Kaplan, Helen S. *The Evaluation of Sexual Disorders: Psychological and Medical Aspects*. New York: Brunner-Mazel, 1983.

SEXUALLY TRANSMITTED DISEASES

Zinner, Stephen H., M.D. *How to Protect Yourself From STDS*. New York: Summit Books, 1985.

SHINGLES

Thomsen, Thomas Carl. *Shingles*. Cross River, NY: Cross River Press, 1990.

SKIN DISORDERS

Fitzpatrick, Thomas B., ed. *Dermatology in General Medicine*, 3rd ed. New York: McGraw-Hill, 1987.

SLEEP PROBLEMS

Hartman, Ernest, M.D. *The Sleep Book: Understanding & Preventing Sleep Problems in People Over 50*. Glenview, IL: AARP, 1987.

Hauri, Peter, and Shirley Linde. *No More Sleepless Nights: The Complete Program for Ending Insomnia*. New York: Wiley, 1990.

STROKE

Lavin, John H. *Stroke: From Crisis to Victory*. New York: Franklin Watts, 1985.

Sarno, John E., and Martha Taylor Sarno. *Stroke: A Guide for Patients and Their Families*. New York: McGraw-Hill, 1979.

SURGERY, GENERAL

Stern, Edward L., M.D. *Surgery, A Layman's Guide to Common Operations*. Tarzana, CA: Lawman Press, 1989.

Way, Lawrence W., ed. *Current Surgical Diagnosis and Treatment*, 8th ed. Los Altos, CA: Appleton & Lange, 1988.

WOMEN'S HEALTH

Boston Women's Health Book Collective. *The New Our Bodies, Ourselves*. New York: Simon & Schuster, 1985.

Utian, Wulf H., and Ruth S. Jacobowitz. *Managing Your Menopause*. New York: Prentice-Hall, 1990.

Stewart, Felicia Hance. *My Body, My Health: The Concerned Women's Guide to Gynecology*. New York: Bantam, 1987.

Index

The Index includes all the Symptoms, Illnesses and Disorders, Surgeries, Medications and Appendices described in this book. All entries are listed in capital and lower-case letters except for generic drugs, which are in CAPITAL LETTERS.

A

Abdominal Aortic Aneurysm, Removal of, 576
Abdominal Pain, Recurrent Attacks, 2
Abdominal Pain, Sudden Attack, 5
Abdominal Swelling, 8
Abdomino-Perineal Resection, 578
Abdominoplasty, 674
Abscess, Lung, 378
Abscess, Periapical, 536
Abscess, Periodontal, 536
Abscess, Tooth, 536
Abuse of the Elderly, 762
Acceleration-Deceleration Cervical Injury, 570
ACE Inhibitors, 686
ACEBUTOLOL, 715
ACETAMINOPHEN, 684
ACETAZALOMIDE, 718
Acetazolam, 718
ACETAZOLAMIDE, 703
ACETOHEXAMIDE, 698
Achromycin, 690
Acne Rosacea, 160
Acquired Immune Deficiency Syndrome, 162
Actidil, 704
Actifed, 704
ACYCLOVIR, 710
ACYCLOVIR (Topical), 712
Addiction and Drug Abuse, 255
Addison's Disease, 161
Adenomatosis, 267
Adenomyosis, 267
Adepin, 697
Adrenal Insufficiency, 161
Adrenalin, 716
Adsorbocarpine, 703
Adult Acne, 160
Advil, 729
Aerolone, 716
Agranulocytosis, 571
AIDS, 162
AIDS-Related Complex, 182
Air Sickness, 395
Ak-Sulf, 690
Ak-Tate, 719

Ak-Trol, 719
Ak-Zol, 703, 718
Alatone, 722
Alazide, 722
ALBUTEROL, 716
Alcoholism, 163
Aldactazine, 722
Aldactone, 722
Aldoclor, 705, 722
Aldomet, 705
Aldoril, 705, 722
Aldosterone, Excessive, 164
Aller-Chlor, 704
Allerfin, 704
Allergic Shock, 171
Allergy Diet, 740
Allergy, Nasal, 405
Allermine, 704
Alopecia Areata, 192
ALS, 168
Altitude Illness, 165
Alupent, 716
Alzheimer's Disease, 166
AMANTADINE, 706, 710
Amen, 723
AMILORIDE, 722
AMINOPHYLLINE, 716
Amitril, 697
AMITRIPTYLINE, 697
AMOBARBITAL, 714
Amoeba Infections, 167
AMOXAPINE, 697
AMOXICILLIN, 692
AMPHOTERICIN B (Topical), 701
AMPICILLIN, 692
Amputation, 580
Amyotrophic Lateral Sclerosis, 168
Anacin, 684
Anal Fissure, 169
Anal Itching, 170
Analgesics (Narcotic), 685
Anaphylaxis, 171
Anaprox, 729
Anemia, Aplastic, 172
Anemia, Folic Acid-Deficiency, 173
Anemia, Hemolytic, 174

INDEX

INDEX

Weight Loss, 154
Weight-Reduction Diet, 745
Wen, 478
Westcort, 719
Wheezing, 157
Whiplash, 570
White Blood Cells, Disorders of, 571
Will, Living, 786
Wryneck, 539
Wyanoids, 699, 708

X
Xanax, 688
X-Otag, 706, 728, 780
Xylocaine, 689
Xylocaine with epinephrine, 689

Y
Yeast Infection, Skin, 572
Yeast Infection, Vaginal, 554

Z
Zantac, 709
Zarontin, 695
Zaroxolyn, 722
Zeasorb-AF, 701
Zestril, 686
ZIDOVUDINE, 710
Zinc Deficiency, 573
Zorprin, 713
Zovirax, 710, 712